2017 EDITION AAHIVM FUNDAMENTALS OF HIV MEDICINE FOR THE HIV SPECIALIST™

Release Date: March 3, 2017

Expiration Date: April 30, 2018

Estimated Time To Complete All Chapters: 42.5 Hours

Jointly Provided By Postgraduate Institute For Medicine And American Academy Of Hiv Medicine

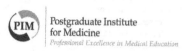

This Activity Is Supported By Independent Educational Grants From Gilead Sciences, Viiv, And Merck.

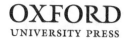

OXFORD
UNIVERSITY PRESS

OXFORD
UNIVERSITY PRESS

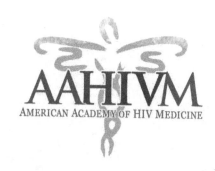

AMERICAN ACADEMY OF HIV MEDICINE

2017 EDITION AAHIVM FUNDAMENTALS OF HIV MEDICINE FOR THE HIV SPECIALIST™

TARGET AUDIENCE

This activity has been designed to meet the educational needs of physicians, nurse practitioners, physician assistants, registered nurses, and pharmacists involved in the care of patients with HIV disease.

OVERALL LEARNING OBJECTIVES

After completing this activity, the participant should be better able to

- describe the evolving epidemiology of HIV disease in the United States, with an emphasis on age, gender, sexuality, race/ethnicity, socioeconomic status, emerging subtypes, and viral resistance;

- implement appropriate laboratory HIV testing methods for screening and diagnosing HIV infections;

- adapt pre- and post-testing patient counseling to best meet patient needs in a variety of situations;

- provide up-to-date HIV care to a broad spectrum of infected patient populations, including pediatrics, adolescents, injection-drug users, incarcerated individuals, and an aging population;

- review the clinical presentation, diagnosis, treatment, and treatment complications of hepatitis B and C in HIV-infected patients;

- adjust treatment based on the various comorbidities that are often found in HIV-infected individuals, including cardiovascular, renal, and neurologic disease; and

- discuss the ethics and legal issues related to caring for HIV-infected individuals.

FACULTY

LEAD EDITOR

W. David Hardy, MD, AAHIVS
Senior Director, Evidence-Based Practices
Whitman–Walker Health
Washington, DC
Adjunct Professor of Medicine
Johns Hopkins University School of Medicine
Baltimore, MD

CO-EDITORS

Jonathan S. Appelbaum, MD, FACP, AAHIVS
Laurie L. Dozier Jr., MD, Education Director and
    Professor of Internal Medicine
Interim Chair, Department of Clinical Sciences
Florida State University College of Medicine
Tallahassee, FL

Roberto C. Arduino, MD
Professor of Medicine
Department of Internal Medicine
Division of Infectious Diseases
McGovern Medical School
The University of Texas Health Sciences
    Center at Houston
Houston, TX

Bruce L. Gilliam, MD
Associate Professor of Medicine
Associate Chief, Division of Infectious Diseases
University of Maryland School of Medicine
Institute of Human Virology
Baltimore, MD

Jeffrey T. Kirchner, DO, FAAFP, AAHIVS
Medical Director – Penn Medicine/LGHP
    Comprehensive Care
Lancaster General Hospital
Lancaster, PA

WRITERS

Saira Ajmal, MD
Infectious Diseases Fellow
Mayo Clinic
Rochester, MN

Lisa Armitige, MD, PhD
Medical Consultant
Heartland National TB Center
San Antonio, TX

Renata Arrington-Sanders, MD, MPH, ScM
Assistant Professor
Medical Director, Pediatric and Adolescent
    HIV/AIDS Program
Division of General Pediatrics & Adolescent Medicine
Johns Hopkins School of Medicine
Baltimore, MD

Jason Baker, MD, MS
Infectious Diseases and HIV Medicine
Hennepin County Medical Center
Associate Professor of Medicine
University of Minnesota
Minneapolis, MN

Ben J. Barnett, MD
Professor of Medicine, Infectious Diseases
McGovern Medical School
The University of Texas Health Science Center
   at Houston
Houston, TX

Tanvir K. Bell, MD, FACP, FIDSA
Adjunct Associate Professor of Internal Medicine
McGovern Medical School
The University of Texas Health Science Center
   at Houston
Houston, TX

Philip Bolduc, MD
Assistant Professor of Family Medicine and
   Community Health
University of Massachusetts Medical School
Worcester, MA
HIV and Viral Hepatitis Program and Fellowship
   Director
Family Health Center of Worcester
Worcester, MA
Co-Clinical Director
New England AIDS Education and Training Center
Boston, MA

Christopher M. Bositis, MD, AAHIVS
Clinical Program Director, HIV and Viral Hepatitis
Greater Lawrence Family Health Center
Lawrence, MA

Christian Brander, PhD
IrsiCaixa AIDS Research Institute
ICREA Senior Research Professor
Hospital Universitari Germans Trias i Pujol
Barcelona, Spain

Christopher Brendemuhl, DMD
Maricopa Integrated Health System
McDowell Dental Clinic
Phoenix, AZ

John P. Casas, MD
Staff Psychiatrist
Albany Stratton VA Medical Center
Albany, NY

Elizabeth Chiao, MD, MPH
Associate Professor of Medicine
Section Infectious Diseases
Scientist
Center for Innovations in Quality, Effectiveness, and Safety
Michael E. DeBakey VA Medical Center
Houston, TX

Carolyn Chu, MD, MSc
Clinical Director
Clinician Consultation Center
Associate Professor of Clinical Family &
   Community Medicine
Department of Family & Community Medicine
University of California at San Francisco
San Francisco, CA

Joseph A. Church, MD
Head
Division of Clinical Immunology and Allergy
Children's Hospital Los Angeles
Professor
Clinical Pediatrics
Keck School of Medicine of USC
Los Angeles, CA

Jennifer Cocohoba, PharmD, MAS, BCPS, AAHIVP
Professor of Clinical Pharmacy
University of California at San Francisco
   School of Pharmacy
Pharmacist
University of California at San Francisco
   Women's HIV Program
San Francisco, CA

Emily Colgate, MD
Primary Care
Community Health Association of Spokane

Dagan Coppock, MD
Post-Doctoral Fellow
Division of Infectious Diseases
Perelman School of Medicine
University of Pennsylvania
Philadelphia, PA

Vishal Dahya, MD
Co-Chief Resident Physician, Teaching Faculty
Internal Medicine Residency
Florida State University College of Medicine
Tallahassee, FL

Elizabeth David, MD
Director
Psychiatry Consult Services
Ben Taub/Harris Health System
Assistant Professor
Department of Psychiatry and Behavioral Sciences
Baylor College of Medicine
Houston, TX

Alejandro Delgado, MD
Attending Physician, Division of Infectious Diseases
Albert Einstein Medical Center

Paul W. DenOuden, MD
Multnomah County HIV Health Services Center
Portland, OR

Madeline B. Deutsch, MD, MPH
Director
UCSF Transgender Care
Associate Professor of Clinical Family &
    Community Medicine
Center of Excellence for Transgender Health
University of California at San Francisco
San Francisco, CA

James P. Dunn, MD
Professor of Ophthalmology
Director, Uveitis Unit
Retina Division
Wills Eye Hospital
Sidney Kimmel Medical College/Thomas
    Jefferson University
Philadelphia, PA

Babatunde Edun, MD
Assistant Professor of Internal Medicine
University of South Carolina School of Medicine
Columbia, SC

Derek M. Fine, MD
Associate Professor of Medicine
Nephrology Fellowship Director
Division of Nephrology
Department of Medicine
Johns Hopkins University School of Medicine
Baltimore, MD

Rajesh T. Gandhi, MD
Director
HIV Clinical Services and Education
Massachusetts General Hospital
Associate Professor
Harvard Medical School
Boston, MA

Bruce L. Gilliam, MD
Associate Professor of Medicine
Associate Chief, Division of Infectious Diseases
University of Maryland School of Medicine
Institute of Human Virology

Michelle K. Haas, MD
Denver Metro Tuberculosis Program
Denver Public Health
Denver, CO
Assistant Professor of Medicine
Division of Infectious Diseases
University of Colorado–Anschutz Medical Campus
Aurora, CO

Dennis Joseph Hartigan-O'Connor, MD, PhD
Assistant Professor
Department of Medical Microbiology and
    Immunology
University of California at Davis
Davis, CA
Core Scientist
California National Primate Research Center
Davis, CA
Assistant Adjunct Professor
Division of Experimental Medicine
Department of Medicine
University of California at San Francisco
San Francisco, CA

Rodrigo Hasbun, MD, MPH
Department of Infectious Diseases
The University of Texas Health Science Center at Houston
Houston, TX

Emily L. Heil, PharmD, BCPS-AQ ID
Assistant Professor
Infectious Diseases Department of Pharmacy
    Practice and Science
University of Maryland School of Pharmacy
Baltimore, MD

Margaret Hoffman-Terry, MD, FACP, AAHIVS
Clinical Assistant Professor of Medicine
Milton S. Hershey Medical Center
Pennsylvania State University College of Medicine
Hershey, PA
Internal Medicine Residency Research Director,
    Chief of Division of HIV Medicine
Lehigh Valley Hospital
Allentown, PA

Jennifer Husson, MD, MPH
Assistant Professor
Institute of Human Virology
University of Maryland School of Medicine
Baltimore, MD

Boris Juelg, MD, PhD
Assistant in Medicine
Infectious Disease Unit
Massachusetts General Hospital
Instructor in Medicine
Harvard Medical School
Boston, MA

Joy H. Kang, DO, MPH, AAHIVS
Assistant Professor
Department of Family and Social Medicine
Montefiore Medical Group
Albert Einstein College of Medicine
Bronx, NY

Joseph S. Kass, MD, JD, FAAN
Associate Professor of Neurology, Psychiatry &
    Medical Ethics
Director, Alzheimer's Disease & Memory
    Disorders Center
Vice Chair for Education, Department of Neurology
Associate Dean of Student Affairs
Baylor College of Medicine
Houston, TX

Carolyn Kramer, MD
Division of Infectious Disease
Hospital of the University of Pennsylvania
Philadelphia, PA

Eurides Lopes, MD
Infectious Disease Fellow
University of Maryland MD

Adrian Majid, MD
Assistant Professor of Medicine
Section of Hospital Medicine
Division of General Internal Medicine
Weill Cornell Medicine
Cornell University
New York, NY

Jose Martagon-Villamil, MD, DTM&H
Attending Physician
Department of Internal Medicine and Infectious Disease
Baystate Medical Center
University of Massachusetts School of Medicine
Springfield, MA

Poonam Mathur, DO, MPH
Infectious Diseases Fellow
University of Maryland Medical Center
Baltimore, MD

Kudakwashe Mutyambizi, MD
Assistant Professor of Dermatology
MD Anderson Cancer Center
The University of Texas Medical School at Houston
Houston, TX

Puja H Nambiar, MD
Transplant Infectious Disease Fellow
Cleveland Clinic Foundation

Naiel N. Nassar, MD, FACP
Professor of Clinical Medicine
Chief, Division of Infectious Diseases
Program Director
Infectious Diseases Fellowship
University of California at San Francisco
Fresno Medical Education Program
Fresno, CA

Karin Nielsen, MD, MPH
Professor of Clinical Pediatrics
Division of Infectious Diseases
David Geffen UCLA School of Medicine
Director
Center for Brazilian Studies
University of California at Los Angeles
Los Angeles, CA

Neha Sheth Pandit, PharmD, AAHIVP, BCPS
Associate Professor Infectious Diseases/Pharmacotherapy
Faculty Fellow
Center for Innovative Pharmacy Solutions
Department of Pharmacy Practice and Science
University of Maryland School of Pharmacy
Baltimore, MD

Rachel Prosser, PhD, APRN, CNP, AAHIVS, FAANP
Hennepin County Medical Center
Minneapolis, MN
University of Minnesota School of Nursing
Minneapolis, MN
Metropolitan University School of Nursing
Centurion
RAAN
Positive Healthcare LLC

Christian B. Ramers, MD, MPH, AAHIVS
Assistant Medical Director, Research/Special
  Populations Director
Graduate Medical Education Family Health
  Centers of San Diego
Clinical Assistant Professor
University of California at San Diego School of Medicine
San Diego, CA

Navid Roder, MD, AAHIVS
Assistant Professor of Family Medicine and
  Community Health
University of Massachusetts Medical School
Worcester, MA

Aroonsiri Sangarlangkarn, MD, MPH
Lead Geriatrician
HIV Netherlands Australia Thailand Research
  Collaboration
Thai Red Cross AIDS Research Centre
Bangkok, Thailand

Jason J. Schafer, PharmD, MPH, BCPS, AAHIVP
Associate Professor
Department of Pharmacy Practice
Jefferson College of Pharmacy
Thomas Jefferson University
Philadelphia, PA

Jeffrey Schouten, MD, JD, AAHIVE
Senior Staff Scientist
Fred Hutchinson Cancer Research Center
Clinical Associate Professor of Surgery and
  Infectious Diseases
University of Washington School of Medicine
Seattle, WA

James D. Scott, PharmD, MEd, FCCP, FASHP, AAHIVP
Associate Dean for Experiential and Professional Affairs
Western University of Health Sciences
Pomona, CA

Rajagopal V. Sekhar, MD
Associate Professor of Medicine
Translational Metabolism Unit
Section of Diabetes, Endocrinology and Metabolism
Baylor College of Medicine
Houston, TX

Peter A. Selwyn, MD, MPH
Professor and Chairman
Department of Family and Social Medicine
Montefiore Medical Center
Albert Einstein College of Medicine
Bronx, NY

Kalpana D. Shere-Wolfe, MD
Clinical Assistant Professor
Department of Medicine
Division of Infectious Diseases
University of Maryland
Baltimore, MD

William R. Short, MD, MPH
Associate Professor of Medicine
Division of Infectious Diseases
Perelman School of Medicine
University of Pennsylvania
Philadelphia, PA

Daniel J. Skiest, MD
Chief
Division of Infectious Diseases
Baystate Medical Center
Springfield, MA

Anthony C. Speights, MD, FACOG, AAHIVS
Assistant Professor and Director of Rural Medical
    Education
Department of Family Medicine and Rural Health
Florida State University College of Medicine
Tallahassee, FL

Gary F. Spinner, PA, MPH, AAHIVS
Southwest Community Health Center
Bridgeport, CT

Zelalem Temesgen, MD, FIDSA, AAHIVS
Professor of Medicine
Executive Director, Mayo Clinic Center for Tuberculosis
Director, HIV Program
Division of Infectious Diseases
Mayo Clinic
Rochester, MN

Ye Thu, MD
Division of Infectious Disease
University of California at San Francisco
Fresno Medical Education Program
Fresno, CA

Karen J. Vigil, MD
Assistant Professor
Department of Internal Medicine
Division of Infectious Diseases
The University of Texas Health Science
    Center at Houston
Houston, TX

Daniel Wlodarczyk, MD
Professor of Clinical Medicine
Department of Medicine
University of California at San Francisco
Attending Physician
San Francisco General Hospital
San Francisco Department of Public Health
San Francisco, CA

David Alain Wohl, MD
Professor
Division of Infectious Diseases
University of North Carolina at Chapel Hill
Chapel Hill, NC

Benjamin Young, MD, PhD
Senior Vice President/Chief Medical Officer
International Association of Providers of AIDS Care
Washington, DC

Thomas P. Young, PhD, NP
T32, Post Doctoral Research Fellow
Assistant Clinical Professor
Community Health Systems
School of Nursing
University of California at San Francisco
San Francisco, CA

Barry Zevin, MD
Medical Director
Homeless Outreach Team
San Francisco Department of Public Health
San Francisco, CA

PHYSICIAN CONTINUING MEDICAL EDUCATION

ACCREDITATION STATEMENT

These activities have been planned and implemented in accordance with the accreditation requirements and policies of the Accreditation Council for Continuing Medical Education (ACCME) through the joint providership of Postgraduate Institute for Medicine and American Academy of HIV Medicine. The Postgraduate Institute for Medicine is accredited by the ACCME to provide continuing medical education for physicians.

CREDIT DESIGNATION

The Postgraduate Institute for Medicine designates these enduring materials for a maximum of 42.5 *AMA PRA Category 1 Credit*(s)™. Physicians should claim only the credit commensurate with the extent of their participation in the activity.

PHARMACIST CONTINUING EDUCATION

ACCREDITATION STATEMENT

Postgraduate Institute for Medicine is accredited by the Accreditation Council for Pharmacy Education as a provider of continuing pharmacy education.

CREDIT DESIGNATION

Postgraduate Institute for Medicine designates these continuing education activities for 41.6 contact hours (4.16 CEUs) of the Accreditation Council for Pharmacy Education.

NURSING CONTINUING EDUCATION

The Postgraduate Institute for Medicine is accredited as a provider of continuing nursing education by the American Nurses Credentialing Center's Commission on Accreditation. These educational activities are designated for 40.0 contact hours by the Postgraduate Institute for Medicine. These activities are designated for 12.9 contact hours of pharmacotherapy credit for Advance Practice Registered Nurses.

CONTENTS

DISCLOSURE OF CONFLICTS OF INTEREST

Postgraduate Institute for Medicine (PIM) requires instructors, planners, managers, and other individuals who are in a position to control the content of this activity to disclose any real or apparent conflict of interest (COI) they may have as related to the content of this activity. All identified COI are thoroughly vetted and resolved according to PIM policy. PIM is committed to providing its learners with high-quality CME activities and related materials that promote improvements or quality in health care and not a specific proprietary business interest of a commercial interest.

The *faculty* reported the following financial relationships or relationships to products or devices they or their spouse/life partner have with commercial interests related to the content of this CME activity:

The *planners and managers* reported the following financial relationships or relationships to products or devices they or their spouse/life partner have with commercial interests related to the content of this CME activity:

The following PIM planners and managers hereby state that they or their spouse/life partner do not have any financial relationships or relationships to products or devices with any commercial interest related to the content of this activity of any amount during the past 12 months: Trace Hutchison, PharmD; Samantha Mattiucci, PharmD, CHCP; Judi Smelker-Mitchek, RN, BSN; and Jan Schultz, MSN, RN, CHCP. The AAHIVM planners and managers have nothing to disclose.

NAME OF FACULTY OR PRESENTER	REPORTED FINANCIAL RELATIONSHIP
Saira Ajmal, MD	Nothing to disclose
Jonathan S. Appelbaum, MD, FACP, AAHIVS	Consulting fees: Merck, Janssen, Gilead
Lisa Armitige, MD, PhD	Nothing to disclose
Renata Arrington-Sanders, MD, MPH, ScM	Nothing to disclose
Jason Baker, MD, MS	Nothing to disclose
Ben J. Barnett, MD	Consulting fees: Gilead, BMS
	Fees for non-CME/CE services: Gilead, Merck
Tanvir K. Bell, MD, FACP, FIDSA	Nothing to disclose
Philip J. Bolduc, MD	Nothing to disclose
Christopher M. Bositis, MD, AAHIVS	Nothing to disclose
Christian Brander, PhD	Nothing to disclose
Christopher Brendemuhl, DMD	Nothing to disclose
John P. Casas, MD	Nothing to disclose
Elizabeth Chiao, MD, MPH	Nothing to disclose
Carolyn Chu, MD, MSc	Nothing to disclose
Joseph A. Church, MD	Contracted research: Gilead, Pfizer, BioProducts Laboratory
Jennifer Cocohoba, PharmD, MAS, BCPS, AAHIVP	Nothing to disclose
Emily Colgate, MD	Nothing to disclose
Dagan Coppock, MD	Nothing to disclose
Vishal Dahya, MD	Nothing to disclose
Elizabeth David, MD	Nothing to disclose
Alejandro Delgado, MD	Nothing to disclose
Paul W. DenOuden, MD	Consulting fees: Gilead
Madeline B. Deutsch, MD, MPH	Nothing to disclose
James P. Dunn, MD	Fees for non-CME/CE services: Speakers Bureau, AbbVie
Babatunde Edun, MD	Nothing to disclose
Derek Fine, MD	Nothing to disclose
Rajesh T. Gandhi, MD	Educational grant to my institution: Gilead, Merck, Viiv
Bruce L. Gilliam, MD	Consulting fees: Viiv Healthcare
Michelle K. Haas, MD	Nothing to disclose
W. David Hardy, MD, AAHIVS	Consulting fees: Gilead, Janssen, GSK/ViiV, Theratechnologies Contracted research: BMS, Gilead, GSK/ViiV, Janssen, Merck
Dennis J. Hartigan-O'Connor, MD, PhD	Nothing to disclose
Rodrigo Hasbun, MD, MPH	Speaker's bureau: Pfizer, Medicine's Company, bioMerieux, BioFire Diagnostics

Emily L. Heil, PharmD, BCPS-AQ ID	Consulting fees: ALK-Abello	William R. Short, MD, MPH	Consulting fees: Gilead, Janssen Fees for non-CME/CE services: Gilead, Janssen
Margaret Hoffman-Terry, MD, FACP, AAHIVS	Consulting fees: Merck, Viiv Fees for non-CME/CE services: Merck, Viiv, Gilead Contracted research: Viiv, Gilead	Daniel J. Skiest, MD	Contracted research: Gilead, Viiv
		Anthony C. Speights, MD, FACOG, AAHIVS	Consulting fees: Gilead
Jennifer Husson, MD, MPH	Contracted research: Merck Investigator Initiated Grant	Gary F. Spinner, PA, MPH, AAHIVS	Consulting fees: Gilead, Viiv Fees for non-CME/CE services: Gilead Ownership interest: Gilead, Sanofi Other: Yale University–speaking fee, New England AIDS Education and Training
Boris Juelg, MD, PhD	Consulting fees: Gilead		
Joy H. Kang, DO, MPH, AAHIVS	Nothing to disclose		
Joseph S. Kass, MD, JD, FAAN	Nothing to disclose		
Jeffrey T. Kirchner, DO, FAAFP, AAHIVS	Nothing to disclose		
Carolyn Kramer, MD	Nothing to disclose	Zelalem Temesgen, MD, FIDSA, AAHIVS	Nothing to disclose
Eurides Lopes, MD	Nothing to disclose	Ye Thu, MD	Nothing to disclose
Adrian Majid, MD	Nothing to disclose	Karen J. Vigil, MD	Contracted research: Merck, Gilead
Jose Martagon-Villamil, MD, DTM&H	Nothing to disclose		
Poonam Mathur, DO, MPH	Nothing to disclose	Daniel Wlodarczyk, MD	Nothing to disclose
Kudakwashe Mutyambizi, MD	Nothing to disclose	David A. Wohl, MD	
Puja H Nambiar, MD	Nothing to disclose		Consulting fees: Gilead, Viiv, Janssen Contracted research: Gilead, Merck
Naiel Nassar, MD, FACP	Nothing to disclose		
Karin Nielsen, MD, MPH	Nothing to disclose		
Neha Sheth Pandit, PharmD, AAHIVP, BCPS	Nothing to disclose	Benjamin Young, MD, PhD	
Rachel A. Prosser, PhD, APRN, CNP, AAHIVS, FAANP	Consulting fees: Gilead Contracted research: Gilead, Viiv, GSK Other: Gilead, Merck, Viiv, BMS		Consulting fees: Gilead, Merck, Viiv Fees for non-CME/CE services: Merck Contracted research: Gilead
Christian B. Ramers, MD, MPH, AAHIVS	Consulting fees: Gilead, BMS Fees for non-CME/CE services: Janssen, Gilead, AbbVie, BMS, Merck	Thomas P. Young, PhD, NP	Nothing to disclose
		Barry Zevin, MD	Nothing to disclose
Navid Roder, MD, AAHIVS	Nothing to disclose		
Aroonsiri Sangarlangkarn, MD, MPH	Nothing to disclose		
Jason J. Schafer, PharmD, MPH, BCPS, AAHIVP	Nothing to disclose		
Jeffrey T. Schouten, MD, JD, AAHIVE	Nothing to disclose		
James D. Scott, PharmD, MEd, FCCP, FASHP, AAHIVP	Nothing to disclose		
Rajagopal V. Sekhar, MD	Consulting fees: Theratechnologies		
Peter A. Selwyn, MD, MPH	Nothing to disclose		
Kalpana D. Shere-Wolfe, MD	Nothing to disclose		

METHOD OF PARTICIPATION AND REQUEST FOR CREDIT

There are no fees for participating and receiving CME/CE credit for this activity. During the period March 2017 through April 30, 2018, participants must read the learning objectives and faculty disclosures and study the educational activity.

PIM supports Green CME by offering your Request for Credit online. If you wish to receive acknowledgment for completing these activities, please complete the post-test and evaluation on **www.cmeuniversity.com**. On the navigation menu, click on "Find Post-test/Evaluation by

Course" and search by course ID **11635**. Upon registering and successfully completing the post-test with a score of 75% or better and the activity evaluation for each activity, your certificate will be made available immediately. Processing credit requests online will reduce the amount of paper used by nearly 100,000 sheets per year.

For pharmacists: Upon successfully completing the post-test with a score of 75% or better and the activity evaluation form, transcript information will be sent to the NABP CPE Monitor Service.
Media
Printed Textbook

DISCLOSURE OF UNLABELED USE

This educational activity may contain discussion of published and/or investigational uses of agents that are not indicated by the FDA. The planners of this activity do not recommend the use of any agent outside of the labeled indications.

The opinions expressed in the educational activity are those of the faculty and do not necessarily represent the views of the planners. Please refer to the official prescribing information for each product for discussion of approved indications, contraindications, and warnings.

DISCLAIMER

Participants have an implied responsibility to use the newly acquired information to enhance patient outcomes and their own professional development. The information presented in this activity is not meant to serve as a guideline for patient management. Any procedures, medications, or other courses of diagnosis or treatment discussed or suggested in this activity should not be used by clinicians without evaluation of their patients' conditions and possible contraindications and/or dangers in use, review of any applicable manufacturer's product information, and comparison with recommendations of other authorities.

1.

EPIDEMIOLOGY AND THE SPREAD OF HIV

*Philip Bolduc, Navix Order, and Emily Colgate**

CHAPTER GOAL

Upon completion of this chapter, the reader should be able to

- provide an overview of the global AIDS pandemic and the US epidemic;

- demonstrate and apply knowledge about the evolving epidemiology of HIV to both individual and population-wide aspects of clinical practice; and

- educate clinicians and patients about factors driving HIV transmission so that they will understand who is at greatest risk and also understand the need to reduce new infections among high-risk groups.

OVERVIEW OF WORLDWIDE PANDEMIC

LEARNING OBJECTIVE

Discuss the global prevalence and geographic distribution of HIV-1 and HIV-2 infections.

WHAT'S NEW

More than 36 million people worldwide are infected with HIV. Although the numbers of new HIV infections and AIDS-related deaths are declining in many regions of the world, including sub-Saharan Africa, there are still certain regions where the incidence of HIV is rising at an alarming rate, most notably in Eastern Europe, Central Asia, the Middle East, and North Africa.

KEY POINTS

- The Joint United Nations Programme on HIV/AIDS (UNAIDS) has identified several demographic subgroups that are at high risk for HIV infection and that are in danger of being left behind by the global AIDS response, including adolescent girls and young women, men who have sex with men, transgender people, people who inject drugs, prisoners, and sex workers.

- HIV occurs as types 1 and 2, with several groups and subtypes comprising HIV-1. Subtype B predominates in the Western Hemisphere and Western Europe, whereas other subtypes and recombinant forms are more prevalent elsewhere. Introduction of other subtypes and recombinant strains is occurring in the Western Hemisphere and Western Europe.

Data from the World Health Organization (WHO) and UNAIDS' *World AIDS Day Report* (2015) show global estimates of HIV continuing to demonstrate a pandemic Figure 1.1. Although the number of newly diagnosed HIV infections is declining in many countries, the number of people living with HIV continues to increase, largely due to improved access to antiretroviral therapy.

Globally, in 2014, there were 36.9 million people living with HIV, 2 million newly diagnosed infections, and 1.2 million deaths due to AIDS-related illnesses (UNAIDS, 2015). The number of new HIV infections has declined by 35% during the past 15 years, and annual AIDS-related deaths have decreased by 42% since the peak of the pandemic in 2004 (UNAIDS Fact Sheet, 2015).

Sub-Saharan Africa remains the region most heavily affected by the AIDS pandemic. However, due to several

---

* All epidemiologic data and figures, unless otherwise noted, were taken from Centers for Disease Control and Prevention HIV/AIDS Resource Library Slide Sets. Available at http://www.cdc.gov/hiv/library/slidesets/index.html. Accessed November 28–December 1, 2015.

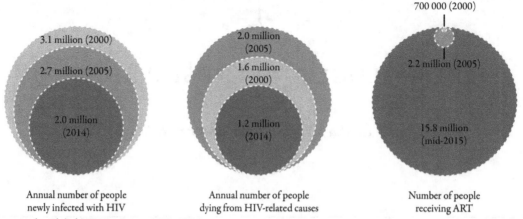

Figure 1.1   Progress in the Global HIV Response, 2000–2015. SOURCE: World Health Organization. Global Health Sector Response to HIV, 2000–2015. Available at http://reliefweb.int/report/world/global-health-sector-response-hiv-2000-2015-focus-innovations-africa-progress-report. Accessed November 28, 2015.

global initiatives, there has been a dramatic decline in the number of new HIV infections in recent years, with a 46% decrease from 2002 to 2014 (2.3 million vs. 1.4 million). There were 34% fewer AIDS-related deaths during the same time period (UNAIDS, 2015). Women continue to be disproportionately affected, accounting for more than half the total number of people living with HIV in sub-Saharan Africa (UNAIDS Fact Sheet, 2015).

Many other regions have experienced similar decreases in the number of new infections. In the Caribbean in 2014, there were 13,000 new infections, a 50% decrease from 2002. In Latin America, there were 87,000 new infections in 2014, a 17% decrease from 2002. In Asia and the Pacific, there were 340,000 new infections in 2014, a 31% decrease from 2002. In Western and Central Europe, as well as North America, the number of new infections has remained fairly stable since 2000; however, AIDS-related deaths have declined by approximately 12% (UNAIDS, 2015).

Unfortunately, there are some regions where the trends are not as encouraging. North Africa, the Middle East, Eastern Europe, and Central Asia have all seen an increase in newly diagnosed HIV since the year 2000. This is most notable in Eastern Europe and Central Asia, where infections have risen by 30% between 2000 and 2014. AIDS-related deaths have more than tripled in Eastern Europe, Central Asia, North Africa, and the Middle East during the past 15 years (UNAIDS, 2015).

Across all countries, several key demographic subgroups have largely missed out on recent progress in the fight against HIV. UNAIDS has identified six populations at higher risk of HIV infection that are in danger of being left behind by the global AIDS response: adolescent girls and young women, men who have sex with men, transgender people, people who inject drugs, prisoners, and sex workers (UNAIDS Numbers, 2015). The importance of each

of these populations varies by region and within countries. For example, in southern Africa, age-disparate intergenerational sexual relationships and transactional sex place adolescent girls and young women at extremely high risk for HIV; in Eastern Europe and Central Asia, most new HIV infections are associated with people who inject drugs; and in the Latin American and Caribbean regions, the largest proportion of new HIV infections is among men who have sex with men.

Despite significant achievements in the global HIV response during the past 15 years, there is still much work to be done. As of June 2015, 15.8 million people were accessing antiretroviral therapy, but there remain 22 million who do not have access to treatment, including 1.8 million children (UNAIDS, 2015). A significant number of people living with HIV are still unaware of their infection (representing ~50% of those living with HIV in 2014), and late initiation of antiretroviral therapy remains common in many areas of the world due to limited access to care and treatment.

HIV DIVERSITY

There are two major types of HIV, designated HIV-1 and HIV-2. Each has a similar but distinct genome with a genetic difference of approximately 60%. The vast majority of clinical cases are caused by HIV-1 (Apetrei, 2004). HIV-2 is found almost exclusively in West Africa and is transmitted at lower rates than HIV-1. It appears to have a longer incubation period, produce lower plasma viral load, and lead to AIDS in fewer patients (Apetrei, 2004). HIV-1 strains are classified into three genetically related groups based on the coding sequence of the envelope gene. Group M (main) is the most common, and groups O and N remain rare (Apetrei, 2004). Group M has at least 11 subtypes, or clades, designated A–K.

Subtype variability may eventually influence how antiretroviral therapy (ART) is used, although studies to date suggest that most antiretroviral agents appear to be equally effective regardless of the viral subtype. Certain subtypes may be less sensitive to or have a greater propensity to develop resistance to antiretroviral drugs or classes of these drugs (Spira, 2003; Gomes, 2002; Wainberg, 2004). A study from Thailand found that discordant viral load results were obtained in persons with non-B subtypes (Hackett, 2004).

There is limited information on the effect of ART for HIV-2 infection, although more clinical studies are becoming available. An in vitro study found that although the HIV-2 isolates tested were susceptible to the antiviral activities of nucleoside reverse transcriptase inhibitors and most protease inhibitors, they were highly resistant to non-nucleoside reverse transcriptase inhibitors (Witvrouw, 2004). Older studies of patients infected with HIV-2 receiving ART found mutations in HIV-2 reverse transcriptase and protease genes associated with HIV-1 drug resistance for each major drug class, including enfuvirtide, although HIV-2 also appears to have reverse transcriptase mutations that are not found in HIV-1 (Witvrouw, 2004; Colson, 2005; Damond, 2005; Rodes, 2000).

A recent in vitro study found that HIV-2 showed susceptibility to several newer antiretroviral agents, including tenofovir, emtricitabine, and the integrase inhibitor elvitegravir (Andreatta, 2013). A small study of five patients with HIV-2 found effective virologic responses and CD4+ cell increases when raltegravir was part of their ART regimen (Peterson, 2012).

Recommended Reading

UNAIDS. Focus on location and population. *World AIDS Day Report 2015*. Available at http://www.unaids.org/en/resources/documents/2015/AIDS_by_the_numbers_2015. Accessed November 28, 2015.
World Health Organization. Global update on the health sector response to HIV, 2014: Executive summary. July 2014. Available at http://www.who.int/hiv/pub/progressreports/update2014/en. Accessed November 28, 2015.

OVERVIEW OF US EPIDEMIC

LEARNING OBJECTIVE

Describe current demographic trends in HIV disease in the United States, especially regarding gender, sexuality, race/ethnicity, age, injection-drug use, socioeconomic status, and recent initiatives.

WHAT'S NEW?

HIV, originally most prevalent in urban areas of the Northeast and California, has moved heavily into the southeastern United States.

KEY POINTS

- HIV incidence and deaths have largely been stable in the past several years, leading to increasing HIV prevalence and the need for more HIV care providers.

- The leading mode of transmission by far continues to be male same-sex contact.

OVERALL US HIV INCIDENCE, DEATHS, AND PREVALENCE

According to the Centers for Disease Control and Prevention (CDC), which reports annually on the prevalence and incidence of HIV and AIDS in the 50 US states and six territories, in 2013 an estimated 1,218,400 persons aged 13 years or older had HIV, including 12.8% who were unaware of their diagnosis, comprising a total US HIV prevalence rate of 18.0 per 100,000 population (CDC. 2015). From 2010 through 2013, the annual number of new HIV diagnoses among men and women was stable or decreasing, but 2014 brought an uptick to an estimated 44,609 new infections that included 81% male and 19% female. This was primarily driven by diagnoses among men who have sex with men (MSM), overcoming decreases in other categories (Figure 1.2), and most dramatically among Black/African American MSM (Figure 1.3). Conversely, from 2008 to 2013, the annual number of deaths among HIV-infected persons declined from 19,421 to 16,281, or from 7.7 to 5.1 per 100,000 population. With new infections consistently outpacing deaths, HIV

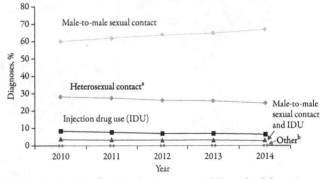

Figure 1.2 Diagnoses of HIV Infection among Adults and Adolescents, by transmission Category,2010-2014 –United states and 6 Dependent areas. SOURCE: CDC HIV/AIDS Resource Library Slide Sets. Available at http://www.cdc.gov/hiv/library/slidesets/index.html. Accessed November 28 2015.

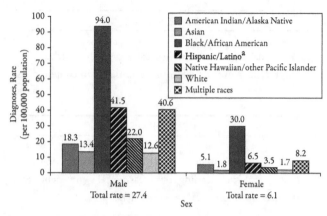

Figure 1.3 SOURCE: CDC HIV/AIDS Resource Library Slide Sets. Available at http://www.cdc.gov/hiv/library/slidesets/index.html. Accessed November 28, 2015.

prevalence continues to rise, with the number of persons living with diagnosed HIV in the United States increasing from 801,411 in 2008 to 950,811 in 2013, or from 319.3 to 355.9 per 100,000 persons. Two important implications of this must not be overlooked, namely that more clinicians will be needed to care for the burgeoning HIV population and more must be done to prevent HIV transmission.

HIV DEMOGRAPHICS ACROSS THE STATES

To take a regional look inside these statistics, Figure 1.4 shows the rates of people living with HIV by state in 2013,

whereas Figure 1.5 displays the annual rate of new HIV diagnoses by state. There is much overlap between these two figures (i.e., new infections still occur most often in areas that already have a high disease burden, such as much of the South, New York, New Jersey, and the Washington, DC, area). However, several states, such as California, Nevada, Illinois, Massachusetts, and the Mid-Atlantic states, have lower relative HIV incidence rankings compared to their prevalence, indicating that these states may be improving HIV transmission prevention. Nevertheless, Figure 1.4 demonstrates that HIV is now widely distributed throughout the United States, sparing no region. To build on the conclusion of the preceding paragraph, more HIV clinicians will be needed, but in newer geographic locations. In addition, HIV prevention and education must expand beyond historically high-prevalence areas to virtually every state and county in the United States to bend the curve of new infections in a way that we have not been able to do thus far.

AIDS REMAINS COMMON

Considering HIV/AIDS diagnoses collectively, it is concerning that the increase in prevalence is not confined to early stage disease, as the number and rate per 100,000 of persons living with AIDS increased from 454,443/180.6 in 2008 to 508,539/194.8 in 2013 (CDC NHHSTP Atlas, 2015). Despite CDC and US Preventive Task Force

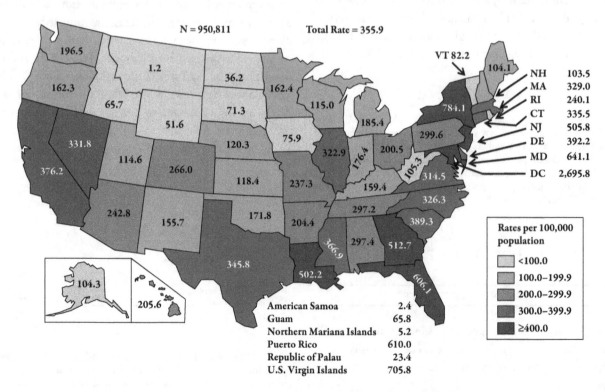

Figure 1.4 SOURCE: CDC HIV/AIDS Resource Library Slide Sets. Available at http://www.cdc.gov/hiv/library/slidesets/index.html. Accessed November 28, 2015.

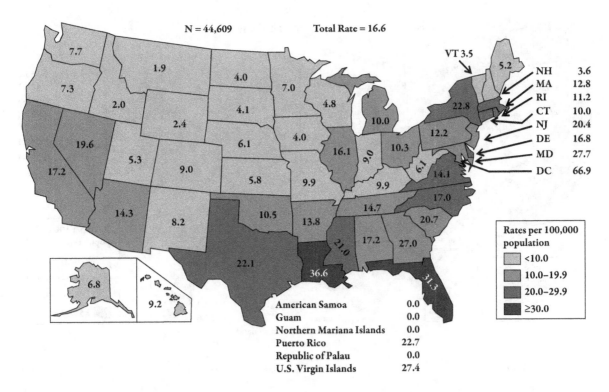

N = 44,609   Total Rate = 16.6

VT	3.5
NH	3.6
MA	12.8
RI	11.2
CT	10.0
NJ	20.4
DE	16.8
MD	27.7
DC	66.9

Rates per 100,000 population

	<10.0
	10.0–19.9
	20.0–29.9
	≥30.0

American Samoa	0.0
Guam	0.0
Northern Mariana Islands	0.0
Puerto Rico	22.7
Republic of Palau	0.0
U.S. Virgin Islands	27.4

Figure 1.5 SOURCE: CDC HIV/AIDS Resource Library Slide Sets. Available at http://www.cdc.gov/hiv/library/slidesets/index.html. Accessed November 28. 2015.

recommendations for routine, opt-out, non-risk factor-based HIV screening, in 2014, 48% of persons newly diagnosed with HIV already had AIDS. This was an improvement from 56% in 2013. There is also a regional trend toward higher rates of AIDS diagnoses in the same areas with the highest HIV incidence. Figures 1.6 and 1.7 display rates of patients who have ever had an AIDS diagnosis and those currently with an AIDS diagnosis, revealing a shift over time concentrating new AIDS diagnoses more heavily in the South and Washington, DC. This highlights areas that need the most focus on screening for occult HIV infection before it progresses to AIDS but also on care linkage, retention, and treatment for those already diagnosed with HIV.

THE US HIV CARE CONTINUUM

The concepts of diagnosis, care linkage and retention, anti-retroviral treatment, and viral suppression are represented in CDC's HIV care continuum (Figure 1.8).

Since the National HIV/AIDS Strategy release in 2010, the HIV treatment community has focused on the care continuum as the leading quality indicator in our health care system's response to HIV. As antiretroviral therapy has become increasingly potent and easier to take, the greatest challenges in suppressing "community viral load" now exist in the first two steps of the continuum, which in 2012

were the number of undiagnosed patients (12.8%) and the number of diagnosed patients who were not receiving medical care (48.1%). Only minor progress was made from 2009 to 2012 in these measures, and in 2012 less than one-third of persons with HIV in the United States were virally suppressed. Providing HIV care across a variety of settings, particularly community health centers and other medical homes that are co-located with and serve affected populations with cultural competence, will be the cornerstone of efforts to improve the HIV care continuum. This is directly reflected in three of the four National HIV/AIDS Strategy goals, which include reducing new HIV infections, increasing access to care and improving health outcomes for people living with HIV infection, and reducing HIV-related health disparities (HIV/AIDS Strategy, 2015).

TRANSMISSION BY MODE AND AGE

Efforts at HIV screening and prevention must consider who is at risk for HIV infection but also how HIV transmissions are occurring and among what age demographics. Figure 1.2 demonstrates an overall MSM transmission increase from 2010 to 2014, whereas heterosexual and injection drug use transmission decreased. Considering all ethnic groups together, same-sex transmission remains the driving force for men (82%), whereas for women, heterosexual infection predominates (87%). This is similar across Blacks/African

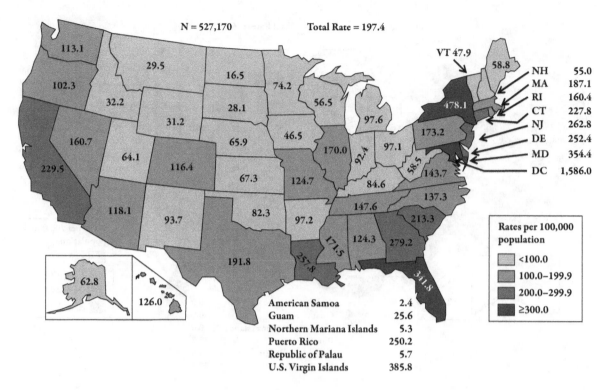

Figure 1.6 SOURCE: CDC HIV/AIDS Resource Library Slide Sets. Available at http://www.cdc.gov/hiv/library/slidesets/index.html. Accessed November 28, 2015.

Americans, Latinos, and Whites, with the exception that injection drug use is a more frequent source of infection in White women compared to the other groups.

Among MSM HIV infections in 2014, an estimated 38% were in Blacks/African Americans and 27% were in Hispanics/Latinos, far exceeding their percentages of the general population (13% and 17%, respectively). Results from CDC's Young Men's Survey (1994–2000) found that many young Black, African American, and Latino MSM who outwardly identify as heterosexual, with female spouses

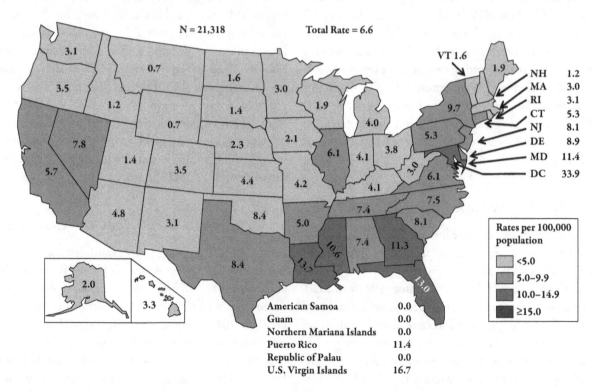

Figure 1.7 SOURCE: CDC HIV/AIDS Resource Library Slide Sets. Available at http://www.cdc.gov/hiv/library/slidesets/index.html. Accessed November 28, 2015.

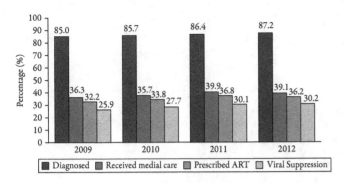

Figure 1.8 SOURCE: CDC HIV/AIDS Resource Library Slide Sets. Available at http://www.cdc.gov/hiv/library/slidesets/index.html. Accessed November 28, 2015.

or partners, also engage in same-sex encounters with other men, and that this high-risk group represents a bridge for transmitting HIV to women (Fitzpatrick, 2004; Millett 2004; Valleroy, 2004). In addition, many poor and/or minority women lack the agency—whether economic, cultural, or otherwise—to leave or at least use condoms with abusive or unfaithful men who engage in high-risk sex with other partners or commercial sex workers. HIV prevention efforts must account for such factors to make inroads against HIV transmission in these highest-risk groups.

When examining HIV transmission by age group, more than half of new infections in 2014 were in persons younger than age 35 years, and 22% were in persons younger than age 25 years. Also worth noting are the 9% of infections in the 55 years old or older cohort, reminding clinicians to screen for HIV well outside the peak demographic of 20- to 40-year-olds. It is clear that HIV prevention measures, which in 2016 included HIV prevention education, HIV treatment as prevention, and HIV pre-exposure prophylaxis, should include a substantial focus on MSM and their female partners as well as teens and older individuals at risk for infection.

Recommended Reading

Centers for Disease Control and Prevention. *HIV Surveillance Report, 2015.* Available at http://www.cdc.gov/hiv/library/reports/surveillance.

SPREAD OF HIV AMONG WOMEN, CHILDREN, AND ADOLESCENTS

WHAT'S NEW?

Twenty-four percent of HIV diagnoses in 2013 in the United States were among women, which represents a slight decrease from 2011. With widespread utilization of antiretroviral therapy, transmission of HIV from mother to child has decreased to less than 2% in the United States.

KEY POINTS

- High-risk heterosexual contact remains the most common risk factor for HIV acquisition among adult women.

- Despite recommendations for universal screening of pregnant women, through 2011, only 23% of pregnant women were tested for HIV during pregnancy.

- Adolescent HIV transmission mirrors adult patterns, with large majorities of males infected via same-sex contact and females via heterosexual contact.

WOMEN

Worldwide, women continue to account for more than half of all HIV-infected persons, largely through heterosexual transmission (amfAR, 2015). However, in the United States, women represented only 24% of HIV diagnoses in 2013, slightly down from 25% in 2010, comprising an estimated 9278 newly diagnosed infections. This disparity is due to the preponderance of male-to-male HIV transmission in the United States. Of these new diagnoses, approximately 6500 were stage 3 (AIDS) classifications, a number that has been declining since 1996, as shown in Figure 1.9. HIV incidence among US women is currently highest in the South; Washington, DC; Illinois; Nevada; and the industrial states of the Northeast (Figure 1.10).

From 2007 through 2013, Black/African American women accounted for the majority of new HIV diagnoses in US females. The seropositivity rate of these women (34.8 per 100,000 persons) was 19 times higher than that of White females (1.8) and 5 times higher than that of Hispanic females (7). Although Black/African American women comprised only 13% of the female population, they accounted for 61% of diagnoses of HIV infection among women. Hispanic/Latino women made up 15% of the female population and accounted for 15% of diagnoses. White women encompassed 65% of the US female population and yet accounted for only 17% of HIV diagnoses in women overall (CDC, 2015).

Factors that increase a woman's risk of acquiring HIV include not knowing her partner's risk factors for HIV infection, having a lack of HIV knowledge, and having a decreased awareness of risk (CDC, 2011). Relationships with their partners play a pivotal role as well. In relationships in which women are physically abused, vulnerability to HIV is increased because they may not insist on condom use due to fear of being harmed. Women with a history of

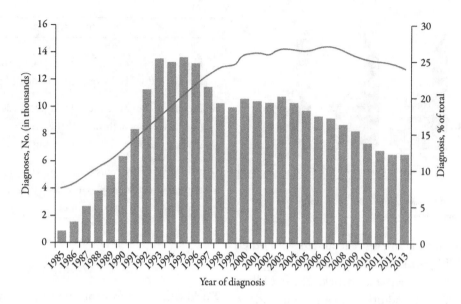

Figure 1.9 SOURCE: CDC HIV/AIDS Resource Library Slide Sets. Available at http://www.cdc.gov/hiv/library/slidesets/index.html. Accessed November 28, 2015.

sexual abuse are more likely to engage in high-risk sexual activity and use drugs compared to women without such behaviors. This includes exchanging sexual activities for drugs and money as well as having difficulty refusing unwanted sex.

As shown in Figure 1.11, the most common mode of transmission for women is high-risk heterosexual contact, followed by injection drug use. Regardless of age, females older than age 13 years are usually infected through heterosexual contact. However, this rate declines as age increases, during which time risk for acquiring HIV through injection drug use increases (CDC, 2015).

Sexual HIV transmission occurs through unprotected vaginal or anal sex, with receptive anal sex posing the highest risk and insertive vaginal sex the lowest. Oral sex is a theoretical risk if there are breaks in the oral and genital mucosa through which blood or genital secretions may pass. Similarly, sexually transmitted infections that disrupt

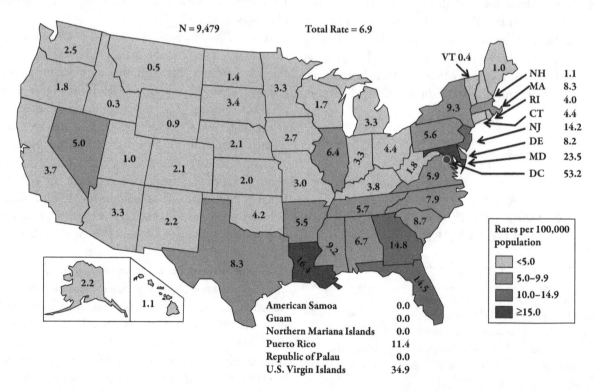

Figure 1.10 SOURCE: CDC HIV/AIDS Resource Library Slide Sets. Available at http://www.cdc.gov/hiv/library/slidesets/index.html. Accessed November 28, 2015.

Stage 3 (AIDS) Classifications among Adult and Adolescent Females, by Transmission Category and Age at Diagnosis 2013—United States and 6 Dependent Areas

Transmission category	Age at Diagnosis (in years)				
	13–19	20–24	25–34	35–44	≥45
	N=147	N=348	N=1,308	N=1,821	N=2,915
	%	%	%	%	%
Injection drug use	2.4	5.2	13	16.4	23.1
Heterosexual contact[a]	39.3	79	85.4	83.4	76.6
Other[b]	58.3	15.8	1.6	0.2	0.3
Total	100.0	100.0	100.0	100.0	100.0

Note: Data include persons with a diagnosis of HIV infection regardless of stage of disease at diagnosis. All displayed data have been statistically adjusted to account for reporting delays and missing transmission category, but not for incomplete reporting.
[a] Heterosexual contact with a person known to have, or to be at high risk for, HIV infection.
[b] Includes blood transfusion, perinatal exposure, and risk factor not reported or not identified.

Figure 1.11 SOURCE: CDC HIV/AIDS Resource Library Slide Sets. Available at http://www.cdc.gov/hiv/library/slidesets/index.html. Accessed November 28, 2015.

genital mucosa and stimulate a local immune response increase the likelihood of acquiring or transmitting HIV. Because gonorrhea and syphilis in particular have a higher rate in women of color compared to white women, this likely plays a role in their heightened risk of HIV acquisition (CDC, 2015). Socioeconomic status also plays a role in HIV risk. In states with higher rates of poverty and limited access to health care, women are more likely to use drugs and exchange sex for drugs or money. These risk factors have been shown to increase risk of HIV, directly or indirectly (CDC, 2015).

CHILDREN

The dramatic reduction in mother-to-child HIV transmission in the United States is a major success of the antiretroviral era (Figure 1.12). In 1992, an estimated 952 pediatric HIV cases were reported in the United States. By 2004, the number declined to 177. In 2011, there were only 53 reported perinatal infections, although this increased to 107 in 2013 (CDC 2014, 2015). The overall rate of perinatal HIV infections reported by the CDC for 2008 was 6.8 per 100,000 live births, and the CDC's goal by the end of 2015 was to reduce this 25% to 5.1 (CDC, 2015).

It bears noting that of all HIV-positive children younger than age 13 years during 2008–2011, less than half (36%) tested positive during their first year of life. This highlights the importance of screening both nonpregnant woman of childbearing age and all women for HIV during pregnancy. The US Public Health Service recommends that all pregnant women be offered HIV counseling and voluntary HIV tests, but through 2011, fewer than 25% were tested during pregnancy (CDC, 2011).

HIV disproportionately affects Black/African American children. While accounting for 66% of diagnoses, they comprised only 14% of the population of US children in 2011, whereas Hispanic (24% of population, 13% of HIV diagnoses) and White (52% of population, 15% of HIV diagnoses) children are infected far less often than their population percentages.

ADOLESCENTS

Of all adolescents and young adults aged 13–24 years diagnosed with HIV infection, 59% were Black/African Americans, again far outpacing their percentage of the general population. Another striking disparity for Black/African American children is that their percentage among

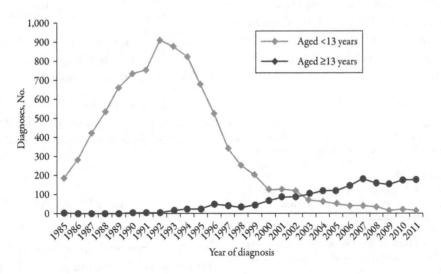

Figure 1.12 SOURCE: CDC HIV/AIDS Resource Library Slide Sets. Available at http://www.cdc.gov/hiv/library/slidesets/index.html. Accessed November 28, 2015.

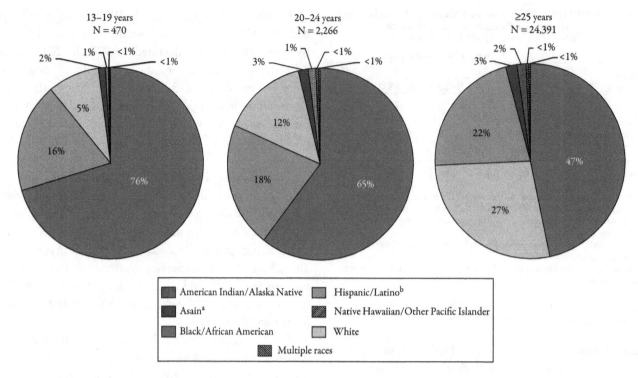

13–19 years
N = 470

20–24 years
N = 2,266

≥25 years
N = 24,391

Legend:
- American Indian/Alaska Native
- Asain[a]
- Black/African American
- Hispanic/Latino[b]
- Native Hawaiian/Other Pacific Islander
- White
- Multiple races

Figure 1.13 SOURCE: CDC HIV/AIDS Resource Library Slide Sets. Available at http://www.cdc.gov/hiv/library/slidesets/index.html. Accessed November 28, 2015.

all children with AIDS increases dramatically with decreasing age, as seen moving right to left in Figure 1.13.

Transmission rates through male same-sex contact increased from 72% to 80% of all transmission from 2009 to 2013 in the adolescent and young adult population, whereas heterosexual infections decreased from 20% to 14%. Infections from injection drug use decreased slightly from 4% to 3%.

In 2013, females comprised 19% of the HIV diagnoses in adolescents (13–19 years) and 11% in young adults (20–24 years) compared to 22% of adults older than 24 years. The mode of HIV transmission varies between sexes in this age group, as it does in adults: Whereas 90% of adolescent and young adult females are infected through heterosexual contact, 90% of males contract HIV through male-to-male sexual contact (CDC 2013).

Recommended Reading

Centers for Disease Control and Prevention. HIV surveillance report: Diagnoses of HIV infection and AIDS in the United States and dependent areas. 2009. Vol. 21. Available at http://www.cdc.gov/hiv/pdf/statistics_2009_HIV_Surveillance_Report_vol_21.pdf. Accessed May 29, 2014.

Centers for Disease Control and Prevention. HIV/AIDS statistics overview. Available at http://www.cdc.gov/hiv/statistics/overview/index.html. Accessed December 1, 2015.

Centers for Disease Control and Prevention. National HIV prevention progress report, 2013 technical notes. Available at http://www.cdc.gov/hiv/pdf/policies_NationalProgressReport.pdf. Accessed November 30, 2015.

SPREAD OF HIV AMONG MEN AND WOMEN IN COMMUNITIES OF COLOR

WHAT'S NEW?

Young Black/African American men who have sex with men have the highest risk for HIV infection of any demographic group in the United States.

KEY POINTS

- Black/African Americans—men who have sex with men, women, and children—are HIV-infected at three to five times higher than their percentage of the US population.

- AIDS and AIDS-related deaths among Black/African Americans and Hispanics are higher than population norms, indicating poorer outcomes with HIV infection.

UNEQUAL BURDENS

Another important perspective of US HIV epidemiologic data is to recognize the ethnic and racial groups hardest hit by HIV infection and deaths, particularly Blacks/

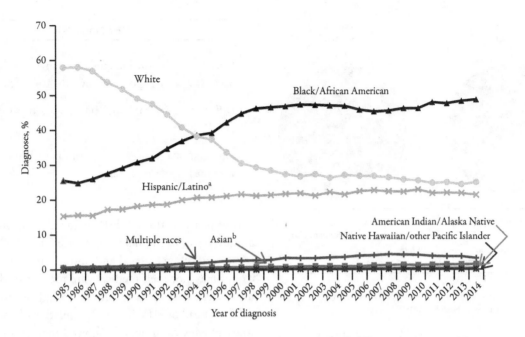

Figure 1.14   SOURCE: CDC HIV/AIDS Resource Library Slide Sets. Available at http://www.cdc.gov/hiv/library/slidesets/index.html. Accessed November 28, 2015.

African Americans. Figure 1.14 shows how this group steadily increased its percentage among AIDS diagnoses early in the epidemic while cases among Caucasians steadily declined, overtaking them in 1995 before leveling off in 2000, continuing to far exceed all other racial groups. Figure 1.15 similarly depicts how Blacks/African Americans continue to be vastly overrepresented among persons living with HIV than in the general population (44% vs. 13%). This is also true, but to a lesser extent, for Hispanics (24% vs. 17%). The current highest risk demographic in the United States is young black MSM who live in the South (Figure 1.16).

Black/African American women are even more impacted by HIV, accounting for 61% of all new diagnoses among women (Figure 1.17), which is 4.7 times the expected population-adjusted rate. Similarly, 64% of all children younger than age 13 years are Black/African American. Death rates are also heavily skewed against Blacks/African Americans with HIV (Figure 1.18), with a nearly eightfold higher death rate than that of HIV-infected Whites. The Hispanic death rate is twice that of Whites, whereas other groups fare the same or better. Regardless of how these data are examined—whether considering HIV diagnoses, AIDS, or deaths—there is a strikingly excessive burden of HIV shouldered in the United States by Blacks/African Americans in particular and somewhat by Hispanics. The National HIV/AIDS Strategy recognizes this in its call to

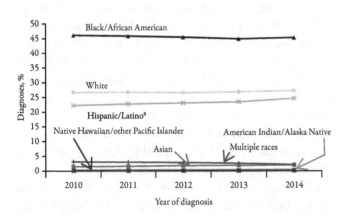

Figure 1.15   SOURCE: CDC HIV/AIDS Resource Library Slide Sets. Available at http://www.cdc.gov/hiv/library/slidesets/index.html. Accessed November 28, 2015.

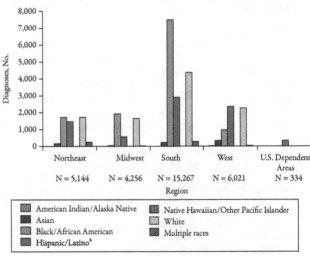

Figure 1.16   SOURCE: CDC HIV/AIDS Resource Library Slide Sets. Available at http://www.cdc.gov/hiv/library/slidesets/index.html. Accessed December 1, 2015.

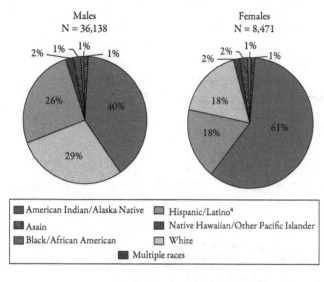

Males
N = 36,138

2% · 1% · 1% · 1%
26%
40%
29%

Females
N = 8,471

2% · 2% · 1% · 1%
18%
61%
18%

■ American Indian/Alaska Native ▧ Hispanic/Latino[a]
▨ Asain ▨ Native Hawaiian/Other Pacific Islander
■ Black/African American □ White
■ Multiple races

Figure 1.17 SOURCE: CDC HIV/AIDS Resource Library Slide Sets. Available at http://www.cdc.gov/hiv/library/slidesets/index.html. Accessed November 28, 2015.

reduce racial disparities in HIV care, and this should be incorporated into the mission of all local, regional, and national HIV programs.

SPREAD OF HIV AMONG IMMIGRANT POPULATIONS

WHAT'S NEW?

- Legal immigrants and refugees from West Africa to the United States may be infected with HIV-2, which has important implications for clinical care.

Deaths of Persons with Diagnosed HIV Infection, by Race/Ethnicity, 2013—United States

Race/ethnicity	No.	Rate
American Indian/Alaska Native	66	2.8
Asian[a]	64	0.4
Black/African American	7,581	19.4
Hispanic/Latino[b]	2,664	4.9
Native Hawaiian/other Pacific Islander	5	0.9
White	5,028	2.5
Multiple races	874	14.1
Total[c]	16,281	5.1

Note: Data include persons with a diagnosis of HIV infection regardless of stage of disease at diagnosis. All displayed data have been statistically adjusted to account for reporting delays, but not for incomplete reporting. Rates are per 100,000 population. Because column totals for estimated numbers were calculated independently of the values for the subpopulations, the values in each column may not sum up to the total column.
[a] Includes Asian/Pacific Islander legacy cases.
[b] Hispanics/Latinos can be of any race.
[c] Includes persons of unknown race/ethnicity

Figure 1.18 SOURCE: CDC HIV/AIDS Resource Library Slide Sets. Available at http://www.cdc.gov/hiv/library/slidesets/index.html. Accessed November 28, 2015.

KEY POINTS

- Since January 2010, immigrants no longer are required to have HIV testing upon entry into the United States.
- Different immigrant populations have widely varying rates of HIV infection.
- Immigrants, legal or not, face many barriers to engagement with the health care system.

A new phase of the US HIV epidemic is evolving among minority groups in many major cities. This includes immigrants and refugees, legal and undocumented, the latter of whom may not seek medical care for fear of deportation. Insufficient data make it difficult to fully assess the potential for spread of HIV in these populations. One binational study of Mexican migrants showed more high-risk behaviors among migrants but also higher condom use rates. However, migrants remain at higher risk for HIV acquisition than Mexicans who do not migrate to the United States. Ideally, a binational surveillance system would be required to assess trends in HIV, sexually transmitted diseases, and tuberculosis and related risk behaviors in the Mexican migrant population between US states such as California and the originating "sending" states such as Mexico (Sanchez 2004; Magis-Rodrigues, 2009).

Since January 2010, refugees are no longer tested for HIV-infection upon arrival to the United States. However, current CDC guidelines recommend universal screening for all persons 13–64 years of age (Branson, 2006). Thus, HIV screening of all refugees is encouraged, along with a consideration of repeat screening 3–6 months following settlement. Specific testing for HIV-2 should be considered for refugees who screen positive for HIV and are native to or have transited through countries with a high prevalence of HIV-2. The new CDC-recommended fourth-generation testing algorithm will differentiate between HIV-1 and HIV-2, although older-generation HIV antibody screening tests generally do not.

Historically, most HIV infections in the United States are HIV-1, whereas HIV-2 largely has been confined to persons in or from West Africa (O'Brien, 1992). The CDC's 2014 surveillance case definition for HIV and AIDS applies to both variants of HIV and has added specific criteria for defining HIV-2 (CDC, 2015). Although the routes of transmission are similar, clinical management may differ (Ntemgwa, 2009). From 1988 to June 2010, only 242 HIV-2 cases were reported to the CDC. Of these, 166 met the case definition for AIDS. The HIV-2 cases were concentrated in the Northeast (66%), including 46% in New York

City. They occurred primarily among persons born in West Africa (81%). No transmission risk factor was identified in most of the cases, and no significant trends in HIV-2 diagnosis were observed (CDC, 2015). Data from 2010 to the present are not available from the CDC, but immigration from West Africa to the United States has continued, so clinicians should be aware of this possibility when caring for these patients.

Variable rates of HIV diagnoses exist within different immigrant populations. In 2012, the annual rate of adults and adolescents living with HIV in the United States for Hispanics/Latinos was 460 per 100,000 persons, which was greater than 2.6 times that for Whites (CDC, 2015). Multiple factors contribute to the risk for HIV infection among Hispanics/Latinos and other immigrants. Migration within and across national borders in search of work may contribute to increased HIV risk behaviors. In addition, change in residence can result in loneliness, isolation, and disruption of social, familial, and sexual relationships that can lead to risk-taking behavior (Organista, 2004). Foreign-born New Yorkers overall are less likely to be diagnosed with HIV than their US-born counterparts (19 vs. 49 per 100,000 persons). However, rates of new HIV diagnoses vary widely by country of birth in this population. In another study, the authors found lack of knowledge regarding HIV risk, social stigma, secrecy, and symptom-driven health-seeking behavior (as opposed to routine preventive care) as factors in delayed HIV presentation in immigrants. Furthermore, compared to US-born patients, immigrants were significantly younger; more likely to present with indicators of more advanced HIV disease, including opportunistic infections; had lower $CD4^+$ counts; and were more likely to be hospitalized at the time of HIV diagnosis (Levy, 2007).

Recommended Reading

US Department of Health and Human Services. AIDSinfo. Available at http://www.aidsinfo.nih.gov/contentfiles/adultandadolescentgl.pdf.

THE EVOLVING ROLE OF THE GAY COMMUNITY IN THE SPREAD OF HIV

WHAT'S NEW?

Whereas the greatest number of HIV infections occur in MSM ages 25–34 years, the greatest percentage increase in HIV diagnoses in recent years has been in MSM older than age 55 years.

KEY POINTS

- Individuals who identify as gay, bisexual, or as other MSM are the only population group in the United States in which new HIV infections have continued to steadily increase since the 1990s, with young Black MSM being disproportionally affected.

- There is limited national data, but it is believed that transgender individuals are at extremely high risk for HIV infection, with reports from other countries indicating that rates of HIV are up to 50 times greater in transgender people compared to the general population.

Since the beginning of the HIV/AIDS epidemic in the United States, MSM have constituted the largest percentage of persons diagnosed with HIV/AIDS. Individuals who identify as gay, bisexual, or other MSM are the only population group in the United States in which new infections have continued to rise steadily since the early 1990s (CDC, 2015). In 2013, an estimated 80.6% (31,023) of all diagnosed HIV infections among adult and adolescent males were attributed to male-to-male sexual contact. The estimated number of diagnoses of HIV infection among adult and adolescent males attributed to male-to-male sexual contact increased by 12%, from 27,668 in 2009 to 31,023 in 2013. Diagnoses of infections attributed to male-to-male sexual contact and injection drug use decreased by 22%, from 1643 in 2009 to 1284 in 2013.

The percentage of HIV cases diagnosed in the gay community differs based on race and ethnicity. From 2009 through 2013, the estimated percentage of MSM diagnosed with HIV infection that were White decreased from 34% to 32%, whereas the percentage of MSM diagnosed with HIV infection that were Hispanic/Latino increased from 23% to 24%. The percentage among those who were Black/African American increased from 38% to 39%.

Differentiating between age groups in MSM, those aged 13–24 and 25–34 years accounted for a significant amount of HIV infections from 2009 to 2013. During this period, the largest number of HIV diagnoses were among MSM aged 25–34 years, increasing by 25%, whereas MSM aged 55 years or older had the greatest percentage increase in diagnoses at 29%. The number of diagnoses among those aged 35–44 years decreased by 13% during this period.

With the high prevalence of HIV in the MSM community, the cumulative risk of contracting or transmitting the virus becomes greater as these individuals age. Being unaware of one's HIV status, especially common among MSM of color and young MSM, increases the risk of transmitting HIV infection as well. A 2008 CDC study showed that among urban MSM from 21 cities, 55% had not been HIV tested in the previous 12 months (MMWR, 2011). According to the latest CDC guidelines, MSM who are high risk for HIV infection should be screened at least annually; this includes those with more than one sex partner since their last HIV test and MSM who are injection drug users (MMWR, 2006).

Transgender individuals comprise one of the highest risk groups in the United States for acquiring HIV infection. Unfortunately, surveillance data on a national level have not been collected in this population, so information is lacking on how many transgender individuals are infected with HIV. However, based on limited data reported by the CDC, in 2010, the highest percentage of newly identified HIV-positive test results was among transgender people. In New York City, from 2007 to 2011, there were 191 new diagnoses of HIV infection among transgender people, 99% of which were among transgender women, with more than 90% being Black/African Americans or Latinos. More than half (52%) of these newly diagnosed transgender women were 20–29 years old. Also, 51% of transgender women had documentation in their medical records of substance use, commercial sex work, homelessness, incarceration, and/or sexual abuse compared with 31% of other people who were not transgender. A review of studies of HIV infection in countries with data available for transgender people estimated that HIV prevalence for transgender women was nearly 50 times greater than that for other adults of reproductive age (CDC, 2015).

Recommended Reading

Centers for Disease Control and Prevention. A web-based survey of HIV testing and risk behaviors among gay, bisexual, and other men who have sex with men—United States, 2012. HIV Surveillance Special Report 14. November 2015. http://www.cdc.gov/hiv/library/reports/surveillance/#panel2. Accessed November 28, 2015.

Centers for Disease Control and Prevention. HIV among transgender people in the United States. November 2013. Available at http://www.cdc.gov/hiv/group/gender/transgender. Accessed November 28, 2015.

References

American Foundation for AIDS Research (amfAR). Statistics: Women and HIV/AIDS. Available at http://www.amfar.org/about-hiv-and-aids/facts-and-stats/statistics--women-and-hiv-aids. Accessed December 1, 2015.

Andreatta K, Miller, MD, White KL. HIV-2 antiviral potency and selection of drug resistance mutations by the integrase strand transfer inhibitor elvitegravir and NRTIs emtricitabine and tenofovir in vitro. J AIDS 2013; 62(4):367–374.

Apetrei C, Marx PA. Simian retroviral infections in human beings. Lancet. 2004;364(9429):137–138.

Branson BM. To screen or not to screen: is that really the question? Ann Intern Med. 2006; 145(11):857–859.

Centers for Disease Control and Prevention. HIV infection among transgender people. November 2013. Available at http://www.cdc.gov/hiv/group/gender/transgender. Accessed November 28, 2015.

Centers for Disease Control and Prevention. HIV surveillance report: Diagnoses of HIV infection and AIDS in the United States and dependent areas. 2009. Vol 21. Available at http://www.cdc.gov/hiv/pdf/statistics_2009_HIV_Surveillance_Report_vol_21.pdf. Accessed May 29, 2014.

Centers for Disease Control and Prevention. HIV surveillance report: Diagnoses of HIV infection and AIDS in the United States and dependent areas, 2014. Vol 26. Available at http://www.cdc.gov/hiv/pdf/library/reports/surveillance/cdc-hiv-surveillance-report-us.pdf. Accessed November 24, 2015.

Centers for Disease Control and Prevention. HIV surveillance report, 2014. Vol. 26. Published November 2015. Available at http://www.cdc.gov/hiv/library/reports/surveillance. Accessed November 28, 2015.

Centers for Disease Control and Prevention. HIV testing among men who have sex with men—21 cities, United States, 2008. MMWR Morb Mortal Wkly Rep. 2011 Jun 3;60(21):694–699.

Centers for Disease Control and Prevention. HIV/AIDS Resource Library Slide Sets. Available at http://www.cdc.gov/hiv/library/slidesets/index.html. Accessed November 30, 2015.

Centers for Disease Control and Prevention. HIV/AIDS Statistics Overview. Available at http://www.cdc.gov/hiv/statistics/overview/index.html. Accessed December 1, 2015.

Centers for Disease Control and Prevention. Monitoring selected national HIV prevention and care objectives by using HIV surveillance data – United States and six dependent areas – 2011. HIV Surveillance Supplemental Report 2013; 18(No.5). Available at http://www.cdc.gov/hiv/library/reports/surveillance. Published October 2013. Accessed May 29, 2014.

Centers for Disease Control and Prevention. National HIV prevention progress report, 2013 Technical Notes. Available at http://www.cdc.gov/hiv/pdf/policies_NationalProgressReport.pdf. Accessed November 30, 2015.

Centers for Disease Control and Prevention. Revised Recommendations for HIV Testing of Adults, Adolescents, and Pregnant Women in Health-care Settings. MMWR September 22, 2006. Available at http://www.cdc.gov/mmwr/preview/mmwrhtml/rr5514a1.htm. Accessed November 28, 2015.

Centers for Disease Control and Prevention. Revised Surveillance Case Definition for HIV- United States, 2014. Recommendations and Reports 2014;63(RR03):1–10. Available at http://www.cdc.gov/mmwr/preview/mmwrhtml/rr6303a1.htm?s_cid=rr6303a1_e. Accessed November 23, 2015.

Colson P, Henry M, Tivoli N, et al. Polymorphism and drug-selected mutations in the reverse transcriptase gene of HIV-2 from patients living in southeastern France. J Med Virol.2005; 75:381–390.

Damond F, Brun-Vezinet F, Matheron S, et al. Polymorphism of the human immunodeficiency virus type 2 (HIV-2 protease gene and selection of drug resistance mutations in HIV-2-infected patients treated with protease inhibitors. J Clin Microbiol. 2005; 43:484–487.

Fitzpatrick LK, Grant L, Eure C, et al. Investigation of HIV transmission among young black men who have sex with men (MSM) in North Carolina: Implications for prevention. In: Program and abstracts of the XV International AIDS Conference; July 11–16, 2004; Bangkok, Thailand. Abstract C10746.

Gomes P, Diogo I, Gonca Ives MF, et al. Different pathways to nelfinavir genotypic resistance in HIV-1 subtypes B and C. In: Program and abstracts of the 9th Conference on Retroviruses and Opportunistic Infections; February 24–28, 2002; Seattle, WA. Abstract 46.

Hackett Jr J, Holzmayer V, Swanson P, et al. Analysis of HIV-1 genetic diversity in London and its impact on the performance of viral load assays. In: Program and abstracts of the XV International AIDS Conference: July 11–16, 2004; Bangkok, Thailand. Abstract 3419.

Levy V, Prentiss D, Balmas G et al. Factors in the delayed HIV presentation of immigrants in Northern California: implications for voluntary counseling and testing programs. J Immig Minor Health. 2007; 9(1):49–54.

Magis-Rodriguez C, Lemp G, Hernandez MT, et al. Going North: Mexican migrants and their vulnerability to HIV. J Acquir Immune Defic Syndr 2009; 51(Suppl 1): S21–S25.

Millett G. Men on the 'down low': more questions than answers. In: Program and abstracts of the 11th Conference on Retroviruses and Opportunistic Infections; February 8-11, 2004; San Francisco, California. Abstract 83.

National HIV/AIDS Strategy for the United States: Update to 2020. https://www.aids.gov/federal-resources/national-hiv-aids-strategy/overview. Accessed November 30, 2015.

Ntemgwa ML, d'Aquin TT, Brenner BG et al. Antiretroviral drug resistance in human immunodeficiency virus type 2. Antimicrob Agents Chemother. 2009; 53(9):3611–3619.

Organista KC, Carillo H, Avala G. HIV prevention with Mexican migrants: review, critique, and recommendations. J Acquir Immune Defic Syndr. 2004; 37(Suppl 4):S227–S239.

O'Brien TR, George JR, Holmberg SD. Human immunodeficiency virus type 2 infection in the United States. Epidemiology, diagnosis, and public health implications. JAMA. 1992; 27(20):2775–2779.

Peterson K, Ruelle J, Vekemans M, et al, The role of raltegravir in the treatment of HIV-2 infections: evidence from a case series. Antivir Ther 2012; 17(6):1097–1099.

Rodes B, Holguin A, Soriano V, et al. Emergence of drug resistance mutations in human immunodeficiency virus type 2-infected subjects undergoing antiretroviral therapy. J Clin Microbiol. 2000:1370–1374.

Sanchez MA, Lemp GF, Magis-Rodriquez C, et al. The epidemiology of HIV among Mexican migrants and recent immigrants in California and Mexico. J Acquir Immune Defic Syndr. 2004; 37(Suppl 4):S204–S214.

Spira S, Wainberg MA, Loemba H, et al. Impact of clade diversity on HIV-1 virulence, antiretroviral drug sensitivity and drug resistance. J Antimicrob Chemother. 2003; 51:229–240.

UNAIDS. AIDS by the Numbers 2015. World AIDS Day Report. Available at http://www.unaids.org/en/resources/documents/2015/AIDS_by_the_numbers_2015. Accessed November 27, 2015.

UNAIDS. Focus on location and population. World AIDS Day Report 2015. Available at http://www.unaids.org/en/resources/documents/2015/FocusLocationPopulation. Accessed November 28, 2015.

UNAIDS. UNAIDS fact sheet 2015. Available at http://www.unaids.org/en/resources/documents/2015/20150714_factsheet. Accessed November 28, 2015.

Valleroy LA, MacKellar D, Behel S, Secura G. The bridge for HIV transmission to women from 15- to 29-year-old men who have sex with men in 7 US cities. In: Program and abstracts of the XV International AIDS Conference; July 11-16, 2004; Bangkok, Thailand. Abstract 1367.

Wainberg MA. HIV-1 subtype distribution and the problem of drug resistance. AIDS. 2004; 18(Suppl 3):S63–S68.

Witvrouw M, Pannecouque C, Switzer VM, et al. Susceptibility of HIV-2, SIV and SHIV to various anti-HIV-1 compounds: implications for treatment and postexposure prophylaxis. Antivir Ther. 2004; 9:57–65.

2.

THE ORIGIN, EVOLUTION, AND EPIDEMIOLOGY OF HIV-1 AND HIV-2

Jeffrey T. Kirchner

CHAPTER GOAL

To explain how HIV evolved from cross-species transmission of strains of simian immunodeficiency virus (SIV) to humans (viral zoonosis), spread out of Africa in the early 20th century, and ultimately resulted in the global AIDS pandemic.

LEARNING OBJECTIVES

- Discuss the distinct origins of HIV-1 and HIV-2 from SIVs and the multiple cross-transmission events from apes to humans.

- Describe the origin of the initial HIV infections in south-central Africa, the key reasons for viral dissemination to other areas of sub-Saharan Africa, and the ultimate global spread of HIV.

- Discuss the diversity of HIV, including viral groups, viral clades, and recombinant forms and their implications for future transmission of HIV, as well as treatments and vaccine developments.

WHAT'S NEW?

The origin of HIV-1 can be traced to the early 1920s from southern Cameroon and then to Kinshasa in what is now the Democratic Republic of Congo. The combination of rapid population growth, changes in sexual behaviors, and the use of unsterilized needles likely contributed to the rapid spread of HIV, especially groups M and O.

KEY POINTS

- All strains of HIV-1 and HIV-2 are genetic descendants of SIVs. Initial cross-species transmission of the virus occurred from butchering and eating of bush meat.

- HIV-1 group M ("main") and associated viral subtypes (A–K) account for approximately 95% of infections globally, with a much smaller number caused by groups N, O, and P.

- HIV-2 and its groups (A–H) are mainly limited to West Africa, but since the discovery of HIV-2 in 1986, cases have been reported in Europe and the United States. HIV-2 represents approximately 3% of all HIV infections, although its prevalence appears to be declining.

- Genetic diversity of HIV, including recombination between subtypes, may continue to present challenges to the development of a globally effective vaccine.

ORIGIN OF HIV AND ENTRY INTO HUMANS

HIV, a retrovirus and member of the lentivirus family, was identified as the cause of AIDS 2 years after the first cases were reported in 1981 (Gottlieb, 1981). Dr. Luc Montaigner in France and Dr. Robert Gallo in the United States are credited respectively with identifying HIV-1 (Gallo, 2003). The pandemic form of HIV, also referred to as group M (for "main"), is responsible for the majority of infections globally, currently estimated to be approximately 75 million. Since the discovery of HIV-1, followed by HIV-2 in 1986, the reasons for its emergence during the 20th century, its transmission to humans, its genetic diversity, and the pathogenesis of the virus have been the subjects of extensive research.

It was first noted in 1999, via genetic sequencing, that the chimpanzee *Pan troglodytes troglodytes* infected with simian immunodeficiency virus (SIV_{cpz}) was likely the primary natural reservoir for HIV-1 (Gao,1999). Later work by Keele determined that HIV-1 in humans began with cross-species transmission and recombination of two SIVs (from red-capped mangabeys and greater spot-nosed monkeys) to chimpanzees that preyed on these animals (Keele, 2006). Keele and his group analyzed mitochondrial DNA and viral-specific antibody from 599 fecal samples from chimpanzees. These samples exhibited a strong and broad cross-reactive Western blot profile indistinguishable from that of HIV-1 human controls. To date, serologic evidence for SIV infection has been identified in more than 45 non-human primate species (NHPS) (Sharp, 2011; Peeters, 2014). The genetic diversity of these viral species is complex and includes coevolution of virus–host, cross-species transmission, and viral recombination.

Like HIV, SIV is sexually transmitted in NHPS and can also be transmitted vertically. In deference to previous thinking, SIV is indeed pathogenic in most NHPS, causing CD4$^+$ T cell depletion (Keele, 2009). Chimpanzees infected with SIV have a 10- to 16-fold increased risk of death compared to those that are uninfected. Fertility and survival of offspring are also decreased in SIV-positive female chimpanzees.

Solid evidence indicated that the first cross-species transmission of HIV to humans that predates emergence of group M occurred in southeast Cameroon (Sharp, 2011). It is not known how humans acquired the zoonotic precursors of HIV-1. However, based on the recognized biology of these viruses, transmission likely arose from cutaneous or mucous membrane exposure to infected chimpanzee blood or body fluid. These exposures often occur in the context of hunting, butchering, and eating of bush meat (Sharp, 2011).

THE SPREAD OF HIV THROUGHOUT AFRICA AND THE WORLD

A 2014 study by Faria and colleagues using phylogenetic analysis and "molecular clocks" (based on the assumption that retroviruses mutate over time at a constant rate) confirmed previous work by Hahn and others regarding the dissemination routes of HIV-1 in West Africa (Sharp, 2011; Cohen, 2014; Faria, 2014). They have also largely determined how group M became the driver of the

AIDS pandemic. It is well established that the first know infections with HIV-1 emerged from Kinshasa (formerly called Leopoldville) in the Democratic Republic of the Congo in approximately 1920. Many refer to Leopoldville/Kinshasa as the cradle of the AIDS pandemic. From this area, the virus spread eastward to other communities via railway lines that carried up to 1 million passengers yearly to other areas of Africa, including the three largest population centers—Brazzaville, Mbuji-Mayi, and Lubumbashi (Cohen, 2014; Faria, 2014). Rivers were major travel and commerce routes and are believed to have enabled the spread of HIV geographically (Figure 2.1).

Sexual transmission is thought to be the primary mode and driver of new HIV infections and resultant dissemination of the virus at this time. Unsterilized injections at clinics in the area may have greatly contributed to the spread of HIV. According to Jaques Pepin, well-intended public health interventions by authorities in the Belgian Congo from 1921 to 1959 to treat trypanosomiasis, syphilis, yaws, malaria, and leprosy resulted in the administration of millions of injections to residents of these communities (Pepin, 2011). The majority of injections were intravenous and administered with syringes that clinicians used repeatedly without sterilization of the needles (Pepin, 2011). Consequently, thousands of these individuals may have acquired HIV iatrogenically. Data suggest similar transmission of hepatitis B and C viruses.

The epidemic histories of HIV-1 groups M and O were similar until approximately 1960, when group M infections underwent an epidemiologic transition and exponential increase, outpacing regional population growth (Faria, 2014). It is unknown why the growth rate of infections with HIV group M nearly tripled at approximately this time, but current explanations include virus-specific factors, population growth factors, and the widespread use of injections (Sharp, 2010; Pepin, 2011).

Tissues samples collected from two patients in Kinshasa in 1959 and 1960 showed that HIV-1 had diversified into different subtypes much earlier than previously believed. Viral sequencing done on plasma from a sailor who died in 1959 is the oldest case of documented HIV-1 infection (Zhu, 1998). Worobey and colleagues amplified and identified HIV-1 from a lymph node specimen obtained in 1960 from a female in Kinshasa (Worobey, 2008). The sizable genetic difference between these two HIV specimens demonstrated that diversification of HIV-1 occurred in Kinshasa at least 20 years before the first AIDS cases were observed in the United States. As HIV-1 group M spread globally, its dissemination led to population bottlenecks

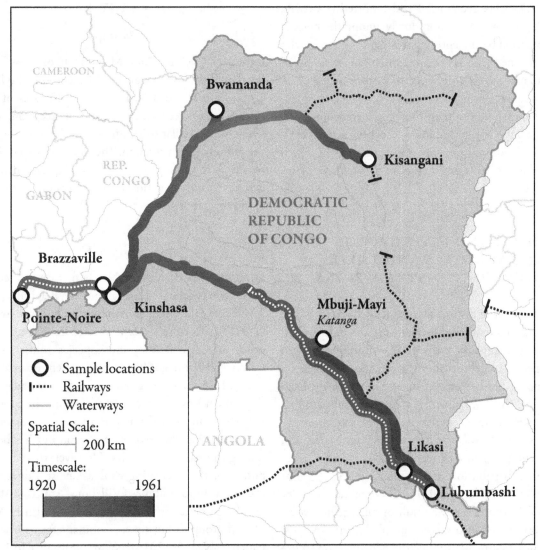

CAMEROON

Bwamanda

REP.
CONGO

GABON

Kisangani

DEMOCRATIC
REPUBLIC
OF CONGO

Brazzaville

Pointe-Noire   Kinshasa

Mbuji-Mayi
Katanga

○ Sample locations
┆┈┈ Railways
│ Waterways

Spatial Scale:
├────────┤ 200 km

Timescale:
1920   1961

ANGOLA

Likasi

Lubumbashi

Adapted from: 1. Faria NR, et al*Science* . 2014 Oct 3; 346(6205): 56–61. 2. Congo Dem Rep Regions Map-es by Burmesedays 2016/CC. 3. Second Congo War 2001 map vector by Don-kun and Uwe Dedering 2013/CC.

Figure 2.1 Spatial dynamics showing the spread of HIV-1 group 1 from Kinshasa in the Democratic Republic of the Congo via rivers and railways that were operational until approximately 1960.

("founder events") that resulted in different lineages, viral subtypes or clades, and circulating recombinant forms (Peters, 2014).

How and when HIV first arrived in the United States remain debatable. The virus first appeared in Haiti between 1960 and 1966. The probable source was Haitian professionals who returned from working in the newly independent Congo. It is estimated that during the 1960s, approximately 4500 skilled Haitian workers were employed by the Congolese government. However, Pepin states that "a single technical assistant infected with HIV-1 subtype B went back to Haiti and stayed long enough to start a local chain of sexual transmission" (Pepin, 2011). Some authorities believe that the selling of sex to American tourists

in Haiti led to HIV infection in individuals who in turn brought the virus back to the United States. Pepin states, "American gay and bisexual men infected Haitian male sex workers."

Work done by Gilbert and colleagues using HIV-1 *gag* gene sequences from five Haitian AIDS patients determined that HIV-1 subtype B definitely arrived in Haiti before it spread to the United States and other Western countries (Gilbert, 2007). The same group of researchers noted that the most recent common ancestor (TMRCA) of HIV-1 subtype B virus appeared in Haiti in 1966 but not in the United States until 1969. Consequently, these data suggest that HIV-1 was circulating cryptically in the United States for approximately 12 years before the 1981 cases of AIDS were recognized and reported (Gottlieb, 1981). The virus was spreading slowly among the heterosexual population before entering the higher risk men who have sex with men (MSM) population, in which it spread much more extensively and began to be recognized clinically. The actual scientific facts will likely never be known; however, Pepin believes that the blood trade in Port-au-Prince exponentially amplified the number of HIV infections in Haiti and possibly other countries in which blood products were sold, including the United States (Pepin, 2011).

HIV-1 AND HIV-2 GROUPS AND SUBTYPES AND THEIR GEOGRAPHIC DISTRIBUTIONS

HIV-1 comprises four distinct lineages termed groups M, N, O, and P. Each has resulted from a distinct and independent cross-species transmission event of SIVs infecting African apes. Using molecular clocks, the most recent common ancestor of group M has been dated to be approximately 1920 (Sharp, 2011). The four known HIV-1 groups share approximately 50–60% homology in their nucleotide sequences.

HIV-1 group M was the first lineage discovered and represents the pandemic form of HIV-1. It has a widespread global distribution and accounts for 90–95% of HIV-1 infections (Sharp, 2011). The genetic diversity within HIV-1 group M is the result of subsequent evolution and spread in humans. Bases on phylogenic analysis, HIV-1 group M can be further divided into nine pure subtypes or clades (A–D, F–H, J, and K) and additional sub-subtypes (A1–A4 and F1–F2). The subtypes share 80% homology in their genetic sequences, meaning they differ genetically by approximately 20%. Subtypes and sub-subtypes can form additional mosaic forms through recombination of different strains inside dually or multiply infected individuals. Some recombinant forms may further achieve epidemic relevance, giving rise to known circulating recombinant forms (CRFs). To date, researchers have identified more than six CRFs and unique recombinant strains (URFs). Globally, subtype C, found mainly in sub-Saharan Africa, represents approximately 50% of HIV-1 infections. This is followed by subtype A (12%), found mainly in central and east Africa. Viral subtype B (11% of infections) is the predominant subtype in the United States and the most geographically dispersed subtype worldwide. Subtypes G and D respectively account for 5% and 2% of infections worldwide (Peters, 2014) (Figure 2.2 and Box 2.1).

HIV-1

Group N

Group N ("N" for "non-M, non-O" or "new") was isolated in 1995 from a woman in Cameroon who had AIDS (Pepin, 2011). To date, fewer than 20 cases of group N infection have been identified, and all except one were from Cameroon. Similar to group M, it is the result of chimpanzee to human transmission. The small number of infections resulting from this group and limited genetic diversity suggest that its introduction into humans did not occur until approximately 1963 (Peters, 2014).

Group O

Group O ("O" for "outlier") was first discovered in 1990 from two Cameroonians living in Belgium (De Leys, 1990) and is thought to represent only approximately 1% all HIV infections. Recent studies have determined that group O originated by cross-species transmission from western lowland gorillas instead of chimpanzees (D'arc, 2015). Like the other groups, it underwent adaptations to the human hosts. A recent study found the prevalence of HIV-1 group O in Cameroon to be approximately 0.6%, indicating that the frequency of group O has been stable during the past few decades. However, the current distribution of the circulating viral strains still does not allow classification as subtypes (Villabona-Arenas, 2015). There are also some reports of dual infections with HIV-1 group M and group O but no recombinant forms in coinfected patients (Ngoupo, 2016). Natural resistance to HIV medications, including integrase inhibitors, has not been identified. This suggests that infection with HIV-1 group O can be adequately managed in countries in which the virus circulates, but this group remains challenging in regard to diagnostic and monitoring strategies.

Group P

Group P was discovered in 2009, isolated from a Cameroonian woman living in France (Plantier, 2009). Despite subsequent screening for more infections caused by this group, only two cases have been identified. It is uncertain when group P virus entered the human population; it is estimated to be any time from 1845 to 1989 (Peters, 2014). In addition, it remains unclear if the source was a chimpanzee or gorilla. The inability to antagonize tetherin protein (human restriction factor) may explain the limited spread of HIV-1 group P in the human population (Sauter, 2011).

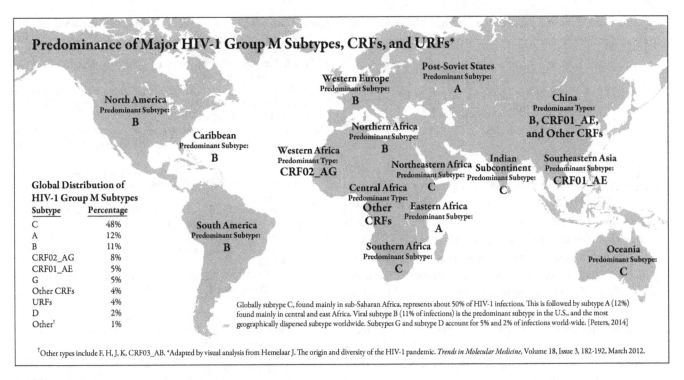

Figure 2.2 The global distribution of HIV-1 group M subtypes.

†Other types include F, H, J, K, CRF03_AB. *Adapted by visual analysis from Hemelaar J. The origin and diversity of the HIV-1 pandemic. *Trends in Molecular Medicine*, Volume 18, Issue 3, 182-192, March 2012.

Box 2.1 DISTRIBUTION OF HIV-1 SUBTYPES

Historically, the distribution of subtypes followed the geographic patterns listed here:

- Subtype A: Central and East Africa as well as Eastern European countries that were formerly part of the Soviet Union

- Subtype B: West and Central Europe, the Americas, Australia, South America, and several Southeast Asian countries (Thailand and Japan), as well as northern Africa and the Middle East

- Subtype C: Sub-Saharan Africa, India, and Brazil

- Subtype D: North Africa and the Middle East

- Subtype F: South and Southeast Asia

- Subtype G: West and Central Africa

- Subtypes H, J, and K: Africa and the Middle East

HIV-2

In 1986, a morphologically similar but antigenically distinct virus was found to cause AIDS in persons living in western Africa and was termed HIV-2 (Clavel, 1986, 1987). This virus has only approximately 30–40% genetic homology with HIV-1; thus, it is considered a different virus and not another HIV-1 group (Pepin, 2011). It was determined that HIV-2 originated in sooty mangabeys with blood-born transmission to humans, similar to HIV-1 (Chen, 1997; Gao, 1992). Molecular clock research has determined that the most common recent ancestor for HIV-2 dates to 1940 and 1945 for the first two groups—A and B (Pepin, 2011).

HIV-2 has been found mainly in Guinea-Bissau, Gambia, Senegal, Cote d'Ivoire, Mali, Nigeria, Senegal, and Sierra Leone. With widespread immigration, cases have been reported throughout Europe, the United States, and other areas of the world (Campbell-Yesufu, 2011).

Since its initial discovery, phylogenic analysis has identified eight different lineages of HIV-2 (groups A–H). As for HIV-1, each group represents a different host transfer of SIV from nonprimate species (mangabeys) to humans. However, unlike HIV-1, only types A and B have spread to humans to any significant degree. The other groups only represent individual human cases. Of note clinically, persons infected with HIV-2 often have lower viral loads compared to those with HIV-1 (Campbell-Yesufu, 2011). There is also less genital shedding in semen and cervical secretions. This likely accounts for decreased infectivity. It has also been observed that persons infected with HIV-2 infection have a longer asymptomatic phase and slower progression to AIDS than those with HIV-1. However, in the absence of treatment, the same progressive decline in immune function and resultant disease complications will occur.

THE FUTURE OF HIV REGIONAL AND GLOBAL GENETIC DIVERSITY

By combining historical, phylogenetic, molecular evolutionary, and epidemiological perspectives, researchers have been able to reconstruct the history of the AIDS pandemic and many unique aspects of HIV-1 and HIV-2. It is hoped that this information will be of value for HIV vaccine research and development that takes into account the genetic diversity discussed previously. It may also determine how strains of HIV may continue to spread and colonize new geographic regions and host populations. It also raises numerous questions: Given the fact that there are many other nonhuman primates infected with SIV, should there be concern for future zoonotic infections from cross-species transmissions? Will the growing prevalence of sexually transmitted infections continue to facilitate the dissemination and adaptation of HIV-1 and HIV-2? May there be a therapeutic role for host-restriction factors? Will it be possible to develop an HIV vaccine that will be effective against all HIV groups and subtypes?

Recommended Reading

Faria NR, Rambaut A, Suchard MA, et al. The early spread and epidemic ignition of HIV-1 in human populations. *Science*. 2014; 346(6205):56–61.

Pepin J. *The Origins of AIDS*. New York, NY: Cambridge University Press; 2011.

Quammen D. *The Chimp and the River: How AIDS Emerged from an African Forest*. New York, NY: Norton; 2015.

References

Campbell-Yesufu OT, Gandhi RT. Update on human immunodeficiency virus (HIV)-2 infection. Clin Infect Dis. 2011; 52(6):780–787. doi:10.1093/cid/ciq248

Chen Z, Lucky A, Sodora DL, et al. Human immunodeficiency virus type 2 (HIV-2) seroprevalence and characterization of a distinct subtype within the range of SIV-infected sooty mangabeys. J Virol. 1997; 71:3953–3960.

Clavel F, Guétard D, Brun-Vézinet F. Isolation of a new human retrovirus from West African patients with AIDS. Science. 1986; 233(4761):343–346.

Clavel F, Mansinho K, Chamaret S. Human immunodeficiency virus type 2 infection associated with AIDS in West Africa. Engl J Med. 1987; 316:1180–1185.

Cohen, J. Early AIDS virus may have ridden Africa's rails. Science. October 2014; 346:21–22.

D'arc, M, Ayouba A, Esteban A, et al. Origin of the HIV-1 group O epidemic in western lowland gorillas. Proc Natl Acad Sci USA. 2015 Mar 17; 112(11):E1343–E1352.

De Leys R. Isolation and partial characterization of an unusual HIV retrovirus from two persons of west-central Africa origin. J Virol. 1990; 64:1207–1216.

Faria, NR, Rambaut A, Suchard MA, et al. The early spread and epidemic ignition of HIV-1 in human populations. Science. 2014; 346(6205):56–61.

Gallo RC, Montagnier L. The discovery of HIV as the cause of AIDS. N Engl J Med. 2003; 349:2282–2285.

Gao F, Bailes E, Robertson DL, et al. Origin of HIV-1 in the chimpanzee Pan troglodytes troglodytes. Nature. February 4, 1999; 397:436–441.

Gao F, Yue L, White AT, et al. Human infection by genetically diverse SIVsm-related HIV-2 in West Africa. Nature. 1992; 358:495–499.

Gilbert MTP, Rambaut A, Wlasiuk G, et al. The emergence of HIV/AIDS in the Americas and beyond. Proc Natl Assoc Sci USA. Nov. 20, 2007; 104(47):18566–18570.

Gottlieb MS, Schanker HM, Fan PT, et al. Pneumocystis pneumonia–Los Angeles. MMWR. June 5, 1981; 30(21):1–3.

Keele BF, Jones JH, Terio KA, et al. Increased mortality and AIDS-like immunopathology in wild chimpanzees infected with SIV$_{cpz}$. Nature. July 2009; 460:515–519.

Keele BF, Van Heuverswyn F, Li Y, et al. Chimpanzee reservoirs for pandemic and nonpandemic HIV-1. Science. 2006 Jul 28; 313(5786):523–526.

Ngoupo PA, Sadeu, MB, Alain S, et al. First evidence of transmission of an HIV-1 M/O intergroup recombinant virus. AIDS. January 2016; 30(1):1–8.

Peeters M, D'Arc M, Delaporta E. The origin and diversity of human retroviruses. AIDS Rev. 2014; 16(1):23–34.

Pepin J. The Origins of AIDS. Cambridge University Press, New York, NY. 2011.

Plantier JC, Leoz, M, Dickerson JE. A new immunodeficiency virus derived from gorillas designated group "P." Nature Med. 2009; 15:871–872.

Sauter D, Hué S, Petit S, et al. HIV-1 group P is unable to antagonize human tetherin by Vpu, Env or Nef. Retrovirology. 2011; 8:103.

Sharp PM, Hahn BH. Origins of HIV and the AIDS pandemic. Cold Spring Harbor Perspect Med. 2011; 1:1–22.

Villabona-Arenas CJ, Domyeum J, Mouacha F, et al. HIV-1 group O infection in Cameroon from 2006–2013: Prevalence, genetic diversity, evolution, and public health challenges. Infect Gener Evo. 2015; 36:210–216. Epub Sept 11, 2015.

Worobey M, Gemmel M, Teuwen DE, et al. Direct evidence of extensive diversity of HIV-1 in Kinshasa by 1960. Nature. 2008 October 2; 455(7213):661–664.

Zhu T, Korber BT, Nahmias AJ, et al. An African HIV-1 sequence from 1959 and implications for the origin of the epidemic. Nature. 1998; 391(6667):594–597.

3.

MECHANISMS OF HIV TRANSMISSION

Puja Nambiar and William R. Short

LEARNING OBJECTIVES

- Describe the relative risk of acquiring HIV infection based on various types of sexual activity; viral load quantity and its relationship to transmission risk.

- Explain the impact of co-occurring sexually transmitted diseases; factors impacting HIV transmission; risk from a needle stick injury and how use of different kinds of drugs impacts the likelihood of HIV infection.

- Discuss the risk of HIV transmission to infants during breast-feeding.

WHAT'S NEW?

- Clinical trial data demonstrate that treatment of HIV infection is also prevention.

- It has been shown that occupational transmission is extremely rare in the United States.

KEY POINTS

- The risk of HIV transmission to a receptive partner remains higher than that to an insertive one; however, both are at risk.

- Anything that compromises the integrity of mucous membranes, such as sexually transmitted infections, may increase the risk of transmission.

- Although not 100% effective, keeping an infected partner's viral load low reduces the risk of transmission to an HIV-negative partner.

- Maternal transmission is a larger concern in developing countries due to lack of access to perinatal treatment with antiretroviral drugs.

SEXUAL TRANSMISSION

HIV is a sexually transmitted infection (STI). According to data gathered by the Centers for Disease Control and Prevention (CDC), most new HIV infections in the United States are the result of sex. It is rare for HIV to be transmitted through oral sex (CDC, 2010). HIV can be readily found in semen and in vaginal fluid from infected persons. There is a strong correlation between high plasma viral load and the amount of virus in genital secretions. Thus, acutely infected individuals with very high viral loads are at the highest risk of transmitting the virus. However, up to 20% of men and women have been found to have HIV in their genital tract despite an undetectable plasma viral load, so there is discordance.

During anal sex, HIV is present in the blood, semen, and preseminal fluids. Unprotected anal sex is considered a very high-risk behavior that can result in infection of either the insertive or the receptive sex partner. However, the person receiving the infected semen is at highest risk of contracting the infection. This is believed to be the case because of the single cell layer of epithelium lining the rectum, which can be easily disrupted, permitting the entry of the virus across the rectal mucosa. The insertive partner is also at significant risk because HIV can enter the penis through the urethra; the mucosa of the nonkeratinized portions of foreskin; or through cuts, abrasions, or open sores on the penis. Circumcision has been demonstrated to significantly reduce the risk of HIV acquisition but not of transmission (Dosekun, 2010).

Worldwide, the AIDS epidemic is being driven by new infections occurring in women of childbearing age. During unprotected intercourse (vaginal sex), both partners are at risk of contracting HIV, although there is a higher risk of a woman contracting HIV from an infected man than a man contracting HIV from an infected woman. As indicated previously, HIV is present in the blood, semen, and preseminal fluid of an infected partner. How HIV enters the body through the relatively well-protected muco-sal membranes lining the vagina is still not completely understood. Although the risk of men acquiring HIV through heterosexual vaginal or anal intercourse is lower, HIV is abundantly present in vaginal secretions, and the anatomic sites of potential infection in the penis are the same as those described previously for anal intercourse (Dosekun, 2010).

Of significant importance is the role of STIs in HIV transmission. Genital ulcer disease (i.e., syphilis, chancroid, and herpes simplex infections) and diseases causing muco-sal inflammation (i.e., gonorrhea and chlamydia) have been shown to increase HIV transmission. This increase is most likely due to both heightened infectivity and susceptibility. Early diagnosis of STIs has the potential to significantly reduce HIV incidence in general, especially if applied to high-risk populations. Another potential factor is the use of hormonal contraception in women because it may thin the vaginal mucosa, making it more susceptible to tears and trauma. However, large randomized clinical trials have provided conflicting results, and currently it is not clear whether or not hormonal contraception has any effect on HIV transmission.

Limiting viral replication and thus viral load in genital secretions is a logical approach to preventing HIV acquisition. Recently, sexual HIV transmission has been shown to be dramatically reduced in serodiscordant couples in which the seropositive partner is receiving suppressive antiretroviral treatment. Specifically, the HPTN 052 clinical trial showed that men and women infected with HIV have a reduced risk of transmitting the virus to their regular or linked, HIV-uninfected sexual partners through early initiation of antiretroviral therapy (ART) (Cohen, 2011). The results of the study showed a sustained, overall 93% reduction of HIV transmission among linked couples when the HIV-infected partner was taking ART and had a suppressed viral load (Cohen, 2015). The PARTNERS study is an ongoing, prospective, international observational study investigating the risk of HIV transmission within serodiscordant couples who are intentionally not using condoms, pre- or post-exposure prophylaxis, and in which the HIV-positive partner is reliably receiving ART and maintaining s an undetectable viral load. Thus far, there have been no transmissions in the PARTNERS study; however, that does not mean there is a zero chance of transmission. Final results of the study will be available by 2017 (Rodger, 2014). Developing novel approaches for the rapid detection and diagnosis of HIV infection and increasing ART coverage are the next important steps in realizing the potential public benefits of these discoveries.

TRANSMISSION IN THE HEALTH CARE SETTING

The risk of occupational transmission of HIV is relatively small, but it has occurred in a variety of settings. Needle stick and other sharp instrument injuries are relatively common in health care. However, in developed countries, only a small fraction of these involve HIV-infected blood. In settings in which HIV incidence is high, such as sub-Saharan Africa, this risk is significantly higher, thus increasing the potential for transmission. Other types of health care-related procedures that can potentially cause transmission involve the use of vascular cannulas and introducers, suture needles, scalpels, and other sharp or cutting instruments. The risk of HIV transmission after puncture with a large-gauge, hollow-bore needle contaminated with HIV-positive blood has been estimated to be 0.3%. There is virtually no risk of HIV transmission via contact of HIV-infected body fluids with intact skin. However, there is an increased risk of transmission when non-intact skin or mucus membranes are involved. The risk of transmission after exposure of a mucous membrane has been estimated to be 0.09% (CDC, 2008).

In addition to blood, some other bodily fluids are also considered potentially infectious, including cerebrospinal fluid, synovial fluid, amniotic fluid, pleural fluid, peritoneal fluid, and pericardial fluid. Of significance, urine, feces, and saliva are not considered to be infectious. Semen and cervicovaginal secretions have been shown to contain both infectious-free virus and virus-infected cells, and they should be considered infectious. Note that several factors can influence the possibility of transmission. Transmission risk is expected to be higher when there are higher levels of virus in blood or body fluids, such as with those from persons during or suspected to have acute HIV infection as well as those at late stages of disease with unsuppressed viremia (CDC, 2008).

Although not common, there have been several documented transmission events from health care workers to patients during routine medical or dental care; poor adherence to infection control procedures has been documented as a likely cause. Furthermore, although increasingly less frequent, there have been documented cases of patient-to-patient transmission, most of which involved the use of contaminated instruments or syringes. Use of universal precautions during all health care procedures and encounters cannot be overemphasized.

Since 1991, the CDC has investigated all cases of HIV infection reported as acquired occupationally by health care workers. There have been a total of 58 confirmed occupationally acquired HIV infections. The majority were in nurses (41%), followed by laboratory clinicians (35%), physicians (10%), and other health-related workers (14%). Since 1999, there has been only one case of occupationally acquired HIV (a laboratory technician who sustained a needle puncture while working with high-titer HIV cultures in 2008) (Joyce, 2015). In cases in which risk of HIV transmission can be determined, specific guidelines exist for the use of antivirals for post-exposure prophylaxis (PEP). Occupational exposures require urgent medical evaluation and initiation of PEP ideally within the first 2 hours of exposure because it has been estimated to reduce the risk of infection by approximately 80%. The preferred initial PEP regimen is tenofovir/emtricitabine plus raltegravir because of its ease of administration, proven potency against established HIV, and good tolerability. Zidovudine is no longer recommended in the preferred PEP regimen due to its side effects. Although originally approved only for health care workers exposed to HIV, PEP's use has been expanded to non-occupational exposures. The recommended duration of PEP is 28 days. However, the medications can have serious side effects that can make it difficult to complete the program. CDC recommendations indicate that PEP should be considered only in settings in which HIV exposure is known. Most important, based on strong animal model data indicating time-dependent efficacy, PEP administration should not be delayed for HIV test results but, rather, should be started empirically and discontinued later if tests are negative (Kuhar, 2013).

TRANSMISSION THROUGH THE USE OF INJECTION DRUGS

Injection drug use has contributed to more than one-third of all HIV infections in the United States. The use of clean needles and syringes is the safest and most effective approach to limit transmission. Use of syringes with small dead volume also can reduce the possibility of transmission. Blacks/African Americans and Hispanics/Latinos account for more than two-thirds of all diagnoses of HIV infection due to injection drug use in the United States. Among women, injection drug use accounts for more than 20% of all infections.

Syringe exchange programs (SEPs) provide free sterile needles and syringes and collect used syringes from injection drug users (IDUs) to reduce transmission of HIV, hepatitis C virus, hepatitis B virus, and other blood-borne infections. SEPs exist in at least 36 states. Most SEPs also provide preventive health and clinical services.

Providing comprehensive prevention services and medical and/or addiction treatment referrals to IDUs can help increase access to health care and substance use treatment (CDC, 2008).

Individuals who use recreational crystal methamphetamine (by a number of routes of ingestion) are at increased risk of contracting HIV. However, there is no clear evidence that methamphetamine itself increases HIV transmission or acquisition. Amphetamine users, in general, report several behaviors known to be risk factors for HIV transmission, including greater number of sex partners, reduced use of condoms, exchange of sex for money or drugs, sex with IDUs, and/or a history of STDs. Furthermore, they are more likely to have unprotected anal or vaginal sex with partners of unknown HIV status. Individuals abusing other mind-altering drugs, such as alcohol, can also be at increased risk for HIV infection (CDC, 2007).

MOTHER-TO-CHILD TRANSMISSION

Pediatric HIV infection is associated with an accelerated course of disease and high mortality. In the absence of antiretroviral therapy, only 65% of HIV-infected children survive until their first birthday, and less than half will reach 2 years of age. Mother-to-child transmission can occur during pregnancy, labor and delivery, or breast-feeding. In the absence of breast-feeding and with no ART, the risk of perinatal transmission is 25%. Up to 20% more children can become infected through breast-feeding. In the United States, the rate of perinatal transmission of HIV has drastically declined to less than 2% with the implementation of prenatal HIV screening; the use of antiretrovirals before, during, and after pregnancy; scheduled cesarean delivery when necessary; and the avoidance of breast-feeding. These interventions are not available worldwide, and in areas such as sub-Saharan Africa, AIDS remains a major cause of infant death.

Most children acquire HIV from their mother in utero, intrapartum, or during breast-feeding. In developed countries, the incidence of mother-to-child transmission of HIV is extremely low. In these countries, HIV-infected women receive antiretroviral therapy before and during pregnancy and delivery, and they are advised to abstain from breast-feeding. Furthermore, their children receive antiretroviral prophylaxis at birth and for several weeks thereafter. The majority of HIV-infected children live in sub-Saharan Africa, where HIV-positive women have limited access to antiretroviral drugs and the health benefits of breast-feeding outweigh the risk of HIV transmission. (For more details about this topic, see Chapter 27.)

Despite the presence of innate factors in human breast milk that display strong HIV inhibitory activity in vitro, up to 44% of HIV infections in children can be attributed to breast-feeding. The risk of acquiring HIV after a single day of breast-feeding is extremely low (0.00028 per day of breast-feeding) (Richardson, 2003). However, after ingesting liters of breast milk over a span of several months to years (~250 liters per year), 5–20% of infants born to HIV-infected women will eventually become infected with HIV in the absence of any preventative measures (WHO, 2008). Elevated levels of HIV particles (cell-free virus) and HIV-infected cells (cell-associated virus) in breast milk of HIV-positive women are associated with an increased risk of HIV transmission during breast-feeding. Although it has been reported that a 10-fold increase in cell-free or cell-associated HIV in breast milk is associated with a 3-fold increase in transmission, it is still unclear whether cell-free virus and/or cell-associated virus are transmitted during breast-feeding. Furthermore, it is not known if the frequency of cell-free and cell-associated HIV transmission varies at different stages of lactation (i.e., colostrum, early breast milk, and mature breast milk).

References

Centers for Disease Control and Prevention. Methamphetamine use and risk for HIV/AIDS. January 2007. http://www.cdc.gov/hiv/resources/factsheets/meth.htm. Accessed December 20, 2015.

Centers for Disease Control and Prevention. Recommendations for post-exposure interventions to prevent infection with hepatitis B virus, hepatitis C virus, or human immunodeficiency virus, and tetanus in persons wounded during bombings and other mass-casualty events—United States, 2008. MMWR. August 1, 2008/57(RR06);1–19.

Centers for Disease Control and Protection. HIV transmission. March 25, 2010. http://www.cdc.gov/hiv/resources/qa/transmission.htm. Accessed December 20, 2015.

Cohen MS, Chen YQ, McCauley M, et al. Prevention of HIV-1 infection with early antiretroviral therapy. N Engl J Med. 2011; 365:493–505.

Cohen MS, et al. Final results of the HPTN 052 randomized controlled trial: Antiretroviral therapy prevents HIV transmission. IAS 2015, 19–22 July 2015, Vancouver. MOAC0101LB.

Dosekun O, Fox J. An overview of the relative risks of different sexual behaviours on HIV transmission. Curr Opin HIV AIDS. 2010; 5:291–297.

Fox J, Fidler S. Sexual transmission of HIV-1: Antiviral Res. 2010; 85:276–285.

Joyce MP, Kuhar D, Brooks JT. Occupationally acquired HIV infection by healthcare personnel—United states, 1985–2013. 22nd Conference on Retroviruses and Opportunistic Infections, Seattle, Abstract 1027, 2015.

Kuhar DT, Henderson DK, Struble KA, et al. Updated US Public Health Service guidelines for the management of occupational exposures to human immunodeficiency virus and recommendations for postexposure prophylaxis. Infect Control Hosp Epidemiol. 2013 Nov; 34(11):1238.

Richardson BA, John-Stewart GC, Hughes JP, et al. Breast-milk infectivity in human immunodeficiency virus type 1-infected mothers. J Infect Dis. 2003; 187:736–740.

Rodger A, Cambiano V, Bruun T, et al. HIV transmission risk through condomless sex if HIV+ partner on suppressive ART: PARTNER study. 21st Conference on Retroviruses and Opportunistic Infections, Boston, Abstract 153LB, 2014.

WHO, UNICEF, UNFPA, and UNAIDS HIV transmission through breastfeeding: A review of available evidence: 2007 update. Geneva: World Health Organization; 2008.

4.

HIV TRANSMISSION PREVENTION

Carolyn Chu and Christopher M. Bositis

INTRODUCTION

Similar to combination HIV treatment using multiple medications alongside other interventions, multifaceted approaches to HIV prevention are required to effectively reduce transmission risk. Prevention strategies encompass a broad range of specific behavioral, structural, and biomedical interventions, and high-quality evidence exists for many of these approaches. HIV pre-exposure prophylaxis has been recently introduced as a new clinical tool. Other novel agents and interventions continue to be investigated and may significantly improve the ability to prevent HIV transmission and acquisition in the near future. Nevertheless, there are still considerable challenges in motivating fundamental individual- and community-level behaviors and overcoming structural obstacles that affect access to prevention resources. These need to be sustainably addressed in order to successfully reduce the global burden of HIV (Figure 4.1).

BEHAVIORAL INTERVENTIONS

LEARNING OBJECTIVES

Provide an overview of behavioral issues surrounding HIV transmission, including the strategies that have been developed in response to reduce HIV exposure risk.

WHAT'S NEW?

Behavioral interventions continue to be developed and evaluated to determine their effectiveness at preventing HIV and HIV-associated risk behaviors. Combination interventions targeted to specific at-risk groups may be more effective than broad prevention measures for the general population due to (1) various social and cultural subtleties and (2) HIV-related health disparities unique to particular communities.

KEY POINTS

- Providers should elicit comprehensive and detailed sociobehavioral histories from all patients to identify areas of HIV risk so that appropriate HIV testing can occur and specific, effective prevention strategies can be shared.

- Various combinations of behavioral strategies will be effective for different risk groups and should be tailored to an individual's and a community's needs.

Behavioral interventions to prevent HIV transmission include both general educational campaigns about sexual health, drug use, and risk reduction and specific messages tailored to special at-risk populations and individuals known to be HIV positive ("prevention with positives"). Condom promotion and skills training and condom distribution services have been mainstays for many sex education and HIV prevention programs. Others have encouraged sexual abstinence or monogamy and fidelity. Studies estimate that condoms reduce HIV transmission by greater than 70% when used consistently by serodiscordant heterosexual partners and men who have sex with men (MSM) (Giannou, 2015; Smith, 2015; Weller, 2002). A growing body of research also cites sexual partnering practices such as partner concurrency and age-discrepant partnering as underrecognized drivers of HIV risk, particularly in specific communities (Adimora, 2014; Anema, 2013; Harrison, 2008). Although in theory such harm reduction strategies should prevent infection, in practice each carries a different and uncertain level of risk due to a range of biological and contextual factors (Wei, 2011), including a low rate of accurate HIV status representation between partners.

Adolescents and adult women may be especially vulnerable to transmission not only from sociocultural factors (e.g., sexual coercion and violence, partner alcohol/drug use, and difficulty negotiating condom use) but also from biological factors such as mucosal and immunological features unique

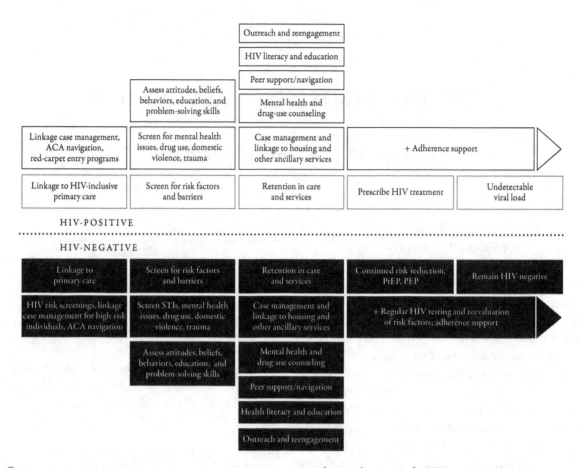

Figure 4.1 Component prevention interventions to promote engagement in care and optimal outcomes for HIV-positive and HIV-negative populations. SOURCE: Treatment Action Group.

to the female genital tract (Kaushic, 2010). Behavioral interventions targeted to young people have attempted to reduce HIV risk by delaying sexual debut, promoting consistent condom use, and reducing partner concurrency and/or changes. Methods include school-based and/or peer-led approaches as well as novel cash transfer programs (to increase financial independence) and social media campaigns to reduce stigma and discrimination (Pettifor, 2013). Similarly, interventions targeted to at-risk women have used group-based, skills training sessions focused on healthy decision-making and mental wellness, aiming to empower women to build balanced relationships free of harmful power dynamics. Older adults are another population requiring unique consideration. Many exhibit risk behaviors similar to those of younger people, but they may be less knowledgeable about HIV, less likely to use condoms, more isolated from their peers, and less inclined to discuss risky activities with a health care provider. Age-related physiologic changes such as decreased vaginal lubrication and vaginal epithelial thinning can put older, postmenopausal women at especially high risk. Older men using erectile dysfunction medications may also demonstrate increased capacity

for risky sexual activities. (Brooks, 2012). Older adults are more likely to be diagnosed with HIV infection late in the course of disease. One study found that median CD4$^+$ T cell counts at first presentation to care were consistently lower for persons aged 50 years or older compared to younger adults by approximately 15% and that a greater proportion of older adults had an AIDS-defining diagnosis at or within 3 months of initial presentation (Althoff, 2010). Therefore, provider awareness and HIV testing are especially important for this often-overlooked population. The Centers for Disease Control and Prevention (CDC) currently maintains the *Compendium of Evidence-Based Interventions and Best Practices for HIV Prevention*, which includes more than 80 HIV risk reduction behavioral interventions at the individual, couple, group, and community levels; several are tailored for specific HIV risk categories (e.g., people who inject drugs and heterosexual adults), by race/ethnicity, and by sex. Many interventions are rooted in the "health belief model," one of several social psychological frameworks used to develop behavioral interventions (Bonell, 2001; Kaufman, 2014). Despite a growing number of evidence-based strategies, one group that remains critically understudied is

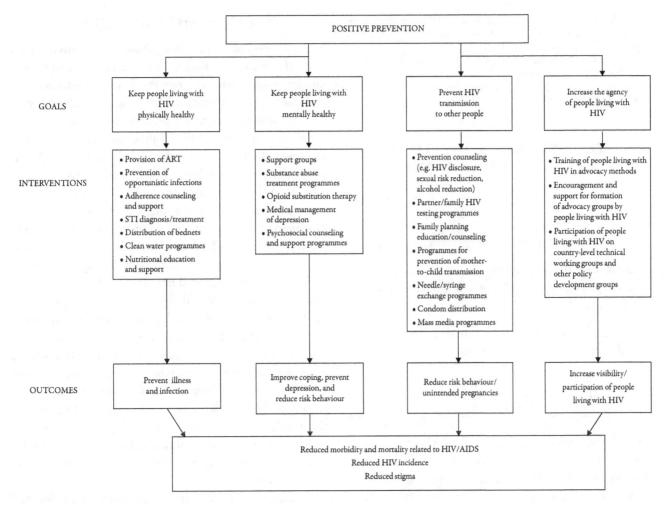

Figure 4.2 Conceptual framework of "prevention with positives" showing select goals, interventions, and outcomes. SOURCE: WHO.

transgender populations. Transgender communities experience some of the highest rates of HIV infection globally, with prevalence estimates range from 8% to 68%. (World Health Organization, 2011), but relatively little data have accumulated on effective prevention options. Transgender female sex workers in particular face unique structural, interpersonal, and individual vulnerabilities that contribute to an extremely high level of HIV risk. Providers should be sensitive to a person's gender identity and avoid making assumptions about sexual orientation and behavior based solely on identity because there is great diversity in this population. Targeted prevention approaches that acknowledge and respond to specific individual needs while empowering transgender communities to take a principal role in addressing population-level, structural concerns may be the most effective. Finally, many behavioral interventions emphasize regular HIV and sexually transmitted infections (STIs) screening as a cornerstone of prevention for all. Widespread efforts to expand HIV counseling and testing can help decrease HIV transmission risk by (1) ensuring that people

living with HIV (PLWH) know their status, (2) supporting safe disclosure to sexual partners, (3) encouraging increased condom use, and (4) assisting with linkage to HIV care.

During the past several years, accumulating evidence has shown that PLWH are central to HIV prevention. Effective interventions targeting PLWH are likely to have a greater and more immediate impact on reducing HIV incidence than changing the behaviors of millions of people who are negative but at risk (CDC, 2014). These "prevention with positives" efforts are often built around the HIV care continuum and include discrete goals such as improving linkage to (and retention in) quality HIV care, initiating early antiretroviral therapy, screening for and treating concurrent STIs, addressing mental health and substance use, providing family planning and partner notification counseling, and achieving durable virologic suppression (Figure 4.2).

Recommended Reading

Centers for Disease Control and Prevention. High-impact HIV prevention: CDC's approach to reducing HIV infections in the United States. Available at http://www.cdc.gov/hiv/library/reports/index.html.

Centers for Disease Control and Prevention. HIV prevention in the United States: At a critical crossroads. Available at http://www.cdc.gov/hiv/library/reports/index.html.

Kaufman M, Cornish F, Zimmerman RS, et al. Health behavior change models for HIV prevention and AIDS care: Practical recommendations for a multi-level approach. *J Acquir Immune Defic Syndr*. 2014; 66(Suppl. 3):S250–S258.

STRUCTURAL AND SYSTEMS-LEVEL INTERVENTIONS

LEARNING OBJECTIVES

• Describe the safety and monitoring of the US blood supply,

• Recognize HIV risk associated with injection drug use (IDU) and interventions that prevent IDU-related HIV transmission

• Discuss additional structural/systems-level interventions that aim to decrease HIV transmission.

WHAT'S NEW?

Data continue to accumulate on the complex issues surrounding injection and non-injection drug use and their impact on HIV transmission. Biomedical advances in substance use treatment (e.g., coordinated opioid substitution and antiretroviral therapies) and renewed public health efforts offer particularly promising strategies to improve IDU-associated HIV outcomes.

KEY POINTS

• The US blood supply remains one of the safest in the world. This is largely a result of multiple layers of safety involving comprehensive screening, testing, and quality assurance practices.

• Although the proportion of HIV infections in the United States attributable to injection drug use has declined overall, recent epidemics in previously low-prevalence areas highlight the need for providers to recognize HIV risks associated with both prescription and nonprescription substance use and to implement effective preventive measures, including harm reduction services and routine, integrated HIV testing for people who inject drugs.

SAFETY OF THE BLOOD SUPPLY

Multiple organizations throughout the United States (e.g., the American Red Cross and hospital and community blood banks) contribute to population-level and local procurement and donation of blood products. Establishments that collect and process blood are ultimately responsible for individual product safety. However, the US Food and Drug Administration (FDA) is responsible for regulating how donations are collected and blood is transfused. It does so by ensuring transfusion recipients are protected through multiple, overlapping safeguards. These specific measures encompass five main "layers" of safety: (1) donor screening for diseases that could be transmitted via transfusion; (2) approval of all testing platforms that evaluate donated blood for infections, including HIV and viral hepatitis; (3) quarantine of donated specimens until testing verifies suitability; (4) donor deferral registries; and (5) required reporting and subsequent investigations and corrective actions when product deviations occur. The FDA also regularly inspects collection centers to confirm that they are adhering to quality standards and best practices. In addition, the CDC plays a role in monitoring blood safety by assisting state and local health departments and hospitals in investigating reports of potential infectious disease transmission.

Widespread HIV-1 antibody screening of donated blood began in the United States in 1985. HIV-2 antibody screening was introduced in 1992. Since 1999, donations have also been pooled and tested for HIV-1 RNA. HIV RNA testing allows for the detection of acute HIV infection because antibodies to HIV typically do not develop until approximately 3 weeks after HIV acquisition. By incorporating HIV-1 RNA testing into the routine evaluation of donated blood products, centers are able to identify donors who might have been recently infected (Busch, 2003; Kleinman, 2009). As a result of these various improvements in screening and testing practices, the modeled risk for HIV infection from transfusion of blood products in the United States declined from 1 in 450,000–600,000 donations in 1995 to 1 in 2,135,000 donations from in 2001. The most recent population-based estimate of the risk for acquiring HIV infection through US blood transfusion is 1 in 1,467,000 (Zou, 2010). In 2010, a description of the most recent reported case of transfusion-transmitted HIV infection was published: This was the first reported occurrence since 2002 (CDC, 2010).

PREVENTION OF HIV RELATED TO INJECTION DRUG USE

Injection drug use has long been associated with HIV transmission. Despite a decrease in the overall number of HIV infections due to IDU, recent CDC estimates indicate that less than 10% of new infections in the United States are attributed to IDU (CDC, 2015). It remains an important transmission risk factor worldwide. Equipment used for injecting can be an effective vector for spreading virus. Blood is often drawn back into the needle and syringe pre- and post-injection; therefore, equipment recently used on an HIV-positive individual can contain a considerable amount of blood that contains HIV. Although HIV generally degrades quickly outside the body under certain conditions, studies indicate it can survive for longer periods of time (up to 6 weeks) within a sealed syringe (Heimer, 2000). Higher levels of HIV present in the blood injected, larger volume of injected blood, and/or higher injection frequency may increase risk of transmission. Estimates of infection risk from IDU on a per-act basis range from 0.63% to 2.4% (Baggaley, 2006). In addition to direct sharing of needles/syringes, various drug preparation practices can "indirectly" lead to HIV transmission, including sharing water used to flush blood out of a needle/syringe, reusing filters, and sharing other equipment that has not been sufficiently disinfected. Finally, although HIV risk has been demonstrated most clearly for intravenous administration of illicit substances, any parenteral exposure to unsterilized equipment can potentially lead to transmission (this includes subcutaneous and intramuscular injections), and HIV infections have been associated with injection of prescription medications, namely opioids.

Prevention of IDU-related HIV transmission has recently re-emerged as a public health priority for various reasons, including local outbreaks of HIV attributed to IDU in communities previously thought to be low prevalence areas (rural Indiana, Kentucky, and West Virginia). Many experts believe a "one size fits all" public health prevention strategy will not be fully effective, and they advocate for a multifaceted approach including (1) broad access to needle exchange and other harm reduction-oriented programs, (2) improved screening and recognition of substance use along with widespread HIV testing, and (3) expanded access to health services and providers who offer medications (i.e., opioid agonists) and other therapies that help mitigate the negative clinical consequences associated with IDU (Strathdee, 2015).

Harm Reduction Approaches to IDU and HIV Prevention

Harm reduction is a concept whereby programs and providers prioritize the prevention or reduction of adverse effects associated with certain behaviors over absolute cessation of the behavior. As applied to substance use (specifically IDU), harm reduction values minimizing substance-related impairment as much as, if not more than, eliminating substance use itself. Since the early 1990s, multiple harm reduction strategies—both biomedical and non-biomedical—have demonstrated effectiveness at decreasing IDU-related HIV transmission risk. Studies have specifically evaluated needle and syringe exchange programs (NSEPs), peer-based education and outreach, opioid substitution therapies, and both pre- and post-exposure prophylaxis (see sections on pre- and post-exposure prophylaxis) (Abdul-Quader, 2013; Aspinall, 2014; Garfein, 2007; MacArthur, 2012; Medley, 2009). NSEPs provide new needles/syringes, generally at no cost, in exchange for used equipment. Programs sometimes also distribute items such as alcohol swabs, sterile water/saline, mixing vessels, filters, and condoms. Other distribution models have been employed, including pharmacy sales and vending machines (MacArthur, 2014). In 2004, the World Health Organization (WHO) published an extensive report, concluding "there is compelling evidence that increasing the availability and utilization of sterile injecting equipment . . . reduces HIV infection substantially" and is cost-effective (WHO, 2004). Since then, evaluations from multiple agencies, such as the Institute of Medicine (IOM) and US Department of Health and Human Services/CDC, have also supported NSEPs as an integral, evidence-based component of comprehensive HIV prevention (CDC, 2012; IOM, 2007). Another non-biomedical prevention strategy, outreach and education, offers basic HIV education and risk reduction counseling; training on safer injecting and sexual practices; overdose prevention education and training (sometimes with naloxone distribution); counseling regarding drug treatment; and, occasionally, drug treatment referrals. Peer-driven and community-based models are particularly effective at engaging difficult to reach populations. They have successfully led to behavior changes such as decreased drug use, reduced equipment sharing, increased condom use, increased HIV testing, and increased enrollment in drug treatment (Garfein, 2007; Latkin, 2009; Medley, 2009; Needle, 2005). Research has also suggested that medically supervised, safer injection facilities are feasible and can play a meaningful role in reducing harms associated with HIV infection among people who inject drugs (PWID) (Kerr, 2007).

Substance Use Screening and Expanded HIV Testing

Screening, brief intervention, and referral to treatment (SBIRT) is a widely adopted public health approach to early identification and delivery of services for people with certain risky health behaviors. Although its effectiveness in reducing alcohol misuse and smoking has been verified, findings on its application to other substances have not been conclusive (Saitz, 2014). In 2008, the US Preventive Services Task Force (USPSTF) stated that evidence is "insufficient to assess the balance of benefits and harms of screening . . . for illicit drug use." Nevertheless, some proponents cite a growing body of supporting evidence (Agerwala, 2012; Humeniuk, 2008; Substance Abuse and Mental Health Services Administration, 2011) and encourage continued efforts to identify optimal approaches for widespread SBIRT implementation in clinical practice.

Since 2006, the CDC has recommended that PWID be screened for HIV at least annually because some studies estimate that greater than 15% of HIV-positive PWID do not know their status (Branson, 2006; Chen 2012). HIV-positive PWID also tend to have lower rates of retention in care and virologic suppression compared to other risk groups (Celentano, 2007; Lourenco, 2014), highlighting important health disparities and opportunities. A recent report describing IDU participants in the National HIV Behavioral Surveillance System indicated that a majority had been tested for HIV at some point in their lifetime, but only half had undergone testing during the previous 12 months (Spiller, 2015). Interventions (including public health campaigns) that can reinforce the importance of regular screening and facilitate timely disclosure of results (i.e., rapid HIV testing) play key roles in identifying and linking HIV-positive PWID with care. Testing can also help prevent additional transmissions because HIV-positive individuals who know their status are significantly more likely to reduce risky behaviors in order to protect HIV-negative contacts (Marks, 2005). Furthermore, testing integrated with services that already focus on PWID—for example, NSEPs—offers a community-based, patient-centered alternative to testing at traditional medical facilities (Heimer, 2007; Strathdee, 2012).

Medical Management of IDU and HIV Prevention

Treatment of substance use, particularly IDU, can be challenging. It often requires a comprehensive, coordinated approach of multiple-component interventions across various dimensions: behavioral, psychological, social, and biomedical. Despite these complexities, multiple biomedical (i.e., pharmacologic) therapies have proven their role in reducing IDU and the subsequent transmission of HIV (MacArthur, 2012; Metzger, 2010; Vlahov, 2010). Opioids continue to be the most commonly injected drugs, and a number of medications are now available to manage opioid dependence, including both agonists (also referred to as opioid substitution therapies (OST)) and antagonists. Methadone, an opioid agonist, is the most widely used agent internationally. In the United States, it has been the mainstay of OST for decades and is available from licensed treatment programs that have attained special accreditation and are highly regulated. Buprenorphine, a partial opioid agonist, can be offered from a broader variety of settings (including primary care facilities), but trained prescribers must obtain special education and designation from the Drug Enforcement Administration. With buprenorphine, patients can be seen in practices not specifically identified as substance use treatment centers. This may help offset some of the stigma surrounding drug use and its treatment. Naltrexone (an opioid antagonist) is used mainly in relapse prevention, often subsequent to detoxification. Naloxone is another opioid antagonist and is commonly used to reverse the effects of opioids, especially in overdose. It is distributed as a co-formulation with buprenorphine to reduce potential for buprenorphine abuse. For HIV-positive PWID, effective treatment for drug use improves adherence to antiretroviral therapy and leads to sustained viral suppression, which then helps reduce the risk of forward transmission to uninfected partners (Metzger, 2010). Recent work also suggests that combined OST and antiretroviral therapy may yield the best clinical outcomes compared to either intervention alone (Nosyk, 2015).

In addition to heroin and other opioids, other substances are frequently injected and have been implicated in HIV transmission. Crystal methamphetamine (CM) in particular is a highly addictive stimulant that increases sexual arousal while also decreasing social inhibitions. Similar to cocaine, people who use CM are at risk not only through sharing equipment but also via certain sexual practices (e.g., engaging in unprotected and/or transactional sex and having multiple partners) that increase the likelihood of HIV transmission or acquisition. Although CM use and subsequent HIV risk have been mostly associated with MSM, the population of CM users is very diverse, and novel approaches to treatment and HIV prevention are needed to address multiple complexities surrounding its use (Degenhardt, 2010; HRSA, 2009).

Legal Considerations Surrounding HIV Prevention with IDU

As stated in the WHO's 2004 report, "HIV infection among [PWID] is more likely to occur in legal environments where sterile injection equipment is more severely restricted." Public facilitation of access to sterile equipment has faced significant controversy from law enforcement agencies and policymakers for decades. Historically, the United States has had among the most severe restrictions of any country. Use of federal funds for NSEPs was banned in 1988, lifted in 2009, and reinstated in 2011. Lack of a central funding mechanism has thus hampered scale up of NSEPs in the United States, and programs are largely funded through a mix of state and local government monies with some additional support by private donations. At the state level, some laws expressly prohibit possessing injection equipment, whereas others require a physician's prescription for purchase. In areas where carrying used needles/syringes could be a prosecutable offense, PWID are often disincentivized from utilizing NSEPs despite their availability (for fear of arrest outside programs). Individual programs also represent a broad spectrum of structure and access: They can be fixed or mobile, with highly variable hours of operation. As of April 2015, 16 states and the District of Columbia explicitly authorized syringe exchange programs. A number of other states have laws that either decrease barriers to clean needle distribution or remove syringes altogether from the list of drug paraphernalia (Law Atlas, 2015). In states such as Connecticut and New York where restrictions on syringe access were repealed, some encouraging trends have been noted: Equipment sales through pharmacies have increased, self-reported needle-sharing has declined, and HIV incidence and prevalence have also declined (WHO, 2004).

In addition to the existence of drug control laws, enforcement of these laws influences individual behaviors, community stigma surrounding IDU, and the overall risk environment for PWID. In areas and situations perceived to be threatening, PWID may respond in ways that actually increase risk of acquiring or transmitting HIV—for example, injecting in a hurried manner, visiting unsupervised "shooting galleries," and improperly disposing of used equipment that can then be picked up and used by someone else (Burris, 2011). Although PWID might try to balance risks and opportunities associated with obtaining new equipment, multiple economic, sociocultural, and political/regulatory limitations in the local environment undoubtedly shape decision-making and subsequently influence people's actions.

ADDITIONAL STRUCTURAL AND SYSTEMS-LEVEL CONSIDERATIONS

In order to design feasible prevention interventions at the systems level, several other structural factors have been evaluated to determine how they affect HIV risk. These factors represent an extensive landscape of physical, economic, sociocultural, policy, and organizational dynamics. Physical factors such as proximity to—and convenience of—HIV services can play important roles in determining whether an individual is motivated to seek health care. Settings that offer co-located services (e.g., prevention counseling with STI/HIV testing and additional on-site medical care) and across expanded hours can be especially effective at linking people to, and retaining them in, quality care (Rothman, 2007). Stable housing and safety of the local community are other extremely important physical determinants of health and HIV risk. Many studies have found that unsafe and inadequate housing are significant barriers to receiving quality care and also increase risk of forward transmission (Aidala, 2015; Garcia 2015). In addition to specific substance use-associated HIV risks detailed previously, the intersections between behavioral/mental health and HIV have been well described (HRSA, 2015; Sikkema, 2010). Integrating behavioral and mental health services into prevention and treatment programs may help ensure coordinated delivery of comprehensive care for vulnerable populations. If possible, providers should elicit a thorough mental health history as well as screen for prior/current trauma and violence when caring for at-risk and HIV-positive individuals, and they should be able to do so in a sensitive manner. Clinicians should also approach substance use and sexual practices in a patient-centered, nonjudgmental manner in order to counsel effectively on HIV prevention and testing.

Economic factors are closely intertwined with HIV: A disproportionate burden of disease exists in less developed countries and among resource-limited communities. Such discrepancies directly and indirectly involve poverty and gender inequality, economic instability, labor migration, access to education and health resources, substance use, drug policies and enforcement, and so on (Zanakis, 2007). Low socioeconomic status has been linked to riskier health behaviors such as earlier initiation of sexual activity and less frequent condom use (Adler, 2006).

The epidemiology of incarceration closely reflects that of HIV. Many have cited socioeconomic marginalization as a common element that fuels these overlapping epidemics and results in correctional facilities bearing disproportionately high rates of HIV (National Minority AIDS Council and Housing Works, 2013). Challenges include lack of resources for testing and treatment in home communities as well as correctional facilities. Particularly in jails, rapid turnover of incarcerated individuals often limits widespread screening and evaluation.

Health insurance status is another economically related determinant affecting access to primary care and preventive services. Medical costs are prohibitive for the large number of people at risk for or living with HIV. In 2010, the Affordable Care Act (ACA) was signed into law. This had many significant HIV-related implications, including the following: (1) Individuals could not be denied coverage due to pre-existing health conditions including HIV, (2) states were given an option to expand Medicaid eligibility, (3) community health centers received increased support to provide HIV care, and (4) USPSTF-recommended HIV screening became reimbursable. Although it has been in effect for only a few years, early research predicts the ACA "may increase the number of people getting tested for HIV by nearly 500,000 by 2017" and that among people living with HIV who gain insurance through the ACA, the proportion of those unaware will decline by greater than 20% (Wagner, 2014). Even prior to the ACA, the majority of states (and the District of Columbia) already had public health HIV testing laws consistent with CDC testing recommendations, with many specific statutes encouraging HIV risk management and partner counseling/referral services in conjunction with testing.

Values and normative behaviors are shaped by sociocultural networks with which an individual identifies. They also often influence attitudes and beliefs regarding HIV risk. High levels of fear and lack of knowledge surrounding HIV, as well as negative perceptions/disapproval toward populations it most visibly affects, have propelled HIV-related stigma and discrimination since the 1980s. As a result, both PLWH and those at risk often feel isolated, becoming increasingly marginalized from family members, peers, and communities. Some individuals have also described negative experiences with health care providers (Anderson, 2009). Fear of stigma and discrimination continue to be major reasons why people are reluctant to discuss risky behaviors, get tested, and disclose their HIV status to social contacts as well as service providers (Valdiserri, 2002). One approach that multiple organizations have attempted is to expand public health awareness through large-scale, mass media campaigns (including social media) that foster greater knowledge of HIV/AIDS and improved attitudes and behaviors including testing. These and other efforts directed at health literacy aim to empower individuals and increase both self-efficacy and self-care behaviors. Community building and mobilization are other important components to scaling up prevention interventions because social networks play a key role in delivering peer-to-peer information and support (Latkin, 2013; Mahajan, 2008). Finally, antidiscrimination policies and laws such as the 2009 US repeal of the HIV travel and immigration ban (resulting from decades of advocacy and education) can help reduce HIV-related stigma and advance universal human rights. In jurisdictions in which same-sex relationships and/or transactional sex are criminalized, MSM and sex workers may feel less inclined to access condoms and/or present for HIV testing for fear of discrimination and legal punishment.

Recommended Reading

Busch MP, Kleinman SF, Nemo GJ. Current and emerging infectious risks of blood transfusions. *JAMA.* 2003; 289(8):959–962.

Metzger DS, Zhang Y. Drug treatment as HIV prevention: Expanding treatment options. *Curr HIV/AIDS Rep.* 2010; 7(4):220–225.

Strathdee SA, Shoptaw S, Dyer TP, et al.; Substance Use Scientific Committee of the HIV Prevention Trials Network. Towards combination HIV prevention for injection drug users: Addressing addictophobia, apathy and inattention. *Curr Opin HIV AIDS.* 2012; 7(4):320–325.

MEDICAL INTERVENTIONS FOR HIV TRANSMISSION PREVENTION

LEARNING OBJECTIVES

- Define what it means to be at high risk for HIV acquisition, and identify patients who meet these criteria.

- Describe the screening and evaluation process necessary prior to starting pre-exposure prophylaxis (PrEP), occupational post-exposure prophylaxis (oPEP), and non-occupational post-exposure prophylaxis (nPEP).

- Describe the monitoring process for patients on PrEP, nPEP, and oPEP, including visit, laboratory, and counseling recommendations, and describe the common side effects, toxicities, and other potential risks associated with their use.

WHAT'S NEW?

- The CDC, the New York State Department of Health AIDS Institute, and WHO have released clinical practice guidelines on PrEP.

- Real-world observational data have found PrEP to be highly effective at preventing HIV transmission outside the clinical trial setting and have failed to demonstrate significant risk compensation as a result of PrEP use.

- All patients who are determined eligible to receive PEP (oPEP or nPEP) should receive a three-drug regimen for 28 days. Two-drug regimens are no longer recommended in published practice guidelines.

INTRODUCTION

Medical interventions used to prevent HIV transmission and acquisition among patients at risk include PrEP, oPEP and nPEP, STI screening and treatment, voluntary medical male circumcision, vertical transmission prevention, and treatment as prevention (TasP).

PRE-EXPOSURE PROPHYLAXIS

PrEP is the use of antiretroviral medication before HIV exposure as a means to prevent HIV acquisition in at-risk, HIV-negative individuals. For the purposes of this section, PrEP should be understood to mean daily oral antiretroviral prophylaxis. Other routes and schedules (e.g., vaginal antiretroviral therapy (ART)-containing gel and intermittent PrEP) have been and/or are being studied but are discussed in the section Investigational Interventions.

Data: Clinical Trials and Real-World Effectiveness

Studies evaluating this strategy have found that, when taken consistently, PrEP is very effective at reducing the rate of HIV acquisition in those at highest risk, including MSM, transgender women who have sex with men, PWID, and coupled and single women and men engaging in heterosexual sex (see Table 4.1). Although the benefit varied slightly across the various studies, with reductions in the rate of HIV infection ranging from 44% to 75%, several common features should be highlighted. First, it was most effective among those who were most adherent. In the iPrEx study, for example, the relative risk of HIV infection was 92% lower among those with detectable levels of study drug compared to those without (Grant, 2010), and in the Bangkok Tenofovir study it was 70% lower (Choopanya, 2013). Furthermore, in the two negative PrEP trials to date, adherence was extremely poor (<30%) based on drug-level testing (Marrazzo, 2015; van Damme, 2012), again underscoring the importance of adherence for PrEP to be beneficial. Second, it was generally well tolerated, with fewer than 10% of patients reporting serious adverse events (US Public Health Service, 2014). Third, risk behaviors generally decreased during the study period; in both the iPrEx and the Partners PrEP studies, for example, the percentage

Table 4.1 SUMMARY OF RANDOMIZED, CONTROLLED PREP TRIALS

TRIAL	*N*, STUDY POPULATION; SETTING	INTERVENTION	EFFECT—HAZARD RATIO [ESTIMATED REDUCTION IN HIV ACQUISITION] (95% CI)	REFERENCE
iPrEX	2499 MSM, transgender women, United States, South America, Thailand, South Africa	TDF/FTC	0.56 [44%] (15–63)	Grant (2010)
Partners PrEP	4747 heterosexual women and men; Kenya and Uganda	TDF TDF/FTC	0.33 [67%] (0.19–0.56) 0.25 [75%] (0.13–0.45)	Baeten (2012)
TDF 2	1219 heterosexual women and men; Botswana	TDF/FTC	0.38 [62%] (0.22–0.83)	Thigpen (2012)
Thai IDU	2413 PWIDs; Thailand	TDF	0.51 [49%] (0.1–0.72)	Choopanya (2013)
FemPrEP	2120 heterosexual women; Africa	TDF/FTC	0.94 [6%] (0.59–1.52)	Van Damme (2012)
VOICE	5029 heterosexual women; Africa	TDF TDF/FTC	1.49 [−49%] (0.97–2.29) 1.04 [−4%] (0.73–1.49)	Marrazzo (2015)

FTC, emtricitabine; MSM, men who have sex with men; PWID, people who inject drugs; TDF, tenofovir disoproxil fumarate.

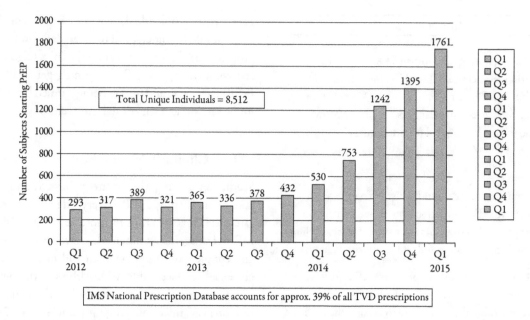

Figure 4.3 Number of new PrEP starts over time. SOURCE: Bush (2015).

of patients who reported unprotected intercourse decreased significantly during the study period (Baeten, 2012; Grant, 2010).

Since the publication of these study data, the number of at-risk patients taking PrEP has increased substantially (Figure 4.3). Effectiveness of PrEP in the "real world" has not yet been studied exhaustively. However, data from the Kaiser group in San Francisco are highly encouraging: Among 657 PrEP initiators in an 18-month period, no new infections occurred during 388 person-years of follow-up, despite the fact that data from similar populations would predict an infection rate of 8.9/100 person-years—suggesting that as many as 34 new infections may have been averted through PrEP use (Volk, 2015). In addition, data from the PROUD study in the United Kingdom, which was designed to mimic real-world settings, showed a relative reduction in HIV incidence among MSM receiving PrEP of 86%, corresponding to a number needed to treat of just 13 in order to prevent 1 new HIV infection (McCormack, 2015).

Eligibility

According to the CDC's 2014 guidelines, PrEP (using tenofovir disoproxil fumarate/emtricitabine (TDF/FTC)) is recommended as a prevention option for adults at substantial risk of acquiring HIV infection, including MSM, heterosexually active women and men, and injection drug users (Table 4.2) (CDC, 2014). The guidelines do not define what constitutes a "high number" of sex partners, nor do they define what constitutes a "high prevalence area or

network"; however, note that recent data from the National Health and Nutrition Examination Survey (NHANES) indicate that the lifetime prevalence of HIV is almost twice as high for individuals reporting 5–9 lifetime sexual partners, and nearly fivefold higher among those reporting 10 or more, compared to those reporting 4 or fewer (Woodring, 2015). Regarding the definition of "high prevalence," the majority of PrEP studies were conducted in populations in which the background HIV incidence was at least 3 per 100 person-years, and the International Antiviral Society–USA panel therefore recommends PrEP for those in which the background incidence is greater than 2% (Marrazzo, 2014).

The New York State Department of Health AIDS Institute also released PrEP guidelines in 2015 (New York State Department of Health, 2015). These guidelines define patients at substantial, ongoing risk for HIV acquisition as follows:

- MSM who engage in unprotected anal intercourse

- Individuals who are in a serodiscordant sexual relationship with a known HIV-infected partner

- Male-to-female and female-to male transgender individuals engaging in high-risk sexual behaviors

- Individuals engaging in transactional sex, such as sex for money, drugs, or housing

- Injection drug users who report any of the following behaviors: sharing injection equipment (including to inject hormones among transgender individuals), injecting one or more times per day, injecting cocaine or methamphetamine, and engaging in high-risk sexual behaviors

- Individuals who use stimulant drugs associated with high-risk behaviors, such as methamphetamine

- Individuals diagnosed with at least one anogenital sexually transmitted infection in the past year

- Individuals who have been prescribed nPEP who demonstrate continued high-risk behavior or have used multiple courses of nPEP

WHO recently released its updated guidelines on PrEP, which simply state that "oral PrEP containing TDF should be offered as an additional prevention choice for people at substantial risk of HIV infection as part of combination HIV prevention approaches" (WHO, 2015). WHO defines substantial risk as HIV incidence greater than 3 per 100 person-years in the absence of PrEP (WHO, 2015).

It is important to emphasize that PrEP should not be prescribed as a sole prevention intervention in those at risk but, rather, it should be part of a comprehensive HIV prevention plan, including behavioral and other prevention strategies.

How PrEP Should Be Prescribed

Prior to initiating PrEP in eligible patients, providers must document the following:

- Absence of acute or chronic HIV infection

- Normal renal function (CrCl ≥60 ml/min)

- Hepatitis B immunity or infection and vaccination status

To document absence of acute or chronic HIV infection, the CDC recommends following the algorithm shown in Figure 4.4. Oral rapid HIV testing should not be used due to its lower sensitivity for detecting HIV compared to blood tests (CDC, 2014), and a negative (preferably fourth-generation) test result should be documented within the week before initiating PrEP. Additional testing, such as viral load testing, should also be done for anyone who reports signs or symptoms of acute HIV infection within the previous 4 weeks and for those with high-risk exposures within 4 weeks prior to initiating PrEP (CDC, 2014; New York State Department of Health, 2014).

Current CDC guidelines state that eligible patients meeting appropriate clinical criteria should receive tenofovir/emtricitabine (TDF 300 mg/FTC 200 mg) once daily.

Table 4.2 SUMMARY GUIDELINES FOR PREP USE

	MEN WHO HAVE SEX WITH MEN	HETEROSEXUALLY ACTIVE WOMEN AND MEN	INJECTION DRUG USERS
Those at substantial risk of acquiring HIV	HIV-infected sexual partner Recent bacterial STI High number of sex partners Inconsistent or no condom use History of engaging in commercial sex work	HIV-infected sexual partner Recent bacterial STI High number of sex partners Inconsistent or no condom use History of engaging in commercial sex work Being in a high-prevalence area or network	HIV-positive injecting partner History of sharing injection equipment History of recent drug treatment (but currently injecting)
Clinically eligible if	Documented negative HIV test No signs/symptoms of acute HIV infection Normal renal function (CrCl ≥60 ml/min) No contraindicated medications Documented hepatitis B virus infection and vaccination status		
Prescription	TDF/FTC (FDC) once daily No more than 3-month supply		
Other services	Follow-up visits at least every 3 months to provide HIV test, medication adherence counseling, behavioral risk reduction support, side effect assessment, and STI symptom assessment At 3 months and every 6 months thereafter, assess renal function Every 6 months, test for bacterial STIs		
	Do oral/rectal STI testing	Assess pregnancy intent; pregnancy test every 3 months	Access to clean needles/syringes and drug treatment services

FDC, fixed-dose combination; FTC, emtricitabine; STI, sexually transmitted infection; TDF, tenofovir disoproxil fumarate.

SOURCE: Adapted from CDC (2014).

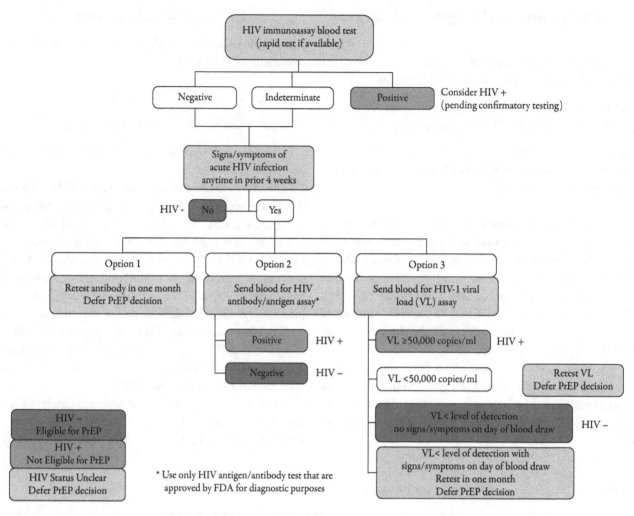

Figure 4.4 Assessment for acute/chronic HIV infection prior to PrEP initiation. SOURCE: CDC (2014).

Whereas the CDC states that daily TDF alone may be given as an alternative to PWID and heterosexually active women and men, WHO lists daily TDF as the preferred PrEP regimen (CDC, 2014; WHO, 2015). The CDC recommends that patients be given no more than a 3-month supply of medications at one time. Recommended follow-up and testing for PrEP toxicity and comorbid conditions are detailed in Table 4.2.

PrEP Risks

PrEP has generally been very well tolerated in both clinical studies and real-world settings, with fewer than 10% of recipients experiencing serious adverse events (CDC, 2014). The most commonly reported side effects are gastrointestinal, such as nausea, flatulence, headache, and weight loss. Sometimes referred to as "startup syndrome," most resolve within the first month of treatment and can usually be managed symptomatically with over-the-counter medications (CDC, 2014).

More serious potential PrEP toxicities include acute and/or chronic kidney injury and bone demineralization. Analyses from the iPrEX study indicate that PrEP recipients experience a small but statistically significant decline in creatinine clearance (CrCl) that is nonprogressive and reversible upon PrEP discontinuation (Solomon, 2014). Similarly, patients from the same study who received PrEP experienced a small but statistically significant decrease in bone mineral density (BMD) compared to those who received placebo. However, there was no increase in fracture risk, no one with low BMD, and observed decreases in vertebral BMD were reversible with PrEP discontinuation (Mulligan, 2015).

For patients who become infected with HIV while on PrEP, there has been concern about the possible development of drug resistance. To date, such resistance has been rare, and it has been primarily observed in patients who had acute seronegative HIV infection, underscoring the importance of screening patients for possible acute HIV before initiating PrEP (CDC, 2014). When it does occur, resistance mutations to FTC appear to be more common than those to TDF (Lehman, 2015).

Concern that PrEP use will lead to an increase in risky sexual behavior ("risk compensation") so far has not been borne out in either clinical trial or "real-world" settings. In both the iPrEx and the Partners PrEP studies, the percentage of patients who reported having sex without a condom decreased during the study period (Baeten, 2012; Grant, 2010). "Real-world" data from the aforementioned Kaiser cohort and PROUD studies also failed to demonstrate evidence of risk compensation based on the number of reported sexual partners, condom use, and rates of STIs (McCormack, 2015; Volk, 2015). Last, while adherence to PrEP was greatest among those reporting condomless anal intercourse in the ATN 110 study, which is an open-label feasibility study in young MSM ages 18–22 years, overall rates of sexual risk behavior as measured by the number of male partners, instances of condomless receptive anal intercourse, and instances of condom breakage during receptive anal intercourse remained stable (Hosek, 2015).

For patients who are chronically infected with hepatitis B virus (HBV) as evidenced by a positive hepatitis B surface antigen (sAg) test, the CDC recommends evaluation by a clinician experienced in the treatment of chronic HBV. Such patients who are given PrEP should be counseled that there is a potential risk of a flare in their HBV infection should they abruptly discontinue TDF-containing PrEP, although this has not yet been reported in HBV-positive, HIV-negative patients (CDC, 2014; Grant, 2010).

Women of childbearing age who wish to become pregnant or breast-feed while taking PrEP should be counseled that the PrEP studies to date excluded women who were or who became pregnant; however, data from the Antiviral Pregnancy Registry demonstrate no evidence of harm to fetuses exposed to these medications (Antiretroviral Pregnancy Registry, 2015). Furthermore, it should be emphasized that HIV-uninfected women who wish to conceive with an HIV-infected partner are at increased risk for HIV acquisition, and current US perinatal guidelines permit the use of PrEP for such patients (US Department of Health and Human Services, 2015). Although data are limited, the use of PrEP during lactation appears to be safe (CDC, 2014).

Discontinuing PrEP

PrEP should be discontinued in patients who acquire HIV infection; experience unacceptable side effects or toxicities, including renal disease; are unable to adhere to the prescribed regimen or follow-up visit schedule; or change their risk status such that PrEP is no longer indicated (CDC, 2014; New York State Department of Health AIDS Institute, 2014). Patients who acquire HIV while taking PrEP should be initiated on combination ART based on genotypic testing results and in accordance with current HIV treatment guidelines.

Unanswered Questions

Although PrEP has clearly been shown to be beneficial in the appropriate settings, unanswered questions remain. It is not clear, for example, how long PrEP can be safely prescribed. The CDC guidelines state that it should not be given for life but, rather, only during times of highest risk of HIV acquisition; however, many PrEP-eligible patients can be expected to remain so for extended periods of their lives (CDC, 2014).

The role of "on-demand" PrEP has also not yet been elucidated. Although data from the IPERGAY study conducted in France demonstrated high rates of protection when taken before and after sex (Molina, 2015), this strategy was not as effective as daily PrEP among the US-based cohort of the HPTN 067/ADAPT trial (Mannheimer, 2015).

Last, the role of PrEP for patients in serodiscordant relationships in which the HIV-infected partner is on suppressive ART is not clear. Data from the HPTN 052 trial demonstrated that no linked transmissions occurred among couples when the infected partner was suppressed on ART (Cohen, 2015). However, concerns persist that HIV transmission may still be possible due to daily variations in viral load, as well as potential discordance between serum viral load and that in genital and rectal secretions (Hosein, 2011). In addition, HIV-negative patients in such relationships may have other partners whose HIV status is unknown or who are HIV infected but not yet on treatment. This possibility was highlighted by the fact that nearly 40% of transmissions in the HPTN 052 study were unlinked (i.e., they came from someone other than their identified serodiscordant partner) (Cohen, 2015). PrEP is likely to be beneficial for such patients.

OCCUPATIONAL AND NON-OCCUPATIONAL POST-EXPOSURE PROPHYLAXIS

Ethical considerations prohibit the evaluation of either oPEP or nPEP using randomized controlled trials. The data to support its use largely derive from animal models, inference from postnatal prophylaxis studies, observational studies, and one retrospective case–control study that showed an 81% reduction in the risk of infection among health care workers who took zidovudine after exposure (Cardo, 1997; Lunding, 2015; Otten, 2000;Shih, 1991; Young, 2007).

oPEP

The use of ART to prevent transmission of HIV for health care personnel who experience a high-risk occupational exposure was first recommended in 1990, and the US Preventive Health Service released its most recent oPEP guidelines in 2013 (Kuhar, 2013).

The risk of HIV acquisition after exposure in the health care setting appears to be directly related to the size of the viral inoculum, which is in turn influenced by the stage of disease of the source patient, as well as the quantity of blood to which the worker was exposed (Kuhar, 2013).

Current guidelines emphasize the following:

- The HIV status of the source patient should be determined whenever possible to guide the need for initiating and/or maintaining oPEP.

- When indicated, it should be started as soon as possible, preferably within 72 hours from the time of exposure.

- All oPEP regimens should include three antiretroviral medications and should be taken for 4 weeks (Table 4.3).

- Expert consultation, with either local experts or through the national HIV Post-Exposure Prophylaxis Hotline, is recommended in certain situations (Table 4.4).

- Close follow-up services, including counseling, repeat HIV testing, and monitoring for drug toxicity, should be provided. HIV follow-up testing should be done 6 weeks, 12 weeks, and 4 months (if using a fourth-generation combination HIV antibody–p24 antigen test) or 6 months after the exposure (Table 4.5).

It is also important to remember that health care workers who experience an occupational exposure should be screened for hepatitis B and C virus infections. All hepatitis B-susceptible individuals should initiate the hepatitis B vaccine series, and those exposed to a patient with known acute or active HBV should be given hepatitis B immune globulin as well. There is currently no effective prophylaxis for hepatitis C infection.

nPEP

The CDC's most recent nPEP guidelines were published in 2016 (Dominguez, 2016). The New York State Department of Health AIDS Institute released comprehensive guidelines on the use of antiretroviral medications following non-occupational exposures, including for victims of sexual assault, in 2014 (New York State Department of

Table 4.3 RECOMMENDED OPEP REGIMENS—ALL TO BE TAKEN ×4 WEEKS

Preferred regimen	NRTI backbone	Base
	Truvada 1 PO daily (TDF 300 mg/FTC 200 mg FDC)	Raltegravir 400 mg twice daily
Alternatives	One of following	With one of following
	Tenofovir DF (Viread; TDF) + emtricitabine (Emtriva; FTC) available as Truvada	Raltegravir (Isentress; RAL)
	or	*or*
	Tenofovir DF (Viread; TDF) + lamivudine (Epivir; 3TC)	Darunavir (Prezista; DRV) + ritonavir (Norvir; RTV)
	or	*or*
	Zidovudine (Retrovir; ZDV; AZT) + lamivudine (Epivir; 3TC); available as Combivir	Etravirine (Intelence; ETR)
	or	*or*
	Zidovudine (Retrovir; ZDV; AZT) + emtricitabine (Emtriva; FTC)	Rilpivirine (Edurant; RPV)
		or
		Atazanavir (Reyataz; ATV) + ritonavir (Norvir; RTV)
		or
		Lopinavir/ritonavir (Kaletra; LPV/RTV)
	or	
	Tenofovir + emtricitabine + elvitegravir + cobicistat (TDF/FTC/EVG/cobi, Stribild)	

FDC, fixed-dose combination; FTC, emtricitabine; TDF, tenofovir disoproxil fumarate.

SOURCE: Adapted from Kuhar (2013).

Table 4.4 SITUATIONS IN WHICH EXPERT CONSULTATION FOR OPEP IS RECOMMENDED

SCENARIO	COMMENTS
Delayed (i.e., later than 72 hours) exposure report	Interval after which benefits from PEP are undefined.
Unknown source (e.g., needle in sharps disposal container or laundry)	Use of PEP to be decided on a case-by-case basis. Consider severity of exposure and epidemiologic likelihood of HIV exposure. Do not test needles or other sharp instruments for HIV.
Known or suspected pregnancy in the exposed person	Provision of PEP should not be delayed while awaiting expert consultation.
Breast-feeding in the exposed person	Provision of PEP should not be delayed while awaiting expert consultation.
Known or suspected resistance of the source virus to antiretroviral agents	If source person's virus is known or suspected to be resistant to one or more of the drugs considered for PEP, selection of drugs to which the source person's virus is unlikely to be resistant is recommended. Do not delay initiation of PEP while awaiting any results of resistance testing of the source person's virus.
Toxicity of the initial PEP regimen	Symptoms (e.g., gastrointestinal symptoms and others) are often manageable without changing PEP regimen by prescribing antimotility or antiemetic agents. Counseling and support for management of side effects is very important because symptoms are often exacerbated by anxiety.
Serious medical illness in the exposed person	Significant underlying illness (e.g., renal disease) or an exposed provider already taking multiple medications may increase the risk of drug toxicity and drug–drug interactions.

Expert consultation can be made with local experts or by calling the National Clinicians' Post Exposure Prophylaxis Hotline (PEPline) at 1-888-448-4911

SOURCE: Adapted from Kuhar (2013).

Health, 2014). Key points from these guidelines include the following:

- For sexual assault victims, important considerations before initiating PEP include whether or not a significant exposure occurred during the assault; whether the victim is ready and willing to complete a PEP regimen; and knowledge of the alleged assailant's HIV status, although a lack thereof should not delay PEP initiation when warranted based on the nature of the exposure.

  - Exposure types warranting PEP include direct contact of the vagina, penis, anus, or mouth with the semen, vaginal fluids, or blood of the alleged assailant, with or without physical injury, tissue damage, or the presence of blood at the site of the assault; when broken skin or mucous membranes of the victim have been in contact with blood, semen, or vaginal fluids from the alleged assailant; and in cases of bites that result in visible blood.

  - Baseline HIV testing should be performed for the victim, as should a pregnancy test for female victims.

  - When indicated, PEP should be initiated within 2–36 hours after the exposure.

- Prophylactic treatment to prevent gonorrheal and chlamydial infections should also be offered, as should emergency contraception for female victims.

- For patients with other potential non-occupational exposures to HIV, determination of the level of risk from the exposure is critical; nPEP is generally only indicated for patients with higher risk exposures (Table 4.6). Other key points include the following:

  - HIV testing of the source patient should be performed when possible.

  - All exposed patients should have the following done at baseline: HIV testing, site-specific testing for gonorrhea and chlamydia, testing for syphilis, and pregnancy testing for women.

  - When indicated, PEP should be initiated within 2–36 hours after the exposure.

  - Risk-reduction counseling should also be provided, including referrals for mental health and/or substance use disorder treatment programs when indicated, as well as discussion of future PrEP use for individuals with ongoing risk behavior.

Table 4.5 RECOMMENDED FOLLOW-UP OF HEALTH CARE PERSONNEL EXPOSED TO KNOWN OR SUSPECTED HIV-POSITIVE SOURCES

TIME FROM EXPOSURE	RECOMMENDED SERVICES	
	COUNSELING	TESTING
Baseline	Transmission prevention (condom use; avoidance of blood/tissue donation; avoid breast-feeding if possible) Possible drug toxicities Possible drug interactions Importance of adherence	HIV antibody testing (preferable fourth-generation combined antibody/p24 antigen test) Complete blood count Liver function TESTS Renal function tests
72 hours	Even if not taking PEP—to review additional information about exposure or the source patient if available *If on PEP* Transmission prevention (condom use; avoidance of blood/tissue donation; avoid breast-feeding if possible) Possible drug toxicities Possible drug interactions Importance of adherence	
2 weeks	Transmission prevention Possible drug toxicities Possible drug interactions Importance of adherence	Complete blood count Liver function tests Renal function tests
6 weeks	Transmission prevention	HIV antibody testing (preferable fourth-generation combined antibody/p24 antigen test)
If fourth-generation HIV testing is used		
4 months		HIV antibody testing (if negative, HIV infection is excluded)
If fourth-generation HIV testing is not used		
12 weeks	Transmission prevention	HIV antibody testing
6 months		HIV antibody testing (if negative, HIV infection is excluded)

SOURCE: Adapted from Kuhar (2013).

Table 4.6 LEVEL OF RISK BASED ON EXPOSURE TYPE FOR CONSIDERATION OF NPEP

High-risk exposures—nPEP should be recommended	Receptive and insertive vaginal or anal intercourse with a partner who is HIV positive, or when the partner's HIV status is unknown Needle sharing with a partner who is HIV positive, or when the partner's HIV status is unknown Injuries with exposure to blood or other potentially infected fluids from a source known to be HIV-infected or HIV status is unknown (including needle sticks with a hollow-bore needle, human bites, and accidents)

Lower risk exposures—require case-by-case evaluation for nPEP	Oral–vaginal contact (receptive and insertive)
	Oral–anal contact (receptive and insertive)
	Receptive penile–oral contact with or without ejaculation
	Insertive penile–oral contact with or without ejaculation
	Factors that increase risk (nPEP should be offered)
	    Source person is known to be HIV-infected with high viral load
	    An oral mucosa that is not intact (e.g., oral lesions, gingivitis, and wounds)
	    Blood exposure
	    Presence of genital ulcer disease or other sexually transmitted infections

Exposures that do *not* warrant nPEP	Kissing Oral-to-oral contact without mucosal damage (mouth-to-mouth resuscitation) Human bites not involving blood Exposure to solid-bore needles or sharps not in recent contact with blood (e.g., tattoo needles and lancets) Mutual masturbation without skin breakdown or blood exposure

SOURCE: Adapted from New York State Department of Health AIDS Institute (2014).

New York State's recommended nPEP regimen is as follows:

Tenofovir 300 mg + emtricitabine 200 mg (Truvada) once daily

Plus

Raltegravir 400 mg twice daily *or* dolutegravir 50 mg once daily

For 28 days

As with patients who experience occupational exposures, those with non-occupational exposures should be screened for hepatitis B and C infections and be given appropriate treatment and follow-up as described previously.

SCREENING AND TREATMENT FOR SEXUALLY TRANSMITTED INFECTIONS

The link between STIs and an increased risk for HIV transmission/acquisition has been established for some time. This is supported by both biologic plausibility (e.g., genital tract inflammation leading to increased viral shedding in infected partners and increased access of HIV to subepithelial target cells) and epidemiologic synergy (Mayer, 2011; Ward, 2010). However, multiple confounders have made it difficult to estimate just how much these contribute to increased risk, and STI treatment studies to date have failed to consistently demonstrate any reduction in HIV transmission (Mayer, 2011; Ward, 2010). The Mwanza study from Tanzania stands out as the one notable exception: It demonstrated a 38% reduction in HIV incidence with syndromic STI management (Grosskurth, 1995). Nonetheless, the strong link between the two argues for the importance of regular screening and treatment for STIs in those at risk because those who screen positive are likely to benefit from PrEP and risk reduction counseling in general. This point is highlighted by an analysis from New York City that demonstrated that 1 in 20 MSM with a new syphilis diagnosis were diagnosed with HIV within 1 year (Prathela, 2015).

VOLUNTARY MEDICAL MALE CIRCUMCISION

Three large randomized trials performed in sub-Saharan Africa demonstrated that voluntary circumcision of HIV-uninfected men led to an approximate risk reduction for heterosexual HIV acquisition of 50% (Auvert, 2005; Bailey, 2007; Gray, 2007; Siegfried, 2009). This prevention benefit does not appear to extend to the female partners of circumcised HIV-infected men (Weiss, 2009). Although observational data suggest that circumcision may be beneficial for MSM who practice primary insertive anal intercourse, there is currently insufficient evidence to determine whether or not this is the case in general for MSM (Wiysonge, 2011).

VERTICAL TRANSMISSION PREVENTION

This is reviewed in detail in Chapter 26.

TREATMENT AS PREVENTION

This is reviewed in detail in Chapter 23.

Recommended Reading

New York State Department of Health AIDS Institute. HIV prophylaxis following non-occupational exposure. Available at http://www.hivguidelines.org/clinical-guidelines/post-exposure-prophylaxis/hiv-prophylaxis-following-non-occupational-exposure.

Siegfried N, Muller M, Deeks JJ, et al. Male circumcision for prevention of heterosexual acquisition of HIV in men. *Cochrane Database Syst Rev.* 2009;2:CD003362. DOI: 10.1002/14651858.CD003362.pub2

US Public Health Service. Preexposure prophylaxis for the prevention of HIV infection in the United States–2014: A clinical practice guideline. Available at http://stacks.cdc.gov/view/cdc/23109.

INVESTIGATIONAL INTERVENTIONS

LEARNING OBJECTIVES

Describe three investigational biomedical interventions for HIV prevention and how they complement existing, proven interventions.

WHAT'S NEW?

- The use of on-demand and time-driven dosing strategies for oral PrEP, as well as long-acting injectable formulations, is under active investigation.

- Drug-eluting vaginal rings, some of which are co-formulated with hormonal contraception, are being evaluated and could offer promise as a novel woman-driven HIV prevention method.

- New vaccine strategies, such as the use of broadly neutralizing antibodies per se and the use of bioinformatically developed antigens, are also being evaluated.

INTERMITTENT AND ON-DEMAND PRE-EXPOSURE PROPHYLAXIS

As previously mentioned, currently approved PrEP regimens require the daily use of antiretrovirals. Alternative dosing schedules, including on-demand and time-driven use of oral formulations as well as the use of long-acting injectable formulations, are under active investigation. Also as mentioned previously, mixed results have been obtained from studies evaluating non-daily oral PrEP use. The IPERGAY study conducted in France, Quebec, Canada, and other French-speaking countries evaluated event-driven PrEP in high-risk MSM. Participants in the intervention arm of this prospective, randomized, placebo-controlled trial took two tablets of TDF/FTC 2–24 hours before sex, 1 tablet 24 hours after sex, and an additional tablet 48 hours after the first dose. This on-demand approach was highly effective, with an 86% reduction in the risk of HIV seroconversion among those in the intervention arm compared to placebo (Molina, 2015). On the other hand, in the HPTN 067/ADAPT Harlem study, which compared daily PrEP with time-driven (one dose twice weekly plus one dose after sex) and event-driven (one dose before and one dose after sex) dosing schedules among MSM and transgender women in the United States, the daily strategy provided better coverage of reported sex acts and higher overall adherence compared to the other two (Mannheimer, 2015). It is also important to note that there are concerns about the use of nondaily strategies in different populations based on varying levels of drug penetration into different tissue categories. For example, oral tenofovir appears to concentrate more quickly in rectal compared to vaginal mucosa (Hendrix, 2013), which could limit the applicability of event- and time-driven PrEP in women.

Another investigational strategy is the use of long-acting injectable antiretrovirals for PrEP. Both cabotegravir, a novel integrase strand transfer inhibitor, and the non-nucleoside reverse transcriptase inhibitor rilpivirine can be formulated for depot injection and could potentially be given every 3 months as single agents, or in combination, for prevention (Ford, 2013; Snyder, 2014; Spreen, 2014). Concerns about dosing due to pharmacokinetic variability and the potential to select for HIV drug resistance as patients discontinue these drugs remain (Jackson, 2015; Penrose, 2015). Phase II trials (HPTN 076, HPTN 077, and HPTN 083) are currently underway or will soon be enrolling to further investigate the pharmacokinetics, safety, and tolerability of these agents (Krakower, 2015; see www.hptn.org).

Microbicides

Microbicides are products that are applied locally to the vaginal or rectal mucosa to reduce the risk of HIV, and other STI, acquisition. There was great optimism for this strategy when the results of the CAPRISA 004 trial were released. This study examined the effectiveness and safety of coitally dosed (one dose within 12 hours before sex and a second dose as soon as possible within 12 hours after sex) 1% tenofovir vaginal gel in sexually active South African women aged 18–40 years. It was found that use of this gel resulted in a 39% reduction overall in the risk of HIV acquisition and a 54% reduction in those who used the gel at least 80% of the time (Abdool Karim, 2010). However, this optimism was dampened by the failure of two subsequent studies, VOICE and FACTS 001, to show any reduction in HIV acquisition among women using this same tenofovir gel (Marrazzo, 2015; Rees, 2015). Note that HIV acquisition was reduced by approximately 50% among women who used the gel consistently, as measured by plasma TDF levels in both studies (Dai, 2015; Rees, 2015).

Despite the previously mentioned disappointment, the use of microbicides or other local drug-delivery devices such as vaginal rings has several theoretical benefits. First, they deliver high concentrations of the drug to the desired tissue with minimal systemic exposure (Hendrix, 2013). As such, they have the potential to provide on-demand protection, especially considering the time delay that occurs between oral TDF dosing and drug penetration of the vaginal mucosa. These products also may be given to women, who comprised almost half of new HIV infections globally in 2014 (WHO, 2015), and represent an additional HIV preventive option that they can control. Last, they have the potential to be co-formulated with other medications and as such may provide protection against other STIs and pregnancy. Ongoing studies currently evaluating novel microbicide approaches include several examining drug-eluting vaginal rings that can be left in the vagina for up to 1 month at a time and that contain TDF, darunavir, maraviroc, or dapivirine, with or without a hormonal contraceptive, usually levonorgestrel; and another study evaluating the use of a rectal gel for MSM and women who engage in receptive anal intercourse (Krakower, 2015). Importantly,

Table 4.7 SUMMARY OF HIV VACCINE EFFICACY TRIALS

TRIAL	VACCINE PRODUCT	STUDY POPULATION; SITE	RESULTS	REFERENCE
Vax 003	Recombinant gp120 (B/E)	Male and female PWID; Thailand	No efficacy	Pitisuttithum (2006)
Vax 004	Recombinant gp120 (B/B′)	Heterosexual women and MSM; United States and the Netherlands	No efficacy	Flynn (2005)
HVTN 502	Recombinant Ad5 (Clade B gag/pol/nef)	MSM, heterosexual women and men; North and South America, Caribbean, Australia	No efficacy	Buchbinder (2008)
HVTN 503	Recombinant Ad5 (Clade B gag/pol/nef)	Heterosexual women and men; South Africa	No efficacy	Gray (2011)
HVTN 505	6-plasmid DNA vaccine and rAd5 vector boost	MSM; United States	No efficacy	Hammer (2013)
RV 144	ALVAC: Canarypox (gag, pol, env) + AIDSVAX B/E recombinant gp120	Heterosexual women and men; Thailand	31% reduction in acquisition	Rerks-Ngarm (2009)

MSM, men who have sex with men; PWID, people who inject drugs.

SOURCE: Adapted from Tieu (2013) and Rubens (2015).

results of the MTN-020/ASPIRE trial, which evaluated the efficacy of a monthly dapivirine-eluting vaginal ring for HIV prevention in at-risk African women, were recently released and demonstrated a modest 27% reduction in the incidence of new HIV infections among women who received the study ring compared to those who received placebo. Adherence was again an important factor because the efficacy of the ring increased to 37% when data from two study sites with reduced rates of adherence and retention were excluded (Baeten, 2016). Although the overall protective effect was not as great as seen with other PrEP methods, this study offers hope for women-controlled prevention options.

Vaccines

Multiple challenges, both biomedical and social, have impeded the development of an effective HIV vaccine. These include HIV viral diversity and pathogenesis, identification of appropriate immune correlates of protection, community preparedness and concerns about vaccine-induced positivity, and, more recently, the expanded use of PrEP (Hammer, 2015). With the exception of the modestly positive Thai vaccine trial, which demonstrated a 31% reduction in new infections among vaccine recipients, clinical trials of HIV preventive vaccines have had disappointing results (Table 4.7). However, the pursuit of an effective vaccine remains as important as ever. Even with the promise of ART-mediated control of the epidemic through TasP and PrEP, an effective vaccine is essential for timely, sustainable control to occur, given the complexities of human behavior and the risk that programs supporting treatment-based interventions could

be defunded over time (Fauci, 2014). The ability of a vaccine to elicit broadly neutralizing antibodies (BNAbs), or antibodies that can protect against multiple pathogenic HIV strains by binding to highly conserved regions of the virus, is crucial for its success but thus far has been elusive. Recent advances in the identification and understanding of BNAbs have injected new hope into HIV vaccine development. One such antibody product, VRC01, is currently under investigation in the AMP study, a collaborative HVTN/HPTN study expected to begin enrollment in late 2015/early 2016 (see http://ampstudy.org). The use of bioinformatically developed mosaic antigens to elicit antibody responses that are protective against all clades of HIV is another novel approach that is under investigation in the HIV-V-A004 trial (Barouch, 2013; see http://www.avac.org/trial/hiv-v-a004ipcavd-009-approach).

Recommended Reading

Fauci AS, Marston HD. Ending AIDS—Is an HIV vaccine necessary? *N Engl J Med.* 2014;370(6):495–498.

Krakower DS, Mayer KH. Pre-exposure prophylaxis to prevent HIV infection: Current status, future opportunities and challenges. *Drugs.* 2015;75:243–251.

CONCLUSION

Tremendous progress has been made in the field of HIV transmission prevention. Although recent attention has focused on ART-based interventions such as TasP and PrEP, a truly multifaceted approach that includes behavioral, structural, and novel biomedical interventions will be needed to have a significant, lasting impact on the global incidence of HIV.

References

Abdool Karim Q, Abdool Karim SS, Frohlich JA, et al. Effectiveness and safety of tenofovir gel, an antiretroviral microbicide, for the prevention of HIV infection in women. *Science* 2010; 329(5996): 1168–1174.

Abdul-Quader AS, Feelemyer J, Modi S, et al. Effectiveness of structural-level needle/syringe programs to reduce HCV and HIV infection among people who inject drugs: a systematic review. *AIDS Behav* 2013; 17(9): 2878–2892.

Adimora AA, Hughes JP, Wang J, et al. Characteristics of multiple and concurrent partnerships among women at high risk for HIV infection. *J Acquir Immune Defic Syndr* 2014; 65(1): 99–106.

Adler NE. Overview of health disparities. In: GE Thompson, F Mitchell, M Williams, eds. *Examining the health disparities research plan of the National Institutes of Health: Unfinished business.* Washington, DC: National Academic Press, 2006; 129–188.

Agerwala SM, McCance-Katz EF. Integrating Screening, Brief Intervention, and Referral to Treatment (SBIRT) into clinical practice settings: A brief review. *J Psychoactive Drugs* 2012; 44(4): 307–317.

Aidala AA, Wilson MG, Shubert V, et al. Housing status, medical care, and health outcomes among people living with HIV/AIDS: A systematic review. *Am J Public Health* 2015; 106: e1–e23.

Althoff KN, Gebo KA, Gange SJ, et al. CD4 count at presentation for HIV care in the United States and Canada: Are those over 50 years more likely to have a delayed presentation? *AIDS Res Ther* 2010; 7: 45.

Anderson BJ. HIV stigma and discrimination persist, even in health care. *AMA J Ethics* 2009; 11(12): 998–1001.

Anema A, Marshall BD, Stevenson B, et al. Intergenerational sex as a risk factor for HIV among young men who have sex with men: A scoping review. *Curr HIV/AIDS Rep* 2013; 10(4): 398–407.

Antiretroviral Pregnancy Registry International Interim Report for 1 January 1989–31 January 2015. Available at http://www.apregistry.com/forms/exec-summary.pdf. Accessed November 29, 2015.

Aspinall EJ, Nambiar D, Goldberg DJ, et al. Are needle and syringe programs associated with a reduction in HIV transmission among people who inject drugs: A systematic review and meta-analysis? *Int J. Epidemiol* 2014; 43(1): 235–248.

Auvert B, Taljaard D, Lagarde E, Sobngwi-Tambekou J, Sitta R, et al. Randomized, controlled intervention trial of male circumcision for reduction of HIV infection risk: The ANRS 1265 trial. PLoS Med 2005; 2(11): e298.

Baeten JM. Donnell D, Ndase P, et al. Antiretroviral prophylaxis for HIV prevention in heterosexual men and women. N Engl J Med 2012; 367: 399–410.

Baeten JM, Palanee-Phillips T, Brown ER, et al. Use of a Vaginal Ring Containing Dapivirine for HIV-1 Prevention in Women. *N Engl J Med.* 2016 Feb 22. [Epub ahead of print]

Baggaley R, Boily M-C, White RG, et al. Risk of HIV-1 transmission for parenteral exposure and blood transfusion: a systematic review and meta-analysis. *AIDS* 2006; 20(6): 805–812.

Bailey RC, Moses S, Parker CB, et al. Male circumcision for HIV prevention in young men in Kisumu, Kenya: a randomised controlled trial. Lancet 2007; 369: 643

Barouch DH, Stephenson KE, Borducchi EN et al. Protective efficacy of a global HIV-1 mosaic vaccine against heterologous SHIV challenges in rhesus monkeys. *Cell* 2013; 155(3):531–539.

Bonell C, Imrie J. Behavioral interventions to prevent HIV infection: rapid evolution, increasing rigor, moderate success. *Br Med Bull* 2001; 58(1): 155–170.

Branson BM, Handsfield HH, Lampe MA, et al.; Centers for Disease Control and Prevention. Revised recommendations for HIV testing of adults, adolescents, and pregnant women in health-care settings. *MMWR Recomm Rep* 2006; 55(RR-14): 1–17.

Brooks JT, Buchacz K, Gebo K, et al. HIV infection and older Americans: The public health perspective. *Am J Public Health* 2012; 102(8): 1516–1526.

Buchbinder SP, Mehrotra DV, Duerr A, et al. Efficacy assessment of a cell-mediated immunity HIV-1 vaccine(the Step Study): A double-blind, randomised, placebo-controlled, test-of-concept trial. *Lancet* 2008; 372(9653): 1881–1893.

Burris S, Chiu J. Punitive Drug Law and the Risk Environment for Injecting Drug Users: Understanding the Connections. Working paper prepared for the Third Meeting of the Technical Advisory Group of the Global Commission on HIV and the Law, 7–9 July 2011. Available at http://hivlawcommission.org/index.php/working-papers?view=document&id=98&tmpl=component. Accessed November 17, 2015.

Busch MP, Kleinman SF, Nemo GJ. Current and emerging infectious risks of blood transfusions. *JAMA* 2003; 289(8): 959–962.

Bush S, Ng L, Magnuson D, et al. Significant Uptake of Truvada for Pre-exposure Prophylaxis (PrEP) Utilization in the US in Late 2014–1Q2015. In: Abstracts of the 10th International Conference on HIV Treatment and Prevention Adherence, Miami, FL, 2015. Abstract 74. Available at http://iapac.org/AdherenceConference/presentations/ADH10_OA74.pdf. Accessed November 29, 2015.

Caceres CF, Gerbase A, Lo YR, et al. *Prevention and Treatment of HIV and Other Sexually Transmitted Infections Among Men Who Have Sex with Men and Transgender People: Recommendations for a Public Health Approach.* Geneva: World Health Organization Document Production Services, 2011.

Cardo DM, Culver DH, Ciesielski CA, et al.; Centers for Disease Control and Prevention Needlestick Surveillance Group. A case control study of HIV seroconversion in health care workers after percutaneous exposure. *N Engl J Med* 1997; 337(21):1485–1490.

Celentano DD, Lucas G. Optimizing treatment outcomes in HIV-infected patients with substance abuse issues. *Clin Infect Dis* 2007; 45 (Suppl. 4): S318–S323.

Centers for Disease Control and Prevention. HIV transmission through transfusion—Missouri and Colorado, 2008. *MMWR Morb Mortal Wkly Rep* 2010; 59: 1335–1339.

Centers for Disease Control and Prevention. Integrated prevention services for HIV infection, viral hepatitis, sexually transmitted diseases, and tuberculosis for persons who use drugs illicitly: Summary guidance from CDC and the U.S. Department of Health and Human Services. *MMWR* 2012; 61(RR-5): 1–46.

Centers for Disease Control and Prevention, Health Resources and Services Administration, National Institutes of Health, American Academy of HIV Medicine, Association of Nurses in AIDS Care, International Association of Providers of AIDS Care, the National Minority AIDS Council, and Urban Coalition for HIV/AIDS Prevention Services. *Recommendations for HIV Prevention with Adults and Adolescents with HIV in the United States, 2014.* December 11, 2014. Available at http://stacks.cdc.gov/view/cdc/26062.

Centers for Disease Control and Prevention. HIV and Injection Drug Use in the United States. Available at http://www.cdc.gov/hiv/risk/idu.html. Accessed November 11, 2015.

Chen M, Rhodes PH, Hall HI, et al. Prevalence of undiagnosed HIV infection among persons aged ≥13 years—National HIV Surveillance System, United States, 2005–2008. *MMWR Suppl.* 2012; 61(02): 57–64.

Choopanya K, Martin M, Suntharasamai P, et al. Antiretroviral prophylaxis for HIV infection in injecting drug users in Bangkok, Thailand (the Bangkok Tenofovir Study): A randomised, double-blind, placebo-controlled phase 3 trial. *Lancet* 2013; 381: 2083–2090.

Cohen MS, Chen YQ, McCauley M, et al. Antiretroviral treatment prevents HIV transmission: final results from the HPTN 052 randomized controlled trial. Program and abstracts of the 8th IAS Conference on HIV Pathogenesis, Treatment & Prevention; July 19-22, 2015; Vancouver, Canada. Abstract MOAC0101LB.

Dai JY, Hedrix CW, Richardson BA, et al. Pharmacological measures of treatment adherence and risk of HIV infection in the VOICE study. *J Infect Dis.* DOI: 10.1093/infdis/jiv333. [Epub ahead of print]

Degenhardt L, Mathers B, Guarinieri M, et al. Meth/amphetamine use and associated HIV: Implications for global policy and public health. *Int J Drug Policy* 2010; 21(5): 347–358.

Dominguez K, Smith DK, Vasavi T, et al. Updated Guidelines for Antiretroviral Postexposure Prophylaxis After Sexual, Injection Drug Use, or Other Nonoccupational Exposure to HIV—United States, 2016. U.S. Centers for Disease Control and Prevention. Available at http://stacks.cdc.gov/view/cdc/38856. Accessed April 25, 2016.

Fauci AS, Martson HD. Ending AIDS—Is an HIV vaccine necessary? *N Engl J Med* 104; 370(6):495–498.

Flynn NM, Forthal DN, Harro CD, et al. Placebo-controlled phase 3 trial of a recombinant glycoprotein 120 vaccine to prevent HIV-1 infection. *J Infect Dis* 2005; 191(5):654–665.

Ford SL, Gould E, Chen S, et al. Lack of pharmacokinetic interaction between rilpivirine and integrase inhibitors dolutegravir and GSK1265744. *Antimicrob Agents Chemother* 2013; 57(11):5472–5477.

Garcia J, Parker C, Parker RG, et al. "You're really gonna kick us all out?" Sustaining safe spaces for community-based HIV prevention and control among black men who have sex with men. *PLoS One* 2015; 10(10): e0141326.

Garfein RS, Golub ET, Greenberg AE, et al. A peer-education intervention to reduce injection risk behaviors for HIV and hepatitis C virus infection in young injection drug users. *AIDS* 2007; 21: 1923–1932.

Giannou FK, Tsiara CG, Nikolopoulos GK, et al. Condom effectiveness in reducing heterosexual HIV transmission: A systematic review and meta-analysis of studies on HIV serodiscordant couples. *Expert Rev Pharmacoecon Outcomes Res* 2015; 1–11.

Grant RM., Lama JR, Anderson PL, et al. Preexposure chemoprophylaxis for HIV prevention in men who have sex with men. *N Engl J Med* 2010; 363:2587–2599.

Gray GE, Allen M, Moodie Z, et al. Safety and efficacy assessment of the HVTN 503/Phambili Study: A double-blind randomized placebo-controlled test-of-concept study of a Clade B-based HIV-1 vaccine in South Africa. *Lancet Infect Dis* 2011; 11(7): 507–515.

Gray RH, Kigozi G, Serwadda D, et al. Male circumcision for HIV prevention in men in Rakai, Uganda: A randomised trial. Lancet 2007; 369: 657–666.

Grosskurth H, Mosha F, Todd J, et al. Impact of improved treatment of sexually transmitted diseases on HIV infection in rural Tanzania: Randomised controlled trial. *Lancet* 1995; 346: 530–536.

Hammer SM. Advances in preventive HIV vaccines: Efficacy trial evolution. ID Week 2015; October 7-11, 2015; San Diego, California. Oral session 0021.

Hammer SM, Sobieszczyk ME, Janes H, et al. Efficacy trial of a DNA/rAd5 HIV-1 preventive vaccine. *N Engl J Med* 2013; 369: 2083–2092.

Harrison A, Cleland J, Frohlick J. Young people's sexual partnerships in KwaZulu/Natal, South Africa: Patterns, contextual influences, and HIV risk. *Studies Fam Planning* 2008; 39(4): 295–308.

Heimer R, Abdala N. Viability of HIV-1 in syringes: Implications for interventions among injection drug users. *AIDS Reader* 2000; 10(7).

Heimer R, Grau LE, Curtin E, et al. Assessment of HIV testing of urban injection drug users: Implications for expansion of HIV testing and prevention efforts. *Am J Public Health* 2007; 97(1): 119–116.

Hendrix CW, Chen BA, Guddera V, et al. MTN-001: Randomized pharmacokinetic cross-over study comparing tenofovir vaginal gel and oral tablets in vaginal tissue and other compartments. *PLoS One* 2013; 8(1): e55013. doi:10.1371/journal.pone.0055013.

Hosein SR and Wilson DP. Decision-making by people living with HIV requires communications from clinicians about the risk of transmission despite undetectable plasma viral load. *HIV Med* 2011; 12(8):516.

HRSA CARE Action [newsletter]. Methamphetamines and HIV. June 2009. Available at http://hab.hrsa.gov/newspublications/careactionnewsletter/june2009.pdf. Accessed November 15, 2015.

HRSA CARE Action [newsletter]. Impact of mental illness on people living with HIV. January 2015. Available at http://hab.hrsa.gov/deliverhivaidscare/mentalhealth.pdf. Accessed November 24, 2015.

Hosek S, Rudy B, Landowitz R, et al. An HIV pre-exposure prophylaxis (PrEP) demonstration project and safety study for young men who have sex with men in the United States (ATN 110). Program and abstracts of the 8th IAS Conference on HIV Pathogenesis, Treatment & Prevention; July 19-22, 2015; Vancouver, Canada. Abstract TUAC0204LB.

Humeniuk, R, Dennington V, Ali R; WHO ASSIST Phase III Study Group. The effectiveness of brief intervention for illicit drugs linked to the alcohol, smoking and substance involvement screening test (ASSIST) in primary health care settings: a technical report of phase III findings of the WHO ASSIST randomized controlled trial. Geneva: World Health Organization Document Production Services, 2008.

Institute of Medicine. *Preventing HIV Infection Among Injecting Drug Users in High-Risk Countries: an Assessment of the Evidence.* Washington, DC: National Academies Press, 2007.

Jackson A, McGowan I. Long-acting rilpivirine for HIV prevention. *Curr Opin HIV AIDS* 2015; 10(4):253–257.

Kaufman M, Cornish F, Zimmerman RS, et al. Health behavior change models for HIV prevention and AIDS care: Practical recommendations for a multi-level approach. *J Acquir Immune Defic Syndr.* 2014; 66 (Suppl 3): S250–S258.

Kaushic C, Ferreira VH, Kafka JK, et al. HIV infection in the female genital tract: Discrete influence of the local mucosal microenvironment. *Am J Reprod Immunol* 2010; 63(6): 566–575.

Kennedy CE, Medley AM, Sweat MD, et al. Behavioral interventions for HIV positive prevention in developing countries: A systematic review and meta-analysis. *Bull World Health Organization* 2010; 88: 615–623.

Kerr T, Kimber J, Debeck K, et al. The role of safer injection facilities in the response to HIV/AIDS among injection drug users. *Curr HIV/AIDS Rep* 2007; 4(4): 158–164.

Kleinman SH, Lelie N, Busch MP. Infectivity of human immunodeficiency virus-1, hepatitis C virus, and hepatitis B virus and risk of transmission by transfusion. *Transfusion* 2009; 49(11): 2454–2489.

Krakower DS, Mayer KH. Pre-exposure prophylaxis to prevent HIV infection: Current status, future opportunities and challenges. *Drugs* 2015; 75:243–251.

Kuhar DT, Henderson DK, Struble KA et al. Updated USPHS guidelines for the management of occupational exposures to human immunodeficiency virus and recommendations for post-exposure prophylaxis. *Infect Control Hosp Epidemiol.* 2013 Sept; 34(9):875–892.

Latkin CA, Davey-Rothwell MA, Knowlton AR, et al. Social network approaches to recruitment, HIV prevention, medical care, and medication adherence. *J Acquir Immune Defic Syndr* 2013; 63 (Suppl 1): S54–S58.

Latkin C, Donnell D, Metzger D, et al. The efficacy of a network intervention to reduce HIV risk behaviors among drug users and risk partners in Chiang Mai, Thailand and Philadelphia, US. *Soc Sci Med* 2009; 68(4): 740–748.

LawAtlas: The Policy Surveillance Portal. Report—Syringe Distribution Laws (April 2015). Available at http://lawatlas.org/files/upload/20150421_SyringeD_Report.pdf. Accessed November 17, 2015.

Lehman DA, Baeten JM, McCoy CO, et al. Risk of drug resistance among persons acquiring HIV within a randomized clinical trial of single- or dual-agent prophylaxis. *J Infect Dis* 2015; 211:1211–1218.

Lourenco L, Colley G, Nosyk B, et al.; STOP HIV/AIDS Study Group. High levels of heterogeneity in the HIV cascade of care across different population subgroups in British Columbia, Canada. *PLoS One* 2014; 9(12): e115277.

Lunding S, Katzenstein TL, Kronborg G, et al. The Danish PEP Registry: Experience with the use of post-exposure prophylaxis following blood exposure to HIV from 1999-2012. *Infect Dis (Lond).* 2015 Nov 3:1-6. [Epub ahead of print].

MacArthur GJ, Minozzi S, Martin N, et al. Opiate substitution treatment and HIV transmission in people who inject drugs: systematic review and meta-analysis. *BMJ* 2012; 345: e5945.

MacArthur GJ, van Velzen E, Palmateer N, et al. Interventions to prevent HIV and hepatitis C in people who inject drugs: A review of reviews to assess evidence of effectiveness. *Int J Drug Policy* 2014; 25(1): 34–52.

Mahajan AP, Sayles JN, Patel VA, et al. Stigma in the HIV/AIDS epidemic: A review of the literature and recommendations for the way forward. *AIDS* 2008; 22 (Suppl 2): S67-S79.

Mannheimer S, Hirsch-Moverman Y, Loquere A, et al. HPTN 067ADPAT study: A comparison of daily and intermittent Pre-exposure prophylaxis (PrEP) for HIV prevention in men who have sex with men and transgender women in New York City. 8th IAS Conference on HIV Pathogenesis, Treatment, and Prevention. 2015; Vancouver, Canada. Abstract MOAAC0305LB.

Marks G, Crepaz N, Senterfitt JW, et al. Meta-analysis of high-risk sexual behavior in persons aware and unaware they are infected with HIV in the United States: Implications for HIV prevention programs. *J Acquir Immune Defic Syndr* 2005; 39(4): 446–453.

Marrazzo JM, del Rio C, Holtgrave DR, et al. HIV prevention in clinical care settings: 2014 recommendations of the International Antiviral Society—USA Panel. *JAMA* 2014; 312(4):390–409.

Marrazzo JM, Gita R, Richardson BA, et al. Tenofovir-based preexposure prophylaxis for HIV infection among African women. *N Engl J Med* 2015; 372: 509–518.

Mayer KH, Venkatesh KK. Interactions of HIV and other sexually transmitted diseases, and genital tract inflammation facilitating local pathogen transmission and acquisition. *Am J Reprod Immunol* 2011; 65: 308–316.

McCormack S, Dunn DT, Desai M, et al. Pre-exposure prophylaxis to prevent the acquisition of HIV-1 infection (PROUD): Effectiveness results from the pilot phase of a pragmatic open-label randomised trial. *Lancet* 2015 Sep 9. pii: S0140-6736(15)00056-2. doi: 10.1016/S0140-6736(15)00056-2.

Medley A, Kennedy C, O'Reilly K, et al. Effectiveness of peer education interventions for HIV prevention in developing countries: A systematic review and meta-analysis. *AIDS Educ Prev* 2009; 21(3): 181–206.

Metzger DS, Zhang Y. Drug treatment as HIV prevention: Expanding treatment options. *Curr HIV/AIDS Rep* 2010; 7(4): 220–225.

Molina JM, Capitant C, Charreau I, et al. On demand PrEP with oral TDF/FTC in MSM: Results of the ANRS Ipergay trial. *N Engl J Med* 2015; 373:2237–2246.

Mulligan K, Glidden DV, Anderson PL, et al. Effects of emtricitabine/tenofovir on bone mineral density in HIV-negative persons in a randomized, double-blind, placebo-controlled trial. *Clin Infect Dis* 2015; 61(4):572–580.

Needle RH, Burrows D, Friedman SR, et al. Effectiveness of community-based outreach in preventing HIV/AIDS among injecting drug users. *Int J Drug Pol* 2005; 16 (Suppl): S45–S57.

New York State Department of Health AIDS Institute. Guidance for the use of pre-exposure prophylaxis (PrEP) to prevent HIV transmission, Oct 2015 revision. Available at http://www.hivguidelines.org/clinical-guidelines/pre-exposure-prophylaxis/guidance-for-the-use-of-pre-exposure-prophylaxis-prep-to-prevent-hiv-transmission. Accessed November 25, 2015.

New York State Department of Health AIDS Institute. HIV prophylaxis following non-occupational exposure. Available at http://www.hivguidelines.org/clinical-guidelines/post-exposure-prophylaxis/hiv-prophylaxis-following-non-occupational-exposure. Accessed October 26, 2015.

New York State Department of Health AIDS Institute. HIV prophylaxis for victims of sexual assault. Available at http://www.hivguidelines.org/clinical-guidelines/post-exposure-prophylaxis/hiv-prophylaxis-for-victims-of-sexual-assault.

Nosyk B, Min JE, Evans E, et al. The effects of opioid substitution treatment and highly active antiretroviral therapy on the cause-specific risk of mortality among HIV-positive people who inject drugs. *Clin Infect Dis* 2015; 61(7): 1157–1165.

Otten RA, Smith DK, Adams DR, et al. Efficacy of postexposure prophylaxis after intravaginal exposure of pig-tailed macaques to a human-derived retrovirus (human immunodeficiency virus type 2). *J Virol* 2000; 74(20):9771–9775.

Panel on Antiretroviral Guidelines for Adults and Adolescents. Guidelines for the use of antiretroviral agents in HIV-1-infected adults and adolescents. Department of Health and Human Services. Available at http://www.aidsinfo.nih.gov/ContentFiles/AdultandAdolescentGL.pdf. Accessed April 15, 2015.

Penrose K, Parikh UM, Hamanishi KA, et al. Selection of rilpivirine resistant HIV-1 in a seroconverter on long-acting rilpivirine (TMC278LA) from the lowest dose arm of the SSAT040 trial. *J Infect Dis* 2015; [Epub ahead of print]

Pettifor A, Bekker L-G, Hosek S, et al. Preventing HIV among young people: Research priorities for the future. *J Acquir Immune Defic Syndr* 2013; 63 (Suppl 2): S155-S160.

Pitisuttithum P, Gilbert P, Gurwith M, et al. Randomized, double-blind, placebo-controlled efficacy trial of a bivalent recombinant glycoprotein 120 HIV-1 vaccine among injection drug users in Bangkok, Thailand. *J Infect Dis* 2006; 194:1671–71.

Prathela P, Braunstein SL, Blank S, et al. The high risk of an HIV diagnosis following a diagnosis of syphilis: a population-level analysis of New York City men. *Clin Infect Dis* 2015; 61(2):281–287.

Rees H, Delany-Moretlwe SA, Lombard C, et al. FACTS 001 phase III trial of pericoital tenofovir 1% gel for HIV prevention in women. Program and abstracts of the 2015 Conference on Retroviruses and Opportunistic Infections; February 2015; Seattle, Washington. Abstract 26LB.

Rerks-Ngarm S, Pitisuttithum P, Nitayaphan S, et al. Vaccination with ALVAC and AIDSVAX to prevent HIV-1 infection in Thailand. *N Engl J Med* 2009; 361:2209–2220.

Rothman F, Rudnick D, Slifer M, et al. Co-located substance use treatment and HIV prevention and primary care services, New York State, 1990–2002: A model for effective service delivery to a high-risk population. *J Urban Health* 2007; 84(2): 226–242.

Rubens M, Ramamoorthy V, Saxena A, et al. HIV vaccine: Recent advances, current roadblocks, and future directions. *J Immunol Res* 2015; 2015: Epub 2015 Oct 22.

Saitz R. Screening and brief intervention for unhealthy drug use: Little or no efficacy. *Fron Psychiatry* 2014; 5: 121.

Shih CC, Kaneshima H, Rabin L, et al. Post exposure prophylaxis with zidovudine suppresses human immunodeficiency virus type 1 infection in SCID-hu mice in a time-dependent manner. *J Infect Dis* 1991; 163(3):625–627.

Shubert G; for the National Minority AIDS Council and Housing Works. Mass Incarceration, Housing Instability, and HIV/AIDS: Research Findings and Policy Recommendations. February 2013.

Siegfried N, Muller M, Deeks JJ, et al. Male circumcision for prevention of heterosexual acquisition of HIV in men. *Cochrane Database Syst Rev* 2009;2:CD003362. DOI: 10.1002/14651858.CD003362.pub2

Sikkema KJ, Watt MH, Drabkin AS, et al. Mental health treatment to reduce HIV transmission risk behavior: A positive prevention model. *AIDS Behav* 2010; 14(2): 252–262.

Smith DK, Herbst JH, Zhang XJ, et al. Condom effectiveness for HIV prevention by consistency of use among men who have sex with men (MSM) in the US. *J Acquir Immune Defic Syndr* 2015; 68(3): 337–344.

Snyder O, Vincent H, Lachau-Durant S, et al. Preclinical evaluation of TMC-278 LA, a long-acting formulation of rilpivirine, demonstrates significant protection from vaginal HIV infection. *AIDS Res Hum Retroviruses* 2014; 30 (Suppl 1): A11–A12.

Solomon MM, Lama JR, Glidden DV, et al. Changed in renal function associated with oral FTC/TDF use for HIV pre-exposure prophylaxis. *AIDS* 2014;28:851–859

Solomon MM, Schechter M, Liu AY, et al. The safety of tenofovir-emtricitabine for HIV pre-exposure prophylaxis (PrEP) in individuals with active hepatitis B. *J Acquir Immune Defic Syndr* 2015 Sep 21. [Epub ahead of print].

Spiller MW, Broz D, Wejnert C, et al.; Centers for Disease Control and Prevention; National HIV Behavioral Surveillance System Study Group. HIV infection and HIV-associated behaviors among persons who inject drugs—20 cities, United States, 2012. *MMWR Morb Mortal Wkly Rep* 2015; 64(10): 270–275.

Spreen B, Rinehart A, Smith K, et al. HIV PrEP dose rationale for cabotegravir (GSK 1265744) long-acting injectable nanosuspension. *AIDS Res Hum Retroviruses* 2014; 30(Suppl 1):A12.

Strathdee SA, Beyrer C. Threading the needle—How to stop the HIV outbreak in rural Indiana. *N Engl J Med* 2015; 373: 397–399.

Strathdee SA, Shoptaw S, Dyer TP, et al.; Substance Use Scientific Committee of the HIV Prevention Trials Network. Towards combination HIV prevention for injection drug users: Addressing addictophobia, apathy and inattention. *Curr Opin HIV AIDS* 2012; 7(4): 320–325.

Substance Abuse and Mental Health Services Administration. *White Paper on Screening, Brief Intervention and Referral to Treatment (SBIRT) in Behavioral Healthcare- 2011*. Rockville, MD, 2011.

Thigpen MC, Kebaabetswe PM, Paxton LA, et al. Antiretroviral prophylaxis for heterosexual HIV transmission in Botswana. *N Engl J Med* 2012; 367:423–434.

Tieu HV, Rolland M, Hammer SM, et al. Translational research insights from completed HIV vaccine efficacy trials. *J Acquir Immune Defic Syndr* 2013; 63:S150–S154.

US Public Health Service. Preexposure prophylaxis for the prevention of HIV infection in the United States—2014: A clinical practice guideline. http://stacks.cdc.gov/view/cdc/23109.

Valdiserri RO. HIV/AIDS stigma: An impediment to public health. *Am J Public Health* 2002; 92(3): 341–342.

Van Damme L, Corneli A, Ahmed K, et al. Preexposure prophylaxis for HIV infection among African women. *N Engl J Med.* 2012; 367: 411–422.

Vlahov D, Robertson AM, Strathdee SA. Prevention of HIV infection among injection drug users in resource-limited settings. *Clin Infect Dis* 2010; 50(Suppl 3): S114–S121.

Volk JE, Marcus JL, Phengrasamy T, et al. No new HIV infections with increasing use of HIV preexposure prophylaxis in a clinical practice setting. *Clin Infect Dis* 2015; 61(10):1601–1603.

Wagner Z, Wu Y, Sood N. The Affordable Care Act my increase the number of people getting tested for HIV by nearly 500,000 by 2017. *Health Aff (Millwood)* 2014; 33(3): 378–385.

Ward H, Rönn M. The contribution of STIs to the sexual transmission of HIV. *Curr Opin HIV AIDS* 2010; 5(4): 305–310.

Wei C, Fisher Raymond H, Guadamuz TE, et al. Racial/ethnic differences in seroadaptive and serodisclosure behaviors among men who have sex with men. *AIDS Behav* 2011; 15(1): 22–29.

Weiss HA, Hankins CA, Dickson K. Male circumcision and risk of HIV infection in women: A systematic review and meta-analysis. *Lancet Infect Dis* 2009; 9: 669–677.

Weller S, Davis K. Condom effectiveness in reducing heterosexual HIV transmission. *Cochrane Database Syst Rev* 2002; 1: CD003255.

Wiysonge CS, Kongnyuy EJ, Shey M, et al. Male circumcision for prevention of homosexual acquisition of HIV in men. *Cochrane Database Syst Rev* 2011;6.CD007496. DOI:10.1002/14651858. CD007496.pub2

Wodak A, Cooney, A. *Effectiveness of Sterile Needle and Syringe Programming in Reducing HIV/AIDS Among Injecting Drug Users.* Geneva: World Health Organization Document Production Services, 2004.

Woodring J, Kruszon-Moran D, McQuillan G. HIV infection in U.S. household population aged 18–59: Data from the National Health and Nutrition Examination Survey, 2007–2012. *Natl Health Stat Report* 2015 Sep 24;(83):1–13

World Health Organization. Global Summary of the AIDS Epidemic, 2014. Available at http://www.who.int/hiv/data/en. Accessed November 29, 2015.

World Health Organization. Guideline on when to start antiretroviral therapy and on pre-exposure prophylaxis for HIV, 2015. Available at http://www.who.int/hiv/pub/guidelines/earlyrelease-arv/en. Accessed November 8, 2015.

Young TN, Arens FJ, Kennedy GE, et al. Antiretroviral post-exposure prophylaxis (PEP) for occupational HIV exposure. *Cochrane Database Sys Rev.* 2007;1:CD002835.

Zanakis SH, Alvarez C, Li V. Socio-economic determinants of HIV/AIDS pandemic and nations efficiencies. *Eur J Operational Res* 2007; 176: 1811–1838.

Zou S, Dorsey KA, Notari EP, et al. Prevalence, incidence, and residual risk of human immunodeficiency virus and hepatitis C virus infections among United States blood donors since the introduction of nucleic acid testing. *Transfusion* 2010; 50(7): 1495–1504.

5.

IMMUNOLOGY

Dennis J. Hartigan-O'Connor and Christian Brander

CHAPTER GOAL

Upon completion of this chapter, the reader should be able to demonstrate knowledge of the evolving science describing the interaction between HIV and the immune system in order to effectively counsel and educate patients and their communities about the disease.

MECHANISMS OF CD4⁺ T CELL DECLINE

LEARNING OBJECTIVE

Describe the processes contributing to CD4⁺ T cell decline and immune activation in untreated HIV infection.

WHAT'S NEW?

Chronic inflammation in HIV disease may have its origins in translocation of microbial products across a Th17 cell-deficient mucosal barrier. Collagen deposition in lymph nodes contributes to T cell loss by interrupting homeostasis.

KEY POINTS

- Cytopathic infection alone is insufficient to explain CD4⁺ T cell loss in HIV infection.

- Chronic inflammation is strongly associated with CD4⁺ T cell loss in pathogenic lentiviral infection such as HIV, but it is not seen in nonpathogenic infections.

- Translocation of microbial constituents and lymph node scarring have been recognized as likely contributors to CD4⁺ T cell decline.

The prototypic outcomes associated with HIV infection are progressive CD4⁺ T cell decline, consequent immunodeficiency, and chronic inflammation. In untreated disease, circulating memory CD4⁺ T cells, some of which are infected, are both dividing and dying at an accelerated rate (Hellerstein, 1999). In addition, CD4⁺ T cells that are resident in the gastrointestinal mucosa are important early targets of infection and are decimated early in disease (Guadalupe, 2003; Heise, 1994; Veazey, 1998). Although direct cytopathic infection contributes to CD4⁺ T cell loss, many *uninfected* CD4⁺ T cells are dividing and dying in HIV disease. Thus, other mechanisms must be invoked to fully explain CD4⁺ T cell decline. The death of infected cells is likely due to exposure to tat, gp120, or other toxic proteins (all of which can induce apoptosis) and/or adaptive immune clearance of HIV-infected cells (Lenardo, 2002). HIV can also impair CD4⁺ T cell regeneration by destroying the immunologic niches that are required for T cell homeostasis, by depleting essential hematopoietic progenitor cells, and by inhibiting the regenerative process through production of immune mediators (Douek, 2003; Grossman, 2002).

Chronic inflammation and immune activation have also been shown to be associated with CD4⁺ T cell decline. It has been shown, for example, that pathogenic lentiviral infections (e.g., HIV infection) and nonpathogenic infections (e.g., lentiviral infections of many nonhuman primates) are each associated with robust virus replication. Immune activation, however, is observed only in the pathogenic models, suggesting that this mechanism is directly responsible for disease progression (Silvestri, 2003).

Chronic inflammation and CD4⁺ T cell decline have recently been linked in a self-perpetuating cycle that may underlie progressive T cell loss in HIV infection. It has been shown that CD4⁺ Th17 cells are among those cells lost from the gastrointestinal tract in early simian immunodeficiency virus (SIV) and HIV infection (Brenchley, 2008; Favre, 2009). Th17 cells are important for maintenance of the "mucosal barrier" between gut luminal contents and circulation. When these cells are depleted, microbial constituents and even whole microbes can migrate from the gut into circulation (Brenchley, 2006; Raffatellu, 2008). These pro-inflammatory microbial products vigorously activate the immune system, resulting in activation-induced cell death and/or altered homeostasis. This cycle is initiated early in SIV infection (Hirao, 2014) and appears to be an important driver of disease progression because the presence of sufficient Th17 cells before infection can limit viral replication (Hartigan-O'Connor, 2012).

Another increasingly recognized self-perpetuating cycle pertains to the impact of HIV-associated inflammation on lymphoid structures. The inflammatory response generated by HIV results in upregulation of certain countervailing "regulatory" responses, including production of transforming growth factor-β, which stimulates collagen deposition (Estes, 2008). The scarring of the lymph nodes, which appears to be irreversible, prevents normal T cell homeostasis and antigen presentation. The immunodeficiency that results can lead to excess burden of a variety of microbes, including cytomegalovirus (CMV), gut microbes, and perhaps HIV itself. This microbial burden contributes to the cycle by causing even more inflammation and scarring (Arthos, 2008).

Recommended Reading

Douek, DC, Picker, LJ, Koup, RA. T cell dynamics in HIV-1 infection. *Annu Rev Immunol.* 2003; 21:265–304.

EFFECTS OF HIV ON THE WHOLE IMMUNE SYSTEM

LEARNING OBJECTIVE

Demonstrate knowledge of the effects of HIV on immune cells other than CD4+ T cells.

KEY POINTS

- HIV has broad effects on many immune cell types, including many cells that are not infected by the virus.

- HIV disrupts the entire lymphoid system through its effects on secondary lymphoid organs such as lymph nodes.

Although HIV is tropic for CD4+ T cells, it is clear that many manifestations of HIV infection result from direct or indirect effects on other immune cell types. One example is the high death rate and turnover of CD8+ T cells, as well as numerical depletion of naive CD8+ T cells, even in the asymptomatic phase of infection (Roederer, 1995). HIV also has direct or indirect effects on antigen-presenting cells, B cells, and natural killer (NK) cells (Hamada, 2009; Kader, 2009; Klatt, 2010; Nigam, 2011; Zhou, 2015).

One factor that likely mediates some of the effects of HIV on the broader immune system, particularly in late disease, is the destruction of lymphoid tissue architecture. In early disease, as antigen-presenting cells are activated and initiate immune responses within lymph nodes, CD4+ T cells are retained within the nodes while activated CD8+ T cells migrate into circulation. This process contributes to CD8+ lymphocytosis and inversion of the CD4:CD8 ratio (Bishop, 1990; Bujdoso, 1989). In later disease, there is structural damage to primary and secondary lymphoid organs resulting from fibrotic scarring (Estes, 2008). Naive T cells, including CD8+ T cells, require access to lymph node paracortical T cell zones for access to critical homeostatic signals and growth factors, including interleukin-7 (IL-7) (Link, 2007). Presumably, therefore, lymphoid tissue scarring is one factor that contributes to failure to fully reconstitute CD4+ and CD8+ T cells despite complete virologic suppression.

HIV-1 can also infect myeloid cells, including macrophages and dendritic cells, both of which can express the chemokine receptor CCR5. However, compared to CD4+ T cells, myeloid cells are relatively resistant to *productive* infection with HIV (Coleman, 2009). The relative inability of SIV and HIV-2 to cause productive infection of these cells is mediated by the cellular restriction factor SAMHD1 (Hrecka, 2011; Laguette, 2011). The viral accessory protein Vpx blocks this cellular response, thus allowing infection. Because HIV-1 lacks this accessory protein, it remains unclear how this virus might productively infect macrophages (Hrecka, 2011; Laguette, 2011; Manel, 2010).

Natural killer T (NKT) cells are also rapidly and selectively depleted in HIV infection (Sandberg, 2002; van der Vliet, 2002). NKT cells may be broadly divided into those that are CD4+ and those that are CD4−, with the former population secreting both Th1 and Th2 cytokines and likely providing B cell help or carrying out immunoregulatory functions. The latter population (CD4−) produces mainly Th1 cytokines and has stronger cytolytic activity. The CD4+ NKT population is depleted more rapidly in HIV infection compared to the CD4− population, but it is restored more slowly after treatment with antiretroviral therapy (ART) (Li, 2008). HIV also interferes with the activation of NKT cells by downregulating expression of CD1d (a major histocompatiblity complex (MHC)-related protein that presents glycolipid antigens to NKT cells) on antigen-presenting cells (Hage, 2005). This downregulation appears to be mediated mainly by the viral Nef protein (Cho, 2005).

There is considerable interest in the effect of HIV and other agents of chronic infection on NK cells, particularly subsets with expanded functional capacity, including "memory" NK cells (Hwang, 2012; Lee, 2015; Lopez-Verges, 2011; Sun, 2009; Zhang, 2013). Such cells are considered to be innate cells with adaptive features, including more robust and rapid responses to pathogen encounter (Sun, 2009). To date, limited evidence has been presented demonstrating that HIV infection drives expansion of memory NK cells (Zhou, 2015). Human CMV infection, however, which is common in HIV-positive people, is thought to be the most important driver of memory NK cell expansion (Brodin, 2015; Lopez-Verges, 2011; Zhang, 2013). People co-infected with HIV and CMV may therefore present unique immunologic features.

Recommended Reading

Brodin P, Jojic V, Gao T, et al. Variation in the human immune system is largely driven by non-heritable influences. *Cell*. 2015; 160:37–47.
Zhou J, Amran FS, Kramski M, et al. An NK cell population lacking FcRgamma is expanded in chronically infected HIV patients. *J Immunol*. 2015; 194:4688–4697.

MECHANISMS OF CHRONIC INFLAMMATION IN HIV DISEASE

LEARNING OBJECTIVE

Demonstrate knowledge of the mechanisms contributory to T cell activation and chronic inflammation in HIV disease.

WHAT'S NEW?

Multiple mechanisms contribute to chronic inflammation in HIV disease.

KEY POINTS

- Innate immune responses that result in production of type I interferons are important drivers of inflammation in early disease.

- Early depletion of CD4+ T cells from the gastrointestinal mucosa likely contributes to chronic, persistent immune activation.

- CMV and other chronic infections are important contributors to T cell activation in co-infected individuals.

It was first demonstrated more than 15 years ago that T cell activation was associated with shorter survival in advanced HIV disease (Giorgi, 1999). One might imagine that chronic T cell activation is simply the inevitable consequence of ongoing viral replication, and that more T cell activation is indicative of more active disease. However, it is clear from studies of nonpathogenic lentiviral infections that chronic, high-level virus replication can occur without eliciting massive immune activation (Silvestri, 2003). Indeed, in the natural hosts of SIV, the rapid reduction in immune activation appears to protect against subsequent CD4+ T cell decline and disease progression. The mechanism by which HIV-1 causes a sustained and partially irreversible increase in immune activation remains a strong focus of ongoing research.

The virion itself elicits innate immune responses via activation of toll-like receptors (TLRs) 7, 8, and 9 within antigen-presenting cells. TLR engagement results in production of type I interferons, including interferon-α (IFN-α). Indeed, a spike of IFN-α production is observed in acute HIV and SIV infection (Favre, 2009; Stacey, 2009), which doubtless shapes the ensuing adaptive immune responses. Binding of virion components to signaling molecules such as CD4+ and CCR5 may also stimulate cells directly, and viral proteins such as Tat and Nef have been shown to have pro-inflammatory effects (Decrion, 2005). After the first 2 weeks of infection, the adaptive immune response to HIV proteins contributes to T cell activation, although many of these activated T cells are specific for CMV and other chronic pathogens rather than HIV (Doisne, 2004; Papagno, 2004). Less appreciated is the fact that lymphopenia alone can lead to T cell activation; for example, resting T cells spontaneously become activated and proliferate when introduced into T cell-deficient hosts (Srinivasula, 2011; Surh, 2008). Thus, the progressive loss of CD4+ T cells can be both a consequence and a cause of immune activation (Jone, 2009; King, 2004).

In addition to these general effects of lymphocyte depletion, the field has recently begun to appreciate the implications of early and profound lymphocyte depletion from the gastrointestinal mucosa (Heise, 1994; Veazey, 1998). Among the lymphocytes lost in early infection are CD4+ Th17 cells, which have an important structural role in maintenance of the tight junctions between intestinal epithelial cells (Brenchley, 2008; Favre, 2009). Loss of these cells contributes to a breakdown in the physical barrier separating the gut lumen from general circulation, which allows bioactive microbial products such as lipopolysaccharide (LPS) into the blood (Brenchley, 2006), whereas maintenance of sufficient Th17 cells is associated with reduced viral replication

(Hartigan-O'Connor, 2012). Mucosal barrier breakdown and pro-inflammatory processes such as tryptophan catabolism, in turn, are associated with disturbance ("dysbiosis") of the gut-resident microbial community (Vujkovic-Cvijin, 2013). Persistent microbial dysbiosis may help to drive further immune dysregulation and inflammation.

Both occult and symptomatic opportunistic infections also contribute to chronic inflammation in HIV disease. In particular, the prevalence of CMV co-infection among HIV-infected persons is at least 90% (Berry, 1988; Lang, 1989). Furthermore, CMV infection has been associated with T cell activation in HIV-uninfected people (Lenkei, 1995). Indeed, CMV-specific T cells account for nearly 10% of the circulating memory T cell pool in seropositive individuals, suggesting that CMV replication can have a major influence on the immune system even in healthy individuals who are not immunocompromised (Sylwester, 2005). CMV appears to have an even stronger effect on T cell remodeling in untreated and treated HIV infection (Naeger, 2010). A pilot study tested the possibility that chronic immune activation in HIV disease could be reduced by treatment of CMV infection, randomizing 30 individuals on ART to treatment with valganciclovir or placebo (Hunt, 2011). A significant 20% reduction in the percentage of activated $CD8^+$ T cells was demonstrated in the valganciclovir group, suggesting that CMV infection (or infection with other valganciclovir-sensitive herpesviruses) is a significant contributor to T cell activation in treated HIV and CMV co-infected individuals.

IMMUNOLOGIC EFFECTS OF ANTIRETROVIRAL THERAPY AND ROLE OF PERSISTENT IMMUNE DYSFUNCTION DURING THERAPY ON CLINICAL OUTCOMES

LEARNING OBJECTIVE

Demonstrate knowledge of the effect of antiretroviral therapy on immune function.

WHAT'S NEW?

Antiretroviral therapy does not fully restore immune function in many patients. Suboptimal $CD4^+$ T cell gains and chronic inflammation during treatment have both been implicated in subsequent disease progression.

KEY POINTS

- A small but clinically important subset of treated patients exhibit suboptimal $CD4^+$ T cell gains.

- Chronic inflammation, lymphoid fibrosis, hematopoietic progenitor cell loss, and thymic dysfunction all likely contribute to failure of normal T cell homeostasis.

- Chronic inflammation during treated disease has been associated with subsequent disease progression.

Combination ART results in complete or near-complete suppression of HIV replication. As a consequence, many of the factors that cause progressive immunodeficiency are reversed. Prevention of continued $CD4^+$ T cell destruction (via both direct and indirect effects) and homeostatic regeneration results in eventual restoration of $CD4^+$ T cell numbers in blood and tissues. The increase in peripheral $CD4^+$ T cell counts during therapy appears to be biphasic (Pakker, 1998). A robust increase of approximately 50–100 cells/mm^3 is often observed in the first several weeks. Because memory cells account for most of the increase, it has long been assumed that the redistribution of cells from tissues to the periphery accounts for this rapid increase. After this early phase, $CD4^+$ T cell counts increase slowly (at a rate of approximately 50 cells/mm^3/year) until they achieve a normal range (i.e., >500 cells/mm^3) (Mocroft, 2007). The augmented $CD4^+$ T cell population includes naive cells and hence is thought to reflect true immune reconstitution. Although less well studied, $CD4^+$ T cell gains also occur in tissues during effective therapy.

Although nearly everyone exhibits some degree of immune reconstitution during therapy, the outcome is highly variable. A small but clinically important subset of patients fail to achieve normal peripheral $CD4^+$ T cell counts, even after many years of ART. These so-called immunologic "failures" or "nonresponders" remain at relatively high risk for cancer, heart disease, liver failure, and other non-AIDS complications, but they usually achieve sufficient restoration of immune function to prevent AIDS-related complications. Patients who are older and who start therapy during late disease (e.g., low $CD4^+$ nadir) are at higher risk of exhibiting suboptimal gains during therapy. In one study, approximately 40% of patients who delayed therapy until their $CD4^+$ T cell count was less than 200 cells/mm^3 failed to achieve a normal $CD4^+$ T cell count after several years of viral suppression (Kelley, 2009). Other factors that have been associated with blunted $CD4^+$ T cell gains include hepatitis C virus co-infection, high levels of T cell activation, the use of certain nucleoside analogues (particularly the older combination of stavudine and didanosine), and the use of efavirenz-based regimens (compared to maraviroc-, raltegravir-, and protease inhibitor-based regimens).

Given its clinical importance, there is intense interest in determining the pathogenesis of immunologic failure (defined variably). In untreated disease, HIV-mediated destruction of hematopoietic stem cells, thymic tissue, lymphoid tissue, and central memory cells contributes to progressive CD4+ T cell loss. Treatment-mediated suppression of HIV replication partially restores these factors. Persistent lymph node fibrosis, thymic dysfunction, and loss of cells with stem-like properties have all been associated with CD4+ T cell regeneration failure and suboptimal gains during therapy (McCune, 2001; Sauce, 2011; Schacker, 2002; Teixeira, 2001).

Untreated HIV infection is associated with heightened levels of immune activation. Long-term suppression of HIV replication dramatically reduces most measures of immune activation, but this effect is often incomplete because inflammatory markers typically remain higher in treated HIV-infected adults than in age-matched uninfected adults (Neuhaus, 2010). Persistent inflammation during therapy is associated with excess risk of non-AIDS complications, including heart disease, cancer, liver disease, kidney disease, bone disease, and neurologic complications (Deeks, 2011; Kuller, 2008; Phillips, 2008). Persistent CMV replication may be an important cause of continued inflammation while on therapy because higher anti-CMV IgG antibody levels are associated with increased prevalence of carotid artery lesions among HIV-infected women who achieve HIV suppression on antiretroviral therapy but not among viremic or untreated women (Parrinello, 2012).

Persistent and possible irreversible damage to the infrastructure that supports T cell homeostasis may account for much of the persistent immunodeficiency and inflammation often observed during therapy. Theoretically, collagen deposition and scarring of the lymphoid system during untreated disease result in a loss of the regulatory pathways (particularly those involving IL-7) that control T cell regeneration (Zeng, 2012). This disruption results in persistently low CD4+ T cell counts and an inability to generate effective memory T cells in response to acute or chronic infections. Loss of lymphoid structures may also result in loss of immune surveillance and development of malignancies, as a well as a loss of key anti-inflammatory regulatory responses and, as a result, autoimmune-related clinical syndromes. In a self-perpetuating "vicious" cycle that persists in the absence of any HIV replication, persistent immunodeficiency results in a reduced capacity of host responses to

clear pathogens. The resulting burden of these pathogens contributes to more inflammation, which in turn continues to damage the lymphoid tissues. The collective outcome is a combination of low CD4+ T cell counts and chronic inflammation. It is hoped that knowledge about these pathways will lead to novel interventions aimed at preventing or reversing this immunodeficient and pro-inflammatory environment.

Recommended Reading

Deeks SG, Tracy R, Douek D. Systemic effect on inflammation on health during chronic HIV infection. *Immunity*. 2013; 39(4):633–645.

PATHOGENESIS OF IMMUNE RECONSTITUTION INFLAMMATORY SYNDROME

LEARNING OBJECTIVE

Demonstrate knowledge of the leading hypotheses explaining the pathogenesis of immune reconstitution inflammatory syndrome (IRIS), including antigen persistence and immune dysregulation.

WHAT'S NEW?

The presence of a greater inflammatory environment in untreated HIV disease is associated with IRIS episodes after treatment. Data on the role of regulatory CD4+ T cells (Tregs) in IRIS have been unclear.

KEY POINTS

- IRIS is seen most commonly in patients initiating ART with low CD4+ T cell counts, high viral loads, and preexisting opportunistic infections.

- Many IRIS symptoms are localized to sites of previous infection, suggestive of the presence of persistent microbial antigen.

- Development of IRIS is associated with increased T cell activation prior to initiation of treatment with ART.

A subset of AIDS patients who are immunorestored with ART develop inflammatory conditions known collectively as immune reconstitution inflammatory syndrome (IRIS) (Price, 2009). A meta-analysis showed that 16% of patients starting ART developed an IRIS event (Muller, 2010). Patients most likely to be affected are those initiating ART with low CD4 counts and preexisting opportunistic infections (Muller, 2010; Price, 2009). The symptoms of IRIS are often localized to sites of previous infection (Lawn, 2007), which led to the suggestion that IRIS is caused by adaptive immune responses to persistent pathogen-derived antigens (Muller, 2010). For example, IRIS in patients with a history of CMV retinitis can manifest as inflammation of the posterior uveal tract of the eye (Nussenblatt, 1998). The most frequent clinical manifestation of cryptococal IRIS, by contrast, is aseptic meningitis (Boulware, 2010).

The hypothesis that an IRIS is caused by the host immune response to persistent antigen (in the form of intact organisms, dead organisms, or debris) has the appeal of simplicity, but there are surprisingly few data available to support this idea. One study demonstrated that among patients with recent cryptococcal meningitis who were placed on ART, those developing cryptococcal IRIS had fourfold higher titers of cryptococcal antigen in serum (Boulware, 2010). In cases of *Mycobacterium tuberculosis* or *Mycobacterium avium* complex-associated IRIS, patients normally convert to skin test positivity, suggesting that at a minimum, the disease is mediated by pathogen-specific CD4+ T cells (French, 2004). In the case of CMV immune recovery uveitis, however, the presence of CMV antigens has not been demonstrated in affected patients.

A number of studies have suggested that a pretherapy inflammatory environment predicts IRIS. For example, Antonelli and colleagues showed that individuals who presented with an IRIS episode had a higher proportion of activated CD4+ T cells before starting ART compared with those who did not develop IRIS (Antonelli, 2010). These activated T cells had a Th1/Th17 skewed cytokine profile before therapy began. Furthermore, IRIS patients displayed higher serum IFN-γ levels near the time of their IRIS events. Understanding of the importance of Tregs in controlling immune responses to self-antigens has prompted the suggestion that failure to reconstitute these anti-inflammatory cells predisposes to IRIS (Seddiki, 2009). However, data to support this hypothesis have been inconsistent (Bourgarit, 2006; Hartigan-O'Connor, 2011). Other groups have argued that poorly regulated innate immune responses may be central to IRIS. Pretherapy and early treatment-mediated changes in various nonspecific inflammatory biomarkers (including C-reactive protein, IL-6, TNF-α, and D-dimers) have been associated with increased risk of IRIS and mortality during the first several months of effective ART (Barber, 2012; Boulware, 2010).

In summary, pathogenesis of IRIS seems dependent on the presence of both lymphopenia and antigen-specific CD4+ T cells. These T cells may be responding to persistent pathogen-derived antigens, self-antigens, or unrelated foreign antigens. In these latter cases, the opportunistic pathogen may be viewed as the trigger rather than the target of the pathogenic T cell response. Lymphopenia establishes a dysregulated environment in which either the response of the antigen-specific T cells or the effect of that response on the host is exaggerated.

Recommend Reading

Barber DL, Andrade BB, Sereti I, et al. Immune reconstitution inflammatory syndrome: The trouble with immunity when you had none. *Nat Rev Microbiol.* 2012; 10(2):150–156.

Boulougoura A, Sereti I. HIV infection and immune activation: The role of coinfections. *Curr Opin HIV AIDS.* 2016; 11(2):191–200.

MECHANISMS AND CONSEQUENCES OF VIRUS CONTROL IN "ELITE" CONTROLLERS

LEARNING OBJECTIVE

Demonstrate knowledge of how some individuals maintain durable control of HIV in the absence of antiretroviral therapy.

WHAT'S NEW?

Multiple mechanisms contribute to durable "elite" HIV control in untreated individuals.

KEY POINTS

- HIV-specific CD8+ T cells contribute to durable control of HIV in elite controllers.

- Despite the lack of readily detectable HIV RNA in plasma, elite controllers have higher than normal levels of immune activation, which may contribute to slow disease progression.

Approximately 1% of antiretroviral-untreated, chronically infected adults have no readily detectable HIV RNA in their plasma. These individuals are generally referred to as "elite" controllers, although other terms, including "long-term non-progressors," have been used to define this or similar groups of individuals keeping viral replication low in the absence of treatment. Given that the host mechanisms that might account for virus control in these individuals could inform both vaccine and cure research, there has been long-term intense interest in enumerating their mechanisms of control as well as in describing the degree to which controllers exhibit any evidence of disease progression.

Most investigators interested in determining the mechanisms of HIV control in these individuals have assessed specific candidate host factors in controllers and non-controllers. These studies have generally been cross-sectional, making it difficult to determine if a given host response is a cause or a consequence of virus control (Deeks, 2007). Some recent efforts have been made to follow individuals closely during the pre-HIV infection period both to capture information about the earliest events after infection and to study dynamic changes that may be important for eventual control (Ndhlovu, 2015).

Although no one study design is optimal, the collective data support a central role for potent HIV-specific $CD8^+$ T cells and, to a lesser degree, $CD4^+$ T cells in maintaining virus control. This is also supported by the fact that most genetic predictors of virus control are found on chromosome 6 in the HLA region that governs the antigenic specificity of T cells (Pereyra, 2010). Recent studies on SIV-infected monkeys further support the importance of virus-specific cytotoxic T lymphocyte responses in virus control, although at least in the RhCMV-vectored vaccine setting, their MHC class I restriction may not be universal, and there may be a significant contribution of MHC class II-restricted $CD8^+$ T cells (Hansen, 2013a, 2013b). Similarly, the role of the Th17 cell compartment in sustaining viral replication has been highlighted in recent monkey studies and will need to be investigated in the human HIV setting (Hartigan-O'Connor, 2012). Other factors that have been associated with virus control include (1) strong NK cell responses (Martin, 2007; Sips, 2012), (2) prevention of apoptosis/cell death in central memory cells (van Grevenynghe, 2008), (3) intrinsic intracellular restriction to HIV replication mediated by p21 (Chen, 2011) and other as yet poorly characterized factors (O'Connell, 2011; Saez-Cirion, 2011), and (4) acquisition of a replication-deficient virus. However, care must be taken not to confuse causative, functional markers of virus control with simple correlates of controlled infection. For instance, biomarkers such as proliferative capacity of HIV-specific T cells may be the consequence of otherwise controlled/uncontrolled HIV infection rather than its physiological cause. Longitudinal studies, identifying infected people within days of infection and following them in the absence of treatment, may be clinically and ethically challenging but could prove highly informative in defining true causes of control in vivo.

Given that controllers are being studied as a potential model for "functional cure," the consequences of long-term, host-mediated virus control on overall health are also of interest (Migueles, 2010). HIV persists at very low levels in nearly all controllers and appears to be replicating (Hatano, 2009; Men, 2010). Persistent virus production generates a sustained inflammatory environment (Hunt, 2008), which in turn might cause end-organ damage, including cardiovascular disease (Hsue, 2009). In addition, potential alterations in the gut microbiota of chronically infected individuals may contribute to or be the result of ongoing viral replication, even in elite controllers, and may impact on therapeutic vaccine outcomes (Williams, 2015). These considerations suggest that even elite controllers might benefit from antiretroviral drugs. Studies addressing this hypothesis are in progress.

Recommend Reading

Deeks SG, Walker BD. Human immunodeficiency virus controllers: Mechanisms of durable virus control in the absence of antiretroviral therapy. *Immunity*. 2007; 27:406–416.

Okulicz JF, Lambotte O. Epidemiology and clinical characteristics of elite HIV controllers. *Curr Opin HIV AIDS*. 2011; 6(3):163–168.

FUTURE OF IMMUNE-BASED THERAPEUTICS IN HIV DISEASE

LEARNING OBJECTIVE

Demonstrate knowledge of experimental approaches to chronic inflammation in antiretroviral-treated disease.

WHAT'S NEW?

Many promising immune-based therapeutics are now being tested in small clinical trials.

KEY POINTS

- Proving that HIV-associated inflammation is causally associated with disease progression will ultimately require a clinical end point study involving immune-based therapies that directly affect these pathways.

- Several promising drugs are currently being tested in small, pathogenesis-oriented studies.

Much of the effort of clinical investigators during the past two decades has focused on the development and optimization of combination ART. With the development of several highly effective and well-tolerated ART regimens for both initial treatment and "salvage" therapy, the need for new antiretroviral drugs has declined. Now that most individuals with access to ART can achieve and maintain undetectable HIV RNA levels for years, it is increasingly apparent that in order to fully restore health, other adjunctive therapies may be needed. Given the consistent observation that inflammation is elevated during otherwise effective therapy and that the degree of inflammation predicts disease progression, there has been a recent shift from aggressively developing new antiretroviral drugs to testing existing agents for potentially beneficial effects on inflammation in conjunction with suppressed viremia or to developing entirely new approaches that will modify the inflammatory process (Fumaz, 2012; Perez-Matute, 2015).

A number of immune-based therapeutics have been tested in the clinic. The results have been largely disappointing. Prednisone, hydroxyurea, cyclosporine, and mycophenoate acid have all be studied in clinical trials. Although there were some promising early results, these drugs proved to be either too toxic or to lack efficacy, and there is hence limited interest in using nonspecific drugs that globally affect immune responses. The only exception thus far to this idea is the HMG-CoA reductase inhibitors ("statins"). These drugs are known to have broad anti-inflammatory effects (although the mechanism for these effects remains controversial) and are generally safe and well tolerated. Recent pilot data from HIV-infected adults suggest that these drugs might reduce HIV-associated T cell activation and hence prove beneficial in patients for reasons independent of their effects on lipids (Ganesan, 2011). A large clinical end point study similar to those done in the general population will likely be needed to prove that these drugs have unique roles in treated HIV-infected patients who might not otherwise require a statin for lipid or cardiovascular disease management.

Multiple factors contribute to persistent immune activation during therapy, including (1) irreversible breakdown of gut mucosa and subsequent microbial translocation; (2) excess CMV burden and/or enhanced immune responses to CMV (and perhaps other herpesviruses); (3) loss of immunoregulatory cells such as T regulatory cells; (4) antiretroviral treatment toxicity, including generation of pro-inflammatory lipids and development of metabolic syndrome; and (5) lymphoid fibrosis, hematopoietic stem cell dysfunction, and thymic dysfunction. Many, if not all, of these mechanisms can be addressed

therapeutically. For example, a number of drugs, including rifaximin (an antibiotic that is not absorbed systemically), sevelamer (which binds LPS/endotoxin in vivo), colostrum-related products (which bind LPS/endotoxin in the gut), chloroquine (which blocks LPS-mediated TLR signaling in myeloid cells), and mesalamine (which is an aspirin-like anti-inflammatory drug used in ulcerative colitis), have been or are being tested as means to reduce the inflammatory consequences of microbial translocation (Byakwaga, 2011; Gori, 2011; Murray, 2010; Piconi, 2011). Interventions that aim to restore certain bacterial species to the gut microbiota are also being studied, although a complete characterization of alterations in gut microbiota and related confounders is needed before such approaches can be effective (Noguera, 2016). Valganciclovir-mediated reduction in CMV has been shown to reduce immune activation in HIV disease (Hunt, 2011). Growth hormone enhances thymic function and could in theory result eventually in generation of effective immunity (Napolitano, 2008). Perfenidone and angiotensin-converting enzyme inhibitors, among other drugs, are being studied in nonhuman primates and humans as a means to prevent and/or reverse fibrosis. IL-7 has shown promise in a number of studies as a means to enhance immune function during treated disease (Levy, 2009). Although these studies will provide important insights into the mechanisms of chronic immune activation, it remains unclear how such drugs will eventually be tested in phase III clinical trials. Given the lack of a valid surrogate marker for inflammation and immunodeficiency, clinical end point studies will be needed. These studies are large and expensive, and they would be considered very high risk given the experience with the IL-2 clinical end point studies (Abrams, 2009). A relevant trial that has overcome some of these hurdles is that of tocilizumab, an IL-6 receptor-blocking antibody that has the potential to interfere at a crucial point in the pro-inflammatory cascade (Fumaz, 2012; Rodriguez, 2014).

Given the role of chronic inflammation in heart disease and aging, it is hoped that the management of inflammation in HIV-infected adults might be informed by what is happening in those other disciplines. The following can all have anti-inflammatory effects: daily exercise; a balanced diet rich in fish, legumes, grains, and fresh vegetables (e.g., the Mediterranean diet); prevention of excess weight gain; and aggressive management of traditional risk factors such as hypertension, hyperlipidemia, and lipid levels.

Recommended Reading

Funderburg NT, Jiang Y. Rosuvastatin reduces vascular inflammation and T-cell and monocyte activation in HIV-infected subjects on antiretroviral therapy. *J Acquir Immune Defic Syndr*. 2015; 68(4):396–404.

Funderburg NT, Jiang Y, Debanne SM, et al. Rosuvastatin treatment reduces markers of monocyte activation in HIV-infected subjects on antiretroviral therapy. *Clin Infect Dis.* 2014; 58(4):588–595.

References

Abrams, D, Levy, Y., Losso, M.H., et al. Interleukin-2 therapy in patients with HIV infection. N Engl J Med 2009; 361, 1548–1559.

Antonelli, L.R., Mahnke, Y., Hodge, J.N., et al. Elevated frequencies of highly activated CD4+ T cells in HIV+ patients developing immune reconstitution inflammatory syndrome. Blood 2010; 116, 3818–3827.

Arthos, J., Cicala, C., Martinelli, E., et al. HIV-1 envelope protein binds to and signals through integrin alpha4beta7, the gut mucosal homing receptor for peripheral T cells. Nat Immunol 2008; 9, 301–309.

Barber, D.L., Andrade, B.B., Sereti, I., Sher, A. Immune reconstitution inflammatory syndrome: The trouble with immunity when you had none. Nat Rev Microbiol. 2012; 10(2), 150–156.

Berry, N.J., Burns, D.M., Wannamethee, G., et al. Seroepidemiologic studies on the acquisition of antibodies to cytomegalovirus, herpes simplex virus, and human immunodeficiency virus among general hospital patients and those attending a clinic for sexually transmitted diseases. J Med Virol 1988; 24, 385–393.

Bishop, D.K., Ferguson, R.M., Orosz, C.G. Differential distribution of antigen-specific helper T cells and cytotoxic T cells after antigenic stimulation in vivo: A functional study using limiting dilution analysis. J Immunol 1990; 144, 1153–1160.

Boulware, D.R., Meya, D.B., Bergemann, T.L., et al. Clinical features and serum biomarkers in HIV immune reconstitution inflammatory syndrome after cryptococcal meningitis: A prospective cohort study. PLoS Med 2010; 7, e1000384.

Bourgarit, A., Carcelain, G., Martinez, V., et al. Explosion of tuberculin-specific Th1-responses induces immune restoration syndrome in tuberculosis and HIV co-infected patients. AIDS 2006; 20, F1–F7.

Brenchley, J.M., Paiardini, M., Knox, K.S., et al. Differential Th17 CD4 T-cell depletion in pathogenic and nonpathogenic lentiviral infections. Blood 2008; 112, 2826–2835.

Brenchley, J.M., Price, D.A., Schacker, T.W., et al. Microbial translocation is a cause of systemic immune activation in chronic HIV infection. Nat Med 2006; 12, 1365–1371.

Brodin, P., Jojic, V., Gao, T., et al. Variation in the human immune system is largely driven by non-heritable influences. Cell 2015; 160, 37–47.

Bujdoso, R., Young, P., Hopkins, J., et al. Non-random migration of CD4 and CD8 T cells: changes in the CD4:CD8 ratio and interleukin 2 responsiveness of efferent lymph cells following in vivo antigen challenge. Eur J Immunol 1989; 19, 1779–1784.

Byakwaga, H., Kelly, M., Purcell, D.F., et al. Intensification of antiretroviral therapy with raltegravir or addition of hyperimmune bovine colostrum in HIV-infected patients with suboptimal CD4+ T-cell response: A randomized controlled trial. J Infect Dis 2011; 204, 1532–1540.

Chen, H., Li, C., Huang, J., et al. CD4+ T cells from elite controllers resist HIV-1 infection by selective upregulation of p21. J Clin Invest 2011; 121, 1549–1560.

Cho, S., Knox, K.S., Kohli, L.M., et al. Impaired cell surface expression of human CD1d by the formation of an HIV-1 Nef/CD1d complex. Virology 2005; 337, 242–252.

Coleman, C.M., Wu, L. HIV interactions with monocytes and dendritic cells: Viral latency and reservoirs. Retrovirology 2009; 6, 51.

Decrion, A.Z., Dichamp, I., Varin, A., Herbein, G. HIV and inflammation. Curr HIV Res 2005; 3, 243–259.

Deeks, S.G. HIV infection, inflammation, immunosenescence, and aging. Annu Rev Med. 2011; 62, 141–155.

Deeks, S.G., Walker, B.D. Human immunodeficiency virus controllers: Mechanisms of durable virus control in the absence of antiretroviral therapy. Immunity 2007; 27, 406–416.

Doisne, J.M., Urrutia, A., Lacabaratz-Porret, C., et al. CD8+ T cells specific for EBV, cytomegalovirus, and influenza virus are activated during primary HIV infection. J Immunol 2004; 173, 2410–2418.

Douek, D.C., Picker, L.J., Koup, R.A. T cell dynamics in HIV-1 infection. Annu Rev Immunol 2003; 21, 265–304.

Estes, J.D., Haase, A.T., Schacker, T.W. The role of collagen deposition in depleting CD4+ T cells and limiting reconstitution in HIV-1 and SIV infections through damage to the secondary lymphoid organ niche. Semin Immunol 2008; 20, 181–186.

Favre, D., Lederer, S., Kanwar, B., et al. Critical loss of the balance between Th17 and T regulatory cell populations in pathogenic SIV infection. PLoS Pathog 2009; 5, e1000295.

French, M.A., Price, P., Stone, S.F. Immune restoration disease after antiretroviral therapy. AIDS 2004; 18, 1615–1627.

Fumaz, C.R., Gonzalez-Garcia, M., Borras, X. Psychological stress is associated with high levels of IL-6 in HIV-1 infected individuals on effective combined antiretroviral treatment. Brain Behav Immun 2012; 26, 568–572.

Ganesan, A., Crum-Cianflone, N., Higgins, J., et al. High dose atorvastatin decreases cellular markers of immune activation without affecting HIV-1 RNA levels: Results of a double-blind randomized placebo controlled clinical trial. J Infect Dis 2011; 203, 756–764.

Giorgi, J.V., Hultin, L.E., McKeating, J.A., et al. Shorter survival in advanced human immunodeficiency virus type 1 infection is more closely associated with T lymphocyte activation than with plasma virus burden or virus chemokine coreceptor usage. J Infect Dis 1999; 179, 859–870.

Gori, A., Rizzardini, G., Van't Land, B., et al. Specific prebiotics modulate gut microbiota and immune activation in HAART-naive HIV-infected adults: Results of the "COPA" pilot randomized trial. Mucosal immunology 2011; 4, 554–563.

Grossman, Z., Meier-Schellersheim, M., Sousa, AE., et al. CD4+ T-cell depletion in HIV infection: Are we closer to understanding the cause? Nat Med 2002; 8, 319–323.

Guadalupe, M., Reay, E., Sankaran, S., et al. Severe CD4+ T-cell depletion in gut lymphoid tissue during primary human immunodeficiency virus type 1 infection and substantial delay in restoration following highly active antiretroviral therapy. J Virol 2003; 77, 11708–11717.

Hage, C.A., Kohli, L.L., Cho, S., et al. Human immunodeficiency virus gp120 downregulates CD1d cell surface expression. Immunol Lett 2005; 98, 131–135.

Hamada, H., Garcia-Hernandez Mde, L., Reome, J.B., et al. Tc17, a unique subset of CD8 T cells that can protect against lethal influenza challenge. J Immunol 2009; 182, 3469–3481.

Hansen, S.G., Piatak, M., Jr., Ventura, A.B., et al. Immune clearance of highly pathogenic SIV infection. Nature 2013a; 502, 100–104.

Hansen, S.G., Sacha, J.B., Hughes, C.M., et al. Cytomegalovirus vectors violate CD8+ T cell epitope recognition paradigms. Science 2013b; 340, 1237874.

Hartigan-O'Connor, D.J., Abel, K., Van Rompay, K.K., et al. SIV replication in the infected rhesus macaque is limited by the size of the pre-existing TH17 cell compartment. Sci Transl Med 2012; 4, 136ra169.

Hartigan-O'Connor, D.J., Jacobson, M.A., Tan, Q.X., Sinclair, E. Development of cytomegalovirus (CMV) immune recovery uveitis is associated with Th17 cell depletion and poor systemic CMV-specific T cell responses. Clin Infect Dis 2011; 52, 409–417.

Hatano, H., Delwart, E.L., Norris, P.J., et al. Evidence for persistent low-level viremia in individuals who control human immunodeficiency virus in the absence of antiretroviral therapy. J Virol 2009; 83, 329–335.

Heise, C., Miller, C.J., Lackner, A., Dandekar, S. Primary acute simian immunodeficiency virus infection of intestinal lymphoid tissue is associated with gastrointestinal dysfunction. J Infect Dis 1994; 169, 1116–1120.

Hellerstein, M., Hanley, M.B., Cesar, D., et al. Directly measured kinetics of circulating T lymphocytes in normal and HIV-1-infected humans. Nat Med 1999; 5, 83–89.

Hirao, L.A., Grishina, I., Bourry, O., et al. Early mucosal sensing of SIV infection by paneth cells induces IL-1beta production and initiates gut epithelial disruption. PLoS Pathog 2014; 10.

Hrecka, K., Hao, C., Gierszewska, M., et al. Vpx relieves inhibition of HIV-1 infection of macrophages mediated by the SAMHD1 protein. Nature 2011; 474, 658–661.

Hsue, PY, Hunt, P.W., Schnell, A., et al. Role of viral replication, antiretroviral therapy, and immunodeficiency in HIV-associated atherosclerosis. AIDS 2009; 23, 1059–1067.

Hunt, P.W., Brenchley, J., Sinclair, E., et al. Relationship between T cell activation and CD4+ T cell count in HIV-seropositive individuals with undetectable plasma HIV RNA levels in the absence of therapy. J Infect Dis 2008; 197, 126–133.

Hunt, P.W., Martin, J.N., Sinclair, E., et al. Valganciclovir reduces T cell activation in HIV-infected individuals with incomplete CD4+ T cell recovery on antiretroviral therapy. J Infect Dis 2011; 203, 1474–1483.

Hwang, I., Zhang, T., Scott, J.M., et al. Identification of human NK cells that are deficient for signaling adaptor FcRgamma and specialized for antibody-dependent immune functions. Int Immunol 2012; 24, 793–802.

Jones, J.L., Phuah, C.L., Cox, A.L., et al. IL-21 drives secondary autoimmunity in patients with multiple sclerosis, following therapeutic lymphocyte depletion with alemtuzumab (Campath-1H). J Clin Invest 2009; 119, 2052–2061.

Kader, M., Bixler, S., Piatak, M., et al. Anti-retroviral therapy fails to restore the severe Th-17: Tc-17 imbalance observed in peripheral blood during simian immunodeficiency virus infection. J Med Primatol 2009; 38(Suppl 1), 32–38.

Kelley, C.F., Kitchen, C.M., Hunt, P.W., et al. Incomplete peripheral CD4(+) cell count restoration in HIV-infected patients receiving long-term antiretroviral treatment. Clin Infect Dis 2009; 48, 787–794.

King, C., Ilic, A., Koelsch, K., Sarvetnick, N. Homeostatic expansion of T cells during immune insufficiency generates autoimmunity. Cell 2004; 117, 265–277.

Klatt, N.R., Harris, L.D., Vinton, C.L. Compromised gastrointestinal integrity in pigtail macaques is associated with increased microbial translocation, immune activation, and IL-17 production in the absence of SIV infection. Mucosal Immunol 2010; 3, 387–398.

Kuller, L.H., Tracy, R., Belloso, W., et al. Inflammatory and coagulation biomarkers and mortality in patients with HIV infection. PLoS Med 2008; 5, e203.

Laguette, N., Sobhian, B., Casartelli, N., et al. SAMHD1 is the dendritic- and myeloid-cell-specific HIV-1 restriction factor counteracted by Vpx. Nature 2011; 474, 654–657.

Lang, D.J., Kovacs, A.A., Zaia, J.A., et al. Seroepidemiologic studies of cytomegalovirus and Epstein–Barr virus infections in relation to human immunodeficiency virus type 1 infection in selected recipient populations. Transfusion Safety Study Group. J Acquir Immune Defic Syndr 1989; 2, 540–549.

Lawn, S.D., Myer, L., Bekker, L.G., Wood, R. Tuberculosis-associated immune reconstitution disease: Incidence, risk factors and impact in an antiretroviral treatment service in South Africa. AIDS 2007; 21, 335–341.

Lee, J., Zhang, T., Hwang, I., et al. Epigenetic modification and antibody-dependent expansion of memory-like NK cells in human cytomegalovirus-infected individuals. Immunity 2015; 42, 431–442.

Lenardo, M.J., Angleman, S.B., Bounkeua, V., et al. Cytopathic killing of peripheral blood CD4(+) T lymphocytes by human immunodeficiency virus type 1 appears necrotic rather than apoptotic and does not require env. J Virol 2002; 76, 5082–5093.

Lenkei, R., Andersson, B. High correlations of anti-CMV titers with lymphocyte activation status and CD57 antibody-binding capacity as estimated with three-color, quantitative flow cytometry in blood donors. Clin Immunol Immunopathol 1995; 77, 131–138.

Levy, Y., Lacabaratz, C., Weiss, L., et al. Enhanced T cell recovery in HIV-1-infected adults through IL-7 treatment. J Clin Invest 2009; 119, 997–1007.

Li, D., Xu, X.N. NKT cells in HIV-1 infection. Cell Res 2008; 18, 817–822.

Link, A., Vogt, T.K., Favre, S., et al. Fibroblastic reticular cells in lymph nodes regulate the homeostasis of naive T cells. Nat Immunol 2007; 8, 1255–1265.

Lopez-Verges, S., Milush, J.M., Schwartz, B.S., et al. Expansion of a unique CD57(+)NKG2Chi natural killer cell subset during acute human cytomegalovirus infection. Proc Natl Acad Sci USA 2011; 108, 14725–14732.

Manel, N., Hogstad, B., Wang, Y., et al. A cryptic sensor for HIV-1 activates antiviral innate immunity in dendritic cells. Nature 2010; 467, 214–217.

Martin, M.P., Qi, Y., Gao, X., et al. Innate partnership of HLA-B and KIR3DL1 subtypes against HIV-1. Nat Genet 2007; 39, 733–740.

McCune, J.M. The dynamics of CD4+ T-cell depletion in HIV disease. Nature 2001; 410, 974–979.

Mens, H., Kearney, M., Wiegand, A., et al. HIV-1 continues to replicate and evolve in patients with natural control of HIV infection. J Virol 2010; 84(24), 12971–12981.

Migueles, SA., Connors, M. Long-term nonprogressive disease among untreated HIV-infected individuals: clinical implications of understanding immune control of HIV. JAMA 2010; 304, 194–201.

Mocroft, A., Phillips, A.N., Gatell, J., et al. Normalisation of CD4 counts in patients with HIV-1 infection and maximum virological suppression who are taking combination antiretroviral therapy: An observational cohort study. Lancet 2007; 370, 407–413.

Muller, M., Wandel, S., Colebunders, R., et al. Immune reconstitution inflammatory syndrome in patients starting antiretroviral therapy for HIV infection: A systematic review and meta-analysis. Lancet Infect Dis 2010; 10, 251–261.

Murray, S.M., Down, C.M., Boulware, D.R., et al. Reduction of immune activation with chloroquine therapy during chronic HIV infection. J Virol 2010; 84, 12082–12086.

Naeger, D.M., Martin, J.N., Sinclair, E., et al. Cytomegalovirus-specific T cells persist at very high levels during long-term antiretroviral treatment of HIV disease. PLoS One 2010; 5, e8886.

Napolitano, L.A., Schmidt, D., Gotway, M.B., et al. Growth hormone enhances thymic function in HIV-1-infected adults. J Clin Invest 2008; 118(3), 1085–1098.

Ndhlovu, Z.M., Kamya, P., Mewalal, N., et al. Magnitude and kinetics of CD8+ T cell activation during hyperacute HIV infection impact viral set point. Immunity 2015; 43, 591–604.

Neuhaus, J., Jacobs, D.R., Jr., Baker, J.V., et al. Markers of inflammation, coagulation, and renal function are elevated in adults with HIV infection. J Infect Dis 2010; 201, 1788–1795.

Nigam, P., Kwa, S., Velu, V., Amara, R.R. Loss of IL-17-producing CD8 T cells during late chronic stage of pathogenic simian immunodeficiency virus infection. J Immunol 2011; 186, 745–753.

Noguera, J., Rocafort, M., Guillén, Y., et al. Gut microbiota linked to sexual preference and HIV infection. EBioMedicine 2016; 5, 135–146.

Nussenblatt, R.B., Lane, H.C. Human immunodeficiency virus disease: Changing patterns of intraocular inflammation. Am J Ophthalmol 1998; 125, 374–382.

O'Connell, K.A., Rabi, S.A., Siliciano, R.F., Blankson, J.N. CD4+ T cells from elite suppressors are more susceptible to HIV-1 but produce fewer virions than cells from chronic progressors. Proc Natl Acad Sci USA 2011; 108, E689–E698.

Pakker, N.G., Notermans, D.W., de Boer, R.J., et al. Biphasic kinetics of peripheral blood T cells after triple combination therapy in HIV-1 infection: A composite of redistribution and proliferation. Nat Med 1998; 4, 208–214.

Papagno, L., Spina, C.A., Marchant, A., et al. Immune activation and CD8(+) T-cell differentiation towards senescence in HIV-1 infection. PLoS Biol 2004; 2, E20.

Parrinello, C.M., Sinclair, E., Landay, A.L., et al. Cytomegalovirus immunoglobulin G antibody is associated with subclinical carotid artery disease among HIV-infected women. J Infect Dis 2012; 205, 1788–1796.

Pereyra, F., Jia, X., McLaren, P.J., et al. The major genetic determinants of HIV-1 control affect HLA class I peptide presentation. Science 2010; 330, 1551–1557.

Perez-Matute, P., Perez-Martinez, L., Aguilera-Lizarraga, J., et al. Maraviroc modifies gut microbiota composition in a mouse model of obesity: A plausible therapeutic option to prevent metabolic disorders in HIV-infected patients. Rev Esp Quimioter 2015; 28, 200–206.

Phillips, A.N., Neaton, J., Lundgren, J.D. The role of HIV in serious diseases other than AIDS. AIDS 2008; 22, 2409–2418.

Piconi, S., Parisotto, S., Rizzardini, G., et al. Hydroxychloroquine drastically reduces immune activation in HIV-infected, antiretroviral therapy-treated immunologic nonresponders. Blood 2011; 118, 3263–3272.

Price, P., Murdoch, D.M., Agarwal, U., et al. Immune restoration diseases reflect diverse immunopathological mechanisms. Clin Microbiol Rev 2009; 22, 651–663.

Raffatellu, M., Santos, R.L., Verhoeven, D.E., et al. Simian immunodeficiency virus-induced mucosal interleukin-17 deficiency promotes Salmonella dissemination from the gut. Nat Med 2008; 14, 421–428.

Rodriguez, B. (2014). AIDS 347: IL-6 blockade in treated HIV infection. Available at http://www.clinicaltrials.gov.

Roederer, M., Dubs, J.G., Anderson, M.T., et al. CD8 naive T cell counts decrease progressively in HIV-infected adults. J Clin Invest 1995; 95, 2061–2066.

Saez-Cirion, A., Hamimi, C., Bergamaschi, A., et al. Restriction of HIV-1 replication in macrophages and CD4+ T cells from HIV controllers. Blood 2011; 118, 955–964.

Sandberg, J.K., Fast, N.M., Palacios, E.H., et al. Selective loss of innate CD4(+) V alpha 24 natural killer T cells in human immunodeficiency virus infection. J Virol 2002; 76, 7528–7534.

Sauce, D., Larsen, M., Fastenackels, S., et al. HIV disease progression despite suppression of viral replication is associated with exhaustion of lymphopoiesis. Blood 2011; 117(19), 5142–5151.

Schacker, T.W., Nguyen, P.L., Beilman, G.J., et al. Collagen deposition in HIV-1 infected lymphatic tissues and T cell homeostasis. J Clin Invest 2002; 110, 1133–1139.

Seddiki, N., Sasson, S.C., Santner-Nanan, B., et al. Proliferation of weakly suppressive regulatory CD4+ T cells is associated with over-active CD4+ T-cell responses in HIV-positive patients with mycobacterial immune restoration disease. Eur J Immunol 2009; 39, 391–403.

Silvestri, G., Sodora, D.L., Koup, R.A., et al. Nonpathogenic SIV infection of sooty mangabeys is characterized by limited bystander immunopathology despite chronic high-level viremia. Immunity 2003; 18, 441–452.

Sips, M., Sciaranghella, G., Diefenbach, T., et al. Altered distribution of mucosal NK cells during HIV infection. Mucosal Immunol 2012; 5, 30–40.

Srinivasula, S., Lempicki, R.A., Adelsberger, J.W., et al. Differential effects of HIV viral load and CD4 count on proliferation of naive and memory CD4 and CD8 T lymphocytes. Blood 2011; 118, 262–270.

Stacey, A.R., Norris, P.J., Qin, L., et al. Induction of a striking systemic cytokine cascade prior to peak viremia in acute human immunodeficiency virus type 1 infection, in contrast to more modest and delayed responses in acute hepatitis B and C virus infections. J Virol 2009; 83, 3719–3733.

Sun, J.C., Beilke, J.N., Lanier, L.L. Adaptive immune features of natural killer cells. Nature 2009; 457, 557–561.

Surh, C.D., Sprent, J. Homeostasis of naive and memory T cells. Immunity 2008; 29, 848–862.

Sylwester, A.W., Mitchell, B.L., Edgar, J.B., et al. Broadly targeted human cytomegalovirus-specific CD4+ and CD8+ T cells dominate the memory compartments of exposed subjects. J Exp Med 2005; 202, 673–685.

Teixeira, L., Valdez, H., McCune, J.M., et al. Poor CD4 T cell restoration after suppression of HIV-1 replication may reflect lower thymic function. AIDS 2001; 15, 1749–1756.

van der Vliet, H.J., von Blomberg, B.M., Hazenberg, M.D., et al. Selective decrease in circulating V alpha 24+V beta 11+ NKT cells during HIV type 1 infection. J Immunol 2002; 168, 1490–1495.

van Grevenynghe, J, Procopio, F.A., He, Z., et al. Transcription factor FOXO3a controls the persistence of memory CD4(+) T cells during HIV infection. Nat Med 2008; 14, 266–274.

Veazey, R.S., DeMaria, M., Chalifoux, L.V., et al. Gastrointestinal tract as a major site of CD4+ T cell depletion and viral replication in SIV infection. Science 1998; 280, 427–431.

Vujkovic-Cvijin, I., Dunham, R.M., Iwai, S., et al. Dysbiosis of the gut microbiota is associated with hiv disease progression and tryptophan catabolism. Sci Transl Med 2013; 5, 193ra191.

Williams, W.B., Liao, H.X., Moody, M.A., et al. HIV-1 VACCINES. Diversion of HIV-1 vaccine-induced immunity by gp41-microbiota cross-reactive antibodies. Science 2015; 349, aab1253.

Zeng, M., Southern, P.J., Reilly, C.S., et al. Lymphoid tissue damage in HIV-1 infection depletes naive T cells and limits T cell reconstitution after antiretroviral therapy. PLoS Pathog 2012; 8, e1002437.

Zhang, T., Scott, J.M., Hwang, I., Kim, S. Cutting edge: Antibody-dependent memory-like NK cells distinguished by FcRgamma deficiency. J Immunol 2013; 190, 1402–1406.

Zhou, J., Amran, F.S., Kramski, M., et al. An NK cell population lacking FcRgamma is expanded in chronically infected HIV patients. J Immunol 2015; 194, 4688–4697.

6.

HIV CURE STRATEGIES[a]

Boris Juelg and Rajesh Gandhi

LEARNING OBJECTIVES

- Identify key hurdles for HIV eradication strategies.
- Explain how the "kick and kill" approaches might overcome these challenges.

WHAT'S NEW?

Novel strategies to promote HIV latency reversal and approaches to boost HIV-specific immunity are moving into clinical trials aimed at eradicating HIV.

KEY POINTS

- HIV-1 persists quiescently in cellular reservoirs, not detected by the immune system due to the lack of active viral replication; these reservoirs represent the major obstacle for cure approaches.
- Reversal of HIV-1 latency and induction of virus expression by a variety of interventions may render infected cells susceptible to immune recognition and active clearance.
- Strategies to boost immune responses via vaccination, immunomodulation, or gene therapy are being evaluated with the aim of achieving HIV-1 control without antiretroviral therapy if not viral eradication.

WHY SHOULD WE TRY TO CURE HIV?

Although current antiretroviral therapy (ART) is highly effective at controlling HIV-1 replication, it does not eradicate or cure the infection. There are several compelling reasons for trying to cure HIV-1. First, despite efforts to expand access to treatment, the majority of HIV-1-infected individuals worldwide do not receive ART, which leads to ongoing transmission of the virus. Second, because current ART does not eradicate HIV-1, infected patients must take ART for many decades, which may eventuate in difficulties with adherence, substantial cost, and the potential for long-term side effects. Third, HIV-1-infected patients have increased rates of cardiovascular disease, liver disease, neurocognitive disorders, and other non-infectious complications, which may be driven by elevated levels of inflammation that persist despite suppressive ART. Finally, HIV-1 infection continues to be associated with stigma and social isolation, which adversely affect quality of life. Given the limitations of current ART, there is a renewed and concerted effort to find a cure for HIV-1.

Although complete viral eradication, or a "sterilizing cure," is the ultimate goal, the concept of a "functional cure" has been introduced, which includes strategies aimed at achieving host control of the virus without the need for ART. Several clinical observations within the past few years have fueled the belief that one or the other of these types of "cure" might be possible. Certainly, the most compelling example is that of the "Berlin patient," the only person to have been cured of HIV-1. This HIV-1-positive patient with virologic suppression on ART received, as treatment for acute myelogenous leukemia, allogeneic hematopoietic stem cell transplants from a donor who carried a homozygous deletion in CCR5 (Hutter, 2009), the co-receptor for HIV-1, thereby making his new CD4[+] T cells resistant to infection. Following discontinuation of ART, no HIV-1 RNA has been detected in the Berlin patient's peripheral blood; moreover, multiple attempts to detect HIV-1 RNA or proviral DNA in cellular reservoirs

---

[a] This chapter is based on a previous version written by David Margolis MD, University of North Carolina at Chapel Hill.

and other tissue compartments have been negative (Yukl, 2013). Because of the risk of stem cell transplantation, however, this intensive approach is not appropriate in HIV-1-infected patients who do not have a hematologic malignancy. Another notable "proof-of-concept" derived from studies of early initiation of ART during acute HIV-1 infection. The Visconti study identified 14 HIV-1-infected patients whose viremia has remained controlled for years after the interruption of ART that had been initiated during primary infection (Saez-Cirion, 2013). Along these lines, the "Mississippi baby," a child born to an HIV-1-infected mother, was started on ART 30 hours after delivery (Persaud, 2013) and quickly achieved virologic suppression. The child was lost to follow-up, however, and ART was discontinued by the caregiver. Despite stopping ART, the virus remained undetectable for 27 months, but the child ultimately experienced virologic rebound (Luzuriaga, 2015). These examples demonstrate that it is possible, under extraordinary circumstances, to eradicate HIV-1 (in the case of the Berlin patient) or control HIV-1 without ART (in the case of the VISCONTI cohort and, temporarily, the Mississippi child). Now, the challenge is to extend the insights from these remarkable cases to the development of practical interventions that will lead to ART-free remission in the large population of people living with HIV-1.

EARLY ESTABLISHMENT AND PERSISTENCE OF THE LATENT HIV-1 RESERVOIR

In 1995, Chun et al. identified integrated provirus as a persistent reservoir of infection in the resting CD4$^+$ T cells of HIV-1-infected patients (Chun, 1995). Although most activated memory CD4$^+$ T cells are destroyed during viral replication, a small fraction of infected cells survive to return to a resting and memory state. Once converted to a resting memory state, HIV-1 gene expression is shut down, resulting in latently infected CD4$^+$ T cells (Nabel, 1987). Because these infected cells do not express viral proteins, they remain hidden from the host immune response; moreover, without active replication, antiretroviral drugs cannot act against the virus. Although infected resting cells leave the quiescent memory pool at a steady rate, the pool of infected cells persists, perhaps in part because of homeostatic proliferation. It has also been suggested that specific CD4$^+$ T cell memory subsets, including central memory (T$_{CM}$), transitional memory (T$_{TM}$), and memory stem cells (T$_{SCM}$), harbor the majority of integrated HIV-1 DNA and

that eradication therapies may require targeting of specific CD4$^+$ T cell populations (Buzon, 2014).

When latently infected cells are reactivated, viral gene expression is renewed and productive infection is reignited. In patients on long-term ART, the frequency of latently infected cells is extremely low: Less than 1 per 1 million resting memory CD4$^+$ T cells harbors replication-competent HIV-1 (Finzi, 1997; Wong, 1997). Nevertheless, this latent pool decays very slowly: The mean half-life of this reservoir is approximately 44 months, and as a result, suppressive ART would need to be maintained for more than 60 years to achieve viral eradication even if an infected person has only 100,000 latently infected cells (Finzi, 1999). In addition, it is conceivable that latent infection may persist in cells that are not CD4$^+$ T cells; however, this has yet to be proven.

It was initially believed that early suppression of viral replication during primary infection might prevent the reservoir from becoming established. However, Chun et al. demonstrated that ART initiated within 10 days of primary infection did not prevent the generation of latently infected CD4$^+$ T cells (Chun, 1998), pointing toward an early seeding of the reservoir. Newer data from the rhesus macaque model demonstrate that the latent reservoir is established within days of virus exposure, even before virus can be detected in peripheral blood (Whitney, 2014); the implication of this finding is that it will be practically impossible to treat or even diagnose HIV-1 infection early enough to avoid reservoir seeding. Several studies, however, have demonstrated that initiating ART during the acute/early phase of the infection results in a smaller HIV-1 reservoir (Ananworanich, 2012; Hocqueloux, 2013; Saez-Cirion, 2013), suggesting that early treatment could be beneficial by reducing the barrier to cure (Henrich, 2013; Strain, 2005).

The presence and persistence of the HIV-1 latent reservoir represent the major obstacle for cure approaches. For this reason, a deeper understanding of how latency is maintained and how this state can be reversed is critical to inform HIV-1 eradication strategies (Richman, 2009).

"KICK AND KILL"

In order to achieve viral eradication, or at least a state of HIV-1 suppression without requiring continuous ART, different strategies have been proposed, including modification of the host immune response to achieve enhanced control of viral replication, interventions to prevent reactivation of virus latency (Mousseau, 2015), and gene therapy to increase the resistance of target cells to HIV-1 infection

(Tebas, 2014). Currently, the strategy that is receiving the most attention is the "shock and kill" or "kick and kill" approach. In this strategy, the first step is to flush out HIV-1 from the latent reservoir by activating proviral DNA expression in resting cells, leading to de novo viral protein production (the so-called "shock" or "kick"). If this "kick" is successful, the next step is to enhance immune recognition and elimination of infected cells (the "kill"). This two-step approach, however, requires a latency-reversing strategy and an antiviral immune response in order to clear infected cells; both tasks are encumbered by substantial challenges.

LATENCY REVERSAL APPROACHES

The absence of HIV-1 gene expression in patients on suppressive ART enables evasion of latently infected CD4$^+$ T cells from immune surveillance (Hermankova, 2003). Reversal of HIV-1 latency and induction of virus expression may render infected cells susceptible to attack by cytolytic T lymphocytes or to destruction by viral cytopathic effects (Chun, 1997; Deeks, 2012). Several latency-reversing agents (LRAs) have been identified, perhaps the most promising of which are histone deacetylase inhibitors (HDACi) and Toll-like receptor (TLR) agonists. HDACi are currently approved as anticancer drugs, and several agents have been evaluated in ART-suppressed HIV-1-infected individuals for their latency-reversing potential (Archin, 2014; Elliott, 2014; Rasmussen, 2014). Vorinostat, the first HDACi to be studied in HIV-1-infected patients on ART, was found to induce HIV-1 RNA expression by an average of 4.8-fold in resting CD4$^+$ T cells after a single dose (Archin, 2014). Two other HDACi—panobinostat and romidepsin—have also been found to induce virus expression in HIV-1-infected patients on suppressive ART (Rasmussen, 2014; Sogaard, 2015). Following administration of romidepsin, plasma HIV-1 RNA levels became detectable in some patients, suggesting that the LRA was inducing virus production (Sogaard, 2015). However, the size of the HIV-1 reservoir, based on measurements of HIV-1 DNA and virus outgrowth assay, remained unchanged following three weekly infusions of romidepsin, suggesting additional interventions will be needed. A larger trial of romidepsin is currently enrolling to confirm these results (ClinicalTrials. gov Identifier NCT01933594), and combination studies are being planned. Another strategy that is being studied is the use of a TLR agonist, specifically against TLR7, which has been shown to induce transient increases in plasma viral load and decreases in cellular viral DNA levels in simian immunodeficiency virus (SIV)-infected rhesus macaques, suggesting a latency-reversing and reservoir-reducing effect

of this agent (Whitney, 2015). This preclinical observation needs to be confirmed in ART-treated HIV-1-infected humans, and such a trial is currently underway. Overall, it remains uncertain whether a single agent will be sufficient to effectively and completely purge the pool of replication-competent, integrated, latent HIV-1; rather, a combination of latency-reactivating agents targeting distinct pathways, and potentially different cell types, might be required (Laird, 2015).

IMMUNE ENHANCING STRATEGIES

Although latency reversal will be crucial for eradication strategies, inducing viral replication alone will most likely not be sufficient to eliminate the infection. Indeed, in an in vitro model, reversal of latency alone did not result in clearance of infected cells (Shan, 2012). For this reason, it is anticipated that following reactivation, cells harboring the reservoir will need to be actively cleared, most likely through a second line of attack by the host's immune system. Strategies to enhance immune responses via immunization or immunomodulation have been proposed based on the hypothesis that boosting T cell responses will lead to enhanced viral control—similar to that in so-called HIV-1 elite controllers, patients who maintain undetectable viral loads in the absence of ART (Deeks, 2007), in whom antiviral T cells have been associated with viral suppression (Deeks, 2007; McMichael, 2010).

The ability to enhance the host's immune responses by therapeutic vaccination faces several key challenges. The majority of HIV-1-infected individuals have dysfunctional HIV-1-specific effector cells as a result of continuous antigenic stimulation prior to treatment (Sauce, 2013), and ART only incompletely restores T cell functionality. Furthermore, in patients who initiate ART during chronic infection, almost all of the proviral sequences in the latent reservoir contain escape mutations that prevent killing of infected cells by cytotoxic T lymphocytes (Deng, 2015; Papuchon, 2013). The implication is that an effective vaccination strategy, instead of just expanding preexisting responses that already had failed to control the infection, would need to improve the quality and functionality of HIV-1-specific immune response and elicit CD8$^+$ T cell responses against previously untargeted epitopes or unmutated regions of the virus to avoid escape. To achieve this goal, multiple approaches are currently being tested in preclinical and clinical studies, including the following:

- Viral vector-based vaccines, such as adenovirus, poxvirus modified vaccinia Ankara, and modified cytomegalovirus: Some of these approaches to deliver HIV-1 antigens have demonstrated robust immunogenicity, inducing broad and durable cellular immune responses that were able to protect monkeys against SIV infection in preclinical challenge studies (Barouch, 2012, 2013; Hansen, 2011, 2013).

- Plasmid DNA-expressing HIV-1 genes (Hallengard, 2011; Ramirez, 2013; Rodriguez, 2013).

- Dendritic cell-based vaccines to deliver HIV-1 antigens: In one study, this approach was associated with reduced plasma viral load post-treatment interruption (Levy, 2014).

Some of these vaccines have been tested already in humans and are safe and immunogenic, but proof of efficacy in reducing the HIV-1 reservoir has yet to be demonstrated.

Given the challenge that preexisting T cell exhaustion in HIV-1-infected patients poses for therapeutic vaccination strategies, novel immune-modulating concepts have been developed to reverse this state of exhaustion by inhibiting immune checkpoints. During progressive HIV-1 infection with persistent antigen exposure, increased expression of inhibitory receptors such as PD-1 on HIV-1-specific T cells is associated with greater immune dysfunction (Day, 2006; Khaitan, 2011). Inhibiting the PD-1 pathway has shown efficacy in reversing T cell exhaustion in the cancer field (Topalian, 2012), and recent data suggest that PD-1 blockade restores the ability of antiviral T cells to inhibit HIV-1 replication in animal models (Palmer, 2013; Velu, 2009). A dose-escalation trial of an anti-PD-L1 antibody in HIV-1-infected patients has been initiated (ClinicalTrials. gov Identifier NCT02028403), and studies of immune checkpoint inhibitors and their effect on the virus reservoir are being conducted in HIV-1-infected patients with malignancies.

An alternative approach, which circumvents the problem of eliciting immune responses in HIV-1-infected patients with immune dysregulation, is the adoptive transfer of T cells with molecularly cloned high-affinity TCRs and superior antiviral activity targeting conserved and vulnerable regions of the virus (Varela-Rohena, 2008). A phase I clinical study testing the in vivo efficacy of these high-affinity Gag-specific T cells in ART patients has been performed; the results of this study are pending (ClinicalTrials. gov Identifier NCT00991224). Furthermore, chimeric antigen receptor transduced T cells, which combine the specificity of an antibody with the signaling of a TCR, have shown promise in the cancer field (Hombach, 2013) and are now being studied in HIV-1 (Lam, 2013).

The recent identification of novel broadly neutralizing anti-HIV-1 antibodies (bNAbs), which are able to neutralize the majority of viral strains at very low concentrations, may provide another approach to target the HIV-1 reservoir. In preclinical studies, administration of bNAbs was shown to reduce plasma viremia in chimeric simian–human immunodeficiency virus (SHIV)-infected macaques (Barouch, 2013; Shingai, 2013); in fact, one monoclonal antibody, PGT121, also resulted in substantial reductions of proviral DNA in peripheral blood, lymph nodes, and gastrointestinal mucosa (Barouch, 2013). Two bNAbs have been tested so far in HIV-1-infected humans and have shown promising reductions in plasma viremia (Caskey, 2015; Lynch, 2015). However, it remains to be determined what effect bNAbs will have on the viral reservoir in humans, and limitations such as the lack of accessibility of antibodies to certain anatomic reservoir sites (e.g., the central nervous system) will need to be overcome.

Finally, a novel method to combine antibody and T cell activity against HIV-1-infected cells is through bispecific protein constructs, which are designed to latch onto HIV-1 envelope proteins on the surface of infected cells while also binding to CD3 on T cells. This approach directs cytotoxic T cells to eliminate infected cells while obviating the need for the T cells to specifically bind to HIV-1 surface antigens (Pegu, 2015; Sung, 2015). Early in vitro studies of this approach are promising, but additional preclinical work is needed to confirm that these immunomodulatory proteins are safe enough to test in human trials.

GENE MODIFICATION

RENDERING THE HOST'S CD4+ T CELLS RESISTANT AGAINST INFECTION

The finding that the Berlin patient appeared to be cured of HIV-1 after receiving a stem cell transplant from a CCR5-δ32 homozygous donor has inspired attempts to generate HIV-1-resistant cells through gene therapy. Using artificial restriction enzymes such as zinc finger nucleases (ZFN), DNA can be cleaved at specific sites; this approach has been used to disrupt the CCR5 gene (which encodes the HIV-1 co-receptor) in CD4+ T cells (Perez, 2008). Using the ZFN strategy, Tebas et al. modified the CCR5 gene ex vivo in autologous CD4+ T cells in 12 HIV-1-infected subjects and infused the cells back into the autologous donor (Tebas, 2014). The study found that genetically modified cells persisted in vivo with a half-life of nearly 1 year. Although no dramatic difference was seen in viral load set points following interruption of ART in 6 study participants, the modified cells appeared to be protected from HIV-1 infection because unmodified cells showed a faster depletion.

EXCISING THE HIV-1 PROVIRUS FROM THE HOST CELL GENOME

Several research groups have successfully applied this technology to excise HIV-1 provirus from the host cell genome (Ebina, 2013; Hu, 2014; Liao, 2015). Importantly, the disruption of provirus expression not only restricted transcriptionally active provirus but also blocked the expression of latently integrated provirus (Ebina, 2013). Moreover, inserting the stably expressed CRISPR/Cas9 system into a T cell line conferred long-term protection against HIV-1 infection (Liao, 2015). These results from in vitro cell culture models are promising, and this technology may open new avenues to developing antiviral therapies in the future.

CONCLUSIONS

Although antiretroviral medications are able to effectively treat HIV-1 infection, there are many compelling reasons to attempt to cure HIV-1, including the stigma and isolation experienced by many infected patients. The major barrier to HIV-1 cure is the persistence of a long-lived population of latently infected cells in patients on suppressive treatment; because the latent reservoir is established soon after HIV-1 acquisition, even early initiation of ART cannot cure the infection. Current efforts to cure HIV-1 infection are centered on flushing HIV-1 out of the latent reservoir along with enhancing immune mechanisms to clear infected cells. We are still in the early days of this massively difficult undertaking, and it is too soon to determine whether the approaches being pursued now will be effective. However, just as the development of combination ART was based on a series of advances that culminated in our ability to successfully treat HIV-1, the stepwise progress being made today, it is hoped, will lead us to an even greater breakthrough: the capability to eradicate or control HIV-1 without the need for lifelong therapy.

References

Ananworanich J, Schuetz A, Vandergeeten C, et al. Impact of multi-targeted antiretroviral treatment on gut T cell depletion and HIV reservoir seeding during acute HIV infection. PloS One. 2012;7(3):e33948.

Archin NM, Bateson R, Tripathy MK, et al. HIV-1 expression within resting CD4+ T cells after multiple doses of vorinostat. Journal of Infectious Diseases. 2014;210(5):728–735.

Barouch DH, Liu J, Li H, et al. Vaccine protection against acquisition of neutralization-resistant SIV challenges in rhesus monkeys. Nature. 2012;482(7383):89–93.

Barouch DH, Stephenson KE, Borducchi EN, et al. Protective efficacy of a global HIV-1 mosaic vaccine against heterologous SHIV challenges in rhesus monkeys. Cell. 2013;155(3):531–539.

Barouch DH, Whitney JB, Moldt B, et al. Therapeutic efficacy of potent neutralizing HIV-1-specific monoclonal antibodies in SHIV-infected rhesus monkeys. Nature. 2013;503(7475):224–228.

Buzon MJ, Sun H, Li C, et al. HIV-1 persistence in CD4+ T cells with stem cell-like properties. Nature Medicine. 2014;20(2):139–142.

Caskey M, Klein F, Lorenzi JC, et al. Viraemia suppressed in HIV-1-infected humans by broadly neutralizing antibody 3BNC117. Nature. 2015;522(7557):487–491.

Chun TW, Engel D, Berrey MM, et al. Early establishment of a pool of latently infected, resting CD4(+) T cells during primary HIV-1 infection. Proceedings of the National Academy of Sciences of the United States of America. 1998;95(15):8869–8873.

Chun TW, Finzi D, Margolick J, et al. In vivo fate of HIV-1-infected T-cells: quantitative analysis of the transition to stable latency. Nature Medicine. 1995;1(12):1284–1290.

Chun TW, Stuyver L, Mizell SB, et al. Presence of an inducible HIV-1 latent reservoir during highly active antiretroviral therapy. Proceedings of the National Academy of Sciences of the United States of America. 1997;94(24):13193–13197.

Day CL, Kaufmann DE, Kiepiela P, et al. PD-1 expression on HIV-specific T cells is associated with T-cell exhaustion and disease progression. Nature. 2006;443(7109):350–354.

Deeks SG. HIV: Shock and kill. Nature. 2012;487(7408):439–440.

Deeks SG, Walker BD. Human immunodeficiency virus controllers: Mechanisms of durable virus control in the absence of antiretroviral therapy. Immunity. 2007;27(3):406–416.

Deng K, Pertea M, Rongvaux A, et al. Broad CTL response is required to clear latent HIV-1 due to dominance of escape mutations. Nature. 2015;517(7534):381–385.

Ebina H, Misawa N, Kanemura Y, et al. Harnessing the CRISPR/Cas9 system to disrupt latent HIV-1 provirus. Scientific Reports. 2013;3:2510.

Elliott JH, Wightman F, Solomon A, et al. Activation of HIV transcription with short-course vorinostat in HIV-infected patients on suppressive antiretroviral therapy. PLoS Pathogens. 2014;10(10):e1004473.

Finzi D, Blankson J, Siliciano JD, et al. Latent infection of CD4+ T cells provides a mechanism for lifelong persistence of HIV-1, even in patients on effective combination therapy. Nature Medicine. 1999;5(5):512–517.

Finzi D, Hermankova M, Pierson T, et al. Identification of a reservoir for HIV-1 in patients on highly active antiretroviral therapy. Science. 1997;278(5341):1295–1300.

Hallengard D, Haller BK, Maltais AK, et al. Comparison of plasmid vaccine immunization schedules using intradermal in vivo electroporation. Clinical and Vaccine Immunology. 2011;18(9):1577–1581.

Hansen SG, Ford JC, Lewis MS, et al. Profound early control of highly pathogenic SIV by an effector memory T-cell vaccine. Nature. 2011;473(7348):523–527.

Hansen SG, Piatak M Jr, Ventura AB, et al. Immune clearance of highly pathogenic SIV infection. Nature. 2013;502(7469):100–104.

Henrich TJ, Gandhi RT. Early treatment and HIV-1 reservoirs: a stitch in time? Journal of Infectious Diseases. 2013;208(8):1189–1193.

Hermankova M, Siliciano JD, Zhou Y, et al. Analysis of human immunodeficiency virus type 1 gene expression in latently infected resting CD4+ T lymphocytes in vivo. Journal of Virology. 2003;77(13):7383–7392.

Hocqueloux L, Avettand-Fenoel V, Jacquot S, et al. Long-term antiretroviral therapy initiated during primary HIV-1 infection is key to achieving both low HIV reservoirs and normal T cell counts. Journal of Antimicrobial Chemotherapy. 2013;68(5):1169–1178.

Hombach AA, Holzinger A, Abken H. The weal and woe of costimulation in the adoptive therapy of cancer with chimeric antigen receptor (CAR)-redirected T cells. Current Molecular Medicine. 2013;13(7):1079–1088.

Hu W, Kaminski R, Yang F, et al. RNA-directed gene editing specifically eradicates latent and prevents new HIV-1 infection. Proceedings of the National Academy of Sciences of the United States of America. 2014;111(31):11461–11466.

Hutter G, Nowak D, Mossner M, et al. Long-term control of HIV by CCR5 Delta32/Delta32 stem-cell transplantation. New England Journal of Medicine. 2009;360(7):692–698.

Khaitan A, Unutmaz D. Revisiting immune exhaustion during HIV infection. Current HIV/AIDS Reports. 2011;8(1):4–11.

Laird GM, Bullen CK, Rosenbloom DI, et al. Ex vivo analysis identifies effective HIV-1 latency-reversing drug combinations. Journal of Clinical Investigation. 2015;125(5):1901–1912.

Lam S, Bollard C. T-cell therapies for HIV. Immunotherapy. 2013;5(4):407–414.

Levy Y, Thiebaut R, Montes M, et al. Dendritic cell-based therapeutic vaccine elicits polyfunctional HIV-specific T-cell immunity associated with control of viral load. European Journal of Immunology. 2014;44(9):2802–2810.

Liao HK, Gu Y, Diaz A, et al. Use of the CRISPR/Cas9 system as an intracellular defense against HIV-1 infection in human cells. Nature Communications. 2015;6:6413.

Luzuriaga K, Gay H, Ziemniak C, et al. Viremic relapse after HIV-1 remission in a perinatally infected child. New England Journal of Medicine. 2015;372(8):786–788.

Lynch RM, Boritz E, Coates EE, et al. Virologic effects of broadly neutralizing antibody VRC01 administration during chronic HIV-1 infection. Science Translational Medicine. 2015;7(319):319ra206.

McMichael AJ, Borrow P, Tomaras GD. The immune response during acute HIV-1 infection: Clues for vaccine development. Nature Reviews Immunology. 2010;10(1):11–23.

Mousseau G, Kessing CF, Fromentin R, et al. The Tat inhibitor didehydro-cortistatin A prevents HIV-1 reactivation from latency. mBio. 2015;6(4):e00465-15.

Nabel G, Baltimore D. An inducible transcription factor activates expression of human immunodeficiency virus in T cells. Nature. 1987;326(6114):711–713.

Palmer BE, Neff CP, Lecureux J, et al. In vivo blockade of the PD-1 receptor suppresses HIV-1 viral loads and improves CD4$^+$ T cell levels in humanized mice. Journal of Immunology. 2013;190(1):211–219.

Papuchon J, Pinson P, Lazaro E, et al. Resistance mutations and CTL epitopes in archived HIV-1 DNA of patients on antiviral treatment: Toward a new concept of vaccine. PloS One. 2013;8(7):e69029.

Pegu A, Asokan M, Wu L, et al. Activation and lysis of human CD4 cells latently infected with HIV-1. Nature Communications. 2015;6:8447.

Perez EE, Wang J, Miller JC, et al. Establishment of HIV-1 resistance in CD4$^+$ T cells by genome editing using zinc-finger nucleases. Nature Biotechnology. 2008;26(7):808–816.

Persaud D, Gay H, Ziemniak C, et al. Absence of detectable HIV-1 viremia after treatment cessation in an infant. New England Journal of Medicine. 2013;369(19):1828–1835.

Ramirez LA, Arango T, Boyer J. Therapeutic and prophylactic DNA vaccines for HIV-1. Expert Opinion on Biological Therapy. 2013;13(4):563–573.

Rasmussen TA, Tolstrup M, Brinkmann CR, et al. Panobinostat, a histone deacetylase inhibitor, for latent-virus reactivation in HIV-infected patients on suppressive antiretroviral therapy: A phase 1/2, single group, clinical trial. Lancet HIV. 2014;1(1):e14–e21.

Richman DD, Margolis DM, Delaney M, et al. The challenge of finding a cure for HIV infection. Science. 2009;323(5919):1304–1307.

Rodriguez B, Asmuth DM, Matining RM, et al. Safety, tolerability, and immunogenicity of repeated doses of dermavir, a candidate therapeutic HIV vaccine, in HIV-infected patients receiving combination antiretroviral therapy: Results of the ACTG 5176 trial. Journal of Acquired Immune Deficiency Syndromes. 2013;64(4):351–359.

Saez-Cirion A, Bacchus C, Hocqueloux L, et al. Post-treatment HIV-1 controllers with a long-term virological remission after the interruption of early initiated antiretroviral therapy ANRS VISCONTI Study. PLoS Pathogens. 2013;9(3):e1003211.

Sauce D, Elbim C, Appay V. Monitoring cellular immune markers in HIV infection: From activation to exhaustion. Current Opinion in HIV and AIDS. 2013;8(2):125–131.

Shan L, Deng K, Shroff NS, et al. Stimulation of HIV-1-specific cytolytic T lymphocytes facilitates elimination of latent viral reservoir after virus reactivation. Immunity. 2012;36(3):491–501.

Shingai M, Nishimura Y, Klein F, et al. Antibody-mediated immunotherapy of macaques chronically infected with SHIV suppresses viraemia. Nature. 2013;503(7475):277–280.

Sogaard OS, Graversen ME, Leth S, et al. The depsipeptide romidepsin reverses HIV-1 latency in vivo. PLoS Pathogens. 2015;11(9):e1005142.

Strain MC, Little SJ, Daar ES, et al. Effect of treatment, during primary infection, on establishment and clearance of cellular reservoirs of HIV-1. Journal of Infectious Diseases. 2005;191(9):1410–1418.

Sung JA, Pickeral J, Liu L, et al. Dual-affinity re-targeting proteins direct T cell-mediated cytolysis of latently HIV-infected cells. Journal of Clinical Investigation. 2015;125(11):4077–4090.

Tebas P, Stein D, Tang WW, et al. Gene editing of CCR5 in autologous CD4 T cells of persons infected with HIV. New England Journal of Medicine. 2014;370(10):901–910.

Topalian SL, Hodi FS, Brahmer JR, et al. Safety, activity, and immune correlates of anti-PD-1 antibody in cancer. New England Journal of Medicine. 2012;366(26):2443–2454.

Varela-Rohena A, Molloy PE, Dunn SM, et al. Control of HIV-1 immune escape by CD8 T cells expressing enhanced T-cell receptor. Nature Medicine. 2008;14(12):1390–1395.

Velu V, Titanji K, Zhu B, et al. Enhancing SIV-specific immunity in vivo by PD-1 blockade. Nature. 2009;458(7235):206–210.

Whitney JB, Hill AL, Sanisetty S, et al. Rapid seeding of the viral reservoir prior to SIV viraemia in rhesus monkeys. Nature. 2014;512(7512):74–77.

Whitney JB, Lim SY, Osuna CE, et al. Treatment with a TLR7 agonist induces transient viremia in SIV-infected ART-suppressed monkeys. Conference on Retroviruses and Opportunistic Infections, Seattle, WA, 2015.

Wong JK, Hezareh M, Gunthard HF, et al. Recovery of replication-competent HIV despite prolonged suppression of plasma viremia. Science. 1997;278(5341):1291–1295.

Yukl SA, Boritz E, Busch M, B, et al. Challenges in detecting HIV persistence during potentially curative interventions: A study of the Berlin patient. PLoS Pathogens. 2013;9(5):e1003347.

7.

HIV TESTING AND COUNSELING

Alejandro Delgado and William P. Mazur

LEARNING OBJECTIVES

- List the types of HIV testing.

- Present an overview of HIV counseling and how to adapt to counseling to the variety of situations or environments in which these conversations can take place.

WHAT'S NEW?

- During the past decade, the evidence favoring the early institution of therapy for HIV has been steadily growing, showing benefits in virologic control and decreased transmission of HIV.

- The most recent data published in 2015 by the Centers for Disease Control and Prevention (CDC) estimate that approximately 14% of people living with HIV are unaware of their diagnosis. In certain states and among men who have sex with men (MSM), who constitute 60% of new yearly diagnoses, the percentage of people who are unaware of their HIV infection may be as high as 25%. Knowledge of diagnosis is a critical first step toward being linked to care. The World Health Organization and the US Department of Health and Human Services now advocate for universal treatment of patients who are diagnosed with HIV.

- In June 2014, the CDC revised its testing algorithm favoring the use of fourth-generation assays that are capable of early detection of HIV-1 and HIV-2 antibodies as well as the p24 antigen. This has substantially narrowed the window between initial infection and positive test results. For the first time since 1989, the CDC has eliminated the use of confirmation testing with a first-generation Western blot or immunofluorescence assay (Figure 7.1).

KEY POINTS

- HIV testing should be offered as part of routine medical care to all patients. In 2013, the US Preventive Services Task Force formally recommended that clinicians screen all patients between the ages of 15 and 65 years. Testing in younger and older patients should be offered when special circumstances deem this appropriate.

- All persons screened for HIV should be counseled regarding risk-reduction strategies regardless of test result.

- All pregnant women should be screened for HIV at the earliest instance possible.

HIV TESTING: HISTORY AND EVOLUTION

In centuries past, the role of medicine was to aggressively intervene in the event of illness. In addition to more mundane approaches, treatments included bloodletting, purges, starvation, ice baths, and the administration of heavy metals, among other strange concoctions. In the 1820s, there was a dramatic paradigm shift when a group of British and American physicians consciously withheld more aggressive treatments and made note of the subsequent improvement in survival rates. As a more conservative approach to disease developed, the profession of medicine concentrated on the art of diagnosis (Weeks, 2010). The focus on diagnosis reached extraordinary intensity in the early years of the HIV pandemic, producing one of the most accurate screening and diagnostic batteries in medical history (Weeks, 2010).

In 1985, when HIV testing first became available, the main goal of testing was to protect the blood supply. When it was discovered that those who simply wished to learn their

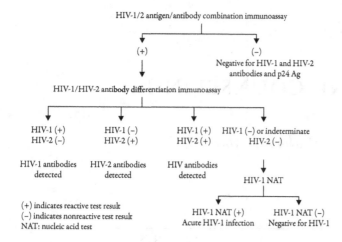

HIV-1/2 antigen/antibody combination immunoassay

(+) / (−) Negative for HIV-1 and HIV-2 antibodies and p24 Ag

HIV-1/HIV-2 antibody differentiation immunoassay

HIV-1 (+) HIV-2 (−) | HIV-1 (−) HIV-2 (+) | HIV-1 (+) HIV-2 (+) | HIV-1 (−) or indeterminate HIV-2 (−)

HIV-1 antibodies detected | HIV-2 antibodies detected | HIV antibodies detected

HIV-1 NAT

HIV-1 NAT (+) Acute HIV-1 infection | HIV-1 NAT (−) Negative for HIV-1

(+) indicates reactive test result
(−) indicates nonreactive test result
NAT: nucleic acid test

Figure 7.1 HIV-1/-2 testing algorithm.

HIV status were using blood donation testing sites, alternative testing sites were implemented. Because at that time no treatment was available and routes of transmission had yet to be established, opinion was divided about the value of testing. By 1987, the implications of a positive HIV serology were clear, and the US Public Health Service issued the first set of guidelines for HIV testing and counseling (Branson, 2006). Periodic revisions informed by the epidemiology of the pandemic extended the outreach and flexibility of testing, culminating in the "Revised Recommendations for HIV Testing of Adults, Adolescents, and Pregnant Women in Health-Care Settings" (Branson, 2006).

Earlier guidelines targeted those in "high-risk groups," but experience taught that a more productive approach focused on behaviors rather than membership in a particular population. Hence, the thrust of the current guidelines is that HIV screening is recommended for all patients aged 13 to 65 years, in all health care settings.

HIV TESTING TYPES AND TERMINOLOGY

Table 7.1 enumerates the various types of HIV testing.

PRE- AND POST-TEST COUNSELING ELEMENTS

PRETEST COUNSELING

Although formal pretest counseling and written informed consent are no longer recommended by the 2006 CDC testing guidelines, considerable debate has occurred on the efficacy of counseling to prevent HIV infection. A prospective randomized study found that brief counseling sessions using personalized risk-reduction plans were effective at reducing the spread of sexually transmitted diseases (STDs) (Kamb, 1998). These results support the practice of individualized counseling; however, results of other studies measuring a reduction in risk behaviors have been equivocal.

Table 7.1 TESTING TERMINOLOGY

TEST TYPE	DESCRIPTION
Anonymous testing	No identifying information links the patient to the test sample. At the time of testing, the patient is handed a code number, and a matching code number is affixed to the sample. No institutional record of the code is kept. Results are given only verbally because no medical record is created. Treatment cannot be instituted based on this form of testing.
Confidential testing	Test remains linked to patient identifiers, and access to results is available for review only by those identified within "need to know" medical standards, including local, state, and national (e.g., CDC) public health agencies.
Screening	Performing an HIV test for all persons in a defined population. For individual patients, screening is most cost-effective through an antibody-based test, the most common of which is the enzyme-linked immunosorbent assay (ELISA).
Opt-in screening	Patient approaches the provider and requests HIV testing.
Opt-out screening	Health care provider offers routine HIV testing to all patients unless refused by patient.
Point-of-care or rapid testing	Simplified antibody-based testing procedure that can give a screening-level result in approximately 20 minutes and that can be implemented by a trained non-health care individual.
Diagnostic testing	Testing prompted by the presence of clinical signs or symptoms. The term may also refer to the antigen-based confirmation of a positive ELISA. In the United States, the validation test formerly used most often was the Western blot analysis. New CDC guidelines now recommend using a fourth-generation HIV Ag/Ab enzyme immunoassay test or HIV RNA test for diagnostic confirmation. The validation testing may also be referred to as confirmatory testing.
Targeted testing	Performing an HIV test on persons perceived to be at higher risk, as defined by behavioral, clinical, or demographic characteristics. Formerly the main strategy for HIV testing, it has been supplanted by the recommendation to treat HIV screening as a routine part of medical care.

This may be due to the quality and delivery of information rather than the presence or absence of counseling.

In addition to informing the patient about the possibility of HIV screening, effectively performed pretest counseling is an interactive process of assessing risk, recognizing specific risk-inducing behaviors, and reviewing risk-reduction strategies. This may be done in a variety of ways—through written material, films, or orally by a variety of trained staff. Of greatest importance is setting a nonjudgmental atmosphere, imparting accurate information in a useful format, offering an opportunity for questions, and maintaining strict confidentiality of personal information.

If deemed to be appropriate, elements of pretest counseling should include the following:

- A functional assessment of the patient's decision-making capacity

- The meaning, sensitivity, and specificity of the test

- The potential ramifications of a positive test result

- A discussion about confidentiality and disclosure of test results by the health care providers to public health authorities and by the patient to sexual and/or drug partners

- A frank discussion of risk-reduction behaviors

- Specific instructions about accessing treatment in the event of a positive result

POST-TEST COUNSELING

Elements of post-test counseling should include the following:

- For a negative result
  - The validity of the negative result
  - Possible retesting if indicated
  - Reinforcement of transmission reduction behaviors (US Department of Veterans Affairs, 2002)
- For a positive result
  - Review of the availability and effectiveness of treatment
  - Reinforcement of disclosure to spouse and/or sexual and/or drug partners

- Reinforcement of transmission reduction behaviors

- An assessment of any intent to harm self or others

- A positive result

- Optimally given during a face-to-face meeting

SPECIAL POPULATIONS AND ENVIRONMENTS

BLOOD SUPPLY SCREENING

Since 1990, all persons desiring to donate blood or plasma are required to undergo testing, as are those donating sperm for artificial insemination or tissue or organs for transplantation. The donor is notified only if the specimen tests positive.

As of January 4, 2010, the US Department of Health and Human Services and the CDC removed HIV infection from the list of diseases that keep people who are not US citizens from entering the United States.

PERINATAL SCREENING

HIV screening should be a routine component of prenatal testing, and it should preferably be repeated in the third trimester (<36 weeks of gestation). An additional third-trimester test should be offered to women in high-incidence areas or those with high-risk behavior. This pattern of testing should be repeated for each successive pregnancy. Women with undocumented HIV status at the time of labor or delivery should be screened with a point-of-care (POC) HIV test unless they opt out. If a mother's HIV status is unknown postpartum, POC testing of the newborn is recommended (and is legally mandated in many states) as soon as possible so that antiretroviral prophylaxis can be offered to HIV-exposed infants. The mother should be informed that the identification of HIV antibodies in the newborn indicates that the mother is infected (Branson, 2006).

TESTING SETTINGS

The essential elements for testing are the same for a standard medical setting and a nontraditional delivery site, and these were discussed previously. The basic difference lies in who conducts the interview. In nontraditional settings, properly trained and supervised "testing counselors" provide high-quality interventions in STD clinics, needle-exchange sites, and other nonmedical venues, such as gay pride parades and homeless "stand-downs." Regardless of the settings, the standards of care remain the same.

A 3-year study utilizing intensified testing was performed in a publicly funded STD clinic in San Francisco. To enhance HIV surveillance, public health officials augmented standard testing by adding a "detuned" enzyme-linked immunosorbent assay (ELISA) test, which can distinguish recent from chronic infection; pooled nucleic acid amplification testing to ELISA-negative samples to identify acute seroconversion; and performed genotypic HIV resistance testing for all new infections. In a sample of 9868 patients, 380 new cases were diagnosed, of which 29 were categorized as acute infections and 128 as recent infections. Transmitted antiretroviral resistance was identified in 47 cases and appeared to increase over time. These findings suggest that intensified testing in high-HIV prevalence areas can enhance best treatment and prophylactic practices. However, the resources for most testing programs would not cover these testing practices. Nevertheless, the study does highlight that more work is needed to optimize the approach to HIV testing in different settings (Truong, 2011).

AREAS OF SPECIAL INTEREST

Several presentations from the 2015 Conference on Retroviruses and Opportunistic Infections described the challenges associated with HIV testing in the United States and identified potential areas for improvement in access to and/or engagement in testing efforts. Wejnert and colleagues presented data from CDC surveys of MSM in 20 US cities (Wejnert, 2016). Black MSM were more likely to be HIV infected than White MSM among all age groups, with greatest differences in the youngest age group. Among MSM aged 18–24 years, 1 in 5 Blacks were HIV seropositive compared to less than 1 in 20 Whites and less than 1 in 13 Latinos. Awareness of HIV serostatus was also considerably lower among Black MSM than White MSM in all age categories younger than 50 years. Overall, less than two-thirds of Black HIV-positive MSM were aware of their serostatus; of those who were younger than age 30 years, less than half of them were aware of their serostatus. Hall and colleagues presented data from the US National HIV Surveillance System on the proportion of new HIV diagnoses that were considered "late" (i.e., presented with a CD4+ count <200 cells/mm³ or an opportunistic infection within 3 months of diagnosis) (Hall, 2016). In 2012, 24% of all new HIV diagnoses met these criteria. The proportion of late diagnoses was higher among injection drug users and heterosexuals than among MSM. Late diagnoses were more common in Blacks than in Whites in 38 of 105 metropolitan statistical areas (MSAs), and late diagnoses were more common in Hispanics than in Whites in 68 MSAs.

Several investigators have attempted strategies to increase HIV testing in emergency departments. Investigators from The Johns Hopkins Hospital Emergency Department performed identity-unlinked HIV virus testing and chart abstraction over a 6- to 8-week period on all adult patients who had blood drawn for other reasons in 1987, 1988, 1992, 2001, 2003, 2007, and 2013 (Kelen, 2016). HIV prevalence peaked at 12% in 1993 and declined to 6% in 2013. Awareness of HIV serostatus increased from 20% in 1987 to 93% in 2013. The investigators also noted an increase in the percentage of individuals linked to care within 90 days of HIV diagnosis from 47% in 2005 to 88% in 2013. Antiretroviral therapy use also increased from 27% in 2007 to 80% in 2013, and viral suppression increased from 22% in 2001 to 60% in 2013. Interestingly, HIV incidence in the area declined during this same time period from 2.5% per year in 2001 to 0.2% per year in 2013.

STRATEGIES TO IMPROVE UPTAKE OF HIV TESTING

HIV screening should be voluntary and undertaken only with the patient's knowledge and understanding. Testing is optimally undertaken with the goal of preventing newly acquired infection in those found to be negative and linkage to care in those found to be positive. The knowledge imparted during testing is an essential part of the screening process. Without knowledge of risk reduction for those who are negative, and linkage to care for those who are positive, screening is of little benefit to the patient (CDC, 2011). The commonality of concurrent STDs in HIV practices argues against the notion that safer sex practices are promoted through knowledge of one's positive status alone. In the highly structured, technical, reimbursement-driven health care environment, a truly successful screening program is not one that is measured by the number of tests performed but, rather, one that takes into account that HIV screening deals with the most elemental and intimate aspects of human existence.

References

Branson BM, Hansfield HH, Lampe MA, et al. Revised recommendations for HIV testing of adults, adolescents, and pregnant women in health-care settings. CDC MMWR Recommendations and Reports, September 22, 2006. Retrieved February 25, 2012, from https://www.cdc.gov/mmwr/preview/mmwrhtml/rr5514a1.htm.
Centers for Disease Control and Prevention. Vital Signs: HIV Prevention Through Care and Treatment, November 29, 2011.

Retrieved February 25, 2012, from https://www.cdc.gov/mmwr/preview/mmwrhtml/mm6047a4.htm.

Centers for Disease Control and Prevention. Laboratory testing for the diagnosis of HIV infection. Updated recommendations published June 27, 2014.

Hall HI, Tang T, Espinoza L. Late diagnosis of HIV infection in metropolitan areas of the United States and Puerto Rico. AIDS Behav. 2016; 20(5):967–972. Available at http://www.ncbi.nlm.nih.gov/pubmed/26542730.

Kamb ML, Fishbein M, Douglas JM, et al. Efficacy of risk-reduction counseling to prevent human immunodeficiency virus and sexually transmitted diseases. Journal of the American Medical Association 1998; 280:1161–1167.

Kelen GD, Hsieh YH, Rothman RE, et al. Improvements in the continuum of HIV care in an inner-city emergency department. AIDS. 2016; 30(1):113–120. Available at http://www.ncbi.nlm.nih.gov/pubmed/26731757.

Truong H. Sentinel surveillance of HIV-1 transmitted drug resistance, acute infection, and recent infection. PLoS One October 6, 2011; 6:e25281.

US Department of Veterans Affairs. The VA Prevention Handbook: A Guide for Clinicians. Washington, DC: Veterans Health Administration; 2002.

Weeks BS, Alcamo EL. AIDS: The Biological Basis. Sudbury, MA: Jones & Bartlett; 2010.

Wejnert C, Hess KL, Rose CE, et al. Age-specific race and ethnicity disparities in HIV infection and awareness among men who have sex with men—20 US cities, 2008–2014. J Infect Dis. 2016; 213(5):776–783. Available at http://www.ncbi.nlm.nih.gov/pubmed/26486637.

8.

LABORATORY TESTING STRATEGIES

DETECTION AND DIAGNOSIS

Thomas P. Young

CHAPTER GOAL

Upon completion of this chapter, the reader should understand the various laboratory testing methods used for screening and diagnosis of HIV infections.

SEROLOGIC TESTING METHODS

LEARNING OBJECTIVE

Explain how available immunoassays can be used for screening and diagnosing of most early and primary HIV infections.

WHAT'S NEW?

- Two fourth-generation immunoassays are approved for screening and diagnosing HIV infections in the United States:

  - Architect HIV Ag/AB Combo (Abbott Diagnostics, Des Plaines, IL)

  - GS HIV Combo Ag/AB EIA (Bio-Rad Laboratories, Hercules, CA)

- These assays test for the presence of both antibodies to HIV-1 and HIV-2 and HIV p24 antigen, thereby allowing earlier detection of acute and primary HIV infection.

KEY POINTS

- Laboratory confirmation of HIV infection is primarily through the detection of HIV antibodies in an individual.

- The classical testing algorithm that had been in use for more than 25 years involved using a sensitive screening immunoassay (an enzyme-linked immunosorbent assay) and confirming any positive tests with a more specific immunoassay, such as a Western blot.

- New testing algorithms have replaced the Western blot immunoassay with other confirmatory assays (e.g., HIV nucleic acid tests).

- The prevalence of HIV-2 is increasing in the United States; thus, it is important to use immunoassays approved for detecting HIV-2 (as well as other non-group M HIV-1 viruses), especially when the clinical history indicates that an HIV-2 infection should be considered.

- Using the current immunoassays and confirmatory testing, false-positive results are exceedingly rare. However, providers should use clinical judgment when interpreting test results and consider additional follow-up testing when appropriate.

- False-negative immunoassays are also exceedingly rare except for individuals who are early in their infection and have yet to produce HIV antibodies that are detectable by current assays.

- Rapid HIV tests have similar testing accuracies as those of currently available immunoassays and can be useful testing options for settings such as health fairs, nonclinical locations, and other situations in which quickly receiving preliminary test results would be beneficial (e.g., pre-exposure prophylaxis and/or post-exposure prophylaxis).

ENZYME IMMUNOASSAYS

Opt-out HIV screening recommendations for all individuals aged 13–64 years in the United States (Centers for Disease Control and Prevention (CDC), 2006) would not have been possible without readily available, accurate, and cost-effective laboratory assays for screening and diagnosing HIV infections. The first enzyme immunoassay (EIA) was licensed in 1985 (CDC, 1990); since then, the number of EIAs has increased, and the quality of available assays has continued to improve.

This approach continues to be the most reliable and cost-effective testing method for most individuals in the United States. Exceptions include screening and diagnostic testing for individuals with acute HIV infections (see Virologic Assays) and screening and diagnostic testing for infants and newborns (see Alternative Algorithms for Screening and Diagnosing HIV Infections). Screening and diagnostic testing for HIV-2 infections, now becoming more common in the United States, require the use of assays that are specifically approved to detect this virus type. Using the appropriate EIA to identify HIV-2 and/or group O HIV-1 would be particularly important for testing in areas with a high prevalence of immigrants who might be infected with HIV. In addition, these assays would be valuable in locations outside the United States (Hackett, 2012; Swenson, 2014).

The timelines for viremia and antibody seroconversion following initial HIV infection have been well characterized (Fiebig, 2003). Acute HIV infection has been described as a flu-like syndrome that occurs after a person contracts HIV-1. The syndrome is characterized by fever, sore throat, headache, skin rash, and swollen glands (lymphadenopathy) (Cohen, 2010; Hecht, 2011).

Figure 8.1 shows the curves for viral RNA, p24 antigen, and HIV antibody development. Following HIV infection, there is a seroconversion "window" that includes an eclipse period and acute infection period in which an HIV infection may not be detectable by immunological assays. Although there is no accepted laboratory definition of an acute HIV infection, a current operational definition is the detection of HIV RNA or p24 antigen in the blood before antibodies have formed (Cohen, 2010). In these individuals,

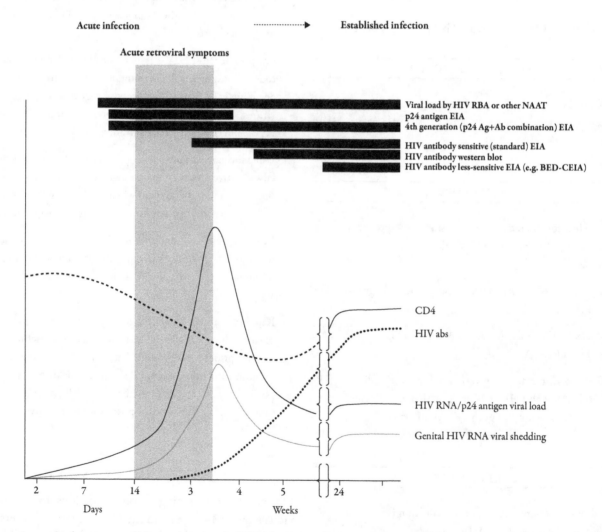

Figure 8.1 Sequence of appearance of laboratory markers for HIV infection. SOURCE: Branson (2010).

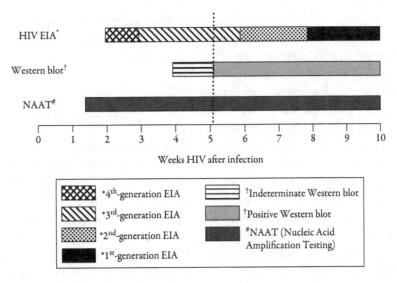

Figure 8.2 Time to detection differences for various generations of EIAs. SOURCE: Modified from Branson (2007) and Patel (2010); data from Fiebig (2003) and Hecht (2011).

nonserologic assays should be used, or follow-up serological testing should be performed after several weeks.

In addition, it is important to understand that viral kinetics and serologic markers may not always be as accurate with non-clade B subtype infections. Additional testing may be necessary to fully understand what is occurring with regard to these markers (Hackett, 2012; Swenson, 2014).

HIV EIAs are described as being from particular "generations," which helps to identify the different technological advancements that have occurred throughout the years, resulting in improved testing accuracy. As shown in Figure 8.2, these improvements have shortened the detection window period substantially. The first-generation EIAs used HIV lysate as an antigen to capture antibodies present in an individual's blood sample. Because cellular protein contamination could occur while preparing the HIV lysate antigen, first-generation EIAs had a relatively high number of false-positive test results (Houn, 1987). First-generation EIAs were also not able to capture antibodies against non-group M strains or HIV-2 (Louie, 2006). For these reasons, and also due to the development of newer assays, first-generation EIAs are no longer available in the United States (Patel, 2010).

Second-generation EIAs use recombinant viral proteins or peptides instead of the viral lysate antigen, which limits cellular protein contamination (Chappel, 2009). Second-generation assays were used to screen blood bank donations in the late 1980s. These assay condensed the window period before antibody detection from 56 to 42 days (Busch, 1997).

Third-generation EIAs were introduced in the 1990s and even further reduced the window period because the binding antigen, created through a "sandwich technique," was able to bind to both IgG and IgM antibodies (late vs. early antibody response, respectively). This reduced the window period to 20–25 days without changing the specificity for more established infections. Many currently available third-generation EIAs detect HIV-1 and HIV-2, as well as group O. Recent additional innovations using third-generation assays include the use of random access sequencing machines, which can generate test results in as few as 58 minutes (Branson, 2007).

Antigen/antibody combination tests, also known as fourth-generation EIAs, have been in use outside of the United States for several years, and two assays are now approved for use in the United States. These assays act as both a third-generation assay and a capture immunoassay, directly detecting the p24 antigen (Weber, 1998). Thus, fourth-generation EIAs reduce the detection window period even further while maintaining the third generation's accuracy (Pandori, 2009; Rosenberg, 2015; Sickinger, 2004).

RAPID HIV TESTS

There are currently eight rapid HIV tests approved by the US Food and Drug Administration (FDA) for use in the United States (Table 8.1). Like EIAs, rapid HIV tests detect HIV antibodies present in a sample or specimen. Third- and fourth-generation EIAs have shorter detection windows compared to the currently available rapid tests, but rapid tests are as accurate and test results are available in less than 30 minutes (Branson, 2007). Persons with a recent potential exposure and those with ongoing high risk for

HIV infection who have negative rapid test results should be counseled to be retested (Delaney, 2011), and additional testing should be considered that is more sensitive for detecting acute HIV infections in these situations. Several rapid tests have received Clinical Laboratory Improvement Amendment (CLIA) waivers, making them attractive for point-of-care testing and screening in settings in which transporting specimens to a laboratory is either not possible or not practical. Rapid tests can use oral fluid, finger-stick blood, or venipuncture whole blood/plasma specimens.

When determining whether to utilize an approved rapid HIV test or EIA testing for screening and/or diagnosing HIV infections, one must take into account the setting in which testing will occur, the cost, and the population being tested. Rapid tests generally will cost more compared to EIA assays, especially if relatively large numbers of tests are being performed. Batch processing of EIA tests using newly available random access machines can produce test results nearly as quickly as rapid tests. However, rapid testing can be particularly useful for public health testing programs outside of clinical settings, such as during health fairs or at social venues where high-risk individuals may be located. Testing women who are in labor is another situation in which rapid HIV testing may be a more suitable choice for compared to EIAs (Merhi, 2005).

WESTERN BLOT ASSAY

The first Western blot assay was approved in 1987; thereafter, it was recommended as a confirmatory assay for positive screening immunoassays (CDC, 1988). A Western blot separates the individual proteins of the HIV-1 lysate into bands that allow for capturing of antibodies specific to selected HIV antigens in an individual's blood or urine. Laboratories report test results as positive, negative, or indeterminate based on established criteria that use the presence of a specific number of specific bands to interpret the test results. Negative Western blot assays have no bands.

Assays are reported positive if the bands present meet an established criterion; assays are reported as indeterminate if bands are detected, but those detected do not meet the criteria for a positive test (CDC, 1989). Indeterminate results could be the result of a false positive or may be from individuals who are in the process of seroconverting (Healey, 1992). Western blot assays generally first begin to be positive after 5 weeks; however, specific bands, including the p24 and gp160 bands, can appear within 30 days of initial HIV infection (Hecht, 2011). Clinical judgment based on a careful history can help determine whether an indeterminate test result indicates a recent infection or a false

positive. Follow-up testing and/or using assays to test for nucleic acids or viral antigens should also be considered in such cases.

INDIRECT IMMUNOFLUORESCENCE ASSAYS

Indirect immunofluorescence assays (IFAs) use a stock of infected cells from immortalized cell lines to capture antibodies present in a sample. Bound antibodies are then conjugated to a molecule that will emit light by fluorescence when exposed to ultraviolet light. Test results are visually evaluated for their degree and pattern of fluorescence (Fluorognost HIV-1 IFA, Sanochemia Pharmazeutika, Vienna, Austria). In the United States, IFAs are less commonly used compared to Western blot assays, but they are used more frequently elsewhere (Bala, 2010). IFAs can be performed on dried blood spot samples, and they are currently used to confirm positive tests for HIV home testing kits (Home Access Health Corporation, Hoffman Estates, IL).

Recommended Reading

Branson BM. State of the art for diagnosis of HIV infection. *Clin Infect Dis*. 2007; 45:S221–S225.

Busch MP, Satten GA. Time course of viremia and antibody seroconversion following human immunodeficiency virus exposure. *Am J Med*. 1997; 102:117–124.

Centers for Disease Control and Prevention. Revised surveillance case definitions for HIV infection among adults, adolescents, and children aged <18 months and for HIV infection and AIDS among children aged 18 months to <13 years—United States, 2008. *MMWR Recommend Rep*. 2008; 57:1–8.

Centers for Disease Control. Laboratory testing for the diagnosis of HIV infection. 2014. Available at http://www.cdc.gov/hiv/pdf/hivtestingalgorithmrecommendation-final.pdf.

VIROLOGIC ASSAYS

LEARNING OBJECTIVE

Discuss when virologic assays should be considered as complementary diagnostics to immunoassays for screening and confirmation of HIV-1 and HIV-2 infections.

WHAT'S NEW?

A nucleic acid amplification test (NAAT) is currently approved for use as an aid to diagnose HIV infections and can be especially useful in diagnosing HIV infections in individuals who may not yet have formed HIV antibodies (acute HIV infections).

- Virologic assays can be useful for diagnosing acute HIV infections and infections in newborns and infants younger than age 18 months.

- Compared to immunoassays, virologic assays are more expensive and have an increased rate of false-positive results; virologic assays may also be falsely negative in individuals with chronic infections, undetectable viral loads, and non-clade B infections.

- To improve cost-effectiveness, several public health laboratories in the United States are pooling negative immunoassay samples and testing the pooled samples using a NAAT. This method increases a screening program's overall accuracy by detecting individuals with acute infections who would have otherwise received a negative test result.

Virologic assays include qualitative and quantitative DNA and RNA assays as well as p24 antigen assays. Fourth-generation antigen/antibody combination immunoassays use the HIV p24 core protein as the antigen component and thus can be considered both a serologic and a virologic assay (Weber, 1998). Stand-alone p24 antigen assays are available, although newer virologic assays such as NAATs are being used more frequently. This is because the p24 antigen rapidly becomes undetectable after antibodies develop, thereby limiting the period during which a p24 antigen assay uniquely provides diagnostic information (see Figure 8.1).

Virologic assays should be considered for the following:

- Diagnosing HIV infection in newborns and infants younger than age 18 months

- Diagnosing acute HIV infections in cases in which, given the history and clinical signs and symptoms, patients would likely not yet have detectable antibodies (see Figure 8.2)

- Enhancing HIV screening programs through the pooling of negative immunoassay samples to detect asymptomatic recent infections that would have otherwise been missed using immunoassays alone

An acute HIV infection is defined as infection during the time from HIV acquisition until seroconversion (Cohen,

Table 8.1 FDA-APPROVED RAPID HIV TESTS

TEST KIT	MANUFACTURER	SPECIMEN TYPE	SENSITIVITY (%)	SPECIFICITY (%)
OraQuick ADVANCE rapid HIV-1/-2 antibody test	OraSure Technologies (http://www.orasure.com)	Oral fluid[a] Whole blood[a,b] Plasma	99.3 (98.4–99.7) 99.6 (98.5–99.9) 99.6 (98.9–99.8)	99.8 (99.6–99.9) 100 (99.7–100) 99.9 (99.6–100)
Reveal G3 rapid HIV-1 antibody test	MedMira (http://www.medmira.com)	Serum Plasma	99.8 (99.2–100) 99.8 (99.0–100)	99.1 (98.8–99.4) 98.6 (98.4–98.8)
Uni-Gold Recombigen HIV-1 test	Trinity BioTech (http://www.trinitybiotech.com)	Whole blood[a,b] Serum Plasma	100 (99.5–100) 100 (99.5–100) 100 (99.5–100)	99.7 (99.0–100) 99.8 (99.3–100) 99.8 (99.3–100)
Multispot HIV 1/2 Rapid test	Bio-Rad Laboratories (http://www.bio-rad.com)	Serum Plasma	100 (99.94–100) 100 (99.94–100)	99.93 (99.79–100) 99.91 (99.77–100)
DPP HIV 1/2	Chembio Diagnostic Systems (http://chembio.com)	Whole blood[a,b] Serum/plasma	99.7 (98.9–100)	99.9 (99.6–100)
HIV 1/2 Stat-Pak Assay (Alere Determine HIV 1/2)	Alere (http://www.alere.com/en/home/product-details/determine-1-2-ag-ab-combo-us.html)	Whole blood[a,b] Serum/plasma	99.7 (98.9–100)	99.9 (99.6–100)
Clearview Complete HIV 1/2	Alere (http://www.alere.com/en/home/product-details/clearview-complete-hiv-1-2.html?c=US)	Whole blood[a,b] Serum/plasma	99.7 (98.9–100)	99.9 (99.6–100)
INSTI HIV-1 antibody test kit	bioLytical Laboratories (http://www.biolyticalus.com)	Whole blood[a,b] Plasma	99.9 (99.5–100) 99.9 (99.5–100)	100 (99.7–100) 100 (99.7–100)

[a]Tests designated as CLIA-waived. Waived Rapid HIV Testing Policy and Quality Assurance Guidelines, June 25, 2014. http://www.cdc.gov/hiv/pdf/testing_nonclinical_clia-waived-tests.pdf.

[b]Blood may be obtained through either finger stick or venipuncture.

SOURCES: FDA website (accessed January 15, 2016) and product package inserts.

2010) or the period after the eclipse phase (see Figure 8.1), in which virologic assays are positive but serologic assays are negative. The serological window period continues to be influenced by the sensitivities of the evolving generations of immunoassays (Owen, 2008; Yerly, 2012).

Because infection transmission risk correlates well with an individual's plasma viral load (Chan, 2012; Quinn, 2000), considerable attention has been given toward detecting acute HIV infections (Cohen, 2010; Hecht, 2002; Patel, 2006, 2010; Pilcher, 2005). Individuals acutely infected will typically have relatively high viral loads before seroconverting (Daar, 1991) and are likely unaware of their infection. Studies have shown that recently infected individuals are likely the source of transmission for up to 50% of all new infections (Yerly, 2012).

QUANTITATIVE ASSAYS FOR DETECTING HIV-1 RNA (VIRAL LOAD ASSAYS)

Several commercially available assays reliably quantify HIV-1 RNA in plasma.:

- Reverse transcription–polymerase chain reaction (RT-PCR)-based technologies

  - Abbott RealTime HIV-1 Amplification Kit (Abbott Molecular, Des Plaines, IL)

  - Roche Amplicor HIV-1 Monitor Test (Roche Molecular Systems, Pleasanton, CA)

  - COBAS AmpliPrep/COBAS TaqMan Version 2.0 HIV-1 Test (Roche Molecular Systems, Pleasanton, CA)

  - Versant HIV-1 RNA 1.0 (kPCR) (Siemens Healthcare Diagnostics, Malvern, PA)

  - Veris^{MDx} (Beckman Coulter, Brea, CA)

  - artus TM HIV-1 QA RGO (QUIAGEN, Waltham, MA)

- NASBA-based technologies

  - Nucli-Sens EasyQ HIV-1 v2.0 (bioMérieux, Marcy-l'Etoile, France)

- Real-time transcription-mediated amplification technologies

  - Panther system (Hologic, Marlborough, MA)

All of these tests reliably quantify plasma HIV-1 RNA with variable dynamic range. These assays detect most HIV-1 subtypes, and although they have become increasingly effective at detecting non-subtype B infections, there is some variability based on clade variations and each assay's performance characteristics. If there is clinical suspicion for underquantification or viral load/immunologic discordance, clinicians should explore a referee assay for viral load confirmation. Both kPCR and RT-PCR assays are proficient at quantitation of many non-clade B strains of HIV-1 (Alvarez, 2015; Elbeik, 2002; Karasi, 2011; Peter, 2004).

Because of the rate of false positives, these quantitative assays must be used with great caution as diagnostic tests, and they were not developed to confirm the presence of an HIV infection. In patients who present with what appears to be symptoms of acute HIV infection but whose antibody tests are negative or indeterminate, these assays may be helpful in diagnosing HIV infection. In this setting, plasma HIV-1 RNA levels are typically very high, whereas levels of false positives tend to be very low (Hecht, 2002).

QUALITATIVE ASSAYS FOR DETECTING HIV-1 RNA

Currently, there is one qualitative virologic assay, frequently referred to as NAAT, approved for use as an aid in the diagnosis of HIV-1 (APTIMA; Gen-Probe, San Diego, CA). This assay can be used to assist with diagnosing an acute HIV infection and as an additional test to confirm an HIV-1 infection when an EIA or rapid test is repeatedly reactive for HIV-1 antibodies. Results for the assay are reported as reactive or nonreactive based on an analytic threshold that gives positive results if a sample contains greater than 90 copies/ml of HIV-1 RNA. Other NAATs not currently approved for use in the United States have detection limits of 20–40 HIV-1 RNA copies/ml (Yerly, 2012).

Although the NAAT assay allows for earlier detection of HIV infections, it should not be used as a standalone screening assay because false-positive results are more likely than with immunoassays, and it is considerably more expensive. Furthermore, long-standing HIV infections may not be reactive because viral loads in some individuals can decrease below the limit of detection even without the use of antiretroviral medications (Migueles, 2010).

To improve the cost-effectiveness of using NAATs, some public health laboratories in the United States have pooled negative EIA samples into a single sample that can then be broken down for further testing if any are positive (Patel, 2006; Pilcher, 2005). By pooling negative samples, the threshold for detection increases, but studies show that 0.1–23% additional acute HIV infections can be detected in this manner (Yerly, 2012). The number of additional HIV infections detected using this method will vary greatly depending on which generation of EIA is used as the initial screening assay. Because third- and fourth-generation assays are being used more frequently, fewer acute infections will likely be missed; thus, the cost-effectiveness of pooled NAAT testing is currently being questioned (Hutchinson, 2010, 2013).

HIV-2 VIROLOGIC ASSAYS

An approved HIV-2 virologic assay is not currently available in the United States. Although some assays may detect a viral load, caution should be exercised when utilizing these results to monitor response to treatment because underquantification is common when viremia is detected (Campbell-Yesufu, 2012). A number of international laboratories use in-house (or laboratory-developed) HIV-2 viral load assays. Some reference laboratories in the United States maintain in-house qualitative HIV-2 PCR assays, but variances between results have been observed, thus limiting their interpretation (Damond, 2011; Gottlieb, 2013). Reference laboratory resources are available by the CDC for public health laboratories evaluating HIV-2 reactive specimens.

ALTERNATIVE ALGORITHMS FOR SCREENING AND DIAGNOSING HIV INFECTIONS

LEARNING OBJECTIVE

Explain the rationale for proposing a new HIV testing algorithm, including how the proposed algorithm would differ from the currently recommended algorithm.

WHAT'S NEW?

Because newer serologic and virologic assays are available, alternative algorithms replacing the Western blot as an confirmatory assay are in development.

KEY POINTS

- Formal recommendation for use of an alternative algorithm for screening and diagnosing HIV infections is likely forthcoming by the CDC after the results of additional clinical trials and public health laboratory input are obtained.

- The proposed alternative algorithm removes the use of the Western blot assay because of its limitations, particularly in confirming acute or recent HIV infections.

- The alternative algorithm would recommend using the most sensitive immunoassay (fourth-generation EIA) as a screening test, as well as following any repeatedly positive results with a different immunoassay that can discriminate between HIV-1 and HIV-2.

- Samples with a positive screening assay but negative confirming assay should be tested using a NAAT.

Currently available EIAs can detect acute or recent infections before a Western blot can provide confirmatory evidence of seropositivity. Key factors driving the evolution of alternative algorithms are the availability of NAAT and the increasing prevalence of HIV-2 infection in the United States (Owen, 2008). At the 2010 HIV Diagnostics Conference, a new algorithm was proposed that would use the most sensitive immunoassays for primary screening along with a confirmatory test that discriminates HIV-1 versus HIV-2 after a repeatedly positive screening test (Pandori, 2010). If the confirmatory test is negative, HIV NAAT should be performed. A positive NAAT would be confirmatory for HIV infection. Figure 8.3 shows the proposed alternative HIV testing algorithm. Early studies

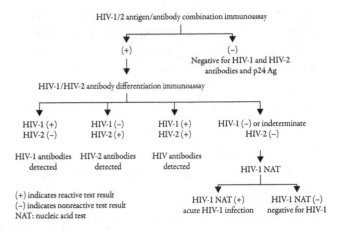

Figure 8.3 Updated testing algorithm for US HIV diagnosis.

(Masciotra, 2011; Zeh, 2011) using the alternative HIV diagnostic algorithm have demonstrated improved or non-inferior sensitivity for detecting acute HIV-1 infections while maintaining the ability to accurately detect established HIV-1 infections.

Currently, the CDC is validating data and obtaining input from laboratories in order to determine whether the alternative algorithm will be formally recommended. It is likely that in the near future, this alternative algorithm will be part of the recommended testing algorithms.

Recommended Reading

Branson BM. The future of HIV testing. *J Acquir Immune Defic Syndr.* 2010; 55:S102–S105.

Brennan CA, Stramer SL, Holzmayer V, et al. Identification of human immunodeficiency virus type-1 non-B subtypes and antiretroviral drug resistant strains in United States blood donors. *Transfusion.* 2009; 49(1):125–133. doi: 10.1111/j.1537-2995.2008.01935.x.

Parker MM, Gordon D, Reilly A, et al. Prevalence of drug-resistant and nonsubtype B HIV strains in antiretroviral naïve HIV-infected individuals in New York State. *AIDS Patient Care STDS.* 2007; 21(9):644–652.

Rosenberg NE, Pilcher CD, Busch MP, et al. How can we better identify early HIV infections? *Curr Opin HIV AIDS.* 2015; 10(1):61–68. doi: 10.1097/COH.0000000000000121.

SCREENING AND DETECTING HIV IN NEWBORNS AND CHILDREN

LEARNING OBJECTIVE

Describe how HIV infection can be diagnosed in newborns and children younger than age 18 months.

WHAT'S NEW?

NAAT and RNA PCR assays are being used more frequently for detecting HIV infection in newborns and infants because they have been shown to have comparable accuracies and are generally more readily available than previously used virologic assays.

KEY POINTS

- Maternal antibodies passed in utero are detectable using current immunoassays, so ruling out HIV infections in newborns requires virologic assay testing.

- HIV testing should be performed within 48 hours of birth, at 1 or 2 months of age, and at 3–6 months of age in infants who are born from HIV-positive women.

- Laboratory confirmation of HIV infection generally requires that more than one test be positive; infections typically can be diagnosed by the age of 1 month and definitively in almost all children at age 6 months.

Because maternal antibodies passed in utero can be detected in uninfected newborns, immunoassays may be positive in uninfected newborns until 18 months of age. Maternal-to-child transmission of HIV infection can occur in utero, at the time of labor and delivery, and through breast-feeding (Kourtis, 2001). Figure 8.4 depicts the HIV RNA levels and antibody response for exposed infants with or without infection.

Thus, when interpreting immunoassay results for an infant, it is important to consider serological window periods after each of these potential exposure events, as well as the presence of maternal antibodies. Non-breast-fed children can be considered presumptively uninfected if there is at least one negative HIV-1 antibody test result at 6 months of age or older, and they can be considered definitively uninfected if there are at least two negative HIV antibody tests from separate specimens obtained at age 6 months or older (CDC, 2008). Virologic assays, however, represent the gold standard for diagnostic testing of infants and children younger than age 18 months (Read, 2007).

A number of virologic studies are currently available for diagnosing infections in newborns, including viral culture, HIV-1 NAAT, HIV-1 DNA assay, HIV-1 RNA assay, and p24 antigen assay. Although HIV-1 culture was once considered the gold standard diagnostic assay, the disadvantages of viral culture (it is labor-intensive, time-consuming, costly, and poses a biohazard risk) (Read, 2007), as well as the availability of other assays, limit its use today. Use of the HIV p24 antigen test is also generally not recommended because of poor sensitivity, especially in the presence of HIV antibodies (CDC, 2008). DNA assays have been used most often to diagnose HIV infection in infants and young children (Read, 2007). However, HIV-1 RNA assays and NAATs are now more commonly used to diagnose HIV-1 in infants because they have comparable sensitivity and specificity to DNA assays (CDC, 2008) and have become more available due to their use in other applications, such as patient treatment monitoring and diagnosing acute HIV infections in adolescents and adults.

Virologic assay testing should be performed on infants born to HIV-infected mothers within the first 48 hours of life, at 1 or 2 months of age, and at 3–6 months of age. If any tests are positive, repeat testing is recommended, and the diagnosis of HIV infection can be made based on two

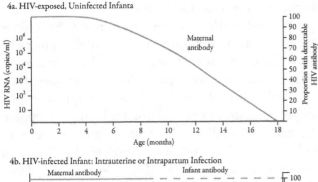

4a. HIV-exposed, Uninfected Infant

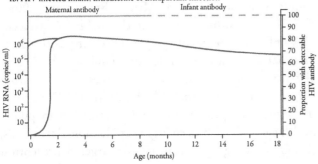

4b. HIV-infected Infant: Intrauterine or Intrapartum Infection

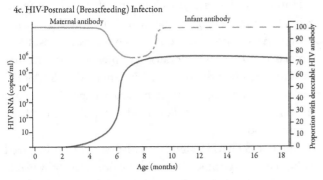

4c. HIV-Postnatal (Breastfeeding) Infection

Figure 8.4 HIV RNA levels and anti-HIV antibody responses among HIV-exposed infants with or without HIV infection. Schematic depiction of the timing of positive HIV-1 antibody testing and RNA levels among HIV-exposed infants. The horizontal axis shows infant age in months. The left vertical axis shows mean HIV-1 RNA level on a logarithmic scale and corresponds to the green lines on each graph. The right vertical axis shows the proportion of infants for whom an HIV antibody test would likely return positive and corresponds to the red lines on each graph. The proportion of infants with a positive antibody test mean RNA levels in all panels are approximate. (a) Results for an HIV-exposed infant who is born without HIV infection and remains uninfected throughout breast-feeding. In this case, HIV RNA level remains zero, and maternal HIV antibody fades with time. (b) Results for infants infected before birth, either during the intrauterine period (IU; resulting in a high RNA level immediately after birth) or during the intrapartum period (IP; resulting in a 1- or 2-week delay before viremia is detectable). Maternal HIV antibody is present at birth; although maternal antibody fades with time, endogenous infant antibody production begins in response to infant infection. (c) Results for an HIV-exposed infant who is uninfected at birth but becomes infected at approximately 6 months of age through breast-feeding. HIV RNA is undetectable while the infant is uninfected but rises rapidly within the first few weeks after infection. Maternal antibody is present at birth and begins to fade with time, but infant antibody production begins after infant infection occurs. SOURCE: From Ciaranello (2011).

separate positive results. A positive virologic test result on one specimen is presumptive for HIV infection (CDC, 2008).

For surveillance purposes, in non-breast-feeding children age 18 months or younger, definitive exclusion of HIV infection can be based on at least two negative virologic test results from separate specimens, both obtained at age 1 month or younger, and one obtained at age 4 months or older. A presumptive exclusion of HIV infection can be based on two negative virologic tests from separate specimens, both obtained at age 2 weeks or older, and one obtained at age 4 weeks or older. One negative virologic test result obtained at age 8 weeks or older also presumptively excludes HIV infection.

For children with a single positive HIV virologic test result, the presumptive exclusion of HIV infection can be based on two subsequent negative virologic test results with at least one performed at age 8 weeks or older. Definitive exclusion of HIV infection is based on two negative virologic tests with one obtained at age 1 month or older and one obtained at age 4 months or older (CDC, 2008).

The laboratory criteria for determining non-HIV infection, both presumptively and definitively as outlined previously, are indicated by the CDC to be for surveillance purposes only and thus must be combined with any clinical evidence of HIV infection before ruling out maternal-to-child transmission (CDC, 2008).

Infants born to HIV-2-infected mothers should be tested with HIV-2-specific virologic assays at time points similar to those used for HIV-1 testing. HIV-2 virologic assays are not commercially available, but the National Perinatal HIV Hotline (1-888-448-8765) can provide a list of sites that perform this testing (Panel on Treatment of HIV-Infected Pregnant Women and Prevention of Perinatal Transmission, 2011).

TESTING NEWBORNS IN RESOURCE-LIMITED SETTINGS

Access to early infant diagnosis of HIV infection is improving in resource-limited settings (Ciaranello, 2011), but key barriers continue to exist. Virologic assays are generally more expensive than immunoassays, and additional barriers such as accurate specimen collection, transport, and laboratory processing can limit their use in these settings. However, multiple RNA and DNA PCR assays are currently being used, and the use of dried blood spots has decreased the phlebotomy requirements. Dried blood spots may be obtained through a finger or heel stick, are heat stable, are non-infectious, and can be shipped via mail or courier (Ciaranello, 2011).

Because breast-feeding may be recommended for children born in resource-limited settings through the age of 12 months, provided the mother and/or child is receiving antiretroviral prophylaxis, clinical and laboratory monitoring for HIV transmission should take into consideration this ongoing exposure risk (World Health Organization, 2010).

Recommended Reading

Centers for Disease Control and Prevention. Revised surveillance case definitions for HIV infection among adults, adolescents, and children aged <18 months and for HIV infection and AIDS among children aged 18 months to <13 years—United States, 2008. *MMWR Recommend Rep*. 2008; 57(RR10):1–8.

New York State Department of Health. Diagnostic, monitoring, and resistance laboratory tests for HIV. Available at http://www.hivguidelines.org/clinical-guidelines/adults/diagnostic-monitoring-and-resistance-laboratory-tests-for-hiv.

Read JS, and the Committee on Pediatric AIDS. Diagnosis of HIV-1 infection in children younger than 18 months in the United States. *Pediatrics*. 2007; 120:e1547–e1562.

ASSAYS FOR INCIDENCE STUDIES

LEARNING OBJECTIVE

Describe population-based serological testing algorithms being used for estimating the incidence of new HIV infections.

WHAT'S NEW?

A number of HIV incidence programs have been implemented throughout the world to more accurately determine the incidence of new HIV infections in populations.

KEY POINTS

- Algorithms for determining recent seroconversions are used for making public health decisions, such as targeting prevention and intervention programs toward emerging trends.

- A number of algorithms using different immunoassay techniques are being used, all of which identify a subset of positive samples likely to be indicative of a recent infection.

- HIV incidence assays have limited use for clinical or diagnostic purposes because they use average rates of serological marker progression and cannot account for the variability in each individual's antibody production and maturation. Also, very late infections may appear as recent infections due to immune system decline.

Important for monitoring the HIV epidemic on a population-based level are Serological Testing Algorithms for Recent HIV Seroconversion (STARHS) programs. STARHS programs are being used in the United States (see http://www.cdc.gov/nchhstp/newsroom/docs/HIV-Infections-2006-2009.pdf and/or http://www.cdc.gov/hiv/statistics/surveillance/index.html), European countries (Haar, 2015; Vu, 2008; http://www.eurosurveillance.org/ViewArticle.aspx?ArticleId=18972), and countries in sub-Saharan Africa (Braunstein, 2009). STARHS algorithms determine the incidence of recent HIV infections by identifying a subset of positive samples that are in a recent infection window period (usually <6 months) versus those samples that are from persons with more established infections. These testing algorithms provide valuable information to public health agencies such as emerging epidemiological trends, thereby creating opportunities for targeted prevention and intervention strategies. Currently, there is little application for these assays for diagnostic or clinical purposes. Most STARHS programs do not report testing results to clinicians and patients because samples used for studies are submitted in a de-identified manner. Also, STARHS methods require significant laboratory expertise and are generally are not available outside of public health or research laboratories.

The first STARHS algorithm (Janssen, 1998) involved testing a blood specimen first with a commercially available enzyme immunoassay, followed by modifications that both diluted the sample and decreased the specimen incubation time. Such steps "detuned" the immunoassay to be less sensitive for HIV antibodies, thus enabling it to differentiate between recent versus chronic HIV infection. Specimens from individuals with early HIV infection would be reactive using the standard assay but nonreactive with the less sensitive or detuned assay. Specimens from individuals with more established infections would be reactive to both the standard and the detuned assay because the affinity for binding to the antigen and the number of antibodies increase over time. This technique could generally recognize infections that occurred within the past 4–6 months versus those that likely came from individuals with a more established infection.

The detuned immunoassay had significant limitations because antibody maturation and production can vary significantly from person to person following initial HIV infection due to host immune and viral factors. Also, specimens from individuals presenting in late stages of infection or on antiviral treatment may have a negative detuned immunoassay result. For these reasons, as well as the technical challenges with performing this algorithm, detuned immunoassays are no longer in use.

The BED-CEIA assay (capture enzyme immunoassay) was developed by the CDC (Dobbs, 2004), and although commercially available, it is intended only for population studies. This immunoassay is based on quantifying the relative proportion of IgG antibody specific for HIV versus the total IgG antibodies in a sample. The advantage of measuring the proportion rather than specific titers is that each test is self-calibrated to a particular individual's antibody levels. Early infections will have fewer antibodies detected. The BED-CEIA assay also contains oligopeptides derived from the gp41 glycoprotein from regions of three different HIV subtypes (B, E, and D), allowing for analysis of antibodies from infections of all three. The mean window period calculated using this immunoassay is 156 days. The BED-CEIA immunoassay was used to adjust the estimated incidence of HIV infections in the United States in 2008 and continues to be used today to estimate the incidence of new infections in this country (Hall, 2008; Prejean, 2011). Like the detuned assay, the BED-CEIA approach can misclassify very late infections as recent infections.

Other methods used to identify recent infections on a population-based level include avidity assays, which measure the maturation of HIV antibodies; the IDE-V3 immunoassay, which is being used as part of the French national screening program; IG3 Anti-HIV; and the Inno-LIA HIV adaptation (Murphy, 2008).

Recommended Reading

Murphy G, Parry JV. Assays for the detection of recent infections with human immunodeficiency virus type 1. *Eurosurveillance*. 2008; 13:4–10.

Pilcher C, Fiscus S, Nguyen T, et al. Detection of acute infections during HIV testing in North Carolina. *N Engl J Med*. 2005; 352:1873–1883.

Prejean J, Song R, Hernandez A, et al. Estimated HIV incidence in the United States, 2006–2009. *PLoS One*. 2011; 6:e17502.

References

Alvarez P, Martin L, Prieto L, et al. HIV-1 variability and viral load technique could lead to false positive HIV-1 detection and to erroneous viral quantification in infected specimens. J Infect. 2015;71(3): 368–376. doi: 10.1016/j.jinf.2015.05.011.

Bala M, Arias J, Deb M, et al. Immunofluorescence assay in India for confirmation of HIV-1 infection using a T-cell line infected with defective HIV-1. Int J Inf Dis. 2010; 14:e1093–e1098.

Branson BM. State of the art for diagnosis of HIV infection. Clinical Infectious Diseases. 2007; 45:S221–S225.

Branson BM. The future of HIV testing. J AIDS. 2010; 55:S102–S105.

Braunstein SL, van de Wijger J, Nash D. HIV incidence in sub-Saharan Africa: A systematic review with implications for surveillance and prevention planning. Abstract 5th IAS Conference on HIV Pathogenesis, Treatment and Prevention, July 19–22, 2009.

Busch MP, Satten GA. Time course of viremia and antibody seroconversion following human immunodeficiency virus exposure. Am J Med. 1997; 102:117–124.

Campbell-Yesufu OT, Gandhi RT. Update on human immunodeficiency virus (HIV)-2 infection. CID. 2011; 52(6):780–787.

Centers for Disease Control and Prevention. Serologic testing for antibody to human immunodeficiency virus. MMWR Morb Mortal Wkly Rep. 1988; 36:509–515.

Centers for Disease Control and Prevention. Interpretation and use of the Western blot assay for serodiagnosis of human immunodeficiency virus type 1 infections. MMWR Morb Mortal Wkly Rep 1989; 38:1–7.

Centers for Disease Control and Prevention. Update: Serologic testing for HIV-1 antibody—The United States, 1988 and 1989. MMWR Morb Mortal Wkly Rep. 1990; 39:380–383.

Centers for Disease Control and Prevention. Revised recommendations for HIV testing of adults, adolescents, and pregnant women in health-care settings. MMWR Morb Mortal Wkly Rep. 2006; 55:1–17.

Centers for Disease Control and Prevention. Revised surveillance case definitions for HIV infection among adults, adolescents, and children aged <18 months and for HIV infection and AIDS among children aged 18 months to <13 years—United States, 2008. MMWR Recommendations and Reports. 2008; 57(RR10):1–8.

Centers for Disease Control and Prevention. Laboratory testing for the diagnosis of HIV infection. 2014. Available at http://www.cdc.gov/hiv/pdf/hivtestingalgorithmrecommendation-final.pdf.

Chan DJ. Can HIV-1 incidence be estimated from plasma viral load and sexual behaviour. Int J STD AIDS. 2012 Oct; 23(10):724–728. doi:10.1258/ijsa.2009.009169.

Chappel RJ, Dax EM, Wilson KM. Immunoassays for the diagnosis of HIV: Meeting future needs by enhancing quality of testing. Future Microbiology. 2009; 48:963–982.

Ciaranello AL, Park JE, Ramirez-Avila L, et al. Early infant HIV-1 diagnosis programs in resource-limited settings: Opportunities for improved outcomes and more cost-effective interventions. BMC Medicine. 2011; 9:1–15.

Cohen MS, Gay CL, Busch MP, et al. The detection of acute HIV infection. JID. 2010; 202:S270–S277.

Daar E, Moudgil M, Meyer R, et al. Transient high levels of viremia in patients with primary human immunodeficiency virus type 1 infection. N Engl J Med. 1991; 324:961–964.

Damond F, Benard C, Jurg Boni M, et al. An international collaboration to standardize HIV-2 viral load assays: Results from the 2009 ACHIEV2E quality control study. J Clin Micro. 2011; 49:3491–3497.

Delaney KP, Branson BM, Uniyal A, et al. Evaluation of the performance characteristics of 6 rapid HIV antibody tests. CID. 2011; 52:257–263.

Dobbs T, Kennedy S, Pau C, et al. Performance characteristics of the Immunoglobulin G-Capture BED-Enzyme immunoassay, an assay to detect recent human immunodeficiency virus type 1 seroconversion. J Clin Micro. 2004; 42:2623–2628.

Elbeik T, Alvord G, Trichavaroj R, et al. Comparative analysis of HIV-1 viral load assays on subtype quantification: Bayer Versant HIV-1 RNA 3.0 versus Roche Amplicor HIV-1 Monitor Version 1.5. J AIDS. 2002; 29:330–339.

Fiebig EW, Wright DJ, Rawal BD, et al. Dynamics of HIV viremia and antibody seroconversion in plasma donors: Implications for diagnosis and staging of primary HIV infection. AIDS. 2003; 17:1871–1879.

Gottlieb, GS. Changing HIV epidemics: What HIV-2 can teach us about ending HIV-1. AIDS. 2013; 27(1):135–137.

Haar K, Amato-Gauci AJ. European men who have sex with men still at risk of HIV infection despite three decades of prevention efforts. Euro Surveill. 2015 Apr 9; 20(14):21087.

Hackett J Jr. Meeting the challenge of HIV diversity: Strategies to mitigate the impact of HIV-1 genetic heterogeneity on performance of nucleic acid testing assays. Clin Lab. 2012; 58(3–4):199–202.

Hall HI, Song R, Rhodes P, et al. Estimation of HIV incidence in the United States. JAMA. 2008; 300:520–529.

Healey D, Maskill W, Howard T, et al. HIV-1 Western blot: Development and assessment of testing to resolve indeterminate reactivity. AIDS. 1992; 6:629–633.

Hecht F, Busch M, Rawal B, et al. Use of laboratory tests and clinical symptoms for identification of primary HIV infection. AIDS. 2002; 16:1119–1129.

Hecht F, Wellman R, Busch M, et al. Identifying the early post-HIV antibody seroconversion period. JID. 2011; 204:526–533.

Houn HY, Pappas AA, Walter EM. Status of current clinical tests for human immunodeficiency virus (HIV): Applications and limitations. Ann Clin Lab Sci. 1987; 17:279–285.L

Hutchinson A, Ethridge S, Wesolowski L, et al. Costs outcomes of laboratory diagnostic algorithms for the detection of HIV. J Clin Virol. 2013 Dec; 58(Suppl 1):e2–e7. doi: 10.1016/j.jcv.2013.10.005

Hutchinson A, Patel P, Sansom S, et al. Cost-effectiveness of pooled nucleic acid amplication testing for acute HIV infection after third-generation HIV antibody screening and rapid testing in the United States: A comparison of three public health settings. PLoS Medicine. 2010; 7:e1000342.,

Janssen RS, Satten GA, Stramer SL, et al. New testing strategy to detect early HIV-1 infection for use in incidence estimates and for clinical and prevention purposes. JAMA. 1998; 280:42–48.

Karasi JC, Dziezuk F, Quennery L, et al. High correlation between the Roche COBAS AmpliPrep/COBAS TaqMan HIV-1, v2.0 and the Abbott m2000 RealTime HIV-1 assays for quantification of viral load in HIV-1 B and non-B subtypes. J Clin Virol. 2011 Nov; 52(3):181–186. doi: 10.1016/j.jcv.2011.07.002.

Kourtis AP, Bulterys M, Nesheim SR, et al. Understanding the timing of HIV transmission from mother to infant. JAMA. 2001; 285:709–712.

Louie B, Pandori M, Wong E, et al. Use of an acute seroconversion panel to evaluate a third-generation enzyme-linked immunoassay for detection of human immunodeficiency virus-specific antibodies relative to multiple other assays. J Clin Micro. 2006; 44:1856–1858.

Masciotra S, McDougal JS, Feldman J, et al. Evaluation of an alternative HIV diagnostic algorithm using specimens from seroconversion panels and persons with established HIV infections. J Clin Virol. 2011; 52S:S17–S22.

Merhi Z, Minkoff H. Rapid HIV screening for women in labor. Exp Rev Mol Diagnostics. 2005; 5:673–679.

Migueles S, Connors M. Long-term nonprogressive disease among untreated HIV-infected individuals. JAMA. 2010; 304:194–201.

Murphy G, Parry JV. Assays for the detection of recent infections with human immunodeficiency virus type 1. Eurosurveillance. 2008; 13:4–10.

Owen SM, Yang C, Spira T, et al. Alternative algorithms for human immunodeficiency virus infection diagnosis using tests that are licensed in the United States. J Clin Microbiol. 2008; 46:1588–1595.

Pandori MW, Branson BM. 2010 HIV Diagnostics Conference. Expert Review of Anti-Infective Therapy. 2010; 8:631–633.

Pandori MW, Hackett J Jr, Louie B, et al. Assessment of the ability of a fourth-generation immunoassay for human immunodeficiency virus (HIV) antibody and p24 antigen to detect both acute and recent HIV infections in a high-risk setting. J Clin Microbiol. 2009 Aug; 47(8):2639–2642. doi: 10.1128/JCM.00119-09. Epub 2009 Jun 17.

Panel on Treatment of HIV-Infected Pregnant Women and Prevention of Perinatal Transmission 2011. Recommendations for use of anti-retroviral drugs in pregnant HIV-1-infected women for maternal health and interventions to reduce perinatal HIV transmission in the United States. 2011. Available at https://aidsinfo.nih.gov/content-files/lvguidelines/perinatalgl.pdf.

Patel P, Klausner J, Bacon O, et al. Detection of acute HIV infections in high-risk patients in California. J AIDS. 2006; 42:75–79.

Patel P, Mackellar D, Simmons P, et al. Detecting acute human immunodeficiency virus infection using 3 different screening immunoassays and nucleic acid amplification testing for human immunodeficiency virus RNA, 2006–2008. Arch Int Med. 2010; 170:66–74.

Peter JB, Sevall JS. Molecular-based methods for quantifying HIV viral load. AIDS Patient Care. 2004; 18:75–79.

Pilcher C, Fiscus S, Nguyen T, et al. Detection of acute infections during HIV testing in North Carolina. N Engl J Med. 2005; 352:1873–1883.

Prejean J, Song R, Hernandez A, et al. Estimated HIV incidence in the United States, 2006–2009. PLoS One. 2011; 6:e17502.

Quinn, TC. Viral load, circumcision and heterosexual transmission. Hopkins HIV Rep. 2000 May;12(3):1, 5, 11.

Read JS; and the Committee on Pediatric AIDS. Diagnosis of HIV-1 infection in children younger than 18 months in the United States. Pediatrics. 2007; 120:e1547–e1562.

Rosenberg NE, Pilcher CD, Busch MP, et al. How can we better identify early HIV infections. Curr Opin HIV AIDS. 2015 Jan;10(1): 61–68. doi: 10.1097/COH.0000000000000121.

Sickinger E, Steiler M, Kaufman B, et al. Multicenter evaluation of a new, automated enzyme-linked immunoassay for detection of human immunodeficiency virus-specific antibodies and antigen. J Clin Microbiol. 2004; 42:21–29.

Swenson LC, Cobb B, Geretti AM, et al. Comparative performances of HIV-1 RNA load assays at low viral load levels: Results of an international collaboration. J Clin Microbiol. 2014 Feb; 52(2):517–523. doi: 10.1128/JCM.02461-13.

Vu SL, Pillonel J, Semaille C, et. al. Principles and uses of HIV incidence estimation from recent infection testing—A review. Eurosurveillance. 2008; 13:11–16.

Weber B, Fall EH, Berger A, et al. Reduction of diagnostic window by new fourth-generation immunodeficiency virus screening assays. J Clin Microbiol. 1998; 36:2235–2239.

Yerly S, Hirschel B. Diagnosing acute HIV infection. Expert Rev Ant Infect Ther. 2012; 10:31–41.

9.

THE MEDICAL HISTORY AND PHYSICAL EXAMINATION OF THE HIV-INFECTED PATIENT

Jose Martagon-Villamil and Daniel J. Skiest

LEARNING OBJECTIVE

Describe key elements of the HIV-oriented history and physical.

WHAT'S NEW?

- This chapter discusses methods to explore sexual or drug-using contacts history to identify potentially exposed persons.

KEY POINTS

- Fostering a strong and empathetic patient–physician relationship is essential for the success of the therapeutic plan.

- A comprehensive understanding of all medical and psychiatric comorbidities, medication history, exposures, risk behaviors, and current state of health is fundamental in caring for the HIV-infected individual.

- The physical exam needs to be comprehensive both for the assessment of current complaints and for baseline comparison with future findings.

THE HIV-ORIENTED MEDICAL HISTORY

The initial office or clinic visit with a new HIV-infected patient, either newly diagnosed or chronically infected, represents a unique opportunity to establish an ongoing beneficial relationship. Establishing a trusting doctor–patient relationship is predictive of future therapeutic success. The following items should be addressed in the initial history of the HIV-infected individual:

- What is the emotional status of the patient? How is he or she coping?

- Has the patient disclosed his or her HIV status to anyone (partner, family member(s), or friends)?

- Which sexual partners may have been exposed? Have they been contacted?

A full history, physical examination, and complete review of systems should be performed during the initial visit (Box 9.1 and Table 9.1). Certain elements of the history, review of systems, and exam that are unique to the HIV-infected patient should be emphasized.

THE MORE THE PATIENT KNOWS, THE BETTER HE OR SHE CAN CARE FOR HIM- OR HERSELF

Knowledge matters, especially for the patient with HIV infection, as studies have demonstrated that patients with more knowledge of their disease status do better over time. Assessing the patient's level of understanding of his or her disease, medications, and risks is essential in the comprehensive care of the HIV-infected individual. The level of sophistication will obviously be different depending on a person's background, level of education, years of infection, and other factors, but any opportunity to emphasize education, understanding, and knowledge of the disease state should be fully embraced.

Open-ended questions such as the following are recommended: "What do you know about HIV?" "What do you think you can do to maintain your health long term?"

Box 9.1 KEY ELEMENTS IN THE HIV-INFECTED INDIVIDUAL'S HISTORY

Current Health Status

- Chief complaint

- HIV history: date of probable/possible seroconversion; date of initial HIV diagnosis; CD4$^+$ nadir (if known); pretreatment CD4$^+$ T cell count and viral load; detailed antiretroviral therapy exposure history, as well as medication-related side effects; all prior resistance tests (if any)

- Hospitalization history

- Comorbidities: thorough understanding of all concurrent diseases (dermatological conditions, cancer, diabetes mellitus, hypertension, hyperlipidemia, heart disease, cerebrovascular disease, kidney disease, endocrine disease, liver disease, etc.)

- Psychiatric history (concomitant mental health diagnosis very common)

- Full medication list, including over-the-counter and herbal supplements and alternative medications

- Drug allergies with specific reaction

- Sexual history, including specific practices and history of sexually transmitted diseases (STDs), reproductive history, HIV status of partner(s)

- Detailed social history, including domestic status, history of abuse, occupational history, travel history, use of tobacco/ethyl alcohol/recreational drugs, employment status, relationship status

- Animal exposures and pets

- Complete family history

- Complete vaccination history

- Prior health care providers/HIV providers/specialists/contact information

- Health care proxy/advance directives/primary contact person in case of emergency, disclosure information

Review of Systems

- General: weight changes, fever, chills, night sweats, fatigue

- Skin: rashes, focal skin lesions, mucosal/genital lesions, psoriasis, lichen planus, seborrheic dermatitis, shingles, folliculitis, hidradenitis

- Head, eyes, ears, nose, and throat (HEENT): vision changes, oral lesions, thrush

- Hemolymphatic: lymphadenopathy/splenic enlargement or splenectomy

- Endocrine: thyroid disorders, diabetes, lipid disorders

- Cardiac coronary artery disease/risk factors/endocarditis

- Pulmonary: asthma/pneumonia/cough/tuberculosis/purified protein derivative (or interferon-γ release assay) status

- Gastrointestinal: hepatitis (including vaccination hepatitis A and B status), pancreatitis, diarrhea, cholelithiasis, peptic ulcer disease/gastroesophageal reflux disease, use of antacid agents

- Genitourinary: kidney disorders/urolithiasis/sexual dysfunction, STDs

- Musculoskeletal: arthritis/osteoporosis/gout

- Neurologic: peripheral neuropathy/headaches/meningitis/cognitive dysfunction, stroke

- Psychiatric: psychiatric disease/hospitalizations/suicidal attempt/sleep disturbance, feelings of depression, suicidality, anxiety

Table 9.1 PHYSICAL EXAM OF THE HIV-INFECTED PATIENT

BODY ORGAN/ SYSTEM	BE ESPECIALLY ATTENTIVE TO
General	• Weight loss, body mass index, blood pressure, pulse, respiration rate, temperature • Pain
Skin	• Rash, seborrheic dermatitis, folliculitis, moles, psoriasis, lichen planus, Kaposi sarcoma lesions • Warts, vesicular lesions, dermatophytes, molluscum contagiosum • Needle marks
HEENT	• Visual acuity • Retinal CMV (hemorrhages and exudates) • HIV retinopathy (cotton-wool spots) • Oral exam: thrush, oral hairy leukoplakia, Kaposi lesions, gingivitis, aphthous ulcers, chancres, dentition • Thyroid exam
Hemolymphatic	• Regional versus generalized lymphadenopathy • Splenomegaly
Cardiac	• Heart sounds, murmurs, gallop
Pulmonary	• Focal or generalized abnormalities
Gastrointestinal	• Jaundice, hepatomegaly • Abdominal masses • Anorectal exam (ulcers, vesicles, chancres, masses, hemorrhoids, warts)

Genitourinary	• Ulcers, warts, chancres, herpetic vesicles
	• Gender-specific exam
	  For women: pelvic exam, cervical exam, Pap smear
	  For men: testicular exam
	  For either: if indicated, anal Pap

Neurologic	• Mental status, cognitive function—consider baseline HIV cognitive assessment (Montreal Cognitive Assessment test) • Cranial nerves, motor strength, sensation, gait, vibratory/proprioceptive exam
Psychiatric	• Depression screen (PHQ-9 or other validated tools) • Evidence of self-injury or self-mutilation • Evidence of abuse

HEENT, head, eyes, ears, nose, and throat.

COMMUNICATION IS KEY

Both HIV infection and the treatments for it will impact other medical conditions. For example, many medications used to treat HIV and its comorbid conditions have drug interactions. Thus, it is essential for the HIV provider (if he or she is not the primary care provider) to be in close communication with the patient's primary care provider and other health care providers involved in the care of the patient. Both the patient and the other health care providers should be aware of the potential for drug interactions before prescribing any new medications, including herbal and over-the-counter products.

SENSITIVE, RESPECTFUL, AND AWARE

HIV providers frequently care for patients with a wide variety of sexual practices, patients who have been victims of abuse, patients who are or have been commercial sex workers, patients who have used intravenous drugs, and individuals in the gay/lesbian/transgender/bisexual communities. Issues of privacy and cultural sensitivity are especially relevant in these encounters. Fostering trust—encouraging truthfulness and openness in the patient–physician relationship—requires special attention to cultivating a nonjudgmental and approachable demeanor. It is important to be sensitive to patients' priorities, be respectful of their individuality, and be aware of their self-perception.

THE HIV-ORIENTED PHYSICAL EXAMINATION

Sir William Osler is credited with the saying, "He who knows syphilis knows medicine." The modern-day equivalent of the old adage is "He who knows HIV knows medicine," because indeed HIV infection and its sequelae can affect every organ system and present in every clinical way possible. The HIV-oriented exam, therefore, needs to be especially comprehensive, both for the assessment of current complaints and for establishing a baseline to compare with future findings.

CULTURAL COMPETENCY ISSUES

In an increasingly globalized and diverse society, clinicians are caring for patients from very different backgrounds, cultures, and places of origin. Training programs are placing more emphasis on cultural competency skills, and the HIV medicine world is no exception.

PATIENT-CENTERED APPROACH

The first step to cultural competency is to avoid generalizations, stereotyping, and assumptions. Not all Latino/Hispanic individuals necessarily share the same culture. All Muslim patients do not have the same needs. The many different Asian cultures are not interchangeable. Explore each individual's sensitivities, expectations, and perspectives. Build trust by developing understanding, showing curiosity, and respecting limits.

TRADITIONS, BELIEFS, AND FAMILY INVOLVEMENT

Different cultures bring to the table different degrees of family and individual involvement in patient care.

Negotiating through a balance of autonomy, informed decision-making, and a culturally acceptable degree of family participation may be fundamental for successful outcomes. Explore beliefs and spirituality, inquire about the use of alternative or non-Western medical approaches, and ask about disease understanding in terms of cultural value systems.

LANGUAGE

Providing HIV care through an interpreter may add another layer of complexity to an already challenging encounter. However, the alternative is certainly less desirable: Language barriers may account for significant misunderstandings in diagnosis and treatment, as well as errors in medication administration, follow-up, and overall clinical care in minorities and immigrants. Clinicians should explore the language competency and literacy of all patients and proactively check for feedback in terms of understanding and comfort with instructions.

Recommended Reading

Aberg JA, Gallant JE, Ghanem KG, et al. Primary care guidelines for the management of persons infected with HIV: 2013 update by the HIV Medicine Association of the Infectious Disease Society of America. *Clin Infect Dis*. 2014; 58:1–34.

10.

INITIAL LABORATORY EVALUATION AND RISK STRATIFICATION OF THE HIV-INFECTED PATIENT

Jose Martagon-Villamil and Daniel J. Skiest

LEARNING OBJECTIVE

Describe the core baseline laboratory evaluation of the recently diagnosed HIV-infected patient.

WHAT'S NEW?

- In stable patients with suppressed viral load, CD4 count monitoring is only required at 6- to 12-month intervals.
- In stable patients with virologic suppression for 2 years or more, viral load monitoring can be decreased to every 6 months.

KEY POINT

- Essential tests include CD4$^+$ count, HIV viral load, HIV resistance assay, and serologic evaluation for certain opportunistic infections.

To adequately understand the HIV-infected individual's stage of disease, risk profile, and management needs, a series of laboratory tests must be performed (Table 10.1). The availability and indication for many of these may be influenced by cost considerations, especially in resource-limited settings.

Table 10.1 BASELINE LABORATORY AND DIAGNOSTIC TESTING FOR THE NEWLY DIAGNOSED HIV-INFECTED PATIENT

TEST	COMMENTS
HIV antibody testing	• Consider repeating if no prior documentation available.
CD4$^+$ count (absolute and percentage)	• Establishes the stage of HIV infection. • Identifies the risk of complications and opportunistic infections, as well as the indications for prophylaxis. • Initially, monitor every 3–6 months; in clinically stable patients with consistent virologic suppression, monitoring is needed only every 6–12 months.
HIV RNA level (viral load)	• Helps predict the rate of CD4 loss and risk of clinical progression. • Consider obtaining two values to establish a firm baseline (viral set point) prior to therapy. • Initially obtain 2–4 weeks after starting or changing ART, and then monitor every 3 or 4 months; can decrease intervals to 6 months in clinically stable, adherent patients with consistent virologic suppression.
Drug resistance testing	• A baseline resistance test should be part of the initial evaluation due to the possibility of transmission of drug-resistant virus (~5–15% in developed countries). • Genotypic tests preferred initially, including screening for integrase strand transfer resistance. • May influence the components of ART. • May be useful in guiding future antiretroviral choices in the event of treatment failure. • Repeat in the event of treatment failure or prior to antiretroviral modification.

(continued)

Table 10.1 CONTINUED

TEST	COMMENTS
Complete blood count with differential	• Screen for anemia, thrombocytopenia, or leukopenia. • Essential for future comparison during therapy. • Eosinophilia may be a clue to parasitic infection, allergy or atopy, eosinophilic folliculitis, or drug-related reactions. • In resource-limited settings, the absolute lymphocyte count may be a surrogate marker for $CD4^+$ count.
Electrolytes and renal function (BUN, creatinine)	• Baseline estimated GFR is essential for adequate drug dosing and choice of initial ART. • Elevated BUN/Cr may be a clue to HIV-associated nephropathy, in itself an indication for therapy.
Liver function tests (AST, ALT, bilirubin, alkaline phosphatase)	• May be a clue to subclinical hepatitis. • May influence the choice of ART.
Hepatitis serology profile	• Screening for hepatitis A–C establishes the need for vaccination and the indication for further workup in terms of active coinfection(s). • May influence the choice of ART.
Fasting blood glucose	• May influence the choice of ART.
Lipid profile	• A baseline is needed to assess the effect of ART on these parameters.
G6PD screen	• Establishes the risk of hemolytic anemia with certain medications, including primaquine and dapsone.
HLA-B5701 screen	• Establishes the risk of abacavir hypersensitivity syndrome and, if positive, represents a contraindication for its use. • Obtain at baseline or prior to prescribing abacavir.
Toxoplasma serology (IgG)	• Identifies need for *Toxoplasma* prophylaxis, when $CD4^+$ count is <100 cells/mm^3. • If negative, may be an indication for counseling, to avoid infection.
Co-receptor tropism assay	• Obtain only prior to prescribing a CCR5 inhibitor.
Syphilis serology	• Screen for latent syphilis. • A positive test may indicate further workup (specific treponemal test) and may be an indication for therapy. • Screen yearly in patients at risk for STDs.
Tuberculosis screening	• A baseline tuberculin skin test (PPD) or IGRA is indicated in all HIV-infected individuals without a history of prior positive test or treatment for latent TB. • Note that a PPD result ≥5 mm induration is considered reactive in HIV-infected patients. • If positive, a chest X-ray should be obtained to rule out active disease along with a careful ROS and exam to rule out extrapulmonary TB.
Sexually transmitted diseases	• Screen all women for trichomoniasis and women age ≤25 years for chlamydia. • Screen men and women for gonorrhea and chlamydia initially. • Screen yearly in patients at risk for STDs. • If positive, this is an indication for treatment and counseling on prevention of STDs.
Cervical Pap smear	• Establishes human papillomavirus infection and risk for neoplastic transformation. • All HIV-infected women should receive a cervical Pap smear (see Chapter 13).
Anal Pap smear	• Consider anal Pap testing in HIV-infected men or women with a history of receptive anal intercourse or abnormal cervical Pap and/or genital warts. However, the optimal follow-up of an abnormal anal Pap has not yet been definitively established.
Age-appropriate health care maintenance	• Breast cancer and colon cancer screening should follow age-appropriate guidelines. • The US Preventive Services Task Force has recommended against routine prostate cancer screening in men using prostate-specific antigen.
DXA	• Baseline bone DXA screening for osteoporosis in postmenopausal women and men age 50 years or older.

ART, antiretroviral therapy; BUN, blood urea nitrogen; DXA, densitometry; GFR, gromerular filtration rate; IGRA, interferon-gamma release assay; PPD, purified protein derivative; ROS, review of systems; STD, sexually transmitted diseases; TB, tuberculosis.

Recommended Reading

Aberg JA, Gallant JE, Ghanem KG, et al. Primary care guidelines for the management of persons infected with HIV: 2013 update by the HIV Medicine Association of the Infectious Disease Society of America. *Clin Infect Dis*. 2014; 58:1–34.

US Department of Health and Human Services, Panel on Antiretroviral Guidelines for Adults and Adolescents. Guidelines for the use of antiretroviral agents in HIV-1-infected adults and adolescents. Available at http://www.aidsinfo.nih.gov/ContentFiles/AdultandAdolescentGL.pdf. Accessed November 20, 2015.

11.

CLINICAL SYNDROMES AND DIFFERENTIAL DIAGNOSIS IN THE HIV-INFECTED PATIENT

Jose Martagon-Villamil and Daniel J. Skiest

CLINICAL PRESENTATION OF ACUTE RETROVIRAL INFECTION

The acute retroviral syndrome (or primary HIV infection) has been variously compared to a "mononucleosis-like" syndrome, a "generalized viral illness," or a "fever–myalgia–rash" syndrome. In one series, in which patients with suspected mononucleosis who had a negative Monospot test underwent HIV testing, the incidence of acute HIV syndrome was 2% (Rosenberg, 1999). The true incidence of acute HIV illness has been difficult to determine accurately. Published series estimate that the incidence of symptomatic, acute retroviral syndrome ranges from 40% to 90% (Kassutto, 2004), depending on the definition and which symptoms are considered attributable to acute HIV infection.

The clinical presentation of acute HIV may include most commonly fever, myalgia, pharyngitis/sore throat, lymphadenopathy, rash, diarrhea, and headache, in various combinations (Table 11.1). The rash tends to be erythematous/maculopapular, nonpruritic, and involves most commonly the trunk and extremities and, occasionally, the face, palms, or soles. A subset of patients may present with aseptic meningitis. In some cases, patients may present with disease severe enough to warrant hospitalization, including hypotension; ulcerative disease of oral, genital, or rectal areas; hemophagocytic syndrome; and, rarely, a full-blown opportunistic infection, including oropharyngeal candidiasis and/or esophagitis, *Pneumocystis* pneumonia, or gastrointestinal cytomegalovirus disease. In one large series,

Table 11.1 SIGNS AND SYMPTOMS OF ACUTE RETROVIRAL ILLNESS

SIGNS AND SYMPTOMS	APPROXIMATE INCIDENCE (%)
Fever	48–88
Pharyngitis/sore throat	21–51
Lymphadenopathy	36–45
Rash	12–47
Oral ulcers	12–17
Myalgia/arthralgia	28–46
Diarrhea	17–35
Headache	34–44
Hepatosplenomegaly	10–15
Oral/oropharyngeal or vaginal candidiasis	10+
Weight loss	21–39
Neurologic syndromes Aseptic meningitis Peripheral neuropathy Guillain–Barré syndrome	Approximately 10+

30% of patients with acute retroviral syndrome presented with atypical signs and symptoms of an acute opportunistic infection (Braun, 2015).

Laboratory abnormalities that may point to acute retroviral illness include thrombocytopenia, leukopenia/lymphopenia, and a mild transaminitis, especially if seen in conjunction with the previously discussed symptoms.

The key factor in diagnosing acute HIV infection remains an accurate and thorough history and exam, especially eliciting a suggestive exposure history—for example, risk behaviors including sexual activity or blood-borne exposure (sharing needles in the case of injecting drug use). Patients with concomitant sexually transmitted diseases are more likely to acquire HIV.

When acute HIV illness is suspected, the clinician should keep in mind that conventional (third-generation) serologic tests (HIV enzyme-linked immunosorbent assay/Western blot) may be negative or indeterminate because antibodies may take 3 or 4 weeks to be measured, and the person may be in the "window period" for developing a positive test. Therefore, if the HIV antibody test is negative or indeterminate, an HIV RNA should be ordered to rule out the presence of replicating virus. However, the fourth-generation HIV antibody–antigen complex is more sensitive in the setting of recently acquired infection because it measures both HIV antibodies and p24 antigen and can detect HIV within 2 weeks of infection. Currently, this is the screening/diagnostic test recommended by the Centers for Disease Control and Prevention (CDC).

Recommended Reading

Braun DL, Kouyos RD, Balmer B, et al. Frequency and spectrum of unexpected clinical manifestations of primary HIV-1 infection. *Clin Infect Dis.* 2015; 61:1013–1021.

Kassutto S, Rosenberg S. Primary HIV type 1 infection. *Clin Infect Dis.* 2004; 38:1447–1453.

Quinn TC. Acute primary HIV infection. *JAMA.* 1997; 278:58–62.

CLINICAL PRESENTATION OF CHRONIC INFECTION

In 2006, the CDC recommended universal voluntary screening for HIV in adults as part of "usual" medical care. Although the number of undiagnosed individuals has declined since then, the CDC estimates that up to 13% of persons infected with HIV in the United States may be unaware of their status (a decrease from 20% in 2003).

Even today, patients may present with manifestations of advanced AIDS at the time of their initial diagnosis. Clinicians should maintain a high index of suspicion in patients with known risk behaviors, and they should screen for HIV on a regular basis. Specific symptoms and signs that may suggest chronic HIV infection and should warrant testing include the following:

• Oral ulcers/aphthous stomatitis

• Oral hairy leukoplakia

• Oral candidiasis

• Unexplained weight loss

• Unexplained chronic fatigue

• Persistent or difficult-to-control seborrheic dermatitis

• Persistent or difficult-to-control vaginal candidiasis

• Unexplained/persistent fevers

• Herpes zoster/shingles (especially if more than one dermatome or recurrent, and especially in young people)

• Chronic diarrhea

• Persistent night sweats

• Persistent generalized lymphadenopathy

• Severe or difficult-to-control psoriasis

• Chronic or persistent herpes simplex infection of the genital tract or perianal region

Likewise, some laboratory findings may clue the clinician to the possibility of chronic HIV infection:

- Chronic thrombocytopenia
- Leukopenia
- Anemia of chronic inflammation, especially without an alternative explanation
- Low lipid levels (low cholesterol, high-density lipoprotein (HDL), and low-density lipoprotein (LDL)), with elevated triglycerides; this has been attributed to chronic inflammatory cytokines (Grunfeld, 1992)
- Elevated globulin:albumin ratio, indicating polyclonal gammopathy
- Persistent or intermittent unexplained transaminitis
- Low albumin or pre-albumin, especially if wasting is present
- Decreased renal function with proteinuria (HIV nephropathy)

Also, a new diagnosis of certain diseases should prompt an HIV test because their incidence is increased in HIV-infected individuals:

- Active tuberculosis
- Non-Hodgkin lymphoma or Hodgkin disease
- Cervical carcinoma in situ
- Listeriosis in an otherwise non-immune-suppressed or pregnant patient
- Extraintestinal salmonellosis
- Recurrent bacterial pneumonia
- Bacteremic pneumococcal pneumonia

HIV WASTING SYNDROME

DIAGNOSIS

HIV wasting syndrome is an AIDS-defining condition and is defined as weight loss of greater than 10%, plus either chronic diarrhea or chronic weakness, for more than 30 days in the absence of an alternative explanation.

In 2004, Polsky et al. published an updated definition, describing HIV wasting as any one of the following (Consensus Development Panel Meeting, 2000):

- 10% unintentional weight loss over 12 months
- 7.5% unintentional weight loss over 6 months
- 5% body cell mass (BCM) loss within 6 months
- Body mass index (BMI) <20 kg/m^2
  - In men: BCM <35% body weight and BMI <27 kg/m^2
  - In women: BCM <23% body weight and BMI <27 kg/m^2

BCM (defined as fat-free mass without bone mineral mass and extracellular water) can be measured by body composition testing, either underwater weighing in research settings or, more commonly in clinical practice, total body potassium or bioelectrical impedance analysis. However, this is rarely done in the ART era. In the pre-ART era, wasting was a common AIDS-related presentation, estimated to occur in approximately 20% of patients. Although much less common in the ART era, when present, it can be an important and challenging condition; its presence has been associated with increased morbidity and mortality and more rapid disease progression.

The cause of HIV wasting is not known, but it is likely multifactorial. Many patients likely have a combination of inadequate caloric intake and an increased rate of metabolism due to increased resting energy expenditure in untreated HIV infection. When wasting is suspected, treatable causes need to be ruled out, especially opportunistic diseases, infectious causes of diarrhea/malabsorption, thyroid dysfunction, malignancy, protein-calorie malnutrition (especially from economic or financial factors), hypogonadism, and psychiatric disease (especially depression). The workup for these should be tailored according to each person's signs and symptoms. In males, measurement of morning serum testosterone (free and total) is recommended, especially if there are signs of hypogonadism. It is important to differentiate wasting from lipodystrophy or lipoatrophy in the setting of ART. Peripheral lipoatrophy due to nucleoside analogs (especially stavudine, didanosine, and zidovudine, which are currently rarely used), can be confused with wasting. However, neither the presence of lipodystrophy nor the use of ART rule out the possibility of wasting.

MANAGEMENT

The management of HIV-associated wasting should include the following (Polsky, 2004):

- Prompt recognition/diagnosis
- Targeted workup for treatable causes
- Commencement of or optimization of ART

Table 11.2 NONPHARMACOLOGIC INTERVENTIONS FOR HIV-ASSOCIATED WASTING

INTERVENTION	COMMENTS
Treatment of underlying causes	• Targeted workup according to each patient's clinical presentation. • Infectious and opportunistic diseases should be ruled out.
Nutritional supplements	• Targeted caloric supplementation is encouraged. • Dietary assessment and counseling should be an integral part of the treatment plan. • Swallowing evaluation may be needed in select cases. • Alternative routes of feeding may be considered in select cases (nasogastric, gastric or jejunal tubes, and parenteral nutrition). • Glutamine replacement (40 g daily in divided doses) and antioxidants may help patients gain weight and body cell mass (Shabert, 1999).
Addressing psychosocial and life stressors	• Financial realities may be an important component to malnutrition in indigent, homeless, migrant, or otherwise vulnerable populations. • Depression and anxiety may be significant contributors to weight loss.
Exercise	• As an adjunct to nutritional support, may improve function, quality of life, and lean body mass.

Table 11.3 PHARMACOLOGIC INTERVENTIONS FOR HIV-ASSOCIATED WASTING

INTERVENTION	DOSE	COMMENTS
ART	Specific to each regimen	• The best and most effective regimen should be selected for each individual patient, with the goal of maintaining an undetectable viral load. • ART should not be thought of as the sole solution to wasting because weight loss and loss of body mass may still occur despite therapy, with or without adequate virologic control.
Appetite stimulators		• Both agents are effective for appetite stimulation and modest weight gain in patients with appetite loss. Not effective in patients with wasting but normal appetite.
Megestrol acetate (Megace)	400–800 mg/day	• Most weight gain is fat (e.g., not lean body mass).
Dronabinol (Marinol)	2.5 mg twice a day	• Megace (progestin analogue) can be associated with hyperglycemia, diarrhea, rash, adrenal insufficiency, erectile dysfunction, gynecomastia, and, over longer periods of time, hypogonadism. • Marinol can cause fatigue and central nervous system side effects, including confusion, dizziness, euphoria, paranoia, somnolence, and anxiety. • There is no benefit to the use of both drugs combined. • Both are US Food and Drug Administration (FDA) approved for weight loss in HIV/AIDS.
Testosterone replacement therapy		• Indicated for males only because there are minimal data for females. • Testosterone free and total levels should be checked in the morning due to diurnal variation.
Cypionate injection	200 mg every 2 weeks	• If low, testosterone replacement may be indicated, which improves lean body mass, energy, libido, and quality of life.
Enanthanate injection	2–6 mg/day	• A digital rectal exam and prostate-specific antigen test are recommended at baseline and every 3–6 months. • Not a specific FDA-approved indication.
Transdermal patch (Androderm)	Dose varies	
1% gel	No specific dosing data in HIV-positive patients	
1.62% gel		
Subcutaneous pellet implanted at 3- to 6-month intervals		
Buccal form		
Anabolic steroids		• May have a role in patients with wasting but normal testosterone levels, but they are not more effective than testosterone (Corcoran et al., 1999).
Nandrolone	100–150 mg IM every 2 weeks	• Role in women unclear.
Oxandrolone	40 mg PO daily	• Weight gain and improved muscle mass.
Oxymetholone	50 mg PO two or three times/day	• Long-term use may be associated with decrease in HDL, increase in LDL, prostate hypertrophy, hypogonadism, liver dysfunction, mood swings, increased hematocrit, acne, hair loss, sleep apnea, and, over time, increased risk of breast and prostate cancer. • Oxandrolone is FDA approved for weight gain in chronic infections.

Table 11.3 CONTINUED

INTERVENTION	DOSE	COMMENTS
Recombinant human growth hormone (rHGH)	35–45 kg: 4 mg SC daily 45–55 kg: 5 mg SC daily >55 kg: 6 mg SC daily	• Multiple trials have documented benefits, including weight gain, increase in lean body mass, decrease in fat, and increased quality of life. • No significant changes observed beyond 12 weeks of therapy, although weight gain can be maintained. • Adverse effects may include edema, myalgia/arthralgia, glucose intolerance, pancreatitis, and carpal tunnel syndrome. • Cost issues may be a barrier to use. • FDA approved indication (Serostim).
Thalidomide	100–200 mg PO daily	• Thought to cause weight gain by cytokine modulation, increase in tumor necrosis factor-α. • Side effects may include neutropenia, rash, peripheral neuropathy, and severe teratogenicity for the fetus, so its use in women of childbearing age mandates reliable contraception. • Access is very restricted, requiring extensive documentation from the prescribing physician. • Rarely used. • Not an FDA-approved indication.
Cannabis	N/A	• Not legal in every state. • Very limited actual data for wasting syndrome in HIV. A Cochrane review (2013) failed to show benefit.
Tesamorelin (Egrfta)	2 mg SC qd	• Growth hormone-releasing factor analogue. • Not an FDA-approved indication. • May cause hyperglycemia.

HDL, high-density lipoprotein; LDL, low-density lipoprotein.

• Corrective measures for the weight loss, including dietary/nutritional assessment and support, with supplements as needed

• Additional therapeutic interventions as needed in each individual case to target appetite stimulation and weight gain (specifically lean body mass)

• Proactively addressing psychosocial and lifestyle issues, especially depression, financial stressors, and transportation

Nonpharmacologic and pharmacologic interventions for HIV-associated wasting are shown in Tables 11.2 and 11.3, respectively.

References

Braun DL, Kouyos RD, Balmer B, et al. Frequency and spectrum of unexpected clinical manifestations of primary HIV-1 infection. *Clin Infect Dis*. 2015; 61:1013–1021.

Consensus Development Panel Meeting. Treatment guidelines for HIV-associated wasting. New York, 2000.

Corcoran C, Grinspoon S. Treatments for wasting in patients with the acquired immunodeficiency syndrome. N Engl J Med. 1999: 340:1740–1750.

Grunfeld C, Pang M, Doerrler WT, et al. Lipids, lipoproteins, triglyceride clearance, and cytokines in human immunodeficiency virus infection and the acquired immunodeficiency syndrome. J Clin Endocrinol Metab. 1992; 74:1045–1052.

Kassutto S, Rosenberg S. Primary HIV type 1 infection. Clin Infect Dis. 2004; 38:1447–1453.

Polsky B, Kotler D. Treatment guidelines for HIV-associated wasting. HIV Clinical Trials. 2004; 5:50–61.

Rosenberg E, Caliendo A, Walker B. Acute HIV infection among patients tested for mononucleosis. N Engl J Med. 1999; 340:969.

Shabert JK, Winslow C, Lacey J, et al. Glutamine-antioxidant supplementation increases body cell mass in AIDS patients with weight loss: A randomized, double-blind controlled trial. Nutrition. 1999; 15:860–864.

12.

HEALTH MAINTENANCE

Babatunde Edun, Michelle K. Haas, Christopher Brendemuhl,

Jason V. Baker, and Anthony C. Speights

PRIMARY CARE NEEDS OF THE HIV INFECTED PATIENT

LEARNING OBJECTIVE

Provide a framework for incorporating a health maintenance flowsheet into the electronic health record.

The most recent guidelines for HIV infection recommend therapy for all those willing to start treatment regardless of CD4 count (INSIGHT START Study Group, 2015). The introduction of highly potent antiretroviral agents has transformed HIV from a disease with a once dismal prognosis to a manageable chronic medical condition. The life expectancy of a newly infected person who is started on therapy in a timely manner now approaches that of the uninfected individual. Persons living with HIV now live longer but are also at increased risk for certain cardiovascular and renal diseases (Althoff, 2015; Freiberg, 2013; Mills, 2012). As a result of these changes, the primary care needs of the HIV-infected patient have increased. The primary care provider as well as the HIV care provider must now focus on aspects of preventive medicine that improve the quality of life and life expectancy of the HIV-infected person. The Health Resources and Services Administration HIV/AIDS Bureau (HRSA) now mandates reporting of several aspects of HIV care as core performance measures for HIV programs that receive federal funding (HRSA, 2013). Certain Centers for Medicare and Medicaid Services (CMS) quality. Reporting and payment programs such as the Medicare and Medicaid Electronic Health Record (EHR) Incentive Program for Eligible Professionals also require reporting of certain metrics and provide incentives to eligible hospitals

and professionals when they demonstrate meaningful use of certified EHR technology. CMS also imposes penalties on health care programs not meeting the set targets for meaningful use of EHR technology (CMS, 2015). Through the use of flowsheets, the EHR provides a valuable method for ensuring that the salient aspects of care are not omitted and that the appropriate information is obtained for various reporting agencies.

Although most EHR systems allow for customized disease-specific flowsheets, at a minimum every flowsheet should have four parts: basic demographics, the specifics of the disease being managed, recommended routine vaccines, and important laboratory data. For HIV in particular, the flowsheet should include serial CD4$^+$ counts and viral load measurements. The recommended age and disease-specific vaccines and laboratory values such as the rapid plasma reagin (RPR), hepatitis serology, tuberculosis skin or blood tests, and important data on medication allergies, smoking history, and glucose-6-phosphate dehydrogenase (G6PD) deficiency should be included in the flowsheet. Documentation of any drug-resistance profiles should also be made. Individuals whose HIV status is unknown should be tested at least once and then subsequently based on risk factors. Ideally, the flowsheet should serve as a clinical reminder for the practitioner.

Patient demographic data, such as name, gender, date of birth, next of kin, and health care proxy, and insurance carrier information are usually obtained during the registration process and are available on the chart coversheet or patient summary section. Patient allergies and information at each visit such as vital signs, weight, body mass index (BMI), and height should also populate this screen. Tables 12.1–12.4 show examples of a health care maintenance flowsheet addressing HIV and primary health care.

Table 12.1 HEALTH CARE MAINTENANCE FLOWSHEET

HIV DIAGNOSTIC INFORMATION

    i. Date of HIV diagnosis

   ii. HIV risk group:

       a. MSM

       b. IDU

       c. Heterosexual

       d. MSM/IDU

       e. Blood transfusion/iatrogenic

       f. Not known

  iii. CD4 T lymphocyte cell count (CD4 count) at diagnosis

  iv. Current HIV regimen and date started

	CD4 COUNT	HIV VL (HIV RNA PCR)
Date (most recent)		
Date		
Date		
. . .		

ANNUAL SCREENING FLOWSHEET		
	DATE	RESULT
RPR/syphilis screen		
TB skin test/interferon-gamma release assay		
Pap smear		
Rectal exam		
Mammogram (flag if >40 years)		
Eye exam		
Dental evaluation		
Colon cancer screening		
Urinalysis		
Lipid panel (Chol, Trig, LDL, HDL)		
HIV knowledge assessment		
Risk reduction counseling		
Mental health screening		
Hepatitis C Ab (repeat if risk factors present)		

Table 12.2 IMMUNIZATION HISTORY FLOWSHEET

IMMUNIZATION HISTORY

	DATE(S) OFFERED	ADMINISTERED/DECLINED
Pneumovax (PPSV23)		
Prevnar (PCV13)		
Twinrix series		
Hepatitis A series		
Hepatitis B series		
TD		
Tdap		
Influenza vaccine		
...		

ANTIBODY TITERS (PREPOPULATE FROM LABS IF AVAILABLE)

Hepatitis Bs Ag
Hepatitis Bs Ab
Hepatitis Bc IgM
Hepatitis Be Ag
Hepatitis Be Ab
Hepatitis A total Ab
Hepatitis A IgM Ab

Table 12.3 MEDICAL HISTORY/PROBLEM LIST FLOWSHEET

MEDICAL HISTORY/PROBLEM LIST

	DATE DIAGNOSED/DATE OF SURGERY
AIDS defining illnesses	
(allow multiple entries)	
Medical problems (current); e.g., hypertension, diabetes mellitus	
Medical history (non-active or "closed"); e.g., latent TB status post treatment	
Previous surgeries (allow multiple entries)	

Table 12.4 HIV DIAGNOSTICS FLOWSHEET

HIV DIAGNOSTICS

	DATE	RESULT
HLA B*5701		
Tropism test		
G6PD level		
Toxoplasma titer (IgG)		
CMV serology		
HIV resistance testing (allow multiple entries)		

References

Althoff KN, McGinnis KA, Wyatt CM, et al. Comparison of risk and age at diagnosis of myocardial infarction, end-stage renal disease, and non-AIDS-defining cancer in HIV-infected versus uninfected adults. *Clin Infect Dis.* 2015; 60(4):627–638.

Centers for Medicare and Medicaid Services. An introduction to the Medicare EHR incentive program for eligible professionals April 2015. Available at https://www.cms.gov/Regulations-and-Guidance/Legislation/EHRIncentivePrograms/downloads/beginners_guide.pdf. Accessed December 17, 2015.

Freiberg MS, Chang CC, Kuller LH, et al. HIV infection and the risk of acute myocardial infarction. *JAMA Intern Med.* 2013; 173(8):614–622.

Health Resources and Services Administration HIV/AIDS Programs. HAB HIV performance measures. November 2013. Available at http://hab.hrsa.gov/deliverhivaidscare/habperformmeasures.html. Accessed December 17, 2015.

INSIGHT START Study Group. Initiation of antiretroviral therapy in early asymptomatic HIV infection. *N Engl J Med.* 2015; 373(9):795–807.

Mills EJ, Bärnighausen T, Negin J. HIV and aging—Preparing for the challenges ahead. *N Engl J Med.* 2012; 366(14):1270–1273.

TUBERCULOSIS SCREENING AND ASSESSMENT

LEARNING OBJECTIVE

Describe tuberculosis screening indications (including exposure history) and assessment methods (including selection, interpretation, and limitations of screening tests in HIV-infected patients).

WHAT'S NEW?

Interferon-gamma release assays (IGRAs) are an alternative to tuberculin skin tests (TSTs) for detection of *Mycobacterium tuberculosis* infection and are preferred for individuals aged 5 years or older who are Bacillus Calmette–Guerin (BCG) vaccinated.

KEY POINTS

- Due to immunodeficiency, HIV-positive individuals are at increased risk for developing active tuberculosis (TB) disease and thus should be routinely screened for TB.

- HIV-positive individuals also frequently have other indications for TB screening, including contact with persons from areas of the world where there is a high incidence of TB and high-risk exposures in correctional and residential facilities.

- In HIV-positive individuals, TSTs or IGRAs should be performed at the time of initial HIV diagnosis. For persons who are initially TST or IGRA negative, testing should be repeated in those who have experienced improvement in immune function due to antiretroviral therapy (ART). Annual testing may be considered in persons with ongoing or repeated exposure to TB.

- TST responses of ≥5 mm in duration are considered positive in persons with HIV. However, even negative TST or IGRA results may warrant preventive therapy in the setting of high-risk exposures.

- Chest radiography is indicated regardless of TST or IGRA results in HIV-positive individuals with recent exposure to patients with active TB, or a history of symptoms consistent with TB, as well as in any HIV-infected person with a positive test result.

HIV-associated immune compromise is associated with an increased incidence of TB among HIV-infected individuals, with a relative risk of 10 times that of HIV-negative persons (Horsburgh, 2011). As with other opportunistic infections, there has been a substantial decrease in the incidence of TB among persons receiving ART. However, untreated TB is one of the few opportunistic infections transmissible to others and thus has additional public health implications for control and prevention.

HIV-infected individuals are at increased risk for developing active disease by reactivation of untreated latent TB infection (LTBI), at an estimated rate of 3–16% *per year* compared to 5–10% *lifetime* risk in HIV-negative persons with no other risk factors. Once infection with *M. tuberculosis* occurs, there can be rapid progression of newly acquired infection to disease—for example, within the first month following exposure to an infectious person. Similarly, reactivation disease may also progress rapidly, particularly in highly immunocompromised individuals. The majority of HIV-negative individuals infected with TB who develop active disease in the United States were born, previously lived, or traveled for extended periods of time in TB endemic areas. Currently, 8% of individuals with active TB have underlying HIV disease. However, prior to the advent of ART, in the United States, the proportion of individuals with TB who had underlying HIV was nearly 50%. TB outbreaks were identified among individuals living with HIV in US institutional settings, including health care facilities, correctional facilities, and homeless shelters. Although transmission in institutional settings in the United States is now rare, there is substantial risk in resource-limited settings in which TB is endemic in the general population. HIV-infected individuals who are employees or volunteers in settings identified as high risk by local health authorities should be advised of their risk of exposure to TB and offered alternate sites of work. HIV-infected health care workers who intermittently work or volunteer in TB endemic countries should be similarly advised about their risk. The health care provider should help the patient assess the level of risk by evaluating factors such as the prevalence of TB in that community, the precautions against transmission that are in place, and the patient's specific duties in those settings.

HIV-infected individuals, especially those with CD4$^+$ cell counts <200/μl, are more likely to present with extrapulmonary TB, miliary pulmonary disease, and disseminated TB compared to HIV-uninfected persons. Persons with HIV may have active pulmonary TB with normal chest radiographs. Similarly, HIV–TB co-infected patients may present with negative acid-fast bacilli (AFB) sputum in up to 70% of cases (Getahun, 2007). In a high-incidence setting and active case-finding study of patients with culture-positive TB, up to 32% had normal chest radiographs; of those who were AFB smear-negative and had normal chest radiographs, 8% had TB, 5% had CD4$^+$ cell counts ≥350/μl, and 10% had CD4$^+$ cell counts <350/μl (Cain, 2010). Nucleic acid amplification tests such as Gene Xpert MTB/RIF are more sensitive than AFB smear, and they may identify up to 70% of smear-negative, culture-positive cases (Boehme 2010).

INDICATIONS FOR LATENT TUBERCULOSIS INFECTION SCREENING

Many indications for LTBI screening may be present concurrently in HIV-infected patients, which represent conditions with higher risk of development of TB than those without these conditions, or in situations that pose high risks of exposure or recent infection with *M. tuberculosis*. Indications for screening include the following:

- Foreign-born persons, or persons in close contact with recent immigrants or refugees, from regions with high rates of TB—that is, Africa, Asia, Latin America, Russia, and countries of the former Soviet Union

- Other medical conditions—that is, diabetes mellitus, silicosis, chronic renal failure, being underweight (≤10% below normal), gastrectomy, injection drug use, malignancies (lymphoma, leukemia, and head and neck cancer), cardiac and renal transplantation, or use of immunosuppressive therapies (especially tumor necrosis factor-α inhibitors)

- Persons from situations with a high risk for person-to-person transmission—for example, those working or residing in correctional facilities (3% of TB cases in the United States), homeless shelters (6% of TB cases in the United States), and other congregate settings (American Thoracic Society, Centers for Disease Control and Prevention, and Infectious Diseases Society of America, 2005)

- Close contacts of person with active TB, 30–40% of whom will be found to have LBTI, and 1% or 2% of whom will have active disease

- Children born to HIV-infected mothers who have TB or who are at high risk for possible LBTI (e.g., close contacts of persons with active disease)

Persons previously treated for latent or active TB who are re-exposed to someone with active TB can become reinfected, particularly in hyperendemic settings.

SCREENING TESTS FOR *MYCOBACTERIUM TUBERCULOSIS* INFECTION

Tuberculin Skin Testing

The time-honored method for diagnosis of *M. tuberculosis* infection is the TST, which measures a polycellular delayed-type hypersensitivity response at the site of injection following the administration of purified protein derivative (PPD), an admixture of mycobacterial antigens. The preferred skin test is the intradermal, or Mantoux, method. It is administered by injecting 0.1 ml of 5 tuberculin units (TU) PPD intradermally into the dorsal or volar surface of the forearm. Tests should be read 48–72 hours after test administration, and the diameter of induration transverse to the long axis of the arm should be recorded in millimeters. Multiple puncture tests (i.e., Tine and Heaf) and PPD strengths of 1 and

250 TU are not sufficiently accurate and should not be used (American Thoracic Society/Centers for Disease Control and Prevention, 2000). Induration of ≥5 mm in HIV-infected individuals indicates a positive TST. TSTs require two visits to perform and confirm the results of the test and experience in intradermal placement of the test. There is some subjectivity in its interpretation, and false-positive results may occur from exposure to nontuberculous mycobacteria or prior vaccination with *M. bovis* BCG. A positive TST has been shown to be predictive of progression to active TB in HIV-infected individuals, who benefit from preventive therapy with a reduction in TB incidence.

Interferon-Gamma Release Assays

IGRAs are blood tests that measure interferon-gamma (IFN-γ) secreted by sensitized T lymphocytes after exposure to TB-specific antigens ESAT-6 and CFP-10. Two tests are currently approved by the US Food and Drug Administration (FDA) and in use for the detection of *M. tuberculosis* infection: QuantiFERON-TB Gold In-Tube (QFT) and T-SPOT TB test (T-Spot). QFT measures IFN-γ concentration using an enzyme-linked immunosorbent assay (ELISA), whereas the T-Spot enumerates T cells releasing IFN-γ using an ELISPOT assay. QFT requires fresh blood to be incubated for 18–24 hours with plasma separation, ELISA testing, and comparison to negative and positive mitogen control antigens (phytohemaglutanin). T-Spot assays must be done on fresh blood specimens, processed within 12 hours, and incubated overnight. IGRAs require a single visit, are less subjective in interpretation than TSTs, and are more specific for detection of *M. tuberculosis* infection—that is, less cross-reactivity to nontuberculous mycobacteria (except *M. kansasii*, *M. szulgai*, and *M. marinum*) and BCG (Centers for Disease Control and Prevention (CDC), 2010).

Current evidence suggests that IGRAs have higher specificity (92–97%) compared to TSTs (56–95%) (NIH-CDC-HIVMA/IDSA, 2013). TSTs are more likely to identify persons with long-standing cellular immune responses to TB antigens, and IGRAs are more likely to be positive in persons with recent *M. tuberculosis* infection (Horsburgh, 2011). For diagnosis of LTBI, the correlation between TSTs and IGRAs is poor to moderate among persons with HIV infection (Cattamanchi, 2011). For HIV-infected individuals with active TB, in one study, sensitivity was low for both QFT-GIT and TST (63% and 55%, respectively) and was inversely correlated with low CD4+ cell counts (Raby, 2008). In HIV-infected patients at low risk of TB exposure, false-positive tests with QFT have also been reported, suggesting the need to repeat a positive QFT test to confirm the diagnosis of LTBI when patients are at low risk of exposure (Gray, 2012). There have been no definitive comparisons of TSTs and IGRAs for LTBI screening of persons with HIV infection in low-incidence settings.

Either TSTs or IGRAs are appropriate for TB screening among HIV-infected individuals in the United States. Some experts have suggested using both the TST and an IGRA to screen for LTBI, but the predictive value of this approach is not clear, and use of this strategy would be more expensive and more difficult to implement. The routine use of both TSTs and IGRAs to screen for LTBI in the same patient is not recommended in the United States (NIH-CDC-HIVMA/IDSA, 2013).

Testing Frequency

HIV-infected individuals should receive a test for LTBI at the time of initial HIV diagnosis, with repeat testing considered for those who are TST or IGRA negative initially with advanced HIV infection (CD4+ cell counts <200/μl) and who have improvement in immune function due to ART (CD4+ cell counts ≥200/μl). Annual testing may also be considered in those who have ongoing or repeated exposure to TB, such as individuals who travel for extended periods of time to hyperendemic TB settings. Intercurrent testing should be done based on recent exposure to a case of active TB, including repeat testing 8–12 weeks after the initial negative test for TB infection because it may take this long for the TST or IGRA to become positive following infection.

Anergy Testing

HIV-infected patients are at increased risk to have impaired delayed-type hypersensitivity responses to skin test antigens due to decreased CD4+ cell counts and, therefore, to have a compromised ability to react to tuberculin skin testing (i.e., to have cutaneous anergy). Anergy testing has not been helpful in attempting to distinguish false-negative TST results due to anergy from true-negative results. Anergy testing is not recommended for routine use in HIV-infected individuals due to problems with test standardization and reproducibility, the variable risk for TB in the setting of anergy, and the lack of demonstrated benefit of preventive therapy in anergic HIV-infected individuals.

Chest Radiography and Symptom Screening in HIV-Infected Patients

In asymptomatic persons with positive tests for LTBI, chest radiography should be done to exclude active TB. Persons with symptoms of TB, such as cough, fever, and night sweats, should be evaluated for TB regardless of IGRA or skin test results. The absence of these symptoms has a high negative predictive value for excluding active TB (Cain, 2010). Chest radiography should also be considered following recent exposure to a person with active TB regardless of skin test or IGRA results. HIV-infected individuals with pulmonary TB are more likely to exhibit atypical radiological presentations, especially those with low CD4+ cell counts and, in some cases, normal chest radiographs (Palmieri, 2002).

Preventive Therapy

Preventive therapy is recommended following exposure to persons with active TB, regardless of initial or repeat TST results, or in persons with TST ≥5 mm and who have not been treated for active or latent TB and have no clinical evidence of active TB. Preventive therapy should be considered in persons with a history of potential exposure in high-risk settings (as listed previously) regardless of results of testing for LTBI.

For further information on evaluation and treatment of active TB disease, see Chapter 32.

Recomm\ended Reading

Centers for Disease Control and Prevention. Anergy skin testing and preventive therapy for HIV-infected persons: Revised recommendations. *MMWR Morb Mortal Wkly Rep.* 1997; 46(RR-15):1–12.

References

American Thoracic Society/Centers for Disease Control and Prevention. Targeted tuberculin testing and treatment of latent tuberculosis infection: Joint statement of the American Thoracic Society and the Centers for Disease Control and Prevention. *Am J Respir Crit Care Med.* 2000; 161:S221–S247.

American Thoracic Society, Centers for Disease Control and Prevention, and Infectious Diseases Society of America. Controlling tuberculosis in the United States. *Am J Respir Crit Care Med.* 2005, 172:1169–1227.

Cain KP, McCarthy KD, Heilg CM, et al. An algorithm for tuberculosis screening and diagnosis in people with HIV. *N Engl J Med.* 2010; 362:707–716.

Cattamanchi A, Smith R, Steingart KR, et al. Interferon-gamma release assays for the diagnosis of latent tuberculosis infection in HIV-infected individuals: A systematic review and meta-analysis. *J Acquir Immune Defic Syndr.* 2011; 56:230–238.

Centers for Disease Control and Prevention. Updated guidelines for using interferon gamma release assays to detect *Mycobacterium tuberculosis* infection—United States, 2010. *MMWR Morb Mort Wkly Rep.* 2010; 59(RR-5):1–26.

Getahun H, Harrington M, O'Brien R, et al. Diagnosis of smear-negative pulmonary tuberculosis in people with HIV infection or AIDS in resource-constrained settings: Informing urgent policy changes. *Lancet.* 2007; 369(9578):2042–2049.

Gray J, Reves R, Johnson S, et al. Identification of false-positive QuantiFERON-TB Gold In-Tube assays by repeat testing in HIV-infected patients at low risk of tuberculosis. *Clin Infect Dis.* 2012; 54:e20–e23.

Horsburgh CR, Rubin EJ. Latent tuberculosis infection in the United States. *N Engl J Med.* 2011: 364:1441–1448.

NIH-CDC-HIVMA/IDSA. Guidelines for prevention and treatment of opportunistic infections in HIV-infected adults and adolescents. 2015. Available at http://aidsinfo.nih.gov/guidelines/html/4/adult-and-adolescent-oi-prevention-and-treatment-guidelines/0.

Palmieri F, Girardi E, Pellicelli AM, et al. Pulmonary tuberculosis in HIV-infected patients presenting with normal chest radiograph and negative sputum smear. *Infection.* 2002; 30(2):68–74.

Raby E, Moyo M, Devendra A et al. The effects of HIV on the sensitivity of a whole blood IFN-gamma release assay in Zambian adults with active tuberculosis. PLOS One. 2008 Jun 18;3(6)e2489.

ACKNOWLEDGMENT

This section is an update from the original version authored by David Cohn, MD, in the previous edition.

DENTAL CARE

LEARNING OBJECTIVE

Discuss the importance of routine dental care for HIV-infected patients and essential information to be included in the treating physician's written referral.

WHAT'S NEW?

A large proportion of HIV-infected patients do not receive needed dental and oral care, despite the high prevalence of such disorders in this population. Referrals for dental care should include information about the patient's risk for secondary infection and bleeding, infectious status, and current medications.

KEY POINTS

- HIV-infected patients are at increased risk for oral and dental problems due to immunodeficiency, salivary gland dysfunction, substance use, tobacco use, poor oral hygiene, and limited access to dental care.

- Oral cavity problems can undermine the success of ART by exacerbating existing medical, nutritional, and psychosocial problems; compromising adherence to treatment regimens; and diminishing quality of life.

- Providers should include basic oral screening in their routine clinic visits and advocate for routine dental care for patients.

- Referrals for dental care should include information about the patient's risk for secondary infection and bleeding, infectious status, and current medications.

Oral health care is an important component of the management of patients with HIV infection. Oral cavity problems can undermine the success of ART by exacerbating existing medical, nutritional, and psychosocial problems; compromising adherence to treatment regimens; and diminishing quality of life (New York State Department of Health AIDS Institute (NYSDOH), 2001).

Oral disease occurs disproportionately in the same individuals most affected by HIV: those of low socioeconomic status, those with limited health care access and use of services, and substance users whose attention to personal health and hygiene is often suboptimal (NYSDOH, 2001). They do not receive the dental care they need. In the HIV Cost and Services Utilization Study, which examined a nationally representative sample of persons in HIV care, 35% of patients had no regular source of dental care, 22% had not received dental care in more than 2 years, 25% had not received needed dental care, and 48% had no dental insurance coverage (Freed, 2005).

Significant proportions of HIV-infected patients have HIV-related oral problems such as untreated caries (39%), gum problems (47%), missing teeth (47%), and xerostomia (dry mouth) (37%) (Freed, 2005). HIV-infected patients with advanced immunosuppression also are at risk for serious systemic opportunistic infections and neoplasms, many of which can manifest in the oral cavity. Examples include candidiasis, hairy leukoplakia, Kaposi's sarcoma, and aphthous ulcerations (Bonito, 2001). The presence of oral candidiasis without medical explanation (e.g., recent antibiotics) is most often related to a low CD4 cell number and is considered a marker for cell-mediated immunodeficiency. Deterioration of oral immunologic functions and changes in salivary flow rate and composition also aid in the development of caries and periodontal diseases, including gingivitis, which can progress to serious necrotizing gingivitis and compromise masticatory functions and nutrition (Bonito, 2001). The presence of necrotizing ulcerative periodontitis, a more aggressive form of periodontal disease, should also be considered a sign of severe immune deterioration. It is a rapidly progressing disease, and treatment should be initiated as early as possible.

Thus, oral health care should be an integral component of primary health care for persons with HIV disease (NYSDOH, 2001). Providers must become familiar with oral conditions that affect HIV-infected persons and include basic oral screening in routine clinic visit exams. Providers also must be aware of and advocate for oral health care and dental services in their communities. Finally, providers must educate patients about the importance of good oral hygiene practices and regular dental care (at least twice annually) (NYSDOH, 2001).

When considering referral to a dental specialist, the main issues of concern are the patient's risk for bleeding, risk for infection, and infectiousness. Accordingly, the following information should be provided in dental referrals:

- Bleeding risk: Platelet count (platelet count <60,000/mm^3 may require platelet transfusion or steroids prior to dental treatment), liver biochemical tests, history of coagulation or other bleeding disorders, history of liver disease, and current hemoglobin (to ascertain risk of anemia should significant bleeding occur)

- Infection risk: Total white blood cell count, absolute neutrophil count, CD4$^+$ cell count, history of valvular or congenital heart disease, and other medical risks for infection (e.g., active intravenous drug use posing a risk for endocarditis)

- Based on the individual need of each patient, antibiotic prophylaxis may be indicated prior to dental care. The need for antibiotic prophylaxis is not based on CD4 counts, viral load, or AIDS diagnosis. Patients with severe neutropenia (neutrophil count <500/mm^3) should be premedicated with antibiotics prior to dental treatment. Otherwise, antibiotic prophylaxis is recommended based on the standard guidelines set forth by the American Heart Association (http://www.aha.org) for the prevention of bacterial endocarditis.

- Concurrent infections: Current HIV viral load, chronic active hepatitis B or hepatitis C infections, and contagious respiratory diseases such as active/untreated tuberculosis

All medications also should be detailed to prevent drug interactions or adverse effects if medications will be used or prescribed as part of the dental care.

Recommended Reading

Freed JR, Marcus M, Freed BA, et al. Oral health findings for HIV-infected adult medical patients from the HIV Cost and Services Utilization Study. *J Am Dental Assoc.* 2005; 136:1396–1405.

Greenspan JS, Greenspan D, Winkler JR. Diagnosis and management of the oral manifestations of HIV infection and AIDS. *Infect Dis Clin North Am.* 1988; 2:373–385.

Integrating HIV Innovating Practices. Implementing oral health care into HIV primary care settings curriculum. December 2013. Available at https://careacttarget.org/library/implementing-oral-health-care-hiv-primary-care-settings-curriculum-0. Accessed November 15, 2015.

Lee KC, Tami TA. Otolaryngologic manifestation of HIV disease. In: Cohen PT, Sande MA, Volberding PA (Eds.), *The AIDS Knowledge Base.* 3rd ed. Philadelphia, PA: Lippincott Williams & Wilkins; 1999: 559–575.

References

Bonito AJ. Management of dental patients who are HIV positive. Summary, evidence report/technology assessment: Number 37. AHRQ Publication No. 01-E041, March 2001. Rockville, MD: Agency for Healthcare Research and Quality. Available at http://www.ncbi.nlm.nih.gov/books/NBK11965. Accessed November 15, 2015.

Freed JR, Marcus M, Freed BA, et al. Oral health findings for HIV-infected adult medical patients from the HIV Cost and Services Utilization Study. *J Am Dental Assoc.* 2005; 136:1396–1405.

New York State Department of Health AIDS Institute. HIV and oral health: General principles. Available at http://www.hivguidelines.org/clinical-guidelines/hiv-and-oral-health/general-principles. Accessed November 15, 2015.

CARDIOPROTECTION AND PREVENTION STRATEGIES

LEARNING OBJECTIVE

Discuss the prevention of cardiovascular disease before clinical presentation among individuals with HIV infection.

WHAT'S NEW?

Most patients with HIV infection engaged in clinical care are receiving effective treatment with ART. Prevention of HIV-related cardiovascular disease (CVD) entails a comprehensive strategy of minimizing toxicity from specific antiretroviral medications, traditional risk factor modification through pharmacotherapies (e.g., blood pressure and cholesterol control), lifestyle modification (e.g., smoking cessation and exercise), and, ultimately, integrating anti-inflammatory strategies as they become available.

KEY POINTS

- HIV-related CVD is a consequence of ART exposure, HIV itself, as well as a higher prevalence of traditional CVD risk factors.

- The profile of metabolic abnormalities among patients with HIV infection typically includes many of the same criteria of the metabolic syndrome.

- The breadth of current antiretroviral medication choices allows providers and patients to tailor ART regimens and greatly minimize metabolic complications.

- Exercise has anti-inflammatory benefits in addition to its accepted effects on traditional risk factors.

- Future research should focus on defining the optimal use of established CVD prevention treatments, specifically among individuals with HIV infection.

Epidemiologic data suggest that individuals with HIV infection are at increased risk for atherosclerotic CVD events, such as acute myocardial infarction and sudden cardiac death, compared to uninfected persons (Freiberg, 2011; Tseng, 2012). Reasons for this excess risk are complex but appear to involve a greater prevalence of traditional risk factors as well as consequences more directly attributable to ART and HIV itself (Friis-Moller, 2007; SMART Study Group, 2006). Rates of cigarette smoking among HIV-infected persons in the United States are typically approximately twice those in the general population. Pro-atherosclerotic disturbances in blood cholesterol are now well-described consequences of ART use and HIV itself (Riddler, 2003). Data also suggest that HIV infection is associated with greater vascular stiffness and endothelial dysfunction (Baker, 2009; Solages, 2006), which has been linked to future risk for development of hypertension as well as CVD events (e.g., myocardial infarction and heart failure). Finally, HIV-related immune activation and inflammation appear to persist despite effective treatment with ART, and this has consequences for the development of premature CVD (Longenecker, 2016). Despite the unique aspects of CVD risk in the context of HIV infection, traditional CVD risk factor modification should remain the centerpiece of current CVD prevention strategies for patients with HIV infection (Petoumenos, 2014).

CARDIOVASCULAR DISEASE RISK ASSOCIATED WITH SPECIFIC ANTIRETROVIRAL MEDICATIONS

Findings from the randomized, controlled, clinical outcomes trial START (Strategic Timing of Antiretroviral Therapy) have demonstrated the clear net clinical benefit of ART treatment for reducing risk for both AIDS and non-AIDS conditions, even at very high CD4$^+$ counts (INSIGHT START Study Group, 2015). Thus, the vast majority of HIV-infected patients will likely spend many decades exposed to ART, when access permits. When considered together with the sentinel finding from the D:A:D (Data collection on Adverse events of anti-HIV Drugs) cohort that risk for myocardial infarction increases with each additional year of ART exposure (with risk largely restricted to protease inhibitors and abacavir use), the CVD-related toxicity from specific antiretrovirals has become a key consideration for both primary and secondary CVD prevention (Worm, 2010). Specifically, much (although not all) of the CVD risk associated with ART use has been attributable to changes in blood cholesterol (Friis-Moller, 2007). Thus, choosing ART regimens associated with the most favorable lipid profiles is one common approach to minimizing CVD risk.

Differences in blood lipid profiles are now an important secondary outcome in trials comparing the effectiveness of specific antiretrovirals. First-line ART medications associated with the most favorable lipid profiles include tenofovir and dolutegravir or raltegravir (Quercia, 2015; Tungsiripat, 2010). Conversely, currently used antiretrovirals associated with the most pro-atherogenic lipid changes include atazanavir or darunavir with ritonavir, or elvitegravir with cobicistat (DeJesus, 2012; Quercia, 2015). Finally, controversy remains with respect to whether current abacavir use increases risk for acute myocardial infarction, with numerous epidemiology studies supporting the presence of an abacavir–CVD link (Choi, 2011; Durand, 2011; INSIGHT/SMART and D:A:D Study Investigators, 2008; Martin, 2009; McComsey, 2012; Obel, 2010; Rotget, 2013; Worm, 2010) and others showing no association (Bedimo, 2011; Cruciani, 2011; Lang, 2010; Ribaudo, 2011).

TRADITIONAL RISK FACTOR MODIFICATION

Hypertension, dyslipidemia, and insulin resistance (or diabetes mellitus) are strong predictors of CVD risk. Targeting these risk factors remains central to any prevention strategy. The consequences of ART toxicity and/or HIV infection itself on increased risk for these conditions are well known. Specifically, persons with ART-treated HIV infection can have a higher prevalence of many of the key features of the metabolic syndrome: elevated blood pressure, elevated triglycerides, low high-density lipoprotein cholesterol (HDL-C), abdominal obesity, insulin resistance, and a pro-inflammatory state. Comprehensive reviews of these data are available elsewhere (e.g., American Heart Association conference proceedings on CVD risk among patients with HIV/AIDS in *Circulation* 2008; 118). The growing use of integrase strand transfer inhibitors as components of first-line ART regimens will likely result in a reduced prevalence of these previously common metabolic abnormalities in the future. However, when present, the treatment strategies and goals of therapy for HIV-infected persons with metabolic abnormalities tend to follow those recommended for the general population.

Historically, the effects of HIV infection on body composition often resulted in low BMI from a loss in lean mass, with additional toxicities from ART in the early era of therapy resulting in lipodystrophy with losses in subcutaneous fat and accumulation of visceral fat. Toxicities have greatly improved with contemporary antiretroviral medications, and HIV-related wasting is much less common, with a high proportion of patients receiving effective ART in the United States. However, data suggest that impaired fasting glucose (>100 mg/dl), and ultimately type 2 diabetes mellitus, is prevalent among patients with HIV infection and is associated with ART exposure (Betene, 2014). Persons at risk of disorders of glucose metabolism should have their ART regimen tailored to minimize any antiretroviral-related toxicity while still maintaining suppression of HIV replication. Ultimately, although the mechanisms of insulin resistance in the context of HIV infection may have unique features, once present, the application of lifestyle modification and pharmacotherapies (e.g., insulin-sensitizing agents and insulin) in clinical practice are similar to those for uninfected persons.

The dyslipidemia associated with ART-treated HIV infection is characterized both by an increase in pro-atherogenic lipids, including low-density lipoprotein cholesterol (LDL-C) and triglycerides, and by a decline in the anti-atherogenic HDL-C that does not fully reverse with ART (Riddler, 2003). Currently, there are no pharmacologic strategies to raise HDL-C that have been associated with corresponding reductions in clinical risk, and the association between triglycerides and CVD risk (when adjusting for other lipoproteins) is believed to be modest at best. Therefore, although unproven, the lipid-lowering properties of HMG-CoA reductase inhibitors (i.e., "statins") are assumed to be at least as clinically protective in the context of HIV-related dyslipidemia as they are in the general population. When also considering the anti-inflammatory effects, statin therapy may be particularly beneficial in the context of HIV-related CVD—a hypothesis that is currently being testing in the REPREIVE clinical trial (Randomized Trial to Prevent Vascular Events in HIV). Until data from REPREIVE are available, goal LDL-C targets applied in the management of HIV-positive individuals remain similar to those established for the general population in the third report of the Adult Treatment Panel III (NIH, 2001): (1) <100 mg/dl for those with known coronary heart disease or risk equivalent, (2) <130 mg/dl for patients with two or more risk factors, and (3) <160 mg/dl for those with one or no risk factors.

The 8th Joint National Committee on the Prevention, Detection, Evaluation and Treatment of High Blood Pressure

(James, 2014) defines a normal blood pressure at <140/ 90 mmHg for persons younger than age 60 years and 150/ 90 mmHg for persons aged 60 years or older. Any reading above that is considered hypertension, and the goal of treatment is then to achieve a blood pressure below these parameters, or <140/90 mmHg among persons with diabetes or chronic kidney disease. Treatment strategies include traditional blood pressure-lowering medications along with lifestyle modifications such as a low-salt diet, weight reduction, physical activity, and/or moderation of alcohol consumption. HIV is not addressed as a special, or high CVD risk, condition in current blood pressure guidelines. However, it is worth noting that the association between lower blood pressure levels and lower CVD risk is present throughout the normotensive range (e.g., systolic blood pressures from 115 to 140 mmHg). Thus, it follows that if HIV-positive individuals remain at increased CVD risk despite optimizing lipid levels and other traditional risk factors, more aggressive blood pressure goals may be a strategy to study in future clinical trials.

In summary, although some important factors contributing to HIV-related CVD risk are unique to HIV infection and/or ART exposure, strategies that target traditional CVD risk factors remain a highly effective and beneficial prevention approach. For example, smoking cessation or reductions in blood cholesterol levels in middle age (e.g., age ~50 years) may significantly reduce subsequent risk for CVD events during a person's lifetime (Petoumenos, 2014).

CIGARETTE SMOKING

Smoking cessation is a critically important clinical goal for patients with HIV infection, given the broad consequences for CVD, lung disease, cancer, infection risk, and overall higher mortality rates among those who smoke cigarettes. An increasing number of pharmacotherapy aids are now available and are generally believed to be the cornerstone of smoking cessation strategies. Both nicotine replacement therapy and non-nicotine medications (e.g., varenicline) have demonstrated success in clinical trials within the general population, although the durability of smoking cessation may remain a question (Ebber, 2015; Koegelenberg, 2014; Schnoll, 2015). More data are needed to establish effective smoking cessation strategies for persons with HIV infection, for whom unique challenges often exist related to a higher prevalence of socioeconomic barriers, multiple comorbidities, and coadministration of ART. Currently, a simple brief option to effectively start the process of smoking cessation in the context of a routine clinic visit entails asking about tobacco use, advising to quit, and referring patients who are receptive to available resources.

LIFESTYLE MODIFICATIONS

Lifestyle factors that are emphasized as potential cardioprevention strategies typically include those related to physical activity, moderation of alcohol intake, smoking cessation, and a healthy diet (e.g., high in fruits and vegetables and low in saturated fats and trans-fatty acids). These factors are also an important component of a broader strategy to counteract obesity and achieve and maintain a desirable weight (e.g., BMI ~19–25 kg/m^2) through caloric restriction and increased energy expenditure. There is also a growing appreciation that psychosocial factors such as depression and anxiety have consequences for CVD risk. Depression is both associated with a physiologic response that may be detrimental for cardiovascular health and may also exacerbate CVD risk through co-association with unhealthy behaviors. Without question, an emphasis on a healthy lifestyle should be a central component of CVD prevention for patients with HIV infection.

The benefits of exercise may be particularly important for persons with HIV infection. Beyond its role in counteracting obesity, insulin resistance, dyslipidemia, and elevated blood pressure, exercise has anti-inflammatory effects that make it attractive for both preventing and treating HIV-related CVD. This may result from a combination of reducing visceral fat mass (known to be pro-inflammatory) and triggering the release of anti-inflammatory mediators during the exercise event (Gleeson, 2011). Furthermore, beyond CVD, exercise may reduce risk for cancer, dementia, and other end-organ diseases.

CLINICAL QUESTIONS FOR FUTURE RESEARCH

Inflammation is a key factor in the pathogenesis of CVD and a hallmark of HIV infection that persists despite effective treatment with ART. In this context, adjunct anti-inflammatory strategies are needed to improve HIV-related CVD prevention, whether or not they target HIV-specific mechanisms or downregulate inflammatory pathways more broadly. One approach may be to take advantage of the pleiotropic anti-inflammatory properties of traditional CVD medications (e.g., statins). Data from the ongoing randomized, placebo-controlled, clinical outcomes trial of pitavastatin (REPRIEVE trial) will provide essential information on the absolute and relative CVD benefits of statin therapy at low to moderate LDL-C levels among persons with HIV infection.

In addition to novel pharmacotherapy approaches, an important clinical question is whether individual treatment goals for blood pressure and cholesterol levels should be more aggressive than they are for the general population or whether HIV infection should potentially be approached as a CVD-risk equivalent, analogous to the case that has been made for diabetes. A related question is whether indications for medicines such as aspirin should be expanded for all persons with HIV infection, for whom the antiplatelet and anti-inflammatory properties may be uniquely beneficial but clinical data from HIV studies are lacking.

Finally, changes in the spectrum of CVD manifestations and the availability of new antiretroviral medications will also be important considerations in managing HIV-related CVD risk in the future. As the armamentarium of antiretroviral agents continues to expand and toxicity improves, ART comparative effectiveness trials will need to include the effects on CVD risk markers, inflammation, metabolic abnormalities, as well as potential interactions with traditional CVD prevention pharmacotherapies. With reduced ART-related CVD toxicity and improved (and potentially more aggressive) risk factor modification among persons with HIV infection in resource-rich countries, atherosclerotic-related clinical complications may continue to decline. Concurrent with such changes, important questions may arise related to risk for other CVD manifestations such as heart failure, which may increase as a result of preventing clinical myocardial infarctions as well as HIV-associated changes in both systolic and diastolic function (Remick, 2014).

Recommended Reading

Franklin BA, Cushman M. Recent advances in preventive cardiology and lifestyle medicine (a themed series). *Circulation.* 2011; 123:2274–2283.

Longenecker CT, Sullivan C, Baker JV. Immune activation and cardiovascular disease in chronic HIV infection. *Curr Opin HIV AIDS* 2016; 11(2):216–225.

Person TA, Blair SN, Daniels SR, et al. AHA guidelines for primary prevention of cardiovascular disease and stroke: 2002 update. Consensus panel guide to comprehensive risk reduction for adult patients without coronary or other atherosclerotic vascular diseases. *Circulation.* 2002; 106:388–391.

Petoumenos, K., P. Reiss, L. Ryom, M. et al. Increased risk of cardiovascular disease (CVD) with age in HIV-positive men: a comparison of the D:A:D CVD risk equation and general population CVD risk equations. *HIV Med.* 2014; 15(10):595–603.

Stein JH, Hadigan CM, Brown TT, et al. Prevention strategies for cardiovascular disease in HIV-infected patients: Working group 6. *Circulation.* 2008; 118(2):e54–e60.

References

Baker JV, Duprez D, Rapkin J, et al. Untreated HIV infection and large and small artery elasticity. *J Acquir Immune Defic Syndr.* 2009; 52:25–31.

Bedimo RJ, Westfall AO, Drechsler H, et al. Abacavir use and risk of acute myocardial infarction and cerebrovascular events in the highly active antiretroviral therapy era. *Clin Infect Dis.* 2011; 53:84–91.

Betene ADC, De Wit S, Neuhaus J, et al. Interleukin-6, high sensitivity C-reactive protein, and the development of type 2 diabetes among HIV-positive patients taking antiretroviral therapy. *J Acquir Immune Defic Syndr.* 2014; 67:538–546.

Bloomfield GS, Alenezi F, Barasa FA, et al. Human immunodeficiency virus and heart failure in low- and middle-income countries. *JACC Heart Fail.* 2015; 3:579–590.

Choi AI, Vittinghoff E, Deeks SG, et al. Cardiovascular risks associated with abacavir and tenofovir exposure in HIV-infected persons. *AIDS.* 2011; 25:1289–1298.

Cruciani M, Zanichelli V, Serpelloni G, et al. Abacavir use and cardiovascular disease events: A meta-analysis of published and unpublished data. *AIDS.* 2011; 25:1993–2004.

Dejesus E, Rockstroh JK, Henry K, et al. Co-formulated elvitegravir, cobicistat, emtricitabine, and tenofovir disoproxil fumarate versus ritonavir-boosted atazanavir plus co-formulated emtricitabine and tenofovir disoproxil fumarate for initial treatment of HIV-1 infection: A randomised, double-blind, phase 3, non-inferiority trial. *Lancet.* 2012; 379:2429–2438.

Durand M, Sheehy O, Baril JG, et al. Association between HIV infection, antiretroviral therapy, and risk of acute myocardial infarction: A cohort and nested case–control study using Quebec's public health insurance database. *J Acquir Immune Defic Syndr.* 2011; 57:245–253.

Ebbert JO, Hughes JR, West RJ, et al. Effect of varenicline on smoking cessation through smoking reduction: A randomized clinical trial. *JAMA.* 2015; 313:687–694.

Freiberg M, McGinnis K, Butt A, et al. HIV is associated with clinically confirmed myocardial infarction after adjustment for smoking and other risk factors. 18th Conference on Retroviruses and Opportunistic Infections, 2011, Boston, MA.

Friis-Moller N, Reiss P, Sabin CA, et al. Class of antiretroviral drugs and the risk of myocardial infarction. *N Engl J Med.* 2007; 356:1723–1735.

Gleeson M, Bishop NC, Stensel DJ, et al. The anti-inflammatory effects of exercise: Mechanisms and implications for the prevention and treatment of disease. *Nat Rev Immunol.* 2011; 11:607–615.

INSIGHT START Study Group. Initiation of antiretroviral therapy in early asymptomatic HIV infection. *N Engl J Med.* 2015; 373:795–798.

INSIGHT/SMART and DAD Study Investigators. Use of nucleoside reverse transcriptase inhibitors and risk of myocardial infarction in HIV-infected patients. *AIDS.* 2008; 22:F17–F24.

James PA, Oparil S, Carter BL, et al. 2014 Evidence-based guideline for the management of high blood pressure in adults: Report from the Panel Members Appointed to the Eighth Joint National Committee (JNC 8). *JAMA.* 2014;311(5):507–520.

Koegelenberg CF, Noor F, Bateman ED, et al. Efficacy of varenicline combined with nicotine replacement therapy vs. varenicline alone for smoking cessation: A randomized clinical trial. *JAMA.* 2014; 312:155–161.

Lang S, Mary-Krause M, Cotte L, et al. Impact of individual antiretroviral drugs on the risk of myocardial infarction in human immunodeficiency virus-infected patients: A case–control study nested within the French Hospital Database on HIV ANRS cohort CO4. *Arch Intern Med.* 2010; 170:1228–1238.

Longenecker CT, Sullivan C, Baker JV. Immune activation and cardiovascular disease in chronic HIV infection. *Curr Opin HIV AIDS.* 2016; 11(2):216–225.

Martin A, Bloch M, Amin J, et al. Simplification of antiretroviral therapy with tenofovir–emtricitabine or abacavir–lamivudine: A randomized, 96-week trial. *Clin Infect Dis.* 2009; 49:1591–1601.

McComsey GA, Kitch D, Daar ES, et al. Inflammation markers after randomization to abacavir/lamivudine or tenofovir/emtricitabine with efavirenz or atazanavir/ritonavir. *AIDS.* 2012; 26:1371–1385.

National Institutes of Health Adult NCEP Treatment Panel III. Detection, evaluation, and treatment of high blood cholesterol in adults (Adult Treatment Panel III). NIH Publication No. 01-3670, May 2001.

Obel N, Farkas DK, Kronborg G, et al. Abacavir and risk of myocardial infarction in HIV-infected patients on highly active antiretroviral therapy: A population-based nationwide cohort study. *HIV Med.* 2010; 11:130–136.

Petoumenos K, Reiss P, Ryom L, et al. Increased risk of cardiovascular disease (CVD) with age in HIV-positive men: A comparison of the D:A:D CVD risk equation and general population CVD risk equations. *HIV Med.* 2014; 15:595–603.

Quercia R, Roberts J, Martin-Carpenter L, et al. Comparative changes of lipid levels in treatment-naive, HIV-1-infected adults treated with dolutegravir vs. efavirenz, raltegravir, and ritonavir-boosted darunavir-based regimens over 48 weeks. *Clin Drug Invest.* 2015; 35:211–219.

Remick J, Georgiopoulou V, Marti C, et al. Heart failure in patients with human immunodeficiency virus infection: Epidemiology, pathophysiology, treatment, and future research. *Circulation.* 2014; 129:1781–1789.

Ribaudo HJ, Benson CA, Zheng Y, et al. No risk of myocardial infarction associated with initial antiretroviral treatment containing abacavir: Short and long-term results from ACTG A5001/ALLRT. *Clin Infect Dis.* 2011; 52:929–940.

Riddler SA, Smit E, Cole SR, et al. Impact of HIV infection and HAART on serum lipids in men. *JAMA.* 2007; 289:2978–2982.

Rotger M, Glass TR, Junier T, et al. Contribution of genetic background, traditional risk factors, and HIV-related factors to coronary artery disease events in HIV-positive persons. *Clin Infect Dis.* 2013; 57:112–121.

Schnoll RA, Goelz PM, Veluz-Wilkins A, et al. Long-term nicotine replacement therapy: A randomized clinical trial. *JAMA Intern Med.* 2015; 175:504–511.

Solages A, Vita JA, Thornton DJ, et al. Endothelial function in HIV-infected persons. *Clin Infect Dis.* 2006; 42:1325–1332.

SMART Study Group. CD4+ count-guided interruption of antiretroviral treatment. *N Engl J Med.* 2006; 355:2283–2296.

Tseng ZH, Secemsky EA, Dowdy D. Sudden cardiac death in patients with human immunodeficiency virus infection. *J Am Coll Cardiol.* 2012; 59:1891–1896.

Tungsiripat M, Kitch D, Glesby MJ, et al. A pilot study to determine the impact on dyslipidemia of adding tenofovir to stable background antiretroviral therapy: ACTG 5206. *AIDS.* 2010; 24:1781–1784.

Worm SW, Sabin C, Weber R, et al. Risk of myocardial infarction in patients with HIV infection exposed to specific individual antiretroviral drugs from the 3 major drug classes: The Data Collection on Adverse Events of Anti-HIV Drugs (D:A:D) study. *J Infect Dis.* 2010; 201:318–330.

CONTRACEPTION AND PRECONCEPTION CARE

LEARNING OBJECTIVE

Discuss family planning and preconception care considerations in serodiscordant and seroconcordant HIV-infected couples.

WHAT'S NEW?

- Patients living with HIV should achieve long-term, maximal suppression of viral load prior to attempts at conception. Some experts now recommend pre-exposure prophylaxis (PrEP) for serodiscordant couples as an additional tool to reduce transmission risk to the uninfected partner during the conception process.

- HIV infection does not preclude the use of any methods of hormonal contraception; however, providers must make themselves aware of any potential drug–drug interactions between hormonal contraceptive methods and combination antiretroviral therapy (cART).

- Emergency contraception, including emergency contraceptive pills or the copper intrauterine device (Cu-IUD), may be offered to HIV-infected women when clinically appropriate. Drug–drug interactions must be considered when using hormonal emergency contraception in combination with antiretroviral drugs (ARVs).

KEY POINTS

- Health care providers need to be proactive in addressing issues related to preconception care and contraception in HIV-infected individuals of childbearing age.

- Family planning for HIV-infected individuals should include condoms to prevent transmission of HIV and other sexually transmitted diseases.

- Patients living with HIV should achieve long-term, maximal suppression of viral load prior to attempts at conception. Some experts now recommend PrEP for serodiscordant couples as an additional tool to reduce transmission risk to the uninfected partner during the conception process.

- HIV infection does not preclude the use of any methods of hormonal contraception; however, providers must make themselves aware of any potential drug–drug interactions between hormonal contraceptive methods and cART.

- Emergency contraception, including emergency contraceptive pills or the Cu-IUD, may be offered to HIV-infected women when clinically appropriate. Drug–drug interactions must be considered when using hormonal emergency contraception in combination with ARVs.

Women now account for approximately 30% of HIV- and AIDS-infected patients in the United States (American College of Obstetricians and Gynecologists (ACOG), 2015). As such, there is continued emphasis placed on family planning and preconception care. The goals of family planning and preconception care are to promote pregnancy planning; reduce unintended pregnancy; and support safer conception and pregnancy for mother, fetus/infant, and uninfected partners. All HIV-infected women of childbearing age should be offered comprehensive family planning and preconception care as part of routine primary medical care (ACOG, 2015; see https://aidsinfo.nih.gov/contentfiles/PerinatalGL.pdf).

THE IMPORTANCE OF FAMILY PLANNING AND PRECONCEPTION CARE

It is increasingly important for health care providers to be proactive in addressing issues related to preconception care and contraception with HIV-infected individuals of childbearing age. In areas in which antiretroviral drugs are widely available and accessible, HIV has become a chronic disease with life expectancy comparable to that of uninfected persons (van Sighem, 2010), and perinatal transmission rates have been reduced to less than 1% (ACOG, 2015). Fertility desires among women with HIV in most recent studies show little difference from those among HIV-uninfected women (Craft, 2007; Finocchario-Kessler, 2012; Loutfy, 2009; Nattabil, 2009; Squires, 2011). In the Women's Interagency HIV Study (WIHS) cohort, there was a 150% increase in live birth rates among HIV-infected women in the ART era compared to the pre-ART era (Sharma. 2007). Studies among women living with HIV suggest that the rate of unintended pregnancies is approximately 50% or higher (Craft, 2007; Loutfy, 2009; Massad, 2004). Many pregnancies among women with HIV occur despite use of contraception (Massad, 2004), implying that the pregnancies were unintended and highlighting the importance of adequate and accurate counseling about use of effective birth control. Women living with HIV express the desire to talk about reproductive plans with their health care providers; however, data suggest that such counseling does not often occur until after conception (Finorcchario-Kessler, 2010; Panozzo, 2003; Squires, 2011). Approximately 50% of HIV-infected individuals are in serodiscordant relationships (Chen, 2001). Finally, recent data suggest that effective ARV therapy may restore or improve fertility (Makumbi, 2011; Myer, 2010). In the WIHS cohort, among HIV-infected women, there was a 150% increase in live birth rates in the highly active antiretroviral therapy (HAART_ era compared to the pre-HAART era (Sharma, 2007).

COUNSELING AND ASSESSMENT ABOUT CHILDBEARING AND CONTRACEPTION

Because they may change over time, childbearing desires and intentions, including desired timing of pregnancy,

should be assessed during the initial evaluation and at intervals throughout the course of care. A comprehensive HIV, medical, and OB/GYN history and understanding of patient goals are important to focus counseling and assist in decision-making. Women who wish to prevent or delay pregnancy should receive information about contraceptive options, their efficacy, adverse effects, and other advantages or disadvantages, including noncontraceptive benefits (Hoyt, 2012). Women who wish to conceive should be given information about risk, rates, and prevention of perinatal transmission and the potential effects of HIV or its treatment on pregnancy course and outcomes. Safer sex practices, including condom use, should be discussed and reinforced both in women who desire to prevent or delay pregnancy and in those wishing to conceive to reduce HIV transmission or superinfection, as well as to prevent transmission and acquisition of other sexually transmitted diseases (STDs). A meta-analysis demonstrated an 80% reduction in the transmission risk of HIV through consistent use of male condoms alone in serodiscordant couples (ACOG, 2015). Also, for couples in serodiscordant relationships, the infected partner should be counseled about the benefits of ART in reducing HIV transmission (Cohen, 2011).

Disclosure and/or knowledge of HIV status for both partners are particularly important when conception is planned and should be encouraged and supported. It is also important to reinforce with patients that there may be legal ramifications for nondisclosure in certain jurisdictions. Knowledge of the disclosure laws in one's area is suggested for review with patients during counseling sessions.

CARE FOR WOMEN WISHING TO CONCEIVE

Interventions for women who wish to conceive include the following:

- Overall health should be optimized, with attention to standard primary care and management of chronic diseases, as well as treatment of drug and alcohol abuse.

- The benefits of smoking cession for mother and developing fetus should be reviewed, and referrals to cessation services should be offered.

- All current medications, including prescription, over-the-counter, and complementary/alternative medications, should be reviewed, and potential adverse effects associated with use of these drugs in pregnancy should be assessed.

- The need to initiate or modify an ARV regimen should be evaluated for all women with HIV prior to conception. For women on ART, a stable, maximally suppressed maternal viral load should be achieved prior to conception. The choice of ART regimen should take into account current adult treatment guidelines, what is known about the use of specific drugs in pregnancy, and the risk of teratogenicity or other adverse effects. The current guidelines for ART management during conception and the prenatal period can be found at https://aidsinfo.nih.gov/contentfiles/lvguidelines/PerinatalGL.pdf.

- Both partners should be screened for genital tract infections, and these should be treated if present. Genital tract inflammation is associated with genital tract shedding of HIV, even in the setting of fully suppressed HIV viral load, and may also increase plasma viremia.

- Immunizations should be given as indicated, and folic acid supplementation should be started.

HIV SEROCONCORDANT COUPLES

In couples in which both partners are HIV positive, a crucial aspect of the reproductive effort is ensuring that both partners have optimized their individual health. This should be accomplished from both the general and the HIV perspective. This includes the aforementioned visits to the primary care provider, gynecologist, and HIV specialist for the female partner and evaluation by a primary care provider and HIV specialist for the male partner. In both cases, sustained optimal viral suppression through cART is critical. Each partner should be evaluated and treated for sexually transmitted infection because their presence can cause inflammation, which can lead to genital tract shedding of the virus even when the plasma viral load is undetectable. Unprotected intercourse should be timed to coincide with ovulation.

A semen analysis should be strongly considered for any HIV-infected male partner prior to attempting conception. Semen abnormalities have been noted in male patients with HIV, including motility abnormalities, low sperm count, low volume of ejaculate, and abnormal morphology (Cardona-Maya, 2009). These abnormalities are thought to arise from ART use and/or as a consequence of viral exposure. Early detection of semen abnormalities can identify potential infertility issues and thus limit the risk of viral mutation from unprotected intercourse.

In addition to discussions aimed at identifying potential fetal risks and benefits during pregnancy, it is important to counsel patients on psychosocial issues. Although there have been advances to allow couples to conceive with significantly lower risk of superinfection or viral mutation, other issues remain. Medication compliance, genetics, and other factors may still result in the death of one or both HIV-infected parents prior to the child becoming an adult (ASRM, 2015). By itself, this is not enough to counsel against conception, but it should be a part of conversations on the risk and benefits of conception in HIV-positive parents.

HIV SERODISCORDANT COUPLES

In couples in which one partner is HIV uninfected, the goal is to achieve pregnancy while minimizing the risk of HIV transmission to the uninfected partner. It is estimated that the risk of transmission to an uninfected partner is approximately 1 in 500–1000 episodes of unprotected intercourse. The risk depends on the viral load of the infected partner (Mandelbrot, 1997). The use of ART has been shown to reduce the risk of transmission during attempted conception, but it has not completely eliminated the risk (Loutfy, 2013). In light of this, the HIV-infected partner should receive ART to achieve sustained, maximal viral suppression prior to attempting conception. Some experts recommend the use of PrEP for HIV-uninfected partners as an additional tool to reduce the risk of transmission from the infected partner.

HIV-Infected Female Partner

In cases in which the female partner is living with HIV, it is advised that artificial insemination is the safest route of conception. This may be achieved through consultation with a physician, or the patient may choose to inseminate herself during her ovulatory window. Timed, unprotected intercourse may also provide a lower transmission risk if the female partner has maintained optimal viral suppression on ARVs and/or the male utilizes PrEP (ASRM, 2015).

HIV-Infected Male Partner

In cases in which the male partner has HIV, consultation with a reproductive health specialist may be beneficial for identifying the options available to the couple. As previously mentioned, a semen analysis is recommended for HIV-infected males prior to attempts at conception to evaluate for abnormalities.

The safest option for conception is insemination with a donor sperm. If this method is unacceptable or undesirable, techniques such as intrauterine insemination or in vitro fertilization with intracytoplasmic sperm injection utilizing sperm that have gone through preparatory techniques may be suitable alternatives (ASRM 2015). Each of these options provides an excellent chance for fertility, with low risk of seroconversion of the mother and fetus. Unprotected intercourse timed only around ovulation has also been used as a method of conception, but it is not recommended due to the inherent risk of transmission. Consistent use of ARVs to fully suppress viral load in the male partner has been shown to decrease this risk but has not eliminated it (Cohen, 2011). The use of PrEP during the periconception period may also further limit the risk of exposure to the female patient (ASRM, 2013). A 2011 study demonstrated no seroconversion of uninfected female patients who used oral tenofovir during conception attempts. In the trial, two doses of tenofovir were administered, the first at the luteinizing hormone peak and the second 24 hours later. The pregnancy rate reached 75% after 12 attempts (Vernazza, 2011).

The FDA has only approved daily dosing of combination tenofovir/emtricitabine for use as PrEP. In serodiscordant couples, the CDC recommends that the uninfected partner begin treatment with daily combination tenofovir/emtricitibine 1 month prior to attempting conception and continue for 1 month beyond attempted conception. As in patients who are using PrEP for routine HIV prophylaxis, baseline HIV and pregnancy testing should be drawn and repeated in 3-month intervals and renal function at baseline and 6-month intervals.

CARE FOR WOMEN WISHING TO PREVENT OR DELAY PREGNANCY

In 2014, an expert panel from the World Health Organization (WHO) reviewed the evidence on currently available methods of hormonal contraception and reaffirmed its 2009 statement that women with HIV can potentially use all existing hormonal contraceptive methods without restriction (WHO, 2014). However, special care must be taken to address any potential drug–drug interactions and alterations in pharmacokinetics that may occur when ARVs and contraceptives are used together.

The WHO and the CDC state that with the use of methods involving spermicides containing nonoxynol-9, risk generally outweighs advantages of the method because of potential disruption of cervical mucosa, which may increase viral shedding and HIV transmission to uninfected partners. Both the Cu-IUD and the levonorgestrel-containing IUD can be initiated or continued in women with HIV, including those with AIDS, who are clinically doing well on ARV therapy. Pharmacokinetic interactions between hormonal contraceptives (primarily studied with combined estrogen–progestin oral contraceptives) and some protease inhibitors and non-nucleoside reverse transcriptase inhibitors may modify steroid levels and potentially decrease contraceptive effectiveness or increase risk of adverse effects, although the true clinical effect is not clear. An additional or alternative contraceptive method is generally advised if hormonal contraception is considered (Cohn, 2007; El-Ibiary and Cocohoba, 2008; USPHS, 2012; Vogler, 2010).

Most studies have found no association between the use of hormonal contraception and HIV disease progression (Morrison, 2011; Polis, 2010: Stringer, 2009). There are conflicting data on the role of hormonal contraception in HIV susceptibility or infectiousness. A recent secondary analysis of data from a large prevention trial found an increased risk of HIV seroconversion (both transmission and acquisition) associated with hormonal contraception (primarily depot medroxyprogesterone acetate) among more than 3700 serodiscordant African couples (Heffron, 2012). A WHO expert group reviewed all available evidence and concluded that the data were not sufficient to warrant a change in the current guidance on the use of hormonal contraception for women at risk of HIV infection (WHO, 2012).

Emergency contraception, including emergency oral contraceptives or the Cu-IUD, may be offered to HIV-infected women if clinically appropriate. When oral contraceptives (either combination or levonorgestrel only) are used with ARVs, the potential for drug interactions seems to be similar to that when they are used for routine contraception.

Currently, there are no data on interactions between ARVs and ulipristal acetate, but interactions should be anticipated due to the metabolism of ulipristal acetate through the CYP3A4 pathways.

INFERTILITY

HIV can adversely affect fertility in HIV-infected patients, regardless of symptom status, in terms of reduced pregnancy rates, increased pregnancy loss, and longer intervals between births. A study from Spain found that almost one-third of HIV-infected women undergoing fertility assessment had evidence of tubal occlusion (Coll, 2007), likely reflecting past infection with gonorrhea or chlamydia. Another potential contributing factor to subfertility in

HIV-infected women is a possible increase in menstrual dysfunction, particularly with lower CD4$^+$ cell counts (Cetjin, 2006; Ezechi, 2010; Harlow, 2000; Massad, 2006). Higher viral loads have also been independently associated with decreased fertility (Ngyuen, 2006). Women with HIV who are unable to conceive should receive fertility evaluation and management. HIV-infected patients should not be denied access to fertility services solely based on their HIV status (Phelps, 2007).

Recommended Reading

American Society for Reproductive Medicine. Human immunodeficiency virus (HIV) and infertility treatment: A committee opinion. *Fertil Steril.* 2015; 104:e1–e8

Panel on Treatment of HIV-Infected Pregnant Women and Prevention of Perinatal Transmission. Recommendations for use of antiretroviral drugs in pregnant HIV-1-infected women for maternal health and interventions to reduce perinatal HIV transmission in the United States. 2015. Available at http://aidsinfo.nih.gov/contentfiles/lvguidelines/PerinatalGL.pdf.

References

American College of Obstetricians and Gynecologists. Gynecologic care for women with human immunodeficiency virus: Practice Bulletin No. 117. *Obstet Gynecol.* 2015; 117:1492–1509.

American Society for Reproductive Medicine. Recommendations for reducing the risk of viral transmission during fertility treatment with the use of autologous gametes: A committee opinion. *Fertil Steril.* 2013; 99:340–346.

American Society for Reproductive Medicine. Human immunodeficiency virus (HIV) and infertility treatment: A committee opinion. *Fertil Steril* 2015; 104:e1–e8.

Anderson J. HIV and reproduction. In: Anderson JR (Ed.), *A Guide to the Clinical Care of Women with HIV/AIDS, 2015 Edition.* Rockville, MD: Department of Health and Human Services, Health Resources and Services Administration, HIV/AIDS Bureau; 2005. Available at http://hab.hrsa.gov/deliverhivaidscare/files/clinicalcareguide2005.pdf. Accessed July 20, 2006.

Cardona-Maya W, Velilla P, Montoya CJ, et al. Presence of HIV-1 DNA in spermatozoa from HIV-positive patients: Changes in the semen parameters. *Curr HIV Res.* 2009; 7(4):418–424.

Centers for Disease Control and Prevention. Trials of pre-exposure prophylaxis for HIV prevention. 2006. Available at http://www.cdc.gov/hiv/resources/factsheets/PDF/prep.pdf. Accessed August 16, 2006.

Centers for Disease Control and Prevention. U.S. medical eligibility criteria for contraceptive use, 2010. *MMWR Recomm Rep.* 2010; 59(RR-4):1–86.

Cohen MS, Chen YQ, McCauley M, et al. Prevention of HIV-1 infection with early antiretroviral therapy. *N Engl J Med.* 2011; 365:493–505.

Hoyt MJ, Storm DS, Aaron E, et al. Preconception and contraceptive care for women living with HIV. *Infect Dis Obstet Gynecol.* 2012; 2012:604183.

Loutfy MR, Blitz S, Zhang Y, et al. Self-reported preconception care of HIV-positive women of reproductive potential: A retrospective study. *J Int Assoc Providers AIDS Care* 2014; 13(5):424–433.

Mandelbrot L, Heard I, Henrion-Geeant E, et al. Natural conception in HIV-negative women with HIV-infected partners. *Lancet.* 1997; 349:850–851.

Vernazza PL, Graf I, Sonnenberg-Schwan U, et al. Preexposure prophylaxis and timed intercourse for HIV-discordant couples willing to conceive a child. *AIDS.* 2011; 25:2005–2008.

Wang CC, Reilly M, Kreiss JK. Risk of HIV infection in oral contraceptive pill users: A meta-analysis (Erratum in: *J Acquir Immune Defic Syndr.* 1999; 21:428). *J Acquir Immune Defic Syndr.* 1999; 21:51–58.

World Health Organization. Hormonal contraceptive methods for women at high risk of HIV and living with HIV: 2014 guidance statement. 2014. Geneva, Switzerland: World Health Organization.

ACKNOWLEDGMENTS

We acknowledge Jean Anderson, MD, FACOG, AAHIVS. She provided the bulk of the material covered in this section in the 2012 edition. We have updated the more recent changes, in line with current treatment goals, strategies, and guidelines published since the previous edition. This was an outstanding section, and we hope that our contributions will only make it better.

CERVICAL PAP SMEARS

LEARNING OBJECTIVE

Discuss the recommended frequency and specimen collection technique for cervical Pap smears in HIV-infected women, the role of human papillomavirus (HPV) testing, and indications for specialist referral for colposcopy.

WHAT'S NEW?

The cervical cancer screening guidelines have been updated by the US Department of Health and Human Services and are more in line with the 2012 cervical cancer guidelines for the HIV non-infected. The changes are categorized into two groups: those for HIV-infected women younger than age 30 years and those for HIV-infected women older than age 30 years.

KEY POINTS

- In HIV-infected patients younger than age 21 years, cervical cancer screening (with liquid-based Pap alone) should begin within 1 year of the onset of sexual activity and no later than age 21 years. If normal, the test is repeated in 12 months. If the patient has three consecutive normal screenings, testing interval should be increased to every 3 years.

- In HIV-infected women older than age 30 years, cervical cancer screening with either Pap alone or combined with HPV co-testing may be offered. The appropriate interval of follow-up screening is determined by the type of screening performed and the results returned.

- Unlike the general population, women with HIV should continue lifelong cervical cancer screening.

CERVICAL HPV INFECTION IN HIV-INFECTED WOMEN

In general, infection with HPV, the cause of cervical cancer, is very common in the United States, with an estimated 24.9 million 14- to 59-year-old women infected (Dunne, 2007). Compared with HIV-uninfected women, HIV-infected women have a higher prevalence and incidence of HPV (Ahdieh, 2001; Branca, 2003), longer persistence of HPV (Ahdieh, 2001; Sun, 1997), higher HPV levels (Jamieson, 2002), higher prevalence of multiple HPV subtypes (Firnhaber, 2009; Jamieson, 2002; Sahasrabuddhe, 2007), and higher prevalence of oncogenic subtypes (Firnhaber, 2009; Minkoff, 1998; Volkow, 2001). In addition, there is increased HPV prevalence and persistence of high-risk HPV with decreasing $CD4^+$ cell counts (Denny, 2008; Palefsky, 1999) and increasing HIV RNA levels (Palefsky, 1999). Also, compared to HIV-uninfected women, HIV-infected women are more likely to have abnormal cervical cytology (Denny, 2008; Ellerbrock, 2000), and both frequency and severity of cervical dysplasia increase with declining $CD4^+$ cell counts (Davis, 2001; Massad, 2001, 2008). Recurrent cervical dysplasia after treatment is more common among HIV-infected women (Boardman, 1999; Fruchter, 1996; Holcomb, 1999; Massad, 2001; Six, 1998). Rates of cervical cancer are also significantly higher among HIV-infected women compared to women in the general population (Chaturvedi, 2009; Clifford, 2005; Dal Maso, 2009; Grulich, 2007). Several HPV subtypes have been associated with the development of squamous intraepithelial lesions and cervical cancer, including most commonly HPV 16 (found in almost half of all cervical cancers) and HPV 18 (found in 10–12% of cervical cancers) and less commonly HPV 31, 33, 35, 39, 45, 51, 52, 56, 58, 59, and 68 (each accounting for <5% of cervical cancers) (Castle, 2009; Schiffman, 2009).

CERVICAL PAP SMEARS

Due to the high level of HPV infection and higher prevalence of oncogenic subtypes, it is critical for HIV-infected women to be regularly screened for cervical dysplasia. Although a single Pap smear has historically been associated with high false-negative rates (10–25%), regular screening can significantly improve accuracy (Anderson, 2012), and Pap smear screening programs have been associated with marked reductions in cervical cancer incidence (Eddy 1990; Nygard, 2002).

The frequency and type of testing recommended for HIV infected women have changed. The new Cervical Cancer Screening Recommendations reflect the paradigm shift in testing noted with non-HIV-infected women in the 2012 recommendations. The following sections present a summary of the cervical cancer screening recommendations from the NIH-CDC-HIVMA/IDSA (2015). The recommendations are categorized into two groups: those for HIV-infected women younger than age 30 years and those for HIV-infected women older than age 30 years.

HIV-Infected Women Younger Than Age 30 Years

Liquid-based Pap screening (with reflex HPV testing if atypical squamous cells of undetermined significance (ASCUS)) should be the primary method of testing. HPV co-testing is not recommended because of the high prevalence of HPV in this age group.

In patients younger than age 21 years, the initial cervical screening should begin within 1 year of the onset of sexual activity. If a patient has not begun sexual activity by the age of 21 years, routine screening should begin at that time. This recommendation holds true regardless of the method of exposure to the virus. In women ages 21–29 years, a baseline Pap should be done at the time of the patient's initial HIV diagnosis. If the Pap is normal, a repeat screen should be done 12 months later (some experts recommend a test 6 months after the baseline). If the patient has three consecutive normal tests, the screening interval should be increased to every 3 years.

If the result of ACS-US with positive high-risk HPV is returned, the patient should be referred for colposcopy. Pap screening should be repeated in 6–12 months for patients in which HPV results are not available. For any result ASCUS or greater on repeat cytology, the patient should be referred for colposcopy. Regardless of HPV screening results (if done), any result low-grade squamous intraepithelial lesion (LGSIL) or greater should be referred for colposcopy.

HIV-Infected Women Older Than Age 30 Years

Pap screening alone or in combination with HPV testing is acceptable.

If Screening with Pap Alone

Pap should be done as a baseline at the time of diagnosis and then every 12 months. Some experts recommend a repeat screen 6 months after the baseline exam. As with the younger group, if the results are negative on three consecutive exams, then subsequent screens should be carried out every 3 years.

Pap Screen Plus HPV Co-testing

Co-testing (Pap smear plus HPV testing) should begin at the age of 30 years or at the time of diagnosis (if available). When Pap screen and HPV co-testing are performed together, results should be reviewed. If the Pap is normal and HPV is negative, the co-test screening can be repeated in 3 years.

If the Pap screen is normal but HPV is positive, the appropriate follow-up is dictated by the HPV subtype(s) identified. If the subtype is HPV 16 or HPV 16/18, the patient should be referred for colposcopy. If HPV is identified but is of any other subtype, follow-up should be carried out in 1 year with a repeat of Pap and HPV testing. On repeat exam, if HPV testing remains positive or Pap is abnormal, then the patient should be referred for colposcopy.

If the result of ACS-US with positive high-risk HPV is returned, the patient should be referred for colposcopy. Pap screening should be repeated in 6–12 months for patients in which HPV results are not available. For any result ASCUS or greater, the patient should be referred for colposcopy.

For results LGSIL or greater, the patient should be referred for colposcopy, regardless of HPV results.

Unlike the general population, who may end cervical cancer screening at the age of 65 years under ideal circumstances, Pap screening should continue for HIV-infected women throughout their lifetime.

TEST INTERPRETATION AND FOLLOW-UP

- *Unsatisfactory for evaluation*: Repeat the Pap smear, with particular attention paid to adequacy of endocervical sampling.

- *Partially obscuring—inflammation*: Evaluate for infection and consider repeating the Pap smear.

- *Atypical glandular cells (AGC)*: Follow up with colposcopy, endocervical sampling; with endometrial sampling if older than age 35 years or abnormal bleeding; cervical conization recommended if initial evaluation negative and cytology favors neoplasia.

- *Atypical squamous cells of undetermined significance (ASCUS) and atypical squamous cells—cannot exclude HSIL (ASC-H)*: Follow up with colposcopy, biopsy if indicated; endocervical sampling if unsatisfactory colposcopy; follow with Pap smear every 6 months, consider repeat colposcopy annually if Pap smear unchanged. May resume annual Pap smears after two successive negatives.

- *Low-grade squamous intraepithelial lesion (LSIL, CIN1)*: Follow up with colposcopy, biopsy if indicated; endocervical sampling if unsatisfactory colposcopy; then follow with a Pap smear every 6 months. Consider repeat colposcopy annually, if Pap smear is unchanged.

- *High-grade squamous intraepithelial lesion (HSIL, CIN2–3, carcinoma in situ)*: Follow up with colposcopy, biopsy, endocervical sampling; and treat with loop excision or conization.

- *Invasive carcinoma*: Follow up with colposcopy with biopsy or conization to confirm diagnosis; treat confirmed invasive disease with surgery or radiation (referral to gynecologic oncologist needed).

- Where economically feasible, HPV vaccine may be of particular use in low-resource settings with limited cervical cancer screening capabilities.

Recommended Reading

American College of Obstetricians and Gynecologists. Gynecologic care for women with human immunodeficiency virus. ACOG Practice Bulletin No. 117. December 2010. Reaffirmed 2015.

Anderson J. Gynecologic problems. In: Anderson JR (Ed.), *A Guide for Clinical Care of Women with HIV/AIDS, 2013 Edition*. Rockville, MD: US Department of Health and Human Services, Health Resources and Services Administration, HIV/AIDS Bureau.

Panel on Opportunistic Infections in HIV-Infected Adults and Adolescents. Guidelines for the prevention and treatment of opportunistic infections in HIV-infected adults and adolescents: Recommendations from the Centers for Disease Control and Prevention, the National Institutes of Health, and the HIV Medicine Association of the Infectious Diseases Society of America. Available at http://aidsinfo.nih.gov/contentfiles/lvguidelines/adult_oi.pdf.

References

Ahdieh L, Klein RS, Burk R, et al. Prevalence, incidence, and type-specific persistence of human papillomavirus in human immunodeficiency virus (HIV)-positive and HIV-negative women. *J Infect Dis*. 2001; 184:1682–1690.

Boardman LA, Peipert JF, Hogan JW, et al. Positive cone biopsy specimen margins in women infected with the human immunodeficiency virus. *Am J Obstet Gynecol*. 1999 Dec;181(6):1395–1399.

Boehme CC, Nabeta P, Hillemann D, et al. Rapid molecular detection of tuberculosis and rifampin resistance. *N Engl J Med*. 2010 Sep 9; 363(11):1005–1015.

Branca M, Garbuglia AR, Benedetto A, et al.; DIANAIDS Collaborative Study Group. Factors predicting the persistence of genital human papillomavirus infections and Pap smear abnormality in HIV-positive and HIV-negative women during prospective follow-up. *Int J STD AIDS*. 2003; 14(6):417–425.

Centers for Disease Control and Prevention (CDC). Human papillomavirus: HPV information for clinicians. 2006 [CDC pamphlet] Available at: http://www.cdc.gov/std/hpv/common-infection/CDC_HPV_ClinicianBro_LR.pdf. Accessed April 2006.

Chaturvedi AK, Madeleine MM, Biggar RJ, et al. Risk of human papillomavirus-associated cancers among person with AIDS. *J Natl Cancer Inst*. 2009 Aug 19; 101(16):1120–1230.

Clifford GM, Polesel J, Rickenbach M, et al. Cancer risk in the Swiss HIV Cohort Study: associations with immunodeficiency, smoking and highly active antiretroviral therapy. *J Natl Cancer Inst*. 2005 Mar 16; 97(6):425–432.

Davis AT, Chakraborty H, Flowers L, et al. Cervical dysplasia in women infected with the human immunodeficiency virus (HIV): a correlation with HIV viral load and CD4+ count. *Gynecol Oncol*. 2001 Mar; 80(3):350–354.

Ellerbrock TV, Chiasson MA, Bush TJ, et al. Incidence of cervical squamous intraepithelial lesions in HIV-infected women. *JAMA*. 2000 Feb 23;283(8):1031–1037.

Dunne EF, Unger ER, Sternberg M, et al. Prevalence of HPV infection among females in the United States. *JAMA*. 2007; 297(8):813–819.

Firnhaber C, Zungu K, Levin S, et al. Diverse and high prevalence of human papillomavirus associated with a significant high rate of cervical dysplasia in human immunodeficiency virus-infected women in Johannesburg, South Africa. *Acta Cytol*. 2009 Jan–Feb;53(1):10–17.

Fruchter RG, Maiman M, Sedlis A, et al. Multiple recurrences of cervical intraepithelial neoplasia in women with the human immunodeficiency virus. *Obstet Gynecol*. 1996; 87:338–344.

Holcomb K, Matthews RP, Chapman JE, et al. The efficacy of cervical conization in the treatment of cervical intraepithelial neoplasia in HIV-positive women. *Gynecol Oncol*. 1999 Sep;74(3):428–431.

Jamieson DJ, Duerr A, Burk R, et al. Characterization of genital human papillomavirus infection in women who have or are at risk for having HIV infection. *Am J Obstet Gynecol*. 2002 Jan;186(1):21–27.

Massad LS, Ahdieh L, Benning L, et al. Evolution of cervical abnormalities among women with HIV-1: Evidence from surveillance cytology in the Women's Interagency HIV study. *J Acquir Immune Defic Syndr*. 2001; 27:432–442.

Massad LS, Seaberg EC, Wright RL, et al. Squamous cervical lesions in women with human immunodeficiency virus: long-term follow-up. *Obstet Gynecol*. 2008 Jun; 111(6):1388–1393.

Minkoff H, Feldman J, DeHovitz J, et al. A longitudinal study of human papillomavirus carriage in human immunodeficiency virus-infected

and human immunodeficiency virus-uninfected women. *Am J Obstet Gynecol*. 1998; 178:982–986.

NIH-CDC-HIVMA/IDSA. Guidelines for prevention and treatment of opportunistic infections in HIV-infected adults and adolescents. 2015. Available at https://aidsinfo.nih.gov/contentfiles/lvguidelines/adult_oi.pdf.

Palefsky JM. Cervical human papillomavirus infection and cervical intraepithelial neoplasia in women positive for human immunodeficiency virus in the era of highly active antiretroviral therapy. *Curr Opin Oncol*. 2003; 15:382–388.

Palefsky JM, Holly EA, Ralston ML, et al. Effect of highly active antiretroviral therapy on the natural history of anal squamous intraepithelial and anal human papillomavirus infection. *J Acquir Immune Defic Syndr*. 2001; 28:422–428.

Panel on Opportunistic Infections in HIV-Infected Adults and Adolescents. Guidelines for the prevention and treatment of opportunistic infections in HIV-infected adults and adolescents: Recommendations from the Centers for Disease Control and Prevention, the National Institutes of Health, and the HIV Medicine Association of the Infectious Diseases Society of America. Available at http://aidsinfo.nih.gov/contentfiles/lvguidelines/adult_oi.pdf. Accessed December 6, 2015.

Sahasrabuddhe VV, Mwanahamuntu MH, Vermund SH, et al. Prevalence and distribution of HPV genotypes among HIV-infected women in Zambia. *Br J Cancer*. 2007 May 7; 96(9):1480–1483.

Six C, Heard I, Bergeron C, et al. Comparative prevalence, incidence and short-term prognosis of cervical squamous intraepithelial lesions amongst HIV-positive and HIV-negative women. *AIDS*. 1998; 12:1047–1056.

Sun XW, Kuhn L, Ellerbrock TV, et al. Human papillomavirus infection in women infected with the human immunodeficiency virus. *N Engl J Med*. 1997 Nov 6; 337(19):1343–1349.

Volkow P, Rubí S, Lizano M, et al. High prevalence of oncogenic human papillomavirus in the genital tract of women with human immunodeficiency virus. *Gynecol Oncol*. 2001; 82:27–31.

ACKNOWLEDGMENTS

We acknowledge Jean Anderson, MD, FACOG, AAHIVS. She provided the bulk of the material discussed in this section in the 2012 edition. We have updated the more recent changes, in line with current treatment goals, strategies, and guidelines published since the previous edition. This was an outstanding section, and we hope that our contributions will only make it better.

13.

ISSUES IN SPECIFIC PATIENT POPULATIONS

Gary F. Spinner, Jean R. Anderson, Joseph A. Church, Renata Arrington-Sanders,

Aroonsiri Sangarlangkarn, Paul W. DenOuden, Madeline B. Deutsch, Daniel Wlodarczyk,

Barry Zevin, Rachel A. Prosser, and Vishal Dahya

DIVERSITY AWARENESS

CHAPTER GOAL

The goal of this chapter is to provide an understanding of the diversity of patients with HIV, the complexity of their unique cultures that are shaped by a multitude of factors, and the importance of becoming competent in developing a clinician–patient relationship across cultural differences.

LEARNING OBJECTIVES

- Relate how a patient's values, beliefs, and judgments may create barriers to successful treatment if the HIV provider does not competently navigate the cultural differences between the patient and the health care provider.

- Recognize the challenges in addressing racial and ethnic disparities in health care and in HIV in particular.

- Discuss the impact that culture, ethnicity, immigration status, sexual orientation, religion, gender, and behavioral health problems may have on the care of HIV-infected patients.

WHAT'S NEW?

It is estimated that 61% of new HIV infections are transmitted by patients who have either dropped out of care or are not taking their medications. In order to improve patient adherence and retention-in-care, efforts to enhance trust in health care providers require a broader understanding of the diversity and cultures of many different groups of patients with HIV.

KEY POINT

- Patients with HIV come from diverse backgrounds and are often mistrustful of health care providers.

LOSS OF RETENTION-IN-CARE

Retaining patients in care requires culturally competent staff at all levels of an organization. It could be easy for the busy HIV specialist to focus more intensely on the complex medical aspects of HIV medicine and relegate the issues of diversity and cultural competence as "soft areas" that are of lesser importance than learning resistance mutations or developing expertise in the use of the latest antiviral drugs. However, to do so runs the risk of failing to adequately comprehend how a patient's behaviors, beliefs, and the characteristics of his or her unique social, ethnic, racial, religious, gender identity, or country of origin may affect his or her engagement with the health care system. Failing to understand the important cultural context from which a patient interacts with the health care system often leads to poor patient adherence with treatment, misunderstandings about the treatment plan, or, worse, loss of retention from care. To successfully treat patients and to achieve the goals of treatment, we need to do our best to understand the unique context of our diverse group of patients and to provide care that acknowledges the cultural values that may impact acceptance of treatment.

A recent Centers for Disease Control and Prevention (CDC) analysis (Skarbinski, 2015) estimated that patients with previously diagnosed HIV infection who were out of care were responsible for 61% of new HIV infections in the United States. Furthermore, a statewide study from North Carolina that analyzed patients with acute HIV infection found that most transmission events (77%) were attributable to partners with previously diagnosed infection, of whom only 23% were reportedly in care and taking antiviral medication within the time that transmission was likely to have occurred (Cope, 2015). This is compelling evidence that the system of HIV care in the United States is failing to treat and retain many patients already diagnosed with HIV. There are likely many reasons for lack of success in patient retention, but it underscores the crucial need to improve the ways health care providers interact with patients in order to successfully keep them engaged in care and adherent with their antiviral medications. Developing competence in understanding the attributes of a diverse patient population is challenging, but failure to do so will allow greater numbers of HIV-infected patients to lose contact with care. The greater challenge in becoming culturally competent is for each health care provider to develop self-awareness of his or her own values, beliefs, and attitudes and what biases may be inherent in the provider's own culture.

DIVERSITY OF PATIENTS WITH HIV

An HIV provider caring for patients with HIV is likely caring for a diverse population of patients from racial or ethnic groups different from his or her own. In the United States, people with HIV are disproportionately African American and Hispanic, and regardless of race or ethnicity, they are often affected by poverty, drug or alcohol abuse, mental health problems, lack of employment, lack of permanent housing, histories of incarceration, inadequate education, and sexual preferences different from those of the general population. Some patients may be immigrants or refugees whose language and cultural differences may cause barriers to acceptance of health care services from a system of care culturally different from that of their own. Understanding how a patient's spiritual and religious values may impact his or her health care decision-making is important when caring for a diverse group of patients. However, in our attempt to develop cultural understanding of their diversity, it is critical to avoid stereotyping patients, which also creates barriers to acceptance of treatment. The values, beliefs, and judgments of patients may differ from those of their health care provider, and unless the health care provider is able to withhold his or her own judgment of a patient's circumstances, a trusting relationship may never develop.

THE IMPORTANCE OF TRUST

Trust is a critically important component of a successful patient–clinician relationship. Without trust, a patient is less likely to adhere to a treatment plan. Patients who do not trust their health care provider or the health care system will be less likely to take prescribed medications, keep scheduled appointments, or accept the advice of their clinician.

Mistrust by certain racial and ethnic minorities in the United States is common. A telephone survey by the Kaiser Family Foundation (Kaiser, 1999) found that one-third of African Americans and one-third of Hispanics reported experiencing unfair treatment by the health care system compared to less than half those numbers of Whites (James, 1999). African Americans were used without their informed consent in medical experimentation by the US Public Health Service from 1932 to 1972 in the notorious Tuskegee syphilis study, which created a legacy of mistrust (CDC, 2015). Mistrust has led to conspiracy theories about the origin of HIV. In 2005, a national telephone survey of 500 African Americans (Bogart, 2015) found that 53% agreed that "there is a cure for AIDS, but it is being withheld from the poor," 27% agreed that "AIDS was produced in a government laboratory," and 16% agreed that "AIDS was created by the government to control the Black population."

DISPARITIES IN HEALTH CARE

The HIV epidemic in the United States is characterized by significant racial and ethnic disparities. In 2013, the rate of new diagnoses of HIV was 6.6 per 100,000 persons for Whites, 18.7 per 100,000 for Hispanic/Latinos, and 55.9 per 100,000 for Blacks/African Americans (CDC, 2013). For many patients, the route of HIV transmission carries significant stigma. Among Black/African American men, for whom 76% contracted the disease by male-to-male sexual contact, being gay or bisexual carries a stigma that is prevalent both in the general population and within the African American community. Stigma creates barriers that keep many men from being tested for HIV or connecting to care once identified as being HIV positive. Understanding the effect of stigma and developing nonjudgmental ways to communicate effectively with patients require that we first acknowledge that patients may enter their relationship with a health care provider assuming the health care provider harbors the same biases as the general population. Becoming culturally competent requires clinicians to develop strategies with each patient to allay the patient's fear of disapproval by his or her health care provider as well as to provide reassurance that the patient's personal health information will be protected and kept confidential.

With significant racial and ethnic disparities concerning who is infected with HIV, the need to provide culturally appropriate care is evident. Failing to adequately understand a patient's culture—best defined as the unique set of beliefs, characteristics, and behaviors formed by the communities in which a patient resides—can create a barrier between patient and health care provider. A lack of trust by the patient may prevent successful treatment. Mistrust of health care providers occurs particularly if patients believe they will receive unequal treatment. Many studies across all disease states have documented the unequal treatment provided to Blacks and Hispanics. According to the Institute of Medicine (Smedley, 2001), racial and ethnic minorities often receive a lower quality of health care services even when insurance status and income are the same as those for non-minorities. Blacks are less likely to be referred for coronary artery revascularization compared to Whites when the same degree of disease severity exists for both (Sheifer, 2000). Other studies have shown that African Americans are less likely than Whites to receive antiviral therapy (Moore, 1995) or prophylaxis for pneumocystis pneumonia (Shapiro, 1999).

Sometimes racial and ethnic disparities result from patient choice or socioeconomic situation, as in cases in which minorities are more likely to refuse recommended treatment services or to delay seeking treatment (Mitchell, 1997). Health care clinicians need to understand what objections a patient may have to the recommended treatment in an effort to help the patient understand potential consequences that may occur without treatment. Clinicians need to take the time to ask patients open-ended questions. Asking questions such as "What are your concerns about taking this medication?" allows the patient to express his or her concerns and the health care provider the opportunity to address them.

BIAS IN HEALTH CARE

Cultural competence requires taking time to learn what cultural barriers might exist. The ethnocentric health care provider only views a patient's culture from the perspective of his or her own culture and risks losing patient trust. Health care providers are not immune from the same biases that exist in the general population. Bias can be subtle and unconscious. Weisse found that White males were twice as likely to be prescribed analgesics for pain as Black males, whereas female physicians prescribed higher doses for Blacks than for Whites (Weisse, 2001). A study examining how patient race affects physician perceptions found that physicians rated Black patients as less intelligent, less educated, more likely to abuse drugs and alcohol, and less likely to adhere to treatment even when taking into account the patient's income and education (van Ryn, 2000). These studies show how racism and personal bias can lead to unequal care.

Bias can be either overt or covert. Derogatory comments made by either providers or office staff about particular "types" of patients are an example of bias. Judgmental comments about "how frequently certain patients develop sexually transmitted infections," "use the emergency room," "look for pain medications," and "had too many uncared for children" are examples of overt bias and stereotyping. Such comments, in addition to be highly unprofessional and judgmental, may reinforce among medical staff involved in patient care that bias and judgment are an acceptable form of professional conduct. Negative comments about a patient, especially if overheard by other patients, can transmit to patients that they may be the unwanted topic of conversation. Health care organizations need to make certain that staff at all levels and functions within the institution become culturally competent. Recognizing the cultural differences that might exist between a patient and a health care provider is an essential step to welcoming each patient with acceptance and understanding. Only by attempting to recognize and to understand these differences can a health care provider best comprehend what may be needed to best inspire patient trust in the provider, the institution, and the plan of treatment.

WOMEN AND HIV

There are 16 million women worldwide living with HIV, and in the United States, one in four persons with HIV are women (CDC, 2013; UNAIDS, 2015). The vast majority of women diagnosed with HIV (84%) acquire the virus through heterosexual sex (CDC, 2015). African American women are disproportionately infected with HIV, with 63% of US women with HIV being Black (CDC, 2013). Women with HIV experience intimate partner violence at twice the national average (Gruskin, 2014). The meta-analysis by Gruskin et al. (Gruskin, 2014) showed that 55% of women with HIV in the United States have experienced trauma and violence. HIV-positive women and transgender women who have experienced trauma and violence had a fourfold higher likelihood of nonadherence to antiviral therapy (Machinger, 2012), The HIV provider should inquire about a history of violence and abuse and should refer the patient to appropriate crisis and domestic violence services as needed. Health care providers should understand that many women who are victims of domestic abuse feel powerless and trapped because of economic dependency, primary responsibility for children, and fear of being homeless. Many women may be slow or unwilling to seek help. A careful mental health and depression screening should be done, and referral to appropriate mental health services should be made when indicated.

LESBIAN, GAY, BISEXUAL, AND TRANSGENDER PATIENTS

Many lesbian, gay, bisexual, and transgender (LGBT) patients do not feel welcome by their health care providers. Many LGBT people do not seek medical care because they have had bad experiences with health care providers (National LBGT Health Education Center, 2015). One recent study of African American men who have sex with men found that 29% experienced racial and sexual stigma from their health care providers and 48% reported mistrust of the health care system (Eaton, 2015). If patients feel uncomfortable speaking about their sexual orientation, they are far more likely to withhold important information. Ways to help LGBT patients feel more welcome include using gender-neutral pronouns, allowing LGBT patients to be called by their preferred name (even if their legal name may be different), and training staff to have a nonjudgmental attitude. Learning and using the language that patients use may make patients feel more comfortable. For example, patients may use the terms "top" or "bottom" to describe insertive anal sex or receptive anal sex. Asking patients if they "have sex with men, women, or both" is an appropriate way to learn patients' sexual orientation. Avoidance of words that imply a patient has a relationship with someone of the opposite sex is also important. "Do you have a partner?" or "Are you in a relationship?" are more appropriate questions than "Do you have a husband or wife?" A patient who feels accepted by his or her care provider is more likely to return for care. Conversely, a patient who perceives disapproval of his or her lifestyle, sexual orientation, or practices will feel uncomfortable and is much more likely to not return.

BEHAVIORAL HEALTH PROBLEMS

The HIV Costs and Services Utilization Study found that nearly 50% of adults treated for HIV have symptoms of a psychiatric disorder—a four to eight times higher prevalence than the general population (Bing, 2001). In the general population, there is a 10- to 20-year reduction in life expectancy in people with severe mental health disorders (Chang, 2001). According to the World Health Organization (WHO), the vast majority of these deaths are due to chronic illnesses such as cardiovascular, respiratory,

and infectious diseases, diabetes, and hypertension (WHO, 2015). Mental illness caries a risk of mortality greater than that of smoking (Chesney, 2014).

Identifying patients with mental illness or addiction is crucial in caring for patients with HIV disease. A careful history followed by referral to mental health services as needed is important because patients with mental illness have been reported to have lower levels of adherence (Patterson, 2000). Stigma about mental health diagnoses may keep many patients from accessing mental health services. On-site behavioral health services increase the likelihood that patients will connect to treatment. Many patients with substance abuse problems may experience a sense of rejection when they reveal that they have chemical dependency or are participating in a substance abuse treatment program. They may assume that mentioning pain will be perceived as drug-seeking by their health care provider—a common stereotype of health care providers. Cultural competence requires communicating with patients openly and without judgment. It requires efforts to develop trust and to help reduce the stigma that most drug users have about their chemical dependency.

CARING FOR IMMIGRANTS AND REFUGEES

Refugees are people who have experienced or been at risk of being persecuted due to race, religion, nationality, membership in a particular social group, or political opinion and have become emigrants fleeing their home country of origin to seek safety. Of the approximately 42 million displaced people in the world, approximately 16 million have sought asylum. The number of refugees accepted into the United States is projected to increase, and many health care providers may see additional refugees in the coming years (*The New York Times*, 2015). Refugees are often victims of physical and emotional trauma. Many immigrants from sub-Saharan Africa have walked hundreds of miles to refugee camps, often while witnessing deaths of family members and becoming victims of violence and sexual trauma. Others have been separated from family. To provide adequate care, it is important for the health care provider to understand both the physical and the emotional trauma the patient has experienced and to provide services that respect the culture, gender roles, and family structure of the patient. Finding culturally and linguistically appropriate counseling or specialty care for immigrants and refugees can be difficult. The use of translation services is often necessary when caring for immigrants and refugees. The diagnosis of HIV for many refugees and immigrants carries great stigma. The HIV provider will need to pay particular attention to understanding how the patient's culture may impact the patient's acceptance of his or her illness and the need to take antiviral medications.

LANGUAGE AND COMMUNICATION

Language comprehension and communication are essential to patient understanding and, ultimately, to good adherence. Many HIV patients speak languages other than English. Language barriers can interfere with the success of treatment. Exit interviews of emergency room patients found that Spanish-speaking patients were less likely to understand their discharge instructions or carry out follow-up plans (Crane, 1997). Another survey found that one in five Spanish-speaking patients delayed or refused medical treatment because of language barriers, underscoring the need to provide linguistically appropriate services to HIV patients who will need lifelong care (Bass, 2000).

Hiring bilingual and bicultural staff is important in a culturally competent organization when there are significant numbers of patients in the local population who speak a particular language. The culturally competent clinical practice needs to make use of professional interpreter services for patients who do not speak the language of the health care provider. The use of family members or friends may inhibit patient honesty when asked to discuss personal information. Telephone interpreter services, although costly, are a necessary tool when on-site interpretation is unavailable. This is especially important for immigrant populations, for which linguistic barriers, often combined with significant cultural differences, may greatly impede the delivery of health care. Patients who used the interpreter services received significantly more recommended preventive services, made more office visits, and had more prescriptions written and filled (Jacobs, 2004).

RELIGION AND SPIRITUALITY

A 2014 Gallup survey found that 81% of Americans identify with a particular religion (Newport, 2014). Patients turn to religion in times of illness, and this often influences the way a person perceives and copes with his or her situation. Many patients with HIV have strong religious affiliations (Cotton, 2006). A patient's faith may sometimes conflict with medical advice, which can lead to a lack of adherence to treatment. It is important to ask patients about their religious and spiritual beliefs and how those beliefs may affect their perception of illness and acceptance of treatment.

CREATING A CULTURALLY COMPETENT HIV PRACTICE

Racial and ethnic diversity in health care leadership and staff is a priority in building culturally competent health care organizations. Including community members and consumer representatives on governing boards, as is done at Federally Qualified Health Centers (FQHCs), can help hold an organization accountable for providing culturally competent care to a diverse patient population. Providing materials that are linguistically appropriate to the population being served at a literacy level appropriate to the level of most patients is important.

Changing the model of care from the traditional physician-centered practice to a model that places the patient in the center of the relationship—the patient-centered medical home (PCMH) model—can improve the quality of care. This model relies on reorganizing care to ensure that it is comprehensive, with integrated physical and mental health services. Care that is patient-centered supports patients' efforts to manage their own care to whatever degree they may choose. It is coordinated so that there is a smoother transition across levels of care, such as primary care, hospital care, and specialty care. Services are accessible, with after-hours access to a health care provider, along with flexible office hours. Last, there is a focus on quality and safety, using evidence-based standards and data for performance improvement (Agency for Healthcare Research and Quality, 2015). Cultural- and linguistic-appropriate services are offered. In one study, retention-in-care for HIV patients was improved with the PCMH model (Sitapati, 2013).

Patients want health care providers who communicate with them and who are empathic. Better health care outcomes have been associated with providers with whom patients can share their feelings and thoughts. Patients of empathic and communicative health care providers are far more likely to comply with their treatment plans (Sitapati, 2013).

The patient-centered approach incorporates cultural competency interventions in order to better address the racial, ethnic, and cultural differences between provider and patient, and it offers training to providers and to all staff who interact with patients in order to make them more culturally competent (Kim, 2004). Health care provider training to improve providers' knowledge and attitudes about diverse populations is essential to creating a culturally competent system of care.

Perhaps most important, aspiring culturally competent health care providers must raise their individual self-awareness of their own cultural beliefs, values, and attitudes and any biases that may be inherent in them. Consciousness of one's own cultural biases and an honest attempt to transcend them will allow the HIV provider to communicate effectively, with empathy, and without prejudgment, facilitating an improved and mutually satisfying relationship with each patient.

Recommended Reading

Anderson LM, Scrimshaw SC, et al. Culturally competent healthcare systems: A systematic review. *Am J Prev Med.* 2003; 24(3S):68–79.

Betancourt JR. Cultural competence in health care: Emerging frameworks and practical approaches: Field Report 2002. The Commonwealth Fund. Available at http://www.commonwealthfund.org/usr_doc/betancourt_culturalcompetence_576.pdf. Accessed December 1, 2015.

Institute of Medicine. Unequal treatment: What healthcare providers need to know about Racial and ethnic disparities in healthcare 2002. National Academy of Sciences. Available at https://www.nationalacademies.org/hmd/~/media/Files/Report%20Files/2003/Unequal-Treatment-Confronting-Racial-and-Ethnic-Disparities-in-Health-Care/Disparitieshcproviders8pgFINAL.pdf. Accessed December 1, 2015.

Institute of Medicine. *Unequal Treatment: Confronting Racial and Ethnic Disparities in Health Care* (full printed version). Washington, DC: National Academies Press; 2003. doi:10.17226/10260.

National LGBT Health Education Center. Providing welcoming services and care for LGBT people—A learning guide for health care staff. January 2015. Available at http://www.lgbthealtheducation.org/wp-content/uploads/Learning-Guide.pdf. Accessed December 1, 2015.

References

Agency for Healthcare Research and Quality. Improving cultural competence to reduce health disparities for priority populations. 2005. Available at http://content.healthaffairs.org/content/24/2/354.full?firstpage=354. Accessed December 1, 2015.

Agency for Healthcare Research and Quality. Defining the PCMH. 2015. Available at https://www.pcmh.ahrq.gov/page/defining-pcmh.

Bass M. Language barriers and illiteracy can affect patient health care. 2000; Robert Wood Johnson Foundation. Available at http://www.rwjf.org/en/library/research/2000/12/language-barriers-and-illiteracy-can-affect-patient-heath-care.html. Accessed December 1, 2015.

Bing EG, Burnam A, Longshore D, et al. Psychiatric disorders and drug use among HIV-infected adults in the US. Arch Gen Psychiatry. 2001; 58:721–728.

Bogart LM, Thorburn S. Are HIV/AIDS conspiracy beliefs a barrier to HIV prevention among African-Americans? J Acquir Immune Defic Syndr. 2005; 38(2):213–218.

Centers for Disease Control and Prevention. HIV surveillance report: Diagnosis of HIV infection in the United States and dependent areas 2013—HIV by race/ethnicity through 2013; Vol. 25. August 2013.

Centers for Disease Control and Prevention. Surveillance report 2013. Available at http://www.cdc.gov/hiv/library/reports/surveillance. Accessed December 1, 2015.

Centers for Disease Control and Prevention. HIV surveillance report 2013. Available at http://www.cdc.gov/hiv/pdf/library/reports/surveillance/cdc-hiv-surveillance-report-vol-25.pdf. Accessed December 1, 2015.

Centers for Disease Control and Prevention. U.S. Public Health Service Study of Syphilis at Tuskegee. Available at http://www.cdc.gov/tuskegee/index.html. Accessed November 8, 2015.

Centers for Disease Control and Prevention. HIV among women. 2015. Available at http://www.cdc.gov/hiv/group/gender/women/index.html. Accessed December 1, 2015.

Chang CK, Hayes RD, Perera G, et al. Life expectancy at birth for people with serious mental illness and other major disorders from a secondary mental health care case register in London. PLoS One 2011; 10:1371.

Chesney E, Goodwin GM, Fazel S. Risks all-cause and suicide mortality in mental disorders: A meta-review. World Psychiatry 2014 Jun; 13(2):153–160.

Cope AB, Power KA, Kuruc JD, et al. Ongoing HIV transmission and the HIV care continuum in North Carolina. PLoS One 2015; 10(6):e0127950.

Cotton S. Spirituality and religion in patients with HIV/AIDS. Gen Intern Med. 2006; 12;21(Suppl. 5):S5–S13.

Crane JA. Patient comprehension of doctor–patient communication on discharge from the emergency department. Emerg Med. 1997 Jan-Feb; 15(1):1–7.

Eaton LA, Driffin DD, Kegler C, et al. The role of stigma and medical mistrust in the routine health care engagement of black men who have sex with men. Am J Public Health 2015; 105(2):75–82.

Gordon MR, Smale A, Lyman R. U.S. will accept more refugees as crisis grows. New York Times, September 20, 2015.

Gruskin S, Safreed-Harmon K, Moore CL, et al. HIV and gender-based violence: Welcome policies and programmes, but is the research keeping up? Reproductive Health Matters 2014; 22(44):174–184.

Jacobs EA, Shepard D, Suaya JA, et al. Overcoming language barriers in health care: Costs and benefits of interpreter services. American Journal of Public Health 2004; 94(5):866–869.

James C. Race ethnicity and medical care: A survey of public perceptions and experiences. Kaiser Family Foundation, September, 1999.

Kim SS, Kaplowitz KS. The effects of physician empathy on patient satisfaction and compliance. Eval Health Prof. 2004; 27(9):237–251.

Machinger EL, Haberer JE, Wilson TC, et al. Recent trauma is associated with antiretroviral failure and HIV transmission risk behavior among HIV-positive women and female-identified transgenders. AIDS and Behavior 2012; 16(8):2160–2170.

Mitchell JB, McCormack LA. Time trends in late-stage diagnosis of cervical cancer: Differences by race/ethnicity and income. Medical Care 1997; 35(12):1220–1224.

Moore RD, Stanton D, Gopalan R, et al. Racial differences in the use of drug therapy for HIV disease in an urban community. N Engl J Med. 1994; 330(11):763–768.

National LGBT Health Education Center. Providing welcoming services and care for LGBT people. 2015. Available at http://www.lgbthealtheducation.org/wp-content/uploads/Learning-Guide.pdf. Accessed December 1, 2015.

Newport F. Three-quarters of Americans identify as Christian. Gallup.com, December, 2014. Available at http://www.gallup.com/poll/180347/three-quarters-americans-identify-christian.aspx. Accessed December 1, 2015.

Paterson DL Swindells S. Adherence to protease inhibitor therapy and outcomes in patients with HIV infection. Ann Intern Med 2000; 133:21–30.

Shapiro MJ, Morton SC, McCaffrey D, et al. Variations in the care of HIV-infected adults in the United States: Results from the HIV Vost and services utilization study. JAMA 1999; 281:2305–2375.

Sheifer SE, Escarce JJ. Race and sex differences in the management of coronary artery disease. Am Heart J. 2000; 139(5):848–857.

Sitapati AM, Limneos J, Bonet-Vázquez M, et al. Retention: Building a patient-centered medical home in HIV primary care through PUFF (patients unable to follow-up found). J Health Care Poor Underserved 2012; 23(3 Suppl):81–95.

Skarbinski J, Rosenberg E, Paz-Bailey G, et al. Human immunodeficiency virus transmission at each step of the care continuum in the United States. JAMA Intern Med 2015; 175(4):596–597.

Smedley D, Stith A, Nelson A (Eds.). *Unequal Treatment—Confronting Racial and Ethnic Disparities in Healthcare*. Institute of Medicine, The National Academies Press, Washington, DC, 2003.

UNAIDS. How AIDS changed everything—MDG6: 15 years, 15 lessons of hope from the AIDS response. July 2015. UNAIDS Secretariat, Geneva, Switzerland. Available at https://issuu.com/unaids/docs/mdg6_executivesummary_en. Accessed December 1, 2015.

van Ryn M, Burke J. The effect of patient race and socioeconomic status on physicians' perceptions of patients. Social Sci Med. 2000; 50:813–828.

Weisse CS, Sorum PC, Sanders KN, et al. Do gender and race affect decisions about pain management? J Gen Intern Med. 2001; 16(4):211–217.

World Health Organization. HIV/AIDS fact sheet. Available at http://www.who.int/mediacentre/factsheets/fs360/en. Accessed November 12, 2015.

CARING FOR HIV-INFECTED WOMEN[1]

LEARNING OBJECTIVE

Discuss issues unique to the management of HIV-infected women.

WHAT'S NEW?

Efavirenz is contraindicated in women wanting to become pregnant or not using effective contraception; it should be used with caution in women of childbearing potential who are not intending to become pregnant. Truncal fat accumulation and certain antiretroviral therapy (ART)-associated toxicities, such as lactic acidosis and nevirapine-induced rash and hepatotoxicity, seem to be more common in women than in men.

KEY POINTS

- The incidence and range of HIV-related illnesses and rates of progression to AIDS are similar in women and men; exceptions include gynecologic manifestations of HIV and low rates of Kaposi's sarcoma.

- Women appear to have lower mean viral loads compared to men with similar CD4$^+$ cell counts; differences are most apparent early in the course of HIV infection and diminish over time. Current US guidelines for starting ART are the same for men and women.

- Hormonal contraceptives—including oral, local, and parenteral—may be used in HIV-infected women, but they do not provide protection against acquisition or transmission of HIV or other sexually transmitted infections (STIs). In addition, drug interactions with certain antiretroviral agents may decrease hormonal contraceptive efficacy or decrease antiretroviral blood levels. For all of these reasons, condom use should always be recommended.

1. This section has not been updated from the 2012 text. Only the references to guidelines have been revised as appropriate.

- Efavirenz should not be included as an ART component in women wanting to become pregnant, and it should be used with caution in women of childbearing potential who are not intending to become pregnant.

- Women on ART appear to have increased rates of lipodystrophy/fat maldistribution, and they seem particularly prone to truncal obesity compared with men. Certain ART-associated toxicities also appear to be more common in women, including lactic acidosis and nevirapine-induced rash and hepatotoxicity.

DIFFERENCES BETWEEN WOMEN AND MEN

The incidence and range of HIV-related illnesses are generally similar in women and men (Prins, 1999; Sterling, 1999); the exceptions are gynecologic manifestations of HIV and low rates of Kaposi's sarcoma (Hessol, 2005). Most studies show similar rates of disease progression and survival in women and men if they have the same access to treatment (Collazos, 2007; Currier, 2010; Fardet, 2006). In general, predictors of progression are the same in women and men (Anastos, 1999), and ART is the strongest predictor of survival. Women tend to have higher CD4$^+$ cell counts when corrected for stage of disease (Anastos, 2000; Collazos, 2007; Prins, 1999), and they also tend to have lower mean viral loads early in the course of infection when controlled for CD4$^+$ cell counts (Gandhi, 2002; Napravnik, 2002; Sterling, 1999, 2001). However, once ART is initiated, viral suppression does not appear to differ by sex, and sex differences in outcome generally disappear when adjusted for treatment (Losina, 2009; Perez-Hoyas, 2007; Porter, 2003). Current US recommendations for initiation of ART are the same for men and women (US Department of Health and Human Services (DHHS), 2015).

HORMONAL CONTRACEPTIVES

Hormonal contraceptives—including oral, local, and parenteral forms—may be used in HIV-infected women without medical contraindications for their use (CDC, 2013); however, they do not provide protection against the transmission or acquisition of HIV or STIs, and they should consistently be used in conjunction with male or female condoms. Most studies have found no association between the use of hormonal contraception and HIV disease progression (Morrison, 2011; Polis, 2010; Stringer, 2009). There are conflicting data on the role of hormonal contraception in HIV susceptibility or infectiousness (Morrison, 2012). A secondary analysis of data from a large prevention trial found a twofold increased risk of HIV seroconversion (both transmission and acquisition) associated with hormonal contraception (primarily depot medroxyprogesterone acetate) among more than 3700 serodiscordant African couples (Heffron, 2012). HIV-infected women using hormonal contraception had higher genital HIV RNA concentrations compared to women not using hormonal contraceptives. Oral contraceptive (OC) use was not significantly associated with transmission of HIV, but the number of women using OCs in this study was insufficient to adequately assess risk. It is important to note that other studies have not shown a link between hormonal contraception and transmission or acquisition of HIV and that individuals in this study were not receiving ART (Blish, 2011; Morrison, 2012).

Noncontraceptive benefits of combined estrogen–progestin contraceptives include a decrease in iron deficiency anemia, increased menstrual regularity (not seen with progestin-only methods), protection of bone density, decreased risk of pelvic inflammatory disease, and a decrease in endometrial and ovarian cancer (Hatcher, 2012). In addition to oral daily formulations, alternate delivery routes of hormonal contraception include the estrogen–progestin vaginal ring or patch, as well as progestin-only methods (e.g., Depo-Provera and Implanon), which do not require daily administration. Although data on the levonorgestrel-releasing intrauterine device are relatively limited, it is considered safe to use in HIV-infected women, including those with AIDS, who are clinically doing well on ART (CDC, 2013; Heikinheimo, 2009, 2011; Lehtovirta, 2007).

Pharmacokinetic interactions between hormonal contraceptives (primarily studied with combined estrogen–progestin oral contraceptives) and some protease inhibitors (PIs) and non-nucleoside reverse transcriptase inhibitors (NNRTIs) (EFV, NVP, ATV/r, DRV/r, FPV/r, LPV/r, SQV/r, TPV/r, ATV alone, and NFV) may result in a decrease or increase in blood levels of the estrogen and progestin components of the hormonal contraceptive, potentially decreasing contraceptive effectiveness or increasing risk of adverse effects, although the true clinical effect is not clear. An additional or alternative contraceptive method is generally advised if hormonal contraception is considered. Unboosted FPV should not be coadministered with oral contraceptives because of a concomitant decrease in FPV level (Cohn, 2007; El-Ibiary, 2008; USPHS, 2015; Vogler, 2010). In small studies of HIV-infected women receiving injectable depot-medroxyprogesterone acetate (DMPA) while on ART, there were no significant interactions

between DMPA and EFV, NVP, NFV, or NRTI drugs (Cohn, 2007; Nanda, 2008; Watts, 2008). Contraceptive failure of the etonogestrel implant in two patients on EFV-based therapy has been reported (Leticee, 2011).

OCs may also interact with other drugs commonly used in HIV-infected individuals, such as rifampin/rifabutin and several anticonvulsants (Hatcher, 2012). Health care providers should discuss the available options for hormonal contraception, as well as other contraceptive methods. Concerns about pharmacokinetic interactions between hormonal contraceptives and antiretrovirals (ARVs) should not prevent clinicians from prescribing hormonal contraceptives for women on ART.

MEDICATION EFFECTS AND ADVERSE EFFECTS

A number of studies have suggested that gender may influence the frequency, presentation, and severity of selected ARV-related adverse events (Clark, 2005). Women with $CD4^+$ cell counts >250/mm^3 or with elevated baseline transaminase levels appear to be at greatest risk for nevirapine-related symptomatic and often rash-associated liver toxicity in ARV-naive individuals (Baylor, 2004; Dieterich, 2004; Leith, 2005; Wit, 2008). It is generally recommended that NVP not be prescribed to ARV-naive women who have $CD4^+$ counts >250 cells/mm^3 unless there is no other alternative and the benefit from NVP outweighs the risk of hepatotoxicity (DHHS, 2015). Women are also at increased risk for symptomatic and even fatal lactic acidosis associated with prolonged exposure to NRTIs (Lactic Acidosis International Study Group, 2007). In terms of metabolic complications associated with ARV use, HIV-infected women are more likely to experience increases in central fat with ART and are less likely to have triglyceride elevations on treatment (Galli, 2003; Thiebaut, 2001). Women have an increased risk of osteopenia/osteoporosis, particularly after menopause, and this risk is exacerbated by HIV and ART (Brown, 2007; Yin, 2005).

Although data are limited, there is also evidence that pharmacokinetics for some ARV drugs may differ between men and women, possibly due to variations by sex in factors such as body weight, plasma volume, gastric emptying time, plasma protein levels, cytochrome P (CYP) 450 activity, drug transporter function, and excretion activity (Floridia, 2008; Gandhi, 2004; Ofotokun, 2007).

Efavirenz is currently the only antiretroviral agent associated with teratogenic risk (US Food and Drug Administration category D), based on preclinical primate data and retrospective case reports after first-trimester

Table 13.1 ABSOLUTE CONTRAINDICATIONS
TO ORAL CONTRACEPTIVE USE (ESTROGEN/
PROGESTIN COMBINATIONS)

- History of thromboembolic disease or known thrombogenic mutations
- Age >35 years and smoker ≥15 cigarettes/day
- Hypertension with systolic ≥160 mm Hg or diastolic ≥100 mm Hg
- Diabetes mellitus and >20 years' duration; or <20 years' duration with nephropathy, retinopathy, neuropathy, or other vascular disease
- Coronary artery disease
- Complicated valvular heart disease
- Peripartum cardiomyopathy with moderately or severely impaired cardiac function
- Cerebrovascular disease
- Major surgery with prolonged immobilization
- Systemic lupus erythematosus (+) antiphospholipid antibodies
- Migraines with focal neurologic signs or aura
- Breast cancer
- Acute viral hepatitis or flare; severe cirrhosis; or benign or malignant liver tumor
- Graft failure or rejection after solid organ transplant

SOURCE: Adapted from Centers for Disease Control and Prevention. U.S. medical eligibility criteria for contraceptive use, 2010. *MMWR.* 2010; 59:1–85.

human exposure; however, recent data suggest that the risk is likely to be quite low (Ford, 2011) (Table 13.1). EFV-containing regimens should be avoided in women who are trying to conceive or who are or may engage in sexual activity that could result in pregnancy (DHHS, 2015). The most vulnerable period in fetal organogenesis is early in gestation, often before pregnancy is recognized.

Recommended Reading

Centers for Disease Control and Prevention. U.S. medical eligibility criteria for contraceptive use, 2010. *MMWR.* 2010; 59:1–85.

Hatcher RA, Trussell J, Nelson AL, et al. (Eds.). *Contraceptive Technology,* 20th ed. New York, NY: Ardent Media, 2012.

Public Health Service Task Force. Recommendations for use of antiretroviral drugs in pregnant HIV-1-infected women for maternal health and interventions to reduce perinatal HIV-1 transmission in the United States. Update available at https://aidsinfo.nih.gov/content-files/lvguidelines/PerinatalGL.pdf.

US Department of Health and Human Services. Guidelines for the use of antiretroviral agents in HIV-1 infected adults and adolescents. 2012. Available at http://aidsinfo.nih.gov/ContentFiles/AdultandAdolescentGL.pdf.

References

Anastos K, Kalish LA, Hessol N, et al. The relative value of CD4 cell count and quantitative HIV-1 RNA in predicting survival in HIV-1-infected women: results of the women's interagency HIV study. AIDS. 1999; 13(13):1717–1726. [Erratum in AIDS 2000 May 5; 14(7):891]

Anastos K, Gange SJ, Lau B, et al. Association of race and gender with HIV-1 RNA levels and immunologic progression. J Acquir Immune Defic Syndr. 2000 Jul 1; 24(3):218–226.

Baylor MS, Johann-Liang R. Hepatotoxicity associated with nevirapine use. J Acquir Immune Defic Syndr. 2004 Apr 15; 35(5): 538–539.

Blish CA, Baeten JM. Hormonal contraception and HIV-1 transmission. Am J Reprod Immunol. 2011 Mar; 65(3):302–307. doi:10.1111/j.1600-0897.2010.00930.x

Brown TT, Qaqish RB. Response to Berg et al. "Antiretroviral therapy and the prevalence of osteopenia and osteoporosis: A meta-analytic review." AIDS. 2007 Aug 20; 21(13):1830–1831.

Centers for Disease Control and Prevention. Hormonal contraception and HIV. September 2013. Accessed at http://stacks.cdc.gov/view/cdc/21848.

Clark R. Sex differences in antiretroviral therapy-associated intolerance and adverse events. Drug Saf. 2005; 28(12):1075–1083.

Cohn SE, Park JG, Watts DH, et al. Depo-medroxyprogesterone in women on antiretroviral therapy: Effective contraception and lack of clinically significant interactions. Clin Pharmacol Ther. 2007 Feb; 81(2):222–227.

Collazos J, Asensi V, Cartón JA. Sex differences in the clinical, immunological and virological parameters of HIV-infected patients treated with HAART. AIDS. 2007 Apr 23; 21(7):835–843.

Currier J, Averitt Bridge D, Hagins D, et al. Sex-based outcomes of darunavir-ritonavir therapy: A single-group trial. Ann Intern Med. 2010 Sep 21; 153(6):349–357. doi:10.7326/0003-4819-153-6-201009210-00002

Dieterich DT, Robinson PA, Love J, et al. Drug-induced liver injury associated with the use of nonnucleoside reverse-transcriptase inhibitors. Clin Infect Dis. 2004 Mar 1; 38(Suppl 2):S80–S89.

El-Ibiary SY, Cocohoba JM. Effects of HIV antiretrovirals on the pharmacokinetics of hormonal contraceptives. Eur J Contracept Reprod Health Care. 2008 Jun; 13(2):123–132. doi:10.1080/13625180701829952

Fardet L, Mary-Krause M, Heard I, et al. Influence of gender and HIV transmission group on initial highly active antiretroviral therapy prescription and treatment response. HIV Med. 2006 Nov; 7(8):520–529.

Floridia M, Giuliano M, Palmisano L, et al. Gender differences in the treatment of HIV infection. Pharmacol Res. 2008 Sep–Oct; 58(3–4):173–182. doi:10.1016/j.phrs.2008.07.007

Ford N, Calmy A, Mofenson L. Safety of efavirenz in the first trimester of pregnancy: An updated systematic review and meta-analysis. AIDS. 2011 Nov 28; 25(18):2301–2304. doi:10.1097/QAD.0b013e32834cdb71

Galli M, Veglia F, Angarano G, et al. Gender differences in antiretroviral drug-related adipose tissue alterations: Women are at higher risk than men and develop particular lipodystrophy patterns. J Acquir Immune Defic Syndr. 2003 Sep 1; 34(1):58–61.

Gandhi M, Bacchetti P, Miotti P, et al. Does patient sex affect human immunodeficiency virus levels? Clin Infect Dis. 2002 Aug 1; 35(3):313–322. [Erratum in Clin Infect Dis 2002 Dec 1; 35(11):1455]

Hatcher AM, Turan JM, Leslie HH, et al. Predictors of linkage to care following community-based HIV counseling and testing in rural Kenya. AIDS Behav. 2012 Jul; 16(5):1295–1307. doi:10.1007/s10461-011-0065-1

Heffron R, Donnell D, Rees H, et al. Use of hormonal contraceptives and risk of HIV-1 transmission: A prospective cohort study. Lancet Infect Dis. 2012 Jan; 12(1):19–26. doi:10.1016/S1473-3099(11)70247-X [Erratum in: Lancet Infect Dis. 2012 Feb; 12(2):98]

Heikinheimo O, Lähteenmäki P. Contraception and HIV infection in women. Hum Reprod Update. 2009 Mar–Apr; 15(2):165–176. doi:10.1093/humupd/dmn049

Heikinheimo O, Lehtovirta P, Aho I, et al. The levonorgestrel-releasing intrauterine system in human immunodeficiency virus-infected women: A 5-year follow-up study. Am J Obstet Gynecol. 2011 Feb; 204(2):126.e1–e4. doi:10.1016/j.ajog.2010.09.002

Hessol NA, Fuentes-Afflick E. Ethnic differences in neonatal and post-neonatal mortality. Pediatrics. 2005 Jan; 115(1):e44–e51.

Lactic Acidosis International Study Group. Risk factors for lactic acidosis and severe hyperlactataemia in HIV-1-infected adults exposed to antiretroviral therapy. AIDS. 2007 Nov 30; 21(18):2455–2464.

Lehtovirta P, Paavonen J, Heikinheimo O. Experience with the levonorgestrel-releasing intrauterine system among HIV-infected women. Contraception. 2007 Jan; 75(1):37–39.

Leith J, Piliero P, Storfer S, et al. Appropriate use of nevirapine for long-term therapy. J Infect Dis. 2005 Aug 1; 192(3):545–546; Author reply 546.

Leticee N, Viard JP, Yamgnane A, et al. Contraceptive failure of etonogestrel implant in patients treated with antiretrovirals including efavirenz. Contraception. 2012 Apr; 85(4):425–427. doi:10.1016/j.contraception.2011.09.005

Losina E, Schackman BR, Sadownik SN, et al. Racial and sex disparities in life expectancy losses among HIV-infected persons in the United States: Impact of risk behavior, late initiation, and early discontinuation of antiretroviral therapy. Clin Infect Dis. 2009 Nov 15; 49(10):1570–1578. doi:10.1086/644772

Morrison CS, Chen PL, Nankya I, et al. Hormonal contraceptive use and HIV disease progression among women in Uganda and Zimbabwe. Acquir Immune Defic Syndr. 2011 Jun 1; 57(2):157–164. doi:10.1097/QAI.0b013e318214ba4a

Morrison CS, Nanda K. Hormonal contraception and HIV: An unanswered question. Lancet Infect Dis. 2012 Jan; 12(1):2–3. doi:10.1016/S1473-3099(11)70254-7

Nanda K, Amaral E, Hays M, et al. Pharmacokinetic interactions between depot medroxyprogesterone acetate and combination antiretroviral therapy. Fertil Steril. 2008 Oct; 90(4):965–971.

Napravnik S, Poole C, Thomas JC, et al. Gender difference in HIV RNA levels: A meta-analysis of published studies. J Acquir Immune Defic Syndr. 2002 Sep 1; 31(1):11–19.

Ofotokun I, Chuck SK, Hitti JE. Antiretroviral pharmacokinetic profile: A review of sex differences. Gender Med. 2007 Jun; 4(2): 106–119.

Panel on Antiretroviral Guidelines for Adults and Adolescents. Recommendations for use of antiretroviral drugs in pregnant HIV-1-infected women for maternal health and interventions to reduce perinatal HIV transmission in the United States. Department of Health and Human Services. Available at https://aidsinfo.nih.gov/contentfiles/lvguidelines/PerinatalGL.pdf.

Panel on Antiretroviral Guidelines for Adults and Adolescents. Guidelines for the use of antiretroviral agents in HIV-1-infected adults and adolescents. Department of Health and Human Services. Available at https://aidsinfo.nih.gov/contentfiles/lvguidelines/AdultandAdolescentGL.pdf.

Perez-Hoyos S, Rodríguez-Arenas MA, García de la Hera M, et al. Progression to AIDS and death and response to HAART in men and women from a multicenter hospital-based cohort. J Womens Health (Larchmt). 2007 Sep; 16(7):1052–1061.

Polis CB, Wawer MJ, Kiwanuka N, et al. Uganda. AIDS. 2010 Jul 31; 24(12):1937–1944. doi:10.1097/QAD.0b013e32833b3282

Porter K, Babiker A, Bhaskaran K, et al. Determinants of survival following HIV-1 seroconversion after the introduction of HAART. Lancet. 2003 Oct 18; 362(9392):1267–1274.

Prins M, Robertson JR, Brettle RP, et al. Do gender differences in CD4 cell counts matter? AIDS. 1999 Dec 3; 13(17):2361–2364.

Sterling TR, Lyles CM, Vlahov D, et al. Sex differences in longitudinal human immunodeficiency virus type 1 RNA levels among seroconverters. J Infect Dis. 1999 Sep; 180(3):666–672.

Stringer EM, Giganti M, Carter RJ, et al. Hormonal contraception and HIV disease progression: a multicountry cohort analysis of the MTCT-Plus Initiative. AIDS. 2009 Nov; 23(Suppl 1):S69–S77. doi:10.1097/01.aids.0000363779.65827.e0

Thiébaut R, Dequae-Merchadou L, Ekouevi DK, et al. Incidence and risk factors of severe hypertriglyceridemia in the era of highly active antiretroviral therapy: The Aquitaine Cohort, France, 1996–99. HIV Med. 2001 Apr; 2(2):84–88.

Vogler MA, Patterson K, Kamemoto L, et al. Contraceptive efficacy of oral and transdermal hormones when co-administered with protease inhibitors in HIV-1-infected women: Pharmacokinetic results of ACTG trial A5188. J Acquir Immune Defic Syndr. 2010 Dec; 55(4):473–482. doi:10.1097/QAI.0b013e3181eb5ff5

Watts DH, Park JG, Cohn SE, et al. Safety and tolerability of depot medroxyprogesterone acetate among HIV-infected women on antiretroviral therapy: ACTG A5093. Contraception. 2008 Feb; 77(2):84–90. doi:10.1016/j.contraception.2007.10.002

Wit FW, Kesselring AM, Gras L, et al. Discontinuation of nevirapine because of hypersensitivity reactions in patients with prior treatment experience, compared with treatment-naive patients: The ATHENA cohort study. Clin Infect Dis. 2008 Mar 15; 46(6):933–940. doi:10.1086/528861

Yin M, Dobkin J, Brudney K, et al. Bone mass and mineral metabolism in HIV+ postmenopausal women. Osteoporos Int. 2005 Nov; 16(11):1345–1352.

CARING FOR HIV-INFECTED CHILDREN[2]

LEARNING OBJECTIVE

Identify the diagnostic criteria, laboratory markers, epidemiologic patterns, spectrum of disease manifestations, and unique immunization and therapy issues in HIV-infected children.

WHAT'S NEW?

In 2014, the CDC revised the definitions for and stage classification of HIV infection in persons of all ages.

KEY POINTS

- In the United States, the prevalence of perinatally acquired HIV has declined dramatically.

- Pediatric and adult HIV/AIDS differ in the following areas: AIDS-defining conditions, epidemiology and transmission, pathophysiology, diagnostic challenges, clinical manifestations, and management issues.

---

2. In the following discussion, the definition of "children" encompasses a broader population than that generally appreciated because children's maturation to adolescence varies greatly. There may be some redundancies of HIV-related topics with the section on adolescents.

- In the United States, pediatric HIV/AIDS disproportionately affects ethnic minorities, particularly African Americans.

- Due to pathophysiologic differences, untreated HIV-infected children younger than 2 years of age are uniquely susceptible to encephalopathy and routinely have higher viral loads than adults.

- Normal CD4$^+$ T cell counts are higher in healthy infants and children younger than 6 years of age than in adults.

- Infants born to HIV-positive mothers will test positive on routine anti-HIV antibody tests due to placental IgG transport; sequential nucleic acid test (NAT) analysis can identify infected infants usually by 1 month of age.

- Clinical features more common in children include developmental delay, recurrent otitis media and sinobronchial infections, lymphoid interstitial pneumonia, and severe dental carries.

- In children and adults, the general concepts of ART, opportunistic infection (OI) prophylaxis, viral load, and CD4$^+$ T cell count monitoring are similar, but the indications for beginning, the thresholds for changing, and the potential complications of therapy are different.

- Administration of routine immunizations in HIV-infected children is complicated by the use of live virus vaccines (rotavirus; measles, mumps, and rubella (MMR); and varicella zoster virus (VZV)) in standard practice.

- Avoidance of breast-feeding by HIV-infected mothers continues to be advised.

- The HIV-infected child's family needs, both material and psychosocial, are often extraordinarily complex, requiring intensive, community, social services utilization.

- Whenever possible, a pediatric HIV specialist should supervise the management of children younger than age 16 years.

In the United States, the prevalence of perinatally acquired HIV/AIDS has declined dramatically during the past 20 years due to extraordinary public health investments. Despite this, children continue to be born to HIV-infected women and to be infected with HIV. Pediatric and adult HIV/AIDS differ significantly in the following areas: AIDS-defining conditions, epidemiology, pathophysiology, diagnostic challenges, clinical manifestations, and management issues that are unique to children.

DEFINITION

Conceptually, "AIDS" may be considered to be the most serious clinical consequences of HIV-associated immune dysregulation, including immunodeficiency and immune hyperactivation.

In 2014, the CDC and the Council of State and Territorial Epidemiologists revised and combined surveillance case definitions and stage classification for HIV infection into a single entity covering persons of all ages (Selik, 2014). Confirmed cases of HIV infection are classified into stages 0, 1, 2, 3, or unknown.

Stage 0 is defined as the presence of early HIV infection with a negative HIV antibody test. The stage includes "acute HIV infection" or "acute retroviral syndrome" that occurs days to weeks postexposure and presents with flu-like or mononucleosis-like signs and symptoms.

Classification of stages 1, 2, and 3 is based on age-specific CD4$^+$ T lymphocyte count or percentage of total lymphocyte count (Table 13.2) or the diagnosis of an opportunistic condition in the case of stage 3 (Table 13.3). Furthermore, clinical features considered as "mild" or "moderate" HIV-related symptoms are listed in the recent guidelines (see https://aidsetc.org/guide/hiv-classification-cdc-and-who-staging-systems).

EPIDEMIOLOGY

It is estimated that 70% of HIV-infected women are sexually active and 25–30% of HIV-infected women in North America express a desire to have children (Chen, 2001). In the United States, factors that place children at increased risk for HIV infection include being born to an HIV-infected mother, blood transfusion (outside the United States), being fed premasticated food, sexual abuse, and accidental sharps injury.

Remarkably, in contrast to the persistently high incidence of new HIV infection in adults in the United States (an estimated 56,000 new cases per year), the number of HIV-infected children has declined dramatically during the past 20 years (Figure 13.1). This decline has been due to the intense efforts by public health departments and local perinatal HIV centers. Factors contributing to this dramatic change include the following:

- HIV transmission through blood transfusion has been eliminated (except in very rare circumstances) through the screening of all blood products since 1985.

- HIV-infected women are increasingly aware of their HIV-infection status and receive effective ART prior to conception and throughout their pregnancies.

Table 13.2 HIV INFECTION STAGING BASED ON AGE-SPECIFIC CD4+ T LYMPHOCYTE NUMBERS OR PERCENTAGE

| | AGE ON DATE OF CD4+ T LYMPHOCYTE TEST | | | | | |
| | <1 YEAR | | 1–5 YEARS | | ≥6 YEARS | |
STAGE	CELLS/ML	%	CELLS/ML	%	CELLS/ML	%
1	≥1500	≥34	≥1000	≥30	≥500	≥26
2	750–1499	26–33	500–999	22–29	200499	14–25
3	<750	<26	<500	<22	<200	≤14

SOURCE: Reproduced from Centers for Disease Control and Prevention. Revised surveillance care definition for HIV infection—United States, 2014. *MMWR*. 2014; 63(3):1–10.

- HIV screening of pregnant women has allowed the implementation of highly active antiretroviral therapy (HAART) during pregnancy and prior to delivery.

- Rapid HIV testing during labor identifies HIV-infected women, allowing initiation of antiviral therapy during labor and delivery and postnatally to the newborn.

- Treatment of newborns exposed to HIV (e.g., in a mother without prenatal care) can still result in a substantial reduction in transmission when the infant alone is treated. This was the first demonstration of effective post-exposure prophylaxis.

- HIV-infected infants and children treated prior to the development of clinical symptoms and adherent to their treatment regimens rarely develop AIDS-defining conditions.

Despite this extraordinary progress in reducing maternal-to-child transmission, disturbing racial and ethnic disparities among children persist and generally reflect the prevalence of HIV infection in the respective populations. Black and Hispanic children are disproportionately infected with HIV. African Americans comprise more than 50% of newly infected children (Figure 13.2).

From 2010 through 2014, 3 infants were born HIV-infected in Los Angeles County, California. During the same time period, approximately 400 HIV-infected women gave birth in Los Angeles County, resulting in a dramatic <1% maternal-to-child transmission rate. Also during the same time period, 21 HIV-infected children, adopted from outside the United States, entered care in Los Angeles County (data from the Enhanced Perinatal Surveillance (EPS) and Enhanced HIV/AIDS Reporting System (eHARS) as of November 2015, Los Angeles Country Department of Public Health, Division of HIV/STD Programs).

UNIQUE FEATURES OF PEDIATRIC HIV/AIDS PATHOGENESIS

HIV pathogenesis in children differs from that in adults in several ways. Untreated infection during embryologic or perinatal development has the potential to interfere with

Table 13.3 STAGE-3/AIDS-DEFINING CONDITIONS

All ages	• Opportunistic infections (e.g., PJP and severe or disseminated CMV, toxoplasma HSV, mycobacteria) • Selected malignancies (lymphoma, KS) • HIV encephalopathy • HIV wasting
<1 year old	• CD4+ T cell count <750 (<26%)
1–5 years old	• CD4+ T cell count <500 (<22%) • Recurrent bacterial infections
≥6 years old	• CD4+ T cell count <200 (<14%) • Cervical cancer, invasive • Recurrent pneumonia

CMV, cytomegalovirus; HSV, herpes simplex virus; KS, Kaposi's sarcoma; PJP, *Pneumocystis jirovecii* pneumonia.

SOURCE: Adapted from Centers for Disease Control and Prevention. Revised surveillance care definition for HIV infection—United States, 2014. *MMWR*. 2014; 63(3):1–10.

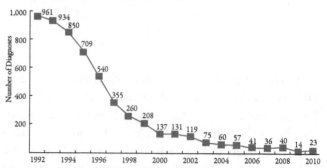

Figure 13.1 Estimated numbers of AIDS diagnoses in children younger than age 13 years, by year of diagnosis, 1992–2010. SOURCE: Reproduced from US Department of Health and Human Services, Health Resources and Services Administration, Maternal and Child Health Bureau. *Child Health USA 2011*. Rockville, MD: US Department of Health and Human Services, 2012. Accessed online November 7, 2015.

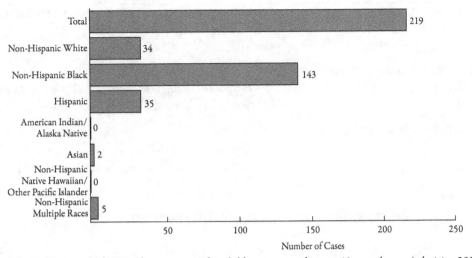

Figure 13.2 Estimated numbers of diagnoses of HIV infection reported in children younger than age 13 years, by race/ethnicity, 2010. SOURCE: Reproduced from US Department of Health and Human Services, Health Resources and Services Administration, Maternal and Child Health Bureau. *Child Health USA 2012*. Rockville, MD: US Department of Health and Human Services, 2013. Accessed online November 7, 2015.

normal neurologic and immunologic developmental processes at critical times during ontogeny. In addition, the blood–brain barrier in children is more permissive to viral entry, and the combination of undiagnosed HIV infection and an opportunistic infection such as *Pneumocystis jirovecii* pneumonia (PCP) may increase trafficking of HIV-infected monocytes to the brain (Nottet, 1996).

HIV infection in infants that occurs prior to the generation of antigen-specific T and B cell repertoires may damage the thymus before these protective immune responses can occur. Furthermore, the "normal" recurrent infection pattern in children may enhance the immunologic activation that is part of the immunopathogenesis of HIV (Sodora, 2008). The combination of these factors can result in unique manifestations of pediatric neuroencephalopathy, immunodeficiency, and pathologic findings.

DIAGNOSIS OF HIV INFECTION IN CHILDREN

Although current fourth-generation HIV antigen/antibody testing algorithms are useful for decreasing the "window" between infection and seropositivity, they are not particularly useful in children. Maternal antibodies are efficiently transported across the placenta, and infants born to HIV-infected mothers have high levels of HIV antibodies that may persist for more than 15 months. Therefore, interpretation of an HIV test result in a particular infant depends on his or her age. A positive HIV antibody test in an infant younger than age 18 month identifies the infant as being "at risk" for HIV infection but not necessarily infected (Husson, 2008) (Box 13.1).

SELECTED CLINICAL FEATURES OF HIV INFECTION IN CHILDREN

Clinical features of HIV infections that are similar in children and adults include opportunistic infections, "opportunistic" malignancies, chronic enteropathy (infectious and non-infectious), hepatosplenomegaly, lymphadenopathy, parotitis, and cardiomyopathy. However, clinical features that are more common in children than in adults include the following (Church, 2000):

- "Torch" syndrome

- Growth failure/short stature

- Developmental delay/mental retardation

- Cerebral palsy

- Aspiration/swallowing dysfunction

- Recurrent otitis media/sinusitis

- Recurrent bacterial pneumonias

- Severe molluscum contagiosum

- Lymphoid interstitial pneumonia

- Bacterial meningitis

- Severe dental caries

- Delayed puberty

Importantly, HIV-infected infants and children without other complicating factors (Box 13.2) treated soon after birth usually will develop few of these features.

Box 13.1 ABBREVIATED SUMMARY OF HIV DIAGNOSTIC AND INFECTION-EXCLUSION CRITERIA

A. **Diagnosis of HIV Infection in Children**

    <24 months of age   Two positive nucleic acid tests (NAT); DNA or RNA PCR preferred

    >24 months of age   Confirmed positive HIV antigen/antibody test

B. **Exclusion of HIV Infection in Children**

    Birth   Negative maternal HIV antigen/antibody test

    <18 months of age   At least two negative virologic tests (DNA or RNA PCR):

    Definitive *exclusion* of HIV infection (in absence   One at >1 month age, and

    of breast-feeding)   One at >4 months of age

    >24 months of age (in absence of breast-feeding)   Negative HIV antigen/antibody test

SOURCE: Reproduced from HHS Panel on Antiretroviral Therapy and Medical Management of HIV-Infected Children. *Guidelines for the Use of Antiretroviral Agents in Pediatric HIV Infection.* 2016. Available at https://aidsinfo.nih.gov/contentfiles/lvguidelines/PediatricGuidelines.pdf.

MANAGEMENT OF HIV-EXPOSED NEWBORNS

HIV-infected pregnant women are best managed in perinatal centers that are highly experienced with this patient population. For newborns at risk of acquiring HIV, the following are recommended (Panel on Treatment of HIV-Infected Pregnant Women and Prevention of Perinatal Transmission, 2016):

- Avoid breast-feeding

- Obtain pretreatment laboratory studies

  - HIV DNA or RNA polymerase chain reaction (PCR)

  - CD4$^+$ T cell count and percentage

  - Complete blood count with differential

  - Cytomegalovirus PCR (oral swab or urine)

- Begin ART (Dose adjustments are necessary for premature infants.)

  - Zidovudine 4 mg/kg q 12 hours for 4–6 weeks

  - Depending on the degree of risk of acquiring HIV (high maternal viral load, lack of ART, or zidovudine-resistant HIV), consider adding additional medications (e.g., nevirapine 2 mg at birth, 48 hours after first dose, and 96 hours after second dose)

- Obtain RNA or DNA PCR within 48 hours of birth; repeat at 2 and 4 weeks and at 4 months; longer if exposure (breast-feeding) continues

- Consult a specialist in pediatric HIV management

MANAGEMENT OF HIV-INFECTED CHILDREN

Combination antiretroviral therapy (cART) has transformed the nature of pediatric HIV/AIDS. When initiated in a timely manner and adherence is maintained, HIV-infected children are now leading near normal lives. Management is best guided at centers experienced in the unique features of pediatric HIV/AIDS. Recommendations for the initiation of ART in children have been developed and revised (Table 13.4).

Recommended ART regimens for HIV-infected children generally contain a 2-NRTI "backbone" with either an NNRTI or a boosted PI. However, a number of alternative regimens may be considered, and treatment should be individualized based on advantages and disadvantages of each regimen, including palatability and availability of safety and pharmacokinetic data for specific ages. Although there are similarities between children and adults with regard to regimen selection and the importance of adherence to ART, there are special considerations for the treatment of infants and children (Panel on Antiretroviral Therapy and Medical Management of HIV-Infected Children, 2016, E1–E4):

- There is the additional goal of maintaining normal physical growth and neurocognitive development.

- Medication doses must be monitored in growing children.

- Liquids, particularly protease inhibitors, have poor palatability. Gastrostomy tube placement may be necessary in selected patients.

- There is a lack of pharmacokinetic and toxicity data for newer drugs.

Maternal High-Risk Behaviors with Newborn Consequences

- Lack of prenatal care
  - ↑ Risk prematurity
  - ↑ Pregnancy, labor, and delivery complications

- Compromised intrauterine environment
  - Malnutrition
  - Illicit drug exposure

- Increased risk of non-HIV congenital infections
  - Toxoplasmosis—Hepatitis B, condylomata (human papillomavirus)
  - Cytomegalovirus—Hepatitis C
  - Herpes simplex virus—Group B β streptococci

Newborn Consequences of Maternal HIV Infection

- HIV transmission
- ↑ Early spontaneous abortions
- Complications of C-section
- Impaired T cell progenitor function
- Exposure to antiretroviral drugs
  - Infection with resistant HIV
  - ↑ Risk prematurity
  - Nucleoside analogues
    - Anemia, neutropenia
    - Mitochondrial toxicity/encephalopathy
    - Premature delivery

SOURCE: Reproduced from HHS Panel on Antiretroviral Therapy and Medical Management of HIV-Infected Children. *Guidelines for the Use of Antiretroviral Agents in Pediatric HIV Infection*. 2016; F2–F7. Available at https://aidsinfo.nih.gov/contentfiles/lvguidelines/Pediatric Guidelines.pdf.

MONITORING

Close psychosocial, clinical, and laboratory monitoring of children before and after initiation of cART is critical (Table 13.5).

Table 13.4 RECOMMENDATIONS FOR INITIATION OF COMBINATION ANTIRETROVIRAL THERAPY (CART) IN INFANTS AND CHILDREN

Recommend urgent treatment	Age <12 months Age >12 month	• All infants • Infants with stage 3 opportunistic illnesses or immunodeficiencies
Recommend treatment	Age >12 months	• Moderately symptomatic children • HIV RNA >100,000 c/ml • Stage 2 immunodeficiency
Consider treatment	Age >12 months	• Mildly symptomatic or asymptomatic *and* stage 1 immunodeficiency

SOURCE: HHS Panel on Antiretroviral Therapy and Medical Management of HIV-Infected Children. *Guidelines for the Use of Antiretroviral Agents in Pediatric HIV Infection*. 2016; F2–F7. Available at https://aidsinfo.nih.gov/contentfiles/lvguidelines/PediatricGuidelines.pdf).

PREVENTION OF SECONDARY INFECTIONS

Primary (PCP prophylaxis with trimethoprim-sulfamethoxazole is recommended for all HIV-infected infants from 4 weeks of age to 1 year, regardless of CD4+ T cell counts or percentages. After 1 year, the need for PCP prophylaxis is determined by the level of immune suppression. The CDC has recommended secondary prophylaxis for selected opportunistic infections in HIV-infected infants and children and for others only if episodes are frequent or severe (Panel on Opportunistic Infections in HIV-Exposed and HIV-Infected Children, 2015, FF1–FF6).

CDC guidelines provide detailed recommendations for the treatment of opportunistic infections in children. However, the effectiveness of ART in children can be remarkable. With consistent adherence, HIV-positive children will rarely experience the types of opportunistic infections listed previously (Table 13.6).

Primary prophylaxis for PCP and *Mycobacterium avium* complex may be discontinued after CD4+ counts exceed the threshold for initiation of prophylaxis.

IMMUNIZATION IN HIV-INFECTED INFANTS AND CHILDREN

- Rotavirus (live) vaccine should be considered in HIV-infected infants (<6 months of age), but it should be withheld if there is a suspicion of severe immunocompromised.

Table 13.5 SAMPLE OF A MONITORING SCHEDULE FOR PEDIATRIC HIV/AIDS

EXAM	PRETHERAPY	1 OR 2 WEEKS ON THERAPY	4–6 WEEKS ON THERAPY	EVERY 3 OR 4 MONTHS
History and physical exam	X	X	X	X
Social and adherence evaluations	X	X	X	X
Complete blood count with differential	X		X	X
Chemistry panel	X		X	X
Urinalysis	X			X
CD4+ T cell count/%	X		X	X
HIV RNA viral load	X		X	X
Resistance testing	X			

SOURCE: HHS Panel on Antiretroviral Therapy and Medical Management of HIV-Infected Children. *Guidelines for the Use of Antiretroviral Agents in Pediatric HIV Infection*. 2016. Available at https://aidsinfo.nih.gov/contentfiles/lvguidelines/PediatricGuidelines.pdf).

- Infants should receive the primary immunization series and "boosters" with inactivated vaccines when age appropriate:

  - Diphtheria, tetanus, and pertussis (DTaP)

  - Inactivated polio vaccine (IPV)

  - *Haemophilus influenzae* type b conjugate vaccine (Hib)

  - Pneumococcal conjugate vaccine (PCV)

- Meningococcal conjugate vaccine (MCV4) at ages 11 and 16 years

- Hepatitis A and B vaccines

- Influenza vaccine (annually)

- MMR and VZV (live) vaccines are recommended for HIV-infected children who are asymptomatic and not "severely immunosuppressed."

Table 13.6 PROPHYLAXIS TO PREVENT OCCURRENCES OR RECURRENCES OF SELECTED OPPORTUNISTIC INFECTIONS AMONG HIV-INFECTED INFANTS AND CHILDREN

PATHOGEN	PROPHYLAXIS INDICATION	FIRST CHOICE AGENT
Pneumocystis jirovecii	Severe immunosuppression	TMP-SMZ
Mycobacterium avium complex	Very severe immunosuppression	Clarithromycin plus ethambutol, plus rifabutin
Toxoplasma gondii	Prior toxoplasma encephalitis	Sulfadiazine plus pyrimethamine plus leucovorin
Cryptococcus neoformans	Prior disease	Fluconazole
Histoplasma capsulatum	Prior disease	Itraconazole
Coccidiodes immitis	Prior disease	Fluconazole
Cytomegalovirus	Prior disease	Ganciclovir
Recommended Only If Subsequent Episodes Are Frequent or Severe		
Invasive bacterial infections	More than two infections in a 1-year period	TMP-SMZ or IVIG
Herpes simplex virus	Frequent or severe recurrences	Acyclovir
Candida (oropharyngeal or esophageal)	Frequent or severe recurrences	Fluconazole

IVIG, intravenous immunoglobulin; TMP-SMZ, trimethoprim–sulfamethoxazole.

SOURCE: Adopted from HHS Panel on Antiretroviral Therapy and Medical Management of HIV-Infected Children. *Guidelines for the Use of Antiretroviral Agents in Pediatric HIV Infection*. 2016. Available at https://aidsinfo.nih.gov/contentfiles/lvguidelines/PediatricGuidelines.pdf).

- Human papillomavirus (HPV) dose series should begin at age 11 years. (Panel on Opportunistic Infections in HIV-Exposed and HIV-Infected Children, 2015, KK1–KK4)

TYPICAL REFERRAL NEEDS OF HIV-INFECTED INFANTS, CHILDREN, AND THEIR FAMILIES

Most HIV-infected children are born into socially and economically disadvantaged families of color and not infrequently are placed in the foster care setting. These children and families require multiple support services, including the following:

- Medical management for HIV, sexually transmitted diseases, and hepatitis
- AIDS prevention case management
- Drug/alcohol abuse prevention/treatment
- Mental health services for the child and family
- Partner counseling and services for parents
- Legal and immigration services
- Housing, food, and transportation needs
- Child care services
- Domestic violence counseling
- Educations programs
- Disclosure counseling
- Adherence counseling

Other issues important to families are illustrated by the following questions:

- When should an HIV-infected child be told of his or her diagnosis?
- Are families obligated, legally or ethically, to disclose their child's diagnosis to other care providers and schools?
- Should HIV-infected children be allowed to participate in contact sports?
- Under what circumstances should post-exposure prophylaxis be offered to an HIV-negative child potentially exposed after sexual abuse or needle stick injury?
- When should an HIV child be removed from parental custody if antiretroviral therapy adherence is poor?
- Can HIV-infected children safely have children of their own?

UNRESOLVED PEDIATRIC ISSUES

Although ART has dramatically improved the longevity and quality of life for HIV-infected children, there are unresolved, long-term questions that remain to be answered, including the following:

- Is neurocognitive development really normal in children treated early in the course of infection?
- Will inadequate bone mineralization in childhood result in increased bone disease later in life?
- What will be the clinical impact of the mitochondrial dysfunction identified in HIV-infected infants and those exposed to antiretroviral agents in utero?
- Will the cardiovascular complication dyslipidemia and long-term immune activation (despite effective viral suppression in the peripheral blood) result in early myocardial infarction or stroke?
- What will be the long-term outcome of HIV-infected children with co-infections including tuberculosis, hepatitis B virus, and hepatitis C virus?

Recommended Resources

AIDS Info website. http://www.aidsinfo.nih.gov/guidelines.
American Academy of Pediatrics. Human immunodeficiency virus infection. In: Kimberlin DW, Brady MT, Jackson MA, et al. (Eds.), *Red Book: 2015 Report of the Committee on Infectious Diseases.* 30th ed. Elk Grove Village, IL: American Academy of Pediatrics; 2015:453–476.
Centers for Disease Control and Prevention website. http://www.cdc.gov/hiv.
HIV InSite website. http://hivinsite.ucsf.edu.
Lala MM, Merchant RH (Eds.). *Principles of Perinatal and Pediatric HIV/AIDS.* New York, NY: Jaypee Brothers; 2011.
National Perinatal Hotline. (888) 449–8765.
Women, Children, and HIV website. http://www.womenchildrenhiv.org.

References

Chen JL, Philips KA, Kanouse DE, et al. Fertility desires and intentions of HIV-positive men and women. *Family Planning Perspectives.* 2001; 33:144–152, 165.
Church JA. HIV disease in children: The many ways it differs from the disease in adults. *Postgrad Med* 2000; 107:163–182.
Husson RN, Comeau AM, Hoff R. Diagnosis of human immunodeficiency virus infection in infants and children. *Pediatrics* 1990; 86:1–10.
Nottet, HSLM, Persidsky Y, Sasseville VG, et al. Mechanisms for the transendothelial migration of HIV-1-infected monocytes into brain. *J Immunol* 1996; 156:1284–1295.

Panel on Antiretroviral Therapy and Medical Management of HIV-Infected Children. Guidelines for the use of antiretroviral agents in pediatric HIV infection. Available at https://aidsinfo.nih.gov/contentfiles/lvguidelines/PediatricGuidelines.pdf. Accessed June 27, 2016.

Panel on Opportunistic Infections in HIV-Exposed and HIV-Infected Children. Guidelines for the prevention and treatment of opportunistic infections in HIV-exposed and HIV-infected children. Available at https://aidsinfo.nih.gov/contentfiles/lvguidelines/oi_guidelines_pediatrics.pdf. Accessed June 27, 2016.

Panel on Treatment of HIV-Infected Pregnant Women and Prevention of Perinatal Transmission. Recommendations for use of antiretroviral drugs in pregnant HIV-1-infected women for maternal health and interventions to reduce perinatal HIV transmission in the United States. Available at https://aidsinfo.nih.gov/contentfiles/lvguidelines/PerinatalGL.pdf. Accessed June 27, 2016.

Selik R, Mokotoff E, Branson B, et al. Revised surveillance case definition for HIV infection—United States, 2014. *MMWR*. 2014; 63(RR03):1–10.

Sodora DL, Silvestri G. Immune activation and AIDS pathogenesis. *AIDS* 2008; 22:439–446.

CARING FOR HIV-INFECTED ADOLESCENTS

LEARNING OBJECTIVE

Describe the developmental, cognitive, social, and environmental factors that may affect treatment adherence and secondary prevention in adolescents.

WHAT'S NEW?

Young men who have sex with men (YMSM) now represent the majority of new cases of HIV infection in adolescents and young adults.

KEY POINTS

- Adolescents are at risk for HIV through risky behaviors; most adolescents acquire HIV through unprotected sex.

- Adolescents in late puberty can be managed according to adult/adolescent guidelines; prepubescent and early pubescent adolescents can be managed according to pediatric guidelines.

- Psychosocial issues that could affect adherence should be addressed before starting treatment.

- Sexual risk behaviors in HIV-infected adolescents should be given special attention.

The period of adolescence (defined as ages 12–24 years) is a critical time of physical, social, emotional, and cognitive growth and development (Sanders, 2013). However, adolescents are the most uninsured and underinsured age group in the United States and the least likely group to use primary care and other outpatient medical services (Kaiser Foundation, 2007). Those with specific health and social problems, as well as those with particular difficulty obtaining appropriate medical care and other services, are at heightened risk for HIV infection. These groups include adolescents who are gay, lesbian, bisexual, or transgender; homeless and runaway individuals; injection drug users; individuals who have a mental illness; and those who have been sexually or physically abused or incarcerated or are in foster care.

Health disparities occur as a result of an individual's interaction with socioenvironmental factors at the interpersonal (e.g., family and social/sexual networks), intermediate structural (e.g., community, social institutions, culture, social norms, and values), and macrostructural (e.g., socioeconomic conditions) levels (McLeroy, 1988) that contribute to high rates of HIV. For example, young Black gay and bisexual men and other MSM were disproportionately impacted by HIV in the United States between 2010 and 2014 (CDC, 2015) (Figures 13.3 and 13.4), and they account for more than half (55%) of all new HIV infections in YMSM (CDC, 2012). Such high rates do not result from increased individual behavior but, rather, the complex interrelationship of multiple social identities—for

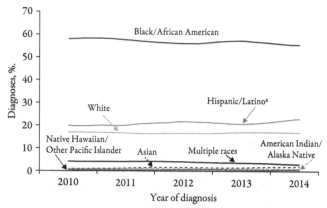

Figure 13.3 Diagnoses of HIV infection among adolescents and young adults aged 13–24 years, by race/ethnicity, 2010–2014—40 states and 5 US-dependent areas. Data include persons with a diagnosis of HIV infection regardless of stage of disease at diagnosis. All displayed data have been statistically adjusted to account for reporting delays but not for incomplete reporting. [a] Hispanic/Latinos can be of any race. SOURCE: Centers for Disease and Control and Prevention. http://www.cdc.gov/hiv/pdf/library/slidesets/cdc-hiv-surveillance-adolescents-young-adults-2014.pdf. Accessed January 31, 2016.

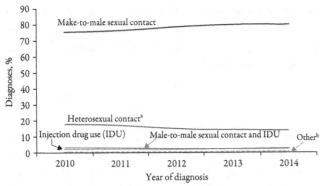

Figure 13.4 Diagnoses of HIV infection among adolescents and young adults aged 13–24 years, by transmission category, 2010–2014—40 states and 5 US-dependent areas. Data include persons with a diagnosis of HIV infection regardless of stage of disease at diagnosis. All displayed data have been statistically adjusted to account for reporting delays and missing risk-factor information but not incomplete reporting. [a]Heterosexual contact with a person known to have, or to be at high risk for, HIV infection. [b]Includes hemophilia, blood transfusion, perinatal exposure, and risk factor not reported or not identified. SOURCE: Centers for Disease and Control and Prevention. http://www.cdc.gov/hiv/pdf/library/slidesets/cdc-hiv-surveillance-adolescents-young-adults-2014.pdf. Accessed January 31, 2016.

example, race, ethnicity, gender, and sexual orientation—that intersect at the individual's experience and reflect larger social-structural inequities experienced on the macro level (Bowleg, 2013; Crenshaw, 1991; Haltikis, 2013).

Although the CDC does not collect data on transgender women, this population has also been demonstrated to have extremely high seroprevalence rates (Garofalo, 2006; Wilson, 2009). A meta-analysis estimated HIV prevalence in transgender women in the United States to be 21.7%, which is a 34-fold increased odds of HIV infection compared to that of all reproductive age adults (Baral, 2013). Transwomen of color are particularly affected. Data from Washington, DC, suggest that rates of HIV are as high as 32% among Black transgender women (Xavier, 2005).

Perinatally infected youth from the 1990s are another group of adolescents and young adults living with HIV. With near universal maternal identification and treatment, this population is small in most high-income countries. The same cannot be said for low-resource countries, in which perinatal transmission continues to be an ongoing concern. Perinatal youth share many common issues with youth infected behaviorally—namely sexuality, disclosure, unplanned pregnancy, nonadherence, and substance misuse and abuse. However, this population generally is on more complicated antiretroviral regimens based on the development of resistance mutations during childhood.

The same socioecologic factors (discrimination, isolation, microaggressions, and minority stress) that contribute to HIV risk predispose youth to comorbidities (high rates of mental health and substance use disorders) and medical

nonadherence in care. Differences in the treatment cascade of care by age have been hypothesized as an explanation for the increase in HIV infections by at-risk youth nationally (Zanoni, 2014). Less than half (40%) of those aged 13–29 years are aware of their HIV status, and best estimates suggest that only 62% of those are connected to care within their first year of diagnosis (Zanoni, 2014). Other studies have suggested that adolescents have much lower linkage rates, ranging from 29% to 73% successfully linked within the first year of diagnosis (Craw, 2008; Torian, 2008). The CDC and the US Preventive Services Task Force recommend routine HIV screening for all youth (Branson, 2006; Moyer, 2013). Annual screening is recommended based on risk, and gay and bisexual youth should be screened every 3–6 months (CDC, 2015). Venue-based and social networking testing is another effective strategy to reach high-risk youth and increase the identification and linkage of youth into care (Barnes, 2010; Boyer, 2013; Straub, 2011). Once diagnosed with HIV, special efforts to improve engagement in care are often necessary to maximize youth accessing care.

DEVELOPMENTAL ISSUES

Adolescents face the same barriers to treatment adherence as adults, but they have additional challenges due to their developmental stage and legal circumstances (Table 13.7). Social stigma, fear of alienation from peer groups, medication side effects, lack of transportation, dependence on parents or other caregivers, growing autonomy, and "feeling fine" are major contributors to nonadherence (Futterman, 2005; HRSA, 2014; Radcliff, 2010).

MEDICAL MANAGEMENT

Currently, most adolescents who acquire HIV are infected through sexual transmission and unaware of their diagnosis, making them excellent candidates for prevention counseling, linkage to and engagement in care, and initiation of ART (DHHS, 2016). The mean HIV viral load in a cohort of adolescents from 15 HIV sites was 94,398 copies/ml (Ellen, 2014). In addition, studies suggest that approximately 18% of newly infected youth have multiclass resistance at time of diagnosis, suggesting a transmission dynamic that includes older partners who have been on medications (Agwu, 2012). Data extrapolated from the START and TEMPRANO trials favor initiating ART in all individuals who are able and willing to commit to treatment, understand the benefits and risks of therapy, and understand the importance of adherence (DHHS, 2016). The course of disease in youth is similar to that in adults,

Table 13.7 BARRIERS TO ADOLESCENT ADHERENCE

Barriers for the General Population

- Complexity of medical regimen
- Lack of social support
- Adverse effects of treatment
- Distrust of health care providers
- Lack of understanding about the medication
- Difficulty coming to terms with a life-threatening illness
- Sense of invulnerability

Additional Barriers: Developmental Capacities of Adolescence

Early Adolescence

- Concrete, not yet abstract, thinking (undeveloped problem-solving skills)
- Preoccupation with self and questions about pubertal changes

Middle Adolescence

- Need for acceptance from peers (desire not to appear different)
- Present orientation (decreased ability to plan for future doses and future implications of disease)
- Busy, unstructured lives (difficulty remembering to take pills)

Late Adolescence

- Establishment of independence (the need to challenge authority figures and restructure regimens)
- Feelings of immortality (disbelief that HIV can hurt them)
- Simultaneous increase in risk perception with greater emotional satisfaction with risk-taking behavior

Additional Barriers for Adolescents with HIV

- For most, fear of disclosure of their HIV status to family and friends
- For many, lack of adult or peer support to reinforce their adherence
- For youth establishing independence, the conflict between the need to challenge authority figures and the need to depend on adult providers for support in taking antiretroviral therapy (ART)
- For asymptomatic adolescents, difficulty accepting the implications of a serious illness when they still feel well
- For some who still think concretely, difficulty grasping the concept that there is a connection between strict adherence to ART and prevention of disease progression
- For youth who live in the inner city, fear that they will die from violence, not AIDS
- For homeless and transient youth, lack of refrigeration or a place to store medicines and lack of a daily routine

SOURCE: Adapted from Schietinger et al. (1999).

and they generally should be treated according to the same guidelines (DHHS, 2016). Medications should be dosed on the pediatric schedule for early puberty or prepubescent adolescents and on the adult schedule for postpubertal adolescents. Antiretroviral medication regimens that are more forgiving of poor adherence should be considered in youth at high risk for nonadherence.

SEXUAL RISK

Youth living with HIV continue to engage in sexual behavior that may predispose them to sexual risk. Studies suggest that youth living with HIV experience high rates of unintended pregnancy (Nachman, 2009), STIs (Trent, 2007), and condomless sex (Clum, 2009; Weiner, 2007). This, combined with rates of screening for STIs that lag in HIV clinics compared to non-HIV clinics, can promote high rates of STI and transmission of HIV (Barry, 2015). In addition, recent work suggests that in females living with HIV, overall self-efficacy (B = –0.15, p = 0.01), self-efficacy to discuss safe sex with one's partner (B = –0.14, p = 0.01), and self-efficacy to refuse unsafe sex (B = –0.21, p = 0.01) are related to condomless vaginal and anal intercourse episodes (Boone, 2015). In young men, alcohol may be a key contributor to condomless sex with HIV-negative or unknown status partners (Bruce, 2013). Other studies suggest a complicated relationship with psychological stress, substance use, and mental health that contributes to condomless sex (Nugent, 2009). Disclosure is complicated by HIV stigma and fear of rejection personally with partners and publically (Toska, 2015).

There is a need to regularly address the risk for pregnancy, acquiring STIs, and the secondary spread of HIV to partners. The CDC recommends screening for STIs in women younger than age 25 years because of the high rates of STIs in this age range. In YMSM, screening for STIs is recommended from extragenital body sites because oropharyngeal, rectal, and urethral infections are commonly present in this population (Workowski, 2015). The CDC provides complete screening guidelines for youth living with HIV. Clinic-based motivational interviewing can improve condom use (Chen, 2011; Naar-King, 2006). Referrals to mental health and substance abuse treatment may be key interventions to consider for appropriate youth.

SUBSTANCE ABUSE

In a large AIDS Treatment Network (ATN) study of 1712 youth, 61% of males and 45% of females scored 2 or higher on the CRAFT screener (data presented at the October 2011 ATN meeting). Daily use of cannabis was 33% for males and 25% for females. Daily use of alcohol was reported for 5% of males and 2.6% of females. As stated previously, substance use during sex was common. The regular assessment of substance abuse with appropriate counseling and referral is a key requirement in care.

MENTAL HEALTH

In the ATN study of 1712 youth, 21% had a positive screen for depression and 15% for anxiety. Fifteen percent of the cohort had reported seriously considering suicide, and 14% were prescribed psychotropics. Seventy percent of the cohort recalled seeing a mental health provider while in care, and 38% of men and 42% of women reported currently wanting to receive mental health services (data presented at the October 2011 ATN meeting). These data suggest that regular screening and referral for mental health disorders is crucial. Stigma is another common concern for youth living with HIV (Dowshen, 2009; Swenderman, 2010) and can relate to HIV, sexual identity, or racial/ethnic minority. Stigma can lead to risky behaviors, including unsafe sex and nonadherence to medications, and counseling may be required to adequately address this issue.

MEDICATION ADHERENCE

Youth living with HIV are particularly at risk for nonadherence because of the aforementioned psychosocial, developmental, and cognitive factors. Several studies have documented nonadherence in youth living with HIV (Belzer, 2008, 1999; Reisner, 2009). Rates of adherence to HIV meds during the past 30 days range from 28% to 70% (Reisner, 2009). Barriers include medical, psychological, and logistic. Medical barriers include an AIDS diagnosis (Martinez, 2012; Murphey, 2003), a difficult ART regimen (Buchanan, 2012), the absence of symptoms, and an unwelcoming medical environment (Philbin, 2014). Psychological barriers include depression, anxiety (Tanney, 2012; Wagner, 2011), stigma associated with the diagnosis or transmission history (Rao, 2007), and lack of social support (Williams, 2006). In addition, behavioral problems impact 50% of youth living with HIV (Bing, 2001). Positive self-efficacy and outcome expectancy were associated with better adherence, and logistical barriers such as lack of housing, insurance, and transportation were associated with poorer adherence (Rudy, 2008). Comprehensive systems of care are required to serve the medical, logistical, and psychosocial needs of youth living with HIV. Individually tailored interventions that address social and psychological factors (e.g., substance use, lack of insurance despite universal access to care, and lack of social support) and structural barriers (e.g., housing and insurance instability) will need to be developed in order to better meet the needs of youth living with HIV. Attention to potential barriers to adherence prior to treatment initiation is likely to improve outcomes.

CARE MODELS

Based on the high rates of psychosocial problems reviewed previously, developmentally based care models that utilize interdisciplinary care teams are preferable. When a one-stop shopping care model is not available, it becomes imperative that the management of complex youth with behavioral problems be facilitated by close communication among physicians, nurses, social workers or case managers, and behavioral health providers. Avoiding potentially catastrophic health outcomes, including rapid HIV progression, multiclass drug resistance, depression and suicide, chronic homelessness, prolonged incarceration, drug addiction, and secondary transmission of HIV, may require intensive attention to psychosocial issues. At times, a temporary approach of delaying early antiretroviral initiation may improve outcomes by allowing time to focus on developmental and social barriers.

TRANSITION TO ADULT CARE

Finally, clinicians must plan for the transition of HIV-infected adolescents into adult care. In a joint statement, the American Academy of Pediatrics, the American Academy of Family Physicians, the American College of Physicians, and the American Society of Internal Medicine affirmed that all adults, including those with special medical needs, benefit from care by doctors who are trained in adult medicine (Cohen, 2002). They recommend that an identified health care provider be responsible for the transition, that a portable medical summary be maintained, and that a written transition plan be developed with the patient and family by age 14 years. In addition to these recommendations, Valenzuela et al. (2011) recommends the following:

- Optimizing provider communication between adolescent and adult clinics

- Identifying adult care providers willing to care for adolescents and young adults

- Addressing patient and family resistance to transition of care caused by lack of information, concerns about stigma or risk of disclosure, and differences in practice styles

- Helping youth develop life skills, including counseling them on the importance of appropriate use of a primary care provider, managing appointments, symptom recognition and reporting, and self-efficacy

- Identifying an optimal clinic model based on specific needs

- Implementing ongoing evaluation to measure the success of a selected model

- Engaging adult and adolescent care providers in regular multidisciplinary case conferences

- Implementing interventions that may improve outcomes, such as support groups and mental health consultation

- Incorporating a family planning component into clinical care

- Educating HIV care teams and staff about transitioning

The National Health Alliance also has resources that organize transition into the Six Core Elements. These resources can effectively be used in any clinical setting (see http://www.gottransition.org/providers/index.cfm).

SUMMARY

Adolescents or youth who are living with HIV may have multiple developmental, cognitive, social, and environmental challenges that impact their identification, linkage, and engagement with care. Attention to the factors noted previously will likely improve the care, treatment, and adherence of youth living with HIV and, potentially, will result in the avoidance of them falling through the cracks.

References

Agwu AL, Bethel J, Hightow-Weidman LB, et al. Substantial multi-class transmitted drug resistance and drug-relevant polymorphisms among treatment-naive behaviorally HIV-infected youth. AIDS Patient Care STDS. Apr 2012; 26(4):193–196.

Baral SD, Poteat T, Stromdahl S, et al. Worldwide burden of HIV in transgender women: A systematic review and meta-analysis. Lancet Infect Dis. 2013; 13:214–222.

Barnes W, D'Angelo L, Yamazaki M, et al. Identification of HIV-infected 12–24-year-old men and women in 15 cities through venue based testing. Arch Pediatr Adolesc Med. 2010; 164:273–276.

Belzer ME, Fuchs DN, Luftman GS, et al. Antiretroviral adherence issues among HIV-positive adolescents and young adults. J Adolesc Health. 1999. Nov; 25(5):3316–3319.

Belzer ME, Olson J. Adherence in adolescents: A review of the literature. Adolescent medicine: State of the art reviews. Evaluation and management of adolescent issues. Am Acad Pediatr. 2008; 19:99–117.

Bing EG, Burnam MA, Longshore D, et al. Psychiatric disorders and drug use among human immunodeficiency virus-infected adults in the United States. Arch Gen Psychiatr 2001; 58:721–728.

Boone MR, Cherenack EM, Wilson PA, et al. Self-efficacy for sexual risk reduction and partner HIV status as correlates of sexual risk behavior among HIV-positive adolescent girls and women. AIDS Patient Care STDS. 2015 Jun; 29(6):346–353.

Bowleg, L., "Once you've blended the cake, you can't take the parts back to the main ingredients": Black gay and bisexual men's descriptions and experiences of intersectionality. Sex Roles 2013; 68(11–12):754–767.

Boyer CB, Hightow-Weidman L, Bether J, et al. An assessment of the feasibility and acceptability of a friendship-based social network recruitment strategy to screen at-risk African American and Hispanic/Latina young women for HIV infection. JAMA Pediatr. 2013 Mar 1; 167(3):289–296.

Branson B, Handsfield H, Lampe M, et al. Revised recommendations for HIV testing of adults, adolescents, and pregnant women in health-care settings. MMWR. 2006; 55(RR14):1–17.

Bruce D, Kahana S, Harper G, et al. Alcohol use predicts sexual risk behavior with HIV-negative or partners of unknown status among young HIV-positive men who have sex with men. AIDS Care: Psychological and Socio-medical Aspects of AIDS/HIV. 2013; 25(5):559–565.

Buchanan AL, Montepiedra G, Sirois PA, et al. Barriers to medication adherence in HIV-infected children and youth based on self- and caregiver report. Pediatrics 2012; 129:e1244–e1251.

Centers for Disease Control and Prevention. HIV surveillance report, 2014; vol. 26. Available at http://www.cdc.gov/hiv/pdf/library/reports/surveillance/cdc-hiv-surveillance-report-us.pdf. Accessed January 30, 2016.

Centers for Disease Control and Prevention. Estimated HIV incidence in the United States, 2007–2010. HIV Surveillance Supplemental Report 2012; 17(4).

Chen X, Murphy DA, Naar-King S, et al. A clinic-based motivational intervention improves condom use among subgroups of youth living with HIV. J Adolescent Health 2011; 49:193–198.

Clum G, Chung S, Ellen J. Mediators of HIV related stigma and risk behavior in HIV infected young women. AIDS Care 2009; 21:1455–1462.

Cohen D, Farley T, Taylor S, et al. When and where do youths have sex? The potential role of adult supervision. Pediatrics. 2002; 110:1–6.

Craw JA, Gardner LI, Marks G, et al. Brief strengths-based case management promotes entry into HIV medical care: Results of the antiretroviral treatment access study-II. J Acquir Immune Defic Syndr. 2008; 47(5):597–606.

Crenshaw K. Mapping the margins: Intersectionality, identity politics, and violence against women of color. Stanford Law Review 1991; 43:1241–1299.

Dowshen N, Binns HJ, Garofalo R. Experiences of HIV-related stigma among young men who have sex with men. AIDS Patient Care and STDs 2009; 23:371–376.

Ellen JM, Kapogiannis B, Fortenberry JD, et al. HIV viral load levels and CD4+ cell counts of youth in 14 cities. AIDS. May 15 2014; 28(8):1213–1219.

Futterman D. HIV in adolescents and young adults: Half of all new infections in the United States. Top HIV Med. 2005. Aug–Sep; 13(3):101–105.

Garofalo R, Deleon J, Osmer E, et al. Overlooked, misunderstood and at-risk: Exploring the lives and HIV risk of ethnic minority male-to-female transgender youth. J Adolescent Health 2006; 38:230–236.

Halkitis PN, Wolitski RJ, Millett GA. A holistic approach to addressing HIV infection disparities in gay, bisexual, and other men who have sex with men. Am Psychologist 2013; 68(4):261.

Kaiser Family Foundation. *Key Facts: Race, Ethnicity, and Medical Care.* Menlo Park, CA: Kaiser Family Foundation; 2007.

Martinez J, Harper G, Carleton RA, et al. The impact of stigma on medication adherence among HIV-positive adolescent and young adult females and the moderating effects of coping and satisfaction with health care. AIDS Patient Care STDS 2012; 26:108–115.

McLeroy KR, Bibeau D, Steckler A, et al. An ecological perspective on health promotion programs. Health Educ Q 1988; 15(4):351–377.

Moyer VA; US Preventive Services Task Force. Screening for HIV: US Preventive Services Task Force recommendation statement. Ann Intern Med. 2013 Jul 2; 159(1):51–60.

Murphy DA, Sarr M, Durako SJ, et al. Barriers to HAART adherence among HIV-infected adolescents. Arch Pediatr Adolesc Med. 2003; 157:249–255.

Naar-King S, Wright K, Parsons JT, et al. Health choices: Motivational enhancement therapy for health risk behaviors in HIV-positive youth. AIDS Education Prevention 2006; 18:1–11.

Nachman SA, Cheroff M, Gona P, et al. Incidence of noninfectious conditions in perinatally HIV-infected children and adolescents in the HAART era. Arch Pediatr Adolesc Med. 2009; 163:164–171.

National Alliance to Advance Adolescent Health. Got transition. http://gottransition.org/providers/index.cfm. Accessed January 31, 2016.

Nugent NR, Brown LK, Belzer M, et al. Youth living with HIV and problem substance use: Elevated distress is associated with nonadherence and sexual risk. J Int Assoc Phys AIDS Care 2010 Mar-Apr; 9(2):113–115.

Philbin MM, Tanner AE, Duval A, et al. Linking HIV-positive adolescents to care in 15 different clinics across the United States: Creating solutions to address structural barriers for linkage to care. AIDS Care. Jan 2014; 26(1):12–19.

Radcliff J, Doty N, Hawkins LA, et al. Stigma and sexual risk in HIV-positive African American young men who have sex with men. AIDS Patient Care and STDs 2010; 24:493–499.

Rao D, Kekwaletswe TC, Hosek S, et al. Stigma and social barriers to medication adherence with urban youth living with HIV. AIDS Care 2007; 19:28–33.

Reisner S, Mimiaga MJ, Skeer M, et al. A review of HIV antiretroviral adherence and intervention studies among HIV-infected youth. Int AIDS Soc USA Topics HIV Med. 2009; 17:1425.

Rudy BJ, Murphy DA, Harris DR, et al. Patient-related risks for nonadherence to antiretroviral therapy among HIV-infected youth in the United States: A study of prevalence and interactions. AIDS Patient Care and STDs. 2008; 23:1–10.

Sanders RA. Adolescent psychosocial, social, and cognitive development. Pediatr Rev. 2013 Aug; 34(8):354–358; quiz 358–359.

Schietinger H, Schechter C. Examining medical coverage for Medicare beneficiaries with HIV/AIDS. AIDS Public Policy J. 1999 Summer; 14(2):68–79.

Straub DM, Arrington-Sanders R, Harris DR, et al. Correlates of HIV testing history among urban youth recruited through venue-based testing in 15 US cities. Sex Transm Dis. 2011 Aug; 38(8):691–696.

Swenderman D, Rotherman-Borus MJ, Comulada S, et al. Predictors of HIV-related stigma among young people living with HIV. Health Psychology 2006; 25:501–509.

Tanney MR, Naar-King S, MacDonnell K. Depression and stigma in high-risk youth living with HIV: A multi-site study. J Pediatr Health Care 2012; 26:300–305.

Torian LV, Wiewel EW, Liu K, et al. Risk factors for delayed initiation of medical care after diagnosis of human immunodeficiency virus. Arch Intern Med. 2008; 168(11):1181–1187.

Toska E, Cluver LD, Hodes R, et al. Sex and secrecy: How HIV-status disclosure affects safe sex among HIV-positive adolescents. AIDS Care. 2015 Dec; 27(Suppl 1):47–58.

Trent M, Chung SE, Ellen JM, et al. New sexually transmitted infections among adolescent girls infected with HIV. Sexually Transmitted Infections 2007; 83:468–469.

US Department of Health of Human Services. Guidelines for the use of antiretroviral agents in HIV-1-infected adults and adolescents. https://aidsinfo.nih.gov/guidelines/html/1/adult-and-adolescent-treatment-guidelines/0. Accessed January 28, 2016.

US Department of Health and Human Services, Health Resources and Services Administration, HIV/AIDS Bureau. Guide for HIV/AIDS clinical care. 2014. http://hab.hrsa.gov/deliverhivaidscare/2014guide.pdf. Accessed February 12, 2016.

Valenzuela JM, Buchanan CL, Radcliffe J, et al. Transition to adult services among behaviorally infected adolescents with HIV—A qualitative study. J Pediatr Psychol. Mar 2011; 36(2):134–140.

Wagner GJ, Goggin K, Remien RH, et al. A closer look at depression and its relationship to HIV antiretroviral adherence. Ann Behav Med 2011; 42:352–360.

Weiner LS, Battles HR, Wood LV. A longitudinal study of adolescents with perinatally or transfusion acquired HIV infection: Sexual knowledge, risk reduction self efficacy and sexual behavior. AIDS and Behavior 2007; 11:471–478.

Williams PL, Storm D, Montepiedra G, et al. Predictors of adherence to antiretroviral medications in children and adolescents with HIV infection. Pediatrics 2006; 118:e1745–e1757.

Wilson EC, Garofalo R, Harris DR, et al. Transgender female youth and sex work: HIV risk and a comparison of life factors related to engagement in sex work. AIDS Behav 2009 Oct; 13(5):902–913.

Workowski K, Bolan G. Sexually transmitted diseases treatment guidelines, 2015. MMWR Recomm Rep 2015; 65(3).

Xavier J, Bobbin M, Singer B, et al. A needs assessment of transgendered people of color living in Washington, DC. Int J Transgenderism 2005; 8:31–47.

Zanoni BC, Mayer KH. The adolescent and young adult HIV cascade of care in the United States: Exaggerated health disparities. AIDS Patient Care STDS 2014; 28(3):128–135.

CARING FOR OLDER HIV-INFECTED PATIENTS

LEARNING OBJECTIVE

Describe the differences in HIV care and management for patients who are 50 years or older.

WHAT'S NEW?

- 13-Valent pneumococcal conjugate vaccine (PCV13) is recommended in adults 65 years old or older.

- High-dose inactivated influenza vaccine (IIV) serves as an equivalent option to standard-dose IIV in adults 65 years old or older, regardless of HIV status.

- Goal blood pressure in older adults may be affected by the Systolic Blood Pressure Intervention Trial (SPRINT) trial, which was halted early due to benefits of lowering systolic blood pressure to below 120 mm Hg.

KEY POINTS

- Each HIV-infected older adult is a unique and complex individual, and disease-centric guidelines should not be applied the same way in every patient.

- Management of diseases in older HIV-infected patients should be guided by aging phenotypes, interactions with multimorbidity, and patient preferences.

> • The Veterans Aging Cohort Study (VACS) index may be used to identify aging phenotypes and can provide prognostic information to help prioritize interventions and guide shared decision-making with patients and caregivers.

There are increasing proportions of older individuals living with HIV. It is estimated that currently more than 50% of HIV-infected patients in the United States are 50 years or older (Brooks, 2012). This group is composed of individuals who have aged with chronic HIV infection, but a large proportion consists of individuals with new HIV diagnosis, with almost 20% of all new HIV infection in 2013 diagnosed in patients aged 50 years or older (CDC, 2015).

Although many of the recommendations on the management of HIV infection are not age-specific, HIV-infected patients older than age 50 years differ from their younger counterparts in many aspects, including diagnostic considerations, immune response to ART, and multimorbidity. In the following sections, these differences are outlined, a strategy for caring for this unique population is presented, and special considerations for the problem-based management of HIV-infected adults older than age 50 years are discussed.

DIFFERENCES IN OLDER HIV-INFECTED ADULTS COMPARED TO THE YOUNGER HIV-INFECTED POPULATION

Diagnostic Considerations

The most common mode of HIV transmission among adults 50 years old or older is through sexual contact (CDC, 2013). Among men, male-to-male sexual contact is the most common transmission risk (CDC, 2015), whereas heterosexual contact is the most common risk among women. This may be due to a false sense of security among older patients, who view sexually transmitted disease (STD) as a condition of the young and may forgo safe sex practices based on this perception (Pilowsky, 2015). They may also forgo barrier contraceptives when unwanted pregnancy is no longer a concern. Although sexual exposure is the most common mode of HIV transmission among HIV-infected patients 50 years old or older, research has found that health care professionals often underestimate the level of sexual activity among older adults and their risk of STD exposure (Lindau, 2007; Pilowsky, 2015). Injection drug use remains a significant risk factor for transmission of HIV in older adults.

Moreover, many symptoms of early HIV infection mimic those of old age and may be difficult for clinicians to tease apart. Symptoms of acute HIV infection, such as headache, loss of energy, loss of appetite, flu-like symptoms, and weight loss, are common in older adults and can be caused by a myriad of conditions associated with old age, such as malignancy or frailty.

With inaccurate perception of HIV exposure risk and symptom mimicry, underdiagnoses and late diagnoses of HIV infection are common among older adults (Dai, 2015; Pilowsky, 2015). Late diagnosis is associated with delayed treatment, impaired response to ART, increased morbidity and mortality, lost opportunity to prevent onward transmission, and increased cost of health care (British HIV Association, 2015). As a result, it is essential that clinicians maintain a high suspicion and routinely screen older adults for HIV, regardless of risk perception. Although guidelines from the CDC recommend routine screening up to the age of 64 years (CDC, 2015), the rationale or research evidence for this age cutoff was not included, and we recommend routine screening for all older adults because risk perception may be inaccurate in this population.

Immune Response to ART

Despite successful viral suppression with ART, older adults have less robust immunologic recovery compared to their younger counterparts, with associated increased mortality (Semeere, 2014; Vinikoor, 2014). Consequently, early HIV diagnosis and treatment are of great importance.

Multimorbidity

Older HIV-infected adults are at increased risk of multimorbidity (Guaraldi, 2014), defined as the development of multiple chronic conditions that do not simply coexist but, rather, together interact to worsen health outcomes. Compared to the uninfected, older HIV-infected adults have higher burdens of cardiovascular, metabolic, pulmonary, renal, bone, and malignant diseases (Schouten, 2012). Both lifestyle risk factors and chronic HIV infection likely contribute to multimorbidity, with longer duration of severe immunodeficiency (CD4$^+$ counts <200 cells/μl) correlating with higher comorbidity burden (Schouten, 2012).

Multimorbidity has important ramifications on health outcomes. It is associated with self-reported poor health, declines in self-rated health status, and increased mortality (adjusted odds ratio, 11.87; 95% confidence interval, 5.72–24.62) (Korourkian, 2015). With increasing disease burden, HIV-infected patients with multimorbidity are also at risk of fragmentation in care due to involvement of multiple clinicians in multiple settings. Guidelines for one disease may clash with those of another because most are disease-centric recommendations based on the ideal patient without multimorbidity (Tinetti, 2012). Treatments for one disease may inadvertently worsen other conditions, and increased treatment burden stemming from efforts to adhere to all relevant disease-centric guidelines without prioritization may not result in improvement in mortality or quality of life.

MANAGEMENT STRATEGY FOR THE CARE OF OLDER HIV-INFECTED ADULTS

Each HIV-infected older adult is a unique and complex individual. These adults cannot be described fully by one-dimensional classifications, such as chronological age or single disease entities. Aging occurs at different rates in different individuals, and within the same individual in different organs (Division of Geriatric Medicine, Emory University, 2015), resulting in different aging phenotypes that cannot be predicted by chronological age alone. In addition, viewing HIV-infected patients by a single disease entity ignores the importance of multimorbidity and the often multifactorial nature of their diseases. Most important, different patients have different goals and preferences. Consequently, applying disease-centric guidelines uniformly to every patient without taking into account aging phenotypes, multimorbidity, or individual preference ignores the unique care needs of each patient and likely will not lead to desirable patient-centered outcomes.

Understanding that not all 50-year-old HIV-infected patients should be approached the same way, clinicians may utilize the VACS index (Justice, 2013) to distinguish between those who are aging well and those who may appear phenotypically older than their chronological age. The VACS index has been shown to correlate with functional status (Malcolm, 2014), provide insight into clinician assessment of severity of illness (Justice, 2013), and predict cause-specific (Justice, 2012) as well as all-cause mortality (Justice, 2013). Based on prognosis predicted by the VACS index, clinicians can elicit patient preferences, identify diseases and risk factors that affect these goals, calculate the likely effects and lag time to benefit (Lee, 2013) of various disease-centric guidelines on these goals, and use this information to prioritize interventions and guide shared decision-making with patients and caregivers (Tinetti, 2012).

SPECIAL CONSIDERATIONS FOR PROBLEM-BASED MANAGEMENT OF HIV-INFECTED ADULTS AGED 50 YEARS OR OLDER

Immunizations

Live attenuated varicella vaccination approved for uninfected adults older than age 50 years can be given to adult HIV-infected patients without evidence of immunity with $CD4^+$ counts ≥ 200 cells/μl (CDC, 2010) because no transmission of vaccine strain VZV has been documented in HIV-infected persons with $CD4^+$ counts above this threshold (Shafran, 2016). Although the CDC has no recommendation on zoster vaccine in HIV-infected adults older than age 60 years with $CD4^+$ count ≥ 200 cells/μl, it may be reasonable to vaccinate this group of patients (Aberg, 2014).

A recent study showed superior immunogenicity in adults aged 65 years or older who received high-dose IIV compared to standard dosing. Similar results were shown in a small clinical trial among HIV-infected patients aged 18 years or older (McKittrick, 2013). Currently, the CDC recommends high-dose IIV as an equivalent option to standard-dose IIV in adults aged 65 years or older regardless of HIV status (CDC, 2010).

HIV-infected adults aged 19 years or older should receive both PCV13 and 23-valent pneumococcal polysaccharide vaccine (PPSV23). However, the interval between the two types of vaccine and the number of doses needed differ for HIV-infected adults aged 65 years or older. In pneumococcal vaccine-naive persons, PCV13 should be given first, followed by PPSV23 at least 1 year later. In persons who previously received PPSV23 at age 65 years or older, only PCV13 should be given at the interval of at least 1 year after the prior dose of PPSV23. In persons who previously received PPSV23 before age 65 years, PCV13 should be given at least 1 year after the prior dose of PPSV23, followed by a second dose of PPSV23 at least 1 year after PCV13 and at least 5 years after the prior dose of PPSV23 (CDC, 2015).

Polypharmacy

Older HIV-infected adults are at increased risk of polypharmacy (Hughes, 2015), defined as prescribing medications that are inappropriate for the patient's medical condition, using medications that cause adverse drug events, or underutilizing beneficial therapy. Polypharmacy in older HIV-infected adults is contributed by increased multimorbidity, multiple HIV-related factors affecting cytochrome P450 isoenzymes and renal function, and few pharmacokinetic studies conducted in older HIV-infected adults.

To avoid polypharmacy, we recommend a medication review at every visit and a medication reconciliation annually (American Academy of HIV Medicine (AAHIVM), 2015). Routine use of an up-to-date electronic resource such as Epocrates, Lexi-Comp, and Tarascon will help the clinician monitor the array of drug–drug interactions and needed dose modifications based on renal or hepatic function. Of note, although CKD-EPI glomerular filtration rate estimate is the most accurate for use in HIV-infected adults on stable ART (Vrouenraets, 2012), the Crockcroft–Gault calculated creatinine clearance remains the standard of care for medication dosing. Last, patients should be encouraged to utilize a single pharmacy, preferably specializing in HIV with an integrated computer network.

Diabetes

Although primary care guidelines for the management of persons infected with HIV by the Infectious Disease Society of America (IDSA) did not include age-specific glycemic goals for HIV-infected patients, AAVHIM recommends a target hemoglobin A1C of 8% for aging HIV-infected patients with frailty, less than 5-year life expectancy, a high risk for hypoglycemia, or a high risk for polypharmacy (AAHIVM, 2015). This recommendation mirrors the guideline on standards of medical care in diabetes from the American Diabetes Association (2015).

Malignancy

As with the general population, age is a risk factor for multiple types of malignancies among HIV-infected adults. According to IDSA, mammography should be performed annually in HIV-infected women aged 50 years or older, and colorectal cancer screening should be performed at age 50 years in asymptomatic HIV-infected adults with average risk and greater than 10-year life expectancy (Aberg, 2014).

Bone

Certain lifestyle and HIV-related factors place HIV-infected adults at higher risk of osteoporosis, including smoking, alcohol abuse, glucocorticoid therapy, low consumption of calcium and vitamin D, low physical activity, immune dysfunction and persistent inflammation, and side effects of antiretroviral medications (Castronuovo, 2015). Modifiable risk factors should be addressed, and viral suppression should be achieved with ART. IDSA recommends

baseline bone densitometry (DEXA) screening for osteoporosis in HIV-infected postmenopausal women and men aged 50 years or older (Aberg, 2014). Vitamin D levels should also be checked; if low, supplementation with vitamin D, calcium, and bisphosphonates may be considered, with a follow-up DEXA 1 year afterward to monitor response to therapy.

Hypertension

Goal blood pressure for hypertensive patients in the general population remains controversial and presents a challenge for clinicians, with even less evidence to guide management among the HIV-infected population. Although the SPRINT was halted in September 2015 due to benefits of lowering systolic blood pressure to below 120 mm Hg (Ambrosius, 2014), full results are not yet available and current hypertension guidelines have not taken these results into account. Currently, the Eighth Joint National Committee (JNC8) recommends a blood pressure goal of <150/90 mm Hg in hypertensive adults aged 60 years or older and a goal of <140/90 mm Hg for all hypertensive adults with diabetes or nondiabetic chronic kidney disease (James, 2014). In older adults, the risk of overtreatment of hypertension is greater than the risk of undertreatment. However, there are no specific guidelines for the HIV-infected population.

Neurocognitive Disorders

Age is a risk factor for cognitive impairment associated with HIV as well as other causes (Chan, 2014). Although the CDC and IDSA do not offer guidelines on HIV-associated neurocognitive impairment, the European AIDS Clinical Society (2015) guideline provides an algorithm for its diagnosis and management.

Age is also a risk factor for peripheral neuropathy (Kaku, 2014). As a result, pain should be considered the fifth vital sign and should be assessed at every visit. Currently, trials on symptomatic and disease-modifying treatments for HIV-associated distal symmetric polyneuropathy have had limited success, and currently there are no US Food and Drug Administration-approved treatments.

Age-Related Sexual Changes

Age-related sexual changes in HIV-infected patients include menopause in women and hypogonadism in men.

The IDSA guideline advises that although hormone replacement therapy may be considered in patients with severe menopausal symptoms, it should be used only for a limited period of time at the lowest effective dose. This is because hormone replacement therapy has been associated with a small increased risk of breast cancer, cardiovascular disease, and thromboembolic morbidity (Aberg, 2014).

Morning serum testosterone level may be assessed in aging HIV-infected men with decreased libido, erectile dysfunction, reduced bone mass or low trauma fractures, hot flashes, or sweats. Low levels should be confirmed with repeat testing. Full recommendations are included in the IDSA guidelines (Aberg, 2014).

Advance Care Planning

With increased risk of neurocognitive impairment and debility from multimorbidity, advance care planning is essential among aging HIV-infected adults (Sangarlangkarn, 2015). Without appropriate documentation of surrogate decision-maker for health care and finances, decisions regarding emergent or end-of-life care may be legally deferred to estranged family members who are unaware of the patient's preferences or HIV status. Although there are no specific guidelines for HIV-infected patients, the DHHS recommends advance care planning for all patients with chronic life-limiting illness or anyone older than age 55 years, regardless of health status (Agency for Health Research and Quality, 2015).

CONCLUSION

There is an increasing proportion of older individuals living with HIV, and they differ from their younger counterparts in many ways, including the risk for late or underdiagnoses, decreased immunologic recovery, and increased multimorbidity. However, each HIV-infected older adult is a unique and complex individual, and disease-centric guidelines should not be applied the same way for every patient. Management of diseases in older HIV-infected patients should be guided by aging phenotypes, interactions with multimorbidity, and patient preferences. The VACS index may be used to identify aging phenotypes and can provide useful prognostic information to help prioritize interventions and guide shared decision-making with patients and caregivers.

Recommended Reading

American Academy of HIV Medicine. Recommended treatment strategies for clinicians managing older patients with HIV. Available at http://hiv-age.org/wp-content/uploads/2013/11/HIVandAgingConsensusProject051815.pdf.

Boyd CM, Lucas GM. Patient-centered care for people living with multimorbidity. *Curr Opin HIV AIDS*. 2014; 9(4):419–427.
Calcagno A, Nozza S, Muss C, et al. Aging with HIV: A multidisciplinary review. *Infection*. 2015; 43(5):509–522.

References

Aberg JA, Gallant JE, Ghanem KG, et al. Primary care guidelines for the management of persons infected with HIV: 2013 update by the HIV medicine association of the Infectious Diseases Society of America. Clin Infect Dis. 2014; 58(1):e1.
Agency for Health Research and Quality, National Guideline Clearinghouse. Advanced care planning guideline. Available at http://www.guideline.gov/content.aspx?id=47803. Accessed October 18, 2015.
Ambrosius WT, Sink KM, Foy CG, et al. The design and rationale of a multicenter clinical trial comparing two strategies for control of systolic blood pressure: The Systolic Blood Pressure Intervention Trial (SPRINT). Clin Trials. 2014; 11(5):532–546.
American Academy of HIV Medicine. Recommended treatment strategies for clinicians managing older patients with HIV. Available at http://hiv-age.org/wp-content/uploads/2014/02/12.-Diabetes-Mellitus-in-HIV-and-Aging.pdf. Accessed October 18, 2015.
American Diabetes Association. Standards of medical care in diabetes—2015 abridged for primary care providers. Clin Diabetes. 2015; 33(2):97–111.
British HIV Association. UK national guidelines for HIV testing. Public Health. 2015.
Brooks J, Buchacz K, Gebo KA, et al. HIV infection and older Americans: The public health perspective. Am J Public Health. 2012; 102(8):1516–1526.
Castronuovo D, Pinzone MR, Moreno S, et al. HIV infection and bone disease: A review of the literature. Infect Dis Trop Med. 2015; 1(2):E116.
Centers for Disease Control and Prevention. HIV surveillance report, 2013; vol. 25. Available at http://www.cdc.gov/hiv/pdf/library/reports/surveillance/cdc-hiv-surveillance-report-vol-25.pdf. Accessed October 18, 2015.
Centers for Disease Control and Prevention. Diagnoses of HIV infection among adults aged 50 years and older in the United States and dependent areas, 2007–2010. HIV Surveillance Supplemental Report 2013; 18(No. 3). Available at https://www.cdc.gov/hiv/topics/surveillance/resources/reports/#supplemental. Accessed October 18, 2015.
Centers for Disease Control and Prevention. Revised recommendations for HIV testing of adults, adolescents, and pregnant women in health-care settings. Available at https://www.cdc.gov/mmwr/preview/mmwrhtml/rr5514a1.htm. Accessed October 18, 2015.
Centers for Disease Control and Prevention. Recommended adult immunization schedule: United States, 2010. Ann Intern Med. 2010; 152(1):36–39.
Centers for Disease Control and Prevention. Intervals between PCV13 and PPSV23 vaccines: Recommendations of the Advisory Committee on Immunization Practices (ACIP). Available at https://www.cdc.gov/mmwr/preview/mmwrhtml/mm6434a4.htm. Accessed October 18, 2015.
Chan P, Brew BJ. HIV associated neurocognitive disorders in the modern antiviral treatment era: Prevalence, characteristics, biomarkers, and effects of treatment. Curr HIV/AIDS Rep. 2014; 11(3):317–324.
Dai SY, Liu JJ, Fan YG, et al. Prevalence and factors associated with late HIV diagnosis. J Med Virol. 2015; 87(6):970–977.
Division of Geriatric Medicine and Gerontology, Emory University. The Emory "BIG 10" basics in geriatrics. Available at http://medicine.emory.edu/documents/geriatrics-big10.pdf. Accessed July 7, 2015.
European AIDS Clinical Society. Guidelines Version 7.1 Available at http://www.eacsociety.org/files/guidelines-7.1-english.pdf. Accessed October 18, 2015.

Guaraldi G, Silva AR; Stentarelli C, et al. Multimorbidity and functional status assessment. Curr Opin HIV AIDS. 2014; 9(4):386–397.

Hughes CA, Tseng A, Cooper R, et al. Managing drug interactions in HIV-infected adults with comorbid illness. Can Med Assoc J. 2015; 187(1):36.

James PA, Oparil S, Carter BL, et al. 2014 evidence-based guideline for the management of high blood pressure in adults: Report from the panel members appointed to the Eighth Joint National Committee (JNC8). JAMA. 2014; 311(5):507.

Justice AC, Modur S, Tate JP, et al. Predictive accuracy of the Veterans Aging Cohort Study Index for Mortality with HIV infection: A North American Cross Cohort Analysis. J Acquir Immune Defic Syndr. 2013; 62(2)149–163.

Justice AC, Tate JP, Brown ST, et al. Can the Veterans Aging Cohort Study Index improve clinical judgment for both HIV infected and uninfected veterans? J Gen Intern Med. 2013; 28:S39–S39.

Justice AC, Tate JP, Freiberg MS, et al. Reply to Chow et al. Clin Infect Dis. 2012. Published online June 5, 2012.

Kaku M, Simpson D. HIV neuropathy. Curr Opin HIV AIDS. 2014;9(6):521–526.

Koroukian SM, Warner D, Owusu C, et al. Multimorbidity redefined: Prospective health outcomes and the cumulative effect of co-occurring conditions. Prev Chronic Dis. 2015; 12:E55.

Lee SJ, Leipzig RM, Walter LC. Incorporating lag time to benefit into prevention decisions for older adults. JAMA. 2013; 310(24):2609–2610.

Lindau ST, Schumm LP, Laumann EO, et al. A study of sexuality and health among older adults in the United States. N Engl J Med 2007; 357(8):762–774.

Malcolm J, Hessol N, Hare BC, et al. Veterans Aging Cohort Study (VACS) Index, functional status, and other patient reported outcomes in old HIV-positive (HIV+) adults. Open Forum Infectious Diseases. 2014; 1(1):S428–S429.

McKittrick N, Frank I, Jacobson JM, et al. Improved immunogenicity with high-dose seasonal influenza vaccine in HIV-infected persons: A single-center, parallel, randomized trial. Ann Intern Med. 2013; 158(1):19–26.

Pilowsky DJ, Wu LT. Sexual risk behaviors and HIV risk among Americans aged 50 years or older: A review. Subst Abuse Rehabil. 2015; 6:51–60.

Sangarlangkarn A, et al. Advance care planning and HIV in the antiretroviral therapy era: A narrative review. Topics Antiviral Med. 2015;23(5):174–180.

Schouten J, Wit FW, Stolte IG, et al. Cross-sectional comparison of the prevalence of age-associated comorbidities and their risk factors between HIV-infected and uninfected individuals: The AGEhIV cohort study. Clin Infect Dis. 2014; 59(12):1787–1797.

Semeere AS, Lwanga I, Sempa J, et al. Mortality and immunological recovery among older adults on antiretroviral therapy at a large urban HIV clinic in Kampala, Uganda. J Acquir Immune Defic Syndr. 2014; 67(4):382–389.

Shafran SD. Live attenuated herpes zoster vaccine for HIV-infected adults. HIV Med. 2016; 17(4):305–310.

Tinetti ME, Fried TR, Boyd C, et al. Designing health care for the most common chronic condition—Multimorbidity. JAMA. 2012; 307(23):2493–2494.

Vinikoor MJ, Joseph J, Mwale J, et al. Age at antiretroviral therapy initiation predicts immune recovery, death, and loss to follow-up among HIV-infected adults in urban Zambia. AIDS Res Hum Retroviruses. 2014; 30(10):949–955.

Vrouenraets SM, Fux CA, Wit FW, et al. A comparison of measured and estimated glomerular filtration rate in successfully treated HIV-patients with preserved renal function. Clin Nephrol. 2012; 77(4):311–320.

ANTIRETROVIRALS DURING AND AFTER HOSPITALIZATION

LEARNING OBJECTIVE

Discuss issues in determining the relative priority of initiating and/or maintaining ART in the context of the hospitalized HIV patients with significant comorbid conditions, as well as issues of continuity of care after discharge from the inpatient setting.

WHAT'S NEW?

- An Updated link to a reference table of available ART formulations is provided.

- New ART agents since last publication are incorporated.

- No new large trials have been performed that have changed the current understanding of hospitalized patient management.

KEY POINTS

- Understanding the evolving drivers for hospitalization in the ART era

- Appropriately weighing the decision to start ART in newly diagnosed or nonadherent patients during hospitalization

- Balancing issues of ART continuation in terms of disease severity, tolerability, and drug–drug interactions while hospitalized

Patients with HIV have higher rates of hospitalization for multiple reasons. In the pre-ART era, progressive OIs and end-stage AIDS were the main causes of recurrent hospitalizations. Hospitalization rates dramatically declined in the ART era, but in the current period there has been evidence that hospitalizations continue to occur at higher than average rates, often for different causes (Crum-Cianflone, 2010). Recent drivers for hospitalization have diversified, with non-AIDS-related comorbidities being the most common causes of admission; examples include methicillin-resistant *Staphylococcus aureus* and other non-AIDS infections; chronic end-organ diseases, particularly liver disease as well as cardiovascular disease; malignancies; and surgical issues. Higher than average rates of substance abuse and psychiatric disorders in the HIV-infected population are also important drivers for hospital admission. There are many considerations in the use of ART during hospitalization, and this issue can be divided into two main categories.

The first category consists of patients not on ART at the time of admission. This may be due to nonadherence or having not been diagnosed with HIV until the hospitalization (usually via presentation with an OI). The main issue in this situation is whether and when to start ART during hospitalization. Concerns regarding additional pill burden, increased potential for side effects and drug interactions, and possible immune reconstitution inflammatory syndrome complications must be weighed against faster OI improvement and ultimate morbidity/mortality benefits. A 2009 randomized controlled trial helped inform the issue, concluding that early ART initiation resulted in less AIDS progression/death with no increase in adverse events or loss of virologic response compared to deferred ART (Zolopa, 2009). A critical additional factor in deciding whether to initiate ART during hospitalization is the importance of ensuring that the patient will be able to access and continue ART upon discharge to prevent lapses in adherence and potential resistance. This issue involves both the immediate availability of ART on discharge (i.e., if the patient has access to outpatient medications via insurance coverage or ADAP programs) and whether the patient is in a position to continue with successful adherence (i.e., housing stability, substance abuse treatment needs, mental health care optimization, and willingness to take ART). In all cases, it is essential to ensure that patients will have streamlined access to ongoing outpatient HIV specialty care and that patients are linked before discharge to prevent adherence lapses.

The second category consists of patients with a known HIV diagnosis who are on ART at the time of admission. Patients who are on stable ART and admitted to the hospital should continue taking their regimen, with few exceptions. Issues that impact ART continuation include the reason for admission and if it impacts the ability to take oral medications—that is, severe gastrointestinal (GI) disturbances such as intractable vomiting or diarrhea or obstruction, and so on. In such cases, ART use may need to be temporarily suspended until the patient's GI symptoms resolve sufficiently to tolerate oral medications again to avoid intermittent absorption and subtherapeutic drug levels predisposing to resistance. In addition, temporary ART discontinuation may need to be considered in presentations of severe lactic acidosis, pancreatitis, severe hepatic enzyme elevations, obtundation, or emergent surgical issues. ART dosing should be resumed as soon as safely possible when the patient clinically improves from these initial severe presentations.

If possible, patients who are nil per os (NPO) should continue ART with water unless there is an acute GI problem that is rendering them NPO. Patients with nasogastric tubes should be given all ART in liquid form, when available, or crushed and reconstituted if no liquid form is available. An updated reference table based on a literature review for ARV that can be crushed or sprinkled and also information on liquid formulation availability can be found at http://www.hiv-druginteractions.org/data/ExtraPrintableCharts/ExtraPrintableChartID10.pdf.

Drug interaction issues need to be considered routinely during hospitalization. Any new medications given need to be checked for interactions with the patient's current ART regimen, and dose adjustments or medication changes should be made as needed, ideally in concert with a HIV specialty pharmacist. Particular attention should be paid to proton pump inhibitor (PPI) interactions because PPIs are often started for ulcer prophylaxis or other reasons during hospitalization. Atazanavir and rilpivirine are particularly susceptible to subtherapeutic drug levels due to PPI interaction; therefore, extra care should be taken to mitigate problematic interactions.

Some other ART considerations during hospitalization include formulary availability, especially at smaller hospitals with less HIV/AIDS experience, and adequate stock of all agents because the number and classes of ART medications have dramatically increased. It is important to work with the pharmacy to ensure that correct ART is available without delay in the correct dosing form and that if there are any supply problems, appropriate class substitutions are given in consultation with an HIV expert. If a patient is on an investigational medication via a research study, it is imperative that the treating physician and the research team administering the investigational drug are notified of the patient's hospital admission because they must make arrangements to bring the drug to the hospital and arrange for its administration by the staff there. Currently, multiple long-acting injectable ART medications are being investigated; if and when these come into clinical use, they may play a significant role in the management of the hospitalized patient in terms of expanding treatment options while decreasing pill burden.

Recommended Reading

Mobula L, Barnhart M, Malati C, et al. Long-acting, injectable antiretroviral therapy for the management of HIV infection: An update on a potential game-changer. *J AIDS Clin Res.* 2015; 6:466.

Nyberg C, Patterson BY, Williams MM. When patients cannot take pills: Antiretroviral drug formulations for managing adult HIV infection. *Topics Antiviral Med.* 2011; 19(3):126–131.

Zucker J, Mittal J, Jen S, et al. Impact of stewardship interventions on antiretroviral medication errors in an urban medical center: A 3-year, multiphase study. *Pharmacotherapy.* 2016; 36(3):245–251.

References

Crum-Cianflone N, Grandits G, Echols S, et al. Trends and causes of hospitalizations among HIV-infected persons during the late HAART era: What is the impact of CD4⁺ counts and HAART use? *J AIDS.* 2010; 54(3):248–257.

Zolopa AR, Andersen J, Powderly W, et al. Early antiretroviral therapy reduces AIDS progression/death in individuals with acute opportunistic infections: A multicenter randomized strategy trial. *PLoS One.* 2009; 4(5):e5575. doi:10.1371/journal.pone.0005575

PERIOPERATIVE CARE AND SURGICAL ISSUES

LEARNING OBJECTIVE

Describe important considerations in the perioperative care of an HIV-infected patient.

WHAT'S NEW?

A 2014 study on perioperative complications after total hip arthroplasty showed a very slight increase in HIV-infected patients (2.9% vs. 2.7%).

KEY POINTS

- The balance of data shows no worsening of operation-associated morbidity and mortality in HIV-infected patients in general.

- Perioperative complications may be more frequent or severe in very immunosuppressed AIDS patients.

- There are some specific anesthesia considerations in HIV-infected patients.

There are evolving data that indicate that overall, operation-associated morbidity and mortality in HIV-infected patients are not different than those in uninfected patients. Most of the studies conducted on surgical complications in HIV-infected patients are descriptive, retrospective, and so inconsistent that many fields of surgery have published reports documenting both favorable and unfavorable postoperative outcomes (Rose, 1998). Given the available data,

however, it seems that HIV infection does not increase the postoperative risk for complications or death (Cacala, 2006; Evron, 2004), especially in the ART era. Due to improvements in outcomes and overall OI reduction in the early ART era, the number of operations for AIDS-related surgical illnesses has decreased considerably (Saltzman, 2005). However, given the vastly improved survival and longevity of patients in the current ART era and the ongoing comorbidities that increase with an aging HIV population, the need for surgical operations and anesthesia has become far more commonplace overall.

POSTOPERATIVE COMPLICATIONS AND HIV INFECTION

HIV infection may influence postoperative wound healing and complication rates (Rose, 1998). Advanced HIV infection accompanied by opportunistic infections or malignancies may complicate the perioperative course and management. This may be due to debility and wasting as much as immunosuppression. A CD4⁺ count and viral load measurement are useful when calculating surgical risks and developing a prognosis in the HIV-infected patient (Evron, 2004; Saltzman, 2005). Postoperative CD4⁺ counts of 200 cells/mm³ or less are associated with higher mortality rates (Saltzman, 2005). Irrespective of surgical procedure, there is a 13.3% mortality rate with a CD4⁺ count less than 50 cells/mm³ and a 0.8% mortality rate with the CD4⁺ count greater than 200 cells/mm³ 6 months postoperatively (Evron, 2004). Postoperative viral loads greater than 75,000 RNA copies/ml are associated with higher complication and mortality rates (Saltzman, 2005). A 2006 Kaiser retrospective study showed that viral load suppression to less than 30,000 copies/ml reduced surgical complications (Harberg, 2006).

In a comprehensive literature review, wound infection rates varied widely, especially for abdominal, anorectal, and general surgeries and central venous catheter insertions, whereas documented ophthalmologic surgery and splenectomies had consistently low morbidity rates (Rose, 1998). In 33% of the reports, complication rates were significantly higher in patients with late-stage HIV compared to early stage patients. One study of dental extractions found that complication rates did not significantly differ by CDC stage of disease. A study of cesarean sections found that complication rates were not significantly different between CDC stages of disease but were significantly associated with patients' CD4⁺ cell counts (Rose, 1998).

To mitigate operative complications, patients with a history of or signs of cardiac or pulmonary dysfunction should undergo a more thorough evaluation prior to surgery (e.g., blood gases, pulmonary function tests, echocardiography, further cardiac testing, or even cardiac catheterization as appropriate). Relevant history of past treatment with potentially cardiotoxic therapies, such as chemotherapy for Kaposi's sarcoma or lymphoma, should be considered in assessing operative risk. HIV-infected patients may be in a relatively hypercoagulable state, with accelerated coronary atherosclerosis and possibly decreased left ventricular contractility (Evron, 2004).

ANESTHETIC CONSIDERATIONS AND DRUG INTERACTIONS

Information about the relative general hazards of anesthesia and surgery for HIV-infected patients is scarce (Evron, 2004). Most antiretrovirals interact directly with anesthetic drugs and can cause side effects that directly influence which anesthetics are used and how they will be administered (Evron, 2004; Hughes, 2004). This issue is continually evolving; currently, there are more than 30 antiretrovirals in six distinct classes.

Specific considerations when administering general anesthesia to HIV-infected patients include the possible effects of anesthesia and opioids on the immune system, the cardiopulmonary and neurologic status of the patient, and possible interactions with ART medications:

- Opioids: Although there is laboratory evidence that opioids may detrimentally affect immune function, the clinical significance of short-term opioid administration during general anesthesia is unclear, and not enough clinical data are available to justify its avoidance.

- Neurologic considerations: Neurologic manifestations, such as overt dementia, may impair the ability of the patient to provide preoperative consent and may increase brain sensitivity to sedative or psychoactive drugs such as opioids, benzodiazepines, and neuroleptics.

- General central nervous system (CNS): Increased intracranial pressure (ICP) and CNS infections (i.e., meningitis, encephalopathy, or myelopathy) are contraindications to neuraxial anesthesia.

- Cerebrospinal fluid analysis and nerve or muscle biopsy may be required, and radiological studies of the spinal cord should be performed as part of the neurological evaluation to exclude compressive lesions in symptomatic patients. Opportunistic infections may be associated with increased ICP, especially in the case of toxoplasmosis. Because these infections respond rapidly to medical therapy, surgery should be postponed whenever possible if they are present.

- Pulmonary considerations: Pulmonary complications can occur as a consequence of many opportunistic infections, leading to respiratory distress and hypoxemia.

Regional anesthesia has been shown to be associated with reduced morbidity and mortality in a wide range of patients, including HIV-positive patients having cesarean delivery under spinal anesthesia. However, a high motor block with intercostal muscle paralysis may not be tolerated (Evron, 2004). Regional anesthesia is less likely to interfere with immune function or interact with antiretroviral drugs. Sepsis and platelet abnormalities are contraindications to regional anesthesia, and neuropathy may also interfere. Post-dural puncture headache may occur after regional anesthesia and may necessitate epidural blood patch. No increase in neurologic abnormalities in six HIV patients receiving an epidural blood patch during a follow-up period of 2 years was observed, and there is no evidence to contraindicate the use of blood patch in HIV-infected patients (Evron, 2004; Tom, 1992).

Nevirapine and efavirenz induce cytochrome P450 enzyme (CYP3A3/4) and may decrease serum levels of some anesthetic or sedative drugs, such as midazolam and fentanyl (Evron, 2004), although these antivirals are not used as frequently. Etomidate, atracurium, remifentanil, and desflurane are not dependent on CYP450 hepatic metabolism and may be preferable in patients using ART (Evron, 2004).

Protease inhibitors are primarily metabolized by the cytochrome P450 isoform 3A4 (CYP3A4). Because PIs often inhibit, but can sometimes also induce, this enzyme, they may increase or decrease the effects of other drugs metabolized by cytochrome P450, so any anesthetics used concomitantly should be carefully titrated. Ritonavir is the most potent inhibitor of CYP3A4 and CYP2D6. Another more recent CYP3A inhibitor, cobicistat, has been approved for use as an ART boosting agent and needs to be taken into consideration when dosing other drugs. Fentanyl is metabolized mainly by CYP3A4 (Evron, 2004). Ritonavir can reduce fentanyl clearance by up to 67%. This strong interaction suggests that fentanyl and other anesthetic dosing should be adjusted in patients on a boosting agent. Also, respiratory monitoring should be maintained because the risk of respiratory depression for a longer period of time will most likely be higher (Hughes, 2004).

References

Cacala SR, Mafana E, Thomson SR, et al. Prevalence of HIV status and CD4 counts in a surgical cohort: Their relationship to clinical outcome. Ann R Coll Surg Engl. 2006; 88(1):46–51.

Desai DM, Kuo PC. Perioperative management of special populations: Immunocompromised host (cancer, HIV, transplantation). Surg Clin North Am. 2005;85(6):1267–1282, xi–xii.

Evron S, Glezerman M, Harow E, et al. Human immunodeficiency virus: Anesthetic and obstetric considerations. Anesth Analg. 2004; 98(2):503–511.

Hughes SC. HIV and anesthesia. Anesthesiol Clin North Am. 2004; 22(3):379–404.

Naziri Q, Boylan M, Issa K, et al. Does HIV infection increase the risk of perioperative complications after THA? A nationwide database study. Clin Orthop Relat Res. 2015; 473(2):581–586.

Rose D, Collins M, Kelban R. Complications of surgery in HIV-infected patients. *AIDS*. 1998; 12:2243–2251.

Saltzman DJ, Williams RA, Gelfand DV, et al. The surgeon and AIDS: Twenty years later. Arch Surg. 2005; 140(10):961–967.

HIV AND TRANSGENDER POPULATIONS

LEARNING OBJECTIVE

Equip providers with the knowledge and skill to develop and provide gender-affirming primary and HIV care and prevention for transgender persons.

WHAT'S NEW?

It is increasingly recognized that the development of transgender-specific programs and interventions and avoiding grouping transgender people with MSM populations result in improved care and prevention outcomes. Biomedical interactions between hormones and antiretrovirals are unlikely, but transgender people may have poorer HIV outcomes or adherence to pre-exposure prophylaxis (PrEP) due to unique behavioral factors.

KEY POINTS

- Transgender people have a range of identities and sexual orientations as well as transition-related goals; each transgender patient should be approached as an individual.

- Transgender people and programs should not be aggregated with MSM; programs and materials should be developed specifically for transgender populations using a culturally grounded approach.

- Gender-affirming hormone therapy with estrogens and androgen blockers is generally safe and compatible with ART regimens. Hormone therapy and other gender-affirming interventions may improve HIV outcomes and reduce risk.

- Transgender patients require ongoing primary and preventive care, as do non-transgender patients; it is important to tailor such care based on the hormonal status and individual organ inventory of each patient.

- Providers should maintain a high index of suspicion for injected silicone and other fillers and related morbidity.

EPIDEMIOLOGY, DEMOGRAPHICS, AND TERMINOLOGY

"Transgender" is an umbrella term used to describe persons whose gender identity and/or expression of gender is different than that which they were assigned at birth. Some transgender persons may seek only gender-affirming hormone therapy (HT), whereas others may seek surgical interventions such as genital reassignment surgery or other procedures on the face, breast, or body. Still other transgender persons may present with a more complex gender identity; some may choose to seek HT or surgical treatments but continue to live part- or full-time in their birth gender, whereas others may assume a fluid gender expression that is not categorizable in either polar gender (Deutsch, Bhakri, 2015). Table 13.8 presents a description of selected terminology and identities. The sexual orientations of transgender persons also lie on a spectrum, with a 2005 Chicago study finding that 30% of transgender women identified as heterosexual and 26% as "other" (Kenagy, 2005). In most cases, transgender persons define their sexual orientation based on their affirmed gender. For example, a transgender man who has sex with men would identify as gay. However, this also varies across cultural and linguistic lines, and the most effective method for determining the sexual history and health of a patient is to ask, "What kind of people do you have sex with? Men? Women? Are any of them transgender people? A mix? What kind of genitals do they have? A penis? A vagina?" Allowing transgender persons to define their own identity and experience, and viewing them as individuals rather than as a stereotype, will enhance the patient–provider relationship and may serve to improve adherence with ART and other care (Melendez, 2009).

The World Professional Association for Transgender Health's *Standards of Care for the Health of Transsexual,*

Table 13.8 DESCRIPTION OF SELECTED
TERMINOLOGY AND IDENTITIES

TERM	DESCRIPTION
Transgender	Umbrella term for gender-nonconforming persons; more "modern" and inclusive term, preferred by many
Transsexual	Older, more clinical term, some use to identify those seeking medical or surgical treatment
Trans	Colloquial term increasingly used in place of "transgender," especially among younger populations
Cross-dresser	Individual who wears clothing of the opposite gender for personal expression, entertainment, or sexual purposes only; "transvestite" now considered a pejorative term
Travestí	Term used by some Latina/Spanish-speaking transgender women
Gay	Term used by some Latina/Spanish-speaking transgender women with complex gender/sexual identities
Transgender woman	Person with a feminine gender identity who was assigned male birth sex
Transgender man	Person with a masculine gender identity who was assigned female birth sex

Transgender and Gender Non-Conforming People, seventh version (SOCv7), states (Coleman, 2012),

> Gender nonconformity refers to the extent to which a person's gender identity, role, or expression differs from the cultural norms prescribed for people of a particular sex. ... Gender dysphoria refers to discomfort or distress that is caused by a discrepancy between a person's gender identity and that person's sex assigned at birth (and the associated gender role and/or primary and secondary sex characteristics).

SOCv7 further states (Coleman, 2012),

> Transsexual, transgender, and gender nonconforming individuals are not inherently disordered. Rather, the distress of gender dysphoria, when present, is the concern that might be diagnosable and for which various treatment options are available. The existence of a diagnosis for such dysphoria often facilitates access to health care and can guide further research into effective treatments. Research is leading to new diagnostic nomenclatures, and terms are changing in both the DSM ... and the ICD.

Epidemiologic surveillance in transgender populations has been limited due to inconsistencies in the collection of gender identity data. Incomplete or inconsistent identification of transgender populations represents a significant structural determinant of the health disparities seen in transgender populations. Best practice for the collection of gender identity data involves the use of the "two-step" method, which records both the current gender identity and the birth assigned sex (Cahill, 2013, 2014; Deutsch, 2013). This method has been found to identify twice as many transgender people as a "one-step" method in which a single "sex/gender" question is asked (Tate, 2012). A population-based statewide telephone survey in Massachusetts found a prevalence of 0.5% (Conron, 2012).

A 2012 meta-analysis found an HIV prevalence of 19.1% among transgender women living in the United States (Baral, 2013). This striking rate is driven by interactions between structural, personal, behavioral, and biological risks unique to transgender women. Structural factors include a lack of legal recognition or protections that often result in survival sex work. Personal factors include the higher rates of mood disorders seen in transgender populations as a result of ongoing discrimination as well as drive for gender affirmation; the model of gender affirmation describes the relationship between denial of gender affirmation (through lack of access to medical interventions or legal rights such as the ability to change one's name and gender on identity documents) and high-risk sexual behavior (Sevelius, 2013). Other behavioral factors include increased rates of condomless sex with primary male partners and anecdotes of increased earnings from sex work when no condom is used. Biological factors have not been explored in depth, but they could include changes to the anal epithelium in the presence of feminizing hormones, reduced erectile function resulting in impaired condom effectiveness, and unknowns such as HIV transmission through receptive vaginal sex in those who have undergone vaginoplasty (Poteat, 2015). Few data exist on HIV risks and prevalence among transgender men, although some data suggest an increased risk (Green, 2015). A 2010 San Francisco study found that 61% of transgender men engaged in sex with other men (TMSM), with 51% participating in vaginal receptive sex and 39% participating in anal receptive sex.

INITIATING HORMONE THERAPY

Gender-affirming HT has been found to have a number of benefits on quality of life and on symptoms of depression, anxiety, and poor social functioning (Colton, 2011; Gómez-Gil, 2011). SOCv7 defines hormonal and surgical treatment as medically necessary and states that it is unethical to deny surgical care solely on the basis of HIV or hepatitis B or C serostatus. SOCv7 departs from prior practices that uniformly required a mental health referral "letter" prior to initiating gender-affirming HT. There are no minimums with regard to time spent in psychotherapy prior to HT, and it is also stated that primary care providers with adequate skill and experience may make their own determination of readiness for initiation of HT. This "informed consent" pathway destigmatizes and depathologizes transgender identities, and it overcomes several perceived or actual barriers to accessing HT; a rigorous mental health screening process may neither be available (lack of resources or lack of trained/willing providers) nor culturally applicable (language barriers and cultural differences between Western-oriented psychotherapy and persons of Latino, African, Aboriginal, or Asian background) (Deutsch, 2012). It is also appropriate to offer physician-supervised HT to those patients who may otherwise turn to unprescribed sources of hormones (Internet and street purchase) or who have already fully adjusted and socially transitioned to the affirmed (new) gender. A 2009 study of transgender women in New York City found that 10% receiving physician-supervised HT were also obtaining hormones from other sources and that patients were frequently taking two or three concomitant hormone regimens. This same study reported as barriers to accessing physician-supervised HT a lack of a knowledgeable provider (32%), lack of a transgender-friendly provider (30%), cost (29%), location (18%), and language (13%) (Sanchez, 2009). It is important that transgender persons have reasonable and realistic expectations about what HT and other treatments can and cannot do. Effectiveness of treatment relates to the age at initiation and the overall health state of the individual, as well as genetic factors. Once gender-affirming hormones have begun, there should be continued monitoring for underlying psychosocial factors or mental health conditions, with interventions as indicated.

FEMINIZING HORMONE REGIMENS

Feminizing hormone therapy involves testosterone blockade in combination with estrogen replacement and also the possible use of a progestogen. The most commonly used testosterone blocker in the United States is spironolactone, a potassium-sparing diuretic taken in divided doses of 50–300 mg twice daily. Caution must be used with patients on angiotensin-converting enzyme inhibitors or those with impaired renal function. Concomitant use of ART medications that may affect renal function, such as tenofovir,

is a theoretical risk; however, no case reports exist of spironolactone causing or worsening renal function in these patients. Fosamprenavir and amprenavir are the only antiretrovirals known to have interactions with estrogens that result in lower antiretroviral drug levels, but these antiretrovirals are rarely used. Side effects of spironolactone are mainly orthostatic hypotension and polyuria, both of which tend to resolve after several weeks. Routine monitoring of potassium and renal function (baseline, 2–4 weeks, and then q 3–6 months thereafter) is reasonable. Creatinine levels should be compared to the male normal range. In patients with contraindications to spironolactone, 5-α-reductase inhibitors such as finasteride 5 mg daily or dutasteride 0.5 mg daily may be used. Some transgender women, especially those whose only opportunity for income is sustenance sex work, prefer to retain erectile function and may choose to avoid or use lower doses of testosterone blockers (Hembree, 2009).

Estrogen treatment may be via an oral, transdermal, or injectable route. Transdermal routes of estradiol (50- to 200-μg patch changed one or two times per week) has been studied extensively and is very safe with respect to risk of thromboembolic disease: A 2008 meta-analysis of vascular thrombotic events (VTEs) in postmenopausal hormone therapy found a relative risk of VTEs in users of transdermal estradiol of 1.1 versus non-user controls. This same review found a 2- to 3-fold increased risk of VTEs among users of any type of oral estrogen in the first year of treatment only; however, this increase translates to only an additional 1.5 VTEs per 1000 woman-years (Canonico, 2008). The transdermal route also delivers fairly constant and physiologic serum estradiol levels, which helps minimize common estrogenic symptoms such as migraine, weight gain, or mood swings; however, transdermal preparations tend to be expensive, may irritate the skin, and are not always included in HIV formularies. Oral 17β-estradiol in divided doses of 2–4 mg twice daily also delivers a constant and physiologic dose and is well-tolerated. Some providers recommend administering oral estradiol sublingually to minimize first-pass metabolism and effects on clotting factors. Prior studies reporting 20- to 40-fold increases in VTE risk in transgender women involved the use of high-dose, highly thrombogenic synthetic ethinyl estradiol, which is no longer used in cross-sex treatment (Asscheman, 1989; van Kesteren, 1997). More recent outcome studies of patients using 17β-estradiol have not found significantly increased rates of thromboembolism (Asscheman, 2011).

Many patients may arrive at clinic requesting, or even demanding, injectable estrogens. Although estradiol valerate 20–40 mg intramuscular or estradiol cypionate 2.5–5 mg twice monthly have been used historically, these routes may deliver supraphysiologic estrogen levels that can vary widely over the injection cycle. Almost no data exist on the short- or long-term effects of this route, although anecdotally it is well-tolerated. This route may be useful in a harm-reduction setting in which there is concern that a patient may turn to unprescribed hormone sources if an injected medication is not prescribed. This route may also be useful in patients who have low psychosocial functioning or to provide an opportunity to bundle HIV-related and other care with frequent hormone administration visits (Ickovics, 2008). Fluctuation of levels may be minimized by dividing the dose into weekly injections and, if needed, titrating peak and trough serum estradiol levels to manage any estrogenic side effects. Furthermore, changes in the hormonal milieu can lead to changes in the balance of Th1–Th2 T lymphocyte function and theoretical alterations in cellular immunity, furthering the argument in favor of constant and physiologic dosing of estrogen.

Interactions between estrogen HT and ART medications are complex and inconsistent, and no studies have been conducted. Data from contraceptive studies are mixed with regard to findings that PI and NNRTI medications may cause changes in serum estrogen and progesterone levels (Kearney, 2009; Marrazzo, 2015). However, should a patient previously on a stable HT regimen begin to experience symptoms of estrogen excess (migraines, weight gain, and mood swings) or deficiency (hot flashes) after a change in ART regimens, it is reasonable to check serum estradiol levels and/or adjust HT dosages empirically. In addition to the previously mentioned tests, monitoring of transgender women using HT should include baseline fasting glucose and lipid profiles, with subsequent monitoring as clinically indicated.

Progestogens have been suggested to enhance breast development and feminization of the body contours, and they may play a role in improving libido and mood. Patients may have a wide range of emotional responses to progestagens, with some patients preferring its effects and others feeling worse. It is reasonable to attempt a trial of oral medroxyprogesterone acetate 5–10 mg orally at bedtime in patients who request this medication, including those with limited breast development, or for those experiencing unpleasant mood or libido changes. Although prior studies on medroxyprogesterone combined with conjugated equine estrogens showed increased risk of thrombogenicity, the risk is minimized when specifically medroxyprogesterone is used in combination with estradiol via the oral, transdermal, or injected routes. Oral micronized progesterone 100–200 mg orally at bedtime may also be used and may be better tolerated, although this medication has a substantially higher cost.

MASCULINIZING HORMONE REGIMENS

Female-to-male treatment primarily involves testosterone administration. Routes include intramuscular testosterone cypionate or enanthate at 50–100 mg once a week or transdermal routes such as patches or gel (5–10 mg daily). Recently, many providers have begun using the subcutaneous route, which is less painful and traumatic and has been found to be non-inferior (Olson, 2014). Dosing can be adjusted to 100–200 mg every 2 weeks; however, this may result in wide fluctuations in hormone levels. This treatment is well-tolerated, with a minimum of side effects in most cases. Dose is titrated to cessation of menses and progression of virilization. Prior concerns about hepatic injury are currently unfounded with the use of non-oral, nonsynthetic androgens. Monitoring should include baseline and periodic (every 6–12 months) fasting serum lipids, glucose, and hematocrit. Due to the lack of menstruation and hematopoietic influence of testosterone, hematocrit should be compared to male normal ranges.

SURGICAL CONSIDERATIONS

SOCv7 requires a readiness and capacity to provide informed consent by a mental health provider prior to most gender-affirming surgical procedures. Common surgical procedures and recommendations from SOCv7 for referral to surgery are listed in Table 13.9. Expanded insurance coverage for gender-affirming surgeries under the Affordable Care Act, in some states MediCal, and by executive order (for providers accepting any federal payment for health care services) has made such procedures available to patients with lower levels of psychosocial functioning and health literacy. Providers should consider additional and ongoing assessments of such perioperative essentials as housing, social support, transportation, and ability for self-care, and they should provide resources and support to address identified needs or gaps (Asscheman, 2011). Patients may also present with a history of any number of surgical procedures. In some cases, the surgery may have been performed in another state or even overseas; as such, local primary care providers may be called upon to provide postoperative care. Most surgeons are willing to work with local physicians and when contacted may ask for photographs to be transmitted by email. For those patients with a complex wound care

Table 13.9 COMMON SURGICAL PROCEDURES AND
RECOMMENDATIONS FOR REFERRAL TO SURGERY

SURGERY	REQUIREMENTS
Transgender women	
Vaginoplasty	Referral from two mental health providers; 12 months continuous full-time living in a gender role congruent with their identity
Orchiectomy or oophorectomy/hysterectomy	Referral from two mental health providers
Augmentation mammoplasty	Referral from a single mental health provider (many surgeons waive this requirement)
Facial feminization procedures	No mental health referral required
Rhinoplasty	
Jaw/mandible contouring	
Reduction thryocondroplasty (Adam's apple reduction) Forehead reconstruction/ hairline advancement	
Female-to-male	
Mastectomy (male chest reconstruction, "top surgery")	Referral from two mental health providers (many surgeons waive this requirement)
Hysterectomy ± oophorectomy	Referral from two mental health providers
Metoidioplasty (removal of clitoral hood and ligaments)	Referral from two mental health providers; 12 months continuous full-time living in a gender role congruent with their identity
Phalloplasty	Referral from two mental health providers; 12 months continuous full-time living in affirmed gender role

issue and remote surgeon, referral to a local wound care center may be a reasonable alternative approach.

Care of transgender women with a history of silicone or saline implant breast augmentation is identical to that of non-transgender persons. More than 90% of vaginoplasties are performed using a penile-inversion technique; the erectile tissue is removed and a "neovagina" is created inverting the penile skin into a pocket created in the pelvis. A clitoris is created using the glans penis, and labia are created with scrotal and possibly urethral skin. The neovagina requires lifelong periodic dilation and/or sexual activity to maintain depth and girth, and an artificial lubricant is required for penetration. Diseases of the neovagina are usually a result of remaining or recurrent granulation tissue (which may be cauterized using silver nitrate) or mixed-skin flora or sebum and debris conditions resulting from a deep inverted pocket of keratinized skin. Candidal infections are uncommon,

and the pH would not be expected to be acidic as in a natal vagina (Weyers, 2009). Although it is not possible to perform a Pap smear on a neovagina, providers should maintain a reasonable index of suspicion for occult penile conditions such as Bowen's disease. A small minority of transgender patients receive a vaginoplasty, in which a self-lubricating vagina is created using a segment of sigmoid colon. These patients must be monitored for possible malignancy or inflammatory bowel disease of the neovagina. Due to the anatomical differences of the surgically constructed neovagina, an anoscope may facilitate improved visualization and better patient tolerance compared to a vaginal speculum. The prostate is not removed during the vaginoplasty procedure; examination of the prostate in a patient who has undergone vaginoplasty may be more effective when performed endovaginally.

PRIMARY CARE

Transgender persons require the same general primary and preventive care considerations as do non-transgender persons. However, it is important to take an inventory of organs on a patient-by-patient basis. For example, transgender women will retain their prostate after vaginoplasty, and some transgender men may have a hysterectomy but retain their ovaries or cervix, necessitating Pap screening. All organ screening should be based on a combination of age and risk factors, maintaining sensitivity to the patient's anxiety, which may be provoked due to examinations and studies on organs related to the birth sex. Screening for breast cancer in transwomen has not been studied; case series exist showing a possible increased risk above that of non-transgender men but lower risk than that of non-transgender women (Brown, 2015; Gooren, 2013). Some experts recommend that after 5–10 years of HT, patients should be considered for breast cancer screening, as are their age-matched non-transgender peers. Overall, providers should attribute HT as the etiology of any new health condition only after other more common causes have been excluded. Solid, long-term health outcome data are lacking. The largest population-based study is a retrospective series in the Netherlands of more than 2000 transgender men and women. In this study, overall mortality among transgender women was increased in comparison to that of the general Dutch population; however, most of this increase was due to HIV, suicide, and substance abuse. Transgender men did not have an increased overall mortality compared to the general population, but they had a 25-fold increased mortality relating to substance abuse (Asscheman, 2011).

HIV CARE AND PREVENTION CONSIDERATIONS

HIV prevention, care, and research programs have historically grouped transgender women with MSM. This linkage fails to recognize the significant behavioral and social differences between these two groups, not the least of which is that transgender women are not men (Poteat, 2015). Other than the possible negative impact of estrogens on amprenavir and fosamprenavir, and theoretical renal interaction between tenofovir and spironolactone, there are no clear biomedical differences in the prevention or management of HIV in transgender persons (El-Ibiary, 2008). The most important considerations are ensuring that programs and clinic settings are culturally appropriate; electronic medical record systems should have the capacity to record and display preferred name and pronoun, social marketing and recruitment materials should include imaging and messaging appropriate for transgender populations, waiting rooms should have transgender-oriented pamphlets and wall art, and clinic bathroom policies should be inclusive and clearly posted. Providers and clinic staff should have adequate cultural fluency and sensitivity (Sevelius, 2014).

HIV PrEP in transgender women has not been studied in depth. The only published study to date of PrEP in transgender women is a subgroup analysis of the iPrEx trial that found no efficacy on an intention-to-treat basis. However, none of the transgender women who seroconverted had detectible drug levels at the time of HIV detection. Hormone use was associated with lower drug levels overall, as well as lower likelihood of having therapeutic drug levels, but the relationship between specific drug levels and HIV risk was identical between MSM and transgender women. It remains to be determined if reduced drug levels in transgender women using hormones are due to a direct interaction or to other confounders, such as increased pill burden or personal fear of interaction between hormones and antiretrovirals (Deutsch, Glidden, 2015).

SILICONE

The use of injected silicone and other soft tissue fillers (pumping) has become an increasingly prevalent practice, particularly among transgender women of color and sex workers. Unscrupulous practitioners, medical assistants, or laypersons will inject up to 1 liter or more of medical- or industrial-grade silicone, lubricant oil, insulating caulk, tire sealant, and other chemicals with the intent of bringing drastic and rapid changes to the physique (Silva-Santisteban, 2013). Most patients are unaware of exactly what is being injected, and the colloquial "silicone" may refer to any one of a number of injected fillers. In addition to the risks associated with the injected material, risks of acute bacterial infections and sepsis as well as transmission of HIV and hepatitis are high under these uncontrolled operating conditions. Some patients may have a sterile systemic inflammatory response mimicking sepsis or suffer embolization syndromes. Long-term risks include chronic pain and disfigurement as the injected material migrates and calcifies.

This procedure is sought due to a variety of factors; in addition to peer pressure and a lack of understanding of the risks, more complex factors of survival are at play. Patients engaging in survival sex work may believe that they need to obtain a hyperfeminine figure in order to be competitive—and therefore pay for food and rent. Others may place a priority on erectile function and avoid HT, using silicone as their sole method of body feminization. Still others may live in neighborhoods in which they do not feel safe being identified as a transgender person, and they believe that silicone will assist them in blending in as a non-transgender person (Clark, 2008).

Treatment of silicone-related morbidities is limited and mostly supportive. Two case reports describe improved symptoms with subcutaneous etanercept 25 mg twice weekly; however, the applicability of etanercept when chemicals other than silicone are used, as well as its safety in HIV-positive patients, is unclear (Desai, 2006; Pasternack, 2005; Rapaport, 2005). An additional concern is subcutaneous or intramuscular medications used in HIV-positive patients, such as penicillin and enfuvirtide, and how these injections may be affected by or complicate preexisting soft tissue fillers. One case report described the safe and successful use of subcutaneous enfuvirtide in a patient with extensive migratory silicone material under ultrasound guidance (Gabrielli, 2010).

CONCLUSION

Most of the special considerations in the care of transgender people living with HIV relate to provider and staff cultural competency, tone and content of messaging, using the correct name and pronoun, and avoiding categorizing transgender women together with MSM. Gender affirmation through hormone and surgical treatment improves quality of life and, when bundled with HIV care or prevention efforts, may have synergistic benefits. More study is needed to evaluate the role of PrEP in transgender communities.

References

Asscheman, H., Giltay, E. J., Megens, J. A. J., et al. (2011). A long-term follow-up study of mortality in transsexuals receiving treatment with cross-sex hormones. *European Journal of Endocrinology, 164*(4), 635–642. http://doi.org/10.1530/EJE-10-1038

Asscheman, H., Gooren, L. J. G., & Eklund, P. L. E. (1989). Mortality and morbidity in transsexual patients with cross-gender hormone treatment. *Metabolism, 38*(9), 869–873.

Baral, S. D., Poteat, T., Strömdahl, S., et al. (2013). Worldwide burden of HIV in transgender women: a systematic review and meta-analysis. *The Lancet Infectious Diseases, 13*(3), 214–222. http://doi.org/10.1016/S1473-3099(12)70315-8

Brown, G. R., & Jones, K. T. (2015). Incidence of breast cancer in a cohort of 5,135 transgender veterans. *Breast Cancer Research and Treatment, 149*(1), 191–198. http://doi.org/10.1007/s10549-014-3213-2

Cahill, S., & Makadon, H. (2013). Sexual orientation and gender identity data collection in clinical settings and in electronic health records: A key to ending LGBT health disparities. *LGBT Health.* Retrieved from http://online.liebertpub.com/doi/abs/10.1089/lgbt.2013.0001

Cahill, S., & Makadon, H. J. (2014). Sexual orientation and gender identity data collection update: U.S. Government takes steps to promote sexual orientation and gender identity data collection through meaningful use guidelines. *LGBT Health.* http://doi.org/10.1089/lgbt.2014.0033

Canonico, M., Plu-Bureau, G., Lowe, G., et al. (2008). Hormone replacement therapy and risk of venous thromboembolism in postmenopausal women: Systematic review and meta-analysis. *BMJ, 336*(7655), 1227.

Clark, R. F., Cantrell, F. L., Pacal, A., et al. (2008). Subcutaneous silicone injection leading to multi-system organ failure. *Clinical Toxicology, 46*(9), 834–837. http://doi.org/10.1080/15563650701850025

Coleman, E., Bockting, W., Botzer, M., et al. (2012). Standards of care for the health of transsexual, transgender, and gender-nonconforming people, version 7. *International Journal of Transgenderism, 13*(4), 165–232. http://doi.org/10.1080/15532739.2011.700873

Colton Meier, S. L., Fitzgerald, K. M., Pardo, S. T., et al. (2011). The effects of hormonal gender affirmation treatment on mental health in female-to-male transsexuals. *Journal of Gay & Lesbian Mental Health, 15*(3), 281–299. http://doi.org/10.1080/19359705.2011.581195

Conron, K. J., Scott, G., Stowell, G. S., et al. (2012). Transgender health in Massachusetts: Results from a household probability sample of adults. *American Journal of Public Health, 102*(1), 118–122. http://doi.org/10.2105/AJPH.2011.300315

Desai, A. M., Browning, J., & Rosen, T. (2006). Etanercept therapy for silicone granuloma. *Journal of Drugs in Dermatology, 5*(9), 894–896.

Deutsch, M. B. (2012). Use of the informed consent model in the provision of cross-sex hormone therapy: A survey of the practices of selected clinics. *International Journal of Transgenderism, 13*(3), 140–146. http://doi.org/10.1080/15532739.2011.675233

Deutsch, M. B., Bhakri, V., & Kubicek, K. (2015). Effects of cross-sex hormone treatment on transgender women and men. *Obstetrics and Gynecology, 125*(3), 605–610. http://doi.org/10.1097/AOG.0000000000000692

Deutsch, M. B., Glidden, D. V., Sevelius, J., et al.(2015). HIV pre-exposure prophylaxis in transgender women: a subgroup analysis of the iPrEx trial. *The Lancet HIV.* http://doi.org/10.1016/S2352-3018(15)00206-4.

Deutsch, M. B., Green, J., Keatley, J., et al. (2013). Electronic medical records and the transgender patient: Recommendations from the World Professional Association for Transgender Health EMR Working Group. *Journal of the American Medical Informatics Association, 2012,* 001472. http://doi.org/10.1136/amiajnl-2012-001472

El-Ibiary, S. Y., & Cocohoba, J. M. (2008). Effects of HIV antiretrovirals on the pharmacokinetics of hormonal contraceptives. *European Journal of Contraception and Reproductive Health Care, 13*(2), 123–132. http://doi.org/10.1080/13625180701829952

Gabrielli, E., Ferraioli, G., Ferraris, L., et al. (2010). Enfuvirtide administration in HIV-positive transgender patient with soft tissue augmentation: US evaluation. *New Microbiologica, 33,* 263–265.

Gómez-Gil, E., Zubiaurre-Elorza, L., Esteva, I., et al. (2012). Hormone-treated transsexuals report less social distress, anxiety and depression. *Psychoneuroendocrinology, 37*(5), 662–670.

Gooren, L. J., van Trotsenburg, M. A. A., Giltay, E. J., et al. (2013). Breast cancer development in transsexual subjects receiving cross-sex hormone treatment. *Journal of Sexual Medicine, 10*(12), 3129–3134. http://doi.org/10.1111/jsm.12319

Green, N., Hoenigl, M., Morris, S., et al. (2015). Risk behavior and sexually transmitted infections among transgender women and men undergoing community-based screening for acute and early HIV infection in San Diego. *Medicine, 94*(41), e1830. http://doi.org/10.1097/MD.0000000000001830

Hembree, W. C., Cohen-Kettenis, P., Delemarre-van de Waal, H. A., et al. (2009). Endocrine treatment of transsexual persons: An Endocrine Society clinical practice guideline. *Journal of Clinical Endocrinology and Metabolism, 94*(9), 3132–3154. http://doi.org/10.1210/jc.2009-0345

Ickovics, J. R. (2008). "Bundling" HIV prevention: Integrating services to promote synergistic gain. *Preventive Medicine, 46*(3), 222–225. http://doi.org/10.1016/j.ypmed.2007.09.006

Kearney, B. P., & Mathias, A. (2009). Lack of effect of tenofovir disoproxil fumarate on pharmacokinetics of hormonal contraceptives. *Pharmacotherapy, 29*(8), 924–929. http://doi.org/10.1592/phco.29.8.924

Kenagy, G. P., & Bostwick, W. B. (2005). Health and social service needs of transgender people in Chicago. *International Journal of Transgenderism, 8*(2–3), 57–66. http://doi.org/10.1300/J485v08n02_06

Marrazzo, J. M., Ramjee, G., Richardson, B. A., et al. (2015). Tenofovir-based preexposure prophylaxis for HIV infection among African women. *New England Journal of Medicine, 372*(6), 509–518. http://doi.org/10.1056/NEJMoa1402269

Melendez, R. M., & Pinto, R. M. (2009). HIV prevention and primary care for transgender women in a community-based clinic. *Journal of the Association of Nurses in AIDS Care, 20*(5), 387–397. http://doi.org/10.1016/j.jana.2009.06.002

Olson, J., Schrager, S. M., Clark, L. F., et al. (2014). Subcutaneous testosterone: An effective delivery mechanism for masculinizing young transgender men. *LGBT Health.* http://doi.org/10.1089/lgbt.2014.0018.

Pasternack, F. R., Fox, L. P., & Engler, D. E. (2005). Silicone granulomas treated with etanercept. *Archives of Dermatology, 141*(1), 13.

Poteat, T., Wirtz, A. L., Radix, A., et al. (2015). HIV risk and preventive interventions in transgender women sex workers. *Lancet, 385*(9964), 274–286. http://doi.org/10.1016/S0140-6736(14)60833-3

Rapaport, M. J. (2005). Silicone granulomas treated with etanercept. *Archives of Dermatology, 141*(9), 1171. http://doi.org/10.1001/archderm.141.9.1171-a

Sanchez, N. F., Sanchez, J. P., & Danoff, A. (2009). Health care utilization, barriers to care, and hormone usage among male-to-female transgender persons in New York City. *American Journal of Public Health, 99*(4), 713.

Sevelius, J. M. (2013). Gender affirmation: A framework for conceptualizing risk behavior among transgender women of color. *Sex Roles, 68*(11–12), 675–689. http://doi.org/10.1007/s11199-012-0216-5

Sevelius, J. M., Patouhas, E., Keatley, J. G., et al. (2014). Barriers and facilitators to engagement and retention-in-care among transgender women living with human immunodeficiency virus. *Annals of Behavioral Medicine, 47*(1), 5–16. http://doi.org/10.1007/s12160-013-9565-8

Silva-Santisteban, A., Segura, E. R., Sandoval, C., et al. (2013). Determinants of unequal HIV care access among people living with HIV in Peru. *Globalization and Health, 9*(1), 22. http://doi.org/10.1186/1744-8603-9-22

Subcutaneous administration of testosterone—A pilot study report. (2006). *Saudi Medical Journal, 27*(12), 1843–1846.

Tate, C. C., Ledbetter, J. N., & Youssef, C. P. (2012). A two-question method for assessing gender categories in the social and medical sciences. *Journal of Sex Research, 50*, 1–10. http://doi.org/10.1080/00224499.2012.690110

van Kesteren, P. J., Asscheman, H., Megens, J. A., et al. (1997). Mortality and morbidity in transsexual subjects treated with cross-sex hormones. *Clinical Endocrinology, 47*(3), 337–342.

Weyers, S., Verstraelen, H., Gerris, J., et al. (2009). Microflora of the penile skin-lined neovagina of transsexual women. *BMC Microbiology, 9*(1), 102. http://doi.org/10.1186/1471-2180-9-102.

HOMELESS POPULATIONS

LEARNING OBJECTIVE

Describe special considerations affecting the medical management of homeless or displaced individuals.

WHAT'S NEW?

- Four single-pill combination regimens for HIV treatment currently available should enhance adherence and reduce pill burden and complexity.

- Innovative programs for linkage and retention-in-care are operational.

- Text messaging may be an important tool for retention-in-care.

- Opioid reversal (naloxone) programs are life-saving.

- Needle exchange programs are essential in preventing clusters of HIV and hepatitis infections in injection drug users.

KEY POINTS

- HIV and homelessness are overlapping epidemics.

- Poverty, mental illness, substance use, and discrimination are barriers to care for both.

- Establishing mutual trust is paramount.

- Linkage to care and retention-in-care require enhanced teamwork.

Homelessness and HIV are two overlapping epidemics that each lead to worse health outcomes. They share many of the same risk factors of poverty, mental illness, substance use, racism, homophobia, stigmatization, and other forms of discrimination. Linkage to care and retention-in-care are challenging and are best met with establishment of a trusting relationship, outreach, case management, partnering with supportive housing programs, and client-centered innovative local programs to reduce the barriers to care.

The federal government estimates that there are approximately 578,424 people who are homeless on any given night. Advocates point to 2 to 3 million persons experiencing homelessness annually (National Law Center on Homelessness and Poverty, 2015). HIV prevalence among homeless populations exceeds national averages. It is estimated that 3.4% of homeless people are HIV infected, compared to less than 1% nationally (Allen, 1994). In certain areas, the HIV prevalence among homeless people is much higher. In San Francisco, 11% of new HIV infections occur in people who are currently homeless. It has also been estimated that one-third to one-half of people with AIDS are either homeless or at imminent risk of homelessness. Rising costs of housing, diminishing stock of single-room occupancies and public housing, and low wages make it nearly impossible to maintain stable housing in many cities.

Obtaining information about housing status and stability should be a routine part of obtaining a psychosocial history for HIV-infected patients. Questions phrased in the vein of "What is your living situation?" are readily understood and are preferable to "Are you homeless?" A follow-up question on the stability of current living arrangements can also give insight into a patient's housing status. If the patient is marginally housed or homeless, knowing how to contact the patient is extremely important. Be aware of any contact phone numbers, as well as places they usually visit, including any agencies that they use, case managers, and food lines and stores that they frequent. This will allow one to contact them in case of abnormal labs, important appointments, and if they are lost to follow-up. Some social service agencies provide free voice mail, which can be a confidential way for the patient to receive messages. Free cell phones, referred to as "Obama phones," are available for low-income individuals. Text messages relaying appointment reminders and motivating messages have been shown to increase attendance at appointments. In Kenya, text messages significantly improved adherence and viral suppression (Lester, 2010). In another African study, text messages were shown to improved attendance to postpartum clinics and early infant diagnosis in HIV pregnant women.

Health status is poorer in homeless populations than in the general population. A recent systematic review that included 152 studies representing 139,757 patients found that worse housing status was independently associated with worse outcomes among people with HIV/AIDS

(Aidala, 2016). The issue of tuberculosis (TB) exposure and transmission is a serious problem for HIV-infected homeless people, and transmission in shelters is well-documented (McElroy, 2003). Aggressive screening for TB is recommended. Louse-borne and rat-borne infections are probably underrecognized given that the seroprevalence of rickettsial and other related infections is as high as 50% in homeless populations studied both in the United States and in Europe (Brouqui, 2005). Body lice can transmit a variety of bacterial infections, including relapsing fever caused by *Borrelia recurrentis*, trench fever caused by *Bartonella quintana*, epidemic typhus caused by *Rickettsia prowazekii*, and bacillary angiomatosis caused by *Bartonella henselae* and *Bartonella quintana*. Bacillary angiomatosis occurs in severely immunosuppressed HIV-infected individuals; infestation with body lice is an important factor in transmission of *Bartonella*, the causative organism (Foucault, 2006).

PREVENTION, MORTALITY, AND MORBIDITY

Homelessness remains an important risk factor for HIV transmission (San Francisco Department of Public Health, 2015; Sypsa, 2015). Current prevention strategies including post-exposure prophylaxis and PrEP have not been well studied in homeless populations, but indications are positive that these would be effective and acceptable (Doblecki-Lewis, 2016). The success of efforts to eliminate transmission by reducing community viral loads will almost certainly pivot on the ability to reach and assure adherence in homeless and multiply diagnosed populations.

Although death rates for HIV have steadily declined since their peak in 1995, homeless people experience excess mortality compared to the general population. Among the homeless in Boston, the mortality rate was 9-fold higher in 25- to 44-year-olds and 4.5-fold higher in 45- to 64-year-olds. One-third of the deaths were due to drug overdoses (Baggett, 2013). Among a cohort of 300 homeless women in San Francisco, half of whom were HIV infected, the mortality rate was 10 times higher than that of the general population. Cocaine-related intoxication, rather than HIV-related complications, was the leading cause of death in these women. Overall, leading causes of death among HIV-infected persons in high-income countries are AIDS-related (29%), liver-related (13%), cardiovascular disease (11%), non-AIDS-related cancer (15%), invasive bacterial infections (7%), suicide (4%), and overdose (3%) (Smith, 2014). Studies suggest that substance use treatment, opiate reversal programs, treatment of hepatitis C and B, cancer

screening, and supportive housing may be life-saving in homeless HIV-infected persons.

Harm reduction measures such as needle exchange programs and naloxone distribution programs can be life-saving. In May 2015, the CDC (2015) reported that in a rural county in Indiana, 135 persons were diagnosed with HIV in a community of 4200. The cases were linked to syringe-sharing partners injecting oxymorphone. Co-infection with hepatitis C was found in 114 patients. A public health emergency was declared, and a needle exchange program was authorized by the governor. Needle exchange programs are important for reducing the spread of HIV and hepatitis C, as well as linking persons to substance use programs and methadone treatment. In a report on more than 10,000 opioid reversals, the CDC stated that making training in the use and distribution of naloxone available to opioid drug users is a strategy that reduces overdose deaths (CDC, 2012). Opioid reversal programs using naloxone have been credited with saving numerous lives. Patients who are prescribed opioids or who use them or are on methadone or buprenorphine should have access to naloxone and training on how to use it.

Clearly, team-based care is essential to address the multiple needs of homeless patients. Randomized controlled trials have shown that HIV-infected homeless people randomized to intensive case management linked to housing were more likely to obtain permanent housing and achieve an undetectable viral load than those who received usual hospital discharge planning (Buchanon, 2009). San Francisco has a respite unit with medical and social services. Homeless patients can have their medications administered, wound care provided, and follow-up appointments tracked. They also may be able to transition into permanent housing. Results from the Seattle Eastlake "wet housing" project showed that heavy alcohol users who were admitted and allowed to drink in the housing significantly decreased their heavy drinking days, reduced their daily intake from 21 to 11 drinks per day, had a major decrease in withdrawal tremors, and saved the city $4 million in the first year (Collins, 2012). Street medicine and mobile health care programs such as Homeless Outreach Team (SF HOT) and HIV Homeless Outreach Mobile Engagement (HHOME) in San Francisco assertively provide continuity to patients who would otherwise be lost from the health care system aside from high-cost acute services. Ironically, cities with budget deficits may find that providing more care and housing can save money. Failure to do so can result in disastrous increases in HIV infection and morbidity and mortality, as has happened as a result of the austerity measures in Athens, Greece (Sypsa, 2015). Some cities have directly observed antiretroviral therapy (DOT) as part of methadone maintenance. Researchers in New York City found that the odds of an undetectable viral load were threefold greater in DOT patients compared to those receiving usual care (Berg, 2011). Methadone clinics can also work with HIV providers to track important appointments and represent an easy way to contact otherwise difficult-to-reach patients. Case management programs can coordinate the comprehensive wraparound services that complex patients need; administrators can accompany these patients to important appointments and find them in the field when necessary. Nevertheless, in recognition of the large disparities that continue to exist for homeless HIV-infected individuals, the Health Resources and Services Administration (HRSA) has initiated a multisite demonstration project called Building a Medical Home for Multiply Diagnosed HIV-Positive Homeless Populations that will evaluate and disseminate information on best practices in caring for this population (HRSA, 2015).

Recent research has demonstrated the pervasive occurrence of chronic pain in this population (Miaskowski, 2011) and the complexity of managing pain in these patients (Hansen, 2011). The National Health Care for the Homeless Clinicians Network has developed a useful guideline for care of homeless patients with chronic pain (Wismer, 2011). Efforts to develop innovative and comprehensive programs to manage pain and co-occurring mental health and chemical dependency in this population are underway in San Francisco and other locations.

With the availability of electronic medical records, quality improvement programs can track measures such as missed appointments; lost to follow-up; detectable viral loads; show-up rates for new patients; or various health care maintenance measures, including Pap smears, mammograms, and colorectal cancer screening. Causes for poor performance can be studied locally, and solutions can be tested with quality improvement methods.

HIV TREATMENT

Although homeless people may face challenges to adherence and compliance that housed individuals may not face, homelessness should not be a limiting factor in the decision to prescribe ART. A 12-month prospective study of 148 HIV-infected homeless individuals on ART in San Francisco showed that one-third discontinued their medications (Moss, 2004). Predictors of discontinuation were depressive symptoms, injection drug use (IDU), African American ethnicity, and poor early adherence. In the group that continued with ART, the average adherence by unannounced pill count was 74%, and 55% of these patients had an undetectable viral load. Predictors of lower adherence were African American ethnicity and use of crack cocaine, but not IDU; MSM had higher adherence. These adherence rates, although not optimal, were similar to those of other population-based studies. A study of HIV-infected injection drug users on ART in Miami showed that homeless subjects had higher rates of anxiety and perceived stress, but they had similar rates of depression as housed subjects (Waldrop-Valverde, 2005). In the study, depression was significantly related to lower adherence, although housing status was not. Sixty-three percent of homeless subjects reported 100% adherence. Both studies showed that depression is a potent predictor of nonadherence, suggesting that HIV-infected homeless individuals should be screened and treated for depression (Moss, 2004; Waldrop-Valverde, 2005).

Strategies to improve adherence in homeless people are similar to those recommended for general populations. There are several additional strategies, including building on existing routines, such as those related to shelter, meals, or even drug-using routines. To assist patients, providers must ask about and understand these routines when prescribing and providing adherence counseling.

We recommend single-pill combination regimens (SPCs), if possible, to prevent running out of part of the regimen and to ease pill burden. In choosing an ART regimen, there are some special considerations, such as whether medications should be taken on an empty stomach or have particular food restrictions, requirements for dose timing that may be difficult to maintain, as well as food times and types that may not be under a person's control. Medications that have CNS side effects, such as efavirenz, may cause sedation and decreased awareness of one's environment and may affect street safety or worsen underlying psychiatric problems. Large numbers of pill bottles or weekly pill boxes are recognizable and difficult to conceal in a shelter setting; as a result, stigmatization, discrimination, or theft of medications may occur. Medication bottles can be kept by a case manager or program director, and small pill boxes that can be refilled frequently may be useful in these cases. Currently, there are four single-pill combination regimens, and more are likely to become available in the future. Coformulated efavirenz, emtricitabine, and tenofovir (Atripla) can cause CNS side effects and can lower methadone levels. The second tricoformulated pill containing rilpivirine, emtricitabine, and tenofovir (Complera) lacks the CNS side effects of Atripla, but it must be taken with a 500-calorie meal (see Complera website for sample meals) because nutritional supplements are not adequate. Furthermore, proton pump inhibitors cannot be used, and Complera is less effective than Atripla as an initial treatment regimen in those with a baseline viral load greater than 100,000 copies/ml. A third SPC regimen of quad-coformulated emtricitabine, cobisistat, tenofovir, elvitegravir (Stribild) is recommended as first-line therapy in the 2015 US guidelines for CrCL >70 ml/min. Cobicistat is a CYP3A inhibitor, and there are multiple drug interactions; it is also an inhibitor of several of the transporter systems. It is recommended that it be taken with food. The fourth SPC regimen is dolutegravir, lamivudine, and abacavir (Triumeq). The patient must be HLA B5701 negative before starting. It may be taken with or without food.

THE MODEL OF CARE

There are more than 100 health care programs for the homeless (HCH) throughout the United States. Linking with a local program or getting advice from a national HCH organization is helpful to HIV providers working with homeless people. Shelter staff are also key resource providers in education and prevention efforts as well as support. Providing housing, particularly supportive housing targeted to formerly homeless people, is a critical health service function.

HIV-infected homeless people have a high prevalence of mental health disorders, especially depression, which is associated with poorer adherence to medications. Histories of both physical and sexual assault are common, especially among homeless women and transgender individuals. In one study, 32% of women and 38% of transgendered persons reported a history of either sexual or physical assault in the previous year. It has also been reported that African American women with a history of childhood abuse have an increased risk of being homeless and using crack cocaine (Wechsberg, 2003).

Building a trusting relationship and providing a non-judgmental medical home in which patients can feel that they are valued as individuals is of utmost importance. The health care team should be able to recognize and treat post-traumatic stress disorder, depression, and other psychiatric disorders. A harm reduction approach is recommended. An effective program will also need to coordinate services with local jails and prisons because incarceration is more common among the homeless and those with HIV. Many homeless people are devoted to their pets and will not take care of their own health needs unless their pets are safe. Some cities have a special arrangement with the local humane society or have special services for pets.

In San Francisco, the Positive Health Access to Services and Treatment (PHAST) team works to encourage testing in the inpatient setting, emergency room, and urgent care and primary care clinics. The PHAST team provides easy linkage to care and actively works with newly HIV-infected people or people who have fallen out of care, meeting them in the emergency room or in their inpatient room. PHAST works to stabilize patients, navigate them through often complex health care and benefits systems, and works on their barriers as defined by the patients. Patients are followed closely to link them and retain them in care. The key is not giving up on the patients; it may take a long time for them to fully engage. The San Francisco Department of Public Health's LINCS program (Linkage, Navigation, Integration, and Comprehensive Services) takes referrals for all San Francisco clients who would benefit from connecting or reconnecting with services. LINCS has outreach workers who search for both newly diagnosed patients and patients lost to follow-up.

Recommended Reading

Buchanan DB, Kee R, Sadowski LS, et al. The health impact of supportive housing for HIV-positive homeless patients: A randomized controlled trial. *Am J Public Health.* 2009; 99(6):S675–S680.

O'Connell, J. *Stories from the Shadows: Reflections of a Street Doctor.* Boston, MA: BHCHP Press; 2015.

Wismer B, Amann T, Diaz R, et al. (Eds.). *Adapting Your Practice: Recommendations for the Care of Homeless Adults with Chronic Non-malignant Pain.* Nashville, TN: Health Care for the Homeless Clinicians' Network, National Health Care for the Homeless Council; 2011:119.

References

Aidala AA, Wilson MG, Shubert V, et al. Housing status, medical care, and health outcomes among people living with HIV/AIDS: A systematic review. American Journal of Public Health 2016; 106:e1–e23. http://doi.org/10.2105/AJPH.2015.302905

Allen DM, Lehman JS, Green TA, et al. HIV infection among homeless adults and runaway youth, United States, 1989-1992. Field Services Branch. *AIDS.* 1994 Nov; 8(11):1593–1599.

Baggett, TP, Hwang SW, O'Connell JJ, et al. Mortality among homeless adults in Boston: Shifts in causes of death over a 15 year period. JAMA Intern Med 2013; 173:189–195.

Berg KM, Litwin A, Li X, et al. Directly observed antiretroviral therapy improves adherence and viral load in drug users attending methadone maintenance clinics: A randomized controlled trial. Drug Alcohol Dependence 2011; 113(2–3):192–199.

Brouqui P, Stein A, Dupont HT, et al. Ectoparasitism and vector-borne diseases in 930 homeless people from Marseilles. *Medicine (Baltimore).* 2005 Jan; 84(1):61–68.

Buchanan DB, Kee R, Sadowski LS, et al. The health impact of supportive housing for HIV-positive homeless patients: A randomized controlled trial. American Journal of Public Health 2009; 99(6):S675–S680.

Centers for Disease Control and Prevention. Community based opioid overdose prevention programs providing naloxone—United States. MMWR 2012; 61:101–105.

Centers for Disease Control and Prevention. Community outbreak of HIV infection linked to injection drug use of oxymorphone—Indiana. MMWR 2015; 64:443–444.

Collins SE, Malone DK, Clifasefi SL, et al. Project-based housing first for chronically homeless individuals with alcohol problems: Within-subjects analyses of 2-year alcohol trajectories. American Journal of Public Health 2012; 102(3):511–519.

Doblecki-Lewis S, Lester L, Schwartz B, et al. HIV risk and awareness and interest in pre-exposure and post-exposure prophylaxis among sheltered women in Miami. International Journal of STD & AIDS 2016; 27(10):873–881. http://doi.org/10.1177/0956462415601304.

Hansen L, Penko J, Guzman D, et al. Aberrant behaviors with prescription opioids and problem drug use history in a community-based cohort of HIV-infected individuals. J Pain Symptom Management 2011; 42(6):893–902.

Health Resources and Services Administration HIV/AIDS Programs (HRSA SPNS). (n.d.). Building a medical home for multiply diagnosed HIV-positive homeless populations. Available at http://hab.hrsa.gov/abouthab/special/homeless.html. Accessed November 16, 2015.

Lester RT, Ritvo P, Mills E, et al. Effects of a mobile phone short message service on antiretroviral treatment adherence in Kenya (WelTel Kenya1): A randomized trial. Lancet 2010; 376:1838–1845.

Miaskowski C, Penko JM, Guzman D, et al. Occurrence and characteristics of chronic pain in a community-based cohort of indigent adults living with HIV infection. J Pain 2011; 12(9):1004–1016.

Moss AR, Hahn JA, Perry S, et al. Adherence to highly active antiretroviral therapy in the homeless population in San Francisco: a prospective study. *Clin Infect Dis.* 2004 Oct 15; 39(8):1190–1198.

National Health Care for the Homeless Council and Clinicians Network. Adapted clinical guidelines. Available at https://www.nhchc.org/resources/clinical/adapted-clinical-guidelines.

National Health Care for the Homeless Council and Clinicians Network. https://www.nhchc.org.

National Law Center on Homelessness and Poverty (2015, January). Homelessness in America: Overview of data and causes. Available at http://www.nlchp.org/documents/Homeless_Stats_Fact_Sheet. Accessed November 16, 2015.

San Francisco Department of Public Health Population Health Division (SFDPH). (2015, August). HIV-Epidemiology Annual Report-2014. Retrieved November 16, 2015, from https://www.sfdph.org/dph/files/reports/RptsHIVAIDS/AnnualReport2015-20160831.pdf.

Smith, CJ, Ryom, L, Weber R, et al. Trends in underlying causes of death in people with HIV from 1999 to 2011 (D:A:D): A multicohort collaboration. Lancet 2014; 384:241–248.

Sypsa V, Paraskevis D, Malliori M, et al. Homelessness and other risk factors for HIV infection in the current outbreak among injection drug users in Athens, Greece. *Am J Public Health.* 2015 Jan; 105(1):196–204.

Waldrop-Valverde D, Valverde E. Homelessness and psychological distress as contributors to antiretroviral nonadherence in HIV-positive injecting drug users. *AIDS Patient Care STDS.* 2005 May; 19(5):326–334.

Wismer B, Amann T, Diaz R, et al. (Eds.). *Adapting Your Practice: Recommendations for the Care of Homeless Adults with Chronic Non-malignant Pain.* Nashville, TN: Health Care for the Homeless Clinicians' Network, National Health Care for the Homeless Council; 2011.

Wechsberg WM, Lam WK, Zule W, et al. Violence, homelessness, and HIV risk among crack-using African-American women. *Subst Use Misuse.* 2003 Feb–May; 38(3–6):669–700.

INCARCERATED POPULATIONS

LEARNING OBJECTIVE

Discuss the provision of HIV care and release planning in the context of correctional facilities.

WHAT'S NEW?

In light of the 2015 DHHS ART guidelines, which recommend treating everyone who is HIV positive with ART irrespective of pretreatment CD4+ T cell count, correctional facilities may need to re-evaluate and prioritize their antiretroviral formulary list. The splitting of coformulated tablets into their respective components and generic drug preferences may become more common practice as part of efforts to treat more HIV-infected inmates while being fiscally prudent. Caution is urged that correctional facilities do not stray from the DHHS-recommended regimens for treatment-naive individuals.

KEY POINTS

- The United States has the highest incarceration rate in the world.

- Persons of color are disproportionately incarcerated.

- Rates of HIV infection and AIDS diagnoses are 5 and 2.5 times higher, respectively, in state and federal correctional facilities compared to the general public.

- Correctional facilities pose unique barriers to ART adherence.

- Strategies for successful release planning may include having an appointment with an HIV provider soon after release and working with case managers/social workers to obtain medical coverage and referrals to community HIV organizations.

According to US Department of Justice statistics, approximately 6,937,600 offenders were under the supervision of correctional systems at the end of 2012. Of these individuals, 4,781,300 were supervised via probation or parole systems. The remaining individuals were living in jails or state or federal prisons. The number of individuals who are incarcerated in the United States has been declining slowly since 2009. At the end of 2012, 1 in every 35 adults in the United States was under some form of correctional observation. This is the lowest rate observed since 1997.

The risk factors associated with acquiring HIV infection and having an interaction with the criminal justice system are similar. In 2014, approximately half of federal inmates and 16% of state inmates were serving time for drug-related offenses. Black, non-Hispanic males have a 3.8–10.5 times higher rate of incarceration compared to their White, non-Hispanic counterparts. Similarly, Black, non-Hispanic females have a 1.6–4.1 times higher rate of incarceration compared to White, non-Hispanic females. In 2014, women accounted for approximately 7% of the total prison population. White women comprise 50% and black women 21% of all incarcerated women. An estimated 7.3% of black men between the ages of 30 and 34 years were in a state or federal correctional facility (Guerino, 2011).

HIV EPIDEMIOLOGY IN CORRECTIONAL FACILITIES

Within state and federal correctional systems, HIV infection prevalence is 5 times higher than that in the general population. Rates of confirmed AIDS cases in prisons are approximately 2.5 times greater than those of non-incarcerated populations (Marucschak, 2006; Spaulding, 2002). Results from studies conducted with HIV-infected inmates demonstrated that being Black or Hispanic, being a man who has sex with men, having a history of IDU, having an STI, or having a psychiatric condition were all positive predictors of HIV infection (Beckwith, 2010).

The prevalence of hepatitis C virus (HCV) co-infection among HIV-infected inmates varies greatly depending on region. Rates of HIV/HCV co-infection in correctional settings have been estimated to be as high as 65–70% (Weinbaum, 2005).

PROBLEMS WITH HIV PREVENTION IN PRISONS

Although risk behaviors such as tattooing, drug use, and sex are forbidden in correctional facilities, these activities are common. Condoms are not available and deemed contraband in most facilities. Not surprisingly, clean needles are not provided, and needle exchange programs do not exist. Thus, prevention programs cannot provide the materials necessary to prevent the spread of sexually transmitted diseases and other illnesses. Fortunately, to date, the actual transmission of HIV within correctional facilities is thought to be relatively low, and it is believed to be lower in comparison to the transmission rates in the general public. However, the true rate of HIV acquisition among inmates is difficult to ascertain because routine HIV testing on entry and exit from correctional facilities is poorly documented. Effective treatment of HIV will further decrease the risk of HIV transmission in correctional settings.

BARRIERS TO HIV TREATMENT IN CORRECTIONAL FACILITIES

Policies governing the provision of care and access to medical testing vary across prisons and jails. For example, some state prisons require HIV testing, and some merely recommend it. The CDC has recommended routine opt-out testing of inmates (CDC, 2009). In 2005, only 33% of state and federal prisons were performing routine mandatory HIV testing (Hammett, 2007). Not surprisingly, routine opt-out testing strategies yield greater numbers of screening and subsequent HIV diagnoses. Jails, as opposed to prisons, typically have an extremely rapid turnover rate, making routine or opt-out HIV screening and follow-up difficult to implement. According to Minton and Sabol (2009), the average weekly turnover rate in jails was 66.5% in 2008.

Facilities may or may not meet national standards; they may or may not have access to HIV specialists and to specialty tests, such as co-receptor tropism assays, integrase inhibitor resistance testing, HLA-B*5701 screening testing, or resistance genotypes (Bernard, 2006).

Similar to the non-incarcerated population, there are many reasons for nonadherence to ART among inmates, but some are unique to correctional facilities. Movement between facilities, being in segregation, and "lockdown" (wings or halls forbid any departures from cells by inmates for periods of time) can cause disruptions in adherence. Facilities not receiving medications in a timely manner or inmates not being alerted to pick up their medications can serve as barriers to adherence. Inmates cannot always keep their own medication ("keep on person" (KOP)), and some are required to pick up medication daily at the pharmacy or infirmary (DOT). Confidentiality can be a major concern, for example, when picking up medications or going for DOT. Sometimes, the exposure of HIV status can have severe consequences in prisons. Getting medications on schedule and meeting food requirements can be difficult. Inmates may be required to attend programs or jobs that interfere with the timely ingestion of medication, especially in DOT situations. Meals are served at specific times that may not coincide with the timing for a particular medication. Taking efavirenz at bedtime may not be possible. DOT regimens do not encourage autonomy on the part of the patient. Facilities that require DOT could consider allowing the more real-life KOP system for a specified time before discharge.

Additional barriers unique to correctional facilities stem from limited budgets and the costs of HIV care. Some facilities may have guidelines or restrictions on when providers can initiate ART. Many correctional facilities have formulary restrictions that appear to be cost-effective. Less expensive ART options often result in more pills daily, twice-daily dosing schedules, and greater side effects (all well-documented correlates of nonadherence). Costs incurred as a result of the need for additional medications to counter common ART side effects are difficult to capture and often not included in cost analyses.

ART USE IN CORRECTIONAL FACILITIES

Providers should include the inmate's length of stay and future transfers in the decision-making process of initiating ART. Often, inmates who are released from prison and violate parole will be brought to a jail and then transferred to prison or brought directly back to prison. This movement often results in missed doses of ART. Note that the selection of ART regimens with a higher barrier to resistance will likely provide greater success of the regimens for persons unable to fulfill ART prescriptions and persons who will be in and out of correctional facilities. In the spirit of cost savings, selection of more durable regimens may prevent the development of drug-resistant HIV. Subsequently, avoiding the development of drug-resistant HIV may save on future lab costs and also costs associated with adding agents to effectively treat drug-resistant strains of HIV. Anecdotally, inmates have reported efavirenz-containing regimens as having "street value" in correctional facilities. The drug can be ground up and huffed or snorted for hallucinogenic effects.

RELEASE PLANNING

A key to success of many programs is collaboration among stakeholders—for example, correctional systems, academic institutions, and medical centers in the community (Braithwaite, 1996). A multitude of resources are available for persons living with HIV. It would behoove individuals working with discharge planning and re-entry to the community of HIV-positive inmates to become familiar with the resources available. In some communities, housing and food supplies are available to persons based solely on their HIV diagnosis.

Additional considerations for successful release to the community are scheduling appointments with an HIV provider soon after release and assisting inmates with the linkage to HIV care. Some facilities provide inmates 1 week of medication and a 30-day prescription at time of release. Without some type of health care coverage in place, many inmates are unable to fill the prescriptions. In fact, only approximately 20% of released inmates fill their ART prescription within 30 days of release (Baillargeon, 2009).

References

Baillargeon J, Giordano T, Rich J, et al. (2009). Accessing antiretroviral therapy following release from prison. Journal of the American Medical Association 301(8):848–857.

Beckwith C, Zaller N, Fu J, et al. (2010). Opportunities to diagnose, treat, and prevent HIV in the criminal justice system. Journal of Acquired Immune Deficiency Syndrome 55(Suppl 1):S49–S55.

Bernard K, Sueker J, et al. (2006, March). Provider perspectives about the standard of HIV care in correctional settings and comparison to the community standard of care: How do we measure up? Infectious Diseases in Corrections Report 9(3):1–2, 4–6.

Braithwaite R, Hammett T, Mayberry R (1996). *Prisons and AIDS: A public health challenge.* San Francisco, CA: Jossey-Bass.

Guerino P, Harrison P, Sabol W (2011). Prisoners in 2010. US Department of Justice, Bureau of Justice Statistics. Available at http://www.bjs.gov.

Hammet T, Kennedy S, Kuck S (2007). National survey of infectious diseases in correctional facilities: HIV and sexually transmitted diseases. US Department of Justice. Available at https://www.ncjrs.gov/pdffiles1/nij/grants/217736.pdf.

Maruschak L (2009). HIV in prisons, 2007–08. US Department of Justice, Bureau of Justice Statics. Retrieved from: http://www.bjs.gov/content/pub/pdf/hivp08.pdf.

Minton T, Sabol W (2009). Jail inmates at midyear 2008—Statistical tables. US Department of Justice, Bureau of Justice Statistics. Available at http://bjs.ojp.usdoj.gov/content/pub/pdf/jim08st.pdf.

Sabol W, West H, Cooper M (2009). Prisoners in 2008. US Department of Justice, Bureau of Justice Statistics. Available at http://bjs.ojp.usdoj.gov/content/pub/pdf/p08.pdf.

Spaulding A, Stephenson B, Macalino G, et al. (2002). Human immunodeficiency virus in correctional facilities. Clinical Infectious Diseases 35:305–312.

Weinbaum C, Sabin K, Santibanez S (2005). Hepatitis B, hepatitis C, and HIV in correctional populations: A review of epidemiology and prevention. AIDS 19(Suppl 3):S41–S46.

RURAL POPULATIONS

LEARNING OBJECTIVE
Describe obstacles to optimal HIV care for patients in rural settings.

WHAT'S NEW?
Studies have revealed that rural populations may be less likely to receive quality health care and HIV treatment compared to urban populations.

- Studies have shown that the epidemiology of HIV/AIDS differs in terms of rural versus urban areas, and some studies even show that some rural populations may be less likely to receive quality health care and HIV treatment compared to urban populations.

- Rural HIV-infected patients experience barriers to optimal care, including long travel distances to receive expert care, lack of transportation, poor access to substance use treatment programs, and greater stigma associated with an HIV-infected diagnosis. Establishing optimal care for rural HIV-infected patients will require innovative programs that address all these issues.

Studies suggest that the quality of HIV health care services differs by geographic location, and smaller studies have even found that rural populations are less likely to receive quality care compared to their urban counterparts. Although these conclusions are noteworthy, the results from these studies must be examined closely because large research trials typically sample more urban patients than rural patients due to accessibility to patients for large academic center trials. A 2011 study researched the relationship of geographic location—in particular, rural, urban, and peri-urban—to the receipt of quality HIV health care services (Wilson, 2011). The study evaluated both clinical outcomes and health care utilization in these patients using data from the HIV Research Network, which is a multistate, multisite research cohort. Researchers concluded that patients living in rural and peri-urban areas who received their health care in urban areas had high-quality HIV care and favorable HIV outcomes (virologic suppression and incidence of AIDS-defining illnesses) compared to those patients living in urban areas. High-quality HIV care included initiating ART, attaining HIV suppression on ART, and beginning prophylaxis therapy for opportunistic illnesses. The study also found that the proportion of patients receiving ART was higher for rural patients than for urban patients and that outpatient utilization was lower among rural patients. Unfortunately, this study was not able to follow a large number of rural HIV-infected patients accessing their HIV care in rural locations, and further studies are necessary to examine this issue more closely (Wilson, 2011).

To define urban and rural regions, the CDC used the metropolitan statistical areas employed by the US Office of Management and Budget, with nonmetropolitan or rural areas being those with a population less than 50,000. Figure 13.5 shows the reported AIDS cases among adults and adolescents in metropolitan and nonmetropolitan areas in 2013, and

although all states have some HIV-infected patients living in rural settings, the southeastern United States continues to have the highest rural AIDS prevalence, followed by Midwestern states. According to the CDC 2013 HIV Surveillance Statistics, 6.9% of diagnosed HIV infections were reported in nonmetropolitan or rural settings (CDC, 2013). This statistic may also underestimate the number of HIV-infected persons living in and accessing care in a rural setting.

Another study found that rural HIV-infected patients were less likely than their urban counterparts to have a provider who had seen more than 10 HIV-infected patients within the past 6 months, less likely to be on effective antiretroviral regimens, and less likely to be using appropriate prophylactic medication for opportunistic infections (Cohn, 2001). One strategy rural HIV-infected patients employ to gain access to expert health care is to travel to the closest urban setting. In one study, 75% of rural HIV-infected patients received their care in urban settings. In addition, more than 25% of these clients had put off health care visits within the previous 6 months because they did not have a way to travel to the HIV provider (Schur, 2002). Other barriers to accessing HIV/AIDS care in rural settings include long distances to travel for any care, greater stigma associated with HIV-infected diagnosis, and lack of available substance use treatment programs (Reif, 2005). In a study of US veterans, delayed entry into care increased mortality for rural compared to urban HIV-infected veterans (Ohl, 2010).

Clearly, to provide state-of-the-art health care to the large rural population of HIV-infected persons, programs are needed that improve social supports and eliminate stigma for HIV-infected patients and that enhance rural

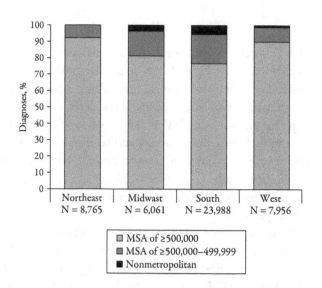

Figure 13.5 Diagnoses of HIV Infection among Adults and Adolescents, by Regions and Population of Areas of Residence, 2013 (United States) SOURCE: Centers for Disease and Control and Prevention. www.cdc.gov/hiv/ppt/2013-Urban-Nonurban-slides_508-REV-5.pptx.

providers' access to expert consultation as they provide care for these patients. Several models exist for providing health care to rural HIV-infected patients (McKinney, 2002):

- Community-based physician networks: Physician-referral networks in which family care practitioners may consult with a network of physicians with HIV/AIDS expertise

- Urban outreach programs: Satellite clinics operated by urban HIV clinics

- Shared care models: HIV specialists partnered with family care practitioners in rural settings for managing HIV/AIDS patient cases

- "Enhanced" clinics: Using Ryan White Care Act funds (Parts B and C) to allow existing clinics to provide more comprehensive HIV care

Outside the United States, other successful models exist for providing care to HIV-infected persons, including a program developed in Haiti using *accompagnateurs* (local community health workers) to provide medications with DOT and to support HIV-infected patients (Koenig, 2004).

Unfortunately, the economic downturn after 2008 has resulted in increased poverty and further access problems throughout rural America. Resources for rural HIV care are available through the National Rural Health Association and the Rural Assistance Center. It is hoped that increased interest in community health centers and implementation of the Affordable Care Act will improve access to basic health care throughout the United States. A web resource is available to locate nearby federally funded community health centers (US Department of Health and Human Resources; available at http://findahealthcenter.hrsa.gov/Search_HCC.aspx).

Recommended Reading

Centers for Disease Control and Prevention, National Center for HIV/ AIDS, Viral Hepatitis, & STD and TB Prevention. HIV/AIDS surveillance in rural and nonurban areas: Slide series (through 2013). 2013. Available at https://www.cdc.gov/hiv/pdf/2013-Urban-Nonurban-slides_508-REV-5_6-5.pdf.
Wilson LE, Korthuis T, Fleishman JA, et al. HIV-related medical service use by rural/urban residents: A multistate perspective. *AIDS Care.* 2011; 23(8):971–979.

References

CDC. *HIV Surveillance Report*, Vol. 23; February 2013. HIV diagnosis data are estimates from all 50 states, the District of Columbia, and 6 U.S. dependent areas. Rates do not include U.S. dependent areas.
Cohn SE, Berk ML, Berry SH, et al. The care of HIV-infected adults in rural areas of the United States. *J Acquir Immune Defic.* 2001 Dec 1; 28(4):385–392.
Koenig SP, Leandre F, Farmer P. Scaling up HIV treatment programmes in resource-limited settings: The rural Haiti experience. *AIDS.* 2004; 18(Suppl 3):S21–S25.
McKinney MM. Variations in HIV epidemiology and service delivery models in the United States. *J Rural Health.* 2002; 18:455–466.
Ohl M, Tate J, Duggal M, et al. Rural residence is associated with delayed care entry and increased mortality among veterans with human immunodeficiency virus infection. *Medicare Care.* 2010; 48:1064–0170.
Reif S, Golin CE, Smith SR. Barriers to accessing HIV/AIDS care in North Carolina: rural and urban differences. *AIDS Care.* 2005 Jul; 17(5):558–565.
Schur CL, Berk ML, Dunbar JR, et al. Where to seek care: an examination of people in rural areas with HIV/AIDS. *J Rural Health.* 2002 Spring; 18(2):337–347.
Wilson LE, Korthuis T, Fleishman JA, et al. HIV-related medical service use by rural/urban residents: A multistate perspective. *AIDS Care.* 2011; 23(8):971–979.

MIGRANT POPULATIONS

LEARNING OBJECTIVE

Discuss limitations in HIV care and special needs among migrant populations or patients with undocumented citizenship.

WHAT'S NEW?

Updated statistics reveal encouraging trends, but more concerted preventative efforts must be made toward at-risk migrant populations.

KEY POINTS

- The CDC only recently began tracking data regarding country of origin, time in the United States, or immigration status, so a more complete picture of the HIV epidemic among immigrants to the United States is just now emerging.

- Research in these populations is challenging due to a myriad of factors, including recruitment issues, ethical challenges, and subgroup differentiation.

- Prevalence and incidence of HIV in Hispanics and African Americans in the United States are higher than those of Whites, and these populations have less access to care and treatment than do Whites.

- Among HIV-infected immigrant populations, the prevalence and presentation of opportunistic infections or co-infections differ from those of US-born HIV-infected individuals.

- Among HIV-infected immigrant populations, the prevalence and presentation of opportunistic infections or co-infections differ from those of US-born HIV-infected individuals.

Migrating populations experience many barriers to accessing appropriate medical care for HIV infection. These barriers include lack of sufficient epidemiologic data on HIV infection among immigrants to the United States, issues of poverty, legal and language barriers to care among undocumented and/or illegal immigrants, and insufficient cultural competence among health care providers caring for immigrants. In addition, the medical presentation of HIV infection in the immigrant may differ in striking ways from that of the native-born US citizen.

Developing an accurate picture of the HIV epidemic among immigrants to the United States has been hampered by a lack of national data. The CDC only recently began tracking country of origin in HIV/AIDS, and currently there is no national publication on the topic. Some reports have been published on AIDS and immigrant populations at the county, city, and state levels. An example is a report from the Massachusetts Department of Public Health (MDPH) on the epidemiologic profile of HIV and AIDS in Massachusetts, which addresses emerging populations (MDPH, 2012). Historically, such local epidemiologic studies have been the predominant method for assessing need and planning services for immigrant populations.

A 2005 study detailed the research challenges posed when attempting to study the migrant and the immigrant Hispanic populations in the United States. These challenges were grouped into four categories: the need to use multilevel theoretical frameworks, the need to differentiate between Hispanic subgroups, challenges to recruitment and data collection, and ethical issues (Deren, 2005). When studying migrant populations, multilevel theoretical frameworks are necessary that incorporate the multiple influences that affect their daily living, including cultural, social, environmental, and individual factors. Differentiation of subgroups is also necessary due to the complexity of each subgroup, including lifestyle behaviors and cultural backgrounds. Recruitment and data collection is a major challenge because follow-up data are difficult to obtain in these populations due to the fact that their residency is commonly transient. Ethical issues are common in conducting these studies because they involve multiethnic populations with communication obstacles, and important consideration should be placed on cultural norms and sensitivities (Deren, 2005).

It is known that Hispanics and African Americans in the United States have higher HIV prevalence and incidence rates than other groups (Kaiser Family Foundation, 2014). In nearly every transmission category, Blacks have annual AIDS incidence and prevalence rates up to twice as high as those of Whites. Black Americans also account for more

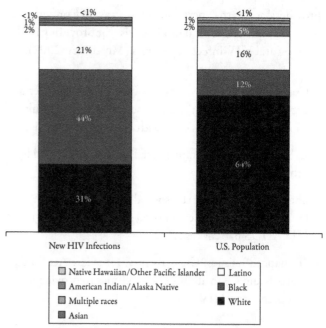

Figure 13.6 New HIV Infections and U.S. Population, by Race/Ethnicity, 2010.

new HIV infections and HIV-related deaths than any other racial/ethnic group in the United States (Kaiser Family Foundation, 2014). Despite these disproportionate statistics, there are declining numbers of new HIV infections among Black women (Figures 13.6 and 13.7). Although these data correspond to all members of these racial/ethnic groups, the numbers of infections among *immigrants* within these groups are unknown.

According to the Kaiser Family Foundation, Latinos represented approximately 16% of the US population but account for 21% of the new HIV infections and 19% of people living with HIV. In 2012, it was reported by the National Center for Health Statistics (NCHS) that the HIV death rate per 100,000 for Latinos was more than twice the rate for Whites (NCHS, 2012). One large study of the Hispanic population in the United States found that up to 28% of

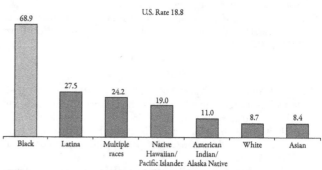

Figure 13.7 Rates of New HIV Infections per 100,000, by Race/Ethnicity, for Adults/Adolescents, 2010.

Hispanic residents live below the poverty level (Hajat, 2000). Because some states require a valid photo identification to receive benefits such as Medicaid, ADAP, or other forms of health insurance, undocumented immigrants are deterred from accessing appropriate HIV care.

Illegal immigrants with HIV infection face additional barriers to accessing health care. The Personal Responsibility and Work Opportunity Reconciliation Act of 1996 greatly restricts the provision of many federal, state, and local public services to undocumented immigrants (Kullgren, 2003). Although the intent of such legislation was to reduce illegal immigration, its main effects have been to burden the public health care system and to threaten overall public health. The recession of 2008 and improved enforcement of immigration laws have created additional obstacles to the provision of adequate HIV care to many immigrant populations. A positive development was the 2010 lifting of the requirement for HIV testing before immigration to the United States. However, undocumented immigrants are prohibited from accessing the benefits of the Affordable Care Act, including Medicaid and subsidized insurance premiums.

Immigrant HIV-infected populations more often present later in the course of their disease than do US-born patients. The medical presentation of HIV infection is different in immigrants compared with native-born US citizens. For example, the prevalence of infection with *Mycobacterium tuberculosis* is higher among immigrants from Africa, Central America, Southeast Asia, India, and other areas where TB is endemic. Therefore, screening HIV-infected persons for TB infection is essential in many immigrant populations. Active TB often occurs in HIV-infected persons with higher T helper cell counts, has more unusual or atypical presentations, and may be the initial presentation of HIV infection. It is more difficult to successfully treat TB in HIV-infected individuals than in HIV-negative individuals, and HIV-infected patients may require prolonged TB treatment.

Among Asian populations, the prevalence of chronic hepatitis B virus (HBV) infection is higher than that among other populations. ART may be more toxic in persons with chronic hepatitis, so the prevalence of HBV infection in Asian populations may complicate attempts to treat HIV. There is evidence that viral subtypes common in Southeast Asia may respond differently to currently available treatments for HBV. Opportunistic infections not usually seen in US-born persons may present in HIV-infected immigrants, reflecting the epidemiology of their country of origin. Examples include *Penicillium marnefii* in persons of Southeast Asian origin and a variety of parasitic diseases in persons of African descent.

In summary, immigrants face many barriers to receiving appropriate and affordable HIV care. Efforts to reduce these barriers should include legislation that will support and enhance the public health system, improved access to HIV services, better epidemiologic data on HIV-infected immigrants to the United States, and enhanced training and support for health care providers who serve immigrant populations. Often crucial to success in working with immigrant populations is the utilization of a team approach involving interpreters, social workers, and case managers; hiring of cultural-appropriate staff; inclusion of peer navigators; networking with local community-based organizations working with the impacted populations; Ryan White Program and 340B Pharmacy access; and legal services. The CDC has a useful website dedicated to immigrant and refugee health issues (see http://www.cdc.gov/immigrantrefugeehealth).

Recommended Reading

Kaiser Family Foundation. Fact sheet: Black Americans and HIV/AIDS. Menlo Park, CA: Henry J. Kaiser Family Foundation; April 2014. Available at http://files.kff.org/attachment/fact-sheet-black-americans-and-hiv-aids.

Kaiser Family Foundation. Fact sheet: Latinos and HIV/AIDS. Menlo Park, CA: Henry J. Kaiser Family Foundation; April 2014. Available at https://kaiserfamilyfoundation.files.wordpress.com/2014/04/6007-11-latinos-and-hiv-aids1.pdf.

References

Centers for Disease Control and Prevention. HIV surveillance report, Vol. 23; February 2013. (HIV diagnosis data are estimates from all 50 states, the District of Columbia, and six US-dependent areas. Rates do not include US-dependent areas.)

Deren M, Shedlin M, Decena CU, et al. Research challenges to the study of HIV/AIDS among migrant and immigrant Hispanic populations in the United States. Journal of Urban Health 2005; 82(3):iii13–iii25.

Hajat A, Lucas JB, Kington R. Health outcomes among Hispanic subgroups: data from the National Health Interview Survey, 1992-1995. *Adv Data*. 2000 Feb 25; (310):1–14.

Kaiser Family Foundation. Fact Sheet: Black Americans and HIV/AIDS. Menlo Park, CA: Henry J. Kaiser Family Foundation; April 2014. Available at http://files.kff.org/attachment/fact-sheet-black-americans-and-hiv-aids.

Kaiser Family Foundation. Fact sheet: Latinos and HIV/AIDS. Menlo Park, CA: Henry J. Kaiser Family Foundation: April 2014. Available at https://kaiserfamilyfoundation.files.wordpress.com/2014/04/6007-11-latinos-and-hiv-aids1.pdf.

Kullgren JT. Restrictions on undocumented immigrants' access to health services: the public health implications of welfare reform. *Am J Public Health*. 2003 Oct; 93(10):1630–1633.

Massachusetts Department of Public Health (MDPH). HIV/AIDS Fact Sheet: Persons Born Outside the U.S. 2012. Accessed at http://www.mass.gov/eohhs/docs/dph/aids/2012-profiles/born-outside-us.pdf.

National Center for Health Statistics. Health, United States, 2012. May 2013.

14.

COMPLEMENTARY AND ALTERNATIVE MEDICINE/INTEGRATIVE MEDICINE APPROACHES

Kalpana D. Shere-Wolfe

LEARNING OBJECTIVES

- Discuss the fundamentals and practice of complementary medicine as it pertains to HIV medicine.

- Describe the established and evolving science of natural products, mind-body practices, and traditional medical systems.

WHAT'S NEW?

This edition contains new information on the effects of micronutrient supplementation on CD4+ T cell counts and HIV disease progression; the effects of probiotics on inflammatory markers and CD4+ T cell counts; and the effect of mind–body practices on expression of genes, biomarkers of stress, and CD4+ T cell counts. In addition, herb–drug interactions are reviewed, with new data presented on interactions with newer antiretroviral medications.

KEY POINTS

- Complementary and alternative medicine (CAM) use is common in patients with HIV. Physicians caring for HIV-infected individuals should be aware of the high prevalence of CAM use and failure of most patients to disclose CAM use. Physicians need to routinely ask about CAM use, particularly herbal medicines and supplements.

- Nutritional supplementation with micronutrients—vitamins A, B, C, and E, zinc, and selenium—has been shown to improve markers of HIV progression and, in some studies, to also affect mortality.

- Natural health products (herbs, vitamins, and supplements) have the potential for significant drug interactions, which may lower the efficacy or increase the adverse effects of antiretroviral therapy.

- Recent trials suggest that probiotics may influence markers of coagulation, inflammation, microbial translocation, and microbiota in HIV-infected individuals.

- Studies suggest that stress, anxiety, and depression can affect HIV progression. Mind–body practices such as meditation, mindfulness, yoga, and tai chi can reduce stress, improve blood pressure, and and improve quality of life. In addition, they may affect adverse health behaviors. The effects of these practices on CD4+ T cell counts and disease progression are currently under investigation.

- Acupuncture may be of benefit in patients with musculoskeletal pain and sleep issues.

WHAT IS CAM AND INTEGRATIVE MEDICINE?

Complementary and alternative medicine (CAM) is a group of diverse medical and health care systems, practices, and products that are not currently considered part of conventional medicine. Although the terms *complementary* and *alternative* are used simultaneous and interchangeably, they refer to different entities. If a non-mainstream practice is used together with conventional medicine, it is considered "complementary." If a non-mainstream practice is used in place of conventional medicine, it is considered "alternative." True alternative medicine is uncommon in developed countries but may be commonly found in resource-limited settings. Most people who use non-mainstream approaches use them along with conventional treatments (see the National Center for Complementary and Integrative Health (NCCIH) website at https://nccih.nih.gov/health/herbsataglance.htm). The term *integrative medicine* is a relatively new but increasingly more common term in use. It refers to the use of CAM modalities with conventional medicine in an evidence-based integrated manner with emphasis on the importance of the relationship between practitioner and patient. Cornerstones of integrative medicine—nutrition, stress management, and exercise/movement—overlap those of conventional medicine but vary in their emphasis and approach.

Complementary and integrative health approaches encompass three broad areas: natural products, mind and body practices, and traditional medical systems. Natural products are herbs or botanicals, vitamins and minerals, and probiotics. They are widely marketed, readily available to consumers, and often sold as dietary supplements. Mind and body practices include a large and diverse group of techniques typically administered by trained practitioner. They include yoga, chiropractic and osteopathic manipulation, meditation, massage therapy, acupuncture, relaxation techniques (e.g., breathing exercises, guided imagery, and progressive muscle relaxation), tai chi, gi qong, healing touch, and hypnotherapy. Traditional medical systems include various types of healers, Ayurvedic medicine, Chinese medicine, homeopathy, and naturopathy. The research on these various modalities varies widely. Although there are many studies on certain herbal products, acupuncture, yoga, spinal manipulation, and meditation, there have been fewer studies on other practices. Moreover, studies using these modalities in HIV-infected patients are limited.

USE OF CAM BY HIV-INFECTED PATIENTS

Historically, CAM was popular in the HIV/AIDS community prior to the development of antiretroviral therapy (ART), and it remains popular. This is true in the United States, Canada, Australia, many European countries, Asia, and Africa. Now that effective treatment options exist for people living with HIV/AIDS and the life expectancy of these patients parallels that of people without HIV, CAM therapies are being sought for general wellness, mood disorders, stress reduction, and reduction of medication-associated side effects, as well as for boosting the immune system (Lorenc, 2013; Thompson, 2012). Importantly, one of the key reasons why CAM is being used by patients is because it enables them to have a more active role in their health care as well as a sense of control. CAM use is a way to shift the focus away or "de-medicalize" HIV management and focus on sense of wellness and normalcy (Littlewood, 2011). Factors that contribute to the increasingly popular concept of wellness include good nutrition, exercise, physical relaxation, and mental ease.

CAM is used by approximately 55–60% of HIV-infected patients; however, when restricted to practitioner-based CAM, the prevalence is approximately 15% or 16% (Dhalla, 2006; Greene, 1999; Josephs, 2007; London, 2003; Lorenc, 2013; Standish, 2001; Visser, 2002). CAM use is predicted by higher levels of education, men who have sex with men, female gender, longer disease duration, symptom severity and time on ART, and financial resources (Agnoletto, 2006; Littlewood, 2008; Lorenc, 2013). Vitamins, herbs, and supplements are most common, followed by prayer, meditation, and spiritual approaches. In developing countries and areas with poor access to conventional HIV treatment, traditional culture-based systems are widely used. In general, patients have a high level of satisfaction with CAM modalities, with 50–70% reporting improvement in malaise, various symptoms, and quality of life (Agnoletto, 2003; Duggan, 2001).

One study found decreased adherence to ART with CAM use (Owen-Smith, 2007). However, most studies have found that CAM users do not have decreased adherence to conventional medication nor do they reject conventional ART. Rather, they use CAM in an integrated manner with their conventional HIV care (Littlewood, 2008, 2014; Liu, 2009; Milan, 2008).

PHYSICIAN ATTITUDES TOWARD CAM

Less in known about physician attitudes, especially among infectious disease (ID) physicians and HIV providers, toward CAM. In one study of 89 HIV care providers, 63% believed that CAM and integrative medicine therapies may be helpful for HIV-infected patients, and 36% had personally used one (Wynia, 1999). A national survey of ID physicians demonstrated that they are familiar with various CAM modalities, including vitamin and mineral supplementation, massage, acupuncture, chiropractic, yoga, and herbal medicine. They most recommended vitamin and mineral supplementation (80%) and massage (62%). Data regarding clinical efficacy, drug interactions, and safety appear to be important factors that influence ID physicians' use of these modalities for their patients (Shere-Wolfe, 2013).

PATIENT DISCLOSURE REGARDING CAM USE

Studies have shown that the majority of physicians do not ask their patients about CAM use and that patients may not disclose CAM use for various reasons unless asked directly (Wynia, 1999). It is important that clinicians caring for patients with HIV/AIDS ask about CAM use to identify any potential drug interactions and safety issues.

CAM use disclosure rates vary across studies from 38% to 90% (Littlewood, 2008). In the Women's Interagency HIV Study, CAM use disclosure was associated with women older than age 45 years who had a college degree and health insurance; nondisclosure was associated with minority racial status. Compared to natural products and body-based practices such as acupuncture and massage, mind–body practices have the lowest prevalence of CAM use disclosure. In one study, CAM use disclosure was also significantly associated with higher ART adherence (Liu, 2009).

Discussing CAM use is important, especially with respect to natural products. Concerns regarding drug interaction are paramount; however, also important are issues related to contamination of natural products. One study found that 21% of Ayurvedic medicines purchased via the Internet contained detectable levels of lead, mercury, and arsenic (Saper, 2008). Similarly, Chinese herbal medicines may have microbial and heavy metal contamination (Ting, 2013). Heavy metal toxicity and testing may be considered in patients with new symptoms after initiating Chinese or Ayurvedic medicines. Other safety issues include side effects from taking extremely large doses of vitamins. High doses of vitamin A can cause liver and bone damage as well as increase the risk of birth defects. High-dose vitamin C apparently increases the risk of kidney stones. High doses of zinc (>75 mg/day) have been linked to copper deficiency.

Questions such as "Are you taking any vitamins, supplements, or herbs?" can be asked immediately after inquiring about conventional medications and compliance. For foreign patients, asking "Are you taking any natural medicines from your country?" may elicit information that might not otherwise be offered. A brief statement such as "This is important as many natural products can interfere with your HIV medication" or "I want to make sure what you are using is safe, even simple things like vitamins can hurt you if you take too much" can help elicit information and foster a partnership relationship. With increasing use of electronic medical records, this information can be included and tracked easily. It is important to ask in a nonjudgmental manner that allows the patient to feel comfortable with disclosure. Many patients may not be well informed about the products they are using. It may be helpful to direct patients to the National Institutes of Health's Medline Plus website for free, easy-to-understand, evidence-based information about many herbal products.

NATURAL HEALTH PRODUCTS TO CONSIDER FOR USE IN HIV-INFECTED PATIENTS

NUTRITIONAL SUPPLEMENTATION

Micronutrients (vitamin and minerals) are important for human development, disease prevention, and well-being. They are not produced in the body and must be derived from the diet. Vitamins A, D, E, C, and B, as well as zinc, iron, and selenium, play an important role in immunity. The HIV-infected population has been found to have various micronutrient deficiencies that are prevalent before symptomatic disease and occur in patients who are ART-naive and in those taking ART (Baum, 1995; Beach, 1992; Hepburn, 2004; Remacha, 2003). Micronutrient supplementation has been shown to improved markers of HIV progression (CD4$^+$ T cell count and viral load (VL)) and mortality in both early stages of HIV (Baum, 2013) and late stages of disease (Filteau, 2015; Jiamton, 2003; Kaiser, 2006; Range, 2006), as well as in pregnant women (Fawzi, 2004). There are very limited and conflicting reports regarding whether micronutrient supplementation increases HIV shedding (Jiamto, 2005; McClelland, 2004; Sudfeld, 2014).

In a large randomized clinical trial of Botswanian HIV-infected (subtype C) ARV-naive individuals with a CD4$^+$ T cell count greater than 350/μl, the effect of multivitamin (MVI; particularly B, C, and E vitamins) with selenium, MVI alone, and selenium alone was compared to placebo in delaying disease progression over 24 months. MVI alone and selenium alone were not statistically different from placebo. MVI plus selenium was found to significantly reduce the risk of reaching a CD4$^+$ T cell count of 250 μl or less and the risk of secondary events of combined outcomes for disease progression (CD4$^+$ T cell count <250/μl, AIDS-defining condition, or AIDS-related death) (Baum, 2013).

The effects of MVI (vitamins A, B, C, and E) on the health status of HIV-positive pregnant women in Tanzania were studied. A double-blind, randomized controlled trial (RCT) found a significantly lower rate of progression to World Health Organization stage 4 AIDS and a significantly lower death rate in the MVI group compared to the placebo group. Multivitamins also resulted in significantly higher CD4+ T cell counts and significantly lower levels of viral load (Fawzi, 2004).

Zinc deficiency is common in HIV-infected adults and is independently associated with disease progression (Baum, 1997, 2003; Beach, 1992; Falutz, 1988; Graham, 1991; Jones, 2006). In a randomized, double-blind, placebo-controlled trial of 231 HIV-infected patients with low plasma zinc levels, zinc supplementation at 12–15 mg of elemental zinc for 18 months resulted in a fourfold decrease in the likelihood of immunological failure, defined as a decrease in CD4+ T cell count to 200 cells/mm^3, compared to placebo. Viral load was not affected by zinc supplementation. Zinc supplementation also significantly reduced diarrhea compared with placebo. Respiratory diseases and HIV-related mortality were not affected by supplementation. Zinc testing and supplementation should be considered in HIV-infected populations with a high prevalence of zinc deficiency, such as drug users, children, men who have sex with men, and populations in developing countries (Baum, 2010).

Another single nutrient that has been studied in the HIV population is selenium. A randomized, double-blind, placebo-controlled trial of 300 HIV-infected individuals in Rwanda with CD4+ T cell counts between 400 and 650 cells/μl demonstrated that selenium supplementation led to a decrease in the rate of CD4+ T cell decline by 43.8% compared to placebo, which was determined to be a difference of approximately 40 cells at the end of 24 months (Kamwesiga, 2015). Another double-blind, randomized, placebo-controlled trial of selenium supplementation in HIV-infected patients showed selenium supplementation to be associated with favorable outcomes on VL and CD4+ T cell count. Selenium responders whose serum level increased significantly had no change in VL compared to placebo and to nonresponders, whose viral load increased. Similarly, CD4+ T cell count increased in the selenium responder group by approximately 30 cells compared to a decrease in CD4+ T cell count in the nonresponders and the placebo group (Hurwitz, 2007). Finally, selenium supplementation was found to have a significant effect on CD4+ T cell decline and hospital admission rates in a randomized clinical trial of HIV-infected individuals (Burbano, 2002). As already reviewed, Baum et al. found no effect of selenium alone on CD4+ T cell count but did find an effect when it was combined with MVI (Baum, 2010). Selenium supplementation should be used with caution in primiparous women not receiving ART because at least one study has shown increased HIV-1 RNA detection in the breast milk of these women with selenium supplementation (Sudfeld, 2014).

Vitamin D deficiency is common among HIV-infected patients and has been reported to be as high as 90%. The causes are likely multifactorial and include ART, especially regimens with efavirenz, which have been shown to interfere with vitamin D metabolism. Vitamin D plays an important role in osteoporosis, cardiovascular disease (CVD), and the immune system (Eckard, 2014). The degree to which vitamin D deficiency contributes to osteopenia and osteoporosis, CVD, and disease progression in the HIV population is unknown. The Endocrine Society recommends that at-risk persons be screened, including all persons receiving ART; the European AIDS Clinical Society recommends initial screening in all HIV-infected patients and follow-up screening in at-risk patients such as those receiving certain ART medications.

A recent trial demonstrated that supplementation with high-dose vitamin D$_3$ (4000 IU) and calcium carbonate (1000 mg) with ART initiation (efavirenz, emtricitabine, and tenofovir) increased 25-(OH)D levels and attenuated increases in bone turnover markers and bone loss at the hip and lumbar spine by approximately 50% at 48 weeks (Overton, 2015). It is unclear if these results can be extrapolated to non-EFV- and TDF-containing regimens.

Given the data in the general population that support the use of vitamin D and calcium supplementation to decrease risk of fractures and improve bone mineral density (BMD), it seems reasonable to screen high-risk, HIV-infected individuals and provide supplementation to minimize HIV-related complications of osteoporosis and, theoretically, to also affect CVD and disease progression.

Obviously, macronutrient and micronutrient supplements are no replacement for proper diet. All patients should be counseled with general dietary recommendations that include adequate consumption of fruits, vegetables, whole grains, low-fat dairy products, and seafood and less consumption of foods high in sodium (salt), saturated fats, trans fats, cholesterol, added sugars, and refined grains. However, given the benefits of micronutrients on CD4+ T cell counts and disease progression in a variety of HIV-infected groups, an MVI supplement that has key micronutrients (vitamins A, B, C, and E, selenium, and possibly zinc in certain populations) seems reasonable in all HIV-infected patients. Vitamin D screening and supplementation should be considered in HIV-infected patients, particularly those who are on ART, which is known to adversely affect BMD.

TEA TREE OIL

Two studies suggest that tea tree oil, *Melaleuca alternifolia*, may be effective in some patients with refractory oral candidiasis. In one study, patients with AIDS and fluconazole-refractory oral candidiasis were treated with melaleuca oral solution. At the 4-week evaluation, 8 of 12 patients showed a response (2 cured and 6 improved), 4 were nonresponders, and 1 had deteriorated (Jandourek, 1998). In a prospective open-label trial of tea tree oil preparations in AIDS patients with fluconazole-refractory oropharyngeal Candida *albicans* infection, 60% of patients showed a clinical response, with 7 patients cured and 8 clinically improved (Vazquez, 2002).

FISH OILS

The HIV-infected population is at increased risk for CVD due to multifactorial reasons. Data show that CVD mortality for the HIV-infected population has increased significantly from 1999 to 2013 (Feinstein, 2016). Omega-3 fatty acids have been shown in epidemiological and clinical trials to reduce the incidence of CVD. Large-scale epidemiological studies suggest that individuals at risk for CHD benefit from the consumption of omega-3 fatty acids. Evidence from prospective secondary prevention studies suggests that eicosapentaenoic acid (EPA) and docosahexaenoic acid (DHA) supplementation ranging from 0.5 to 1.8 g/day (either as fatty fish or as supplements) significantly reduces subsequent cardiac and all-cause mortality in the general population. Based on the scientific evidence prior to 2002, the American Heart Association has recommended that all individuals eat fish at least twice a week to prevent CVD. For individuals with coronary artery disease, the recommended dose of omega-3 polyunsaturated fatty acids (PUFAs) is 1 g of EPA and DHA daily (Kris-Etherton, 2002). Relatively recent randomized clinical trials have questioned the cardiovascular benefits of fish oil (Burr, 2003; Galan, 2010; Kromhout, 2010; ORIGIN Trial Investigators, 2012; Rauch, 2010). In addition, a large meta-analysis of 20 studies including more than 68,000 patients showed no benefit of fish oils in reducing risk of cardiac death, myocardial infarction, or stroke (Rizos, 2012). This analysis has been criticized for (1) including studies that had subtherapeutic doses of fish oils; (2) lack of assessment of co-interventions such as statins, beta-blockers, and acute coronary intervention; and (3) an unusually high level of significance ($p < 0.0063$ vs. $p < 0.05$) (Galli, 2013; Lewis, 2013; Sethi, 2013; Vlachopoulos, 2013). Using the typical standard, the analysis would have concluded that the omega-3 fatty acids were associated with a 9% reduction in cardiac deaths. Several large RCTs are currently in progress to further evaluate the effect of omega-3 fatty acids in CVD. Despite the inconsistencies of some of the data, the data still show a protective effect of omega-3 PUFA supplements in patients with CHD who are not receiving optimal treatment (i.e., statins and beta-blockers) (Kimming, 2013).

Fish oils appear to be beneficial for the treatment of hypertriglyceridemia, although the data for modifying CVD risk are inconsistent and further trials are currently ongoing. Fish oils are also relatively safe and do not have significant drug interactions with ART. In 100 HIV-infected patients receiving ART with hypertriglyceridemia, fish oils at doses of approximately 6 g/day significantly reduced triglyceride concentrations. There was no significant effect of fish oils on CD4$^+$ T cell counts or immune function or on lopinavir trough concentrations (Gerber, 2008). This result was confirmed in another RCT study of 48 HIV-infected patients on ART also receiving fenofibrate (Peters, 2012). Fish oils alone have also been shown to decrease triglyceride levels without adverse effects on immune parameters or antiretroviral pharmacokinetics (De Truchis, 2005). In a study of HIV-infected patients on combination ART with elevated fasting triglycerides, the use of 3.0 g of fish oils combined with diet counseling and exercise resulted in a decrease in triglyceride levels of 25% at 4 weeks versus a 2.8% increase in the control group (Wohl, 2005).

High doses greater than 3 g/day should be used with caution in patients with bleeding disorders or on anticoagulants. Unlike other supplements, fish oils are also available in prescription form as Lovaza (previously Omacor) for use in hypertriglyceridemia. It is reasonable that fish oils—either as supplements or as fatty fish twice a week (salmon, mackerel, herring, lake trout, sardines, and albacore tuna)—be considered in HIV-infected patients with hypertriglyceridemia and possibly those with CVD, especially if they are not medically optimized.

PROBIOTICS

Gut microbiota is changed in HIV-infected people compared to the uninfected healthy population (Dillon, 2014; Dinh, 2015; Lozupone, 2013; Mutlu, 2014; Vujkovic-Cvijin, 2013). In simian immunodeficiency virus (SIV)-infected macaques treated with ART, probiotic and prebiotic supplementation resulted in enhance gastrointestinal (GI) immune function and increased reconstitution of colonic CD4$^+$ T cells and reduced fibrosis of lymphoid follicles in the colon (Klatt, 2012). Recent trials with probiotics in HIV-infected individuals have shown interesting results. They have focused mainly on examining the effect of markers of coagulation (D-dimers), inflammation (interleukin-6 (IL-6)), tumor necrosis factor-α (TNF-α), high-sensitivity C-reactive protein (hs-CRP), interferon-γ (IFN-γ), microbial translocation (lipopolysaccharide-binding protein (LBP) and soluble CD14), and microbial composition.

Stiksrud et al. demonstrated significantly reduced levels of D-dimer and increases in *Bifidobacteria* spp. and *Lactobacilli* spp. in 15 HIV-infected patients treated with multistrain probiotics versus control and placebo groups. There was also a trend toward reduced levels of CRP ($p = 0.05$) and IL-6 ($p = 0.06$) (Stiksrud, 2015). In a randomized, double-blind, placebo-controlled trial of 44 HIV-infected patients with VL <20, *Saccharomyces boulardii* at 6×10^7 yeasts per day for 12 weeks decreased LBP and IL-6. The effect persisted for 3 months after treatment (Villar-Garcia, 2015). In an open-label study of HIV-infected children in India, the probiotic supplement group showed a significant increase in CD4+ T cell counts compared to the control group ($p = 0.0022$) (Gautam, 2014). In a small trial of 20 patients randomized to probiotic, synbiotic (probiotic + prebiotic), prebiotic, or placebo groups, the synbiotic group was noted to have an increased CD4+ T cell count ($p = 0.05$) and a decreased level of IL-6 ($p = 0.016$) (Gonzalez-Hernandez, 2012). In a larger study of 112 HIV-infected patients, the addition of probiotics to a micronutrient-fortified yogurt was well tolerated but was not associated with a further increase in CD4+ T cell count after 4 weeks (Hummelen, 2011). In an African study, probiotic yogurt consumption was reported to improve ability to work, reduce fever incidence, achieve daily nutrient requirements, and have overall lower impact of GI symptoms on routine activities (Irvine, 2011).

There are a small number of case reports describing bacteremia or fungemia attributed to probiotic administration, including one report of *Lactobacillus acidophilus* bacteremia in a patient with AIDS temporally related to excessive consumption of probiotic-enriched yogurt (Haghighat, 2015). However, this complication has not been reported in any clinical trials with probiotics.

Currently, probiotics cannot be recommended for HIV-infected patients; however, they deserve further investigation, particularly as immunomodulators.

INTERACTION OF NATURAL HEALTH PRODUCTS WITH ANTIRETROVIRAL AGENTS

Concurrent use of natural health products (NHPs) with ART is common among HIV-infected patients. Of all the CAM modalities, herbal supplements have the greatest potential for adverse effects in HIV-infected patients due to potential drug interactions. The following considerations add to the complexity and unpredictability of these interactions (MacDonald, 2009):

1. Many herbal remedies are complex products made of many different phytochemicals, some of which may not be fully characterized and standardized.

2. Some NHPs induce and inhibit gastrointestinal and hepatic enzymes simultaneously.

3. Many ART medications are substrates, inhibitors, or inducers of the drug-metabolizing enzymes (CYP family) and drug transporters (P-glycoprotein (P-gp)).

4. In vitro experiments may not predict in vivo effects due to various effects of intestinal enzymes, colonic microflora, and other factors.

5. Because of variations in extraction methods, constituents, and plant type and part, results from one study are not generalizable to other brands and formulation of NHPs.

For these reasons, it is difficult to state with absolute certainty that any NHP is free from the possibility of potential drug interactions. However, certain NHPs are known to interact with ART and should be avoided. Most ART drug interactions occur through the cytochrome P450 pathway and, to a lesser extent, the P-gp efflux drug transporter. The major isoform responsible for protease inhibitor (PI) metabolism is CYP3A4; non-nucleoside reverse transcriptase inhibitors (NNRTIs) are metabolized by CYP3A4 and CYP2B6. Protease inhibitors tend to inhibit CYP3A4, whereas most NNRTIs induce CYP3A4. Integrase strand transfer inhibitors (dolutegravir and raltegravir) neither induce nor inhibit CYP3A4. Also, PIs are substrates for P-gp, whereas NNRTIs usually are not. Exceptions to this include NRTIs and raltegravir. Raltegravir is primarily metabolized via glucuronidation. It is not an inducer, inhibitor, or substrate of CYPs; therefore, drug interactions with herbal medicines that affect CYPs are unlikely. However, the potential for drug interactions exists with any products that are uridine diphosphate glucuronosyltransferase (UGT) inducers. Any medications, supplements, or herbs that interfere with CYP, P-gp, or UGT have the potential to result in changes in concentration of HIV and non-HIV drugs. In addition, ART–herbal interactions are bidirectional, and ART may affect concentrations and efficacy and side effects/adverse effects of herbal medicines (Ladenheim, 2008; Lamorde, 2012).

In addition to herbs and supplements, many plant chemicals, especially flavonoids and polyphenols, inhibit CYP3A4. For example, the flavonoids naringenin and furanocoumarin bergamottin, present in grapefruit, interact with CYP3A4. However, grapefruit does not affect all PIs similarly. Clinical

Table 14.1 GUIDE FOR NATURAL HEALTH PRODUCT–DRUG INTERACTION

LIKELY SAFE	USE CAUTION BASED ON IN VITRO AND CASE REPORTS	AVOID
Cod liver oil	Ginseng[a]	Red yeast rice extract
Flaxseed oil/flaxseed	Gingko	St. John's wort
Fish oils	Cat's claw	Garlic
Vitamin C	Goldenseal	
Aloe vera	Evening primrose oil	
	African potato	
	Milk thistle[a]	
	Echinacea[a]	

[a]Data showing safety with specific ART.

studies with grapefruit juice and PIs show an increase in saquinavir levels but not indinavir or amprenavir (Lee, 2006).

Some commonly used CAM products, such as MVI, cod liver oil, and flax/flaxseed oil, have no known interactions with ART medications. Kava kava (*Piper methysticum*), black cohosh (*Cimicifuga racemose*), valerian (*Valeriana officinalis*), bitter orange (*Citrus aurantium*), saw palmetto (*Serenoa repens*), and Siberian ginseng (*Eleutheroccus senticosus*) have not been found to interact with CYP3A4. Therefore, it is unlikely that clinically significant pharmacokinetic interactions would occur with PIs or NNRTIs, but they may affect other ART (Lee, 2006).

Many CAM products have the potential to interact with ART. These are briefly described here and summarized in Table 14.1:

- Red yeast rice extract (RYRE) is sometimes used by patients to lower cholesterol. It is made by fermenting a type of yeast called *Monascus purpureus* over red rice. RYRE contains several compounds known as monacolins, which block the production of cholesterol. One of these, monacolin K, has the same structure as the drugs lovastatin and mevinolin (Ma, 2000). Lovastatin is exclusively metabolized by CYP3A4 and is contraindicated in patients taking PIs. Red yeast rice was marketed in the United States as the dietary supplement Cholestin. The US Food and Drug Administration banned it in 1998. However, RYREs are still available, and some of them still contain lovastatin. Patients should be cautioned to avoid RYRE if on PIs or statins.

- St. John's wort or *Hypericum perforatum* is an herbal product used for depression. St. John's wort is known to be an inducer of CYP3A4 and P-gp, and it also contains constituents that can affect other CYPs, including CYP2D6. It has been shown to alter levels of nevirapine, rilpivirine, and indinavir (de Maat, 2001; Hafner, 2010; Piscitelli, 2000). St. John's wort should be avoided by patients on ART.

- Echinacea is commonly used for viral infections and immunologic boosting. The two major forms, *Echinacea angustifolia* and *Echinacea purpurea*, affect CYP3A4 activity. *Echinacea purpurea* has been shown to induce CYP3A4 metabolism of darunavir but without effect on overall darunavir or ritonavir pharmacokinetics (Molto, 2011). Echinacea was also not found to affect etravirine concentrations (Molto, 2012) or the pharmacokinetics of lopinavir/ritonavir (LPV/RTV) (Penzak, 2010). The potential for drug interactions with other ART still exists.

- Garlic is often taken to prevent heart disease, high cholesterol, and high blood pressure and also to boost the immune system. Garlic may induce intestinal CYP3A4 or P-gp (Berginc, 2010). In one study, garlic markedly reduced the concentration of saquinavir, although the results suggested that it affected the bioavailability of saquinavir rather than its systemic clearance (Piscitelli, 2002). Garlic should be avoided by patients on ART.

- Silybins, the active component of milk thistle, inhibits CYP3A4 and P-gp activity in vitro; however, milk thistle has not been shown to significantly affect darunavir–ritonavir concentrations (Molto, 2012) or indinavir pharmacokinetics (DiCenzo, 2003; Mills, 2005; Piscitelli, 2002).

- Ginseng may induce CYP3A4 activity in the liver and GI tract. One study of *Panax ginseng* showed no effect on LPV/RTV levels after 2 weeks in healthy volunteers (Calderon, 2014).

- *Ginkgo biloba* was not found to significantly alter raltegravir or LPV/RTV pharmacokinetics in healthy volunteers (Blonk, 2012), but it was reported in two patients to potentially affect the efficacy of efavirenz (Naccarato, 2012; Wiegman, 2009).

- Based on a case report, cat's claw, which is used for a wide variety of ailments including inflammatory and infectious diseases, may interfere with atazanavir, ritonavir, and saquinavir levels (Lopez Galera, 2008).

- Goldenseal has potent CYP3A4 inhibition properties but was not shown to affect indinavir levels in one study (Sandhu, 2003). Patients taking goldenseal should be monitored for increased toxicity of CYP3A4 substrate drugs.

- Fish oil in combination with LPV/RTV showed no significant decrease in ART level (Gerber, 2008).

- Vitamin C does not affect CYP3A4 activity, and high-dose vitamin C did not affect indinavir levels in healthy volunteers (Slain, 2005; Stolbach, 2015).

- Two popular African herbs, *Hypoxis hermerocallidea* (African potato) and *Lessertia frutescens* (Cancer bush), have been shown to inhibit CY3A4 and P-gp in vitro (Awortwe, 2014). However, in a study of 16 patients, coadministration of African potato did not significantly alter the pharmacokinetics of LPV/RTV (Gwaza, 2013).

- Evening primrose inhibits CYP3A4 and CYP2D6, and there is one case report of evening primrose affecting LPV levels (Beukel, 2008).

Lack of high-quality studies in humans and lack of standardization of herbal formulations, among other factors, limit our knowledge on ART and herbal interactions. Other than a few herbal products such as St. John's wort, there is no simple guide to which NHP and ARV combinations clearly have significant clinical interactions. In vitro testing may be helpful for identifying products to screen, but it is limited in its clinical extrapolation. Therefore, caution is advised, and consultation with a pharmacist regarding any NHP and ARV interaction is warranted. Resources for information on natural health products for both clinicians and patients are listed in Table 14.2. Particularly useful for clinicians is the Natural Medicines Database website (formerly known as Natural Standard and Natural Medicine Comprehensive Database), which has an extensive database on herbal medicines with in-depth information as well as a drug interaction checker. The database is available through subscription and is usually also available through most academic libraries; it is available as an app for smartphones. ART–herbal interactions can also be checked at http://www.hiv-druginteractions.org. The NCCIH also has concise evidence-based information on common herbs and links for information on herb–drug interactions.

HERBAL MEDICINES FOR HIV TREATMENT

In a meta-analysis of 12 RCTs involving 881 patients with AIDS, traditional Chinese medicine (TCM) interventions were associated with significantly reduced plasma viral load compared with placebo ($p = 0.04$). Patients receiving TCM interventions had significantly higher CD4$^+$ T lymphocyte counts compared with those on placebo ($p = 0.002$). In addition, TCM interventions were significantly more likely to result in improved clinical symptoms ($p < 0.00001$). TCM interventions conferred a similar risk of adverse events compared with control interventions ($p = 0.29$). However, the reductions in plasma viral load significantly favored conventional Western medical therapy alone over integrated traditional Chinese and Western medical therapy ($p = 0.004$) (Deng, 2014).

MIND–BODY APPROACHES

Mind and body practices include a large and diverse group of procedures or techniques typically administered by trained practitioners or teachers rather than by physicians.

Table 14.2 INTERNET RESOURCES FOR NATURAL HEALTH PRODUCTS INFORMATION AND NATURAL HEALTH PRODUCT–DRUG INTERACTIONS

RESOURCE	WEBSITE
Natural Medicines Database	http://www.naturaldatabase.com
National Center for Complementary and Integrative Health	https://nccih.nih.gov/health/herbsataglance.htm
HIV–Drug Interaction	http://www.hiv-druginteractions.org
National Institutes of Health, Office of Dietary Supplements Dietary Supplement Label Database	http://www.dsld.nlm.nih.gov/dsld/index.jsp
National Institutes of Health, Office of Dietary Supplements	https://ods.od.nih.gov
National Institutes of Health, MedlinePlus Herbs and Supplements Directory	https://nlm.nih.gov/medlineplus/druginfo/herb_All.html
ConsumerLab	http://www.consumerlab.com

They include yoga, chiropractic and osteopathic manipulation, meditation, massage therapy, acupuncture, relaxation techniques (e.g., breathing exercises, guided imagery, and progressive muscle relaxation), tai chi, gi qong, healing touch, and hypnotherapy. Central to these modalities is the elicitation of the relaxation response.

RELAXATION RESPONSE

The relaxation response can be described as a state of deep rest that changes the short- and long-term physical and emotional responses to stress (e.g., decreases in heart rate, blood pressure, rate of breathing, and muscle tension)—it is the opposite of the fight-or-flight response (Benson, 1974). Preliminary studies suggest that this response can affect gene expression and telomere length. One study of 52 healthy people—26 novices and 26 long-term practitioners (yoga/meditation)—showed that one session of relaxation-response practice was enough to enhance the expression of genes involved in energy metabolism and insulin secretion and reduce the expression of genes linked to inflammatory response and stress (Bhasin, 2013). Nobel Laureate Elizabeth Blackburn showed that shortened telomere length and reduced telomerase activity are associated with premature mortality and predict a variety of health risks and diseases (Epel, 2004). She also demonstrated that family dementia caregivers (a typically chronically stressed population) who practiced 12 minutes of daily yogic meditation for 8 weeks had a 43% increase in telomerase activity compared to 3.7% in the passive relaxation group, suggesting an improvement in stress-induced aging (Lavretsky, 2013).

STRESS, DEPRESSION, AND HIV PROGRESSION

HIV infection presents many stresses and challenges—mental, emotional, and physical—that vary from time of diagnosis to coping with adherence and medication-related side effects, aging issues, and dealing with the loss of infected loved ones. Not surprisingly, individuals who are HIV-infected have a higher incidence of depression and anxiety than the uninfected population (Pence, 2006; Whetten, 2008). Psychosocial variables and stress can affect measurable factors such as $CD4^+$ T cell counts and viral loads in a variety of ways, including drug adherence, immune function, and health behaviors.

Stress has been shown in prospective human observational studies, animal studies, and laboratory experiments to be associated with depression, CVD, and progression of HIV/AIDS. This effect is generally thought to be mediated by negative affective states such as anxiety and depression, behavioral patterns (adherence, substance abuse, etc.), and stress-elicited endocrine responses mediated by the hypothalamic–pituitary–adrenocortical axis and the sympathetic–adrenal–medullary system (Cohen, 2007). In HIV-infected populations, some studies have shown that stress may be associated with reductions in natural killer cell and cytotoxic T lymphocyte phenotypes (Leserman, 1997; Stern, 1995).

Results from studies prior to 2000 were inconsistent with respect to the effect of stress and depression on HIV progression. However, several studies after 2000 have suggested a link between stress and HIV progression (Leserman, 2008). Among 96 asymptomatic, HIV-infected gay men not on antiretroviral medication at baseline who were followed every 6 months for up to 9 years, each additional moderately severe stress event increased risk of progression to AIDS by 50% and of developing an AIDS-related clinical condition by 2.5-fold after controlling for demographics, baseline $CD4^+$ T cells and VL, and antiretroviral medications (Leserman, 2002). In a study of 177 HIV-infected men and women, baseline depression and hopelessness predicted slope of $CD4^+$ T cells and VL. High cumulative depression and avoidant coping were associated with approximately twice the rate of $CD4^+$ T cell decline and greater increases in VL (Ironson, 2005).

MEDITATIVE PRACTICES

Meditation is a practice of concentrated focus on a sound, object, visualization, the breath, movement, or attention itself in order to increase awareness of the present moment, reduce stress, promote relaxation, and enhance personal and spiritual growth. Examples include mantra meditation and mindfulness meditation. Yoga, tai chi, and chi gong are forms of breath coordinated movement meditations.

YOGA

Yoga is often practiced for wellness and stress reduction. It has been shown to affect health behaviors. In one large analysis of approximately 35,000 US adults, yoga users reported high rates of health behavior outcomes such as motivation to exercise (~60%), eat healthier (~40%), cut back or stop drinking alcohol (12%), and cut back or stop smoking cigarettes (25%). More than 80% perceived reduced stress as a result of practicing yoga (Stussman, 2015).

Well-designed studies of yoga in the HIV-infected population are lacking. One prospective controlled study of yoga in HIV-infected adults with CVD risk factors showed that 20 weeks of supervised yoga was effective in significantly reducing resting systolic and diastolic blood pressure by an average of 5/3 mm Hg—reductions similar to those achieved with the Dietary Approaches to Stop Hypertension (DASH) diet. Studies suggest that a 10-mm reduction in systolic blood pressure and a 5-mm Hg reduction in diastolic blood pressure predict a 40–50% lower risk of death from CAD. Extrapolating from these data in HIV-uninfected adults, yoga intervention would theoretically translate into a decreased risk of death from CAD by 20–25% in HIV-infected patients. Yoga did not affect body weight, fat mass, proatherogeneic lipids, glucose tolerance, or immune or virologic status (Cade, 2010).

Mantram meditation (repetition of a word or phrase) was found to be effective in reducing anger, improving quality of life (QOL), and improving spiritual well-being in a randomized controlled study of HIV-infected adults (Bormann, 2006).

MINDFULNESS-BASED STRESS REDUCTION

Mindfulness-based stress reduction (MBSR) is a technique that uses cultivation of nonjudgmental awareness in the present moment. It is usually taught as an 8-week structured program. MBSR has been shown to decrease the side effects of ART and alleviate symptoms. In one randomized wait-list controlled study of 76 HIV-infected patients with ART-related side effects, MBSR was found to significantly reduced frequency of symptoms and distress related to symptoms (Duncan, 2012). In another RCT of 117 HIV-infected patients, MBSR was found to result in a reduction in avoidance, higher positive affect, and improvement in depression at 6 months (Gayner, 2012).

Few studies have examined the effect of MBSR on CD4[+] T cell count. One small randomized controlled short-term study of a diverse group of HIV-infected patients suggested that MBSR could buffer CD4[+] T cell decline (Creswell, 2009). In a later RCT of 40 long-term diagnosed and treated HIV-infected patients, mindfulness-based cognitive therapy (which combined elements of MBSR and CBT) patients were found to have decreased stress, anxiety, and depression and also a significantly increased CD4[+] T cell count at week 20 compared to placebo ($p < 0.001$), with no change in viral load (Gonzalez-Garcia, 2014).

TAI CHI

In a small study of 38 HIV-infected patients randomized to tai chi, exercise, and control groups, both tai chi and exercise were found to improve physiologic parameters, functional outcomes, and QOL. These patients were also noted to have improved social interactions (Galantino, 2005).

In a large group of 252 HIV-infected patients, those randomized to three 10-week stress management approaches—cognitive–behavioral relaxation training, focused tai chi training, and spiritual growth—were compared to a wait-listed control group. Both the cognitive–behavioral relaxation and tai chi groups used less emotion-focused coping and had augmented lymphocyte proliferative function. Moreover, the tai chi group had an increase in QOL related mainly to an increase in emotional well-being (McCain, 2008).

Meditative practices can increase QOL; reduce stress, anxiety, and depression; and affect health-related behaviors. These practices have not been shown to have harmful side effects, and they should be considered for interested patients with stress, depression, anxiety, and adverse health behaviors. These practices may also be considered for patients who are unwilling to utilize psychological counseling, support, or cognitive–behavioral therapy. Many meditative practices are available. Which one is best depends on patient preference, which may be influenced by cultural factors, convenience, and finances. The practice most likely to be effective is the one that the patient is most likely to do.

ACUPUNCTURE

Pain is a frequently reported symptom in persons living with HIV/AIDS (Vogl, 1999). Pain may be secondary to peripheral neuropathy or to musculoskeletal issues. Results from a number of studies suggest that acupuncture may help with chronic pain syndromes related to low back pain, neck pain, and osteoarthritis/knee pain (Hinman, 2014; Linde, 2009; Manheimer, 2010; Vickers, 2012; Witt, 2006). Acupuncture may also help reduce the frequency of tension headaches and prevent migraine headaches. Clinical practice guidelines issued by the American Pain Society and the American College of Physicians in 2007 recommend acupuncture as one of several nonpharmacologic approaches that physicians should consider when patients with chronic low back pain do not respond to practices such as remaining active, applying heat, and taking pain-relieving medications (Chou, 2007).

Few studies have examined the effect of acupuncture in HIV-infected patients. A large multicenter, modified double-blind, randomized, placebo-controlled study comparing acupuncture and sham acupuncture for symptomatic treatment of HIV-related neuropathy revealed a modest decrease in average pain scores in both groups but no significant improvement with acupuncture (Shlay, 1998). In another small study of 23 HIV-infected participants with sleep disturbances at least three times per week, patients received acupuncture two evening a week for 5 weeks. Both sleep time and sleep quality were reported as improved (Phillips, 2001).

Although studies of acupuncture in HIV-infected patients are limited, it seems reasonable to consider acupuncture in patients with musculoskeletal pain and perhaps those with sleep disturbances, especially in those who are either reluctant to take or intolerant of conventional medications.

EXERCISE

Substantial evidence indicates that regular physical activity contributes to the primary and secondary prevention of several chronic diseases, such as CVD, osteoporosis, and diabetes, and is associated with a reduced risk of premature death (Warburton, 2006). Moreover, studies have shown that in HIV-infected patients, exercise can improve strength, endurance, time to fatigue, and body composition; increase quality of life and sense of well-being; and decrease depression and anxiety (Dudgeon, 2004; MacArthur, 1993; Rigsby, 1992; Stringer, 1998). Given the increased risk of CVD, muscle wasting, and bone disease, it makes sense that some form of physical activity be encouraged for capable HIV-infected patients. Physicians have an important role in educating and encouraging exercise as a measure for well-being and disease prevention.

MANUAL THERAPIES

Manual CAM therapies include massage, shiatsu, reiki, therapeutic touch, acupressure, and chiropractic manipulation. Manual modalities are often used by patients for their purported effects of increasing circulation, pain alleviation, relaxation, and stimulation of immune function (Power, 2002). One small RCT showed that massage therapy combined with stress management resulted in a decrease in medical care usage and an increase in health perceptions in HIV-infected individuals (Birk, 2000). A Cochrane review of massage in HIV-infected patients showed that there appears to be a positive effect on the quality of life of affected individuals, particularly when massage is combined with other interventions such as meditation and stress management (Hillier, 2010).

TRADITIONAL MEDICINE

It is beyond the scope of this chapter to review the major traditional medical systems of India, China, and Africa. These systems are broad and complex, and they often combine different therapeutic modalities discussed previously in this chapter, such as a combination of herbal remedies and mind–body practices. Reasons for the use of these traditional systems in the HIV-infected population stem from cultural beliefs, economic considerations, and limited accessibility to ART. Data from well-designed clinical trials regarding efficacy and safety of these systems are sparse.

Traditional Indian medicine consisting of Ayurveda, Unani medicine, Siddha medicine, homeopathy, and naturopathy is used by two-thirds of the Indian population—especially in rural areas—for both primary care needs and HIV. One review found only four RCTs evaluating traditional Indian medicine; the trials had significant methodological flaws (Fritts, 2008).

Similarly, in Africa, a large portion of the population uses herbs for primary health care, HIV/AIDS, and HIV-related health problems (Calitz, 2014). Although there is increasing study of herbal medicines and their potential for drug interactions in vitro, clinical trials are lacking.

Traditional Chinese medicine has probably been the most studied of the traditional systems, with data showing potential efficacy of TCM herbs for HIV and HIV-associated conditions. Mind–body approaches such as tai chi and acupuncture have also shown benefit for a varieties of health issues; however, many of these studies were performed on the non HIV-infected population. Many of these were reviewed previously in this chapter.

Given that these systems play such a central role in health care delivery in their respective countries and that there are usually many more traditional health practitioners than allopathic practitioners, collaboration and cooperation among traditional and allopathic practitioners seems indicated. However, conflicts often arise between the two. Allopathic physicians frequently regard traditional medicines and practices as untested, possibly unsafe, and likely ineffective. Traditional practitioners, on the other hand, do not necessarily see the need or benefit of rigorously testing their time-honored practices; some also believe that Western-trained physicians misunderstand traditional medical practice because they continue to view it through the scientific lens of biomedicine. Nevertheless, strides toward some form of partnership are being made in these countries. In Africa, many traditional practitioners have been educated and trained on HIV/AIDS transmission and prevention and have served effectively as community educators (Bodeker, 2006).

To date, no data exist to support the use of these systems as primary treatment for HIV. Some data exist on efficacy, especially of TCM on end points such as CD4$^+$ T cells and VL; however, they have been inferior to ART. There may be a role for these systems in the management of symptoms, HIV-associated conditions, and delaying of HIV progression in those not on ART, but more data are needed with respect to their efficacy and herb–drug interactions.

Other aspects of traditional medical systems excluding herbal medicines, such as spiritual and healing practices and attitudes toward sickness and death (provided they do not harm), should be acknowledged and respected by physicians.

SUMMARY

Complementary, integrative, and alternative modalities are widely used by HIV-infected patients. True alternative medicine for HIV is rare in developed countries but widespread in resource-limited areas. Physicians caring for HIV-infected individuals need to be aware of the prevalence of complementary therapies among their patients, the potential for herbal–drug interactions, and the potential toxicities of herbal medicines.

Physicians can also play an important role in fostering partnerships with their patients who use CAM modalities by the use of nonjudgmental and open communication about their benefits and risks. Some natural health products, such as fish oils and MVI, should be considered for use in HIV-infected individuals. Strategies to delay HIV progression using micronutrients, probiotics, and traditional natural products in HIV-infected populations with high CD4$^+$ T cell counts deserve further research, particularly in resource-limited settings in which access to ART is limited. Many mind–body techniques are useful for reducing stress, anxiety, and depression—all of which may affect HIV disease progression. These techniques may be especially useful in patients with adverse health behaviors who are unwilling to undergo formal therapy. They should also be considered in resource-limited settings as a self-empowering, low-cost means of coping with the emotional and physical challenges associated with HIV.

Treatment of HIV remains complex and multifactorial. Complementary and integrative modalities with low potential for adverse effects, such as mind–body techniques and certain natural products, should be considered in the balanced approach to dealing with the multidimensional aspects of HIV disease. The use of such practices will likely increase in the future. Therefore, it behooves physicians caring for these patients to understand the range of available options, their potential interactions with standard therapeutic regimens, and the ongoing data regarding their potential efficacy and safety.

Recommended Reading

Baum, M. K., Campa, A., Lai, S., et al. (2013). Effect of micronutrient supplementation on disease progression in asymptomatic, antiretroviral-naive, HIV-infected adults in Botswana: A randomized clinical trial. *JAMA, 310*(20), 2154–2163.

Bhasin, M. K., Dusek, J. A., Chang, B., et al. (2013). Relaxation response induces temporal transcriptome changes in energy metabolism, insulin secretion and inflammatory pathways. *PLoS ONE, 8*(5), e62817. doi:10.1371/journal.pone.0062817

Cade, W., Reeds, D. N., Mondy, K. E., et al. (2010). Yoga lifestyle intervention reduces blood pressure in HIV-infected adults with cardiovascular disease risk factors. *HIV Medicine, 11*(6), 379–388.

Dinh, D. M., Volpe, G. E., Duffalo, C., et al. (2015). Intestinal microbiota, microbial translocation, and systemic inflammation in chronic HIV infection. *Journal of Infectious Diseases, 211*(1), 19–27. doi:10.1093/infdis/jiu409

Jiménez-Nácher, I., Alvarez, E., Morello, J., et al. (2011). Approaches for understanding and predicting drug interactions in human immunodeficiency virus-infected patients. *Expert Opinion on Drug Metabolism & Toxicology, 7*(4), 457–477.

Klatt, N. R., Canary, L. A., Sun, X., et al. (2013). Probiotic/prebiotic supplementation of antiretrovirals improves gastrointestinal immunity in SIV-infected macaques. *Journal of Clinical Investigation, 123*(2), 903–907. doi:10.1172/JCI66227

Lavretsky, H., Epel, E., Siddarth, P., et al. (2013). A pilot study of yogic meditation for family dementia caregivers with depressive symptoms: Effects on mental health, cognition, and telomerase activity. *International Journal of Geriatric Psychiatry, 28*(1), 57–65.

Littlewood, R. A., & Vanable, P. A. (2011). A global perspective on complementary and alternative medicine use among people living with HIV/AIDS in the era of antiretroviral treatment. *Current HIV/AIDS Reports, 8*(4), 257–268.

MacDonald, L., Murty, M., & Foster, B. C. (2009). Antiviral drug disposition and natural health products: Risk of therapeutic alteration and resistance. *Expert Opin Drug Metab Toxicol., 5*(6), 563–578. doi:10.1517/17425250902942302

Saper, R. B., Phillips, R. S., Sehgal, A., et al. (2008). Lead, mercury, and arsenic in US-and Indian-manufactured Ayurvedic medicines sold via the Internet. *JAMA, 300*(8), 915–923.

References

Agnoletto, V., Chiaffarino, F., Nasta, P., et al. (2003). Reasons for complementary therapies and characteristics of users among HIV-infected people. *International Journal of STD & AIDS, 14*(7), 482–486. doi:10.1258/095646203322025803

Agnoletto, V., Chiaffarino, F., Nasta, P., et al. (2006). Use of complementary and alternative medicine in HIV-infected subjects. *Complementary Therapies in Medicine, 14*(3), 193–199.

Awortwe, C., Bouic, P. J., Masimirembwa, C. M., et al. (2014). Inhibition of major drug metabolizing CYPs by common herbal medicines used by HIV/AIDS patients in Africa—Implications for herb-drug interactions. *Drug Metabolism Letters, 7*(2), 83–95. doi:DML-EPUB-58874

Baum, M. K., Campa, A., Lai, S., et al. (2003). Zinc status in human immunodeficiency virus type 1 infection and illicit drug use. *Clinical Infectious Diseases, 37*(Suppl. 2), S117–S123. doi:CID30489

Baum, M. K., Campa, A., Lai, S., et al. (2013). Effect of micronutrient supplementation on disease progression in asymptomatic, antiretroviral-naive, HIV-infected adults in Botswana: A randomized clinical trial. *JAMA, 310*(20), 2154–2163.

Baum, M. K., Lai, S., Sales, S., et al. (2010). Randomized, controlled clinical trial of zinc supplementation to prevent immunological failure in HIV-infected adults. *Clinical Infectious Diseases, 50*(12), 1653–1660. doi:10.1086/652864

Baum, M. K., Shor-Posner, G., Lu, Y., et al. (1995). Micronutrients and HIV-1 disease progression. *AIDS, 9*(9), 1051–1056.

Baum, M. K., Shor-Posner, G., Lai, S., et al. (1997). High risk of HIV-related mortality is associated with selenium deficiency. *Journal of Acquired Immune Deficiency Syndromes, 15*(5), 370–374.

Beach, R. S., Mantero-Atienza, E., Shor-Posner, G., et al. (1992). Specific nutrient abnormalities in asymptomatic HIV-1 infection. *AIDS, 6*(7), 701–708.

Benson, H., Beary, J. F., & Carol, M. P. (1974). The relaxation response. *Psychiatry, 37*(1), 37–46.

Berginc, K., Trdan, T., Trontelj, J., et al. (2010). HIV protease inhibitors: Garlic supplements and first-pass intestinal metabolism impact on the therapeutic efficacy. *Biopharmaceutics & Drug Disposition, 31*(8–9), 495–505.

Beukel van den Bout-van den, C.J., Bosch, M. E., Burger, D. M., et al. (2008). Toxic lopinavir concentrations in an HIV-1 infected patient taking herbal medications. *AIDS (London), 22*(10), 1243–1244. doi:10.1097/QAD.0b013e32830261f4

Bhasin, M. K., Dusek, J. A., Chang, B., et al. (2013). Relaxation response induces temporal transcriptome changes in energy metabolism, insulin secretion and inflammatory pathways. *PLoS ONE, 8*(5), e62817. doi:10.1371/journal.pone.0062817

Birk, T. J., McGrady, A., MacArthur, R. D., et al. (2000). The effects of massage therapy alone and in combination with other complementary therapies on immune system measures and quality of life in human immunodeficiency virus. *Journal of Alternative and Complementary Medicine, 6*(5), 405–414.

Blonk, M., Colbers, A., Poirters, A., et al. (2012). Effect of ginkgo biloba on the pharmacokinetics of raltegravir in healthy volunteers. *Antimicrobial Agents and Chemotherapy, 56*(10), 5070–5075. doi:10.1128/AAC.00672-12

Bodeker, G., Carter, G., Burford, G., et al. (2006). HIV/AIDS: Traditional systems of health care in the management of a global epidemic. *J Altern Complement Med, 12*(6), 563–576.

Bormann, J. E., Gifford, A. L., Shively, M., et al. (2006). Effects of spiritual mantram repetition on HIV outcomes: A randomized controlled trial. *Journal of Behavioral Medicine, 29*(4), 359–376.

Burbano, X., Miguez-Bubano, M. J., McCollister, K., et al. (2002). Impact of a selenium chemoprevention trial on hospital admissions of HIV-infected participants. *HIV Clinical Trials, 3*(6), 483–491.

Burr, M. L., Ashfield-Watt, P. A. L., Dunstan, F. D. J., et al. (2003). Lack of benefit of dietary advice to men with angina: Results of a controlled trial. *European Journal of Clinical Nutrition, 57*(2), 193–200.

Cade, W., Reeds, D. N., Mondy, K. E., et al. (2010). Yoga lifestyle intervention reduces blood pressure in HIV-infected adults with cardiovascular disease risk factors. *HIV Medicine, 11*(6), 379–388.

Calderón, M. M., Chairez, C. L., Gordon, L. A., et al. (2014). Influence of panax ginseng on the steady state pharmacokinetic profile of Lopinavir–Ritonavir in healthy volunteers. *Pharmacotherapy: The Journal of Human Pharmacology and Drug Therapy, 34*(11), 1151–1158.

Calitz, C., Steenekamp, J. H., Steyn, J. D., et al. (2014). Impact of traditional African medicine on drug metabolism and transport. *Expert Opinion on Drug Metabolism & Toxicology, 10*(7), 991–1003.

Chou, R., Qaseem, A., Snow, V., et al. (2007). Diagnosis and treatment of low back pain: A joint clinical practice guideline from the American College of Physicians and the American Pain Society. *Annals of Internal Medicine, 147*(7), 478–491.

Cohen, S., Janicki-Deverts, D., & Miller, G. E. (2007). Psychological stress and disease. *JAMA, 298*(14), 1685–1687.

Creswell, J. D., Myers, H. F., Cole, S. W., et al. (2009). Mindfulness meditation training effects on CD4+ T cell T lymphocytes in HIV-1 infected adults: A small randomized controlled trial. *Brain, Behavior, and Immunity, 23*(2), 184–188.

de Maat, M. M., Hoetelmans, R. M., Mathôt, R. A., et al. (2001). Drug interaction between St. John's wort and nevirapine. *AIDS, 15*(3), 420–421.

De Truchis, P., Kirstetter, M., Perier, A., et al. (2005). Treatment of hypertriglyceridemia in HIV-infected patients under HAART, by (n-3) polyunsaturated fatty acids: A double-blind randomized prospective trial in 122 patients [Abstract 39]. Paper presented at the 12th Conference on Retroviruses and Opportunistic Infections, Boston, February 22–25.

Deng, X., Jiang, M., Zhao, X., et al. (2014). Efficacy and safety of traditional Chinese medicine for the treatment of acquired immunodeficiency syndrome: A systematic review. *J Tradit Chin Med., 34*(1):1–9.

Dhalla, S., Chan, K. J., Montaner, J. S., et al. (2006). Complementary and alternative medicine use in British Columbia—A survey of HIV positive people on antiretroviral therapy. *Complementary Therapies in Clinical Practice, 12*(4), 242–248.

DiCenzo, R., Shelton, M., Jordan, K., et al. (2003). Coadministration of milk thistle and indinavir in healthy subjects. *Pharmacotherapy, 23*(7), 866–870.

Dillon, S., Lee, E., Kotter, C., et al. (2014). An altered intestinal mucosal microbiome in HIV-1 infection is associated with mucosal and systemic immune activation and endotoxemia. *Mucosal Immunology, 7*(4), 983–994.

Dinh, D. M., Volpe, G. E., Duffalo, C., et al. (2015). Intestinal microbiota, microbial translocation, and systemic inflammation in chronic HIV infection. *Journal of Infectious Diseases, 211*(1), 19–27. doi:10.1093/infdis/jiu409

Dudgeon, W. D., Phillips, K. D., Bopp, C. M., et al. (2004). Physiological and psychological effects of exercise interventions in HIV disease. *AIDS Patient Care and STDs, 18*(2), 81–98.

Duggan, J., Peterson, W. S., Schutz, et al. (2001). Use of complementary and alternative therapies in HIV-infected patients. *AIDS Patient Care and STDs, 15*(3), 159–167.

Duncan, L. G., Moskowitz, J. T., Neilands, T. B., et al. (2012). Mindfulness-based stress reduction for HIV treatment side effects: A randomized, wait-list controlled trial. *Journal of Pain and Symptom Management, 43*(2), 161–171.

Eckard, A. R., & McComsey, G. A. (2014). Vitamin D deficiency and altered bone mineral metabolism in HIV-infected individuals. *Current HIV/AIDS Reports, 11*(3), 263–270.

Epel, E. S., Blackburn, E. H., Lin, J., et al. (2004). Accelerated telomere shortening in response to life stress. *Proceedings of the National Academy of Sciences of the United States of America, 101*(49), 17312–17315. doi:0407162101

Evans, D. L., Leserman, J., Perkins, D. O., et al. (1995). Stress-associated reductions in cytotoxic T lymphocytes and natural killer cells in asymptomatic HIV infection. *American Journal of Psychiatry, 152*(4), 543–550.

Falutz, J., Tsoukas, C., & Gold, P. (1988). Zinc as a cofactor in human immunodeficiency virus-induced immunosuppression. *JAMA, 259*(19), 2850–2851.

Fawzi, W. W., Msamanga, G. I., Spiegelman, D., et al. (2004). A randomized trial of multivitamin supplements and HIV disease progression and mortality. *New England Journal of Medicine, 351*(1), 23–32.

Feinstein, M. J., Bahiru, E., Achenbach, C., et al. (2016). Patterns of cardiovascular mortality for HIV-infected adults in the united states: 1999–2013. *American Journal of Cardiology, 117*(2), 214–220.

Filteau, S., PrayGod, G., Kasonka, L., et al.; NUSTART (Nutritional Support for Africans Starting Antiretroviral Therapy) Study Team (2015). Effects on mortality of a nutritional intervention for malnourished HIV-infected adults referred for antiretroviral therapy: A randomised controlled trial. *BMC Medicine, 13,* 17-014-0253-8. doi:10.1186/s12916-014-0253-8

Fritts, M., Crawford, C. C., Quibell, D., et al. (2008). Traditional Indian medicine and homeopathy for HIV/AIDS: A review of the literature. *AIDS Research and Therapy, 5,* 25-6405-5-25. doi:10.1186/1742-6405-5-25

Galan, P., Kesse-Guyot, E., Czernichow, S., et al. (2010). Effects of B vitamins and omega 3 fatty acids on cardiovascular diseases: A randomised placebo controlled trial. *BMJ (Clinical Research Ed.), 341,* c6273. doi:10.1136/bmj.c6273

Galantino, M. L., Shepard, K., Krafft, L., et al. (2005). The effect of group aerobic exercise and t'ai chi on functional outcomes and quality of life for persons living with acquired immunodeficiency syndrome. *Journal of Alternative & Complementary Medicine: Research on Paradigm, Practice, and Policy, 11*(6), 1085–1092.

Galera, R. L., Pascuet, E. R., Mur, J. E., et al. (2008). Interaction between cat's claw and protease inhibitors atazanavir, ritonavir and saquinavir. *European Journal of Clinical Pharmacology, 64*(12), 1235–1236.

Galli C., & Brenna J. H. (2013). Omega-3 fatty acid supplementation and cardiovascular disease events [Letter to the Editor]. *JAMA, 309*(1), 27.

Gautam, N., Dayal, R., Agarwal, D., et al. (2014). Role of multivitamins, micronutrients and probiotics supplementation in management of HIV infected children. *Indian Journal of Pediatrics, 81*(12), 1315–1320.

Gayner, B., Esplen, M. J., DeRoche, P., et al. (2012). A randomized controlled trial of mindfulness-based stress reduction to manage affective symptoms and improve quality of life in gay men living with HIV. *Journal of Behavioral Medicine, 35*(3), 272–285.

Gerber, J. G., Kitch, D. W., Fichtenbaum, C. J., et al. (2008). Fish oil and fenofibrate for the treatment of hypertriglyceridemia in HIV-infected subjects on antiretroviral therapy: Results of ACTG A5186. *Journal of Acquired Immune Deficiency Syndromes, 47*(4), 459–466. doi:10.1097/QAI.0b013e31815bace2

Gonzalez-Garcia, M., Ferrer, M. J., Borras, X., et al. (2014). Effectiveness of mindfulness-based cognitive therapy on the quality of life, emotional status, and CD4+ T cell count of patients aging with HIV infection. *AIDS and Behavior, 18*(4), 676–685.

González-Hernández, L. A., Jave-Suarez, L. F., Fafutis-Morris, M., et al. (2012). Synbiotic therapy decreases microbial translocation and inflammation and improves immunological status in HIV-infected patients: A double-blind randomized controlled pilot trial. *Nutr. J., 11,* 90.

Graham, N. M., Sorensen, D., Odaka, N., et al. (1991). Relationship of serum copper and zinc levels to HIV-1 seropositivity and progression to AIDS. *Journal of Acquired Immune Deficiency Syndromes, 4*(10), 976–980.

Greene, K. B., Berger, J., Reeves, C., et al. (1999). Most frequently used alternative and complementary therapies and activities by participants in the AMCOA study. *Journal of the Association of Nurses in AIDS Care, 10*(3), 60–73.

Gwaza, L., Aweeka, F., Greenblatt, R., et al. (2013). Co-administration of a commonly used Zimbabwean herbal treatment (African potato) does not alter the pharmacokinetics of lopinavir/ritonavir. *International Journal of Infectious Diseases, 17*(10), e857–e861.

Hafner, V., Jager, M., Matthee, A. K., et al. (2010). Effect of simultaneous induction and inhibition of CYP3A by St John's Wort and ritonavir on CYP3A activity. *Clinical Pharmacology and Therapeutics, 8*(2), 191–196.

Haghighat, L., & Crum-Cianflone, N. F. (2015, June 30). The potential risks of probiotics among HIV-infected persons: Bacteraemia due to lactobacillus acidophilus and review of the literature. *International Journal of STD & AIDS.* doi:0956462415590725

Hepburn, M. J., Dyal, K., Runser, L. A., et al. (2004). Low serum vitamin B12 levels in an outpatient HIV-infected population. *International Journal of STD & AIDS, 15*(2), 127–133. doi:10.1258/095646204322764334

Hillier, S. L., Louw, Q., Morris, L., et al. (2010). Massage therapy for people with HIV/AIDS. *The Cochrane Library, 1,* CD007502

Hinman, R. S., McCrory, P., Pirotta, M., et al. (2014). Acupuncture for chronic knee pain: A randomized clinical trial. *JAMA, 312*(13), 1313–1322.

Hummelen, R., Hemsworth, J., Changalucha, J., et al. (2011). Effect of micronutrient and probiotic fortified yogurt on immune-function of anti-retroviral therapy naive HIV patients. *Nutrients, 3*(10), 897–909.

Hurwitz, B. E., Klaus, J. R., Llabre, M. M., et al. (2007). Suppression of human immunodeficiency virus type 1 viral load with selenium supplementation: A randomized controlled trial. *Archives of Internal Medicine, 167*(2), 148–154.

Ironson, G., O'Cleirigh, C., Fletcher, M. A., et al. (2005). Psychosocial factors predict CD4+ T cell and viral load change in men and women with human immunodeficiency virus in the era of highly active antiretroviral treatment. *Psychosomatic Medicine, 67*(6), 1013–1021. doi:67/6/1013

Irvine, S. L., Hummelen, R., & Hekmat, S. (2011). Probiotic yogurt consumption may improve gastrointestinal symptoms, productivity, and nutritional intake of people living with human immunodeficiency virus in Mwanza, Tanzania. *Nutrition Research, 31*(12), 875–881.

Jandourek, A., Vaishampayan, J. K., & Vazquez, J. A. (1998). Efficacy of melaleuca oral solution for the treatment of fluconazole refractory oral candidiasis in AIDS patients. *AIDS, 12*(9), 1033–1037.

Jiamto, S., Chaisilwattana, P., & Pepin, J. (2005). A randomized placebo-controlled trial of the impact of multiple micronutrient supplementation on HIV-1 genital shedding among Thai subjects (vol 37, pg 1216, 2004). *Journal of Acquired Immune Deficiency Syndromes, 38*(2), 240–240.

Jiamton, S., Pepin, J., Suttent, R., et al. (2003). A randomized trial of the impact of multiple micronutrient supplementation on mortality among HIV-infected individuals living in Bangkok. *AIDS, 17*(17), 2461–2469.

Jiménez-Nácher, I., Alvarez, E., Morello, J., et al. (2011). Approaches for understanding and predicting drug interactions in human immunodeficiency virus-infected patients. *Expert Opinion on Drug Metabolism & Toxicology, 7*(4), 457–477.

Jones, C. Y., Tang, A. M., Forrester, J. E., et al. (2006). Micronutrient levels and HIV disease status in HIV-infected patients on highly active antiretroviral therapy in the nutrition for healthy living cohort. *Journal of Acquired Immune Deficiency Syndromes, 43*(4), 475–482. doi:10.1097/01.qai.0000243096.27029.fe

Josephs, J., Fleishman, J., Gaist, P., et al. (2007). Use of complementary and alternative medicines among a multistate, multisite cohort of people living with HIV/AIDS. *HIV Medicine, 8*(5), 300–305.

Kaiser, J. D., Campa, A. M., Ondercin, J. P., et al. (2006). Micronutrient supplementation increases CD4+ T cell count in HIV-infected individuals on highly active antiretroviral therapy: A prospective, double-blinded, placebo-controlled trial. *Journal of Acquired Immune Deficiency Syndromes, 42*(5), 523–528. doi:10.1097/01.qai.0000230529.25083.42

Kamwesiga, J., Mutabazi, V., Kayumba, J., et al. (2015). Effect of selenium supplementation on CD4+ T-cell recovery, viral suppression and morbidity of HIV-infected patients in Rwanda: A randomized controlled trial. *AIDS (London), 29*(9), 1045–1052. doi:10.1097/QAD.0000000000000673

Kimmig, L. M., & Karalis, D. G. (2013). Do omega-3 polyunsaturated fatty acids prevent cardiovascular disease? A review of the randomized clinical trials. *Lipid Insights, 6,* 13.

Klatt, N. R., Canary, L. A., Sun, X., et al. (2013). Probiotic/prebiotic supplementation of antiretrovirals improves gastrointestinal immunity in SIV-infected macaques. *Journal of Clinical Investigation, 123*(2), 903–907. doi:10.1172/JCI66227

Kris-Etherton, P. M., Harris, W. S., Appel, L. J., & American Heart Association. Nutrition Committee (2002). Fish consumption, fish oil, omega-3 fatty acids, and cardiovascular disease. *Circulation*, *106*(21), 2747–2757.

Kromhout, D., Giltay, E. J., & Geleijnse, J. M. (2010). n-3 fatty acids and cardiovascular events after myocardial infarction. *New England Journal of Medicine*, *363*(21), 2015–2026.

Ladenheim, D., Horn, O., Werneke, U., et al. (2008). Potential health risks of complementary alternative medicines in HIV patients. *HIV Medicine*, *9*(8), 653–659.

Lamorde, M., Byakika-Kibwika, P., & Merry, C. (2012). Pharmacokinetic interactions between antiretroviral drugs and herbal medicines. *British Journal of Hospital Medicine*, *73*(3), 132–136.

Lavretsky, H., Epel, E., Siddarth, P., et al. (2013). A pilot study of yogic meditation for family dementia caregivers with depressive symptoms: Effects on mental health, cognition, and telomerase activity. *International Journal of Geriatric Psychiatry*, *28*(1), 57–65.

Lee, L. S., Andrade, A. S., & Flexner, C. (2006). Interactions between natural health products and antiretroviral drugs: Pharmacokinetic and pharmacodynamic effects. *Clinical Infectious Diseases*, *43*(8), 1052–1059. doi:CID39658

Leserman, J. (2008). Role of depression, stress, and trauma in HIV disease progression. *Psychosomatic Medicine*, *70*(5), 539–545. doi:10.1097/PSY.0b013e3181777a5f

Leserman, J., Petitto, J., Gu, H., et al. (2002). Progression to AIDS, a clinical AIDS condition and mortality: Psychosocial and physiological predictors. *Psychological Medicine*, *32*(06), 1059–1073.

Leserman, J., Petitto, J. M., Perkins, D. O., et al. (1997). Severe stress, depressive symptoms, and changes in lymphocyte subsets in human immunodeficiency virus-infected men: A 2-year follow-up study. *Archives of General Psychiatry*, *54*(3), 279–285.

Lewis, E. (2013). Omega-3 fatty acid supplementation and cardiovascular disease events [Letter to the Editor]. *JAMA*, *309*(1), 27.

Linde, K., Allais, G., Brinkhaus, B., et al. (2009). Acupuncture for tension-type headache. *Cochrane Database Syst Rev, 1*, CD007587.

Littlewood, R. A., & Vanable, P. A. (2008). Complementary and alternative medicine use among HIV-positive people: Research synthesis and implications for HIV care. *AIDS Care*, *20*(8), 1002–1018.

Littlewood, R. A., & Vanable, P. A. (2011). A global perspective on complementary and alternative medicine use among people living with HIV/AIDS in the era of antiretroviral treatment. *Current HIV/AIDS Reports*, *8*(4), 257–268.

Littlewood, R. A., & Vanable, P. A. (2014). The relationship between CAM use and adherence to antiretroviral therapies among persons living with HIV. *Health Psychology*, *33*(7), 660.

Liu, C., Yang, Y., Gange, S. J., et al. (2009). Disclosure of complementary and alternative medicine use to health care providers among HIV-infected women. *AIDS Patient Care and STDs*, *23*(11), 965–971.

London, A. S., Foote-Ardah, C. E., Fleishman, J. A., et al. (2003). Use of alternative therapists among people in care for HIV in the united states. *American Journal of Public Health*, *93*(6), 980–987.

Lorenc, A., & Robinson, N. (2013). A review of the use of complementary and alternative medicine and HIV: Issues for patient care. *AIDS Patient Care and STDs*, *27*(9), 503–510.

Lozupone, C. A., Li, M., Campbell, T. B., et al. (2013). Alterations in the gut microbiota associated with HIV-1 infection. *Cell Host & Microbe*, *14*(3), 329–339.

Ma, J., Li, Y., Ye, Q., et al. (2000). Constituents of red yeast rice, a traditional Chinese food and medicine. *Journal of Agricultural and Food Chemistry*, *48*(11), 5220–5225.

MacArthur, R. D., Levine, S. D., & Birk, T. J. (1993). Supervised exercise training improves cardiopulmonary fitness in HIV-infected persons. *Medicine & Science in Sports & Exercise*, *25*(6), 684–688.

MacDonald, L., Murty, M., & Foster, B. C. (2009). Antiviral drug disposition and natural health products: Risk of therapeutic alteration and resistance. *Expert Opin Drug Metab Toxicol.*, *5*(6), 563–578. doi:10.1517/17425250902942302

Manheimer, E., Cheng, K., Linde, K., et al. (2010). Acupuncture for peripheral joint osteoarthritis. *Cochrane Database Syst Rev, 1*, CD001977.

McCain, N. L., Gray, D. P., Elswick Jr, R., et al. (2008). A randomized clinical trial of alternative stress management interventions in persons with HIV infection. *Journal of Consulting and Clinical Psychology*, *76*(3), 431.

McClelland, R. S., Baeten, J. M., Overbaugh, J., et al. (2004). Micronutrient supplementation increases genital tract shedding of HIV-1 in women: Results of a randomized trial. *Journal of Acquired Immune Deficiency Syndromes*, *37*(5), 1657–1663.

Milan, F. B., Arnsten, J. H., Klein, R. S., et al. (2008). Use of complementary and alternative medicine in inner-city persons with or at risk for HIV infection. *AIDS Patient Care and STDs*, *22*(10), 811–816.

Mills, E., Wilson, K., Clarke, M., et al. (2005). Milk thistle and indinavir: A randomized controlled pharmacokinetics study and meta-analysis. *European Journal of Clinical Pharmacology*, *61*(1), 1–7.

Molto, J., Valle, M., Miranda, C., et al. (2011). Herb–drug interaction between echinacea purpurea and darunavir–ritonavir in HIV-infected patients. *Antimicrobial Agents and Chemotherapy*, *55*(1), 326–330. doi:10.1128/AAC.01082-10

Molto, J., Valle, M., Miranda, C., et al. (2012). Effect of milk thistle on the pharmacokinetics of darunavir–ritonavir in HIV-infected patients. *Antimicrobial Agents and Chemotherapy*, *56*(6), 2837–2841. doi:10.1128/AAC.00025-12

Molto, J., Valle, M., Miranda, C., et al. (2012). Herb–drug interaction between echinacea purpurea and etravirine in HIV-infected patients. *Antimicrobial Agents and Chemotherapy*, *56*(10), 5328–5331. doi:10.1128/AAC.01205-12

Mutlu, E. A., Keshavarzian, A., Losurdo, J., et al. (2014). A compositional look at the human gastrointestinal microbiome and immune activation parameters in HIV infected subjects. *PLoS Pathog, 10*(2), e1003829.

Naccarato, M., Yoong, D., & Gough, K. (2012). A potential drug-herbal interaction between ginkgo biloba and efavirenz. *Journal of the International Association of Physicians in AIDS Care (Chicago)*, *11*(2), 98–100. doi:10.1177/1545109711435364

National Center for Complementary and Alternative Medicine (2010). *What Is Complementary and Alternative Medicine?*

ORIGIN Trial Investigators (2008). Rationale, design, and baseline characteristics for a large international trial of cardiovascular disease prevention in people with dysglycemia: The ORIGIN trial (Outcome Reduction with an Initial Glargine Intervention). *American Heart Journal*, *155*(1), 26. e1–e26. e13.

Overton, E. T., Chan, E. S., Brown, T. T., et al. (2015). Vitamin D and calcium attenuate bone loss with antiretroviral therapy initiation: A randomized trial. *Annals of Internal Medicine*, *162*(12), 815–824.

Owen-Smith, A., Diclemente, R., & Wingood, G. (2007). Complementary and alternative medicine use decreases adherence to HAART in HIV-positive women. *AIDS Care*, *19*(5), 589–593.

Pence, B. W., Miller, W. C., Whetten, K., et al. (2006). Prevalence of DSM-IV-defined mood, anxiety, and substance use disorders in an HIV clinic in the southeastern United States. *Journal of Acquired Immune Deficiency Syndromes*, *42*(3), 298–306. doi:10.1097/01.qai.0000219773.82055.aa

Penzak, S. R., Robertson, S. M., Hunt, J. D., et al. (2010). Echinacea purpurea significantly induces cytochrome P450 3A activity but does not alter lopinavir–ritonavir exposure in healthy subjects. *Pharmacotherapy*, *30*(8), 797–805. doi:10.1592/phco.30.8.797

Peters, B. S., Wierzbicki, A. S., Moyle, G., et al. (2012). The effect of a 12-week course of omega-3 polyunsaturated fatty acids on lipid parameters in hypertriglyceridemic adult HIV-infected patients undergoing HAART: A randomized, placebo-controlled pilot trial. *Clinical Therapeutics*, *34*(1), 67–76.

Phillips, K. D., & Skelton, W. D. (2001). Effects of individualized acupuncture on sleep quality in HIV disease. *Journal of the Association of Nurses in AIDS Care*, *12*(1), 27–39.

Piscitelli, S. C., Burstein, A. H., Chaitt, D., et al. (2000). Indinavir concentrations and St. John's wort. *Lancet, 355*(9203), 547–548.

Piscitelli, S. C., Burstein, A. H., Welden, N., et al. (2002). The effect of garlic supplements on the pharmacokinetics of saquinavir. *Clinical Infectious Diseases, 34*(2), 234–238. doi:CID010586

Piscitelli, S. C., Formentini, E., Burstein, A. H., et al. (2002). Effect of milk thistle on the pharmacokinetics of indinavir in healthy volunteers. *Pharmacotherapy: The Journal of Human Pharmacology and Drug Therapy, 22*(5), 551–556.

Power, R., Gore-Felton, C., Vosvick, M., et al. (2002). HIV: Effectiveness of complementary and alternative medicine. *Primary Care: Clinics in Office Practice, 29*(2), 361–378.

Range, N., Changalucha, J., Krarup, H., et al. (2006). The effect of multi-vitamin/mineral supplementation on mortality during treatment of pulmonary tuberculosis: A randomised two-by-two factorial trial in Mwanza, Tanzania. *British Journal of Nutrition, 95*(4), 762–770.

Rauch, B., Schiele, R., Schneider, S., et al. (2010). OMEGA, a randomized, placebo-controlled trial to test the effect of highly purified omega-3 fatty acids on top of modern guideline-adjusted therapy after myocardial infarction. *Circulation, 122*(21), 2152–2159. doi:10.1161/CIRCULATIONAHA.110.948562

Remacha, A. F., Cadafalch, J., Sarda, P., et al. (2003). Vitamin B-12 metabolism in HIV-infected patients in the age of highly antiretroviral therapy: role of homocysteine in assessing vitamin B-12 status. *American Journal of Clinical Nutrition, 77*(2), 420–424.

Rigsby, L. W., Dishman, R., Jackson, A. W., et al. (1992). Effects of exercise training on men seropositive for the human immunodeficiency virus-1. *Medicine & Science in Sports & Exercise, 24*(1), 6–12.

Rizos, E. C., Ntzani, E. E., Bika, E., et al. (2012). Association between omega-3 fatty acids supplementation and risk of major cardiovascular disease events. *JAMA, 308*(10), 1024–1033.

Sandhu, R. S., Prescilla, R. P., Simonelli, T. M., et al. (2003). Influence of goldenseal root on the pharmacokinetics of indinavir. *Journal of Clinical Pharmacology, 43*(11), 1283–1288.

Saper, R. B., Phillips, R. S., Sehgal, A., et al. (2008). Lead, mercury, and arsenic in US- and Indian-manufactured Ayurvedic medicines sold via the Internet. *JAMA, 300*(8), 915–923.

Sethi, A., Singh, M., & Arora, R. (2013). Omega-3 fatty acid supplementation and cardiovascular disease events [Letter to the Editor]. *JAMA, 309*(1), 27.

Shere-Wolfe, K. D., Tilburt, J. C., D'Adamo, C., et al. (2013). Infectious diseases physicians' attitudes and practices related to complementary and integrative medicine: Results of a national survey. *Evidence-Based Complementary and Alternative Medicine, 2013*, Article ID 294381.

Shlay, J. C., Chaloner, K., Max, M. B., et al. (1998). Acupuncture and amitriptyline for pain due to HIV-related peripheral neuropathy: A randomized controlled trial. *JAMA, 280*(18), 1590–1595.

Slain, D., Amsden, J. R., Khakoo, R. A., et al. (2005). Effect of high-dose vitamin C on the steady-state pharmacokinetics of the protease inhibitor indinavir in healthy volunteers. *Pharmacotherapy, 25*(2), 165–170.

Standish, L., Greene, K., Bain, S., et al. (2001). Alternative medicine use in HIV-positive men and women: Demographics, utilization patterns and health status. *AIDS Care, 13*(2), 197–208.

Stiksrud, B., Nowak, P., Nwosu, F. C., et al. (2015). Reduced levels of D-dimer and changes in gut microbiota composition after probiotic intervention in HIV-infected individuals on stable ART. *Journal of Acquired Immune Deficiency Syndromes, 70*(4), 329–337. doi:10.1097/QAI.0000000000000784

Stolbach, A., Paziana, K., Heverling, H., et al. (2015). A review of the toxicity of HIV medications II: Interactions with drugs and complementary and alternative medicine products. *Journal of Medical Toxicology, 11*(3), 326–341.

Stringer, W. W., Berezovskaya, M., O'Brien, W. A., et al. (1998). The effect of exercise training on aerobic fitness, immune indices, and quality of life in HIV patients. *Medicine & Science in Sports & Exercise, 30*(1), 11–16.

Stussman, B. J., Black, L. I., Barnes, P. M., et al. (2015). Wellness-related use of common complementary health approaches among adults: United States, 2012. *National Health Statistics Reports, 85*, 1–12.

Sudfeld, C. R., Aboud, S., Kupka, R., et al. (2014). Effect of selenium supplementation on HIV-1 RNA detection in breast milk of Tanzanian women. *Nutrition, 30*(9), 1081–1084.

Thompson, M. A., Aberg, J. A., Hoy, J. F., et al. (2012). Antiretroviral treatment of adult HIV infection: 2012 recommendations of the International Antiviral Society–USA panel. *JAMA, 308*(4), 387–402.

Ting, A., Chow, Y., & Tan, W. (2013). Microbial and heavy metal contamination in commonly consumed traditional Chinese herbal medicines. *Journal of Traditional Chinese Medicine, 33*(1), 119–124.

Vasquez, J. A., Zawawi, A. A. (2002). Efficacy of alcohol-based and alcohol-free melaleuca oral solution for the treatment of fluconazole-refractory oropharyngeal candidiasis in patients with AIDS. *HIV Clinical Trials, 3*(5), 379–385.

Vickers, A. J., Cronin, A. M., Maschino, A. C., et al. (2012). Acupuncture for chronic pain: Individual patient data meta-analysis. *Archives of Internal Medicine, 172*(19), 1444–1453.

Villar-Garcia, J., Hernandez, J. J., Guerri-Fernandez, R., et al. (2015). Effect of probiotics (*Saccharomyces boulardii*) on microbial translocation and inflammation in HIV-treated patients: A double-blind, randomized, placebo-controlled trial. *Journal of Acquired Immune Deficiency Syndromes, 68*(3), 256–263. doi:10.1097/QAI.0000000000000468

Visser, R. D., & Grierson, J. (2002). Use of alternative therapies by people living with HIV/AIDS in Australia. *AIDS Care, 14*(5), 599–606.

Vlachopoulos, C., Richter D., Stefanadis C. (2013). Omega-3 fatty acid supplementation and cardiovascular disease events [Letter to the Editor]. *JAMA, 309*(1), 27.

Vogl, D., Rosenfeld, B., Breitbart, W., et al. (1999). Symptom prevalence, characteristics, and distress in AIDS outpatients. *Journal of Pain and Symptom Management, 18*(4), 253–262.

Vujkovic-Cvijin, I., Dunham, R. M., Iwai, S., et al. (2013). Dysbiosis of the gut microbiota is associated with HIV disease progression and tryptophan catabolism. *Science Translational Medicine, 5*(193), 193ra91. doi:10.1126/scitranslmed.3006438

Warburton, D. E., Nicol, C. W., & Bredin, S. S. (2006). Health benefits of physical activity: The evidence. *Canadian Medical Association Journal, 174*(6), 801–809. doi:174/6/801

Whetten, K., Reif, S., Whetten, R., et al. (2008). Trauma, mental health, distrust, and stigma among HIV-positive persons: Implications for effective care. *Psychosomatic Medicine, 70*(5), 531–538. doi:10.1097/PSY.0b013e31817749dc

Wiegman, D. J., Brinkman, K., Franssen, E. J. (2009). Interaction of Ginkgo biloba with efavirenz. *AIDS, 23*(9), 1184–1185.

Witt, C. M., Jena, S., Brinkhaus, B., et al. (2006). Acupuncture for patients with chronic neck pain. *Pain, 125*(1), 98–106.

Wohl, D. A., Tien, H. C., Busby, M., et al. (2005). Randomized study of the safety and efficacy of fish oil (omega-3 fatty acid) supplementation with dietary and exercise counseling for the treatment of antiretroviral therapy-associated hypertriglyceridemia. *Clinical Infectious Diseases, 41*(10), 1498–1504. doi:CID37106

Wynia, M. K., Eisenberg, D. M., & Wilson, I. B. (1999). Physician–patient communication about complementary and alternative medical therapies: A survey of physicians caring for patients with human immunodeficiency virus infection. *Journal of Alternative and Complementary Medicine, 5*(5), 447–456.

15.

CARE COORDINATION

Joy H. Kang and Peter A. Selwyn

CHAPTER GOAL

Upon completion of this chapter, readers should be able to demonstrate knowledge and practice of interdisciplinary care coordination in HIV patient care.

IMPORTANCE OF AN INTERDISCIPLINARY APPROACH TO HIV PATIENT CARE

LEARNING OBJECTIVE

Describe the importance of an interdisciplinary team approach to the HIV continuum of care.

WHAT'S NEW?

- Interdisciplinary team is an essential comprehensive care strategy to approaching the HIV continuum of care—to help diagnose, link, engage, and successfully treat patients with HIV with effective chronic disease management. The full continuum of care has multiple components, all of which are interdependent and require structured and well-coordinated care to address the full range of medical, psychosocial, and behavioral comorbidities.

KEY POINTS

- Patients infected with HIV are now living longer, and there is a growing prevalence of HIV-related and/or non-HIV-related comorbidities, often with an increasing need for chronic disease management beyond the treatment of HIV infection.

- The barriers to each of the steps in the HIV continuum of care need to be identified, anticipated, and addressed. Often, addressing these barriers entails medical, psychosocial, and other specialized services.

- The interdisciplinary team approach is essential to effective coordination of care for patients with multiple health and service needs.

HIV infection is a preventable and treatable chronic disease. Currently available antiretroviral therapies (ART) have higher efficacy and lower side effect profiles compared to ART available in previous decades. Thus, patients with HIV are living longer than ever before, with projected life spans approaching those of the general population (Samji, 2014; Wada, 2014). A consequence of this prolonged survival, however, is the growing prevalence of HIV-related and/or non-HIV-related comorbidities in this patient population and often an increasing need for chronic disease management beyond the treatment of HIV infection per se (Chu, 2011). In addition, with decreasing overall mortality rates and little, if any, decrease in the incidence of new HIV infections, the total number of patients living with HIV in the United States continues to increase, suggesting the need for care services for a growing population (Centers for Disease Control and Prevention (CDC), 2011).

New HIV infections often occur in high-risk subpopulations (e.g., young men who have sex with men of color), and late diagnosis and/or inconsistent engagement with care may also reflect intrapersonal, interpersonal, and system-based barriers to care (Bauman, 2013; CDC, 2011; Irvine, 2014; Scanlon, 2013). This ultimately results in lower levels of viral suppression and greater drop offs in the "treatment cascade" than those in less vulnerable populations (Gardner, 2011; Whitehouse, 2014). Thus, patients with HIV often have multiple service needs in addition to those for their HIV infection and may require an array of services that are often delivered by different systems and payers.

COMPLEXITY OF HIV PATIENT CARE NEEDS

The following are illustrative case examples of the types of complex comorbidities and chronic conditions that currently characterize the care of patients with HIV infection:

1. A 35-year-old male with a recent diagnosis of HIV who also is currently homeless and opioid dependent. He is in need of ART, housing, drug abuse treatment, and opportunistic infection (OI) prophylaxis all at the same time.

2. An obese 55-year-old female with uncontrolled HIV infection, chronic hepatitis C, and chronic depression who was recently diagnosed with diabetes and osteoarthritis of the knees.

3. A 28-year-old male with HIV/AIDS who is intermittently incarcerated. He is poorly adherent to ART and is in need of stable primary HIV care and health insurance coverage.

4. A perinatally infected 18-year-old female with controlled HIV infection who is establishing care in an adult clinic. She was recently removed from a foster home to live on her own for the first time in her life.

5. A 74-year-old male with stable HIV disease, a history of multiple strokes, and painful peripheral neuropathy who recently began to have mild cognitive decline.

6. A 36-year-old pregnant female with marginal viral suppression who is in an abusive relationship with her boyfriend and presents with vaginal bleeding after an episode of domestic violence.

7. A 66-year-old asymptomatic HIV-infected female on ART who needs to make decisions about hospice care and further ART for her 68-year-old husband, who has advanced HIV disease and is confined to bed following a recent severe stroke.

It has been widely noted, as mentioned previously, that HIV patient care in the United States increasingly involves the care of other related or coexisting comorbidities. Some of these conditions are age-related, whereas others are related to HIV infection or the therapies used to treat it. Comorbid conditions include diabetes, obesity, hypertension and cardiovascular disease, chronic obstructive pulmonary disease, renal disease, liver disease (both infectious and non-infectious), mental health, bone disease, musculoskeletal pain, and other common primary care conditions. In addition, substance use and other psychological and social conditions require more than the narrow focus on the virus or on ART; it is important to recognize that the goal is to always treat the patient, not just the virus, and care systems and coordination need to be oriented to achieve this goal. In addition, complex health care systems and diffuse or uncoordinated medical and social services may limit access and delay timely and effective services to patients (Bauman, 2013; Boyd, 2014; Chu, 2011). Thus, comprehensive, interdisciplinary, and well-coordinated HIV patient care should be well structured within any model of HIV patient care.

THE HIV CONTINUUM OF CARE

The primary goals of HIV patient care are to (1) suppress the virus; (2) decrease HIV-related morbidities; (3) improve immune status, life expectancy, and quality of life; and (4) decrease transmission (US Department of Health and Human Services, 2015). In order to successfully achieve these goals, a series of steps from initial diagnosis through successful viral suppression are needed (CDC, 2014). In 2011, the concept of the "HIV treatment cascade," which graphically reflects the continuum of care from diagnosis to viral suppression, was promulgated to describe and discuss the interdependent steps of this ideal process of care (Figure 15.1) (Gardner, 2011). Based on this, in 2014, the Joint United Nations Programme on HIV/AIDS (UNAIDS) announced a three-part target known as 90–90–90: 90% of all people living with HIV to (1) know their status, (2) receive sustaining treatment, and (3) have viral suppression by 2020 (UNAIDS, 2014). Ultimately, the goal of the HIV continuum of care is the end of the AIDS epidemic.

The first step in the HIV continuum of care is the timely diagnosis of HIV infection. This requires targeted community outreach to high-risk populations as well as routine HIV screening in the general population (CDC, 2006; US Preventive Services Task Force, 2013). Once a patient is diagnosed, he or she should be quickly linked to care. Once engaged in care, it is critical to retain the patient in care while ART is initiated. Once ART is initiated—and potentially for decades to follow—the patient needs to be effectively followed and supported in care to ensure durable virologic suppression. The barriers to each of the steps in the

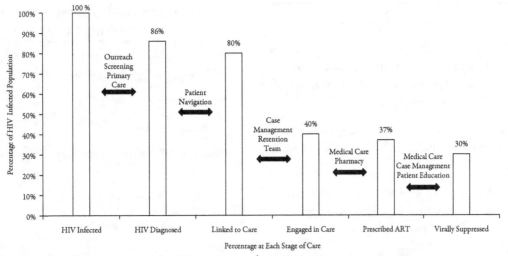

Figure 15.1 Key roles of interdisciplinary care team in the HIV continuum of care. SOURCES: The White House Office of National AIDS Policy. *National HIV/AIDS Strategy: Update of 2014 Federal Actions to Achieve National Goals and Improve Outcomes Along the HIV Care Continuum.* Washington, DC: The White House Office of National AIDS Policy; 2014; and Centers for Disease Control and Prevention. Vital signs: HIV diagnosis, care, and treatment among persons living with HIV—United States, 2011. *MMWR.* 2014; 63(47):1113–1137.

HIV continuum of care need to be identified, anticipated, and addressed. Often, addressing these barriers entails medical, psychosocial, and other specialized services, including substance abuse treatment, case management, patient education, social work, and other necessary services that can be facilitated by an interdisciplinary team working collaboratively (Dombrowski, 2015; Dykeman, 1996).

For example, an obese 55-year-old female with uncontrolled HIV infection, chronic hepatitis C, and chronic depression who was recently diagnosed with diabetes and osteoarthritis of the knees might require a coordinated team approach to care in order to address the following issues:

- Medical: Obesity, diabetes, HIV, and hepatitis C all need chronic treatment and monitoring; osteoarthritis might require pain management, physical therapy, assistive devices, and/or other supportive interventions.

- Psychosocial: The patient's depression needs evaluation and treatment in its own right and/or as a risk factor for nonengagement or loss to follow-up in HIV/medical care. Mental health, social work, and case management services may all be needed to provide psychosocial treatment and support.

- Behavioral/ancillary: Case management and health/adherence education may help support the patient to enhance follow-up and adherence with care and may promote healthier behaviors (e.g., nutrition, exercise, and use of substances) that might improve chronic disease outcomes.

Recommended Reading

Centers for Disease Control and Prevention, Division of HIV/AIDS Prevention. Understanding the HIV care continuum. 2014. Available at https://stacks.cdc.gov/view/cdc/26481. Accessed November 3, 2015.

Chu C, Selwyn PA. An epidemic in evolution: The need for new models of HIV care in the chronic disease era. *J Urban Health.* 2011; 88(3):556–566.

Gardner EM, McLees MP, Steiner JF, et al. The spectrum of engagement in HIV care and its relevance to test-and-treat strategies for prevention of HIV infection. *Clin Infect Dis.* 2011; 52(6):793–800.

KEY PRINCIPLES OF THE INTERDISCIPLINARY HIV PATIENT CARE TEAM

LEARNING OBJECTIVES

- Describe the roles and responsibilities of the interdisciplinary HIV patient care team.

- Discuss strategies for developing an HIV patient care team.

WHAT'S NEW?

- An interdisciplinary team consists of professionals with different expertise and responsibilities who work interdependently, with clearly defined roles and open communication, to achieve a common goal of optimizing the health care of the patient.

- Effective linkage to and engagement in care can be achieved by interdisciplinary HIV care, which may help decrease transmission of new HIV infections and reduce the overall cost of HIV care in the United States.

- The success of an interdisciplinary team depends on effective and open communication and coordination among members.

- Team leadership by a designated professional can provide needed direction on how the team addresses patient needs by ensuring unified goals and communication among interdisciplinary team members.

- Understanding and strategic planning to develop an interdisciplinary team is needed to provide comprehensive health care to patients with HIV and multiple comorbidities.

Box 15.1 MULTIPLE DISCIPLINARY MEMBERS OF HIV PATIENT CARE TEAM

HIV specialist/primary care physician

Nurse practitioner

Physician assistant

Specialists (dental, ophthalmology, cardiology, palliative care, etc.)

Psychiatrist/mental health provider

Substance abuse treatment provider

Psychologist

Nurse

Pharmacist

Health educator

Nutritionist

Adherence counselor

Risk reduction counselor

Patient outreach worker

Social worker

Financial advisor/insurance coordinator

Case manager/coordinator

Health care manager

Patient navigator

Administrative staff

Information and technology specialist

Researcher

Public health worker

Community-based organization worker

Interdisciplinary care among patients with HIV has been associated with improved engagement and retention in care (Conviser, 2002; Magnus, 2001). Recent HIV epidemic and economic analyses have shown that increasing the rates of screening and linkage to care and focused efforts to improve retention of high-risk group would decrease the transmission of new HIV infections and result in overall cost savings in HIV care in the United States (Gopalappa, 2012; Shah, 2016). In addition, shared and coordinated patient care among different disciplines can increase the efficiency of care without duplication of services among multiple health care service providers. Thus, interdisciplinary team care has been emphasized as an essential component of effective HIV patient care (Gallant, 2011; Horberg, 2012).

Interdisciplinary HIV patient care is delivered by multiple disciplinary team members including both clinicians and nonclinicians (Box 15.1) (Bauman, 2013; Gallant, 2011; Horberg; 2012). However, some clinics may not have direct access to or all the potentially necessary members of the HIV patient care team at the same location. Thus, principles for developing an interdisciplinary HIV care team—even if not all members are physically located at one site—are essential, especially in resource-limiting settings or when patients need to be referred out to receive necessary services.

SUCCESSFUL CARE TEAM MODEL

An interdisciplinary team is often described as multiple interdisciplinary or interprofessional members working interdependently to achieve a common goal in an integrated, coordinated, and synergistic collaboration (Nancarrow, 2013; Newhouse, 2010). An interdisciplinary team's members have different expertise and responsibilities, and all work together to achieve a common goal of comprehensive and holistic patient care (Nancarrow, 2013; Newhouse, 2010). Thus, success of a team depends on effective communication and coordination among members. Each team member has a responsibility to

- work together to bring a team of individuals motivated by the common goal of optimal patient care and outcomes;

- meet regularly together as a team to discuss patient care;

- demonstrate respect for each team member's contribution and ensure that all members' concerns are heard and that legitimate issues are allowed to influence patient care;

- help to clarify each member's role(s) and the team's expectations;

- use each member's expertise to provide optimal medical care and allow/encourage other team members to use their expertise in a similar manner; and

- develop and ensure cultural competence and sensitivity to the needs of HIV-infected patient populations.

This can be a challenging task when one person—usually a clinician—may be traditionally accustomed to providing the patient care alone. However, a planned and well-thought-out process of developing a team can both support the overall health care of patients and decrease the team's burden of demanding health care needs. One strategy is to start with a small number of the most needed members of the interdisciplinary patient care team and establish a few prioritized goals to achieve. An example of starting an interdisciplinary patient care team with two members and prioritizing care goals for the patient is presented next.

The patient is a 35-year-old male with a recent diagnosis of HIV who also is currently homeless and opioid dependent. He is in need of ART, housing, drug abuse treatment, and OI prophylaxis all at the same time. The interdisciplinary patient care team for this patient consists of the following:

- Case manager: A case manager can help the patient navigate complex medical and legal systems to apply for stable housing and medical insurance. A case manager can also coordinate appointments and referrals to substance abuse treatment and mental health providers.

- HIV specialist/primary care clinician: A clinician can help the patient by providing education; prescribing ART and OI prophylaxis; and referring the patient to other necessary specialists, including mental health and substance abuse treatment providers.

Regular meetings between the case manager and the clinician can lead to building a more comprehensive interdisciplinary patient care team, including mental health and substance abuse treatment providers.

Establishing care priorities for the previously discussed patient can be challenging given the patient's complex medical and psychosocial needs. However, understanding the patient's perspectives on overall health care can help reveal specific barriers to care, which can improve care coordination and patient outcome because these barriers can hinder linkage, engagement/retention, and ultimately viral suppression:

- Stable housing: "I can't focus on taking meds when I have no place to sleep at night."

- Medical insurance: "I don't have green card and I have no money to buy any medication."

- Substance abuse treatment: "I wonder when I will be getting my next 'high.'"

- Linkage to care: "I cannot remember all these appointments. I miss my appointments because I forget things easily."

- ART and OI prophylaxis: "I have too much going on. Besides, I don't feel sick."

The case manager and the clinician should start to address the patient's housing, medical insurance, and substance abuse treatment. Given the patient's AIDS status (needing OI prophylaxis), the clinician and the case manager should continue to educate and encourage the patient to start OI prophylaxis and ART because another team member, such as an adherence counselor, will soon be, if not already, involved.

TEAM MEMBER RESPONSIBILITIES

There are multiple and potentially duplicating roles of HIV patient care team members. Thus, one person may perform more than one responsibility regardless of his or her professional role (Table 15.1). It is also important to clearly define and modify expected responsibilities of team members to efficiently and effectively provide patient care. Although a team approach can enhance coordination of care, it is often helpful to identify one team member as the primary

Table 15.1 DIFFERENT ROLES OF HIV PATIENT CARE TEAM

KEY ELEMENTS	ROLES	RESPONSIBILITIES	POTENTIALLY INVOLVED PERSONNEL
Diagnosis (prevention)	Community outreach	• Offer HIV screening • Link patients to primary care • Offer pre-exposure prophylaxis if HIV negative	• Public health worker • Researcher • Nurse • Health educator
Linkage to care	Patient navigation	• Arrange appointments • Function as a liaison between patient and the health care provider	• Administrative staff • Nurse • Case manager
Linkage to care Prescribing ART	Insurance/social support	• Link patients to available community resources • Apply for medical insurance, including ADAP • Advocate for patient's needs	• Social worker • Financial advisor • Case manager • Advocacy group liaison
Engagement/retention	Retention/engagement	• Outreach to out-of-care patients • Outreach to public health and community-based organizations • Gather patient data on retention	• Administrative staff • Nurse • Case manager • Public health worker
Engagement/retention	Mental health	• Provide counseling • Provide mental health treatment • Provide psychosocial support	• Social worker • Psychologist • Psychiatrist • Substance abuse counselor
Prescribing ART Viral suppression	Medical care	• Provide medical management • Refer to appropriate specialist(s) • Educate on medication adherence	• HIV specialist or primary care clinician • Pharmacist/local pharmacy worker • Nurse
Viral suppression	Patient education	• Provide education on nutrition, adherence, drug interaction, healthy lifestyle, etc.	• Nurse • Adherence counselor • Nutritionist • Health educator • Pharmacist • HIV specialist or primary care clinician
Linkage Engagement/retention Prescribing ART Viral suppression	Population health management	• Gather data on each step of HIV continuum of care • Conduct quality improvement • Measure patient outcomes • Evaluate projects/programs	• Electronic medical record provider • Administrative staff • Data support staff • Researcher • HIV specialist or primary care clinician • Public health worker
All stages of care	Team lead	• Provide system-based coordination • Develop infrastructure	• Any team member • Commonly done by a clinician

ART, antiretroviral therapy.

informal contact with patients to link and retain patients in care (Gardner, 2014).

LEADERSHIP OF THE TEAM

Team leadership by a designated professional can provide needed direction on how the team addresses patient needs by ensuring focused vision and communication among team members (Nancarrow, 2013). Having multiple clinicians and team members increases the collective ability of the team, but it also increases the possibility for lapses in communication and inaccurate or incomplete information transfer. Therefore, each team should develop or adopt methods to ensure routine communication, documentation, and follow-up (Parry, 2004). A fixed and regularly established meeting schedule among team members can help ensure care coordination and consistency. The team leader's work in facilitating communication among various members of a diverse health care team should entail frequent, regular communication among health care team members to support the goal of quality care for patients.

STRATEGIES FOR DEVELOPING AN INTERDISCIPLINARY HIV PATIENT CARE TEAM

The following are steps for developing an interdisciplinary HIV patient care team:

- Establish a team leader.

- Evaluate available HIV patient care data (e.g., percentage of linkage, retention, viral suppression, and no-show appointments)

- List needed resources (e.g., meeting room, education materials, community organizations, and funding) and personnel (designated HIV nurse, patient navigator, financial advisor, social worker, adherence counselor, etc.).

- Assess available resources and personnel at the facility and outside the facility.

- Gather available/needed resources and personnel.

- Set up an initial meeting with members of the team.

- Discuss goals of the team and define each member's responsibilities.

- Set up regularly scheduled meetings and discuss patient care.

- Continue to evaluate the team structure and clinical outcomes.

- Continue to build relationships and collaborate with public health and community organizations.

- Make appropriate plans, evaluations, and implementations to improve quality of care.

Recommended Reading

Gallant JE, Adimora AA, Carmichael JK, et al. Essential components of effective HIV care: A policy paper of the HIV Medicine Association of the Infectious Diseases Society of America and the Ryan White Medical Providers Coalition. *Clin Infect Dis*. 2011; 53:1043–1050.

Nancarrow SA, Booth A, Ariss S, et al. Ten principles of good interdisciplinary team work. *Hum Resourc Health*. 2013; 11:19.

STRATEGIES FOR SUCCESSFUL REFERRAL

LEARNING OBJECTIVE

Describe the steps for obtaining referrals for HIV-infected patients and strategies that can increase the success of referrals.

WHAT'S NEW?

Patients with multiple service needs in addition to those for their HIV disease often require referral to other services, including medical, psychosocial, and ancillary care. Effective referrals can be handled by a planned and monitored referral process and through established connections with referral sources, requiring ongoing communication and information transfer between service providers and organizations.

KEY POINTS

- Steps for a well-crafted referral include assessment of referral needs, planning of the referral, and management and follow-up of the referral to ensure coordination and delivery of care.

- Referrals are typically handled by case managers or other designated care coordinators who can improve the patient's linkage, engagement, and retention to care.

- Clear and regular communication between the referring organization, the receiving organization, and the coordinating organization can help decrease duplication of services, evaluate gaps in care, and help ensure continuity and quality of care.

Because patients with HIV have chronic and complex medical and psychosocial conditions, clinicians delivering HIV care often require special referrals for services that they may not be able to provide themselves. Thus, an effective referral process for such patients is essential for comprehensive and required care. Referrals can range from specialized medical, dental, mental health, and substance use treatment to home care, peer support groups and other peer services, transportation, housing, financial/legal support, meal deliveries, spirituality services, and end-of-life care and hospice (Family Health International, 2005; Kwait, 2001). Referrals can range from informing patients about other sources to taking additional steps to ensure that a referral is successful by communicating with external agencies about the referred patient. The positive impact of effective referrals is demonstrated in data suggesting that supportive services and an emotionally supportive context can enhance clinical outcomes such as improved adherence to ART (Knowlton, 2006).

Steps that can enhance the success of referrals for patients with HIV are discussed next (CDC, 2001).

ASSESS REFERRAL NEEDS

The first step in managing referrals includes a clear assessment of the patient's referral needs. This should include determining both medical specialty needs and any psychosocial support needs. It is important to not only recognize the patient's own priorities but also objectively evaluate the patient's needs.

PLAN THE REFERRAL

Next, the referral should be planned, with consideration of accessible referral sites, client demographics (e.g., culture, language, and gender), and client factors such as substance abuse and mental health conditions that might complicate completion of referrals (CDC, 2001).

REFERRALS AND PATIENT INFORMATION

When communicating with specialists, clinicians typically need to share relevant clinical information. Health Insurance Portability and Accountability Act (HIPAA) regulations and any local regulations and standards need to be known and followed in all such instances of information sharing between providers and agencies (Office of Civil Rights, 2003).

MANAGE THE REFERRALS

All members of the interdisciplinary patient care team can play a role in coordinating delivery of care and handling and managing referrals. One of the most commonly used methods to refer patients is case management. In the process of coordinating patient care, case management is also involved in ongoing social support for patients. Characteristics of a case management intervention might include work to overcome barriers to care (e.g., fear, lack of readiness, and lack of knowledge about services) and efforts to link the patient to services (e.g., accompanying clients to appointments and arranging transportation to the first medical visit).

Case managers (or coordinators or health care managers) can be helpful in many aspects of coordination and communication in complex cases. In one study, among newly infected HIV patients, 78% of those having case management contact had seen an HIV clinician within the 6-month follow-up period compared to just 60% of those who received only a passive referral to care. When extending the period to 12 months, 64% of the case management patients were still in care, whereas only 49% of

passive referrals were so linked (Gardner, 2005). A study on newly diagnosed patients with case management showed 90.5% engagement to care and 66% viral suppression after 12 months of case management. The same study also showed an increase in retention and re-engagement to care among patients who had been intermittently adherent to care or out of care (Irvine, 2014).

Case management operates under different models, commonly (1) medical case management or (2) community-based services or psychosocial case management. In each, care is usually coordinated, respectively, by a medical professional or by a social worker or psychosocial case manager. Case managers in different settings may also have different clinical backgrounds (e.g., social work, counseling, and health education). Thus, it is important to know the expertise of each team member.

Documenting client receipt and progress of referral services is critical to ensuring that referral services have been provided. It is also a means for assessing the efficacy of referral networks (CDC, 2001; Family Health International, 2005). Documentation can include follow-up to check on the status of the referral and evaluation/feedback of referrals from patients by assessing barriers to completion of referrals and satisfaction with the services provided. Clear communication between the referring organization, the receiving organization, and the coordinating organization can help decrease duplication of services and evaluate gaps in care, and it can also help ensure continuity and quality of care. In addition, a designated person who can coordinate communication between different collaborating services as well as a system-based structure (e.g., paper/electronic referral, periodic updates in the medical record, consultation notes, and regular telephonic or in-person meetings) in the management of referrals can help achieve a successful referral process (Family Health International, 2005, 2005).

BECOME FAMILIAR WITH REFERRAL SOURCES AND SERVICES

Ensuring effective referrals involves knowledge of available services across a spectrum of patient care needs. Most communities have resource guides that list public health and community-based organization (CBO) websites or networks, which can help clinicians determine where to refer patients. In establishing referral networks, CBOs can engage in formal referral agreements to outline working relationships, including specifics of referral procedures, handling of confidential patient information, and available services (Family Health International, 2005; Kwait, 2001).

Regular communications and shared, updated contact and referral information for collaborating CBOs and health care facilities should also be included in the interdisciplinary patient care team approach.

Recommended Reading

Centers for Disease Control and Prevention (CDC). Revised guidelines for HIV counseling, testing, and referral. *MMWR Recomm Rep.* 2001; 50(19):37–40.

Family Health International. Establishing referral networks for comprehensive HIV care in low-resource settings 1-16. 2005. Available at http://pdf.usaid.gov/pdf_docs/Pnadf677.pdf. Accessed November 27, 2015.

Kwait J, Valente T, Celentano, D. Interorganizational relationships among HIV/AIDS service organizations in Baltimore: A network analysis. *J Urban Health.* 2001; 78(3):468–487.

SUSTAINABILITY OF THE INTERDISCIPLINARY HIV PATIENT CARE MODEL

LEARNING OBJECTIVE

Discuss the ongoing need to improve and sustain the interdisciplinary HIV patient care model as the AIDS epidemic evolves.

WHAT'S NEW?

HIV patient care is becoming more ambulatory with rapidly changing and evolving systems of health care financing and delivery. Sustainability of HIV patient care requires ongoing attention to interdisciplinary care team support, quality improvement, adequate funding, and patient-centered models of care, regardless of the sites where care is provided.

KEY POINTS

- Clarification of roles and ongoing communication within the interdisciplinary team can help support the efficiency and effectiveness of patient care.

- Creating a shared patient registry and database is helpful to monitor, measure, and improve patient care across the HIV continuum of care.

- Funding from the Health Resources and Services Administration's Ryan White HIV/AIDS Program is one of the central components of sustaining HIV/AIDS care in the United States.

- Patient- and community-centered care models are necessary to continue providing comprehensive and interdisciplinary care for patients with HIV as the epidemic evolves.

An interdisciplinary approach to HIV patient care is an essential component to diagnose, link, and engage/retain HIV-infected patients and eventually lead to viral suppression (Gallant, 2011; Mugavero, 2011). Ongoing evaluation and efforts to improve and ensure quality of the interdisciplinary HIV patient care model are thus important. Several considerations for sustaining the interdisciplinary HIV patient care model include optimizing the interdisciplinary care team, improving quality of care, ensuring adequate funds, and building patient-centered care models.

INTERDISCIPLINARY CARE TEAM

The interdisciplinary team approach is an important part of the interdisciplinary HIV patient care model. Ongoing communication among the interdisciplinary team and the patient is essential to ensure collaborative and patient-centered care (Gallant, 2011; Nancarrow, 2013). The complexity of the patient's medical and psychosocial needs can often be overwhelming, and learning the patient's priorities and making partnered decisions with the patient can help interdisciplinary coordination of care among health care professionals and the patient (Gallant, 2011; Mugavero, 2011). There are limited data on standardized ways of measuring interdisciplinary team care (Boyd, 2014). However, periodic internal review of the interdisciplinary member responsibilities and infrastructure can help improve and consolidate responsibilities of duplicating tasks and augment the efficiency and effectiveness of the team. The complexity of health care among patients with HIV is increasing as the health care system evolves. Thus, more research on the innovative, clinically relevant, patient-centered, and cost-effective interdisciplinary HIV care team is needed.

QUALITY IMPROVEMENT

The goal of the interdisciplinary HIV patient care model is to optimize patient health, decrease HIV transmission, and end the AIDS epidemic. A clear vision with focused efforts to improve clinical outcomes and quality can help to develop, improve, and sustain effective patient care practices (Gallant, 2011; Mugavero, 2011). An up-to-date and available patient registry with relevant clinical and retention data can help monitor and measure patient care outcomes. Use of available electronic medical record systems is helpful, but creating a separate data tool (e.g., an electronic spreadsheet) would also be beneficial. Examples of relevant clinical and retention data include adherence, missed appointments, recent contact information and outreach, detectable viral load, status of ART, and evidence of failing or failed primary care (e.g., development of antiretroviral resistance, new opportunistic infections, onset or worsening of comorbid conditions, or clinical decline).

In a resource-limited setting, targeted data collection may be beneficial instead of attempting to obtain all data at once. For example, it may be beneficial to prioritize and focus resources to high-risk and vulnerable patients such as those who have been out of care for more than 6 months or have detectable viral load. Available patient registry and data can also support the measurement of and improve patient outcomes by strategizing quality improvement projects. An example is the pneumococcal conjugate vaccine (PCV13) among patients with HIV. Having a registry would assist a team member to contact or collaborate with clinicians to strategize to contact patients by mail, phone call, or during vaccine visits to receive vaccination for PCV13.

In addition to the patient registry, if local or state public health, community, or funding organizations have available patient data, such as detectable viral load, linked or out-of-care patients, enrollment to outside services, or other socioeconomic status, this can help in gathering patient information as to why they are not retained in care and have detectable viral load. Also, some patients may be engaged in a facility while they are still registered as patients at another facility. Thus, sharing of data can help clarify and eliminate duplicating efforts to coordinate care among different health care facilities. Availability of such data may be limited to certain local or state public health, community, or funding organizations. If such data are available, they can also be relevant for both the health care facility and the local and state public health, community, and funding organizations to improve services and monitor outcomes along the HIV continuum of care. Moreover, understanding population-based health outcomes can help in the administration, coordination, and improvement of infrastructure and funding of HIV care in the community (CDC, 2014; Whitehouse, 2015).

FUNDING FOR HIV CARE

Studies have highlighted the failure of the health care system to optimally identify and retain HIV-infected persons in care (Gardner, 2011). Patients who do not know their HIV status and patients who know their HIV status but are not engaged in care with effective virologic suppression are estimated to transmit most of the approximately 40,000–50,000 new HIV infections each year in the United States (CDC, 2014; Gardner, 2011; Whitehouse, 2014). With decreasing overall mortality rates and no decrease in new infections, the population of HIV-infected individuals continues to grow (CDC, 2011). This continues to place an ongoing demand for sustainable funding of HIV care in the United States for the foreseeable future (Gallant, 2011; Health Resources and Services Administration AIDS Drug Assistance Program (HRSA ADAP), 2015; Mugavero, 2011). Currently, there are various HIV/AIDS funding sources in the United States, including the following: the HRSA's Ryan White HIV/AIDS Program, the CDC, the US Department of Housing and Urban Development's Housing Opportunities for Persons with AIDS (HOPWA) program, the Substance Abuse and Mental Health Services Administration (SAMHSA), state and local governments, and nongovernment affiliates. As of 2014, the largest funding source of HIV/AIDS care in the United States was the HRSA's Ryan White HIV/AIDS Program ($1.99 billion/total $3 billion) (The Henry Kaiser Family Foundation, 2014).

Health Resources and Services Administration's Ryan White HIV/AIDS Program

The HRSA's Ryan White HIV/AIDS Program funds continuing health care and services to patients living with HIV. Program funding is distributed among Parts A–F. Part A provides emergency assistance to eligible areas that are most severely affected by HIV/AIDS. Part B provides grants to all 50 states and the US territories or associated jurisdictions. Part C provides outpatient-based comprehensive primary health care for people living with HIV. Part D provides family centered care for women, infants, children, and youth with HIV/AIDS. Part F provides funds for a variety of programs, such as health information technology, social media, and outreach programs. The program also funds dental care, special projects, training programs, and minority AIDS initiatives. The program is known for its "wraparound" services to patients with HIV. However, coverage and requirements of Ryan White-funded programs may vary state to state, and grantees of the program should review eligibility and criteria of renewal (including required data collection and conformance with standards of care) (HRSA, 2015). The Ryan White HIV/AIDS Program is always the "payer of last resort."

In general, patients with HIV can benefit from eligible funds and services via the Ryan White HIV/AIDS Program regardless of their immigration status. Since the implementation of the Affordable Care Act (ACA), patients with HIV are able to enroll in eligible insurance regardless of their HIV diagnosis or chronic medication conditions. However, ACA coverage and funding sources of expanded Medicaid HIV/AIDS services may vary state to state. Some patients may still need extra coverage for co-payments, medical fees, and services that are not covered by patients' insurance but that may be covered by Ryan White HIV/AIDS Program funds (HRSA, 2015; HRSA ADAP, 2015; Sood, 2014).

Moreover, ART is essential and a standard of care in chronic HIV management. The cost of ART for a patient is estimated to be up to $12,000 per year (HRSA ADAP, 2015). Part B of the Ryan White Program includes the HIV/AIDS Treatment Extension Act of 2009 (Public Law 111-87), as known as the AIDS Drug Assistance Program (ADAP). ADAP is likely the most known funding source for patients with HIV. ADAP covers the cost of medications for the treatment of HIV disease, and it may be used to provide services that improve treatment. Different states have varied eligibility criteria and renewal processes, including documentation of income status (15 states established income eligibility at 200% or less of the federal poverty level), diagnosis of HIV, opportunistic infections, chronic medical conditions, and/or other service needs (HRSA ADAP, 2015).

Thus, the Ryan White HIV/AIDS Program is an important component of HIV patient care (HRSA HIV/AIDS, 2015; Sood, 2014). With the evolving health care system in the United States, clinical outcomes and the overall effect on the HIV continuum of care through the Ryan White HIV/AIDS Program and other funding sources are important to ensure allocated HIV patient care funds.

HIV PATIENT CARE MODEL

Effective team-based care for patients with HIV must ultimately be successful and sustainable within a rapidly changing and evolving system of health care financing and delivery. Because HIV patients are living longer with multiple comorbidities, there is a need for comprehensive HIV patient care. Thus, HIV care has increasingly shifted to an ambulatory, chronic disease model—patient-centered medical home or "one-stop shop"—that shares the challenges of underfunding experienced by other adult primary care settings in the United States (Chen, 2006; Gallant, 2011; Mayer, 2006; Mugavero, 2011). As HIV-specific care becomes more routine and widespread, and as comorbidities increase in an overall aging population, HIV care may become increasingly integrated into general primary care health systems rather than having specifically designated HIV services or sites. Thus, building integrated and patient-centered HIV patient care model requires more attention and established guidelines.

Recommended Reading

Boyd CM, Lucas GM. Patient-centered care for people living with multi-morbidity. *Curr Opin HIV AIDS.* 2014; 9(4):419–427.

Health Resources and Services Administration (HRSA HIV/AIDS). The Ryan White HIV/AIDS program. Available at http://hab.hrsa.gov/abouthab/aboutprogram.html. Accessed November 17, 2015.

Mugavero MJ, Norton WE, Saag MS. Health care system and policy factors influencing engagement in HIV medical care: Piecing together the fragments of a fractured health care delivery system. *Clin Infect Dis.* 2011; 52(Suppl 2):S238–S246.

The White House Office of National AIDS Policy. *National HIV/AIDS Strategy: Update of 2014 Federal Actions to Achieve National Goals and Improve Outcomes Along the HIV Care Continuum.* Washington, DC: The White House Office of National AIDS Policy; 2014.

References

Bauman LJ, Braunstein S, Calderon Y, et al. Barriers and facilitators of linkage to HIV primary care in New York City. *J AIDS* 2013; 64(1):S20–S26.

Boyd CM, Lucas GM. Patient-centered care for people living with multi-morbidity. *Curr Opin HIV AIDS.* 2014; 9(4):419–427.

Centers for Disease Control and Prevention. Revised guidelines for HIV counseling, testing, and referral. *MMWR Recomm Rep.* 2001; 50(19):37–40.

Centers for Disease Control and Prevention. Revised recommendations for HIV testing of adults, adolescents, and pregnant women in health-care settings. *MMWR Recomm Rep.* 2006; 55(14):1–17.

Centers for Disease Control and Prevention. HIV surveillance—United States, 1981–2008. *MMWR Recomm Rep.* 2011; 60(21):689–693.

Centers for Disease Control and Prevention, Division of HIV/AIDS Prevention. Understanding the HIV care continuum. 2014. Available at https://stacks.cdc.gov/view/cdc/26481. Accessed November 3, 2015.

Chen RY, Accortt NA, Westfall AO, et al. Distribution of health care expenditures for HIV-infected patients. *Clin Infect Dis.* 2006; 42:1003–1010.

Chu C, Selwyn PA. An epidemic in evolution: The need for new models of HIV care in the chronic disease era. *J Urban Health.* 2011; 88(3):556–566.

Conviser R, Pounds M. The role of ancillary services in client-centered systems of care. *AIDS Care.* 2002; 14(1):S119–S131.

Dombroski JC, Simoni JM, Katz DA, et al. Barriers to HIV care and treatment among participants in a public health HIV care relinkage program. *AIDS Patient Care STDs.* 2015; 29:279–287.

Dykeman M, Sternberg C, Jasek J, et al. A model for the delivery of care for HIV-positive clients. *AIDS Patient Care STDS* 1996; 10:240–245.

Family Health International. Establishing referral networks for comprehensive HIV care in low-resource settings 1-16. 2005. Available at http://pdf.usaid.gov/pdf_docs/Pnadf677.pdf. Accessed November 27, 2015.

Gallant JE, Adimora AA, Carmichael JK, et al. Essential components of effective HIV care: A policy paper of the HIV Medicine Association of the Infectious Diseases Society of America and the Ryan White Medical Providers Coalition. *Clin Infect Dis.* 2011; 53:1043–1050.

Gardner EM, McLees MP, Steiner JF, et al. The spectrum of engagement in HIV care and its relevance to test-and-treat strategies for prevention of HIV infection. *Clin Infect Dis.* 2011; 52(6):793–800.

Gardner LI, Giordano TP, Marks G, et al. Enhanced personal contact with HIV patients improves retention in primary care: A randomized trial in six U.S. HIV clinics. *Clin Infect Dis.* 2014; 59(5):725–734.

Gardner LI, Metsch LR, Anderson-Mahoney P, et al. Efficacy of a brief case management intervention to link recently diagnosed HIV-infected persons to care. *AIDS*. 2005; 19:423–431.

Gopalappa C, Farnham PG, Hutchinson A, et al. Cost effectiveness of the national HIV/AIDS strategy goal of increasing linkage to care for HIV-infected persons. *J AIDS*. 2012; 66(1):99–105.

The Henry Kaiser Family Foundation. Total federal HIV/AIDS grant funding. 2014. Available at http://kff.org/hivaids/state-indicator/total-federal-grant-funding. Accessed November 17, 2015.

Horberg MA, Hurley LB, Towner WJ, et al. Determination of optimized multidisciplinary care team for maximal antiretroviral therapy adherence. *J Acquir Immune Defic Syndr.* 2012; 60(2):183–190.

Health Resources and Services Administration. The Ryan White HIV/AIDS program. Available at http://hab.hrsa.gov/abouthab/about-program.html. Accessed November 17, 2015.

Health Resources and Services Administration AIDS Drug Assistance Program. Part B: AIDS Drug Assistance Program. Available at http://hab.hrsa.gov/abouthab/partbdrug.html. Accessed November 27, 2015.

Irvine MK, Chamberlin SA, Robbins RS, et al. Improvements in HIV care engagement and viral load suppression following enrollment in a comprehensive HIV care coordination program. *Clin Infect Dis.* 2014; 60:298–310.

Joint United Nations Programme on HIV/AIDS (UNAIDS). 90-90-90 An ambitious treatment target to help end the AIDS epidemic. 2014. Available at http://www.unaids.org/sites/default/files/media_asset/90-90-90_en_0.pdf. Accessed November 29, 2015.

Knowlton A, Arnstern J, Eldred L, et al. Individual, interpersonal and structural correlates of effective HAART use among urban active injection drug users. *J Acquir Immune Defic Syndr.* 2006; 41(4):486–492.

Kwait J, Valente T, Celentano, D. Interorganizational relationships among HIV/AIDS service organizations in Baltimore: A network analysis. *J Urban Health*. 2001; 78(3):468–487.

Magnus M, Schmidt N, Kirkhart N, et al. Association between ancillary services and clinical and behavioral outcomes. *AIDS Patient Care STDs* 2001; 15:137–145.

Mayer K, Chagutur S. Penalizing success: Is comprehensive HIV care sustainable? *Clin Infect Dis.* 2006; 42:1011–1013.

Mugavero MJ, Norton WE, Saag MS. Health care system and policy factors influencing engagement in HIV medical care: Piecing together the fragments of a fractured health care delivery system. *Clin Infect Dis.* 2011; 52(Suppl 2):S238–S246.

Nancarrow SA, Booth A, Ariss S, et al. Ten principles of good interdisciplinary team work. *Hum Resour Health.* 2013; 11:19.

Newhouse RP, Spring B. Interdisciplinary evidence-based practice: Moving from silos to synergy. *Nurs Outlook.* 2010; 58(6): 309–317.

Office of Civil Rights. Standards of privacy of individually identifiable health information. U.S. Department of Health and Human Services, 2003; 45 CFR Parts 160 and 164. Available at http://www.hhs.gov/hipaa/for-professionals/privacy/guidance/introduction/index.html. Accessed May 12, 2006.

Parry MF, Stewart J, Wright P, et al. Collaborative management of HIV infection in the community: An effort to improve the quality of HIV care. *AIDS Care.* 2004; 26:690–699.

Samji H, Cescon A, Hogg RS, et al. Closing the gap: Increases in life expectancy among treated HIV-positive individuals in the United States and Canada. *PLoS One* 2014; 8(12):e81355.

Shah M, Risher K, Berry SA, et al. The epidemiologic and economic impact of improving HIV testing, linkage, and retention in care in the United States. *Clin Infect Dis.* 2016;62 (2):220–229.

Sood N, Juday T, Vanderpuye-Orgle J, et al. HIV care providers emphasize the importance of the Ryan White program for access to quality of care. *Health Affairs.* 2014; 33(3):394–400.

US Department of Health and Human Services. Panel on Antiretroviral Guidelines for Adults and Adolescents: Guidelines for the use of antiretroviral agents in HIV-1-infected adults and adolescents. 2015. Available at https://aidsinfo.nih.gov/contentfiles/lvguidelines/AdultandAdolescentGL.pdf. Accessed November 15, 2015.

US Preventive Services Task Force. Screening for HIV: U.S. Preventive Services Task Force recommendation statement. *Ann Intern Med.* 2013; 159(1):51–60.

Wada N, Jacobson LP, Cohen M, et al. Cause-specific mortality among HIV-infected individuals, by CD4+ cell count at HAART initiation, compared with HIV-uninfected individuals. *AIDS.* 2014; 28:257–265.

The White House Office of National AIDS Policy. *National HIV/AIDS Strategy: Update of 2014 Federal Actions to Achieve National Goals and Improve Outcomes Along the HIV Care Continuum.* Washington, DC: The White House Office of National AIDS Policy; 2014.

16.

PALLIATIVE CARE AND END-OF-LIFE SUPPORT

Paul W. DenOuden

Revised by Jonathan S. Appelbaum

CHAPTER GOAL

Upon completion of this chapter, the reader should be able to demonstrate knowledge about palliative and end-of-life care in the context of HIV disease to better counsel and educate patients and their families in an effective, professional, and sensitive manner to engage the range of health care resources appropriate to best patient care.

CARING FOR THE TERMINALLY ILL PATIENT

LEARNING OBJECTIVE

Discuss the clinician's responsibilities in caring for the terminally ill person with HIV.

KEY POINTS

- Both providers and patients benefit when providers remain involved in patient care through all stages of illness, up to and including death.

- Hospice and palliative care principles can be easily learned, and many resources are available.

In the early years of the HIV/AIDS epidemic, caring for the terminally ill patient was a regular and inevitable part of the care of HIV/AIDS patients because the disease would inevitably advance to end stages in the pretreatment era. Most HIV/AIDS clinicians were dealing with terminal illness on a daily basis, and in dealing with multiple and recurrent opportunistic infections, there would come a point to focus on palliative/hospice care. Many US cities had multiple AIDS hospices for terminally ill patients. As treatment evolved and became increasingly successful, and especially in the late 1990s onward as death rates plummeted, many hospices closed or changed their focus to skilled nursing, and the daily focus of clinicians became much more geared toward ongoing care of stable patients. However, given the still significant death rates and changing dynamics of causes of mortality in HIV/AIDS patients, it is still important for HIV/AIDS clinicians to be comfortable with and fluent in caring for patients with terminal illnesses. The numbers of end-stage opportunistic infections have decreased, whereas the numbers of malignancies, end-stage liver disease, cardiovascular disease, and age-related comorbidities have increased.

It is important to not lose focus on maintaining a close provider–patient relationship in the transition to terminal illness; the provider not only has a responsibility to the patient to journey with him or her through chronic illness to recovery, stabilization, or death but also has a responsibility to him- or herself to do so. By caring for the dying and attempting to provide patients with "good" deaths, physicians may feel a sense of professional satisfaction. Providing good end-of-life care may make physicians better communicators, helping them to better understand and treat suffering while offering them a deeper understanding of the nature of life (Block, 2001; Cherny, 1996).

It is important to reassure patients that they will not be abandoned when hospice care has begun. Patients and their families usually prefer their primary physicians to stay in contact until death, even if the main tasks of palliative care are taken on by another clinician (Han, 2005). Maintaining contact throughout the dying process is most likely the best policy, within reasonable bounds of previous clinical involvement (Quill, 1995).

Recommended Reading

Emanuel LL, Ferris FD, von Gunten CF, et al. In *Education in Palliative and End-of-Life Care—Oncology*. Chicago, IL: The EPEC Project; 2005.

HOSPICE CARE

LEARNING OBJECTIVE

Discuss indications, advantages, and disadvantages of hospice care.

KEY POINTS

- Hospice care involves an interdisciplinary approach to diagnosing and managing suffering and addressing the physical, psychosocial, and spiritual needs of patients and their families.

- Hospice care should be considered when no further interventions or treatments can cure or prolong the life of a terminally ill patient with an estimated life expectancy of 6 months or less.

- Making the decision for hospice care is often challenging for the patient, family, and clinicians alike in the antiretroviral therapy (ART) era of HIV treatment.

- There are often various options for hospice, including inpatient and home hospice programs.

DEFINITION OF HOSPICE CARE

Hospice care is defined as a comprehensive system of care for patients with limited life expectancy. This system is mobile and can take place both at home and in institutional settings. Hospice care works from a *biopsychosocial* model rather than a *disease* model, and it focuses on comfort, dignity, and personal growth at life's end. This encompasses biomedical, psychosocial, and spiritual aspects of the dying experience, emphasizing quality of life and healing or strengthening of interpersonal relationships rather than prolonging the dying process at any cost. A quality hospice program comprises an interdisciplinary team of experts that deals with all aspects of the dying process (Emanuel, 2005).

Often, people may interchange the terms "palliative care" and "hospice care." Palliative care is used to address

suffering at any stage of illness, from diagnosis to recovery or death. Hospice is a formal structured environment for delivering quality palliative care at the end of life. In the context of cancer, palliative care has been defined by the World Health Organization (WHO, 1990) as

the active total care of patients whose disease is not responsive to curative treatment. Control of pain, of other symptoms, and of psychological, social, and spiritual problems, is paramount. The goal of palliative care is to achieve the best quality of life for patients and their families.

The subset of palliative care tailored to the terminally ill and associated with hospice care is more accurately termed "end-of-life care."

INDICATIONS FOR HOSPICE CARE

In the early days of the HIV epidemic in the United States, death was common and survival unusual. Advances in ART and treatment of AIDS-related illnesses have resulted in dramatic increases in the life expectancy of HIV-infected people. Unfortunately, several end-stage conditions remain very difficult to treat in patients with extensive antiretroviral resistance or in patients who refuse or cannot tolerate medications. It may be appropriate in these circumstances to discuss end-stage options. In this way, hospice care can focus on comfort and quality of life rather than on treatments with uncomfortable side effects and no further benefit.

One study found that the cause of death of HIV-infected patients in the ART era is increasingly likely to be a chronic medical condition such as hepatic failure or malignancies, with "traditional" opportunistic infections (OIs) declining in importance (Sansone, 2000). Crum and colleagues found that 80% of pre-ART deaths were related to AIDS-defining conditions. This declined to 65% in the early post-ART era and reduced further to 56% in the late post-ART era (Crum, 2006).

Since the advent of ART, the biology of HIV and AIDS has shifted, requiring both patients and health care providers to consider the cumulative impact of chronic HIV infection and the long-term side effects of treatment. With longer life spans, people with HIV have become prone to diseases of aging—such as heart disease, diabetes, and osteoporosis—and to progressive conditions such as chronic viral hepatitis (Highleyman, 2005). Chronic viral hepatitis can lead to end-stage liver damage as patients coinfected with HIV and hepatitis B virus and/or hepatitis C virus live longer. Liver problems can also be related to antiretroviral drug toxicity, and ART can increase the risk of cardiovascular disease due to the blood lipid and glucose elevations associated with therapies that include protease inhibitors (Highleyman, 2005).

These changes in end-stage disease have resulted in changes in the approach that caregivers take to their HIV-infected patients and, thus, how physicians and other clinicians discuss end-of-life options with their patients as they reach the terminal phases of disease. However, it is important to keep in mind that AIDS-defining conditions may still appear, especially toward the end of life, and treatment and amelioration of OIs will still have a role in the end-of-life care (Welch, 2002).

ADVANTAGES OF HOSPICE CARE

Hospice and palliative care comprise an interdisciplinary approach to the diagnosis and management of suffering. Suffering is a multidimensional disorder of consciousness that includes physical, psychosocial, and spiritual elements. The unit of care in palliative care is the patient–caregiver dyad, with the needs of the family and loved ones being addressed along with the needs of the patient (Emanuel, 2005). Given that there is still stigma associated with HIV/AIDS and that, for many reasons, families are sometimes alienated from HIV/AIDS patients, special care needs to be taken with family dynamics issues that often come to the fore in hospice care with this population. As the usefulness of medical treatments diminishes, the effectiveness of psychosocial and spiritual interventions increases (Peterson, 1996).

When a patient becomes progressively weaker despite treatment, it is time to consider hospice care. Early hospice evaluation can provide great comfort to the patient and his or her loved ones. Palliative care clinicians are experts in pain and symptom management and can usually improve the patient's level of comfort. If symptoms do not respond to conventional medical therapy, addressing psychological and spiritual suffering may benefit the patient. Alternative and complementary therapies may be used, including relaxation, music therapy, meditation, herbal therapy, and acupuncture (Chesney, 1994; O'Neill, 1997).

It takes time to prepare for a good death, and the earlier a hospice referral is made, the more likely the patient will be able to benefit. Unfortunately, the average length of stay in hospice is only 2 weeks, which may be an indication of missed opportunities for referral.

Understanding, reconciliation, acceptance, and, for many, spiritual growth at the end of life may provide great comfort. Table 16.1 lists many of the practical issues involved in the care of dying patients (Cherny, 1996).

Table 16.1 PRACTICAL ISSUES TO BE ADDRESSED IN THE CARE OF DYING PATIENTS

ISSUE	SPECIFICS TO BE ADDRESSED
Communication	With patient • With family • With other participating caregivers
Symptom control	Physical • Psychological • Existential
Evaluation of family well-being	Coping • Resources
Evaluation of therapeutic plan	Primary therapies • Supportive pharmacotherapies • Hydration and nutrition
Contingency planning	Crisis planning • Addressing do-not-resuscitate orders
Ongoing care planning	Home/inpatient • Home care backup • Observation • 24-Hour availability of clinician with decision-making authority

SOURCE: Adapted from Cherny et al. (1996) with permission from Elsevier.

Many patients with terminal illnesses prefer to die at home, and patients and their families may want to consider end-of-life care at home using an interdisciplinary care management approach. Home hospice services can be cost-effective and can enhance quality of life for terminally ill AIDS patients (Huba, 1998). Home hospice care usually requires stable housing and willing family/partners/friends to help with the dying process at home. Sometimes this can be challenging to accomplish for many social reasons, even if a patient is interested in pursuing home hospice.

DIFFICULTIES OF HOSPICE IN THE ART ERA

With the use of ART, death is less common and often less anticipated. Poor outcome is often related to nonadherence, and feelings of guilt and other emotional responses can become a major issue for the patient and the caregiver. People dying of AIDS tend to be younger and often suffer from depression and other mental illnesses that need evaluation and treatment.

Several issues can lead to difficult deaths, including the biology of HIV disease, provider and system barriers to accepting hospice care, family issues, and patients' values and choices. Patients can experience dramatic improvement even when close to death; however, deaths from comorbid conditions such as hepatitis and cancer are often more abrupt, unpredictable, and devastating (Karascz, 2003).

Many patients and providers may be very reluctant to abandon research and experimental treatment options, even in the late stages of disease. There is evidence that even patients with severe immunosuppression, very low CD4 cell counts, high viral loads, and/or symptomatic AIDS can still derive significant benefit from ART (Highleyman, 2005). This further complicates the choice to seek hospice care. Many people arrive at the end of life stripped of assets. Although hospice can find community support and provide services not covered by ordinary government and private insurance, most insurance coverage of hospice care, following the lead of Medicare rules, generally prohibits curative options for those seeking coverage for hospice and palliative care at the end of life (Scalia-Foley, 2004).

Patients may face very difficult decisions in choosing to stop ART, both for symptom control and psychological reasons, because so many have been conditioned to stay fully adherent and never stop ART, and the complications with hospice coverage make it more difficult to decide how they and their physicians should best face this challenge (Karasz, 2003). AIDS patients frequently do not fit the cancer model on which hospice often rests. For AIDS patients, an insurance program that requires cessation of ART or will not cover other treatments is often problematic and may result in difficulty in planning and decision-making. Generally, ART is not covered under the Medicare hospice benefit.

Recommended Reading

Sansone GR, Frengley JD. Impact of HAART on causes of death of persons with late-stage AIDS. *J Urban Health*. 2000; 77:166–175.

Welch K, Morse A. The clinical profile of end-stage AIDS in the era of highly active antiretroviral therapy. *AIDS Patient Care STDS*. 2002; 16:75–81.

World Health Organization. Cancer pain relief and palliative care: Report of a WHO expert committee. *World Health Organ Tech Rep Ser*. 1990; 804:1–75.

PALLIATIVE CARE

LEARNING OBJECTIVE

Discuss palliative care for common symptoms in end-stage HIV-infected patients.

KEY POINTS

- Pain control can be achieved via transdermal or subcutaneous infusion routes in palliative care when oral medications cannot be swallowed.

- Treating depression and fatigue symptoms often involves a combination approach of antidepressants, psychostimulants such as methylphenidate (Ritalin), and mental health support, and it can greatly aid quality of life in a palliative setting.

- Dry mouth and oral symptoms may need targeted antifungal or antiviral treatment along with mouthwashes, hydration, and oral swabs.

- Dyspnea is common and worsened by the anxiety it provokes. Treatment is directed and may include diuretics, bronchodilators, oxygen, and morphine, as well as anxiolytics. Also, nausea is a common problem in end-stage HIV disease, and it is often difficult to treat.

- Disturbing terminal respiratory secretions may be minimized with anticholinergic drugs such as scopolamine, hyoscyamine, and atropine to help minimize family distress at end of life.

Palliative care is often a major part of hospice care, but it can and should be used for any suffering patients even if they are not actively in hospice. Many end-stage symptoms can be successfully treated in a palliative care setting, making the end of life as comfortable as possible for terminally ill hospice patients. Common and distressing symptoms in terminally ill patients can often be easily managed.

The use of non-oral routes of medication delivery can be helpful in a palliative setting for other symptom management in addition to pain control. Examples of non-oral administration include rectal administration (prochlorperazine suppositories for nausea and diazepam suppositories for agitation), sublingual administration (lorazepam for hiccups or agitation), or subcutaneous/intramuscular administration (clonazepam or haloperidol for acute agitation) (Enck, 2002; Woodruff, 1999).

PAIN

A common fear of patients is that of pain. There are many medication approaches to pain control, and a common treatment model is given by WHO in its report on cancer pain relief and palliative care (WHO, 1990).

In the terminal phase of disease, oral medications become more difficult for patients, and alternate routes such as the transdermal approach have been shown to be safe and effective in patients with AIDS (Newshan, 2001). Another widely used route for effective pain medication delivery is continuous subcutaneous infusion, which is common in the hospice setting and has many potential advantages, including ease of administration/access, decreased infection site complications, less volume overload, and lower cost (Herndon, 2001).

SEIZURES

In patients whose terminal AIDS condition involves intracerebral masses or central nervous system (CNS) infections such as toxoplasmosis or CNS lymphoma, seizures can be a frequent symptom requiring management. There are several common antiepileptic drugs, and because no one drug has shown superiority over the others, they are often used interchangeably with substitution as needed for lack of effectiveness or side effects (Krouwer, 2000). Adding or increasing corticosteroids to treat related peritumoral edema may be indicated if seizures are occurring with a therapeutic antiepileptic drug level (Krouwer, 2000).

DEPRESSION, FATIGUE, AND SLEEP DISTURBANCE

Depression, fatigue, and sleep disturbance are all common and interrelated symptoms that can be addressed effectively in palliative care. Because fatigue and sleep difficulties are common manifestations of depression, effective standard antidepressant treatment (e.g., with a selective serotonin reuptake inhibitor (SSRI) or other appropriate psychopharmacologics) may need to be instituted (see Chapter 37 on psychiatric complications). Psychostimulants (e.g., methylphenidate (Ritalin) or dextroamphetamine) have been studied in the palliative care setting and have been found to be effective in treating depression, opioid-induced sedation, and fatigue. Often dosed in the morning and early afternoon, psychostimulants may improve the cognition, neuropsychological function, and energy of terminally ill patients and allow for better quality of life and interaction with loved ones during the final days of life (Dein, 2002).

DELIRIUM

Another related CNS symptom that many hospice patients experience is delirium, which is defined as a transient disorder of cognition and attention, often accompanied by disruption of the normal sleep–wake cycle (Enck, 2002). The causes of delirium are broad and include metabolic disturbances; acute infection and fever; brain metastases; hypoxia; and side effects of drugs frequently used in palliation, such as opiates and corticosteroids (Enck, 2002; Woodruff, 1999).

Management should be directed at the suspected cause; for example, if hypoxia is suspected, empiric oxygen can be administered via cannula/mask, and if a drug side effect is implicated, nonessential medications can be discontinued or the opioid changed (Woodruff, 1999). Sedation may be necessary to alleviate severe agitation, and neuroleptics, most commonly haloperidol (which can be given orally, intravenously, or intramuscularly as needed), are effective and can be titrated individually (Woodruff, 1999). In the last few days of life, an agitated delirium often termed "terminal restlessness" occurs in some patients (Woodruff, 1999). Benzodiazepines are commonly used in this situation because they specifically aid in relieving myoclonus, seizure activity, and restlessness. There are many options with varying half-lives and many possible routes of delivery, such as diazepam rectal suppository, sublingual lorazepam, and subcutaneous clonazepam.

PRURITUS

Pruritus is common and may be a symptom of dry skin, underlying organ dysfunction or tumor, or induced by opioid use (Krajnik, 2001; WHO, 1998). Directed treatment often includes topical steroid creams and emollients for dry skin (WHO, 1998). Systemic antihistamines, corticosteroids, and even SSRIs have been found to be of benefit (Krajnik, 2001; WHO, 1998). Nursing care for the skin can include colloidal oatmeal soap or baths and warm compresses for comfort.

DRY MOUTH

Dry mouth or oral mucosa breakdown has many etiologies, and symptom relief can be quite helpful for patient comfort. Often in AIDS, infections contribute to this problem, and treatment is related to the specific cause, for example, antifungals for oral candidiasis or antivirals for herpes simplex ulcers. Mouthwashes, hydration techniques such as use of ice chips or popsicles, and oral hygiene using mouth swabs called toothettes can also lessen discomfort (WHO, 1998). Painful aphthous ulcers can be aided by topical corticosteroid orabase and local analgesic agents (WHO, 1998), such as viscous lidocaine; use of thalidomide has also been shown to be effective in patients with AIDS (Woodruff, 1999).

HICCUPS

Hiccups can be difficult and multifactorial in nature. Promoting gastric emptying with metoclopramide can help (Kinzbrunner, 2002). Treating esophagitis, a common cause of hiccups in AIDS (Albrecht, 1994), can be accomplished with antifungals and antacids as appropriate. Symptomatic treatment often includes chlorpromazine (Thorazine) or baclofen trials to calm the CNS response (Kinzbrunner, 2002).

DYSPNEA

Dyspnea is a common end-of-life symptom and can be an unpleasant sensation causing much anxiety to the patient, which often exacerbates the breathlessness. As with other symptoms, the causes are highly variable, and treatment is always directed to the root cause when known. For example, diuretics may be helpful in cases of congestive heart failure or fluid overload, and significant pleural effusions can be drained for symptom relief. If bronchospasm is noted, inhaled bronchodilators can be used, often in nebulized form with a mask if the patient is unable to use a metered-dose inhaler; systemic corticosteroids can also cause effective bronchodilation. Oxygen therapy is of benefit if the patient is hypoxic (e.g., pulse oximeter saturation <90%) and can be titrated for comfort via either nasal prongs or face mask.

Many patients may remain dyspneic even with oxygen use and other interventions, and the use of morphine may be indicated for the relief of continued respiratory symptoms rather than solely for pain control because morphine has been shown to decrease the respiratory rate and sensation of air hunger. Morphine also has the benefit of administration via the oral, subcutaneous, intravenous, intramuscular, or even the nebulized route. The anxiety that accompanies and often worsens dyspnea can be managed using any of the benzodiazepines via any appropriate route and timing schedule (Enck, 2002; Woodruff, 1999).

The final stages of the dying process are variable but commonly involve irregular or Cheyne–Stokes respirations and difficulty in clearing upper airway secretions. The sounds made by these retained secretions during respiration in this phase, often referred to as "death rattle" or "tracheal secretions," may be quite disturbing to family and caregivers of the terminally ill patient. Standard measures to reduce this potentially disquieting sound include positioning, decreasing parenteral hydration, and gentle suctioning, as well as antisecretory drug therapy. Several anticholinergic drugs have been reported to be successful, including scopolamine, atropine, and hyoscyamine (Levsin) (Wildiers, 2002).

NAUSEA

Intractable nausea is common in end-stage AIDS (Karus, 2005), and often the source of the nausea is elusive. The many possible causes of discomfort, including both side effects from therapies and direct effects of opportunistic infections, make therapies difficult to generalize (Karus, 2005; Reiter, 1996). The most effective method is to begin with a phenothiazine such as prochlorperazine or trimethobenzamide, increase the dose to the highest tolerable level, and then add another agent of a different class. Many classes of antiemetics are effective, including butyrophenones, benzodiazepines, benzamides, and cannabinoids. However, simultaneous use of three or four agents may be needed to provide adequate relief (Reiter, 1996).

CONCLUSION

The techniques described in this chapter can aid in providing maximum comfort to the terminally ill patient and allow for an end-of-life transition as dignified and healing as possible. Achieving this will also have a positive impact on the grief and bereavement process for the loved ones witnessing this final journey.

Recommended Reading

Enck RE. *The Medical Care of Terminally Ill Patients.* 2nd ed. Baltimore, MD: Johns Hopkins University Press; 2002.
Kinzbrunner BM, Weinreb NJ, Policzer JS (Eds.). *Twenty Common Problems in End-of-Life Care.* New York, NY: McGraw-Hill; 2002.
Woodruff R. *Palliative Medicine: Symptomatic and Supportive Care for Patients with Advanced Cancer and AIDS.* Oxford, UK: Oxford University Press; 1999.
World Health Organization. *Symptom Relief in Terminal Illness.* Geneva, Switzerland: World Health Organization; 1998.

References

Block SD. Perspectives on care at the close of life. Psychological considerations, growth, and transcendence at the end of life: the art of the possible. *JAMA.* 2001;285:2898–2905.
Cherny NI, Coyle N, Foley KM. Guidelines in the care of the dying cancer patient. *Hematol Oncol Clin North Am.* 1996;10:261–286.
Chesney MA, Folkman S. Psychological impact of HIV disease and implications for intervention. *Psychiatr Clin North Am.* 1994;17:163–182.
Crum NF, Riffenburgh RH, Wegner S, et al. Comparisons of causes of death and mortality rates among HIV-infected persons: analysis of the pre-, early, and late HAART (highly active antiretroviral therapy) eras. *J Acquir Immune Defic Syndr.* 2006;41:194–200.
Dein S, George R. A place for psychostimulants in palliative care? *J Palliat Care.* 2002;18:196–199.
Han PK, Arnold RM. Palliative care services, patient abandonment, and the scope of physicians' responsibilities in end-of-life care. *J Palliat Med.* 2005;8:1238–1245.

Highleyman L. Mortality trends: toward a new definition of AIDS? *BETA*. 2005;17:18–28.

Huba GJ, Cherin DA, Melchior LA. Retention of clients in service under two models of home health care for HIV/AIDS. *Home Health Care Serv Q*. 1998;17:17–26.

Karasz A, Dyche L, Selwyn P. Physicians' experiences of caring for late-stage HIV patients in the post-HAART era: challenges and adaptations. *Soc Sci Med*. 2003;57:1609–1620.

Karus D, Raveis DH, Alexander C, Hanna B, Selwyn P, Marconi K, Higginson I. Patient reports of symptoms and their treatment at three palliative care projects servicing individuals with HIV/AIDS. *J Pain Symptom Management*. 2005;30:408–417.

Kinzbrunner BM, Weinreb NJ, Policzer JS, eds. *Twenty Common Problems in End-of-Life Care. New York: McGraw-Hill*; 2002

Krajnik M, Zylicz Z. Understanding pruritus in systemic disease. *J Pain Symptom Manage*. 2001;21:151–168.

Krouwer HG, Pallagi JL, Graves NM. Management of seizures in brain tumor patients at the end of life. *J Palliat Med*. 2000;3:465–475.

Newshan G, Lefkowitz M. Transdermal fentanyl for chronic pain in AIDS: a pilot study. *J Pain Symptom Manage*. 2001;21:69–77. Herndon CM, Fike DS. Continuous subcutaneous infusion practices of United States hospices. *J Pain Symptom Manage*. 2001;22:1027–1034.

O'Neill JF, Alexander CS. Palliative medicine and HIV/AIDS. *Prim Care*. 1997;24:607–615.

Peterson JL, Folkman S, Bakeman R. Stress, coping, HIV status, psychosocial resources, and depressive mood in African American gay, bisexual, and heterosexual men. *Am J Community Psychol*. 1996;24:461–487.

Quill TE, Cassel CK. Nonabandonment: A central obligation for physicians. *Ann Intern Med*. 1995;122:368–374.Emanuel LL, Ferris FD, von Gunten CF, Von Roenn J. EPEC-O:Education in Palliative and End-of-Life Care—Oncology. The EPEC(TM) Project, Chicago, IL, 2005.

Reiter GS, Kudler NR. Palliative care and HIV, part II: systemic manifestations and late-stage issues. *AIDS Clin Care*. 1996;8:27–30, 33, 36.

Sansone GR, Frengley JD. Impact of HAART on causes of death of persons with late-stage AIDS. *J Urban Health*. 2000;77:166–175.

Scala-Foley MA, Caruso JT, Archer D, Reinhard SC. Medicare's hospice benefits: when cure is no longer the goal, medicare will cover palliative care. *Am J Nurs*. 2004;104:66–67.

Wildiers H, Menten J. Death rattle: prevalence, prevention and treatment. *J Pain Symptom Manag*. 2002;23:310–317.

Woodruff R. *Palliative Medicine: Symptomatic and Supportive Care for Patients With Advanced Cancer and AIDS*. Oxford: Oxford University Press; 1999 Enck RE, *The Medical Care of Terminally Ill Patients*. 2nd Ed. Baltimore: Johns Hopkins University Press; 2002.

World Health Organization. Cancer pain relief and palliative care. Report of a WHO expert committee. *World Health Organ Tech Rep Ser*. 1990;804:1–75

World Health Organization. Cancer pain relief and palliative care. Report of a WHO expert committee. *World Health Organ Tech Rep Ser*. 1990;804:1–75

World Health Organization (WHO). *Symptom Relief in Terminal Illness*. Geneva: World Health Organization; 1998

17.

HIV VIROLOGY

Schuyler Livingston, Benjamin Young, Martin Markowitz,

Poonam Mathur, and Bruce L. Gilliam

CHAPTER GOAL

Upon completion of this chapter, the reader should be able to demonstrate and apply knowledge about established and evolving science describing HIV virology, both in the cell and in the host, and to effectively counsel and educate patients and their communities regarding HIV virology.

HIV LIFE CYCLE

LEARNING OBJECTIVE

Discuss basic HIV virology and its relevance to current and potential drug targets.

WHAT'S NEW?

Expanded discussion of viral entry and integration into the host genome is presented.

KEY POINTS

- HIV is a member of the lentivirus subfamily of retroviruses.

- HIV enters the cell through use of the CD4 receptor and chemokine co-receptors, primarily CCR5 and CXCR4.

- The viral genome is transcribed from RNA to DNA by reverse transcriptase and integrated into the host genome by integrase.

- The HIV genome encodes 15 proteins comprising three categories: structural, regulatory, and accessory.

- After budding from the host cell, the virus matures into its infectious form through cleavage of viral precursor proteins by protease.

VIRAL CLASSIFICATION

Human immunodeficiency virus is a member of the lentivirus subfamily of retroviruses. Two distinct groups of viruses are pathogenic in humans: HIV-1 and HIV-2. Both are transmitted sexually and known to cause immunodeficiency disease. HIV-2 is less pathogenic and epidemiologically distinct from HIV-1. Subsequent discussion, therefore, focuses on HIV-1 infection and pathogenesis.

HIV-1 can be subclassified into three groups: M (major), O (outlier), and N (non-M, non-O) (Simon, 1998). The vast majority of HIV-1 infections belong to group M. Group M has at least nine known genetically distinct subtypes (or clades): A, B, C, D, F, G, H, J, and K. Occasionally, genetic material from different clades of HIV-1 may recombine within the same host to form hybrid viruses called circulating recombinant forms (Salminen, 1997).

VIRAL STRUCTURE

HIV-1 is an RNA virus, and its basic genomic structure is typical of other retroviruses. The integrated form of HIV is known as the provirus, which is flanked at both ends by a repeated sequence known as the long terminal repeats (LTRs). The genes of HIV are located in the central region of the proviral DNA and encode 15 distinct proteins

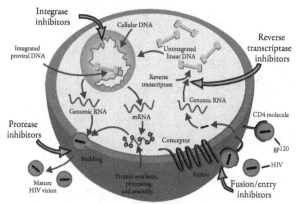

Figure 17.1 HIV life cycle and drug targets. SOURCE: Reproduced from Fauci (2003) with permission from Macmillan Publishers Ltd: *Nat Med*, copyright 2003.

divided into three classes: structural proteins (Gag, Pol, and Env), regulatory proteins (Tat and Rev), and accessory proteins (Vpu, Vpr, Vif, and Nef). In the mature HIV-1 virion, the inner capsid contains the viral RNA and key enzymes necessary for infection: reverse transcriptase, integrase, protease, and accessory proteins. (Figure 17.1). The capsid is surrounded by structural matrix protein, itself contained within the viral envelope. Composed of a phospholipid bilayer derived from the host cell, the envelope contains trimers of the viral glycoproteins gp120 and gp41. The exposed surfaces of gp120 exhibit a high level of variability,

limiting the humoral immune response to circulating virus (Tilton, 2009).

VIRAL ENTRY

HIV gains access to its target cells via multiple interactions of viral proteins with receptors on the cell membrane (Figure 17.2). The viral glycoprotein gp120 binds with high affinity to the CD4 receptor, which normally functions as a co-receptor in the activation of helper T cells. CD4 binding induces a conformational change in gp120, exposing its binding sites for co-receptors on the host cell surface. Viral strains vary in their co-receptor usage. Those that bind the chemokine receptors CCR5 or CXCR4 are classified as R5-tropic or X4-tropic, respectively.

During HIV transmission and early infection, R5-tropic strains predominate. Indeed, individuals who do not express CCR5, by virtue of genetic mutation, are highly resistant to HIV infection. Virus that remains R5-tropic is susceptible to HIV entry inhibitors, which bind CCR5 and alter its interaction with gp120. Through further evolution within the host, some HIV strains become X4-tropic, rendering them resistant to these agents. Following co-receptor binding, the viral glycoprotein gp41 inserts its hydrophobic fusion peptide into the target cell membrane, forming

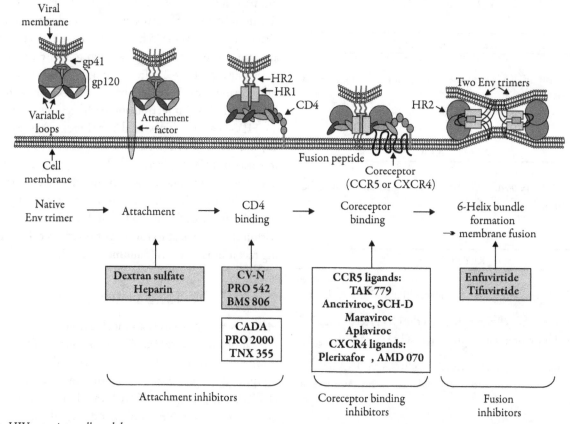

Figure 17.2 HIV entry into cells and drug targets. SOURCE: Reproduced from Reeves and Piefer (2005) with permission from Wolters Kluwer Health.

a pore through which the viral capsid enters (Tavasolli, 2011). This process, known as fusion, is the target of drugs that bind gp41 and prevent formation of the fusion pore.

REVERSE TRANSCRIPTION AND INTEGRATION

After fusion, the viral RNA is released into the host cell cytoplasm, shedding associated proteins in a process known as uncoating. The viral enzyme reverse transcriptase (RT) then produces double-stranded DNA from the viral RNA template. RT is a heterodimer composed of a functional subunit (p66) and a structural subunit (p51). The host enzyme APOBEC3G, a natural antiviral defense mechanism present in CD4$^+$ T cells and macrophages, causes hypermutation in the elongating viral DNA. The viral protein Vif, however, binds APOBEC3G and leads to its degradation (Table 17.1) (Tavasolli, 2011). Current therapies inhibit RT by competitive inhibition (nucleoside/nucleotide reverse transcriptase inhibitors (NRTIs)) or by an allosteric mechanism (non-nucleoside reverse transcriptase inhibitors (NNRTIs)). Pharmacologic agents aimed at blocking the interaction of Vif with APOBEC3G, or preventing dimerization of the RT subunits, may prove effective therapies in the future.

The newly synthesized viral DNA then integrates into the host genomic DNA. First, the viral DNA associates with viral proteins, including HIV integrase and the nuclear localization factor Vpr, to form the preintegration complex. Once in the nucleus, a critical interaction between integrase and the host protein LEDGF/p75 directs this complex to the host DNA, with a preference for actively transcribed genes (Tavasolli, 2011). Integrase then mediates strand transfer, in which covalent bonds link the viral and host DNA. Co-opting host cell proteins, HIV relies on the cell's normal DNA repair mechanism to complete integration. Currently available integrase inhibitors prevent strand transfer; agents targeting the interaction between integrase and LEDGF/p75 are under active investigation.

VIRUS PRODUCTION

Once integrated into the host DNA, the viral genome can remain latent or undergo active expression. In active infection, viral DNA is first transcribed into mRNA. Many of the same transcription factors involved in CD4$^+$ T cell activation also bind to the HIV LTR, promoting expression of the viral genome (Pereira, 2000). The resulting mRNA is spliced, processed, and ultimately translated into viral proteins by the host cell machinery. In a positive feedback loop, the viral protein Tat promotes further viral transcription (Kao, 1987). The viral protein Gag mediates assembly of progeny virions; immature forms then exit the cell in a process known as viral budding. Finally, HIV protease catalyzes the cleavage of the gag-pol precursor polyprotein (p55), yielding the structural proteins that form the mature virion. Protease inhibitors prevent viral maturation and have become critical agents in antiretroviral therapy.

Recommended Reading

Fauci AS. HIV and AIDS: 20 years of science. *Nat Med.* 2003; 9(7):834–843.

Greene WC, Peterlin BM. Molecular insights into HIV biology. *HIV InSite.* Available at http://hivinsite.ucsf.edu/InSite?page=kb-02-01-01. Accessed April 20, 2006.

Moore JP, Kitchen SG, Pugach P, et al. The CCR5 and CXCR4 coreceptors—Central to understanding the transmission and pathogenesis of human immunodeficiency virus type 1 infection. *AIDS Res Hum Retroviruses.* 2004; 20(1):111–126.

Reeves JD, Piefer AJ. Emerging drug targets for antiretroviral therapy. *Drugs.* 2005; 65(13):1747–1766.

HIV NATURAL HISTORY

LEARNING OBJECTIVE

Discuss the course of HIV infection and its dynamics in the host over time.

WHAT'S NEW?

Expanded discussion of acute infection, latent infection, and viral diversity is presented.

KEY POINTS

- In mucosal transmission, HIV crosses the epithelial barrier and establishes an expanding infection at the site of entry.

- During acute infection, HIV disseminates to lymphatic tissue throughout the body.

- The rate of fall in plasma viremia with highly active antiretroviral therapy (HAART) reflects the kinetics of different types of infected host cells.

- HIV exhibits remarkable levels of diversity, both globally and within a single host.

- HIV establishes latent infection in a subset of host cells, allowing it to persist despite HAART.

Table 17.1 VIRAL ACCESSORY AND REGULATORY PROTEIN FUNCTIONS

GENE	FUNCTION
Tat	Transcriptional transactivator
Rev	Allows unspliced viral genomes to leave the nucleus
Nef	Downregulates CD4 receptor and MHC class I, alters T cell activation, aids viral infectivity
Vif	Counters the host restriction factor APOBEC3G
Vpr	Facilitates the nuclear localization of the viral genome
Vpr	Downregulates CD4 receptor, increases viral release

ESTABLISHMENT OF INFECTION

In sexual transmission, HIV must first breach the epithelial barrier of the genital or rectal mucosa. This may occur via physical breaks in the epithelium related to trauma or sexually transmitted infections, particularly herpes simplex virus. HIV may cross intact mucosa via specialized dendritic cells in the genital tract or transcytosis in the gastrointestinal (GI) tract (Morrow, 2008). Upon breaching the mucosa, the virus encounters multiple potential target cells. Initial infection is likely to occur in dendritic cells, components of the innate immune system, which then deliver HIV to CD4+ T cells. In addition, the virus may directly infect local CD4+ T cells. In studies of the closely related simian immunodeficiency virus (SIV), resting CD4+ T cells are the predominant target cells at the site of entry in the vaginal mucosa (Zhang, 2004). This initial step represents a genetic bottleneck in which a large viral inoculum gives rise to a small founder population of infected cells. In heterosexual transmission, infection results from a single viral genotype in 80% of cases, with preference for the CCR5 co-receptor (Haase, 2011).

The eclipse phase refers to the period of approximately 10 days following mucosal exposure to HIV during which the virus remains undetectable in the plasma. Once a founder viral population is established at the portal of entry, it must expand locally before establishing a self-propagating infection in distant draining lymph nodes. In a chain reaction of cell-to-cell signaling, exposure to HIV induces vaginal epithelium to recruit plasmacytoid dendritic cells and ultimately more CD4+ T cells (Haase, 2011). From this locus of infection, dendritic cells may facilitate transport of HIV to draining lymph nodes. These early events may be altered to prevent infection, and they figure prominently in research on microbicides, pre-exposure prophylaxis, and preventative vaccines.

ACUTE INFECTION

Once infection is established in draining lymph nodes, activated CD4+ T lymphocytes become the predominant

source of viral replication. Immune activation increases the pool of susceptible activated CD4+ T cells, creating a positive feedback loop. An exponential increase in plasma viremia ensues, and patients may develop symptoms of the acute retroviral syndrome. HIV disseminates and infects other lymphatic tissues throughout the body. The CD4+ cell count in peripheral blood declines markedly. Meanwhile, a profound depletion of CD4+ T cells occurs in the gut-associated lymphatic tissue, where a large population of CCR5-expressing CD4+ T cells is present. Weakening of the GI mucosal immune response allows an increase in microbial translocation (Haase, 2011). This may provide a further stimulus to systemic immune activation, another positive feedback loop for the virus.

This unfolding of events in acute infection has long-term consequences for the patient. Fibrosis occurs in the lymphoid architecture, leading to incomplete immune reconstitution with HAART (Brenchley, 2004). Damage to the GI epithelium allows continued microbial translocation, likely contributing to chronic immune activation and progression to AIDS. Finally, a reservoir of latently infected cells is established, which later prevents viral eradication with HAART. In the rare cases in which HIV is diagnosed during primary infection, immediate antiretroviral therapy may have potential to limit, although not to reverse, these changes.

VIRAL KINETICS AND LATENCY

Plasma HIV RNA levels reflect a dynamic interplay between the infection of susceptible cells and the destruction of infected cells. With initiation of antiretroviral therapy, susceptible host cells are protected from infection. Consequently, the rate of decline in the viral load following initiation of HAART reveals the kinetics of death of HIV-infected cells (Figure 17.3) (Palmer, 2011).

Viral decay occurs in four distinct phases. The viral load declines dramatically in the first phase, reflecting clearance of activated CD4+ T cells ($t_{1/2}$ = 1 or 2 days), with roughly 90% of the decrease in plasma HIV occurring in these first weeks of therapy (Markowitz, 2003). The second phase, characterized by more gradual decline, correlates with the intermediate half-lives of partially activated CD4+ T cells, macrophages, and possibly dendritic cells. Plasma HIV continues to decline in the third phase, although at levels detectable only by ultrasensitive assays, and finally stabilizes at very low levels (<1–5 copies/ml) in the fourth phase. Research has focused on the resting memory CD4+ T cell as the source of viral replication during these latter stages. Despite fully suppressive HAART, the proportion of resting CD4+ T cells that are latently infected

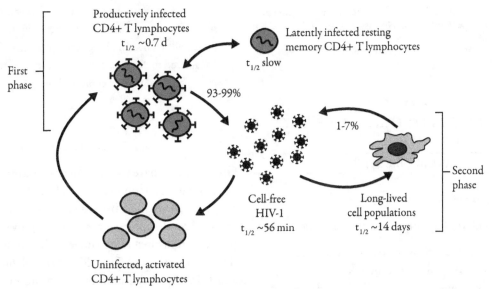

Figure 17.3 Rates of clearance of different cell populations and viral turnover. SOURCE: Reproduced from Simon and Ho (2003) with permission from Macmillan Publishers Ltd: *Nat Rev Microbiol*, copyright 2003.

shows minimal decline over time, yielding an estimated half-life of 44 months (Siliciano, 2003). By this estimate, HIV eradication would require approximately 60 years of uninterrupted HAART.

In light of this problem, increasing attention has turned to the mechanisms that maintain latent infection. Therapies that promote expression of the proviral genome, or activate resting CD4⁺ T cells, have the potential to speed decay of the latent reservoir, leading to eradication of HIV from patients receiving HAART. In latent infection, proviral DNA is integrated into the host genome but remains in a transcriptionally silent, but inducible, state. Several host transcription factors (NF-κB, NFAT, and P-TEFβ) and the viral protein tat promote expression of proviral DNA, but they are present at low levels in resting CD4⁺ T cells. In addition, histone deacetylation and DNA methylation at the HIV LTR alter the local chromatin environment, denying access to the machinery of transcription (Palmer, 2011). Drugs that prevent histone deacetylation (HDAC inhibitors) are under active investigation as a therapy to eradicate latent infection. At the level of the immune system, various cytokines promote the activation of resting CD4⁺ T cells. Ongoing studies are measuring the ability of interleukin-7 to deplete the latent reservoir in patients receiving HAART.

VIRAL DIVERSITY

During untreated infection, HIV replicates at a very high rate, with roughly 10 billion new virions produced each day in a given patient. Reverse transcriptase, in contrast to DNA polymerases, lacks proofreading activity (Taylor, 2008). As a result, frequent mutations occur in the daughter viral

genome, potentially altering the structure and function of viral proteins. The rapid rate of production, combined with frequent mutations, leads to the production of diverse quasispecies. Strikingly, the genetic diversity observed in a single individual after 6 years of HIV infection is roughly equivalent to that observed worldwide in influenza A virus within a given year (Korber, 2001).

This presents a unique challenge for the effort to produce an HIV vaccine. Historically, vaccines have prevented infection by stimulating antibody or cell-mediated immunity in susceptible patients. Both HIV and SIV have been shown to escape from these host immune responses by virtue of their extreme diversity. An effective HIV vaccine may need to elicit broad immune responses that protect against multiple quasispecies and possibly other HIV subtypes. The impact of viral diversity is well known to clinicians engaged in the treatment of HIV. The administration of multiple agents, so-called drug "cocktails," is required to suppress viral replication to levels at which drug-resistant strains are unlikely to emerge. Likewise, viral diversity underpins the importance of strict adherence to HIV therapy. More broadly, the continued evolution of HIV has necessitated the increasing use of resistance testing and the development of antiretrovirals with novel therapeutic mechanisms.

Recommended Reading

Finzi D, Blankson J, Siliciano JD, et al. Latent infection of CD4⁺ T cells provides a mechanism for lifelong persistence of HIV-1, even in patients on effective combination therapy. *Nat Med*. 1999; 5(5):512–517.

Harris RS, Liddament MT. Retroviral restriction by APOBEC proteins. *Nat Rev Immunol*. 2004; 4(11):868–877.

Mehandru S, Tenner-Racz K, Racz P, et al. The gastrointestinal tract is critical to the pathogenesis of acute HIV infection. *J Allergy Clin Immunol*. 2005; 116(2):419–422.

Persaud D, Zhou Y, Siliciano JM, et al. Latency in human immuno-deficiency virus type 1 infection: No easy answers. *J Virol.* 2003; 77(3):1659–1665.

Simon V, Ho DD. HIV-1 dynamics in vivo: Implications for therapy. *Nat Rev Microbiol.* 2003; 1(3):181–190.

OVERVIEW OF ANTIRETROVIRAL THERAPY

LEARNING OBJECTIVES

1. Discuss the goals of antiretroviral treatment.

2. Discuss the rationale for when to initiate antiretroviral therapy.

3. Discuss the current antiretroviral treatment guideline recommendations on which conditions indicate starting an antiretroviral regimen in a HIV-infected and treatment-naive patient.

4. Discuss the principles for antiretroviral regimen selection in HIV-infected, treatment-naive patients.

5. Discuss the principles of switching, or simplifying, antiretroviral therapy.

WHAT'S NEW?

HAART is associated with the potential to decrease both viral-related and non-viral-related comorbidities, as well as reduce levels of population-based HIV transmission. Guidelines for treatment now recommend starting HAART in all who are ready for treatment, regardless of CD4$^+$ cell count, to prevent comorbidities and transmission. Newer antiretroviral agents and regimens can improve tolerability and durable viral suppression in HIV-infected treatment-naive patients.

KEY POINTS

- Untreated and uncontrolled HIV replication is associated with HIV-related inflammation, accelerated aging, and a higher rate of comorbid illnesses that may be reduced with earlier initiation of HAART.

- Recent studies indicate improved clinical outcomes with treatment initiation at CD4$^+$ cell counts greater than 500/mm^3. Based on these studies, treatment is now recommended for all HIV-infected patients regardless of CD4$^+$ cell count.

- Treatment of HIV with HAART can reduce/prevent HIV-1 transmission.

- Choice of regimen is now focused on what is the best suited for the patient and his or her comorbidities to ensure adherence and long-term durability. The factors considered include medication tolerability and toxicities, resistance, and patient comorbidities.

INTRODUCTION

Great strides have been made in antiretroviral therapy since the introduction of zidovudine in 1987. The goals of therapy have evolved from delaying disease progression to maximal viral suppression and to improvements in thera-peutic options including single-tablet regimens. Following the introduction of HAART, AIDS-defining conditions and HIV-associated morbidity and mortality dramatically decreased. Treatment with HAART has been demonstrated to not only suppress viral replication and improve immuno-logic function but also decrease virus-related comorbidities (e.g., HIV-associated nephropathy (HIVAN) and AIDS-defining and non-AIDS-defining malignancies) and reduce HIV transmission. With these advances, many HIV-infected patients can now expect to live a near-normal lifetime.

Paramount to the success of HAART is the patient's willingness and commitment to adhere to lifelong therapy. In the past, acute and long-term adverse effects associated with HAART limited adherence to therapy, leading to treatment failure. However, with the advent of newer agents and better understanding of antiretroviral treatment management, current therapy combinations are now associated with less toxicity, reduced pill burden, and improved potency, allowing many patients to achieve greater than 95% adherence. However, additional concerns that may have a significant impact on antiretroviral treatment success include access to and the cost of long-term HAART (particularly in resource-limited areas); social and economic factors; drug–drug interactions; and comorbid medical conditions such as hepatitis B and C, liver disease, tuberculosis, cardiovascular disease, diabetes, osteoporosis or osteopenia, hyperlipidemia, renal disease, psychological disorders, and chemical dependency. Recognizing and addressing the individual barriers to adherence for each patient prior to initiation of antiretroviral therapy has had a dramatic effect on long-term treatment outcomes.

WHEN TO START ANTIRETROVIRAL THERAPY

Similar to the goals of antiretroviral therapy, the decision of when to start therapy in HIV-infected patients has also evolved over time. Early studies demonstrated a clear benefit of combination antiretroviral therapy in patients with AIDS (defined as a $CD4^+$ cell count <200 cells/mm^3 and/or an AIDS-defining illness) and symptomatic HIV-infection (Cameron, 1998; Hammer, 1997). Subsequent studies demonstrated decreased mortality or reduced risk of disease progression in treated patients with $CD4^+$ cell counts of 201–350 cells/mm^3 (Egger, 2002; Opravil, 2002; Palella, 2003). In addition, although the baseline $CD4^+$ cell count was the predominant marker that significantly predicted the probability of progression to AIDS and/or death, a plasma HIV viral load greater than 100,000 copies/ml was also associated with a higher probability of these risk events (Egger, 2002; Philips, 2004). These and other studies balanced the costs and toxicities of antiretroviral agents and eventually led to recommending initiation of antiretroviral treatment at $CD4^+$ cell counts greater than 350 cells/mm^3.

An analysis of 18 cohort studies in 2009 involving 21,247 patients reported a higher rate of progression to AIDS and death among patients who deferred therapy initiation until their $CD4^+$ cell count dropped below 350 cells/mm^3 compared to those who started HAART with a $CD4^+$ cell count of 351–450 cells/mm^3 (Sterne, 2009). This study advocated for initiation of HAART prior to the minimal threshold of 350 cells/mm^3 but found no significant rate of progression to AIDS and/or death among two groups starting therapy with a $CD4^+$ cell count threshold of 450 cells/mm^3. Meanwhile, the investigators of a large North American Cohort (NA-ACCORD) analyzed data from 17,517 patients with asymptomatic HIV infection and reported a higher risk of death among patients starting therapy with a $CD4^+$ cell count less than 350 cells/mm^3 compared to those who started therapy with a count greater than this threshold (Kitahata, 2009). In addition, these investigators reported a significant reduction in mortality among patients starting HAART with a $CD4^+$ cell count of 351–500 cells/mm^3 compared to patients with a count above this threshold. Although these investigators also found a mortality difference among patients starting HAART with a $CD4^+$ cell count greater than 500 cells/mm^3 (compared to a $CD4^+$ cell count less than this threshold), there were not enough risk events to demonstrate a significant difference between the two groups. Both of these studies demonstrated the benefit of earlier initiation of antiretroviral treatment; however, the results were interpreted differently by different groups globally at that time.

This changed in August 2015 with the publication of the results of the Strategic Timing of Antiretroviral Treatment (START) trial. In this prospective, randomized, controlled trial, asymptomatic HIV-positive adults were randomized to receive HAART at $CD4^+$ T cell levels greater than 500/mm^3 or were started on HAART only after $CD4^+$ T cell levels decreased below 350/mm^3 (the deferred-initiation group). A total of 4685 patients in 35 countries were followed for a mean of 3 years and assessed for a composite end point of serious AIDS-related events and serious non-AIDS-related events, including death from causes other than AIDS, only after $CD4^+$ T cell levels decreased below 350/mm^3. The study was stopped at an interim analysis because a significant benefit was demonstrated in the immediate initiation group. All patients in the deferred initiation group were offered ART. Importantly, no increased rate of adverse effects was observed in the immediate initiation group (START Initiation Group, 2015).

Due to the results of the START trial, the British HIV Association, the European AIDS Clinical Society (EACS), and the World Health Organization joined the US Department of Health and Human Services and the International Antiviral Society–USA in recommending starting all patients with HIV on ART. The data from the START trial prompted a cohesive global recommendation regarding initiation of ART for all patients with HIV/AIDS, eliminating the variability previously present for providers in different nations.

In addition to recent cohort and clinical trial data that support earlier initiation of HAART with respect to the baseline $CD4^+$ T cell count, arguments for initiating earlier HAART also include the following: the risks associated with HIV-mediated chronic immune activation leading to end-organ damage; the risks of increased occurrence and progression of comorbid conditions such as cardiovascular disease, non-AIDS-related infections and malignancies, and liver disease; and continued viral transmission (Cohen, 2011; Donnell, 2010; Ferry, 2009; Granich, 2009; Marin, 2009). In a multicenter cohort study involving 9858 patients (age 16 years or older), investigators suggested that non-AIDS-defining conditions (e.g., cardiovascular disease, non-AIDS-related infections and malignancies, and liver disease) were increased in association with advancing immunodeficiency (defined as a prolonged period below a $CD4^+$ T cell count of 350 cells/mm^3). This study noted that only an increased risk of cardiovascular disease and death were associated with an elevated plasma HIV viral load (>200 copies/ml), regardless of receiving HAART (the plasma viral load is considered a surrogate marker for HIV-related endothelial inflammation). Although there was also an association with liver disease-related deaths and an elevated plasma HIV viral load, patients receiving HAART appeared to have a protective effect. Another cohort of 1281 patients treated with a protease inhibitor-based regimen and followed over a median period of 7.3 years demonstrated that non-AIDS-defining conditions occurred at a higher frequency than HAART toxicities or AIDS-defining conditions (Ferry, 2009). In both of these studies, the investigators suggested that the best strategy for the reduction of non-AIDS-defining morbidity and mortality is earlier initiation of HAART. The earlier implementation of HAART was also demonstrated to reduce sexual transmission of HIV and clinical end points such as tuberculosis, bacterial infections, and death in a large cohort of serodiscordant couples in Africa (Cohen, 2011).

In addition to the recent data promoting earlier initiation of ART, the armamentarium of antiretroviral agents has expanded with many new drugs that have improved toxicity and side effect profiles, lower pill burdens, and easier dosing schedules. At the same time, our understanding of many aspects of HIV has also dramatically increased, including the impact of HIV on comorbid conditions and their effect on HIV progression, the role of mutation threshold of drugs and resistance, the importance of pharmacokinetics and drug–drug interactions, knowledge of side effects/toxicities and how to manage them, and the overwhelming impact of adherence.

CURRENT TREATMENT GUIDELINES

Current US guidelines published by the US Department of Health and Human Services (DHHS, 2016) and the International Antiviral Society–USA (IAS-USA; Gunthard, 2014) are similar and reflect the data and factors discussed previously in their recommendations of and cited level of supporting evidence for treatment in the following patients:

1. Those with symptomatic acute HIV infection, an AIDS-defining condition, and acute opportunistic infections (e.g., *Pneumocystis jiroveci* pneumonia, tuberculosis, or progressive multifocal leukoencephalopathy)

2. Asymptomatic patients with a $CD4^+$ T cell count less than 500 cells/mm^3: DHHS guidelines recommend treating all HIV-infected individuals, with the strength of the recommendation depending on the baseline $CD4^+$ T cell count: $CD4^+$ T cell count <350/mm^3 (AI), $CD4^+$ T cell count of 350–500/mm^3 (AII), and $CD4^+$ T cell count >500/mm^3 (BIII). IAS-USA recommendations are similar.

3. A rapidly declining $CD4^+$ T cell count (>100 cells/mm^3 per year) or a plasma HIV viral load greater than 100,000 copies/ml

4. Pregnant women

5. HIVAN

6. Hepatitis B (HBV) co-infection when treatment is indicated

In addition to the previous recommendations, the IAS-USA guideline also suggests initiation of HAART in patients older than age 60 years, those with active hepatitis C (HCV), and those with active or high-risk cardiovascular disease. The EACS and British HIV Association also recommend treatment in patients with comorbid conditions such as pregnancy and kidney disease. As noted previously, all of the guidelines now focus more on the patient's barriers to adherence and readiness for therapy, as well as the presence of comorbid conditions.

SELECTION OF AN INITIAL ANTIRETROVIRAL REGIMEN

Currently, there are more than 27 different antiretroviral agents that consist of six different mechanisms of action aimed at providing maximal viral suppression when used in combination (DHHS, 2016; Gunthard, 2014). The available classes of agents include NRTIs, NNRTIs, protease inhibitors, fusion inhibitors, CCR5 receptor antagonists, and integrase strand transfer inhibitors (INSTIs). When considering what treatment combination to start, providers should tailor the regimen based on the following factors:

1. Patient readiness and barriers to adherence

2. Cost, convenience (e.g., pill burden), dosing frequency, potential drug toxicities, and potential drug–drug interactions

3. Pregnancy state or potential among women of childbearing age

4. Comorbid conditions (e.g., cardiovascular disease, liver disease, kidney disease, co-infection with HBV and HCV, psychiatric disorder, and chemical dependency)

5. Viral resistance testing results (if available)
   Historically, treatment regimens evolved from the use of one or two NRTIs to a combination of two NRTIs and a third antiretroviral agent. Combination therapy with three or four NRTIs has demonstrated antiviral activity but either lacks comparable data with other regimens or has been shown to be inferior to other combination regimens (DART, 2006; Gulick, 2004). Because most clinical trial data have been based on the use of two

NRTIs, the treatment strategy for the past two decades has consisted of using two NRTIs with a third agent from a different class. Although this has been used with success, recent research has led to different approaches, such as class-sparing regimens. In particular, there has been an interest in nucleoside-sparing regimens to avoid metabolic toxicities and viral resistance while maintaining maximal viral suppression (Riddler, 2008).

Recommendations for antiretroviral regimens are similar among the DHHS (2016) and IAS-USA (Gunthard, 2014) guidelines as well as the British (Ahmed, 2015) and European (EACS, 2015) guidelines. The differences in the recommended agents are based on differing interpretations of clinical data. All of these combination regimens have been demonstrated to be efficacious. However, all individual antiretroviral agents and regimens have different pharmacokinetic profiles, drug–drug interactions, side effects, and toxicities. The optimal choice of agents for a regimen is dependent on the specific needs, situation, and comorbidities of the individual being treated. The critical issues to consider are adherence barriers and lifestyle (e.g., once- vs. twice-daily regimens, need for coadministration with food, and coformulated agents), comorbidities (e.g., hepatitis B, pregnancy, and kidney disease), and tolerability (side effects that the patient can tolerate). The successful regimen will be that which is well-tolerated and well-suited for the individual's lifestyle.

The guidelines have been drafted with the average patient and provider in mind. However, alternative regimens and strategies may also be effective for specific individuals. One of the important issues in the current treatment of HIV is the management of comorbidities and medication toxicities. Combinations listed as alternative or acceptable in the guidelines may be particularly well-suited for specific situations and should not be discouraged for the individual patient with those characteristics. Other treatment regimens may not currently have adequate data to allow them to be recommended as preferred or alternative regimens. Because our knowledge of antiretroviral agents is constantly changing, when new data are available, some agents or combinations may well be recommended or removed from the list of acceptable alternatives. The addition of new classes to our armamentarium also means that we do not yet know about many possible treatment combinations including agents such as the CCR5 antagonists and integrase inhibitors or the best combinations of these and other classes. A recent phase IIb randomized controlled trial with antiretroviral-naive adults showed that the investigational INSTI, cabotegravir, plus NRTIs had potent antiviral activity during 24 weeks of initial treatment compared to treatment with efavirenz.

When these patients switched to cabotegravir plus rilpivirine (NNRTI), antiviral activity was found to be the same as that of dual NRTIs and efavirenz at the end of a 96-week follow-up period. This study adds to the data that suggest that certain two-drug regimens, without NRTIs, might be acceptable for ART-naive patients (Margolis, 2015).

In the future, it is quite possible that the recommended combinations will change based on new data revealing efficacious combinations with the least toxicities (including metabolic, cardiovascular, and renal) and best long-term durability in formulations that facilitate adherence.

WHEN TO SWITCH OR SIMPLIFY ANTIRETROVIRAL THERAPY

Side effects or toxicities due to antiretroviral medications are often encountered in clinical practice. Because patients may have to take antiretroviral medications for a lifetime, side effects and toxicities must be addressed to avoid metabolic complications, decreased adherence, and virologic failure due to nonadherence. With the advent of newer agents with improved toxicity profiles, easier dosing schedules, and fewer pills, providers are often confronted with the question of whether to change individual agents or whole regimens. Although the optimum time for changing therapy remains undetermined, most studies have investigated changes in therapy for patients who have been controlled on a HAART regimen for at least 6 months. Reasons considered for changing therapy in patients controlled on their current regimen include the following (DHHS, 2016):

1. Reduce pill burden or dosing frequency

2. Reduce short- or long-term toxicity and enhance tolerability

3. Change food or fluid requirements

4. Minimize drug–drug interactions

5. Optimize ART regimen for pregnancy or in case of pregnancy

Switching to a simplified, less toxic regimen in patients with an extensive treatment history remains complex. Simply changing one agent may or may not be possible, and a complete review of the patient's treatment history, resistance testing, treatment tolerance, and drug–drug interactions should be conducted prior to designing a new regimen.

In general, two approaches to changing therapy in the virally suppressed patient have been utilized: changing one agent to another agent within the same class (within-class simplification) or changing one agent to an alternate class (out-of-class simplification) (DHHS, 2016). Changing one agent to another agent within the same class can potentially be associated with less toxicity, improved dosing schedule, and lower pill burden with newer and coformulated agents. For example, it is reasonable to change from drugs with higher toxicity rates and more frequent dosing, such as zidovudine or stavudine, to agents with improved toxicity profiles and less frequent dosing, such as tenofovir or abacavir (DHHS, 2016). Although previously viewed as less toxic, the NRTIs tenofovir, abacavir, and lamivudine are not without adverse long-term events. In a 2013 population-based study of approximately 100 patients, these NRTIs (stavudine and didanosine were not studied) were shown to inhibit telomerase activity, leading to accelerated shortening of telomere length in mononuclear cells (tenofovir was found to be the most potent inhibitor). This study suggests that NRTIs are a potential factor in contributing to HIV-associated accelerated aging, and switching patients off NRTI-based regimens may become a higher priority in the future (Leeansyah, 2013).

Other changes, such as switching from one NNRTI to another, may help to reduce toxicities and adverse side effects. In a randomized trial involving 38 men switching from efavirenz to etravirine due to central nervous system toxicity, researchers reported a significant reduction in adverse events in patients whose regimen was changed to etravirine, with all participants maintaining a suppressed viral load at 24 weeks (Waters, 2011). In addition, in a recent analysis of four randomized clinical trials, researchers found that patients on efavirenz were twice as likely to experience suicidal thoughts or attempt to or actually commit suicide as those not receiving efavirenz (Mollan, 2014).

The majority of studies investigating class switches have evaluated the replacement of a protease inhibitor agent to an alternative class, such as an NRTI, NNRTI, or integrase inhibitor. This can be done to reduce the toxicities experienced by the patient or to change to a simple, once-daily coformulated agent. Although this is generally successful in patients without resistance, it can lead to virologic failure in patients with previous underlying resistance, as was demonstrated in the SWITCHMRK study, in which patients who were randomized to change from boosted lopinavir to raltegravir had improved serum lipid concentrations. The study was terminated at 24 weeks due to a higher failure rate than that of those who remained on lopinavir/ritonavir (Eron, 2010).

SUMMARY

Currently, the critical issues in antiretroviral treatment are focused on the individual patient. Adherence and the patient's barriers to adherence remain paramount. These must be addressed prior to treatment initiation in order to achieve treatment success. Once the patient is "ready" for therapy, the key issues in the future will be the patient's medical comorbidities and medication toxicities. The WHO, EACS, and British HIV Association guidelines now recommend treatment of all HIV-infected individuals, regardless of the CD4+ count. The choice of agents/regimen is now dictated by the patient's comorbidities and lifestyle. Switching to newer agents must be done prudently, with careful consideration of the patient's resistance history and comorbidities. Just as there has been enormous progress in the past, it seems probable that we will continue to witness significant change in the future as we seek to find the optimal treatments for our patients.

Recommended Reading

Günthard HF, Aberg JA, Eron JJ, et al.; International Antiviral Society–USA Panel. Antiretroviral treatment of adult HIV infection: 2014 recommendations of the International Antiviral Society–USA Panel. *JAMA.* 2014; 312(4):410–425.

Johnson JA, Sax PE. Beginning antiretroviral therapy for patients with HIV. *Infect Dis Clin North Am.* 2014; 28(3):421–438.

US Department of Health and Human Services, Panel on Antiretroviral Guidelines for Adults and Adolescents. Guidelines for the use of antiretroviral agents in HIV-1-infected adults and adolescents. Available at https://www.aidsinfo.nih.gov/ContentFiles/AdultandAdolescentGL.pdf. Accessed February 10, 2016.

Sellers CJ, Wohl DA. Antiretroviral therapy: When to start. *Infect Dis Clin North Am.* 2014; 28(3):403–420.

Volberding PA, Deeks SG. Antiretroviral therapy and management of HIV infection. *Lancet.* 2010; 376(9734):49–62.

References

Ahmed N, Angus B, Boffito M, et al. British HIV Association guidelines for the treatment of HIV-1 positive adults with antiretroviral therapy 2015. Available at http://www.bhiva.org/guidelines.aspx. Accessed November 5, 2015.

Aiken C, Konner J, Landau NR, et al. Nef induces CD4 endocytosis: requirement for a critical dileucine motif in the membrane-proximal CD4 cytoplasmic domain. *Cell.* 1994 Mar 11;76(5);853–64.

Cameron DW, Heath-Chiozzi M, Danner S, et al. Randomized placebo-controlled trial of ritonavir in advanced HIV-1 disease. *Lancet.* 1998; 351:543–549.

Cohen MS, Chen YQ, McCauley M, et al. Prevention of HIV-1 infection with early antiretroviral therapy. *N Engl J Med.* 2011; 365:493–505.

DART Virology Group and Trial Team. Virological response to a triple nucleoside/nucleotide analogue regimen over 48 weeks in HIV-1-infected adults in Africa. *AIDS.* 2006; 20:1391–1399.

Egger M, May M, Chene G, et al.; the ART Cohort Collaboration. Prognosis of HIV-1 infected patients starting highly active antiretroviral therapy: A collaborative analysis of prospective studies. *Lancet.* 2002; 360:119–129.

Eron JJ, Young B, Cooper DA, et al.; the SWITCHMRK 1 and 2 investigators. Switch to a raltegravir-based regimen versus continuation of a lopinavir–ritonavir-based regimen in stable HIV-infected patients with suppressed viremia (SWITCHMRK 1 and 2): Two multicentre, double-blind, randomized controlled trials. *Lancet.* 2010; 375:396–407.

European AIDS Clinical Society. Guidelines. Version 8.0. October 2015. Available at http://www.eacsociety.org/guidelines/eacs-guidelines/eacs-guidelines.html. Accessed November 5, 2015.

Ferry T, Raffi F, Collin-Filleul F, et al.; the ANRS CO8 (APROCO-COPILOTE) study group. Uncontrolled viral replication as a risk factor for non-AIDS severe clinical events in HIV-infected patients on long-term antiretroviral therapy: APROCO/COPILOTE (ANRS CO8) cohort study. *J Acquir Immune Defic Syndr*. 2009; 23:1743–1753.

Granich RM, Gilks GF, Dye C, et al. Universal voluntary HIV testing with immediate antiretroviral therapy as a strategy for elimination of HIV transmission: A mathematical model. *Lancet*. 2009; 373:48–57.

Gulick RM, Ribaudo HJ, Shikuma CM, et al.; the AIDS Clinical Trials Group Study A5095 Team. Triple-nucleoside regimens versus efavirenz-containing regimens for the initial treatment of HIV-1 infection. *N Engl J Med*. 2004; 350:1850–1861.

Gunthard HF, Aberg J, Eron, J, et al. Antiretroviral treatment of the adult HIV infection: 2014 recommendations of the International Antiviral Society. *JAMA*. 2014; 312(4);410–425.

Hammer SM, Squires KE, Hughes MD, et al. A controlled trial of two nucleoside analogues plus indinavir in persons with human immunodeficiency virus infection and CD4+ cell counts of 200 per cubic millimeter or less. *N Engl J Med*. 1997; 337:725–733.

Heinzinger NK, Bukrinsky MI, Haggerty SA, et al. The Vpr protein of human immunodeficiency virus type 1 influences nuclear localization of viral nucleic acids in nondividing host cells. Proc Natl Acad Sci U S A. 1994 Jul 19;91(15):7311–5.

INSIGHT START Study Group. Initiation of antiretroviral therapy in early asymptomatic HIV infection. *N Engl J Med*. 2015; 373(9):795–807.

Kao SY, Calman AF, Luciw PA, et al. Anti-termination of transcription within the long terminal repeat of HIV-1 by tat gene product. Nature. 1987 Dec 3-9;330(6147):489–93.

Kitahata MM, Gange SJ, Abraham AG, et al.; the NA-ACCORD Investigators. Effect of early versus deferred antiretroviral therapy for HIV on survival. *N Engl J Med*. 2009; 360:1815–1826.

Klimkait T, Strebel K, Hoggan MD, et al. The human immunodeficiency virus type 1-specific protein vpu is required for efficient virus maturation and release. J Virol. 1990 Feb;64(2):621–9.

Leeansyah E, Cameron P, Solomon A, et al. Inhibition of telomerase activity by human immunodeficiency virus (HIV) nucleos(t)ide reverse transcriptase inhibitors: A potential factor contributing to HIV-associated accelerated aging. *J Infect Dis*. 2013; 207:1157–1165.

Luria S, Chambers I, Berg P. Expression of the type 1 human immunodeficiency virus Nef protein in T cells prevents antigen receptor-mediated induction of interleukin 2 mRNA. Proc Natl Acad Sci U S A. 1991 Jun 15;88(12):5326–30.

Margolis D, Brinson C, Smith G, et al. Cabotegravir plus rilpivirine, once a day, after induction with cabotegravir plus nucleoside reverse transcriptase inhibitors in antiretroviral-naive adults with HIV-1infection (LATTE): A randomised, phase 2b, dose-ranging trial. *Lancet Inf Dis*. 2015; 15:1145–1155.

Marin B, Thiebaut R, Bucher HC, et al. Non-AIDS-defining deaths and immunodeficiency in the era of combination antiretroviral therapy. *AIDS*. 2009; 23:1743–1753.

Miller MD, Feinberg MB, Greene WC. The HIV-1 nef gene acts as a positive viral infectivity factor. Trens Microbiol. 1994 Aug;2(8):294–8.

Mollan KR, Smurzynski M, Eron JJ, et al. Association between efavirenz as initial therapy for HIV-1 infection and increased risk for suicidal ideation or attempted or completed suicide: An analysis of trial data. *Ann Int Med*. 2014; 161:1–10.

Opravil M, Ledergerber B, Furrer H, et al.; the Swiss HIV Cohort Study. Clinical efficacy of early initiation of HAART in patients with asymptomatic HIV infection and CD4+ cell count >350 × 10(6)/1. *AIDS*. 2002; 16:1371–1381.

Palella FJ Jr, Deloria-Knoll M, Chmiel JS, et al.; the HIV Outpatient Study Investigators. Survival benefit of initiating antiretroviral therapy in HIV infected persons in different CD4+ cell strata. *Ann Intern Med*. 2003; 138:620–626.

Phillips A, Pezzotti P, and the CASCADE Collaboration. Short-term risk of AIDS according to current CD4+ cell count and viral load in antiretroviral drug-naive individuals and those treated in the monotherapy era. *AIDS*. 2004; 18:51–58.

Riddler SA, Haubrich R, DiRienzo AG, et al.; the AIDS Clinical Trials Group Study A5142 Team. Class-sparing regimens for initial treatment of HIV-1 infection. *N Engl J Med*. 2008; 258:2095–2106.

Schwartz O, Marechal V, Le Gall S, et al. Endocytosis of major histocompatibility complex class I molecules is induced by the HIV-1 Nef protein. Nat Med. 1996 Mar;2(3):338–42.

Sterne JA, May M, Costagliola D, et al.; the When to Start Consortium. Timing of initiation of antiretroviral therapy in AIDS-free HIV-1-infected patients: A collaborative analysis of 18 HIV cohort studies. *Lancet*. 2009; 373:1352–1363.

US Department of Health and Human Services, Panel on Antiretroviral Guidelines for Adults and Adolescents. Guidelines for the use of antiretroviral agents in HIV-1-infected adults and adolescents. Available at https://www.aidsinfo.nih.gov/ContentFiles/AdultandAdolescentGL.pdf. Accessed November 5, 2015.

Waters L, Fisher M, Winston A, et al. A phase IV, double-blind, multicentre, randomized, placebo-controlled, pilot study to assess the feasibility of switching individuals receiving efavirenz with continuing central nervous system adverse events to etravirine. *AIDS*. 2011; 25:65–71.

Willey RL, Maldarelli F, Martin MA et al. Human immunodeficiency virus type 1 Vpu protein regulates the formation of intracellular gp160-CD4 complexes. J Virol. 1992 Jan;66(1):226–34.

World Health Organization. Guideline on when to start antiretroviral therapy and on pre-exposure prophylaxis for HIV. September 2015. Available at http://www.who.int/hiv/pub/guidelines/earlyrelease-arv/en. Accessed November 5, 2015.

ACKNOWLEDGMENTS

The authors thank William Wright, MD, a contributing author of previous editions of this chapter.

18.

PRINCIPLES OF APPLIED CLINICAL PHARMACOKINETICS AND PHARMACODYNAMICS IN ANTIRETROVIRAL THERAPY

Neha Sheth Pandit and Emily L. Heil

LEARNING OBJECTIVE

- Describe the basic pharmacokinetic properties of the main classes of antiretroviral medications

- Explain the benefits of using ritonavir or cobicistat for pharmacokinetic enhancement of protease inhibitors and/or integrase inhibitors where relevant

- Review the potential role for therapeutic drug monitoring for antiretroviral medications

WHAT'S NEW?

- The pharmacokinetics of antiretroviral drugs in anatomical sanctuary sites or reservoirs such as the central nervous system (CNS) and genital tract has been extensively studied for the treatment of HIV-associated neurocognitive disorders (HAND) as well as for insights for disease prevention.

- There is continued interest in individualizing antiretroviral (ARV) dosing based on the genetic polymorphisms that affect metabolism and drug transport, such as cytochrome P450 (CYP) enzymes and P-glycoprotein (P-gp).

- Ongoing development of co-formulated fixed-dose combinations with drugs that share similar half-lives and long-acting formulations to decrease overall medication administration frequency will continue to offer convenient and well-tolerated treatment options that will help ensure adequate drug exposure and help maximize treatment outcomes.

KEY POINTS

- Systemic concentrations of antiretroviral drugs are influenced by the pharmacokinetic properties of absorption, distribution, metabolism, and excretion (ADME).

- Pharmacokinetics and local drug exposure can differ significantly within anatomical sanctuary sites compared with the systemic compartment.

- High variability in interpatient ARV concentrations is common, which makes population pharmacokinetics for ARVs very difficult to interpret. HIV replication is dynamic and requires combination ARV therapy with multiple active agents in order to achieve durable virologic suppression.

- Direct and indirect relationships between drug exposure, efficacy, and/or toxicity are common for most ARVs and can be used to improve overall treatment success.

- Suboptimal adherence can result in inadequate concentrations, drug resistance, and virologic failure.

- Therapeutic drug monitoring can be considered in certain scenarios that should be evaluated on a case-by-case basis.

Understanding the basic principles of applied clinical pharmacokinetics and pharmacodynamics can help the clinician gain insight into contemporary HIV pharmacotherapy and improve therapeutic responses. This information can be used to improve antiretroviral treatment for the individual patient by gaining a fundamental working knowledge of concepts that contribute to the occurrence of drug–drug interactions, adverse drug reactions, poor adherence, decreased efficacy, and the selection of viral resistance.

These factors alone or in combination can lead to treatment failure of antiretroviral therapy (ART) and subsequent progression of HIV disease. This chapter discusses some of the applied clinical pharmacokinetic and pharmacodynamic principles as they relate to the treatment of HIV.

The science of pharmacokinetics studies the amount of drug in various locations or compartments of the body and attempts to explain the effect that the body has on the drug through the assessment of multiple factors, such as (1) absorption or bioavailability of the drug, (2) distribution of the drug throughout body compartments, (3) metabolism of the drug, and (4) elimination or excretion of the drug from the body. Clinical pharmacokinetics is the application of these pharmacokinetic principles to the therapeutic management of a drug in a patient with the goal of enhancing efficacy while minimizing toxicity.

In contrast, pharmacodynamics examines the relationship between the drug concentration and response or the impact that the drug has on the body, which may have an intended or unintended pharmacologic effect. It also attempts to describe how drugs may interact with each other and display an additive effect $(1 + 1 = 2)$, a synergistic effect $(1 + 1 = 3)$, or an antagonistic effect $(1 + 1 = 0)$. An example is the combination of zidovudine and ganciclovir causing additive bone marrow toxicity resulting in neutropenia. The combination of zidovudine and stavudine has also been shown to be antagonistic because these drugs compete for the same site of action on the viral reverse transcriptase target (US Department of Health and Human Services (DHHS), 2016).

PHARMACOKINETICS

ABSORPTION

Absorption of medications highly depends on the route of administration. Oral formulations of ARV medications have varying degrees of bioavailability that affect a patient's serum ARV concentration. Currently, only zidovudine is available in an intravenous formulation, and enfuvirtide is the only ARV available for subcutaneous injection. Long-acting injectable formulations of rilpivirine and an investigational integrase strand transfer inhibitor (INSTI), cabotegravir, are under investigation for intramuscular administration (Margolis, 2015). For the solid dosage forms, tablets or capsules, absorption first requires the dissolution of the tablet or capsule, allowing the drug to be absorbed through the gastrointestinal (GI) tract and then into the systemic circulation from which it will be distributed to its site of action.

Drug absorption is a function of ionization and aqueous solubility, and this can be impacted by factors such as gastric pH, gastric mobility (emptying), absorptive capacity, biliary function, GI enzymes, splanchnic blood flow, CYP enzyme expression in the gut, and transporters such as P-gp. Absorption can be further affected under different patient conditions, such as use of nasogastric or percutaneous endoscopic gastrostomy tubes for medication administration, or when liquid formulations of medications are required, such as for pediatric patients or patients who have difficulty swallowing solid dosage forms. Many ARVs are available in oral solutions or suspensions to facilitate administration in these circumstances. The bioavailability of many ARV medications can be significantly compromised by manipulation of the dosage form, such as crushing tablets or opening up the contents of capsules (Bastiaans, 2014). For example, administration of crushed lopinavir/ritonavir tablets significantly decreased the exposure of both components, with a decrease in area under the plasma drug concentration–time curve (AUC) of 45% and 47%, respectively, compared to swallowing the tablets whole (Best, 2011).

Food can impact the bioavailability and rates of absorption for certain medications because food increases the pH in the stomach and delays gastric emptying to the small intestine, which is the site of absorption for many medications. For example, the relative bioavailability and maximum plasma drug concentration (C_{max}) of efavirenz are increased after a high-fat meal, and it is recommended that the drug be taken on an empty stomach (Sustiva package insert, Bristol-Myers Squibb, 2015). In addition, the solubility of a drug and surface area for absorption can be affected by gastric bypass procedures, which may impact the absorption of ART (Smith, 2011).

Some ARVs require an acidic environment for solubility to occur, and the dissolution of the drug can be impacted by acid-reducing agents. Atazanavir (ATV) is a protease inhibitor whose absorption is dependent on a highly acidic environment (Falcon, 2008). Up to 40 mg by mouth twice daily of famotidine with boosted and unboosted atazanavir was found to decrease atazanavir AUC by approximately 20% (Wang, 2009). A pharmacokinetic study of boosted atazanavir and omeprazole 40 mg reported a 76% reduction in atazanavir AUC and a 79% reduction in atazanavir trough concentration (C_{trough}) compared with boosted atazanavir alone (Agarwala, 2005). Increased gastric pH by acid-reducing agents such as proton pump inhibitors (PPIs) do not cause changes in absorption with other protease inhibitors (PIs), such as lopinavir/ritonavir, darunavir/ritonavir, or fosamprenavir (DHHS, 2016). Increased gastric pH will also decrease rilpivirine absorption, leading to suboptimal concentrations. Rilpivirine 150 mg was given with omeprazole 20 mg to 16 HIV-negative patients. Rilpivirine AUC and C_{max} decreased by 40%. Based on this study, PPIs are contraindicated with rilpivirine use, and H_2 antagonists should be taken 12 hours before or 4 hours after rilpivirine ingestion (Crauwels, 2008).

DISTRIBUTION

After ARVs are absorbed into the bloodstream, they distribute into the interstitial and intracellular fluids depending on the individual physiochemical properties (pK, molecular weight/size, and lipophilicity) of each drug (Minuesa, 2011). Many of the ARVs circulate in the bloodstream reversibly bound to plasma proteins. Albumin primarily binds acidic drugs, and α_1 acid glycoprotein primarily binds basic drugs. Only free, or unbound, drug is pharmacologically active, and the greater the free fraction of the drug, the better it distributes into tissues or compartments. A decrease in plasma protein binding may be seen in patients with cirrhosis or cancer (Morse, 2006). Unbound drug can enter cells or tissue primarily through carrier-mediated transport mechanisms, although some drugs can pass through via transcellular diffusion (Griffin, 2011).

The individual distribution characteristics of ARV compounds are under extensive investigation because each ARV drug may differ in the ability to penetrate into "sanctuary sites" throughout the body. These are areas where HIV can undergo compartmentalized viral replication with the potential to select resistant viral mutations due to suboptimal ARV drug concentrations within these sites. For example, HIV can reside within these anatomical sanctuary sites or reservoirs such as the male and female genital tract and/or the CNS (Pomerantz, 2002; Tseng, 2014). In addition, understanding drug distribution in the genital tract is essential for selecting agents for pre-exposure prophylaxis. Drug distribution to the male and female genital tracts is influenced by many patient factors, including hormonal changes, inflammation, concomitant sexually transmitted infections, and drug factors such as protein binding and lipophilicity (Trezza, 2014).

METABOLISM

Many ARV drugs, including chemokine receptor type 5 (CCR5) inhibitors, non-nucleoside reverse transcriptase inhibitors (NNRTIs), and PIs, are metabolized by CYP enzymes, which are located in the smooth endoplasmic reticulum in cells throughout the body, primarily the liver and intestines. Inhibition of gut CYP3A4 enzymes leads to increased bioavailability, whereas inhibition of liver CYP3A4 metabolism results in delayed elimination and a prolonged elimination half-life. Ritonavir is a highly potent inhibitor of the CYP3A4 enzyme, and coadministration of a subtherapeutic dose (~100 mg) of ritonavir is sufficient to enhance (or "boost") the pharmacokinetic profile of most of the currently licensed PIs (Larson, 2014). Cobicistat, an inhibitor of CYP3A enzymes, is approved by the US Food and Drug Administration (FDA) to provide pharmacokinetic enhancement to the PIs, atazanavir and darunavir, and the INSTI, elvitegravir. Due to its selective inhibition of CYP3A enzymes, cobicistat has less potential for off-target drug–drug interactions. Cobicistat has no anti-HIV activity and is also more soluble than ritonavir, facilitating the development of co-formulated products (Larson, 2014; Shah, 2013).

Pharmacokinetic enhancement of PI concentrations with ritonavir or cobicistat may have a number of benefits, including the following:

- Higher C_{trough} levels, reducing the risk of selection for drug-resistant viral quasispecies

- Higher plasma levels throughout the 24-hour day, minimizing the need for food requirements; reducing or eliminating the significance of interactions with other agents that induce the metabolism of protease inhibitors; and potentially lessening the effects of interpatient variations in drug levels due to factors such as gender, smoking, alcohol consumption, or liver disease

- Increased plasma half-life, resulting in reduced dosing frequency and pill burden

- Increased levels of "forgiveness" with missed or late doses, potentially delaying/preventing the development of viral mutations

P-gp is a cellular protein pump involved in transporting molecules in and out of the cell. P-gp is found extensively in the intestine, and its action is important in drug exposure and bioavailability. Protease inhibitors are known to be substrates for P-gp. Overexpression of P-gp by certain individuals may result in lower intracellular concentrations of some PIs and thus decreased overall drug exposure (Sankatsing, 2004). Ritonavir is a potent inhibitor of P-gp, whereas cobicistat is a weak P-gp substrate and inhibitor that does not lead to clinically relevant interactions (Larson, 2014; Shah, 2013).

EXCRETION

Antiretroviral drugs are eliminated from the body either unchanged by the process of excretion or converted to metabolites that may be more readily excreted. The kidney is the most important organ for the elimination of drugs and their metabolites, whereas the liver is the principal organ responsible for drug metabolism and biliary excretion (Verbeeck, 2009).

Renal and hepatic diseases are common progressive illnesses that occur frequently as comorbidities in the HIV population. Chronic kidney disease is a progressive condition marked by deteriorating kidney function and subsequent decreases in medication elimination. NRTIs are primarily eliminated via the kidney, with the exception of abacavir. If there is a decrease in the glomerular filtration rate (GFR) in chronic kidney disease, it may be necessary to decrease the NRTI dose or increase the dosing frequency interval to prevent high systemic drug concentrations that may lead to adverse drug reactions. It is important for the clinician to routinely check kidney function; it is recommended that kidney function be checked at least every 6 months (DHHS, 2016). The National Kidney Foundation Kidney Disease Outcomes Quality Initiative recommends the use of kidney function estimating equations of either Cockcroft–Gault or the Modification of Diet in Renal Disease (MDRD) for the routine estimation of GFR. Note that most FDA medication package insert dosage guidelines for renal impairment are based on only the Cockcroft–Gault estimating equation. Guidelines for renal dosage adjustments of ARV agents are provided in the most recent version of the DHHS guidelines (DHHS, 2016).

PHARMACODYNAMICS

The need to maintain adequate drug concentrations that are effective in controlling HIV replication and preventing resistance has resulted in considerable interest in the relationship between ARV drug exposure and virologic response or drug-related toxicity. This relationship is better known as therapeutic drug monitoring (TDM), and it is often used to optimize medication dosing to ensure efficacy and to help prevent toxicities. TDM has been well established with certain medications, such as digoxin, vancomycin, aminoglycosides, and immunosuppressants (Pretorius, 2011). However, the use of TDM for the routine management of ART is not without limitations. Specifically, there is a lack of large prospective studies showing improved outcomes, a lack of established therapeutic concentration ranges for antiretroviral agents, intrapatient variability in

concentrations, a lack of availability of Clinical Laboratory Improvement Amendments (CLIA)-compliant clinical laboratories that reliably perform ARV concentrations, and a shortage of experts to assist with analysis and application of ARV concentrations (DHHS, 2016; Pretorius, 2011).

The current strategy for using TDM for ARVs includes patients who may have compromised ADME. For example, absorption may be disrupted in patients with drug–drug interactions or impairment of GI, hepatic, and renal function. Distribution may be affected due to age, weight, and pregnancy. Metabolism may be affected in those who are on concurrent CYP P450 interacting antiretrovirals, and excretion may be compromised, leading to toxicities for patients with hepatic or renal impairment (DHHS, 2016; Pretorius, 2011). For patients who are experiencing virologic rebound, prior to TDM to assess the cause of failure, adherence to their treatment regimen should be thoroughly evaluated because this is the most common cause for treatment failure. Next, the current data on TDM in HIV-infected patients are discussed.

PROTEASE INHIBITORS

Almost all PIs are CYP3A4 substrates (nelfinavir is the exception); thus, there is a risk of drug–drug interactions with commonly used concurrent medications for other disease states, such as dyslipidemia, tuberculosis, and psychiatric conditions, that may induce or inhibit the same CYP enzymes. The most common example of this type of interaction is the boosting effect of ritonavir or cobicistat with other PIs or the INSTI elvitegravir, which was described previously.

A retrospective analysis of 240 HIV-infected patients on boosted and unboosted atazanavir found a direct correlation between ATV plasma concentrations and the incidence and severity of hyperbilirubinemia, percentage increase in triglycerides, and incidence of nephrolithiasis. These toxicities and increased plasma concentrations were seen mostly in the boosted atazanavir group, and the study suggests that concentrations greater than 800 ng/ml are likely the cause (Gervasoni, 2015).

NON-NUCLEOSIDE REVERSE TRANSCRIPTASE INHIBITORS

Similar to PIs, NNRTIs are also substrates of the CYP3A4 enzyme; however, the interactions are different in that they act as inducers as opposed to inhibitors, unlike the PIs. This still places the NNRTIs at high risk for drug–drug interactions and therefore potential candidates for TDM.

Unlike the PIs, NNRTIs have a low barrier to resistance. Single point mutations such as the K103N can cause resistance to first-generation NNRTIs. Second-generation NNRTIs, including rilpivirine, have a higher genetic barrier to resistance (Usach, 2013). The risk of virologic failure with efavirenz-based ART was associated with low efavirenz plasma levels in one small study (Marzolini, 2001). In a larger study, trough levels and AUC_{24} of nevirapine and efavirenz were not predictive of virologic failure, although for efavirenz there was an association between these parameters and virologic failure (Leth, 2006). An analysis of etravirine from the DUET trials failed to show any relationship between etravirine pharmacokinetics and efficacy or toxicities (Kakuda, 2010). Rilpivirine (RPV) is currently being studied as a long-acting subcutaneous injection that could be given at least every 4 weeks. Oral rilpivirine can be given at 25 mg daily, and doses for the long-acting formulation are currently being evaluated at 300, 600, and 1200 mg every 4 weeks. The plasma rilpivirine concentrations seen in the long-acting studies have been similar to those seen with oral RPV use (Williams, 2015).

Efavirenz-induced CNS toxicities have been correlated with elevated plasma concentrations (Marzolini, 2001). Through the use of TDM, elevated plasma efavirenz concentrations were reduced to the recommended therapeutic range while maintaining undetectable viral loads (Mello, 2011). Although subjects in this trial were stable on long-term efavirenz, a significant improvement in anxiety scores and a trend toward lower stress scores were noted with the reduction in concentrations. Efavirenz 400 mg was also compared to the standard 600-mg dose, and it was found that the lower 400-mg dose was non-inferior to the standard 600-mg dose for virologic suppression but was associated with fewer efavirenz-related adverse events (ENCORE1 Study Group, 2015).

INTEGRASE STRAND TRANSFER INHIBITORS

INSTIs are the newest class of ARVs, with the first agent, raltegravir, being approved in 2007. Raltegravir and dolutegravir are metabolized by UGT1A1, whereas elvitegravir acts similar to a PI because it is a substrate of CYP3A4 with the potential for many drug–drug interactions. A study that evaluated raltegravir 800 mg once daily compared to 400 mg twice daily, both given with emtricitabine/tenofovir, in treatment-naive individuals found that although patients in both groups had similar AUCs, a sixfold decrease was seen in C_{trough} in the 800-mg group (Rizk, 2012). Even with the decrease in C_{trough}, similar response rates were seen in

both groups, with a baseline viral load of ≤100,000 copies/ml. The once-daily dosing arm was statistically inferior to the standard twice-daily dosing arm in those patients with a baseline viral load >100,000 copies/ml and a $CD4^+$ T cell count ≤200 mm^3 (Eron, 2011). These findings highlight the importance of maintaining adequate raltegravir concentrations throughout the dosing interval in order to achieve desired virologic outcomes. Dolutegravir (DTG) 50 mg daily has been shown to achieve a 2.5 log decrease in HIV RNA after 10 days of DTG therapy (Lalezari, 2009). Similar results were seen with the use of elvitegravir, which resulted in a >1 log decrease in HIV RNA after once- and twice-daily dosing (DeJesus, 2006).

APPLIED PHARMACOKINETICS AND PHARMACODYNAMICS

CENTRAL NERVOUS SYSTEM EFFECTIVENESS OF ANTIRETROVIRAL DRUGS

The CNS is reached by considerable blood flow, but two anatomical barriers—the blood–brain barrier and the blood–cerebrospinal fluid (CSF) barrier—prevent the free passage of drugs into the brain (Calcagno, 2014). The CNS HIV Antiretroviral Therapy Effects Research (CHARTER) study group developed the CNS Penetration-Effectiveness (CPE) ranking scheme of CNS effectiveness of ARVs based partly on the physiochemical properties of the drug, such as lipophilicity, protein binding, and efflux substrate, that affect penetration into the CNS (Letendre, 2008). Regimens with higher CPE scores may have greater effectiveness in controlling HIV replication in the CSF. However, the use of CPE rankings to affect the course and severity of HAND has not been demonstrated consistently (Caniglia, 2014; Ellis, 2014).

THERAPEUTIC DRUG MONITORING

The combined use of didanosine (ddI) and tenofovir results in tenofovir-induced increases in ddI concentrations as well as a poor $CD4^+$ T cell count response with early virologic failure and rapid selection of resistant mutations (Negredo, 2008). Minimal data exist on the relationship between concentrations of new ARV agents such as dolutegravir, maraviroc, and darunavir and their potential for toxicities. A retrospective study of 1807 samples found that the majority of concentrations for ARVs are above the upper therapeutic threshold and could likely benefit from dose optimization using TDM (Cattaneo, 2014). The current dosing strategy for ARVs is to dose to ensure the highest probability of success despite lower doses with equivalent efficacy. Currently, the only ARV dosed to the lowest efficacious dose is rilpivirine. This dosing strategy has led to post-approval dose reduction in ARVs such as zidovudine, didanosine, and stavudine. Other medications that are efficacious at lower doses include efavirenz, lopinavir, ritonavir, atazanavir, darunavir, and raltegravir (Crawford, 2012).

CONCLUSION

The pharmacokinetic drug properties of ADME will determine the amount of systemic drug concentration that is available for the inhibition of viral synthesis. Other factors, such as drug–drug interactions, drug–food interactions, and concomitant comorbidities contributing to altered GI, renal, and hepatic function, may cause variations in the systemic drug exposure of the ARV agent. Pregnancy, sex differences, and genetic differences can also contribute to pharmacokinetic variability. It is important to note that due to these variables, the same dose of drug does not produce the same drug concentration among patients because of interpatient differences in ADME. Studies are currently underway regarding the use of pharmacogenomics to individualize dosing of ART to improve drug therapy outcomes while minimizing the risk of toxicities (Aceti, 2015; Bonora, 2015). Due to the high interpatient variability of ARV concentrations, it is also important to understand that drug toxicities and efficacy can occur at different plasma concentrations for all patients, and future studies may focus on individualizing treatment strategies.

SCENARIO

Consider the management of a treatment-experienced patient with virologic failure who was prescribed a raltegravir-containing, 3-class regimen in which the other agents are appropriate for once-daily dosing but the patient keeps missing one of the scheduled raltegravir doses. Although raltegravir 800 mg once daily is inferior to 400 mg bid in treatment-naive patients, in this example, for obvious adherence support, it would be acceptable to "compromise" and use the 800-mg once-daily raltegravir because concentrations would be higher than what would be achieved with 400 mg once daily. This would be a practical way to use pharmacokinetic and pharmacodynamic principles to help achieve and/or maintain viral suppression.

Recommended Readings

Pretorius E, Klinker H, Rosenkranz B. The role of therapeutic drug monitoring in the management of patients with human immunodeficiency virus infection. *Ther Drug Monit.* 2011; 33:265–274.

Trezza CR, Kashuba ADM. Pharmacokinetics of antiretrovirals in genital secretions and anatomic sites of HIV transmission: Implications for HIV prevention. *Clin Pharmacokinet.* 2014; 53:611–624.

References

Aceti A, Gianserra L, Lambiase L, et al. Pharmacogenetics as a tool to tailor antiretroviral therapy: A review. *World J Virol.* 2015; 4:198–208.

Agarwala S, Gray K, Wang Y, et al. Pharmacokinetic effect of omeprazole on atazanavir co-administered with ritonavir in healthy subjects [Abstract 658]. In: 12th Conference on Retroviruses and Opportunistic Infections; February 22–25, 2005, Boston, MA.

Bastiaans D, Cressey T, Vromans H, et al. The role of formulation on the pharmacokinetics of antiretroviral drugs. *Expert Opin Drug Metab Toxicity.* 2014; 10:1019–1037.

Best GM, Capparelli EV, Diep H, et al. Pharmacokinetics of lopinavir/ritonavir crushed versus whole tablets in children. *J Acquir Immune Defic Syndr.* 2011; 58:385–391.

Bonora S, Rusconi S, Calcagno A, et al. Successful pharmacogenetics-based optimization of unboosted atazanavir plasma exposure in HIV-positive patients: A randomized, controlled, pilot study (the REYAGEN study). *J Antimicrob Chemother.* 2015; 70:3096–3099.

Calcagno A, Di Perri G, Bonora S. Pharmacokinetics and pharmacodynamics of antiretrovirals in the central nervous system. *Clin Pharmacokinet.* 2014; 53:891–906.

Caniglia EC, Cain LE, Justice A, et al. Antiretroviral penetration into the CNS and incidence of AIDS-defining neurologic conditions. *Neurology.* 2014; 83:134–141.

Cattaneo D, Baldelli S, Castoldi S, et al. Is it time to revise antiretrovirals dosing? A pharmacokinetic viewpoint. *AIDS.* 2014; 28:2477–2479.

Crauwels HM, van Heeswijk RP, Kestens D, et al. The pharmacokinetic interaction between omeprazole and TMC 278, an investigational NNRTI [Abstract P239]. In: 9th International Congress on Drug Therapy in HIV Infection, November 2008, Glasgow, United Kingdom.

Crawford KW, Ripin DHB, Levin AD, et al. Optimising the manufacture, formulation, and dose of antiretroviral drugs for more cost-effective delivery in resource-limited settings: A consensus statement. *Lancet Infect Dis.* 2012; 12:550–560.

DeJesus E, Berger D, Markowitz M, et al. Antiviral activity, pharmacokinetics, and dose response of the HIV-1 integrase inhibitor GS-9137 (JTK-303) in treatment-naïve and treatment-experienced patients. *J Acquir Defic Syndr.* 2006; 43:1–5.

Ellis RJ, Letendre S, Vaida F, et al. Randomized trial of central nervous system-targeted antiretrovirals for HIV-associated neurocognitive disorder. *Clin Infect Dis.* 2014; 58:1015–1022.

ENCORE1 Study Group. Efficacy and safety of efavirenz 400 mg daily versus 600 mg daily: 96-week data from the randomized, double-blind, placebo-controlled, non-inferiority ENCORE1 study. *Lancet Infect Dis.* 2015; 15:793–802.

Eron JJ, Rockstroh JK, Reynes J, et al. Raltegravir once daily or twice daily in previously untreated patients with HIV-1: A randomised, active-controlled, phase 3 non-inferiority trial. *Lancet Infect Dis.* 2011; 11:907–915.

Falcon RW, Kakuda TN. Drug interactions between HIV protease inhibitors and acid-reducing agents. *Clin Pharmacokinet.* 2008; 47:75–89.

Gervasoni C, Meraviglia P, Minisci D, et al. Metabolic and kidney disorders correlate with high atazanavir concentrations in HIV-infected patients: Is it time to revise atazanavir dosage? *PLoS One.* 2015; 10:1–12.

Griffin L, Annaert P, Brouwer KL. Influence of drug transport proteins on the pharmacokinetics and drug interactions of HIV protease inhibitors. *J Pharm Sci.* 2011; 100:3636–3654.

Kakuda TN, Wade JR, Snoeck E, et al. Pharmacokinetics and pharmacodynamics of the non-nucleoside reverse-transcriptase inhibitor etravirine in treatment-experienced HIV-1-infected patients. *Clin Pharmacol Ther.* 2010; 88:695–703.

Lalezari J, Sloan L, DeJesus E, et al. Potent antiviral activity of S/GSK1349572, a next generation integrase inhibitor (INI) in INI-naïve HIV-1-infected patients: ING111521 protocol [Abstract TUAB105]. In: 5th Conference on HIV Pathogenesis, Treatment and Prevention; July 19–22, 2009, Cape Town, South Africa.

Larson KB, Wang K, Delille C, et al. Pharmacokinetic enhancers in HIV therapeutics. *Clin Pharmacokinet.* 2014; 53:865–872.

Letendre S, Marquie-Beck J, Capparelli E, et al. Validation of the CNS penetration-effectiveness rank for quantifying antiretroviral penetration into the central nervous system. *Arch Neurol.* 2008; 65:65–70.

Leth FV, Kappelhoff BS, Johnson D, et al. Pharmacokinetic parameters of nevirapine and efavirenz in relation to antiretroviral efficacy. *AIDS Res Hum Retroviruses.* 2006; 22:232–239.

Margolis DA, Boffito M. Long-acting antiviral agents for HIV treatment. *Curr Opin HIV AIDS.* 2015; 10:246–283.

Marzolini C, Telenti A, Decosterd LA, et al. Efavirenz plasma levels can predict treatment failure and central nervous system side effects in HIV-1-infected patients. *AIDS.* 2001; 15:71–75.

Mello AF, Buclin T, Decosterd LA, et al. Successful efavirenz dose-reduction guided by therapeutic drug monitoring. *Antivir Ther.* 2011; 16:189–197.

Minuesa G, Huber-Ruano I, Pastor-Anglada M, et al. Drug uptake transporters in antiretroviral therapy. *Pharmacol Ther.* 2011; 132:268–279.

Morse GD, Catanzaro LM, Acosta EP. Clinical pharmacodynamics of HIV-1 protease inhibitors: Use of inhibitory quotients to optimise pharmacotherapy. *Lancet Infect Dis.* 2006; 6:215–225.

Negredo E, Garrabou G, Puig J, et al. Partial immunological and mitochondrial recovery after reducing didanosine doses in patients on didanosine and tenofovir-based regimens. *Antivir Ther.* 2008; 13:231–240.

Pomerantz RJ. Reservoirs of human immunodeficiency virus type 1: The main obstacles to viral eradication. *Clin Infect Dis.* 2002; 34:91–97.

Pretorius E, Klinker H, Rosenkranz B. The role of therapeutic drug monitoring in the management of patients with human immunodeficiency virus infection. *Ther Drug Monit.* 2011; 33:265–274.

Rizk ML, Hang Y, Luo WL, et al. Pharmacokinetics and pharmacodynamics of once-daily versus twice-daily raltegravir in treatment-naïve HIV-infected patients. *Antimicrob Agents Chemother.* 2012; 56:3101–3106.

Sankatsing SUC, Beijnen JH, Schinkel AH, et al. P glycoprotein in human immunodeficiency virus type 1 infection and therapy. *Antimicrob Agents Chemother.* 2004; 48:1073–1081.

Shah BM, Schafer JJ, Priano J, et al. Cobicistat: A new boost for the treatment of human immunodeficiency virus infection. *Pharmacotherapy.* 2013; 33:1107–1116.

Smith A, Henrisksen B, Cohen A. Pharmacokinetic considerations in Roux-en-Y gastric bypass patients. *Am J Health Syst Pharm.* 2011; 68:2241–2247.

Trezza CR, Kashuba AD. Pharmacokinetics of antiretrovirals in genital secretions and anatomic sites of HIV transmission: Implications for HIV prevention. *Clin Pharmacokinet.* 2014; 53:611–624.

Tseng A, Seet J, Phillips EJ. The evolution of three decades of antiretroviral therapy: Challenges, triumphs and the promise of the future. *Br J Clin Pharmacol.* 2014; 79:182–194.

US Department of Health and Human Services, Panel on Antiretroviral Guidelines for Adults and Adolescents. Guidelines for the use of antiretroviral agents in HIV-1-infected adults and adolescents. Available at https://www.aidsinfo.nih.gov/ContentFiles/AdultandAdolescentGL.pdf. Accessed February 17, 2016.

Usach I, Melis V, Peris JE. Non-nucleoside reverse transcriptase inhibitors: A review on pharmacokinetics, pharmacodynamics, safety and tolerability. *J Int AIDS Soc.* 2013; 16:1–14.

Verbeeck RK, Musuamba FT. Pharmacokinetics and dosage adjustment in patients with renal dysfunction. *Eur J Clin Pharmacol.* 2009; 65:757–773.

Wang X, Chung E, Mahnke L, et al. Effects of famotidine on the pharmacokinetics of atazanavir when given with ritonavir with or without tenofovir in HIV-infected subjects [Abstract P30]. In: 10th International Workshop on Clinical Pharmacology of HIV Therapy, April 2009, Amsterdam.

Williams PE, Crauwels HM, Basstanie ED. Formulation and pharmacology of long-acting rilpivirine. *Curr Opin HIV AIDS.* 2015; 10:239–245.

19.

CLASSES OF ANTIRETROVIRALS

Benjamin Young

CHAPTER GOAL

After completion of this chapter, the reader should be familiar with the classes of antiretroviral medications and the factors influencing treatment dosing. The reader should also have an understanding of the US Department of Health and Human Services panel's recommended first-line HIV treatments and relevant clinical trials. The chapter also reviews recently approved co-formulated medications, pharmacogenomics, and clinical trials design.

MECHANISMS OF ANTIRETROVIRAL AGENTS

LEARNING OBJECTIVE

Describe the six different mechanisms of action of the antiretroviral classes.

WHAT'S NEW?

Final results of the randomized, international INSIGHT START clinical trial provide definitive proof of the benefit of antiretroviral therapy (ART) initiation in asymptomatic individuals with CD4+ counts greater than 500 cells/mm³.

KEY POINTS

- There are six different classes of antiretroviral agents: two types of reverse transcriptase inhibitors, two types of entry inhibitors, one class of inhibitors of HIV protease, and one class of inhibitors of HIV integrase.

- Combination ART is recommended for all people living with HIV.

Since 2012, the US Department of Health and Human Service (DHHS) panel has recommended combination ART for all people infected with HIV, irrespective of CD4+ cell count or clinical stage. In October 2015, the World Health Organization also strongly recommended the initiation of ART, without regard to CD4+ count. The large, randomized START clinical trial (INSIGHT START Group, 2015) provided conclusive evidence of the benefit of initiation of ART in asymptomatic people with CD4+ cell counts greater than 500 cells/mm³. START randomized treatment-naive individuals with CD4+ counts greater than 500 cells/mm³ to immediate initiation of ART versus delayed initiation when CD4+ counts declined to less than 350 cells/mm³. Overall, among those subjects who immediately initiated ART, there was a statistically significant reduction in progression to AIDS, cancer (Kaposi's sarcoma and non-Hodgkin's lymphoma), tuberculosis, and other serious health end points. This treatment benefit was observed among subjects in high- and low-income countries and did not differ across race or gender.

There are currently 27 unique US Food and Drug Administration (FDA)-approved agents to treat HIV with six different mechanisms of action licensed for treatment of HIV infection. The primary goal of combination ART is to achieve viral suppression (DHHS, 2016). Each antiretroviral class targets a unique step in the replication cycle of HIV-1 (Figure 19.1). The classes include nucleoside/nucleotide reverse transcriptase inhibitors (NRTIs/NtRTIs), non-nucleoside reverse transcriptase inhibitors (NNRTIs), protease inhibitors (PIs), fusion inhibitors (FIs), CCR5 co-receptor antagonists, and integrase strand transfer inhibitors (INSTIs).

NUCLEOSIDE REVERSE TRANSCRIPTASE INHIBITORS

NRTIs inhibit the HIV-encoded reverse transcriptase enzyme in the host cell cytoplasm. This blocks the

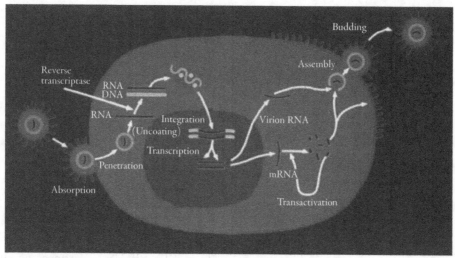

FIGURE 19.1 HIV Replication Cycle.

conversion of single-stranded RNA viral chromosome to double-stranded DNA, ultimately preventing incorporation of HIV genetic material into the host chromosome. NRTIs are nucleoside analogs; when reverse transcriptase incorporates them into the growing DNA, chain elongation is terminated. NRTIs must first be activated in the cell through three phosphorylation steps before they can become active chain terminators. NRTIs are poor substrates for human nuclear DNA polymerases, but some NRTIs can be utilized by human mitochondrial DNA polymerases and can cause toxicity.

NUCLEOTIDE REVERSE TRANSCRIPTASE INHIBITORS

NtRTIs and NRTIs act by the same mechanism; however, parent NtRTI compounds are monophosphorylated and therefore require only two enzymatic reactions to become active triphosphorylated moieties. Tenofovir DF (TDF) and tenofovir alafenamide (TAF) are the NtRTIs approved by the FDA for HIV treatment.

NON-NUCLEOSIDE REVERSE TRANSCRIPTASE INHIBITORS

NNRTIs also inhibit reverse transcriptase in the cytoplasm of the host cell. They act at the same point in the HIV-1 replication cycle as do the NRTIs, but NNRTIs bind the reverse transcriptase adjacent to the active site, causing structural alterations in the enzyme that sterically prevent it from adding any new nucleosides to the growing DNA chain. Because of this different mechanism of action, the viral mutations that encode for resistance to NNRTIs are different from those that encode for resistance to NRTIs.

PROTEASE INHIBITORS

Protease inhibitors act when a nearly mature virion is budding from the surface of the infected host cell. These compounds bind HIV-1 protease, preventing it from cleaving the gag precursor polyprotein, an essential process for HIV core maturation. Thus, the viruses that bud from the cell have immature cores, rendering them defective and unable to infect further host cells. First-line PI regimens that include a pharmacologically boosted PI characteristically are associated with no to very low rates of treatment-emergent drug resistance at the time of virologic failure.

ENTRY INHIBITORS

HIV entry inhibitors disrupt viral attachment or fusion by blocking the interactions between HIV envelope glycoproteins and host receptors. Enfuvirtide, the only FDA-approved fusion inhibitor, binds the HIV envelope protein gp41, preventing virus–cell fusion. Co-receptor inhibitors act by binding to the co-receptors CCR5 or CXCR4, resulting in allosteric changes that prevent HIV binding, attachment, and subsequent fusion. The only FDA-approved entry inhibitor is maraviroc, a CCR5 co-receptor antagonist. Use of maraviroc requires the testing of viral co-receptor utilization. Patients who harbor virus using CXCR4 or mixed co-receptors receive significantly less virological benefit from maraviroc.

INTEGRASE STRAND TRANSFER INHIBITORS

Integrase inhibitors inhibit the viral enzyme integrase, which is responsible for inserting HIV proviral DNA into the host cell's chromosomes. There are three FDA-approved integrase inhibitors (raltegravir, elvitegravir, and dolutegravir); two other integrase inhibitors are in late-stage development. Regimens that include an INSTI are associated with more rapid viral load declines and greater CD4$^+$ cell increases than NNRTI- or PI-based regimens.

Recommended Reading

Coffey S. Antiretroviral drug profiles. In: Peiperl L, Coffey S, Bacon O, et al. (Eds.), HIV InSite Knowledge Base. San Francisco, CA: University of California at San Francisco. Available at http://hivinsite.ucsf.edu/InSite?page=kb-00&doc=ar-drugs. Accessed November 30, 2015.

INSIGHT START Study Group. Initiation of antiretroviral therapy in early asymptomatic HIV infection. *N Engl J Med*. 2015; 373:795–807.

ANTIRETROVIRAL DOSING

LEARNING OBJECTIVE

Describe the usual dosing, dose modifications for weight or impaired renal or hepatic clearance, and food requirements for currently FDA-approved antiretroviral therapies.

KEY POINTS

- The selection of an antiretroviral (ARV) dose should take into consideration the drug concentration that inhibits viral replication and the drug concentration that causes toxicity.

- ARV dosing does not require precise timing; rather, current ARVs are dosed either once or twice daily without need for exact 24- or 12-hour dosing.

- Multiple factors affect drug exposures, including renal and/ or hepatic insufficiency, ARV food requirements, and drug–drug interactions.

The selection of an appropriate dosage of an ARV is based on the amount of drug needed to inhibit viral replication and the ability to physiologically obtain these concentrations without causing significant toxicities. Ideally, the maximum concentration should not cause adverse events, and the minimum drug concentrations at the end of a dosing interval should be in excess of the target concentration needed to inhibit viral replication.

Many antiretroviral agents are metabolized by the liver and/or eliminated by the kidney; thus, changes in hepatic or renal function can cause drug accumulation. This increases the potential for adverse drug events and might necessitate dosing changes. Food requirements are important to ensure optimal drug absorption or minimize adverse drug effects. Appendix B of the 2016 DHHS Guidelines (Adults and Adolescents) lists the standard dose, food requirements, and dosage adjustments in renal and/or hepatic impairment for the FDA-approved antiretrovirals. In those situations in which renal and/or hepatic impairment requires dosage modifications, the use of fixed-dose combinations (e.g., Atripla, Complera, Stribild, Triumeq, Genvoya, Adefsey, and Descovy) may not be possible; these situations may require the use of individual agents with the proper dosage adjustment for each agent.

Counseling patients on optimal dosing and adherence is critical to the success of antiretroviral treatment. Evidence-based guidelines for improving adherence are available and include recommendations for the routine collection of self-reported adherence data and the use of pharmacy refill data adherence monitoring (International Advisory Panel on HIV Care Continuum Optimization, 2015). Nearly all antiretroviral medications currently prescribed are dosed either once or twice daily. Note that this does not imply, nor require, that patients take their medications exactly every 24 or 12 hours but, rather, aim to take their medications within a more generous time window.

Many antiretroviral medications should be taken with food for optimal absorption. Some medications require an acidic stomach environment and may have negative drug–drug interactions with acid-lowering agents such as proton pump inhibitors (e.g., atazanavir and rilpivirine). Others require dietary fat for optimal absorption (e.g., rilpivirine). Counseling and patient adherence to dietary restrictions are important elements for optimal response to ART.

Recommended Reading

International Advisory Panel on HIV Care Continuum Optimization. IAPAC guidelines for optimizing the HIV care continuum for adults and adolescents. *J Int Assoc Provid AIDS Care*. 2015; 14(Suppl. 1):S3–S34. doi:10.1177/2325957415613442

US Department of Health and Human Services, Panel on Antiretroviral Guidelines for Adults and Adolescents. Guidelines for the use of antiretroviral agents in HIV-1-infected adults and adolescents. Available at https://aidsinfo.nih.gov/contentfiles/lvguidelines/adultandadolescentgl.pdf. Accessed January 30, 2016.

RECOMMENDED AND RECENTLY APPROVED ANTIRETROVIRAL AGENTS

LEARNING OBJECTIVE

Describe the DHHS-recommended initial ART regimens and recently FDA-approved antiretroviral agents in terms of their class, dosing requirements, adverse effects, and resistance profile.

WHAT'S NEW?

HIV integrase inhibitors are fast becoming the standard of care for initial therapy. The DHHS HIV treatment guidelines recommend first-line use of six antiretroviral regimens as preferred; five of these regimens are INSTI-based, and one is boosted PI-based. Boosted atazanavir- and NNRTI-based regimens are now classified as alternative. Cobicistat is the second pharmacologic boosting agent and available in new fixed-dose formulations with elvitegravir, darunavir, and atazanavir. Tenofovir alafenamide is a new prodrug of tenofovir that has lower risk of renal and bone adverse effects.

KEY POINTS

- The DHHS recommends one of six regimens for initial treatment of HIV.

- Five of the DHHS-recommended initial regimens include an HIV integrase inhibitor with two NRTIs.

- One DHHS-recommended regimen uses a pharmacologically boosted protease inhibitor with two NRTIs.

- Cobicistat is a new pharmacologic boosting agent.

- Tenofovir alafenamide is a new prodrug of tenofovir with improved pharmacodynamics and lower risk of renal and bone toxicity.

This section reviews and summarizes currently recommended initial ARV regimens and newly FDA-approved ARVs. Today's HIV treatments have revolutionized the prognosis for people living with HIV. Once a typically fatal disease, with care and modern treatment, patients can expect near-normal life expectancy, with low risk of AIDS-related complications and few, if any, significant side effects from medications. HIV treatment is prevention. Recent clinical trials data clearly demonstrate that even in asymptomatic people with normal CD4$^+$ cell counts, ART significantly reduces risk of death, serious illness (including tuberculosis and cancer), and HIV transmission. US and global HIV treatment guidelines now recommend treatment for all people living with HIV, independent of CD4$^+$ count or clinical stage. It is now very clear that the obstacles to achieving these goals are improving access to HIV testing and engagement and retention in care.

The selection of antiretroviral agents for the treatment of HIV is typically aided by evidence-based guidelines (Table 19.1). Among the most rigorous treatment guidelines are the "Guidelines for the Use of Antiretroviral Agents in HIV-1-Infected Adults and Adolescents" issued by the Panel on Antiretroviral Guidelines for Adults and Adolescents of the DHHS (DHHS, 2016).

Based on the results of several large, randomized clinical trials, the DHHS guidelines underwent dramatic revisions in 2015; all six recommended initial regimens include two nucleoside/tide reverse transcriptase inhibitors with either an integrase inhibitor (INSTI; five regimens) or a boosted protease inhibitor (one regimen).

These regimens are as follows (in alphabetical order, based on "third" agent):

- Integrase strand transfer inhibitor-based

  - Dolutegravir/abacavir/lamivudine (DTG/ABC/3TC; Triumeq)

  - Dolutegravir (Tivicay) plus tenofovir disoproxil fumarate/emtricitabine (TDF/FTC; Truvada)

  - Elvitegravir/cobicistat/TDF/FTC (EVG/cobi/TDF/FTC; Stribild)

  - Elvitegravir/cobicistat/FTC/tenofovir alafenamide (EVG/c/FTC/TAF; Genvoya)

  - Raltegravir (RAL; Isentress) plus TDF/FTC

- Protease inhibitor-based

  - Darunavir (Prezista) plus ritonavir (DRV/r) plus TDF/FTC

Previously recommended regimens of atazanavir (Reyataz), ritonavir (RTV, Norvir), and TDF/FTC and the NNRTI regimens efavirenz/TDF/FTC (Atripla) and rilpivirine (RPV)/TDF/FTC (Complera) have been reclassified as alternative regimens because of clinical trials data showing greater rates of treatment discontinuation or toxicity.

The DHHS panel recommends taking into consideration pretreatment conditions in selecting initial

Table 19.1 ANTIRETROVIRAL MEDICATIONS APPROVED BY THE FDA SINCE 2012

TRADE NAME	DRUG/DOSE	ARV CLASS(ES)	DOSE	FOOD REQUIREMENT
Stribild (2012)	EVG (150 mg) COB (150 mg) FTC (200 mg) TDF (300 mg)	1 NRTI + 1 NtRTI + 1 INSTI + 1 PK booster	1 tablet q.d.	Yes
Triumeq (2014)	ABC (600 mg) 3TC (300 mg) DTG (50 mg)	2 NRTI + INSTI	1 tablet q.d.	No
Prezcobix (2015)	DRV (800 mg) COB (150 mg)	PI + 1 PK booster	1 tablet q.d.	Yes
Evotaz (2015)	ATV (300 mg) COB (150 mg)	PI + 1 PK booster	1 tablet q.d.	Yes
Genvoya (2015)	EVG (150 mg) COB (150 mg) FTC (200 mg) TDF (300 mg)	1 NRTI + 1 NtRTI + 1 INSTI + 1 PK booster	1 tablet q.d.	Yes
Dutrebis (2015)	3TC (150 mg) RAL (300 mg)	NRTI + INSTI	1 tablet b.i.d.	No
Viteka (2015)	EVG (85 and 150 mg)	INSTI	1 tablet q.d.	Yes
Tybost (2015)	COB (150 mg)	PK booster	1 tablet q.d. with ARV or DRV	Yes
Adefsey (2016)	RPV (25 mg) + FTC (200 mg) + TAF (25 mg)	NRTI + NtRTI + NNRTI	1 tablet q.d.	Yes
Descovy (2016)	TAF (25 mg) FTC (200 mg)	NRTI + NtRTI	1 tablet q.d.+ at least 1 additional ARV	No

ABC, abacavir; ARV, antiretroviral; ATV, atazanavir; COB, cobicistat; DRV, darunavir; DTG, dolutegravir; EVG, elvitegravir; FTC, emtricitabine; INSTI, integrase strand transfer inhibitor; NRTI, nucleoside reverse transcriptase inhibitor; NNRTI, non-nucleoside reverse transcriptase inhibitor; NtRTI, nucleotide reverse transcriptase inhibitor; PI, protease inhibitor; PK, pharmacokinetic; RAL, raltegravir; RPV, rilpivirine; 3TC, lamivudine; TAF, tenofovir alafenamide; TDF, tenofovir disoproxil fumarate.

ART. For example, in patients with chronic kidney disease or osteoporosis, consider avoiding the use of TDF; in patients with high cardiac risk, avoid the use of ABC (DHHS, 2016).

KEY CHARACTERISTICS AND FINDINGS OF RECENT CLINICAL TRIALS OF DHHS-RECOMMENDED REGIMENS

DOLUTEGRAVIR-BASED REGIMENS

Dolutegravir is the third FDA-approved INSTI. It is commercially available as a stand-alone product (Tivicay) and as a fixed-dose combination with NRTIs abacavir and lamivudine (Triumeq). DTG + TDF/FTC and DTG/ABC/3TC are both DHHS-recommended initial treatment regimens. DTG is generally very well-tolerated, and adverse drug reactions are uncommon. Characteristic adverse effects are diarrhea, nausea, and headache.

DTG is dosed once daily and has no dietary requirements. Oral absorption of INSTIs is affected by divalent cations. Dose separation between DTG and divalent cation (aluminum, magnesium, iron, and calcium)-containing products is recommended. Alternatively, iron- and calcium-containing supplements can be taken with DTG, together, with food. In order to reduce the risk of abacavir hypersensitivity reaction, DTG/ABC/3TC should be administered only to individuals who test negative for the HLA B-5701 allele. DTG causes reversible inhibition of the renal tubular transporter, resulting in decreased tubular excretion of creatinine. This has the effect of increasing serum creatinine levels, without impairment of glomerular filtration.

Three phase 3 clinical trials evaluated DTG-containing treatments (with either TDF/FTC or ABC/3TC) for initial therapy in adults. The SINGLE study was a randomized, double-blind, 144-week study that compared DTG + TDF/FTC to single-tablet EFV/TDF/FTC in approximately 800 treatment-naive adults (Pappa, 2014; Walmsley, 2013). The primary end point demonstrated the statistical superiority of DTG + TDF/FTC, with the difference driven by discontinuations due to side effects related to EFV. There was no significant difference in the rates of viral suppression between treatment groups. The superiority of the DTG study arm was maintained through 144 weeks of follow-up.

The SPRING-2 study was the only powered, head-to-head trial of HIV INSTIs. SPRING-2 was a randomized, double-blind study that compared DTG to RAL (dosed twice daily) with NRTI backbone, ABC/3TC, or TDF/FTC in approximately 800 treatment-naive patients (Raffi, 2013). Overall, the two study arms performed very similarly, with approximately 3% discontinuation due to treatment-related adverse effects and rare treatment-emergent drug resistance (none in the DTG arm), demonstrating non-inferiority between the two INSTIs.

FLAMINGO was an open-label clinical trial comparing DTG to DRV/r (with TDF/FTC or ABC/3TC) in treatment-naive adults (Clotet, 2014; Molina, 2014). The 48- and 96-week results demonstrated the superiority of DTG to DRV/r. The difference between the two study arms was driven by a combination of more frequent virologic and tolerability discontinuations in the DRV/r arm. Changes in fasting lipids were lower among subjects in the DTG arm.

Treatment-emergent resistance to DTG in clinical trials of initial ART is exceptionally rare, with only one case reported with no corresponding decrease in DTG susceptibility (Tivicay package insert, ViiV Healthcare, 2013). Moreover, resistance to NRTI components to initial therapy has not been reported in phase 3 clinical trials. DTG retains activity against some viral strains resistant to other INSTIs, although cross-resistance is possible in isolates harboring resistance mutations at integrase gene codon 148 (in combination with at least two other integrase inhibitor-resistance mutations).

ELVITEGRAVIR-BASED REGIMENS

Elvitegravir was the second INSTI approved for treatment of HIV. EVG requires pharmacologic boosting, typically with co-formulated cobicistat. EVG/c is generally well-tolerated, and adverse drug reactions are uncommon. The characteristic adverse effects of EVG/cobi are gastrointestinal. Two fixed-dose combinations of EVG/cobi are FDA approved: EVG/cobi/TDF/FTC (Stribild) and in combination with the new tenofovir prodrug, tenofovir alafenamide (TAF), EVG/cobi/FTC/TAF (Genvoya). Both fixed-dose combinations are recommended by the DHHS guidelines as initial therapy for the treatment of HIV-infected adults and adolescents. EVG/cobi is usually well-tolerated; its characteristic adverse effects are nausea, diarrhea, and rash.

Cobicistat is a potent CYP3A4 inhibitor and used to boost EVG levels. EVG/cobi can cause a wide range of drug-drug interactions with CYP3A4 substrates. EVG and cobicistat are also available as stand-alone products (Viteka and Tybost, respectively). Cobicistat causes inhibition of the renal tubular transporter, resulting in decreased tubular excretion of creatinine. This has the effect of increasing serum creatinine levels, without impairment of glomerular filtration.

EVG/cobi is dosed once daily and should be taken with food. Oral absorption of INSTIs is affected by divalent cations. Dose separation between EVG and divalent cation (aluminum, magnesium, iron, and calcium)-containing products is recommended. EVG/cobi/TDF/FTC is only recommended for patients with baseline CrCl ≥70 ml/min and should be discontinued if CrCl decreases to <50 ml/min. EVG/cobi/FTC/TAF is approved for use in individuals with an estimated glomerular filtration rate (eGFR) ≥30 ml/min (Gupta, 2015).

EVG/COBI/TDF/FTC

EVG/cobi/TDF/FTC is the first single-tablet INSTI-containing regimen and was FDA approved in 2012. This fixed-dose combination was studied in three large randomized clinical trials in treatment-naive individuals. In a 144-week, randomized, double-blind study of 700 ART-naive individuals comparing two single-tablet regimens, EVG/cobi/TDF/FTC was shown to be statistically non-inferior to EFV/TDF/3TC, with similar virologic effectiveness and rates of treatment discontinuation for adverse events (DeJesus, 2012; Wohl, 2015).

The GS 236-0103 clinical trial randomized 708 ART-naive individuals to receive either EVG/cobi/TDF/FTC or ritonavir-boosted atazanavir + TDF/FTC (Sax, 2015). After 144 weeks, the two study groups showed similar overall results, supporting the finding of non-inferiority of EVG/cobi/TDF/FTC.

WAVES was the first fully powered all-women's phase 3 clinical trial comparing EVG/cobi/TDF/FTC to ritonavir-boosted atazanavir + TDF/FTC in 575 women (Kityo, 2015). After 48 weeks, EVG/cobi/TDF/FTC demonstrated statistical superiority to the ritonavir-boosted protease inhibitor arm, with differences driven by less frequent discontinuations due to adverse events (1.7% vs. 6.6%). Declines in bone mineral density were similar in both treatment arms. No treatment-emergent drug resistance was detected among the EVG/cobi/TDF/FTC-treated patients.

EVG/COBI/FTC/TAF

EVG/cobi/FTC/TAF was FDA approved in late 2015. In two large phase 3 clinical trials, EVG/cobi/FTC/TAF was non-inferior to EVG/cobi/TDF/FTC in approximately 1700 treatment-naive adults (with pretreatment eGFR ≥50 ml/min) at 48 and 96 weeks (Sax, 2015). The study subjects who received TAF had lower declines in eGFR and loss of bone mineral density, suggesting a favorable renal and bone toxicity profile. Lipid parameters were slightly less favorable in the TAF compared with the TDF study arm.

EVG/cobi/FTC/TAF was also studied in an open-label, single-arm study of virologically suppressed patients with mild to moderate renal insufficiency (eGFR, 30–69 ml/min), supporting the FDA indication for the use of EVG/c/FTC/TAF in adults with eGFR ≥30 ml/min (Gupta, 2015).

Resistance to EVG is characterized by mutations at codons T66I/A/K, E92Q/G, T97A, S147G, Q148R/H/K, and N155H in the viral integrase gene. Resistance to EVG commonly confers cross-resistance to RAL and occasionally to DTG.

RALTEGRAVIR-BASED REGIMEN

Raltegravir was the first FDA-approved INSTI (2007). The combination of RAL with TDF/FTC is a DHHS-recommended initial regimen. RAL is generally very well-tolerated, and adverse drug reactions are uncommon. Characteristic adverse effects are diarrhea, nausea, and headache.

RAL is dosed twice daily and has no dietary restrictions. RAL is metabolized by glucuronidation and has no interaction with CYP3A4 substrates. Oral absorption RAL is decreased by divalent cations; co-administration with aluminum- or magnesium-containing antacids is not recommended.

STARTMRK was a 240-week, randomized, double-blind, placebo-controlled study comparing RAL + TDF/FTC compared to EFV/TDF/FTC in 566 ART-naive individuals (DeJesus, 2012). At the primary end point of 48 weeks, RAL + TDF/FTC was non-inferior to EFV/TDF/FTC. The 4- and 5-year analysis showed virologic and immunologic superiority of RAL, with the virologic differences driven by EFV/TDF/FTC discontinuations due to adverse effects (Rockstroh, 2013).

ACTG A5257 was a large randomized open-label trial of more than 1800 treatment-naive subjects that compared twice-daily RAL with once-daily ATV/r or once-daily DRV/r, each administered with TDF/FTC (Lennox, 2014). At week 96, the RAL group was statistically superior to both once-daily PI regimens. Although the regimens had similar virologic suppression rates, there were differences in discontinuations due to side effects and toxicity. Of note, participants receiving RAL had less change in fasting lipids and less decrease in bone mineral density compared to both boosted PI arms.

The SPRING-2 was a double-blind study that randomized treatment-naive subjects to receive RAL or DTG and was discussed previously (Raffi, 2013). Over 96 weeks of follow-up, the two study arms performed nearly identically, demonstrating non-inferiority of the two INSTIs.

Resistance to raltegravir is characterized by mutations at codons 143, 148, and 155 in the viral integrase gene. Resistance to RAL typically confers cross-resistance to EVG and sometimes to DTG. Treatment-emergent resistance to RAL is uncommon. In the STARTMRK and SPRING-2 studies, in individuals initiating ART with RAL + TDF/3TC, INSTI resistance was detected after virologic failure in 4 of 281 (STARTMRK; 240-week data) and 1 of 411 treated individuals (SPRING-2; 96-week data). No INSTI resistance emerged after the first 48 weeks of treatment.

DARUNAVIR-BASED REGIMEN

The regimen containing the ritonavir-boosted protease inhibitor darunavir, with TDF/FTC, is the only non-INSTI-based regimen recommended in the DHHS guidelines. The combination is usually well-tolerated, although characteristic treatment-related adverse effects are gastrointestinal and mild rash. Treatment-emergent drug resistance is very rare among individuals initiating boosted PI ART such as DRV/r. At the time of virologic failure, no emergent PI resistance was detected; there was only rare resistance to the NRTI treatment components.

In the phase III ARTEMIS clinical study, 689 treatment-naive adults were randomized to receive once-daily DRV/r or lopinavir/r with TDF/FTC. Overall, the study showed non-inferiority of DRV/r to lopinavir/r at 48 weeks. DRV/r was statistically superior at 192 weeks. Gastrointestinal side effects and treatment-related discontinuations were more frequent among subjects receiving lopinavir/r (Orkin, 2013).

In recent years, DRV/r was evaluated in randomized clinical trials versus INSTIs in the study ACTG 5257 (vs. RAL) (Lennox, 2014) and the FLAMINGO (vs. DTG) (Clotet, 2014) clinical trials (discussed previously). In both studies, DRV/r was found to be statistically inferior to the INSTI.

DRV is also available as a recently FDA-approved, fixed-dose combination with the pharmacologic booster cobicistat (DRV/c; Prezcobix) for initial treatment (discussed later).

OTHER RECENTLY FDA-APPROVED ANTIRETROVIRAL AGENTS

Reverse Transcriptase Inhibitors

Tenofovir alafenamide (TAF) is a nucleotide reverse transcriptase inhibitor. TAF is a prodrug of tenofovir with pharmacokinetics that result in lower plasma and increased intracellular concentrations over TDF. It is thought that this pharmacodynamic property results in lower risk of renal and bone toxicity compared to TDF (Gupta, 2015; Mills, 2016). TAF is currently available in the EVG/cobi/FTC/TAF and RPV/FTC/TAF single-tablet regimens as well as in the FTC/TAF fixed-dose combination. TAF is categorized by DHHS as an initial ARV for patients with an estimated creatinine clearance ≥30 ml/min.

Protease Inhibitors

Two protease inhibitor fixed-dose combinations with the new pharmacokinetic booster cobicistat were FDA approved in 2015.

Darunavir/cobicistat (DRV/c; Prezcobix) is categorized by DHHS as an alternate initial ARV. FDA approval was based on the similar pharmacokinetic profile of darunavir compared to that of ritonavir-boosted darunavir. DRV/c is generally well-tolerated, and characteristic adverse effects are gastrointestinal. The drug is dosed one tablet, once daily, with food. Like ritonavir, cobicistat is a potent CYP3A4 inhibitor, and DRV/c can cause a wide range of drug–drug interactions with CYP3A4 substrates. DRV/c has a similar virologic and resistance profile as DRV + RTV, with a high genetic barrier to resistance. Treatment-emergent resistance to boosted PIs is rare. A fixed-dose combination of DRV/c with TAF/FTC is currently in late-stage clinical development and will likely receive FDA approval in late 2016 or 2017.

Atazanavir/cobicistat (ATV/c; Evotaz) was FDA approved in 2015. ATV/c is dosed one tablet, once daily and must be taken with food. The medication has interactions with the stomach acid-lowering agents H2-blockers and proton pump inhibitors. Similar to atazanavir when administered with ritonavir, hyperbilirubinemia and jaundice commonly occur in patients taking the medication. Nephrolithiasis and renal adverse events have been reported among individuals taking atazanavir. Like ritonavir, cobicistat is a potent CYP3A4 inhibitor, and ATV/c can cause a wide range of drug–drug interactions with CYP3A4

substrates. ATV/c has a similar virologic and resistance profile as ATV + RTV, with a high genetic barrier to resistance. Treatment-emergent resistance to boosted PIs is rare.

Integrase inhibitors

Elvitegravir (EVG; Viteka), available in fixed-dose combinations with cobicistat, tenofovir, and emtricitabine, was approved in 2015.

Raltegravir/lamivudine (RAL/3TC; Dutrebis) was FDA approved in 2015 for use in combination with other antiretroviral medications. The results of a 106-subject clinical study demonstrated the bioequivalence of the fixed-dose combination with the individual ARV components. RAL/3TC is dosed one tablet, twice daily, but as of December 2015, it was not commercially marketed in the United States.

Pharmacokinetic Booster

Cobicistat (Tybost) is a pharmacokinetic booster that acts through inhibition of CYP3A4. The one notable difference between the other pharmacokinetic enhancer, ritonavir, and cobicistat is that cobicistat has no intrinsic antiretroviral activity. Cobicistat is dosed once daily with food and intended for use to boost the protease inhibitors darunavir and atazanavir. Cobicistat is also contained in several fixed-dose combinations (Stribild, Genvoya, Prezcobix, and Evotaz).

Suggested Reading

US Department of Health and Human Services, Panel on Antiretroviral Guidelines for Adults and Adolescents. Guidelines for the use of antiretroviral agents in HIV-1-infected adults and adolescents. Available at https://aidsinfo.nih.gov/contentfiles/lvguidelines/adultandadolescentgl.pdf. Accessed January 30, 2016.

CO-FORMULATIONS

LEARNING OBJECTIVE

Describe current co-formulations utilized in HIV therapy.

WHAT'S NEW?

Since 2012, eight new co-formulated products have been licensed for the treatment of HIV. Two of these products include the new pharmacologic boosting agent cobicistat and three contain TAF. Notable are single-tablet regimens with INSTIs elvitegravir (Stribild and Genvoya) and dolutegravir (Triumeq).

- Co-formulated medications reduce pill burden and improve adherence to ART.

- There are currently three DHHS panel-recommended single-tablet regimens for initial HIV treatment.

- Phase 1 studies are the earliest clinical trials, focusing mainly on safety and pharmacokinetics.

- Phase 2 studies further evaluate safety and begin to evaluate efficacy and dosing. Dose selection is done in early phase 2.

- Phase 3 studies focus on safety and efficacy in the target population.

- Phase 4 studies, sometimes referred to as postmarketing trials, occur after FDA approval and study the use of the drug in different patient populations and long-term safety.

- Expanded-access programs make a drug available to patients who are in particular need prior to the drug being available commercially. These programs are generally not established until after phase 3 studies have been fully enrolled.

Co-formulated antiretroviral medications have been used for the treatment of HIV since 1997. The rationale to co-formulation is to decrease pill burden, thereby facilitating treatment adherence while decreasing risk of selective nonadherence or supply chain gaps. A recent meta-analysis comparing single-tablet regimens (STRs) to multi-tablet antiretroviral regimens (MTRs) concluded that STRs were associated with statistically significantly more adherence compared to patients on MTRs of any frequency (odds ratio (OR), 2.37; 95% confidence interval (CI), 1.68, 3.35; $p < 0.001$; four studies), twice-daily MTR (OR, 2.53; 95% CI, 1.13, 5.66; $p = 0.02$; two studies), and once-daily MTR (OR, 1.81; 95% CI, 1.15, 2.84; $p = 0.01$; two studies) (Clay, 2015). The relative risk (RR) for 48-week viral load suppression was improved with STRs (RR, 1.09; 95% CI, 1.04, 1.15; $p = 0.0003$; three studies), whereas RR of grade 3 to 4 laboratory abnormalities was lower among patients on STRs (RR, 0.68; 95% CI, 0.49, 0.94; $p = 0.02$; two studies).

As of 2016, there were 15 co-formulations licensed for use in HIV therapy in the United States (Table 19.2). Significant newly approved co-formulated combinations include the integrase inhibitor containing Triumeq (abacavir/lamivudine/dolutegravir, 2014) and Genvoya (tenofovir alafenamide/emtricitabine/cobicistat/elvitegravir, 2015) and cobicistat-boosted protease inhibitors Evotaz (cobicistat/atazanavir, 2015) and Prezcobix (cobicistat/darunavir, 2015) and Adefsey (rilpivirine/emtricitabine/tenofovir alafenamide, 2016) and Descovy (emtricitabine/tenofovir alafenamide, 2016).

Recommended Reading

Clay PG, Nag S, Graham CM, et al. Meta-analysis of studies comparing single and multi-tablet fixed dose combination HIV treatment regimens. *Medicine*. 2015; 94(42):e1677.

CLINICAL TRIALS DESIGN AND ACCESS PROGRAMS

LEARNING OBJECTIVE

Describe the differences between phase 1, 2, 3, and 4 research clinical trials and expanded access programs.

PHASES OF CLINICAL TRIALS

In general, there are four phases to drug development, which are guided by procedures described in the US Code of Federal Regulations 21 CFR 314.126 (FDA, 2001b):

- Phase 1 is the most preliminary clinical work in small numbers of human subjects and helps to determine safety/toxicity (FDA, 2001a). Phase 1 studies usually start as single-dose studies and then progress to multiple-dose studies (mainly using healthy volunteers). They evaluate a range of aspects, such as pharmacokinetics (including drug bioavailability), dosing interval, food effects, tolerability, and toxicity (to define maximum tolerated dose, sentinel adverse effects, and target organ toxicity).

- Phase 2 studies further evaluate toxicity and the effectiveness of the drug for a particular indication in a larger number of patients who have the disease or condition under study, and they potentially establish dosage (FDA, 2001a). This is usually the initial assessment of activity or proof-of-concept study. It includes several doses and a short course of monotherapy or functional monotherapy. It may include randomized dosing and control or may be dose escalating. Phase 2 studies also collect data on pharmacokinetics, dose response, tolerability, and toxicity. In HIV, these studies are usually divided into phase 2a and phase 2b. Phase 2a trials are generally conducted in a small number of

Table 19.2 FDA-APPROVED CO-FORMULATED ANTIRETROVIRAL MEDICATIONS

TRADE NAME	DOSE	CLASSES	DOSE
Combivir (1997)	AZT (300 mg) 3TC (150 mg)	2 NRTIs	1 tablet b.i.d.
Trizivir (2000)	AZT (300 mg) 3TC (150 mg) ABC (300mg) ABC (300 mg)	3 NRTIs	1 tablet b.i.d.
Kaletra (2000)	LPV (200 mg) RTV (50 mg)	2 PIs	2 tablets b.i.d. For treatment-naive patients only: 4 tablets q.d.
Truvada (2004)	FTC (200 mg) TDF (300 mg)	1 NRTI + 1 NtRTI	1 tablet q.d.
Epzicom (2004)	ABC (600 mg) 3TC (300 mg)	2 NRTI	1 tablet q.d.
Atripla (2006)	FTC (200 mg) TDF (300 mg) EFV (600 mg)	2 NRTI + 1 NNRTI	1 tablet q.d.
Complera (2011)	FTC (200 mg TDF (300 mg) RPV (25 mg)	2 NRTI + 1 NNRTI	1 tablet q.d.
Stribild (2012)	EVG (150 mg) COB (150mg) FTC (200 mg) TDF (300 mg)	1 NRTI + 1 NtRTI + 1 INSTI + 1 PK booster	1 tablet q.d.
Triumeq (2014)	ABC (600 mg) 3TC (300 mg) DTG (50 mg)	2 NRTI + 1 INSTI	1 tablet q.d.
Prezcobix (2015)	DRV (800 mg) COB (150 mg)	1 PI + 1 PK booster	1 tablet q.d.
Evotaz (2015)	ATV (300 mg) COB (150 mg)	1 PI + 1 PK booster	1 tablet q.d.
Genvoya (2015)	EVG (150 mg) COB (150mg) FTC (200 mg) TAF (25 mg)	1 NRTI + 1 NtRTI + 1 INSTI + 1 PK booster	1 tablet q.d.
Dutrebis (2015)	3TC (150 mg) RAL (300 mg)	1 NRTI + 1 INSTI	1 tablet b.i.d.
Adefsey (2016)	RPV (25 mg) TAF (25 mg) FTC (200 mg)	NRTI + NtRTI + NNRTI	1 tablet q.d.
Descovy (2016)	TAF (25 mg) FTC (200 mg)	NRTI + NtRTI	1 tablet q.d. + at least 1 additional ARV

ABC, abacavir; ARV, antiretroviral; ATV, atazanavir; AZT, zidovudine; COB, cobicistat; DRV, darunavir; DTG, dolutegravir; EVG, elvitegravir; FTC, emtricitabine; INSTI, integrase strand transfer inhibitor; LPV, lopinavir; NRTI, nucleoside reverse transcriptase inhibitor; NNRTI, non-nucleoside reverse transcriptase inhibitor; NtRTI, nucleotide reverse transcriptase inhibitor; PI, protease inhibitor; PK, pharmacokinetic; RAL, raltegravir; RPV, rilpivirine; RTV, ritonavir; 3TC, lamivudine; TAF, tenofovir alafenamide; TDF, tenofovir disoproxil fumarate.

HIV-infected patients and usually are of short duration. Phase 2b trials usually involve longer term dosing, are almost always in combination with other agents, and have a control arm. Longer term tolerability, toxicity, and effectiveness are important outcomes.

- Phase 3 studies are primarily geared toward large cohort efficacy and (along with the accumulated weight of safety and toxicity studies) form the basis for submission to and approval by the FDA (FDA, 2001a). Phase 3 studies are typically large randomized studies that can provide the main core information for submission and regulatory approval. They frequently include blinded therapy. For antiretrovirals, the end point for the most part has traditionally been some measurement of HIV-1 RNA response.

- Phase 4 studies are postmarketing or post-approval trials and may be mandated by the FDA to further determine long-term toxicities or may serve as vehicles for expanded indications or dosing changes (DHHS, 2005).

Expanded access programs are often created for patients in particular need to make a drug available before it is licensed. These programs are an outgrowth of the expedited review process for HIV drugs and are usually limited in the number of patients enrolled and the duration of availability. Typically, expanded access programs are established after phase 3 studies have been fully enrolled and before drug approval. They are subject to FDA oversight (FDA, 2001a; USC 2002), although considerably less so than are registrational trials. Due to the number of treatment options available today, expanded access programs are much less common than in the past.

MECHANISMS FOR EXPANDED ACCESS

There are five mechanisms for expanded access.

Emergency Investigational New Drug

For an emergency investigational new drug (E-IND), a physician, on behalf of the patient, contacts the FDA and/or pharmaceutical manufacturer. In this type of emergency situation, a written submission is not needed; however, the FDA expects the physician to submit an IND application as soon as possible (FDA, 1998).

Open-Label Protocol

Open-label protocol is designed to account for the time between the completion of a clinical trial and the FDA approval of an investigational drug. This allows for the continuation of treatment and the end of a phase 3 study. Compliance with the patient safeguard processes must also be demonstrated (FDA, 1998).

Treatment Investigational New Drug

The treatment investigational new drug (T-IND) allows patients, most of whom are very ill, access to investigational drugs when there are no alternative therapies. These are sometimes referred to as "compassionate use" studies and are used to collect safety data in very ill patients who use the new therapy (FDA, 1998).

Parallel Track

This mechanism has been developed to expand availability of INDs to patients with AIDS or other related diseases. Patients in a parallel track study, or a study that is being run in parallel with controlled clinical studies for a particular investigational agent, are those who would not otherwise have access to the treatment because of geographical location or because they do not meet the specific entry criteria for the original study. Only patients who cannot enroll in the available original trial and who are not eligible for marketing standard treatment may enroll in these studies (FDA, 1998).

In 2009, the FDA issued two new rules related to expanded access. The first rule, titled "Expanded Access to Investigational Drugs for Treatment Use," clarifies the criteria for access to investigational drugs, enumerates the requirements for access submissions, establishes safeguards to protect patients from adverse side effects, and implements mechanisms for maintaining meaningful data about treatment use and results. Per the rule, those who may be granted access to investigational drugs include individuals with a serious or immediately life-threatening disease and for whom there is no comparable satisfactory alternative therapy, intermediate-size patient populations comprising individuals who are ineligible to participate in clinical trials or whose disease is so rare that a drug is not being developed, and larger populations under a treatment protocol or in a trial conducted as part of an IND application.

The expanded access rule specifies that pharmaceutical companies are responsible for submitting IND safety reports (and annual reports when the protocol continues for 1 year or more) and for providing treating physicians with necessary information to maximize the benefits and minimize the risks of treatment. Physicians who administer the treatments, who are considered "investigators" for purposes of this rule, must report adverse drug events to the sponsor, ensure that informed consent requirements are met, and maintain accurate case histories and drug disposition records. In support of the effort to help seriously ill patients gain access to these therapies, the FDA has a website that provides information for patients and their physicians about options for access to investigational drugs (see http://www.fda.gov/ForConsumers/ByAudience/ForPatientAdvocates/AccesstoInvestigationalDrugs/ucm176098.htm).

The second rule, titled "Charging for Investigational Drugs Under an Investigational New Drug Application," amends the existing rules concerning when drug manufacturers may charge patients for investigational drugs. This rule specifies that a company that wishes to charge a clinical trial participant for a drug must show that the drug may provide a significant advantage over other available treatments (as demonstrated by the trial), that the data from the trial are essential to demonstrating the drug's safety and efficacy, and that charging participants is essential because the cost of the drug is "extraordinary to the sponsor" (FDA, 2009).

Recommended Reading

US Food and Drug Administration. Expanded access to investigational drugs for treatment use. Title 21 CFR Parts 312 and 316. 2009 ed. Available at https://www.gpo.gov/fdsys/pkg/FR-2009-08-13/pdf/E9-19005.pdf. Accessed November 30, 2015.

US Food and Drug Administration. Expanded access to investigational drugs for treatment use—Questions and answers: Guidance for industry. May 2013 ed. Available at http://www.fda.gov/downloads/drugs/guidancecomplianceregulatoryinformation/guidances/ucm351261.pdf. Accessed November 30, 2015.

PHARMACOGENOMICS

LEARNING OBJECTIVE

Demonstrate how pharmacogenomics are applied in the clinical management of HIV-infected patients.

KEY POINTS

- Pharmacogenomics uses genetic information to guide treatment decision-making.

- Drug resistance testing is an example of viral pharmacogenomic testing.

- Patient pharmacogenomic testing for the HLA B5701 haplotype reduces the risk of abacavir hypersensitivity reaction and is recommended prior to the initiation of abacavir-containing therapy.

Pharmacogenomics refers to the concept of using information about genetic variation to individualize therapeutic decision-making. With regard to HIV therapy, pharmacogenomics could be exploited to identify the most effective or tolerated antiretroviral medications for an individual virus or patient. Possible applications of pharmacogenomics can be broadly categorized into the following areas: (1) antiretroviral susceptibility, (2) explaining pharmacokinetic or pharmacodynamic variability, and (3) predicting adverse drug reaction.

The use of genotypic drug resistance testing is well established and recommended prior to the initiation of treatment and after treatment failure. Such viral testing is a well-established example of the use of pharmacogenomics, albeit using genetic markers to predict susceptibility to antiretroviral medications. Management of HIV drug resistance is detailed in Chapter 21.

Efavirenz is associated with characteristic neuropsychological side effects. These side effects correlate with plasma levels of efavirenz. The metabolism of efavirenz is subject to variable metabolism, with higher efavirenz levels associated with genetic polymorphisms of cytochrome CYP2B6 (Rotger, 2007). In one clinical trial from Japan, individuals harboring the CYP2B6*6 or -*26 allele had successful maintenance of plasma efavirenz levels with dose reduction (Gatanaga, 2007).

Atazanavir is occasionally associated with severe hyperbilirubinemia. Genetic polymorphisms in the UGT1A1 gene appear to influence plasma levels of atazanavir (Rotger, 2005) and are weakly associated with the risk of discontinuation of atazanavir among Hispanic recipients (Ribaudo, 2012).

One of the best characterized examples of pharmacogenomic biomarkers is the association between the HLA-B*5701 allele and abacavir hypersensitivity. Without genetic screening, approximately 5–8% of individuals exposed to abacavir develop the hypersensitivity reaction (HSR). Genetic screening identified the HLA-B*5701 allele as a predictor of HSR. The PREDICT study (Mallal, 2008) was a randomized study of HLA screening of 1956 predominantly White individuals who were treated with abacavir-containing ART. The use of genetic screening dramatically reduced clinically suspected HSR from 7.8% to 3.4%. Skin patch test immunologically confirmed HSR was reduced from 2.7% to 0%. In a large, racially diverse group of North American patients, HLA-B*5701 screening resulted in 0.8% of individuals having clinically suspected HSR and no immunologically confirmed cases (Young, 2008). HLA-B*5701 allele screening is now recommended prior to the use of abacavir by multiple national treatment guidelines, including DHHS guidelines (DHHS, 2016).

Recommended Reading

Gatanaga H, Hayashida T, Tsuchiya K, et al. Successful efavirenz dose reduction in HIV type 1-infected individuals with cytochrome P450 2B6*6 and *26. *Clin Infect Dis.* 2007; 45(9):1230–1237.

Haas DW, Tarr PE. Perspectives on pharmacogenomics of antiretroviral medications and HIV-associated comorbidities. *Curr Opin HIV AIDS* 2015; 10(2):116–122.

Phillips E, Mallal S. Successful translation of pharmacogenetics into the clinic: The abacavir example. *Mol Diagn Ther*. 2009; 13(1):1–9.

Ribaudo HJ, Daar ES, Tierney C, et al. Impact of UGT1A1 Gilbert variant on discontinuation of ritonavir-boosted atazanavir in AIDS Clinical Trials Group Study A5202. *J Infect Dis* 2013; 207(3):420–425.

Young B, Squires K, Patel P, et al. First large, multicenter, open-label study utilizing HLA-B*5701 screening for abacavir hypersensitivity in North America. *AIDS*. 2008; 22:1673–1681.

ACKNOWLEDGMENTS

I thank the authors of previous editions of this chapter, Nicholas Bellos, MD, and Amy Keller.

References

Clay PG, Nag S, Graham CM, et al. Meta-analysis of studies comparing single and multi-tablet fixed dose combination HIV treatment regimens. *Medicine*. 2015; 94(42):e1677.

Clotet B, Feinberg J, van Lunzen J, et al.; the ING114915 Study Team. Once-daily dolutegravir versus darunavir plus ritonavir in antiretroviral-naive adults with HIV-1 infection (FLAMINGO): 48 week results from the randomised open-label phase 3b study. *Lancet*. 2014 Jun 28; 383(9936):2222–2231. [Erratum in: *Lancet*. 2015 Jun 27; 385(9987):2576]

DeJesus E, Rockstroh JK, Henry K, et al. Co-formulated elvitegravir, cobicistat, emtricitabine, and tenofovir disoproxil fumarate versus ritonavir-boosted atazanavir plus co-formulated emtricitabine and tenofovir disoproxil fumarate for initial treatment of HIV-1 infection: A randomised, double-blind, phase 3, non-inferiority trial. *Lancet*. 2012; 379(9835):2429–2438.

DeJesus E, Rockstroh JK, Lennox JL, et al. Efficacy of raltegravir versus efavirenz when combined with tenofovir/emtricitabine in treatment-naive HIV-1-infected patients: Week-192 overall and subgroup analyses from STARTMRK. *HIV Clin Trials*. 2012; 13(4):228–232.

Department of Health and Human Services (DHHS). Information on clinical trials and human researchstudies: glossary. 2005. Available at: http://www.clinicaltrials.gov/ct/gui/info/glossary#phasel.

Food and Drug Administration (FDA). Information sheets: 1998 Guidance for Institutional Review Boards and Investigators. 1998. Available at: http://www.fda.gov/oc/ohrt/irbs/drugsbiologics.html.

Food and Drug Administration (FDA). 21 CFR 312.21. Investigational new drug application. In: Food and Drugs. April 1, 2001a. Available at: http://www.access.gpo.gov/nara/cfr/waisidx_01/21cfr312_01.html.

Food and Drug Administration (FDA). 21 CFR 314.126. Applications for FDA approval to market a new drug. In: Food and Drugs. April 1, 2001b. Available at: http://www.access.gpo.gov/nara/cfr/waisidx_01/21cfr314_01.html.

Gatanaga H, Hayashida T, Tsuchiya K, et al. Successful efavirenz dose reduction in HIV type 1-infected individuals with cytochrome P450 2B6*6 and *26. *Clin Infect Dis*. 2007; 45(9):1230–1237.

Gupta S, Pozniak A, Arribas J, et al. Subjects with renal impairment switching from tenofovir disoproxil fumarate to tenofovir alafenamide have improved renal and bone safety through 48 weeks [Abstract TUAB0103]. 8th International AIDS Society Conference on HIV Pathogenesis, Treatment, and Prevention, July 19–22, 2015, Vancouver.

International Advisory Panel on HIV Care Continuum Optimization. IAPAC guidelines for optimizing the HIV care continuum for adults and adolescents. *J Int Assoc Provid AIDS Care*. 2015; 14(Suppl. 1):S3–S34. doi:10.1177/2325957415613442

Kityo C, Squires K, Johnson M, et al. The efficacy and safety of elvitegravir/cobicistat/emtricitabine/tenofovir disoproxil fumarate and ritonavir-boosted atazanavir plus emtricitabine/tenofovir disoproxil fumarate in treatment-naïve women with HIV-1 infection: Week 48 analysis of the phase 3, randomized, double-blind study. EACS 2015 Oct 21–24, Barcelona, Spain—15th European AIDS Conference.

Orkin C, DeJesus E, Khanlou H, et al. Final 192-week efficacy and safety of once-daily darunavir/ritonavir compared with lopinavir/ritonavir in HIV-1-infected treatment-naïve patients in the ARTEMIS trial. *HIV Med*. 2013; 14(1):49–59.

Lennox JL, Landovitz RJ, Ribaudo HJ, et al. Efficacy and tolerability of 3 non-nucleoside reverse transcriptase inhibitor-sparing antiretroviral regimens for treatment-naive volunteers infected with HIV-1: A randomized, controlled equivalence trial. *Ann Intern Med*. 2014; 161(7):461–471.

Mallal S, Phillips E, Carosi G, et al. HLA-B*5701 screening for hypersensitivity to abacavir. *N Engl J Med*. 2008 Feb 7; 358(6):568–579.

Mills A, Arribas JR, Andrade-Villanueva J, et al. Switching from tenofovir disoproxil fumarate to tenofovir alafenamide in antiretroviral regimens for virologically suppressed adults with HIV-1 infection: A randomised, active-controlled, multicentre, open-label, phase 3, non-inferiority study. *Lancet Infect Dis*. 2016; 16(1):43–52.

Molina JM, Clotet B, van Lunzen J, et al. Once-daily dolutegravir is superior to once-daily darunavir/ritonavir in treatment-naive HIV-1-positive individuals: 96 week results from FLAMINGO. *J Int AIDS Soc*. 2014; 17(4 Suppl. 3):19490.

Pappa K, Baumgarten A, Felizarta F, et al. Dolutegravir (DTG) plus abacavir/lamivudine once daily superior to tenofovir/emtricitabine/efavirenz in treatment-naive HIV subjects: 144-week results from SINGLE (ING114467). Paper presented at the Interscience Conference on Antimicrobial Agents and Chemotherapy (ICAAC), 2014, Washington, DC.

Raffi F, Jaeger H, Quiros-Roldan E, et al. Once-daily dolutegravir versus twice-daily raltegravir in antiretroviral-naïve adults with HIV-1 infection (SPRING-2 study): 96 week results from a randomised, double-blind, non-inferiority trial. *Lancet Infect Dis*. 2013; 13(11):927–935.

Ribaudo HG, Daar ES, Tierney C, et al. Impact of UGT1A1 Gilbert variant on discontinuation of ritonavir-boosted atazanavir in AIDS Clinical Trials Group Study A5202. *J Infect Dis*. 2013 Feb 1; 207(3):420–425.

Rockstroh JK, DeJesus E, Lennox JL, et al. Durable efficacy and safety of raltegravir versus efavirenz when combined with tenofovir/emtricitabine in treatment-naive HIV-1-infected patients: Final 5-year results from STARTMRK. *J Acquir Immune Defic Syndr*. 2013; 63(1):77–85.

Rotger M, Tegude H, Colombo S, et al. Predictive value of known and novel alleles of CYP2B6 for efavirenz plasma concentrations in HIV-infected individuals. *Clin Pharmacol Ther*. 2007 Apr; 81(4):557–566.

Sax PE, Wohl D, Yin MT, et al. Tenofovir alafenamide versus tenofovir disoproxil fumarate, coformulated with elvitegravir, cobicistat, and emtricitabine, for initial treatment of HIV-1 infection: Two randomised, double-blind, phase 3, non-inferiority trials. *Lancet*. 2015; 385(9987):2606–2615.

US Code. 21 USC 360bbb. General provisions relating to drugs and devices: expanded access tounapproved therapies and diagnostics. In: Food and Drugs: Drugs and Devices. January 24, 2002. Available at: http://frwebgate.access.gpo.gov/cgi-bin/getdoc.cgi?dbname=browse_usc&docid=Cite:+21USC360bbb.

US Department of Health and Human Services, Panel on Antiretroviral Guidelines for Adults and Adolescents. Guidelines for the use of antiretroviral agents in HIV-1-infected adults and adolescents. Available at https://aidsinfo.nih.gov/contentfiles/lvguidelines/adultandadolescentgl.pdf.

US Food and Drug Administration. Expanded access to investigational drugs for treatment use. Title 21 CFR Parts 312 and 316. 2009 ed. Available at https://www.gpo.gov/fdsys/pkg/FR-2009-08-13/pdf/E9-19005.pdf. Accessed November 30, 2015.

Walmsley SL, Antela A, Clumeck N, et al. Dolutegravir plus abacavir–lamivudine for the treatment of HIV-1 infection. *N Engl J Med.* 2013; 369(19):1807–1818.

Wohl DA, Cohen C, Gallant JE, et al. A randomized, double-blind comparison of single-tablet regimen elvitegravir/cobicistat/emtricitabine/tenofovir DF versus single-tablet regimen efavirenz/emtricitabine/tenofovir DF for initial treatment of HIV-1 infection: Analysis of week 144 results. *J Acquir Immune Defic Syndr.* 2014; 65(3):e118–e120.

Wohl D, Oka S, Clumeck N, et.al. A randomized, double-blind comparison of tenofovir alafenamide vs. tenofovir disoproxil fumarate, each coformulated with elvitegravir, cobicistat, and emtricitabine, for initial HIV-1 treatment: Week 96 results. 15th European AIDS Conference, 2015, Barcelona, Spain.

Young B, Squires K, Patel P, et al. First large, multicenter, open-label study utilizing HLA-B*5701 screening for abacavir hypersensitivity in North America. *AIDS.* 2008; 22:1673–1681.

20.

INITIATION OF ANTIRETROVIRAL THERAPY

WHAT TO START WITH

Saira Ajmal and Zelalem Temesgen

LEARNING OBJECTIVES

Upon conclusion of this chapter, participants should be able to

- discuss categories of regimens for first-line antiretroviral therapy;

- recognize the basis for the US Department of Health and Human Services (DHHS) guidelines for initial antiretroviral therapy; and

- recognize and apply recommended regimens for initiation of antiretroviral therapy.

INTRODUCTION

The benefits of antiretroviral therapy (ART) are becoming increasingly appreciated. The primary goal of therapy is to prevent HIV-associated morbidity and mortality. In addition to the dramatic decline in HIV-related illness and death that has been observed as a result of the introduction and expansion of combination ART, evidence is emerging that uncontrolled HIV replication also has a deleterious impact on conditions that are not conventionally associated with immune deficiency, including cardiovascular disease, kidney disease, liver disease, neurologic complications, and malignancy (Deeks, 2011). Other studies have found an independent association between cumulative exposure to replicating virus over time and mortality (Mugavero, 2011). Emerging data also increasingly support the earlier use of ART (INSIGHT START Study Group, 2015). Although it may still be true that ART is beneficial even when started later in the course of HIV disease, it is becoming clear that the damage by unchecked replication done earlier in the course of HIV disease may be irreparable. It has also been shown that the extent of $CD4^+$ recovery is directly associated with the $CD4^+$ count at initiation of ART. The landmark study, HPTN 052, demonstrated the benefit of ART in preventing HIV transmission to uninfected sexual partners of HIV-infected persons on treatment (Cohen, 2011). Effective ART can reduce viremia and transmission of HIV to sexual partners by more than 96%, making reducing the risk of HIV transmission a secondary goal of ART (Cohen, 2015).

The recommendation to start ART in all HIV-infected patients regardless of pretreatment $CD4^+$ counts has recently been changed to class A1 (strong recommendation based on data from randomized controlled trials) based on the START and TEMPRANO trial results. Both of these randomized controlled trials demonstrated that the clinical benefits of ART were greater when started early with $CD4^+$ counts greater than 500 cells/mm3 than when initiated at a lower $CD4^+$ threshold (INSIGHT START Study Group, 2015; TEMPRANO ANRS 12136 Study Group, 2015).

Currently, there are 27 US Food and Drug Administration (FDA)-approved individual antiretroviral (ARV) drugs classified in six categories based on their mechanism of action: nucleoside/nucleotide analogue reverse transcriptase inhibitors (NRTIs), non-nucleoside analogue reverse transcriptase inhibitors (NNRTIs), protease inhibitors (PIs), fusion inhibitor, CCR5 antagonist, and integrase strand transfer inhibitors (INSTIs). In addition, two drugs (pharmacokinetic boosters (PK)) are used to improve the pharmacokinetic profiles of some ARV drugs.

A panel of leading HIV specialists, convened by the DHHS, has been developing and updating recommendations for use of antiretroviral agents in HIV-infected individuals since the early days of the highly active antiretroviral therapy (HAART) era. The most recent guidelines were revised in 2016 and included key updates to several sections, including changes in recommendations for initial combination regimens for the antiretroviral-naive patient (DHHS, 2016).

FIRST-LINE ANTIRETROVIRAL REGIMENS

In general, an ART regimen is a three-drug regimen consisting of two NRTIs (NRTI backbone) with an INSTI, NNRTI, or PK-enhanced PI as the third drug. Such regimens have resulted in favorable virologic and immunologic outcomes in most patients in clinical trials as well as in clinical practice. The specific regimen should be selected based on each patient's individual requirements, taking into account virologic efficacy, potential adverse effects, pill burden, dosing frequency, drug–drug interaction, patient's resistance profile, comorbid conditions, and cost. A summary of factors to consider when selecting an antiretroviral regimen is provided in Table 20.1.

The recommendations by the DHHS guidelines panel are based primarily on a regimen's efficacy, potency, durability of efficacy, and toxicity profile, as evidenced from published reports of randomized, prospective clinical trial with an adequate sample size and adequate duration. Providers should further individualize selection of an antiretroviral regimen on the basis of other considerations, including potential for drug–drug interactions, comorbid conditions, and resistance test results.

RECOMMENDED NRTI BACKBONES

The NRTI combinations of tenofovir/emtricitabine (TDF/FTC) or abacavir/lamivudine (ABC/3TC) comprise the nucleoside backbone in each of the recommended and alternative regimens. Both NRTI combinations are available as co-formulated, fixed-dose tablets and as components of co-formulated single-tablet regimens. Choosing between the two NRTI pairs is directed mainly by differences between TDF and ABC. Recently, tenofovir alafenamide (TAF), an oral prodrug of tenofovir (TFV), has become available in several co-formulated preparations (TAF/FTC, elvitegravir/cobicistat/TAF/FTC (EVG/c/TAF/FTC), and rilpivirine (RPV)/TAF/FTC) that been approved by the FDA.

In two clinical studies, ACTG 5202 and ASSERT, regimens with ABC/3TC were shown to have an inferior virologic response compared with regimens containing TDF/FTC (Sax, 2009; Post, 2010). ACTG 5202 compared the efficacy and safety of ABC/3TC to that of TDF/FTC when each was used in combination with either EFV or ritonavir-boosted atazanavir (ATV/r); differences in virologic efficacy were noted in those with baseline HIV RNA level greater than 100,000 copies/ml (Sax, 2009). The ASSERT study compared ABC/3TC to TDF/FTC, with each also receiving EFV. The proportion of participants with HIV RNA less than 50 copies/ml was lower among ABC/3TC-treated participants (Post, 2010). However, other studies have documented virologic equivalence between ABC/3TC and TDF/FTC. The HEAT study compared ABC/3TC to TDF/FTC, each in combination with ritonavir-boosted lopinavir (LPV/r); there was no difference in virologic efficacy, including in patients with baseline HIV RNA greater than 100,000 copies/ml (Smith, 2009). Similarly, ABC/3TC has shown comparable virologic efficacy to

Table 20.1 FACTORS FOR CONSIDERATION IN ART REGIMEN SELECTION

PATIENT CHARACTERISTICS	COMORBIDITIES	REGIMEN-SPECIFIC CONSIDERATIONS
Pretreatment HIV RNA level	Cardiovascular disease, hyperlipidemia, renal disease, osteoporosis, psychiatric illness, neurologic disease, drug abuse requiring narcotic replacement therapy	Regimen's genetic barrier to resistance
Pretreatment CD4$^+$ cell count	Pregnancy or pregnancy potential	Potential adverse effects of medications
HIV genotypic drug resistance	Co-infections: Hepatitis C, hepatitis B, tuberculosis	Drug interactions
HLA-B*5701 status		Convenience—pill burden, dosing frequency, availability of fixed-dose combination products, food requirement
Patient's anticipated compliance		Cost
Patient's preference		

TDF/FTC when used in combination with dolutegravir (DTG) (Walmsley, 2013).

ABC has been associated with a hypersensitivity reaction—a systemic illness with fever, rash, constitutional symptoms, and multiorgan involvement—in 5–8% of individuals. Testing for HLA-B*5701 should precede ABC's clinical uses because the risk of an ABC-related hypersensitivity reaction is highly associated with the presence of this allele; ABC is contraindicated in patients who are HLA-B*5701 positive (ViiV Healthcare, 2013).

ABC has also been associated with myocardial infarction (MI) in some observational studies but not in others. No consensus has been reached on the association between ABC use and MI risk or the mechanism for such an association (Monforte, 2013; Palella, 2015; Sabin, 2014; Worm, 2010; Young, 2015).

TDF has been associated with renal impairment. The risk for this adverse event may be greater when TDF is used in regimens containing PIs or elvitegravir boosted with ritonavir or cobicistat (Mocroft, 2015). The use of TDF has also been associated with a decrease in bone mineral density (McComsey, 2011).

TAF is an oral prodrug of TFV that has been designed to achieve higher active metabolite concentrations in peripheral blood mononuclear cells and lower plasma TFV exposures than TDF. This results in comparable antiviral efficacy but less renal and bone mineral adverse effects. The approval of TAF and the two TAF-containing regimens—elvitegravir 150 mg/cobicistat 150 mg/emtricitabine 200 mg/TAF 10 mg (EVG/c/TAF/FTC) and rilpivirine 25 mg/TAF 25mg/FTC 200 mg (RPV/TAF/FTC)—was supported by 48-week data from two pivotal phase III studies in which EVG/c/TAF/FTC was found to be non-inferior to elvitegravir 150 mg/cobicistat 150 mg/emtricitabine 200 mg/TDF 300 mg (EVG/c/TDF/FTC) among treatment-naive adult patients. The safety and efficacy of TAF/FTC were also demonstrated in one switch study of virologically suppressed patients who were randomized to continue TDF/FTC or switch to TAF/FTC (Gallant, 2016; Pozniak, 2016). Bioequivalence studies have demonstrated that stand-alone TAF/FTC achieved the same drug levels of TAF/FTC in the blood as EVG/c/TDF/FTC. Bioequivalence studies have also demonstrated that RPV/TAF/FTC achieved similar drug levels of emtricitabine and TAF in the blood as EVG/c/TAF/FTC and similar drug levels of RPV as stand-alone RPV. Based on these results, EVG/c/FTC/TAF is considered as a recommended initial regimen for ART-naive patients with an estimated creatinine clearance ≥30 ml/min. TAF/FTC is now included as a component of several recommended regimens and offers clinicians an additional NRTI backbone option. Two doses of TAF have been approved: 25 and 10 mg. The 10-mg dose is intended for use in combination with ritonavir or cobicistat; otherwise, the 25-mg dose of TAF is recommended.

CHOOSING BETWEEN AN INSTI, NNRTI, OR PI

The choice of the third drug in an initial ARV regimen between an INSTI, NNRTI, or PI is based on consideration of the regimen's efficacy, genetic barrier to resistance, adverse effects, convenience, comorbidities, and drug–drug interactions. Based on these considerations, the following observations have been noted:

- The efficacy and safety of DTG-based regimens (with either ABC/3TC or TDF/FTC) have been evaluated in three clinical trials (SPRING-2, SINGLE, and FLAMINGO). DTG-based regimens were found to be non-inferior or superior to other INSTI-, NNRTI-, or PI-based regimens. Thus, DTG/ABC/3TC and DTG + TDF/FTC are among recommended first-line ART regimens (Clotet, 2014; Raffi, 2013; Walmsley, 2013).

- The efficacy and safety of RAL (with either TDF/FTC or ABC/3TC) have been evaluated in a number of clinical trials, in which it was shown to be superior to EFV-, ATV/r-, and DRV/r-based regimens and non-inferior to DTG-based regimens (Lennox, 2009, 2014; Raffi, 2013).

- The four-drug, fixed-dose combination product, EVG/c/TDF/FTC, has been evaluated in two randomized clinical trials, in which it was found to be non-inferior to EFV/TDF/FTC or ATV/r plus TDF/FTC (Rockstroh, 2013; Zolopa, 2013).

- Clinical studies of DRV/r + TDF/FTC have shown it to be non-inferior to RAL and superior to LPV/r. Compared to DTG-based regimens in the FLAMINGO study, DRV/r was inferior to DTG, with adverse events being the primary driver for this difference (Clotet, 2014).

- Until recently, EFV, particularly the single-tablet regimen EFV/TDF/FTC, has played a central role in the preferred first-line antiretroviral regimen category. This was based on its demonstrated superiority or non-inferiority to all the regimens against which it was compared. However, recent studies have shown superiority of DTG, RAL, and RPV (in patients with baseline HIV RNA <100,000 copies/ml and

CD4 cell count >200 cells/mm³) to EFV; these results were primarily driven by differences in adverse events. Concern regarding EFV-related adverse events was further enhanced by a possible association with suicidality observed in one analysis of four clinical trials (Mollan, 2014). Thus, EFV/TDF/FTC has been relegated to the alternative first-line ART category.

• Until recently, ATV/r + TDF/FTC was among the preferred first-line antiretroviral regimens based on its virologic efficacy, which is equivalent to that of a number of comparator regimens, including EFV/TDF/FTC, EFV + ABC/3TC, LPV/r + TDF/FTC, and EVG/c/TDF/FTC. However, a recent study, ACTG 5257, compared ATV/r with DRV/r or RAL, each in combination with TDF/FTC. Virologic efficacy was comparable among the three groups; however, more adverse events and treatment discontinuations were noted among patients on ATV/r compared to the other two groups (Lennox, 2015). Thus, ATV/r has been relegated to the alternative first-line ART category.

RECOMMENDED FIRST-LINE ANTIRETROVIRAL REGIMENS

Regimens classified as recommended by the DHHS guidelines are those that have shown optimal and durable virologic efficacy in randomized controlled trials, are easy to use, and have favorable tolerability and toxicity profiles.

There are six recommended regimens for ART-naive patients. Four of these are INSTI-based regimens, and one is a ritonavir-boosted protease inhibitor (PI/r) (Table 20.2.

ALTERNATIVE FIRST-LINE ANTIRETROVIRAL REGIMENS

Alternative regimens are effective regimens with some potential disadvantages (e.g., pill burden, dosing, schedule, toxicity profile, baseline HIV RNA levels, and CD4 cell count) compared to preferred regimens, or they may have less supporting data from randomized clinical trials. However, there may be situations in which an alternative regimen might be preferred in an individual patient (e.g., treatment of a pregnant woman). These alternative regimens are categorized as NNRTI-based regimens and PI-based regimens (Table 20.3).

OTHER FIRST-LINE ANTIRETROVIRAL REGIMENS

These regimens may have reduced virologic activity; lack efficacy from large comparative clinical trials; or have increased toxicity, higher pill burden, increased potential for drug–drug interactions, or limitations for use in certain patient populations (Table 20.4).

INCORPORATING DHHS RECOMMENDATIONS FOR FIRST-LINE ANTIRETROVIRAL REGIMEN INTO CLINICAL PRACTICE: SELECT CLINICAL SCENARIOS

The DHHS guidelines provide an evidence-based menu for selecting an initial antiretroviral regimen. However, it

Table 20.2 **RECOMMENDED INITIAL ART REGIMENS**

INSTI-BASED REGIMENS	PI-BASED REGIMEN
Dolutegravir/abacavir/lamivudine (DTG/ABC/3TC)[a,b]—if HLA-B*5701 negative	Ritonavir boosted darunavir (DRV/r) plus tenofovir/emtricitabine (TDF/FTC)[a,c]
Dolutegravir plus tenofovir/emtricitabine (DTG + TDF/FTC)[a,c]	
Elvitegravir/cobisistat/tenofovir/emtricitabine (EVG/c/TDF/FTC)—if pre-ART CrCl >70 ml/min[b]	
Raltegravir (RAL) plus tenofovir/emtricitabine (TDF/FTC)[a,c]	
Elvitegravir/cobicistat/tenofovir alafenamide/emtricitabine (EVG/c/TAF/FTC)—if pre-ART CrCl ≥30 ml/min[b]	

[a]Lamivudine (3TC) may be interchanged with emtricitabine (FTC) or vice versa.

[b]Single-pill, once-daily regimen.

[c]Fixed-dose co-formulated product for nucleoside backbone.

Table 20.3 ALTERNATIVE ART REGIMENS

NNRTI-BASED REGIMENS	PI-BASED REGIMENS
Efavirenz/tenofovir/emtricitabine (EFV/TDF/FTC)[a,b]	Cobicistat-boosted atazanavir (ATV/c) plus tenofovir/emtricitabine (TDF/FTC)[a,c]—only if pretreatment estimated CrCl ≥70 ml/min
Rilpivirine/tenofovir/emtricitabine (RPV/TDF/FTC)[a,b]—if pretreatment HIV RNA <100000 copies/ml and CD4$^+$ count >200 cells/mm^3	Ritonavir-boosted atazanavir (ATV/r) plus tenofovir/emtricitabine (TDF/FTC)[a,c]
	Cobicistat-boosted darunavir (DRV/c) or ritonavir-boosted Darunavir (DRV/r) plus abacavir/lamivudine (ABC/3TC)[a,c]—if HLA-B*5701 negative
	Cobicistat-boosted darunavir (DRV/c) plus tenofovir/emtricitabine (TDF/FTC)[a,c]—if pretreatment estimated CrCl ≥70 ml/min

[a]Lamivudine (3TC) may be interchanged with emtricitabine (FTC) or vice versa.

[b]Single-pill, once-daily regimen.

[c]Fixed-dose co-formulated product for nucleoside backbone.

Table 20.4 OTHER ART REGIMENS

NNRTI-BASED REGIMEN	PI-BASED REGIMENS	INSTI-BASED REGIMEN
Efavirenz plus abacavir/lamivudine (EFV plus ABC/3TC)[a,b]—if HLA-B*5701 negative and pretreatment HIV RNA <1,000,000 copies/ml	Cobicistat-boosted atazanavir or ritonavir-boosted atazanavir plus abacavir/lamivudine (ATV/c or ATV/r plus ABC/3TC)[a,c]—if HLA-B*5701 negative and pretreatment HIV RNA <100,000 copies/ml	Raltegravir plus abacavir/lamivudine (RAL plus ABC/3TC)[a,c]—if HLAB5701 negative
	Ritonavir-boosted lopinavir (once or twice daily) plus abacavir/lamivudine (LPV/r plus ABC/3TC)[a,c]—if HLAB5701 negative	
	Ritonavir-boosted lopinavir (once or twice daily) plus tenofovir/emtricitabine (LPV/r plus TDF/FTC)[c]	

[a]Lamivudine (3TC) may be interchanged with emtricitabine (FTC) or vice versa.

[b]Single-pill, once-daily regimen.

[c]Fixed-dose co-formulated product for nucleoside backbone.

Table 20.5 BASELINE CHARACTERISTICS

SCENARIO	RECOMMENDED ACTION
Low CD4$^+$ count (<200 cells/mm^3)	Do not use RPV or DRV/r plus RAL.
Pretreatment HIV RNA >100,000 copies/ml	Do not use RPV, ABC/3TC with EFV or ATV/r, or DRV/r plus RAL.

Table 20.6 CONCOMITANT MEDICAL CONDITIONS

SCENARIO	RECOMMENDED ACTION
Cardiac disease	Consider avoiding ABC and LPV/r.
Chronic kidney disease	Avoid TDF, in particular[a] • EVG/c/TDF/FTC • ATV/c with TDF • DRV/c with TDF
HIV-associated dementia	• Avoid EFV because its psychiatric effects may cloud the clinical picture. • Favor use of DRV- or DTG-based regimens due to the possibility of increased central nervous system penetration.
Osteoporosis	Consider avoiding TDF.
Hyperlipidemia	EFV, ABC, PI/r, and EVG/c have been associated with increases in lipids.
Psychiatric illness	Consider avoiding EFV. • It can exacerbate psychiatric symptoms. • It may be associated with suicidality.
Hepatitis B virus co-infection	• Use TDF/FTC or TDF/3TC. • If TDF use is contraindicated, recommend use of FTC or 3TC with entecavir.
Tuberculosis	• If rifampin is used, EFV/TDF/FTC is the recommended regimen. • If a PI/r-based ART regimen is used, rifabutin is the rifamycin of choice in the tuberculosis regimen.
Gastroesophageal reflux disease requiring the use of proton pump inhibitors	Avoid ATV or RPV.
Situations when neither tenofovir nor abacavir can be used	• DRV/r plus RAL • LPV/r plus 3TC

[a]These are regimens for which there are clinical trial data. A combination of other PIs and INSTIs may also result in similar outcomes but has not been tested in clinical studies.

remains the responsibility of clinicians to select the regimen most suited to the clinical scenario at hand. Here, select clinical scenarios are presented to illustrate this point.

BASELINE CHARACTERISTICS

Table 20.5 presents the baseline characteristics.

CONCOMITANT MEDICAL CONDITIONS

Table 20.6 presents the concomitant medical conditions.

Recommended Reading

US Department of Health and Human Services, Panel on Antiretroviral Guidelines for Adults and Adolescents. Guidelines for the use of antiretroviral agents in HIV-1-infected adults and adolescents. Available at https://aidsinfo.nih.gov/guidelines/html/1/adult-and-adolescent-treatment-guidelines/0. Accessed April 20, 2016.

US Department of Health and Human Services, Panel on Antiretroviral Guidelines for Adults and Adolescents. Panel on Antiretroviral Guidelines for Adults and Adolescents includes a fixed-dose combination of elvitegravir/cobicistat/emtricitabine/tenofovir alafenamide among the recommended regimens for antiretroviral treatment-naive individuals with HIV-1 infection. Available at https://aidsinfo.nih.gov/news/1621/evg-c-ftc-taf-statement-from-adult-arv-guideline-panel. Accessed November 22, 2015.

References

Clotet B, Feinberg J, van Lunzen J, et al. Once-daily dolutegravir versus darunavir plus ritonavir in antiretroviral-naive adults with HIV-1 infection (FLAMINGO): 48 week results from the randomised open-label phase 3b study. *Lancet*. 2014 Jun 28; 383(9936):2222–2231.

Cohen MS, Chen YQ, McCauley M, et al. Prevention of HIV-1 infection with early antiretroviral therapy. *N Engl J Med*. 2011; 365:493–505.

Cohen MS, et al. Final results of the HPTN 052 randomized controlled trial: Antiretroviral therapy prevents HIV transmission. Program and abstracts of the 8th IAS Conference on HIV Pathogenesis, Treatment & Prevention; July 19–22, 2015; Vancouver, British Columbia, Canada. Abstract MOAC0101LB.

Deeks SG. HIV infection, inflammation, immunosenescence, and aging. *Annu Rev Med*. 2011; 62:141–155.

Gallant JE, Daar ES, Raffi F, et al. Efficacy and safety of tenofovir alafenamide versus tenofovir disoproxil fumarate given as fixed-dose combinations containing emtricitabine as backbones for treatment of HIV-1 infection in virologically suppressed adults: A randomised, double-blind, active-controlled phase 3 trial. *Lancet HIV*. 2016 Apr; 3(4):e158–e165.

INSIGHT START Study Group. Initiation of antiretroviral therapy in early asymptomatic HIV infection. *N Engl J Med*. 2015; 373:795–807.

Lennox JL, DeJesus E, Lazzarin A, et al. Safety and efficacy of raltegravir-based versus efavirenz-based combination therapy in treatment-naïve patients with HIV-1 infection: a multicentre, double-blind, randomised controlled trial. *Lancet*. 2009 Sep 5; 374(9692):796–806.

Lennox JF, Landovitz RJ, Ribaudo HJ. Three nonnucleoside reverse transcriptase inhibitor-sparing antiretroviral regimens for treatment-naïve volunteers infected with HIV-1. *Ann Intern Med*. 2015 Mar 17; 162(6):461–462.

Lennox JL, Landovitz RJ, Ribaudo HJ, et al. Efficacy and tolerability of 3 nonnucleoside reverse transcriptase inhibitor-sparing antiretroviral regimens for treatment-naive volunteers infected with HIV-1: A randomized, controlled equivalence trial. *Ann Intern Med*. 2014 Oct 7; 161(7):461–471.

McComsey GA, Kitch D, Daar ES, et al. Bone mineral density and fractures in antiretroviral-naive persons randomized to receive abacavir-lamivudine or tenofovir disoproxil fumarate-emtricitabine along with efavirenz or atazanavir-ritonavir: AIDS Clinical Trials Group A5224s, a substudy of ACTG A5202. *J Infect Dis*. 2011; 203(12):1791–1801.

Mocroft A, Lundgren JD, Ross M, et al. Exposure to antiretrovirals (ARVs) and development of chronic kidney disease (CKD). 2015 Conference on Retroviruses and Opportunistic Infections, Seattle, February 23–24, 2015. Abstract 142.

Mollan KR, Smurzynski M, Eron JJ, et al. Association between efavirenz as initial therapy for HIV-1 infection and increased risk for suicidal ideation or attempted or completed suicide: An analysis of trial data. *Ann Intern Med*. 2014 Jul 1; 161(1):1–10.

Monforte Ad, Reiss P, Ryom L, et al. Atazanavir is not associated with an increased risk of cardio- or cerebrovascular disease events. *AIDS*. 2013 Jan 28; 27(3):407–415.

Mugavero MJ, Napravnik S, Cole SR, et al. Viremia copy-years predicts mortality among treatment-naïve HIV-infected patients initiating antiretroviral therapy. *Clin Infect Dis*. 2011 Nov 1; 53(9):927–935.

Palella F, et al. NA-ACCORD: Recent abacavir use and risk of MI. CROI 2015, Seattle, WA, February 23–26, 2015. Abstract 749 LB.

Post FA, Moyle GJ, Stellbrink HJ, et al. Randomized comparison of renal effects, efficacy, and safety with once-daily abacavir/lamivudine versus tenofovir/emtricitabine, administered with efavirenz, in antiretroviral-naive, HIV-1-infected adults: 48-week results from the ASSERT study. *J Acquir Immune Defic Syndr*. 2010; 55(1):49–45.

Pozniak A, Arribas JR, Gathe J, et al. Switching to tenofovir alafenamide, coformulated with elvitegravir, cobicistat, and emtricitabine, in HIV-infected patients with renal impairment: 48-week results from a single-arm, multicenter, open-label phase 3 study. *J Acquir Immune Defic Syndr*. 2016 Apr 15; 71(5):530–537.

Raffi F, Jaeger H, Quiros-Roldan E, et al. Once-daily dolutegravir versus twice-daily raltegravir in antiretroviral-naive adults with HIV-1 infection (SPRING-2 study): 96 week results from a randomised, double-blind, non-inferiority trial. *Lancet Infect Dis*. 2013; 13(11):927–935.

Rockstroh J, DeJesus E, Henry K, et al. A randomized, double-blind comparison of coformulated elvitegravir/cobicistat/emtricitabine/tenofovir DF vs. ritonavir-boosted atazanavir plus coformulated emtricitabine and tenofovir DF for initial treatment of HIV-1 infection: Analysis of week 96 results. *J Acquir Immune Defic Syndr*. 2013; 62(5):483–486.

Sabin C, Reiss P, Ryom L, et al. Is there continued evidence for an association between abacavir and myocardial infarction risk? 21st Conference on Retroviruses and Opportunistic Infections, Boston, 2014. Abstract 747.

Sax P, Tierney C, Collier A, et al. Abacavir–lamivudine versus tenofovir–emtricitabine for initial HIV-1 therapy. *N Engl J Med*. 2009 Dec 3; 361(23):2230–2240.

Smith KY, Patel P, Fine D, et al. Randomized, double-blind, placebo-matched, multicenter trial of abacavir/lamivudine or tenofovir/emtricitabine with lopinavir/ritonavir for initial HIV treatment. *AIDS*. 2009 July 31; 23(12):1547–1556.

The TEMPRANO ANRS 12136 Study Group. A trial of early antiretrovirals and isoniazid preventive therapy in Africa. *N Engl J Med*. 2015; 373:808–822.

US Department of Health and Human Services, Panel on Antiretroviral Guidelines for Adults and Adolescents. Guidelines for the use of antiretroviral agents in HIV-1-infected adults and adolescents. Available at http://aidsinfo.nih.gov/contentfiles/lvguidelines/AdultandAdolescentGL.pdf. Accessed April 30, 2016.

ViiV Healthcare. Ziagen (abacavir) US prescribing information. 2013. Available at http://www.accessdata.fda.gov/drugsatfda_docs/label/2012/020977s025,020978s029lbl.pdf. Accessed April 30, 2016.

Walmsley SL, Antela A, Clumeck N, et al. Dolutegravir plus abacavir–lamivudine for the treatment of HIV-1 infection. *N Engl J Med*. 2013; 369(19):1807–1818.

Worm SW, Sabin C, Weber R, et al.; DAD Study Group. Risk of myocardial infarction in patients with HIV infection exposed to specific individual antiretroviral drugs from 3 major drug classes. *J Infect Dis*. 2010; 201:318–330.

Young J, Xiao Y, Moodier EE, et al. Effect of cumulating exposure to abacavir on the risk of cardiovascular disease events in patients from the Swiss HIV cohort study. *J AIDS*. 2015; 69(4):413–421.

Zolopa A, Sax P, DeJesus E, et al. A randomized double-blind comparison of coformulated elvitegravir/cobicistat/emtricitabine/tenofovir disoproxil fumarate versus favirenz/emtricitabine/tenofovir disoproxil fumarate for initial treatment of HIV-1 infection: Analysis of week 96 results. *J Acquir Immune Defic Syndr*. 2013; 63:96–100.

21.

HIV-1 RESISTANCE TO ANTIRETROVIRAL DRUGS

Ye Thu and Naiel Nassar

LEARNING OBJECTIVE

Discuss the different HIV drug resistance mutations and cross-resistance patterns in each class of HIV medication.

WHAT'S NEW?

In recent years, newer HIV medications have been introduced, and several studies have identified resistance mutations associated with the newer medications.

KEY POINTS

- Previous exposure to antiretroviral (ART) medications has a significant role in the development of drug resistance, especially in patients who are noncompliant with medications.

- Drug resistance testing should be done in the setting of treatment failure because it can help achieve better virologic response.

- There is extensive cross-resistance with first-generation non-nucleoside reverse transcriptase inhibitors and first-generation integrase strand inhibitors.

EPIDEMIOLOGY OF DRUG RESISTANCE

Numerous epidemiologic studies of antiretroviral resistance in both treatment-experienced and treatment-naive individuals have been performed in the potent combination ART era. The development of antiretroviral resistance depends on previous antiretroviral exposure, compliance with the medication, and availability of a fully active antiretroviral regimen for the individual patient. A patients' historical antiretroviral usage will have a major effect on the rate of resistance. For instance, in populations in which a large percentage of patients were previously treated with mono- and dual-nucleoside therapy, there will be higher rates of antiretroviral resistance.

In the developed world, current rates of antiretroviral resistance in treatment-experienced individuals are declining as the rates of virologic failure decrease with the availability of more potent and better tolerated regimens. Also, patients who were previously exposed to suboptimal therapy are becoming a smaller proportion of the total HIV-infected population. According to the Swiss HIV cohort study from 1998 to 2012, the rate of antiretroviral resistance in treatment-experienced patients is declining over time but that in treatment-naive patients is not (Yang, 2015).

In treatment-naive individuals, the rate of transmitted drug resistance (TDR) is related to the prevalence of drug resistance in individuals practicing high-risk behaviors in a community. Thus, rates of TDR can vary widely between locales. Studies of chronically infected individuals in the United States and Western Europe suggest that 8–16% of transmitted viruses will be resistant to at least one antiretroviral, whereas 3–5% of transmitted viruses will have resistance to more than one class of antiretrovirals (Cane, 2005; Ocfemia, 2012; Weinstock, 2004; Wheeler, 2007). In early HIV infection (defined as within 1 year of seroconversion), reported rates of TDR are substantially higher. In New York state, the rate of TDR among recently infected cases increased from 17% in 2006 to 24% in 2013, from 13% to 18% in cases with long-standing infection, and from 13% to 19% in all cases regardless of chronicity of the infection. Prevalence of TDR mutation was significantly higher among recently infected (19% vs. 15%; OR, 1.29; 95% confidence interval, 1.16–1.43) across all subgroups (Wang, 2015). In San Diego, the prevalence of TDR also increased significantly between 1996 and 2013 among recently infected treatment-naive individuals (Panichsillapakit, 2016). There are conflicting reports on the trends of TDR over time. As mentioned previously, the rate of TDR is increasing, especially among the recently infected patients in New York and San Diego. However, according to the UK drug resistance database of the UK collaborative group on HIV drug resistance, the prevalence of TDR in ART-naive individuals tends to be decreasing, especially among the men who have sex with men population (Tostevin, 2015). These differences likely reflect variation in the sampling of infected subjects. Furthermore, the consistent use of the consensus statement on the mutations that should be defined as TDR (versus possible polymorphisms) will aid in the comparison of rates across studies (Bennett, 2009).

GUIDELINES FOR THE USE OF RESISTANCE TESTING

Several expert panels have issued guidelines for the optimal use of resistance testing (Table 21.1) (Asboe, 2012; Hirsh, 2008; US Department of Health and Human Services (DHHS), 2016). All the panels recommend the use of resistance testing in the setting of treatment failure. Several randomized studies have demonstrated that this strategy (regardless of whether genotypic or phenotypic testing is used) leads to superior virologic responses (Baxter, 2000; Cohen, 2002; Durant, 1999). With treatment failure, either genotypic or phenotypic resistance testing is appropriate. In patients with a complex treatment history, the combination of genotypic and phenotypic resistance testing may be helpful. Ideally, resistance testing should be performed while the patient is still on the failing regimen. With removal of drug-selection pressure, wild-type virus will quickly replace the resistant virus as the dominant population circulating in the plasma.

For treatment-naive adults, earlier versions of treatment recommendations only supported resistance testing in early HIV infection. However, studies have shown that TDR can be detected many years after initial infection (Little, 2008). Because patients infected with resistant virus do not have a reservoir of drug-susceptible virus, TDR is only replaced by drug-susceptible virus by back mutation, a process that can require months to years. Furthermore, abundant evidence indicates that TDR, particularly to non-nucleoside reverse transcriptase inhibitors (NNRTIs), leads to suboptimal virologic response (Kuritzkes, 2008; Little, 2002). A cost-effectiveness analysis found baseline genotyping to be cost-effective when the background rate of TDR is 5% or greater (a situation that is likely in most locales in the developed world) (Sax, 2005). Consequently, resistance testing in chronically infected treatment-naive patients is now recommended by all three leading agencies. Resistance testing should be performed when the patient enters clinical care, regardless of whether ART is planned in the near term, because the sensitivity of resistance testing declines with time due to the fact that there is some back mutation to wild-type virus. Due to cost considerations and its improved sensitivity for detecting viral mixtures, genotypic testing is preferred in this setting. Resistance testing is also recommended for treatment-naive pregnant and pediatric patients.

Table 21.1 EXPERT PANEL RECOMMENDATIONS FOR USE OF RESISTANCE TESTING IN THE CLINICAL MANAGEMENT OF HIV-1

SETTING	DHHS[A]	IAS-USA[B]	BHIVA[C]
Primary infection	Recommended	Recommended	Recommended
Chronic infection	Recommended	Recommended	Recommended
Treatment failure	Recommended	Recommended	Recommended
Pregnancy	Recommended	Recommended	Recommended
Pediatric	Recommended	No recommendations	No recommendations

[a]Panel on Antiretroviral Guidelines for Adults and Adolescents (DHHS, 2016).

[b]Hirsh et al. (2008).

[c]The British HIV Association Guidelines 2011 (Asboe et al., 2012).

RESISTANCE TESTING

GENOTYPIC RESISTANCE TESTING: THE TEST AND ITS INTERPRETATION

Genotype testing involves the detection of specific genetic mutations in a patient's dominant viral isolate that are known to be associated with antiretroviral resistance. To perform a genotypic resistance test, polymerase chain reaction (PCR) is used to amplify reverse transcriptase and protease. Many labs can now amplify integrase, if requested. Direct PCR dideoxynucleotide sequencing is performed. Overlapping sequencing reactions are performed in both directions and resolved electrophoretically in a sequencer. The amino acid sequence is then compared to the standard HIV subtype B consensus sequence. Differences in amino acids at positions that have been found to be associated with resistance are reported. With current techniques, there is a high degree of interlab reproducibility in sequencing (Shafer, 2001). However, there is some variability in labs' ability to perform genotypic resistance testing at low viral loads (e.g., between 200 and 1000 copies/ml).

Numerous genotypic interpretation systems (GIS) are available (Table 21.2). In addition, many scores for individual drugs have been created (Pellegrin, 2008; Vingerhoets, 2008). Whereas most GIS are free, the virtual phenotype by Virco (the "Vircotype") uses available genotype–phenotype pairs within the company's database to predict the phenotype based on the genotype. However, there is little evidence that the virtual phenotype outperforms rules-based GIS when predicting virologic response (Torti, 2003).

Although the outputs of the most commonly used GIS are relatively straightforward, there is still a significant role for the expert clinician in deciding on the optimal salvage regimen. The benefit of additional expert advice compared with provider-only interpretation of genotype testing results was clearly demonstrated by the Havana trial (Tural, 2002). Using a factorial design, the investigators

Table 21.2 EXAMPLES OF WIDELY USED WEB-BASED GENOTYPIC INTERPRETATION SYSTEMS

French ANRS (National Agency for AIDS Research)	http://www.hivfrenchresistance.org
International AIDS Society USA Mutation List	http://www.iasusa.org/content/drug-resistance-mutations-in-HIV
Rega Institute	https://rega.kuleuven.be
Stanford University HIV Resistance Database	http://hivdb.stanford.edu

randomized subjects with virologic failure to receive a combination of genotype resistance testing and/or expert advice prior to the choice of the salvage regimen. The study demonstrated that a salvage regimen selected based on both resistance testing and expert advice improved virologic outcomes, and the combination of the two was superior to either one alone.

When comparing the GIS, they are similar in their ability to predict the activity of a drug based on a set of mutations (Grant, 2008). Multiple clinical studies have shown that a genotypic susceptibility score (GSS) created from a GIS is a strong predictor of virologic response (Cooper, 2008; Fätkenheuer, 2008). A GSS that weights the activity of the boosted protease inhibitor in the salvage regimen may have the capacity to improve the predictive value of a GSS derived from a GIS (Fox, 2007).

PHENOTYPIC RESISTANCE TESTING: THE TEST AND ITS INTERPRETATION

Phenotypic resistance testing measures in vitro susceptibility to specific drugs and may complement genotypic testing in complex cases in which there are multiple resistance mutations, especially in protease, that may make it difficult to predict the outcome of mutational interactions.

Phenotypic resistance testing is available as commercial tests from Monogram Biosciences and Virco (Hertogs, 1998; Monogram Biosciences, 2016), both of which use similar methods and require a viral load ≥1000 copies/ml to be performed successfully. However, due to declining demand, since April 2010, the phenotype test from Virco has not been available for routine clinical use. Initially, PCR is used to amplify the reverse transcriptase (RT) and protease (PR) sequences of the patient's virus (and integrase, if requested). This sequence is then transfected into a lab strain of HIV (which has its RT and PR sequences deleted). The chimeric virus is then cultured with CD4 cell lines in the presence of different concentrations of drugs. In the Monogram assay, a reporter gene (luciferase) indicates infection of cells. In the Virco assay, infection of cells is determined by monitoring for viral cytopathic effect. Both assays report a fold change for each drug that is determined by the ratio of the IC_{50} (the concentration of a drug that is required for 50% viral inhibition) from the patient's chimeric virus divided by the IC_{50} of a wild-type virus. A comparison of the two phenotypic assays showed a substantial degree of concordance between their reported outputs for a given isolate. The concordance for the two tests is especially good for the protease inhibitors (PIs) and NNRTIs, but the two tests were less comparable for the nucleoside/nucleotide reverse transcriptase inhibitors (NRTIs), with the Monogram assay showing more sensitivity in detecting drug resistance (Zhang, 2005).

The interpretation of the phenotype is based on defined clinical cut-offs for each drug. There are potentially two important cut-offs for each drug. The lower cut-off would define when the susceptibility begins to decline but the drug still has partial activity, and the upper cut-off would be the fold change at which all drug activity is lost. If these clinical cut-offs have not been defined for a given drug, the clinician is provided a biological cut-off, which is based on the normal variation in fold changes in wild-type virus. If the fold change is above the upper cut-off, it will be reported as decreased susceptibility. However, if the fold change is below the lower cut-off, it will be reported as increased susceptibility.

The PhenoSense assay also reports replication capacity (RC), an attempt to provide a surrogate for in vivo fitness of a virus. Reduced RC measured by this methodology has been associated with slower disease progression in treatment-naive individuals (Goetz, 2007). However, currently, RC plays a relatively limited role in the clinical management of patients.

RESISTANCE TESTING IN RESOURCE-LIMITED SETTINGS

Because of the limited availability of resistance testing in resource-limited settings, it is generally not used to guide therapy choices. The World Health Organization does use a sentinel monitoring system to assess the levels of TDR in various sites in the developing world.

ANTIRETROVIRAL CROSS-RESISTANCE

DEFINITION OF CROSS-RESISTANCE AND FACTORS AFFECTING LIKELIHOOD OF OCCURRENCE

When HIV replicates in the presence of an incompletely suppressive regimen, the viral mutations that are selected by a specific drug may confer resistance to that drug, as well as to other drugs in the same therapeutic class. This phenomenon has been recognized for NRTIs, NNRTIs, PIs, and integrase strand transfer inhibitors (INSTIs). The rate at which cross-resistance develops and the extent to which it affects other drugs in the class vary for the different antiretroviral agents. For the first-generation NNRTIs

and INSTIs, there is a high level of cross-resistance. Among NRTIs, the potential for cross-resistance varies, although there is complete cross-resistance between lamivudine and emtricitabine. Among PIs and second-generation NNRTIs, as more resistance mutations accumulate during virologic failure to drugs in their class, there is an increasing degree of resistance.

CROSS-RESISTANCE PATTERNS IN NRTIS

Nucleoside analogue-associated mutations (NAMs) are a set of reverse transcriptase mutations that confer some degree of resistance to NRTIs and are selected when HIV is exposed to drugs in the NRTI class. These include M41L, E44D, K65R, D67N, 69 insertions, L74V/I, K70R, V118I, Q151M, M184V/I, L210W, T215Y/F, and K219Q/E.

A subset of NAMs that are associated with resistance to zidovudine and stavudine are known as thymidine analogue mutations (TAMs) and occur at positions 41, 67, 70, 210, 215, and 219. An accumulation of TAMs causes loss of susceptibility to the broad NRTI class, independent of the specific mutations associated with resistance to other NRTIs (Whitcomb, 2003).

Two other resistance profiles are also associated with broad NRTI cross-resistance. Q151M usually appears after HIV is exposed to didanosine plus either stavudine or zidovudine. Four other supporting mutations arise afterward (A62V, V75I, F77L, and F116Y), with resulting loss of susceptibility to all NRTIs except tenofovir.

The codon 69 insertion is less common than the Q151M complex. It is composed of a T69S mutation followed by the addition of two amino acids, including serine and usually a second serine, alanine, or glycine. It always arises on a background of TAMs and a few other mutations to create resistance to all currently approved NRTIs.

Most other drug-specific resistance mutations act like the Q151M complex by improving reverse transcriptase's ability to discriminate between NRTIs and the natural nucleoside substrates. For these non-thymidine mutations, the implications of cross-resistance increase when drugs with similar resistance profiles are used together.

K65R confers resistance to the non-thymidine NRTI drugs, including abacavir, didanosine, emtricitabine, lamivudine, and tenofovir. Although uncommon with currently used therapies, K65R developed at high rates in individuals prescribed NRTI-only regimens that lacked a thymidine analogue (e.g., abacavir/lamivudine/tenofovir). The use of thymidine analogues in a regimen appears to decrease the risk of the emergence of K65R because K65R antagonizes the ability of TAMs to facilitate NRTI removal (White, 2006).

The L74V and M184V mutations can also cause cross-resistance. L74V alone causes some decreased susceptibility to abacavir and didanosine. M184V causes resistance to lamivudine and emtricitabine, decreased susceptibility to abacavir and didanosine, and increased susceptibility to tenofovir and zidovudine.

CROSS-RESISTANCE PATTERNS IN NNRTIS

There is extensive cross-resistance between the first-generation NNRTIs (e.g., delavirdine, efavirenz, and nevirapine). Etravirine is unique among currently available NNRTIs in that both in vitro and clinical evidence suggest that it retains antiviral activity in the presence of resistance to first-generation NNRTIs (Madruga, 2007; Vingerhoets, 2008). Rilpivirine has an in vitro profile similar to that of etravirine (Rimsky, 2009). Rilpivirine may also retain antiviral activity in patients with resistance failing treatment with other NNRTIs—efavirenz and nevirapine (Theys, 2015). Rilpivirine-based regimens are well tolerated and associated with fewer virologic failures in full virally suppressed treatment-experienced patients upon switching from other ART regimens for different reasons (Gazaignes, 2014).

Mutations at reverse transcriptase codons 103 or 188 lead to high-level resistance to the first-generation NNRTIs. K103N does not reduce the activity of etravirine, whereas Y188L leads to low-level etravirine resistance. Mutations at position 181 lead to high-level resistance to nevirapine and subsequent rapid development of high-level resistance to efavirenz. The Y181C/I/V mutation also is an important mutation for etravirine and is among the mutations given the greatest weighting within Tibotec's scoring system for etravirine (the others being L100I, K101P, and M230L) (Vingerhoets, 2008).

CROSS-RESISTANCE PATTERNS IN PROTEASE INHIBITORS

Several protease mutations emerge during exposure to a variety of PIs, especially unboosted PIs. The accumulation of four or more mutations at codons 10, 32, 46, 54, 82, 84, and 90 is associated with resistance to most agents in the class. However, darunavir and tipranavir both frequently maintain activity against viruses resistant to older PIs and have shown clinical benefit in patients with extensive drug resistance.

CROSS-RESISTANCE PATTERNS IN INSTIS

There is extensive cross-resistance between the first-generation INSTIs raltegravir and elvitegravir. Raltegravir resistance occurs by three main, occasionally overlapping, mutational pathways: N155H followed by E92Q and other accessory mutations, Q148H/R/K + G140S/A and other accessory mutations, and Y143C/R + T97A and other accessory mutations. With the exception of Y143C/R, most raltegravir-resistance mutations confer cross-resistance to elvitegravir. Likewise, it appears that most elvitegravir-resistance mutations are likely to confer cross-resistance to raltegravir.

Dolutegravir, a second-generation INSTI, has a higher barrier to resistance than raltegravir and elvitegravir. Dolutegravir has good activity against most of the viral strains resistant to raltegravir and elvitegravir. However, the virologic response of dolutegravir is significantly reduced when the Q148 mutation is associated with two or more secondary mutations (G140A/C/S, E138A/K/T, or L74I) compared to no Q148 mutation (Castagna, 2014).

CONSIDERATIONS FOR RESOURCE-LIMITED SETTINGS

In many resource-limited settings, access to resistance testing is limited or unavailable. However, it is still important to understand the implications of resistance when attempting to sequence therapies in these settings. In the absence of resistance testing, a patient who is experiencing virologic failure on an NNRTI-based regimen despite good adherence should be assumed to harbor NNRTI-associated resistance and switched to boosted PI-based regimen, if available.

ANTIRETROVIRAL RESISTANCE MUTATIONS

Figures 21–1 through 21–4 detail the mutations that are associated with resistance to reverse transcriptase, protease, entry, and integrase inhibitors.

Drugs for which a single mutation results in a major change in susceptibility are said to have a low "genetic barrier" to resistance. Examples of such drugs include lamivudine, emtricitabine, enfuvirtide, delavirdine, efavirenz, nevirapine, raltegravir, and elvitegravir. Boosted PIs, etravirine and dolutegravir, have higher genetic barriers to resistance and require multiple mutations that occur

Nucleoside and Nucleotide Analogue Reverse Transcriptaste Inhibitors (nRTIs)[a]

Multi-nRTI Resistance: 69 Insertion Complex[b] (affects all nRTIs currently approved by the US FDA)

M	A	▼	K			L	T	K
41	62	69	70			210	215	219
L	V	Insert	R			W	Y	Q
								I	L

Multi-nRTI Resistance: 151 Complex (affects all nRT is currently approved by the US FDA except tenofovir))

	A		V	F		F	Q
	62		75	77		116	151
	V		I	L		Y	M

Multi-nRTI Resistance: Thymidine Analogue–Associated Mutation (TAMs; affected all nRIS currently approved by the US FDA)

M		D	K				L	T	K
41		67	70				210	215	219
L		N	R				W	Y	Q
									I	L

Abacavir[fa]

	K		L			Y		M
	65		74			115		184
	R		V			I		V

Didanosine[ab]

	K		L
	65		74
	R		V

Emtricitabine

	K					M
	65					184
	R					V
						I
						M

Lamivudine

	K					M
	65					184
	R					V
						I

Stavudine

M		K	D	K			L	T	K
41		65	67	70			210	215	219
L		R	N	R			W	Y	Q
									I	L

Tenofovir[l]

	K		K
	65		70
	R		L

Zidovudine[a]

M		D	K				L	T	K
41		67	70				210	215	219
L		N	R				W	Y	Q
									I	L

Figure 21.1 Mutations in the reverse transcriptase gene associated with resistance to reverse transcriptase inhibitors—NRTIs. SOURCE: Reprinted from the International AIDS Society–USA Drug Resistance Mutations Group update (Wensing, 2015). Reprinted with permission of the IAS-USA.

Nonnucleoside Analogue Reverse Transcriptase Inhibitors (NNRTIs)[a,m]

Efavirenz

L	K	K	V	V			Y		Y	G			P
100	101	103	106	108			181		188	190			225
I	P	N	M	I			C		L	S			H
		S					I			A			

Etravirine[n]

V	A	L	K		V		E		V	Y		G			M
90	98	100	101		105		138		179	181		190			230
I	G	I*	E		I		A		D	C*		S			L
			H				G		F	I*		A			
			P*				K		T	V*					
							Q								

Nevirapine

V	K	K	V	V			Y		Y	G
100	101	103	106	108			181		188	190
I	P	N	A	I			C		C	A
		S	M				I		L	
									H	

Rilpivirine[o]

K			E		V	Y			H	F	M
101			138		179	181			221	227	230
E			A		L	C			Y	C	I
P			G			V					L
			K*								
			Q								
			R								

Figure 21.2 Mutations in the reverse transcriptase gene associated with resistance to reverse transcriptase inhibitors—NNRTIs. SOURCE: Reprinted from the International AIDS Society–USA Drug Resistance Mutations Group update (Wensing, 2015). Reprinted with permission of the IAS-USA.

MUTATIONS IN THE PROTEASE GENE ASSOCIATED WITH RESISTANCE TO PROTEASE INHIBITORS[p,q,r]

Atazanavir +/− ritonavir[r]

Position	10	16	20	24	32	33	34	36	46	48	50	53	54	60	62	64	71	73	82	84	85	88	90	93
Wild-type	L	G	K	L	V	L	E	M	M	G	I	F	I	D	I	I	A	G	V	I	I	N	L	I
Substitution	I F V C	E	R M I T V	I	I	I F V	Q	I L V	I L	V	L	L Y	L V M T A	E	V	L M V	V I T L	C S T A	A T F I	V	V	S	M	L M

Darunavir/ritonavir[t]

Position	11	32	33	47	50	54	74	76	84	89
Wild-type	V	V	L	I	I	I	T	L	I	L
Substitution	I	I	F	V	V	M L	P	V	V	V

Fosamprenavir/ritonavir

Position	10	32	46	47	50	54	73	76	82	84	90
Wild-type	L	V	M	I	I	I	G	L	V	I	L
Substitution	F I R V	I	I	V L	V	L V M	S	V	A F S T	V	M

Indinavir/ritonavir[w]

Position	10	20	24	32	36	46	54	71	73	76	77	82	84	90
Wild-type	L	K	L	V	M	M	I	A	G	L	V	V	I	L
Substitution	I R V	M R	I	I	I	I L	V	V T	S A	V	I	A F T	V	M

Lopinavir/ritonavir[v]

Position	10	20	24	32	33	45	47	50	53	54	63	71	73	76	82	84	90
Wild-type	L	K	L	V	L	M	I	I	F	I	L	A	G	L	V	I	L
Substitution	F I R V	M R	I	I	F	I L A	V A	V	L	V L A M T S	P	V T	S	V	A F T S	V	M

Nelfinavir[u,w]

Position	10	30	36	46	71	77	82	84	88	90
Wild-type	L	D	M	M	A	V	V	I	N	L
Substitution	F I	N	I	I L	V T	I	A F T S	V	D S	M

Saquinavir/ritonavir[u]

Position	10	24	48	54	62	71	73	77	82	84	90
Wild-type	L	L	G	I	I	A	G	V	V	I	L
Substitution	I R V	I	V	V L	V	V T	S	I	A F T S	V	M

Tipranavir/ritonavir[w]

Position	10	33	36	43	46	47	54	58	69	74	82	83	84	89
Wild-type	L	L	M	K	M	I	I	Q	H	T	V	N	I	L
Substitution	V	F	I L V	T	L	V	A M V	E	K R	P	L T	D	V	I M V

Figure 21.3 Mutations in the protease gene associated with resistance to protease inhibitors. SOURCE: Reprinted from the International AIDS Society–USA Drug Resistance Mutations Group update (Wensing, 2015). Reprinted with permission of the IAS-USA.

MUTATIONS IN THE ENVELOPE GENE ASSOCIATED WITH RESISTANCE TO ENTRY INHIBITORS

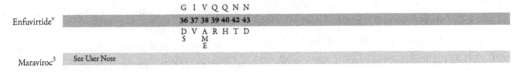

Enfuvirtide[y]

Position	36	37	38	39	40	42	43
Wild-type	G	I	V	Q	Q	N	N
Substitution	D S	V	A M E	R	H	T	D

Maraviroc[z] See User Note

MUTATIONS IN THE INTEGRASE GENE ASSOCIATED WITH RESISTANCE TO INTEGRASE INHIBITORS

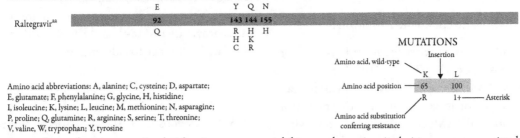

Raltegravir[aa]

Position	92	143	144	155
Wild-type	E	Y	Q	N
Substitution	Q	R H C	H K R	H

MUTATIONS

- Amino acid, wild-type → K
- Insertion → L
- Amino acid position → 65, 100
- Amino acid substitution conferring resistance → R, 1+ ——— Asterisk

Amino acid abbreviations: A, alanine; C, cysteine; D, aspartate; E, glutamate; F, phenylalanine; G, glycine; H, histidine; I, isoleucine; K, lysine; L, leucine; M, methionine; N, asparagine; P, proline; Q, glutamine; R, arginine; S, serine; T, threonine; V, valine; W, tryptophan; Y, tyrosine.

Figure 21.4 Mutations in the envelope gene associated with resistance to entry inhibitors and mutations in the integrase gene associated with resistance to integrase inhibitors. SOURCE: Reprinted from the International AIDS Society–USA Drug Resistance Mutations Group update (Wensing, 2015). Reprinted with permission of the IAS-USA.

in a stepwise manner to confer substantially reduced drug susceptibility.

RESISTANCE ASSOCIATED WITH NRTIS

Mechanisms

As with all enzymatic reactions, reverse transcription exists as an equilibrium between a forward and a reverse reaction. The forward reaction is characterized by attack of the 3′-hyroxyl group of the primer on the α-phosphate of the incoming deoxynucleoside triphosphate (dNTP) to form a phosphodiester bond, releasing pyrophosphate. This extends the length of the primer chain by one base. This process continues to extend the primer until natural completion or until an incoming dNTP is a nucleoside analogue, which lacks the 3′-hydroxyl group and therefore prematurely terminates the chain. The reverse reaction removes the terminal nucleoside monophosphate from the primer by coupling with free pyrophosphate or adenosine triphosphate. This is termed pyrophosphorolysis. If the terminal base is a nucleoside analogue, its removal from the terminated primer will unblock the chain so it can continue extension. This is referred to as primer unblocking.

In general, NRTI-associated resistance mutations cause resistance by either increasing the rate of primer unblocking or decreasing the incorporation of nucleoside analogues compared with the natural dNTPs. Allosteric interference with the incorporation of the nucleoside analogue is the major mechanism by which the mutations M184V, Y115F, Q151M, L74V, V118I, and K65R cause resistance. The TAMs M41L, D67N, K70R, L210W, T215Y/F, and K219Q/E/N enhance primer unblocking. An increase in the number of TAMs proportionally increases the degree of primer unblocking. Insertions at position 69 also enhance primer unblocking, especially in the presence of the TAMs.

Thymidine Analogue Mutations

Zidovudine and stavudine select for mutations at reverse transcriptase positions 41, 67, 70, 210, 215, and 219. Although these TAMs are selected by the thymidine analogues, either alone or in combination with other drugs, increasing numbers of TAMs decrease the in vivo activity of all NRTIs. There are generally two different clusters of evolution among these mutations. The first and most common pathway is M41L, L210W, and T215Y. The second pathway includes D67N, K70R, T215F, and K219Q/E/N. The second pathway results in less phenotypic cross-resistance to other NRTIs compared to the first pathway.

M184V/I

Lamivudine and emtricitabine select for the M184I and V mutations. M184I develops first and then is generally replaced by the M184V mutation due to a fitness advantage. However, in an unusual example of "cross-talk" between the NRTI- and NNRTI-associated mutations, patients with failure to rilpivirine/tenofovir/emtricitabine are more likely to develop M184I (rather than M184V) in combination with E138K (Kulkarni, 2012; Rimsky, 2012). M184V/I is also selected by abacavir and didanosine, and it confers some degree of cross-resistance to these drugs, although this mutation alone is not enough to significantly decrease the response to either. M184V/I reverse TAM-associated resistance to zidovudine, stavudine, and tenofovir.

K65R

K65R is selected by tenofovir and, to a lesser extent, abacavir and didanosine. Interestingly, it also appears more commonly in subtype C virus during failure with stavudine-containing regimens (Doualla-Bell, 2006). K65R confers partial resistance to didanosine, abacavir, tenofovir, lamivudine, emtricitabine, and possibly stavudine. K65R results in in vitro hypersusceptibility to zidovudine, although the clinical relevance of this finding is unclear (Grant, 2010).

L74V

L74V was the most common mutation that arose in patients receiving didanosine monotherapy but also was seen in patients receiving abacavir monotherapy. L74V is rarely selected in combination therapies that include thymidine analogues and didanosine or abacavir; however, it can occur with combination therapies that include didanosine/lamivudine or abacavir/lamivudine. L74V confers resistance or partial resistance to didanosine, lamivudine, emtricitabine, and abacavir. Like M184V and K65R, L74V reduces TAM-associated resistance to zidovudine.

Q151M Complex

Q151M develops in 5–10% of patients treated with thymidine analogue/didanosine combinations and causes moderate resistance to all NRTIs. The Q151M mutation is generally associated with mutations at positions A62V, V75I/F, F77L, and F116Y. Each of these mutations substantially increases the degree of resistance and the fitness of isolates containing Q151M. Tenofovir retains some activity against HIV with this mutational complex, and lamivudine may also have activity.

69 Insertions

Insertions at the fingers region between codons 67 and 70, most commonly two amino acids at position 69, occur in 1% or 2% of patients treated extensively with NRTIs. These inserts are typically found in strains that also contain TAMs. Isolates with insertions at codon 69 and TAMs are highly cross-resistant to all the currently available NRTIs.

E44D/A and V118I

Mutations E44D/A and V118I both occur in untreated patients, but their prevalence increases in subjects who have had extensive exposure to NRTIs. These mutations cause low-level resistance to lamivudine and emtricitabine and probably to each of the other NRTIs.

RESISTANCE ASSOCIATED WITH NNRTIS

Mechanisms

The catalytic domain for reverse transcription has a three-dimensional structure often compared to a right hand. Despite their diverse chemical structure, NNRTIs all bind to a similar location within a hydrophobic pocket in HIV-1 reverse transcriptase outside the active domain of the enzyme. The binding of an NNRTI results in a conformational change in reverse transcriptase, thus resulting in the displacement of the catalytic aspartate residues in relation to the polymerase binding site. Nearly all the NNRTI resistance mutations are within or adjacent to this NNRTI-binding pocket and alter the shape of the NNRTI pocket to exclude the NNRTI. The second-generation NNRTI, etravirine, has a more flexible chemical structure that allows it to bind within the pocket despite the presence of mutations.

K103N

K103N occurs in more than 50% of patients failing efavirenz and also leads to high-level resistance to nevirapine and delavirdine. However, K103N does not affect antiviral response to etravirine and in vitro does not affect susceptibility to rilpivirine.

Y181C

Y181C is often selected for by nevirapine and confers only minimal resistance to efavirenz. However, attempts to sequence drugs using nevirapine followed by efavirenz have resulted in rapid development of resistance to efavirenz, likely due to an emergence of preexisting minority-resistant quasispecies (Lecossier, 2005). Y181C is an important mutation for etravirine and is among the mutations given the greatest weighting within the manufacturer's scoring system for etravirine (Table 21.3).

Y188 C/L/H and G190A/S

Mutations at positions 188 and 190 in reverse transcriptase confer resistance to nevirapine and efavirenz but remain susceptible to delavirdine, although no studies have shown the utility of delavirdine in this setting. Etravirine also maintains activity in the presence of these mutations.

E138K

E138K is the most common mutation selected for by rilpivirine. It is selected less frequently by etravirine and reduces its susceptibility by approximately fivefold. E138K reduces

Table 21.3 **TIBOTEC'S WEIGHTED ETRAVIRINE SCORE**

MUTATION	WEIGHT FACTOR[a]
Y181V/I	3.0
L100I	2.5
K101P	2.5
Y181C	2.5
M230L	2.5
V106I	1.5
E138A	1.5
V179F	1.5
G190S	1.5
V90I	1.0
A98G	1.0
K101E/H	1.0
V179D/T	1.0
G190A	1.0

[a]A weighted mutation score of 0–2, 2.5–3.5, and ≥4 corresponded to response rates of 74% (highest response), 52% (intermediate response), and 38% (reduced response), respectively.

SOURCE: Data from Vingerhoets et al. (2008).

the susceptibility of nevirapine and efavirenz approximately two- to fivefold.

RESISTANCE ASSOCIATED WITH PROTEASE INHIBITORS

Mechanisms

Protease processes the Gag and Gag/Pol polyprotein precursors necessary for viral maturation. The visualization of protease using X-ray crystallography allowed for the development of the PI drug class. Protease exists as a homodimer, with each subunit consisting of 99 amino acids, creating a cleft that is the active site of protease. PIs act as competitive inhibitors, binding within this cleft and disabling the enzyme. Mutations within the cleft can exclude PIs, leading to resistance. Most PI-resistant viruses also require at least one Gag cleavage site mutation to compensate for the altered substrate cleft caused by resistance mutations within protease.

Major Mutations

PI resistance mutations are generally categorized as major mutations (ones that confer significant resistance) and accessory mutations (ones that enhance resistance or viral fitness when a primary resistance mutation is present). Most major mutations lead to some degree of cross-class resistance, but a few signature mutations are not associated with cross-class resistance. The I50L mutation to atazanavir and the D30N mutation to nelfinavir are the best examples of signature mutations that do not lead to class-wide resistance.

The presence of signature mutations in protease that do not lead to cross-resistance led some to advocate for the sequencing of PIs. However, because primary resistance to boosted PIs is very rare in treatment-naive individuals failing boosted PI-based regimens, the argument for the sequencing of boosted PIs is not strong.

The major protease mutations that lead to some degree of cross-class resistance are V32I, M46I/L, G48V/M, I50V, I54V/T/A/L/M, L76V, V82A/T/F/S, I84V, N88S, and L90M. PI cross-resistance is complex as a result of the large number of PI-resistance mutations and the fact that different mutations at the same position can have markedly different effects on PI susceptibility. This is particularly the case for mutations at positions 50, 54, and 82.

Darunavir, however, usually retains activity even in the presence of multiple major PI-associated mutations (Talbot, 2010) and has supplanted lopinavir/ritonavir as first-line treatment in patients harboring extensive PI-associated resistance. In clinical trials, the presence of three or more of the following mutations was associated with a diminished response to darunavir: V11I, V32I, L33F, I47V, I50V, I54L/M, G73S, L76V, I84V, and L89V (De Meyer, 2008).

Tipranavir also has activity against virus with high-level protease resistance. Although genotypic scores have been developed for tipranavir (Scherer, 2007), none of the scores perform well in predicting susceptibility to tipranavir (Talbot, 2010), and a phenotype may be particularly useful when tipranavir is being considered for use. However, tipranavir is rarely used in clinical practice given the preserved activity of darunavir in most cases and tipranavir's multiple drug–drug interactions and concerning side effect profile (US Food and Drug Administration, 2005).

RESISTANCE ASSOCIATED WITH INSTIS

Mechanisms

HIV integrase catalyzes a multistep process that allows the double-stranded HIV cDNA to be irreversibly incorporated within the host DNA. INSTIs inhibit the final step of integration ("strand transfer"), the covalent bonding of the primed viral ends to the cleaved host DNA. INSTIs bind only to integrase bound to viral DNA, attaching closely to the enzyme's active site and disrupting the correct positioning of the viral DNA relative to the active site and the interaction of integrase with the two essential magnesium ions. Although the multiple mutations associated with resistance against INSTIs have been identified, the full-length crystal structure of HIV integrase is still not developed.

N155H

The N155H mutation develops early in the course of virologic failure to raltegravir and is accompanied by E92Q and other accessory mutations. N155H is associated with high-level raltegravir and elvitegravir resistance. However, dolutegravir, a second-generation INSTI, appears to retain activity in the presence of N155H.

Q148H/R/K

Mutations at codon 148 in integrase often develop later in individuals failing raltegravir-based therapy. Mutations at codon 148 are accompanied by mutations at codon 140 and lead to high-level resistance to raltegravir and elvitegravir. When dolutegravir dosed as 50 mg BID provides a good response in patients with resistance to raltegravir/

elvitegravir (Eron, 2011). However, mutations at codon 148 together with two or more secondary mutations (G140A/C/S, E138A/K/T, or L74I) are also associated with low response to dolutegravir (Castagna, 2014).

Y143C/R

Mutations at codon 143 in integrase develop relatively uncommonly with failure to a raltegravir-containing regimen. Site-directed mutagenesis experiments suggest that mutations at codon 143 do not lead to cross-resistance to elvitegravir (Métifiot, 2011), but clinical data are lacking to support elvitegravir's use for this indication.

E92Q

E92Q is the most common integrase mutation that develops during virologic failure to elvitegravir. The mutation leads to cross-resistance with raltegravir, but dolutegravir is expected to maintain activity.

R263K

According to an in vitro study, R263K mutation can lead to low resistance to dolutegravir (Quashie, 2012).

MUTATIONS ASSOCIATED WITH ENTRY INHIBITORS

CCR5 Antagonists

Maraviroc binds to the CCR5 receptor and antagonizes the gp120–CCR5 interaction. Resistance to maraviroc can develop through two distinct mechanisms. Most commonly, the virus can begin using the CXCR4 co-receptor for entry; less commonly, mutations can occur that allow gp120 to bind the bound CCR5 receptor.

When a virus appears to switch from CCR5-tropic to dual/mixed-tropic or CXCR4-tropic, this is more frequently due to outgrowth of a minority variant than a de novo switch. Monogram's second-generation enhanced-sensitivity Trofile assay is more sensitive in detecting these minority variants compared to the first-generation assay. Due to clinicians' experience with the Trofile assay and its use for the evaluation of tropism in clinical trials for maraviroc, this assay remains the gold standard in assessing tropism (Gulick, 2008). However, genotypic interpretation of tropism has been shown to have a high degree of concordance with the Trofile and had a similar ability compared to the first-generation Trofile to predict short-term virologic response to maraviroc (Harrigan, 2009; Raymond, 2008).

When CCR5-tropic viruses become resistant to CCR5 antagonists, they generally show changes in the V3 loop stem in gp120, although changes in gp41 have also been associated with resistance to CCR5 antagonists (Anastassopoulou, 2009). There appears to be a wide variety of mutational patterns in the env gene, and no predictive rules based on genotypic changes have been developed.

Fusion Inhibitors

Currently, enfuvirtide is rarely used, given the frequent injection site reactions that develop with its use. Several mutations in the gp41 envelope gene have been associated with resistance or reduced susceptibility to enfuvirtide, primarily at codons 36–45 of the first heptad repeat (HR1) region.

References

Anastassopoulou CG, Ketas TJ, Klasse PJ, et al. Resistance to CCR5 inhibitors caused by sequence changes in the fusion peptide of HIV-1 gp41. *Proc Natl Acad Sci USA*. 2009; 106:5318–5323.

Asboe D, Aitken C, Boffito M, et al. British HIV Association guidelines for the routine investigation and monitoring of adult HIV-1-infected individuals 2011. *HIV Med*. 2012; 13:1–44.

Baxter JD, Mayers DL, Wentworth DN, et al. A randomized study of antiretroviral management based on plasma genotypic antiretroviral resistance testing in patients failing therapy. *AIDS*. 2000; 14:F83–F93.

Bennett DE, Camacho RJ, Otelea D, et al. Drug resistance mutations for surveillance of transmitted HIV-1 drug-resistance: 2009 update. *PLoS One*. 2009; 4:e4724.

Cane P, Chrystie I, Dunn D, et al. Time trends in primary resistance to HIV drugs in the United Kingdom: Multicentre observational study. *Br Med J*. 2005; 331:1368.

Castagna A, Maggiolo F, Penco G, et al. Dolutegravir in antiretroviral-experienced patients with raltegravir- and/or elvitegravir-resistant HIV-1: 24-Week results of the phase III VIKING-3 study. *J Infect Dis*. 2014; 210(3):354–362.

Cohen CJ, Hunt S, Sension M, et al. A randomized trial assessing the impact of phenotypic resistance testing on antiretroviral therapy. *AIDS*. 2002; 16:579–588.

Cooper DA, Steigbigel RT, Gatell JM, et al. Subgroup and resistance analyses of raltegravir for resistant HIV-1 infection. *N Engl J Med*. 2008; 359:355–365.

De Meyer S, Dierynck I, Lathouwers E, et al. Identification of mutations predictive of a diminished response to darunavir/ritonavir: Analysis of data from treatment-experienced patients in POWER 1, 2, 3 and Duet-1 and Duet-2. Paper presented at the 6th European HIV Drug Resistance Workshop, 2008, Budapest. Abstract 54.

Doualla-Bell FA, Avalos B, Brenner T, et al. High prevalence of the K65R mutation in human immunodeficiency virus type 1 subtype C isolates from infected patients in Botswana treated with didanosine-based regimens. *Antimicrob Agents Chemother*. 2006; 50:4182–4185.

Durant J, Clevenbergh P, Halfon P, et al. Drug-resistance genotyping in HIV-1 therapy: The VIRADAPT randomised controlled trial. *Lancet*. 1999; 353:2195–2199.

Eron J, Kumar P, Lazzari A, et al. DTG in subjects with HIV exhibiting RAL resistance: Functional monotherapy results of VIKING study cohort II. Paper presented at the 18th Conference on Retroviruses and Opportunistic Infections, February 27–March 2, 2011, Boston. Abstract 151LB.

Fätkenheuer G, Nelson M, Lazzarin A, et al. Subgroup analyses of maraviroc in previously treated R5 HIV-1 infection. *N Engl J Med*. 2008; 359:1442–1455.

Fox ZV, Geretti AM, Kjaer J, et al. The ability of four genotypic interpretation systems to predict virological response to ritonavir-boosted protease inhibitors. *AIDS*. 2007; 21:2033–2042.

Gazaignes S, Resche-Rigon M, Yang C, et al. Efficacy and safety of rilpivirine-based regimens in treatment-experienced HIV-1 infected patients: A prospective cohort study. *J Int AIDS Soc*. 2014 Nov 2; 17(4 Suppl 3):19796

Goetz M, Leduc R, Kostman J, et al. HIV replicative capacity is an independent predictor of disease progression in persons with untreated chronic HIV infection. Paper presented at the 4th IAS Conference on HIV Pathogenesis, Treatment and Prevention, July 22–25, 2007, Sydney, Australia. Abstract WEPDB07.

Grant P, Taylor J, Nevins A, et al. Antiviral activity of zidovudine and tenofovir in the presence of the K65R mutation in reverse transcriptase: An international cohort analysis. *Antimicrob Agents Chemother*. 2010; 54:1520–1525.

Grant P, Wong EC, Rode R, et al. Virologic response to lopinavir–ritonavir-based antiretroviral regimens in a multicenter international clinical cohort: Comparison of genotypic interpretation scores. *Antimicrob Agents Chemother*. 2008; 52:4050–4056.

Gulick RM, Lalezari J, Goodrich J, et al. Maraviroc for previously treated patients with R5 HIV-1 infection. *N Engl J Med*. 2008; 359:1429–1441.

Harrigan PR, McGover R, Dong W, et al. Screening for HIV tropism using population based V3 genotypic analysis: A retrospective virological outcome analysis using stored plasma screening samples from MOTIVATE-1. Paper presented at the XVIII International HIV Drug Resistance Workshop, June 9–13, 2009, Fort Myers, FL. Abstract 15.

Hertogs K, de Bethune MP, Miller V, et al. A rapid method for simultaneous detection of phenotypic resistance to inhibitors of protease and reverse transcriptase in recombinant human immunodeficiency type 1 isolates from patients treated with antiretroviral drugs. *Antimicrob Agents Chemother*. 1998; 42:269–276.

Hirsh MS, Gunthard HF, Schapiro JM, et al. Antiretroviral drug testing in adult HIV-1 infection: 2008 Recommendations of an International AIDS Society panel. *Clin Infect Dis*. 2008; 47:266–285.

Kulkarni R, Babaoglu K, Lansdon EB, et al. The HIV-1 reverse transcriptase M184I mutation enhances the E138K-associated resistance to rilpivirine and decreases viral fitness. *J Acquir Immune Defic Syndr*. 2012; 59:47–54.

Kuritzkes DR, Lalama CM, Ribaudo HJ, et al. Preexisting resistance to nonnucleoside reverse-transcriptase inhibitors predicts virologic failure of an efavirenz-based regimen in treatment-naive HIV-1-infected subjects. *J Infect Dis*. 2008; 197:867–870.

Lecossier D, Shulman NS, Morand-Joubert L, et al. Detection of minority populations of HIV-1 expressing the K103N resistance mutation in patients failing nevirapine. *J Acquir Immune Defic Syndr*. 2005; 38:37–42.

Little SJ, Frost SD, Wong JK, et al. Persistence of transmitted drug resistance among subjects with primary human immunodeficiency virus infection. *J Virol*. 2008; 82:5510–5518.

Little SJ, Holte S, Routy JP, et al. Antiretroviral-drug resistance among patients recently infected with HIV. *N Engl J Med*. 2002; 347:385–394.

Madruga JV, Cahn P, Grinsztejn B, et al. Efficacy and safety of TMC125 (etravirine) in treatment-experienced HIV-1 infected patients in Duet-1: 24-Week results from a randomized, double-blind placebo-controlled trial. *Lancet*. 2007; 37:29–38.

Métifiot M, Vandegraaff N, Maddali K, et al. Elvitegravir overcomes resistance to raltegravir induced by integrase mutation Y143. *AIDS*. 2011; 25:1175–1178.

Monogram Biosciences. http://www.monogramvirology.com/hiv-tests/resistance-testing/phenotype. Accessed April 29, 2016.

Ocfemia CB, Kim D, Ziebell R, et al. Prevalence and trends of transmitted drug resistance-associated mutations by duration of infection among persons newly diagnosed with HIV-1 infection: 5 states and 3 municipalities, US, 2006 to 2009. Paper presented at the 19th Conference on Retroviruses and Opportunistic Infections, Seattle, WA, March 5–8, 2012. Abstract 730.

Panichsillapakit T, Smith D, Wertheim T, et al. Prevalence of transmitted HIV drug resistance among recently infected persons in San Diego, California 1996–2013. *J Acquir Immune Defic Syndr*. 2016; 71(2):228–3620.

Pellegrin I, Wittkop L, Joubert LM, et al. Virological response to darunavir/ritonavir-based regimens in antiretroviral-experienced patients (PREDIZISTA study). *Antiviral Ther*. 2008; 13:271–279.

Quashie P, Mespléde T, Han Y, et al. Characterization of the R263K mutation in HIV-1 integrase that confers low-level resistance to the second-generation integrase strand transfer inhibitor dolutegravir. *J Virol*. 2012; 86(5):2696–2705.

Raymond S, Delobel P, Mavigner M, et al. Correlation between genotypic predictions based on V3 sequences and phenotypic determination of HIV-1 tropism. *AIDS*. 2008; 22:F11–F16.

Rimsky L, Vingerhoets J, Van Eygen V, et al. Genotypic and phenotypic characterization of HIV-1 isolates obtained from patients on rilpivirine therapy experiencing virologic failure in the phase 3 ECHO and THRIVE studies: 48-Week analysis. *J Acquir Immune Defic Syndr*. 2012; 59:39–46.

Rimsky LT, Azijn H, Tirry I, et al. In vitro resistance profile of TMC278, a next-generation NNRTI; Evidence of a higher genetic barrier and a more robust resistance profile than first generation NNRTIs. Paper presented at the XVIII International Drug Resistance Workshop, Fort Myers, FL, June 9–13, 2009. Abstract 120.

Sax PE, Islam R, Walensky RP, et al. Should resistance testing be performed for treatment-naive HIV-infected patients? A cost-effectiveness analysis. *Clin Infect Dis*. 2005; 41:1316–1323.

Scherer J, Boucher C, Baxter JD, et al. Improving the prediction of virologic response to tipranavir: The development of a tipranavir weighted score. Paper presented at the 11th European AIDS Conference, 2007, Madrid. P3.4/07.

Shafer RW, Hertogs K, Zolopa AR, et al. High degree of interlaboratory reproducibility of human immunodeficiency virus type 1 protease and reverse transcriptase sequencing of plasma samples from heavily treated patients. *J Clin Microbiol*. 2001; 39:1522–1529.

Talbot A, Grant P, Taylor J, et al. Predicting tipranavir and darunavir resistance using genotypic, phenotypic and virtual phenotypic resistance patterns: An independent cohort analysis of clinical isolates highly resistant to all other protease inhibitors. *Antimicrob Agents Chemother*. 2010; 54:2473–2479.

Theys K, Camacho R, Gomes P, et al. Predicted residual activity of rilpivirine in HIV-1 infected patients failing therapy including NNRTIs efavirenz or nevirapine. *Clin Microbiol Infect*. 2015; 21(6):607. e1–e8.

Torti C, Quiros-Roldan E, Keulen W, et al. Comparison between rules-based human immunodeficiency virus type 1 genotype interpretations and real or virtual phenotype: Concordance analysis and correlation with clinical outcome in heavily treated patients. *J Infect Dis*. 2003; 188:194–201.

Tostevin A, White E, Croxford S, et al. Trends in transmitted drug resistance to HIV-1 in the UK since 2010. British HIV Association Conference (BHIVA), Brighton 2015. Abstract O15.

Tural C, Ruiz L, Holtzer C, et al. Clinical utility of HIV-1 genotyping and expert advice: The Havana trial. *AIDS*. 2002; 16:209–218.

US Department of Health and Human Services, Panel on Antiretroviral Guidelines for Adults and Adolescents. Guidelines for the use of antiretroviral agents in HIV-1-infected adults and adolescents. January 28, 2016. Available at https://aidsinfo.nih.gov/contentfiles/lvguidelines/AdultandAdolescentGL.pdf. Accessed April 29, 2016.

US Food and Drug Administration. New therapy for HIV patients with advanced disease. FDA Patient Safety News, Show 44. October 2005.

Vingerhoets J, Peeters M, Azijn H, et al. An update of the list of NNRTI mutations associated with decreased virologic response to etravirine (ETR): Multivariate analyses on the pooled DUET-1 and DUET-2 clinical trial data. Paper presented at the XVII HIV Drug Resistance Workshop, June 10–14, 2008, Sitges, Spain.

Wang Z, Walits E, Gordon D, et al. Transmitted drug resistance and time of HIV infection, New York State, 2006–2013. Paper presented at the 22nd Conference on Retroviruses and Opportunistic Infections (CROI), February 23–26, 2015, Seattle, WA. Abstract 599.

Weinstock HS, Zaidi I, Heneine W, et al. The epidemiology of antiretroviral drug resistance among drug-naive HIV-1-infected persons in 10 US cities. *J Infect Dis.* 2004; 189:2174–2180.

Wensing AM, Calvez V, Günthard HF, et al. 2015 update of the drug resistance mutations in HIV-1. *Top Antivir Med.* 2015 Oct–Nov; 23(4):132–141.

Wheeler W, Mahle K, Bodnar U, et al. Antiretroviral drug-resistance mutations and subtypes in drug-naïve persons newly diagnosed with HIV-1 infection, US, March 2003 to October 2006. Paper presented at the 14th Conference on Retroviruses and Opportunistic Infections, February 25–28, 2007, Los Angeles, CA. Abstract 648.

Whitcomb JM, Parkin NT, Chappey C, et al. Broad nucleoside reverse-transcriptase inhibitor cross-resistance in human immunodeficiency virus type 1 clinical isolates. *J Infect Dis.* 2003; 188:992–1000.

White KL, Chen JM, Feng JY, et al. The K65R reverse transcriptase mutation in HIV-1 reverses the excision phenotype of zidovudine resistance mutations. *Antivir Ther.* 2006; 11:155–163.

Yang W, Kouyos R, Scherrer A, et al. Assessing the paradox between transmitted and acquired HIV type 1 drug resistance mutations in the Swiss HIV cohort study from 1998 to 2012. *J Infect Dis.* 2015; 212(1):28–38.

Zhang J, Rhee SY, Taylor J, et al. Comparison of the precision and sensitivity of the Antivirogram and PhenoSense HIV drug susceptibility assays. *J AIDS.* 2005; 38:439–344.

ACKNOWLEDGMENTS

We thank the authors of previous editions of this chapter, Philip M. Grant and Andrew R. Zolopa.

22.

MANAGING THE PATIENT WITH MULTIDRUG-RESISTANT HIV

Ye Thu and Naiel Nassar

LEARNING OBJECTIVE

Explain how to construct the antiretroviral regimen for patients with multidrug-resistant HIV.

WHAT'S NEW?

Although it has been general practice to include nucleoside/nucleotide reverse transcriptase inhibitors in salvage regimens, there is not a significant difference in virologic failure rates between regimens containing them versus those that do not.

KEY POINTS

- Treatment guidelines emphasize the need for at least two or preferably three fully active medications in the salvage regimen of patients experiencing virologic failure.

- The new regimen should be started with as little interruption as possible because the structured interruption of treatment in patients with multidrug-resistant HIV infection is associated with greater progression of the disease.

- The pharmacokinetic enhancer, cobicistat, is available as a fixed-dose combination product with antiretroviral medication, which allows the treatment to be simplified and reduces the pill burden.

INTRODUCTION

During the past 15 years, HIV infection has been transformed into a chronic manageable disease primarily due to the effectiveness of antiretroviral therapy. Well-tolerated, potent combination antiretroviral therapy with simpler dosing schedules has led to a reduction in the rates of virologic failure and the proportion of patients harboring multidrug-resistant HIV.

Treatment guidelines emphasize achieving maximal virologic suppression. Given the newer integrase strand inhibitors (e.g., elvitegravir and dolutegravir) and existing classes with extended spectra of activity (e.g., tipranavir, darunavir, and etravirine) and with fewer side effects (e.g., tenofovir alafenamide), it is now possible to achieve maximal virologic suppression in virtually all adherent patients, even those harboring virus with extensive drug resistance. This chapter outlines strategies for managing patients harboring multidrug-resistant virus, including treatment simplification in virologically suppressed patients.

CONSTRUCTING AN ANTIRETROVIRAL DRUG REGIMEN IN PATIENTS EXPERIENCING VIROLOGIC FAILURE

In patients experiencing virologic failure, multiple studies have demonstrated that resistance testing (either genotypic or phenotypic) leads to improved virologic outcomes (Baxter, 2000; Cohen, 2002; Durant, 1999). Treatment guidelines emphasize the need for at least two or preferably three fully active medications in the salvage regimens of patients experiencing virologic failure (US Department of Health and Human Services (DHHS), 2016). In treatment-experienced patients, multiple clinical studies demonstrate higher rates of virologic suppression with an increasing number of active drugs in a salvage regimen (Cooper, 2008;

Fätkenheuer, 2008). However, rates of virologic response plateau when three active drugs are included in a salvage regimen; regimens including four active drugs do not outperform those with three (Cooper, 2008; Staszewski, 1999). In addition, higher baseline CD4[+] T cell count and lower HIV RNA levels predict virologic response (Cooper, 2008; Fätkenheuer, 2008).

OPTIMAL THERAPY FOR "EARLY" SALVAGE

According to the current DHHS guidelines, antiretroviral regimens for treatment-naive patients include either integrase strand inhibitor (INSTI) plus two nucleoside/nucleotide reverse transcriptase inhibitors (NRTIs) or boosted protease inhibitor (PI) plus two NRTIs. Because resistance to boosted PI and INSTIs in treatment-naive patients is relatively rare, most patients have a good virologic response to these regimens. However, if a patient who is already on NRTIs plus non-nucleoside reverse transcriptase inhibitors (NNRTIs) develops virologic failure, switching to boosted PI plus NRTIs has a better response compared to boosted PI alone (Bunupuradah, 2012). Also, based on another study, boosted PI plus INSTI is not inferior to boosted PI plus NRTIs (Boyd, 2013). Therefore, boosted PI plus INSTI can be another reasonable option.

OPTIMAL THERAPY FOR PATIENTS HARBORING VIRUS WITH MORE EXTENSIVE RESISTANCE

As per DHHS guidelines, drug resistance testing should be done for patients with virologic failure. To increase the chance of detecting selected mutations, the test should be done while the patient is taking the failing antiretroviral regimen or within 4 weeks after discontinuation of the treatment. The basic principle is to give at least two or, if possible, three fully active agents. The new treatment regimen should be formulated based on the drug resistance testing and previous drug exposure. The new regimen should be started with as little interruption as possible. One study proved that the structured interruption of treatment in patients with multidrug-resistant HIV infection is associated with greater progression of the disease and does not provide any immunologic or virologic benefit (Lawrence, 2003).

With the availability of medications such as dolutegravir, etravirine, and darunavir that have a higher barrier of resistance, it is easier than in the past to formulate the treatment regimen to achieve the maximum virologic response even for patients with multidrug-resistance HIV.

According to one study, dual therapy with darunavir/ritonavir and etravirine is effective in patients with virologic failure (Bernardino, 2014).

Resistance to INSTI is very rare in patients who are naive to this class of therapy (Doyle, 2015). However, for INSTI-experienced patients with resistance to raltegravir and elvitegravir, a good virologic response can still be achieved with dolutegravir 50 mg twice daily (Castagna, 2014).

For entry inhibitors, maraviroc can be considered fully active in patients with CCR5-tropic virus by the second-generation enhanced-sensitivity Trofile assay (ESTA) or a genotypic tropism assay (Harrigan, 2009). With dual/mixed or CXCR4-tropic viruses, maraviroc should not be expected to provide antiviral activity. Enfuvirtide is rarely required in salvage regimens because usually three other active drugs can be found, but for enfuvirtide-naive patients, it should be considered a fully active drug. For patients with prior ongoing viremia on enfuvirtide, resistance has likely developed, and enfuvirtide cannot be expected to provide residual activity.

Given the availability of the newer drugs, some may question the need for NRTIs in salvage therapy. Previously, general practice was to include NRTIs in salvage regimens, but there is no significant difference in virologic failure rate for salvage regimens without NRTIs compared to regimens containing NRTIs (Tashima, 2015). Examples of these regimens include boosted PIs plus INSTI or boosted PI plus NNRTI (Bernardino, 2014; Boyd, 2013).

SIMPLIFICATION OF ANTIRETROVIRAL THERAPY IN VIROLOGICALLY SUPPRESSED PATIENTS HARBORING MULTIDRUG-RESISTANT HIV

Given the efficacy of modern antiretroviral regimens, fewer patients are now experiencing virologic failure. However, many patients maintain virologic suppression on overly complex or poorly tolerated regimens or on regimens with increased rates of long-term toxicities.

According to DHHS (2016) guidelines, regimen switching in the setting of viral suppression can be considered

to simplify the regimen by reducing pill burden and dosing frequency to improve adherence, to enhance tolerability and decrease short- or long-term toxicity, to change food or fluid requirements, to avoid parenteral administration, to minimize or address drug interaction concerns, to reduce costs.

Treatment simplification requires the clinician to be aware of the patient's antiretroviral treatment history and previous resistance testing. In addition, if previous tropism testing is not available, the ESTA allows one to determine the viral tropism of HIV DNA in virologically suppressed patients so that it can be determined whether maraviroc would be expected to have activity.

In altering established therapy in virologically suppressed patients with a history of virologic failure, regimens should be chosen that would be predicted to be highly active based on the individual's past treatment history and resistance profile (DHHS, 2016). In general, substitutions of medications within the same antiretroviral drug class (generally with co-formulated medications or with newer, better tolerated or potent agents) are straightforward with a low risk of virologic failure (Mallolas, 2009; Martin, 2009).

Many patients with multidrug-resistance HIV take the regimen with boosted PIs because they have a higher barrier of resistance. Previously, ritonavir was the only available pharmacokinetic enhancer for PIs. However, the pharmacokinetic enhancer cobicistat has been recently introduced. The major advantage of cobicistat compared to ritonavir is cobicistat's solubility and dissolution rate, which allow cobicistat as a fixed-dose combination product with antiretroviral medication. This allows the treatment regimen to be simplified and also reduces the pill burden. In one study, darunavir/cobicistat was generally well tolerated and had a similar virologic and immunologic response as that of darunavir/ritonavir (Tashima, 2014).

Cobicistat was also studied as a pharmacokinetic enhancer for integrase inhibitors. It has been demonstrated that co-formulated elvitegravir, cobicistat, emtricitabine (FTC), and tenofovir disoproxil fumarate (TDF) is not inferior to the ritonavir-boosted PI/FTC/TDF regimen (Arribas, 2014; Huhn, 2015). Cobicistat can increase the serum creatinine level and decrease the estimated glomerular filtration rate (GFR). This is due to the effect on renal tubular secretion of creatinine; thus, the actual GFR is not changed with use of cobicistat (German, 2012). However, cobicistat is not recommended for administration with TDF in patients with estimated GFR <70 ml/min because dosage adjustment for TDF has not been established for this regimen. Out-of-class substitutions potentially hold greater risk if not carefully considered. This is especially true when switching a patient off of a PI to another class of medication with a lower barrier to resistance (e.g., a NNRTI or integrase inhibitor). A number of switch studies have shown increased rates of virologic failure when patients with previous histories of virologic failure on PI-based regimens were switched off the PI to a medication class with a lower barrier to resistance (Eron, 2010; Martinez, 2007). Although there are valid reasons to switch patients off PIs, this must be done cautiously in patients with histories of virologic failure and drug resistance.

References

Arribas JR, Pialoux G, Gathe J, et al. Simplification to coformulated elvitegravir, cobicistat, emtricitabine, and tenofovir versus continuation of ritonavir-boosted protease inhibitor with emtricitabine and tenofovir in adults with virologically suppressed HIV (STRATEGY-PI): 48 week results of a randomised, open-label, phase 3b, non-inferiority trial. *Lancet Infect Dis.* 2014; 14(7):581–589.

Baxter JD, Mayers DL, Wentworth DN, et al. A randomized study of antiretroviral management based on plasma genotypic antiretroviral resistance testing in patients failing therapy. *AIDS.* 2000; 14:F83–F93.

Bernardino JI, Zamora FX, Valencia E, et al. Efficacy of a dual therapy based on darunavir/ritonavir and etravirine in ART-experienced patients. *J Int AIDS Soc.* 2014; 17(4 Suppl 3):19787.

Boyd MA, Kumarasamy N, Moore CL, et al. Ritonavir-boosted lopinavir plus nucleoside or nucleotide reverse transcriptase inhibitors versus ritonavir-boosted lopinavir plus raltegravir for treatment of HIV-1 infection in adults with virological failure of a standard first-line ART regimen (SECOND-LINE): A randomised, open-label, non-inferiority study. *Lancet.* 2013 Jun 15; 381(9883):2091–2099.

Bunupuradah T, Chetchotisakd P, Ananworanich J, et al. A randomized comparison of second-line lopinavir/ritonavir monotherapy versus tenofovir/lamivudine/lopinavir/ritonavir in patients failing NNRTI regimens: The HIV STAR study. *Antivir Ther.* 2012; 17(7):1351–1361.

Castagna A, Maggiolo F, Penco G, et al. Dolutegravir in antiretroviral-experienced patients with raltegravir- and/or elvitegravir-resistant HIV-1: 24-Week results of the phase III VIKING-3 study. *J Infect Dis.* 2014; 210(3):354–362.

Cohen CJ, Hunt S, Sension M, et al. A randomized trial assessing the impact of phenotypic resistance testing on antiretroviral therapy. *AIDS.* 2002; 16:579–588.

Cooper DA, Steigbigel RT, Gatell JM, et al. Subgroup and resistance analyses of raltegravir for resistant HIV-1 infection. *N Engl J Med.* 2008; 359:355–365.

Doyle T, Dunn D, Ceccherini-Silberstein F, et al. Integrase inhibitor (INI) genotypic resistance in treatment-naive and raltegravir-experienced patients infected with diverse HIV-1 clades. *J Antimicrob Chemother.* 2015 Nov; 70(11):3080–3086.

Durant J, Clevenbergh P, Halfon P, et al. Drug-resistance genotyping in HIV-1 therapy: The VIRADAPT randomised controlled trial. *Lancet.* 1999; 353:2195–2199.

Eron JJ, Young B, Cooper DA, et al. Switch to a raltegravir-based regimen versus continuation of a lopinavir–ritonavir-based regimen in stable HIV-infected patients with suppressed viremia (SWITCHMRK 1 and 2): Two multicentre, double-blind, randomised controlled trials. *Lancet.* 2010; 375:396–407.

Fätkenheuer G, Nelson M, Lazzarin A, et al. Subgroup analyses of maraviroc in previously treated R5 HIV-1 infection. *N Engl J Med.* 2008; 359:1442–1455.

German P, Liu H, Szwarcberg J, et al. Effect of cobicistat on glomerular filtration rate in subjects with normal and impaired renal function. *J Acquir Immune Defic Syndr.* 2012 Sep 1; 61(1):32–40.

Harrigan PR, McGover R, Dong W, et al. Screening for HIV tropism using population based V3 genotypic analysis: A retrospective virological outcome analysis using stored plasma screening samples from MOTIVATE-1. Paper presented at the XVIII International HIV Drug Resistance Workshop, June 9–13, 2009, Fort Myers, FL. Abstract 15.

Huhn G, Tebas P, Gallant J, et al. Strategic simplification: The efficacy and safety of switching to elvitegravir/cobicistat/emtricitabine/tenofovir alafenamide (E/C/F/TAF) plus darunavir (DRV) in treatment-experienced HIV-1 infected adults (NCT01968551). Paper presented at Infectious Disease Week 2015. Abstract 726.

Lawrence J, Mayers D, Hullsiek KH, et al. Structured treatment interruption in patients with multidrug-resistant human immunodeficiency virus. *N Engl J Med*. 2003; 349:837–846.

Mallolas J, Podzamczer D, Milinkovic A, et al. Efficacy and safety of switching from boosted lopinavir to boosted atazanavir in patients with virological suppression receiving a LPV/r-containing HAART: The ATAZIP study. *J Acquir Immune Defic Syndr*. 2009; 51:29–36.

Martin A, Bloch M, Amin J, et al. Simplification of antiretroviral therapy with tenofovir–emtricitabine or abacavir–lamivudine: A randomized, 96-week trial. *Clin Infect Dis*. 2009; 49:1591–1601.

Martinez E. The NEFA study: Results at three years. *AIDS Rev*. 2007; 9:62.

Staszewski S, Morales-Ramirez J, Tashima KT, et al. Efavirenz plus zidovudine and lamivudine, efavirenz plus indinavir, and indinavir plus zidovudine and lamivudine in the treatment of HIV-1 infection in adults. Study 006 Team. *N Engl J Med*. 1999; 341:1865–1873.

Tashima K, Crofoot G, Tomaka FL, et al. Cobicistat-boosted darunavir in HIV-1-infected adults: Week 48 results of a phase IIIb, open-label single-arm trial. *AIDS Res Ther*. 2014; 11:39.

Tashima K, Smeaton L, Fichtenbaum C, et al. HIV salvage therapy does not require nucleoside reverse transcriptase inhibitors: A randomized, controlled trial. *Ann Intern Med*. 2015; 163(12):908–917.

US Department of Health and Human Services, Panel on Antiretroviral Guidelines for Adults and Adolescents. Guidelines for the use of antiretroviral agents in HIV-1-infected adults and adolescents. Available at https://aidsinfo.nih.gov/guidelines/html/1/adult-and-adolescent-treatment-guidelines/0. Accessed February 22, 2016.

23.

FUTURE ANTIRETROVIRALS, IMMUNE-BASED STRATEGIES, AND THERAPEUTIC VACCINES

Adrian Majid and Bruce L. Gilliam

WHAT'S NEW?

New medications within existing classes of antiretroviral agents are in clinical trials and will likely offer activity against resistant HIV-1 strains and provide alternatives for combination pill therapy. Novel therapeutics including oral attachment inhibitors and monoclonal antibody treatments continue to show efficacy against HIV-1 and progress in clinical trials.

KEY POINTS

- Tenofovir alafenamide is a prodrug that produces higher intracellular levels of tenofovir diphosphate with likely less renal and bone toxicity.

- Among traditional classes of HIV treatment, both doravirine (a non-nucleoside reverse transcriptase inhibitor (NNRTI)) and cabotegravir (an integrase strand inhibitor) are newer agents with activity against resistant virus.

- Maturation inhibitors are a new class of treatment that block protease cleavage, leading to the release of an immature virion.

- Monoclonal antibodies directed against CCR5 (PRO 140) and the CD4 receptor (TNX-355) have shown potency in early clinical trials.

FUTURE DIRECTIONS IN ANTIRETROVIRAL TREATMENT

LEARNING OBJECTIVES

- Discuss new antiretroviral drugs from traditional drug classes in development.

- Describe novel pharmaceuticals that will change HIV treatment in the future.

ANTIRETROVIRAL DRUGS IN DEVELOPMENT

Highly active antiretroviral therapy (HAART) remains the mainstay of treatment for patients chronically infected with HIV. Novel drugs, both within existing classes and new ones, are in various stages of development and testing (Table 23.1). Tenofovir alafenamide (TAF), formerly GS-7340, is a prodrug that produces higher intracellular levels of tenofovir diphosphate than tenofovir disoproxil fumarate (TDF) but lower plasma levels. Therefore, it has been associated with less bone and renal toxicity (Callebaut, 2015). Recent phase III trials have examined a once-daily formulation of TAF combined with elvitegravir, cobicistat, and emtricitabine (EVG/Cobi/FTC). Compared to STRIBILD (EVG/Cobi/TDF/FTC), this regimen showed non-inferiority at 48 weeks for treatment-naive patients and was associated with less of a decline in estimated glomerular filtration

Table 23.1 ANTIRETROVIRAL DRUGS IN CLINICAL TRIALS

AGENT	DESCRIPTION	STAGE OF DEVELOPMENT
NRTIs		
Tenofovir alafenamide (TAF)	Prodrug that is converted to tenofovir diphosphate; may be more effective and with fewer side effects than tenofovir diphosphate	Approved in United States as Genvoya (ELV/Cobi/FTC/TAF), Odefsey (RPV/FTC/TAF), and Descovy (FTC/TAF)
Elvucitabine	L-Cytosine nucleoside analogue that can be used in cases of resistance to FTC or 3TC	Phase II trials completed
NNRTIs		
Doravirine (MK-1439)	May have activity against viral strains resistant to earlier generation NNRTIs (e.g. EFV, RPV)	Phase III
INSTIs		
Cabotegravir (GSK1265744 or GSK744)	Available in both an oral and a long-acting intramuscular formulation; intramuscular formulation being investigated for role in pre-exposure prophylaxis	Phase III scheduled to start fall 2016
GS-9883	Follow-up to elvitegravir that does not require boosting	Phase III
Entry and Fusion Inhibitors		
Fostemsavir (BMS-663068)	Attaches to HIV gp120 to prevent HIV binding and entry into the host cell	Phase III
Cenicriviroc	Once-daily CCR5 antagonist that also has CCR2 activity (anti-inflammatory effect)	Phase II trials specifically examining the use for AIDS dementia complex
HIV Maturation Inhibitor		
BMS-955176	Binds to HIV-1 GAG, inhibiting the last protease cleavage event and resulting in the release of immature, non-infectious virions	Phase IIb trials investigating efficacy of BMS-95176 + ATV
Inhibitors of Rev-Mediated Viral RNA Biogenesis		
ABX464	Enhances viral mRNA splicing by interfering with these Rev-mediated functions (Campos et al., 2015)	Phase II trials

ATV, atazanavir; Cobi, cobicistat; ELV, elvucitabine; FTC, emtricitabine; INSTIs, integrase strand inhibitors; NNRTIs, non-nucleoside reverse transcriptase inhibitors; NRTIs, nucleoside reverse transcriptase inhibitors; RPV, rilpivirine; 3TC, lamivudine.

rate at 48 weeks, less proteinuria, and a smaller decrease in bone mineral density (Sax, 2015; Wohl, 2015). In 2015, the US Food and Drug Administration (FDA) approved this single-pill regimen, now marketed as Genvoya.

Doravirine (MK-1439), an NNRTI, has shown promise in clinical trials for treating drug-naive or NNRTI-resistant patients (Gatell, 2014). It interacts with the backbone of reverse transcriptase, and it has been shown to have activity against viral mutations K103N and Y181C. In phase IIb trials, doravirine performed as well as efavirenz with regard to viral suppression at 24 weeks (73.1% vs. 72.2%, respectively), with fewer discontinuations of treatment and adverse events reported (Gatell, 2015).

Maturation inhibitors are a new class being studied. BMS-955176 works by blocking the cleavage between capsid protein p24 and protein 1 in Gag, which leads to the release of an immature, non-infectious HIV virion (Nowicka-Sans, 2015). It has activity against gag gene variants that conferred resistance to bevirimat, an earlier candidate maturation inhibitor. In recent phase II trials, monotherapy with this drug resulted in a greater than 1 $\log_{10}$ median decline in HIV-1 RNA by day 11 in patients infected with subtype B and subtype C. When used in conjunction with ritonavir (RTV) and atazanavir (ATV), BMS-955176 showed similar rates of viral suppression by day 29 compared to TDF/FTC and ATV/RTV (Hwang, 2015).

New types of entry inhibitors are also being investigated. BMS-663068 (fostemsavir), an oral attachment inhibitor, binds to HIV-1 gp120, blocking viral attachment to host CD4+ T cells. In phase IIa trials of monotherapy in both treatment-naive and treatment-experienced patients over 8 days, it has been shown to decrease viral load and increase CD4+ T cell count (Nettles, 2012). In other recent trials, BMS-663068, when combined with TDF and raltegravir, led to comparable rates of viral suppression as a similar regimen with ATV and RTV (Lalezari, 2015). Because the drug attaches to a viral target, HIV subtype-specific polymorphisms at the gp120 site may contribute to variable efficacy of the drug, an area of further research with this agent. This drug is currently in phase III trials.

Cabotegravir, an investigational integrase strand inhibitor and structural analogue of dolutegravir, is available as both a short-acting daily tablet and a long-acting intramuscular formulation. Cabotegravir has shown similar efficacy at viral suppression to efavirenz as part of an induction regimen with a nucleoside reverse transcriptase inhibitor (NRTI) backbone for antiretroviral-naive patients (Margolis, 2015). When used as part of a dual maintenance regimen with rilpivirine once the HIV-1 RNA is less than 50 copies/ml, it had similar antiviral efficacy as efavirenz with an NRTI backbone. The developers of cabotegravir are conducting a clinical trial on its long-acting injectable formulation, cabotegravir LA, and its use with long-acting rilpivirine as maintenance therapy that would require infrequent dosing. Because of its long-acting duration of activity, cabotegravir LA is also being studied in phase II trials for use as pre-exposure prophylaxis.

Monoclonal Antibodies

During the past decade, multiple monoclonal antibodies (mAbs) have been developed against various viral targets, including viral membrane targets (e.g., gp120 and gp41), the CD4 receptor, and the CCR5 co-receptor (Chen, 2012). Very few of these mAbs have shown clinical benefit, despite efficacy in nonhuman primate models, due, in part, to the challenge of generating broadly neutralizing antibodies against genetically diverse HIV-1 isolates and the virus's ability to rapidly develop resistant variants.

PRO 140, a humanized CCR5 mAb, has been shown to have potent and prolonged antiretroviral activity when given in both intravenous and subcutaneous (SQ) formulations in early clinical trials (Jacobson, 2008, 2010). One of these studies was a randomized, controlled trial of 44 R5-tropic patients with CD4 cell counts >300 cells/μl and HIV-1 RNA >5000 copies/ml off ART for 12 months or longer (Jacobson, 2010). It showed that SQ PRO 140 administered weekly or biweekly produced a dose-dependent and statistically significant reduction in HIV-1 viral load—a more potent effect that was seen even with some of the initial trials of FTC/TDF. PRO 140 is being investigated in clinical trials to determine if weekly subcutaneous dosing can replace oral ART in patients with HIV-1 who are virologically suppressed.

The use of CCR5 mAbs that recognize different epitopes has also been shown to be synergistic with small-molecule CCR5 antagonists such as maraviroc and fusion inhibitors such as enfuvirtide (Murga, 2006; Safarian, 2006).

Clinically relevant mAbs to host cellular receptors have also shown efficacy in clinical trials. Ibalizumab is a humanized mouse mAb directed against the extracellular domains of human CD4 cells aimed at preventing HIV entry into the cell. It has activity against both CCR5 and CXCR4-tropic viruses. Two phase II trials have shown that in treatment-experienced patients, TNX-355 in addition to HAART led to statistically significant reductions in HIV-1 viral load up to 1 year after drug initiation without any significant safety concerns noted to date (Bruno, 2010; Khanlou, 2011). A phase III trial examining the efficacy and safety of ibalizumab in patients with treatment failure is underway, as are trials examining the efficacy and safety of a subcutaneous formulation.

Recommended Reading

Olender, S.A., Taylor B.S., Wong, M., et al. CROI 2015: Advances in antiretroviral therapy. *Top Antivir Med.* 2015; 23(1):28–45.

Pace, P., Markowitz, M. Monoclonal antibodies to host cellular receptors for the treatment and prevention of HIV-1 infection. *Curr Opin HIV AIDS.* 2015; 10(3):144–150.

Richman, D.D., Margolis, D.M., Delaney, M., et al. The challenge of finding a cure for HIV infection. *Science.* 2009; 323(5919):1304–1307.

IMMUNOMODULATORY AGENTS AND GENE THERAPY

LEARNING OBJECTIVES

- Describe different strategies to help restore the immune system in patients chronically infected with HIV-1 and potentially eliminate the latent reservoir.

- Discuss the different gene therapy modalities currently being tested and their potential benefits and limitations to clinical use.

WHAT'S NEW?

A new generation of broadly neutralizing antibodies has demonstrated potency at suppressing HIV-1 viremia in clinical trials and may play a role in immunotherapy and prevention. Latency reversing agents (e.g., histone deacetylase inhibitors) and gene therapy strategies using autologous CD4 T cells and hematopoietic stem cells continue to progress in trials.

Antiretroviral drugs are currently the mainstay of treatment for HIV-1, but these medications do not achieve cure, have potential side effects, and require lifelong adherence. Many HIV-infected patients treated with ART alone also do not achieve immune restoration despite viral suppression. The importance of immune restoration was highlighted by a large trial of HIV-infected adults achieving virologic suppression for 3 years with CD4 counts ≤200 cells/μl (Engsig, 2014). These patients had significantly greater mortality compared to those with CD4 counts >200 cells/μl (adjusted hazard ratio, 2.6). Given significant evidence that CD4 counts have been correlated with normal life expectancy (ART Collaboration Cohort, 2008; Lewden, 2007), attention has turned to strategies to control chronic immune activation and loss of normal T cell homeostasis seen in HIV. This section discusses some of these strategies in further detail, as well as the feasibility for future implementation.

CYTOKINES

IL-2, an autocrine T cell growth factor, is produced by CD4$^+$ T cells and is therefore deficient and dysfunctional in HIV-infected patients. Based on promising phase II trials showing increased CD4$^+$ T cell counts in patients receiving recombinant IL-2 (rIL-2) (Pett, 2010), two phase III trials were performed. In the ESPRIT study, 4111 HIV-infected patients with CD4 counts ≥300 cells/

μl were randomized to receive SQ IL-2 (three 5-day cycles 8 weeks apart) with HAART or HAART alone (Abrams, 2009). Although the rIL-2 group had a significantly higher CD4 count, this difference seemed to decline with time, and clinical outcomes, including opportunistic infection/ death and all-cause mortality, did not significantly differ between the two groups. In addition, there were more grade 4 adverse events in the group receiving IL-2, most notably deep venous thrombosis. Subsequent analysis also raised concern for an increased incidence of pneumonia in patients receiving rIL-2 less than 180 days previously (Pett, 2011).

The SILCAAT study, another phase III trial, randomized 1695 patients with CD4 counts of 50–299 cells/mm^3 to similar treatment arms, except the IL-2 group received six cycles at a lower dose (Abrams, 2009). CD4 cell counts were again higher in the Il-2 group, but statistically significant differences in opportunistic infection/death, all-cause mortality, and grade 4 clinical events were not seen. Both studies do not support an additional clinical benefit to rIL-2 with HAART.

IL-2 has also been studied as a means to eradicate HIV from latently infected CD4 cells and, therefore, reduce the viral reservoir. One randomized trial did not show an impact of rIL-2 with HAART on proviral DNA in blood, lymph nodes, and cerebrospinal fluid compared to HAART alone (Stellbrink, 2002). Other potential uses of rIL-2, such as a means to delay HAART initiation or facilitate HAART treatment interruption or as a vaccine adjunct (discussed later), have been challenged by clinical studies. In the STALWART study, a phase II trial in patients not on HAART with CD4 counts >300 cells/μl, rIL-2 use was associated with more opportunistic disease and death and a statistically significant increase in grade 3 or grade 4 events (Tavel, 2010).

Other cytokines currently being studied for use in HIV include IL-7, IL-15, and IL-21. IL-7 plays a key role in T cell homeostasis, leading to expansion and survival of naive and memory T cells and preventing apoptosis of CD4 and CD8 cells in HIV-infected patients in vitro. In early clinical trials, human recombinant IL-7 therapy was well-tolerated and induced a significant and dose-dependent increase in functional naive and memory CD4 and CD8 cells in lymphopenic patients with HIV on HAART (Levy, 2009; Sereti, 2009). In a randomized, placebo-controlled trial of recombinant IL-7 in antiretroviral drug (ARV)-treated HIV-infected persons, there were brisk CD4 increases of naive and central memory T cells (averaging 323 cells/ μl at 12 weeks) with a durable response seen up to 1 year (Levy, 2012).

In macaque models, IL-21 has improved beneficial immune responses, such as natural killer (NK) and T cell cytotoxicity, with reduced levels of intestinal T cell proliferation and microbial translocation. With this novel profile, it may become a useful treatment for augmenting immune response while ameliorating intestinal immune activation (Palikkuth, 2011, 2013).

IL-15, like IL-2, has lymphocyte stimulatory activity and is significantly increased in HIV patients with a virologic and immunologic response to HAART compared to antiretroviral-naive patients (Forcina, 2004), which has prompted theoretical interest in its role in immune therapy.

OTHER IMMUNOMODULATORY TREATMENTS

Several new classes of medications are being studied for their role in altering immune dysregulation in HIV. Histone deacetylase inhibitors (HDACs), a class of anticancer drugs, have been proposed as latency-reversing agents. There are conflicting data on the ability to HDACs to induce T cell activation and substantial increases in HIV-1 mRNA in latently infected cells. A study that examined panobinostat, vorinostat, and romidepsin did not find any significant increase in HIV-1 production (Bullen, 2014). However, romidepsin has been shown in a single trial to induce a sixfold increase in intracellular RNA levels in latently infected cells, which persisted for 48 hours and correlated with inhibition of cell-associated HDAC activity (Wei, 2014). A recent phase Ib/IIa trial showed that romidepsin, administered intravenously once weekly for 3 weeks to six aviremic HIV-1-infected patients on ART, significantly increased HIV-1 transcription and plasma HIV-1 RNA levels in five of the six patients without decreasing the number of HIV-1-specific T cells or inhibiting T cell cytokine production (Sogaard, 2015).

In combination with protein C agonists, HDACs have also been shown to induce HIV-1 transcription and virus production in ex vivo analysis, contributing to latency reversal without the release of proinflammatory cytokines by resting CD4$^+$ T cells (Laird, 2015). Phase I/II clinical trials of romidepsin are ongoing, as are trials examining its use in conjunction with the therapeutic vaccine Vacc-4x.

Another molecular target is PD-1, a signaling molecule on the surface of CD4 T cells that can be transiently expressed with T cell activation and persistently expressed in a type of cellular dysfunction called T cell exhaustion. This molecule is of specific interest with regard to HIV because it is preferentially expressed by latently infected CD4 T cells, and anti-PD-1 antibodies may be able to restore the function of CD4 and CD8 T cells that have become exhausted

(Porichis, 2012). BMS-936559, a human antibody against PD ligand 1, has been shown in a trial of rhesus macaques to delay viral load rebound after ARV cessation and to significantly lower viral load set point (Mason, 2014). These data have prompted the AIDS Clinical Trial Group (ACTG) and Bristol-Myers Squibb to collaborate on a clinical trial of an antibody that blocks PD-L1. Inhibitors of other checkpoint molecules (e.g., CTLA-4, LAG-3, TIM-3, TIGIT, and 2B4) theoretically may also be effective.

Because T cell activation is controlled by a number of signaling pathways, inhibitors of these pathways may also play a role in reducing the size of the latent viral reservoir. Early preclinical research has shown that mTOR inhibitors (e.g., sirolimus, temsirolimus, and everolimus) may play a role in reducing T cell activation and inflammation (Heredia, 2015; Martin, 2015; Palmer, 2015), although clinical trial data are lacking.

BROADLY NEUTRALIZING MONOCLONAL ANTIBODIES

HIV-1 immunotherapy with first-generation monoclonal antibodies in the preclinical and clinical settings was largely ineffective. A new generation of potent monoclonal antibodies has shown increased potency and breadth of activity, and there has been increased interest in the administration of these antibodies for prevention and immunotherapy. In chronically simian/human immunodeficiency virus (SHIV)-infected rhesus macaques, a cocktail of monoclonal antibodies against the CD4 binding site (3BNC117) and a single N332 glycan-dependent monoclonal antibody (PGT121) led to a rapid decline in plasma viremia (3.1 log decline in 7 days) in addition to reduced proviral DNA in peripheral blood, gastrointestinal mucosa, and lymph nodes (Barouch, 2013). Another SHIV primate model showed viral suppression for 3–5 weeks in macaques infused with a single infusion of antibodies directed against the CD4 binding site and V3 region, with a second infusion helping to control virus rebound (Shingai, 2013). In phase I human trials, a single infusion of 3BNC17 led to a 0.8–2.5 log$_{10}$ reduction in viral load sustained for 28 days (Caskey, 2015). These results will need to be studied further, especially with regard to impact on the latent reservoir and immune dysregulation because chronic antigen stimulation should be reduced by these antibodies.

GENE THERAPY

Gene therapy, also referred to as "intracellular immunization," involves the insertion of protective genes either mechanically or by viral vectors. The goal of gene therapy in HIV is to have the target cells produce gene products that protect them and their progeny from HIV infection. There has been increasing interest in gene therapy after reports of the "Berlin patient," an HIV-positive male with acute myelogenous leukemia who received an allogeneic stem cell transplant from a donor homozygous for the CCR5-delta 32 mutation, known to naturally confer resistance to HIV infection (Hutter, 2009). He successfully engrafted with CCR5 null cells and has remained free of detectable virus for more than 6 years without ART.

Gene therapy research has focused on two areas: the disruption of cellular genes involved in HIV entry, such as the CCR5 co-receptor, and the introduction of genes to disrupt HIV replication. The use of various technologies including ribozymes, aptamers, RNA-based interference strategies, and zinc finger nucleases is currently being investigated.

RIBOZYMES, APTAMERS, AND RNA-BASED INTERFERENCE

Ribozymes are small, catalytically active RNA molecules that can be engineered to target specific RNA sequences. In HIV, they can target viral RNA during uncoating and after transcription, leading to RNA degradation. Although in vitro studies of ribozyme gene therapy have been promising, retroviral vectors delivering ribozymes targeting viral targets (e.g., tat and rev) have been plagued by problems with low transduction efficiency.

The first phase II randomized, controlled trial of an anti-HIV ribozyme was conducted in 74 HIV-1-infected individuals on HAART receiving either autologous stem cells transduced with a ribozyme targeting the overlapping tat and vpr reading frames of HIV-1 (OZ1) or placebo (Mitsuyasu, 2009). No significant adverse events were reported with the infusion, but the subjects also had low engraftment levels and short persistence of the ribozyme. There was a trend, but no statistically significant difference, in HIV-1 viral load at the primary end point; however, after treatment interruption at 40 weeks, patients continuing to express OZ1 RNA had a statistically significant decrease in HIV-1 viral load.

RNA interference utilizes short RNAs that mediate the degradation of mRNAs in a sequence-specific manner. Theoretically, multiple short hairpin RNAs (shRNA) in a single vector are thought to prevent HIV-1 escape. With this strategy, antisense oligonucleotides can bind mRNA and trigger degradation through an RNase H-dependent pathway or block ribosome binding, thus preventing gene expression. Clinical research in this field is evolving, but it

has been limited by difficulty delivering the RNAs to the correct target cells, poor cellular uptake and stability, and viral escape (Zhou, 2011). VRX496 (Lexgenleucel-T), antisense env in a lentiviral vector, has progressed to phase II trials, in which it has been delivered via autologous CD4+ T cell infusion to both patients on failing regimens and patients on a fully suppressive ART regimen. In one trial, 17 patients received Lexgenleucel-T over 16 weeks, with HAART interruption 1 month later in 13 of these patients (Tebas, 2013). Six of 8 patients analyzed were noted to have a decrease in viral load set point. The use of a short-interfering RNA targeting a unique triple repeat of NF-κB has also been shown to achieve long-term suppression of HIV-1 subtype C (Singh, 2014).

Aptamers are single-stranded RNA or DNA molecules that can bind viral proteins, preventing them from carrying out their function in the viral life cycle (Figure 23.1). In clinical trials, when used alone, they have not been shown to be effective. However, strategies combining aptamers, ribozymes, and RNA interference, based on in vitro efficacy, require further investigation because they have been shown to exhibit potent inhibition of HIV-1 in vitro (Centlivre, 2013; ter Brake, 2008).

Theoretically, gene therapy can also be used to inhibit viral fusion. C46, a structurally similar peptide to enfuvirtide, has been engineered to be expressed on autologous T cells and seems to be well-tolerated in clinical trials, although clinical efficacy has not yet been demonstrated (van Lundzen, 2007). Calimmune, a small, public-/private-funded biotech company based in Pasadena, California, has developed Cal-1, an anti-HIV-1 lentiviral vector containing CCR5 shRNA and C46 that has been shown in preclinical studies to be nontoxic and to protect gene-modified cells from both CXCR4- and CCR5-tropic HIV-1 strains (Wolstein, 2014). A phase I/II clinical trial is currently in its final cohort using autologous, Cal-1-modified CD4+ cells and hematopoietic progenitor/stem cells with and without bone marrow condition in HIV-positive patients to test the Cal-1 construct for the treatment of HIV-1.

ZINC FINGER NUCLEASES

Zinc finger nucleases (ZFNs) are engineered proteins with two functional domains—one that recognizes DNA and one that cleaves it. ZFNs can bind specific DNA sequences, produce a double-stranded break, and then lead to permanent gene disruption when cellular repair pathways lead to the addition or deletion of nucleotides at the break site. ZFNs have been shown to disrupt CCR5 expression in human stem cells administered in a mouse model of HIV

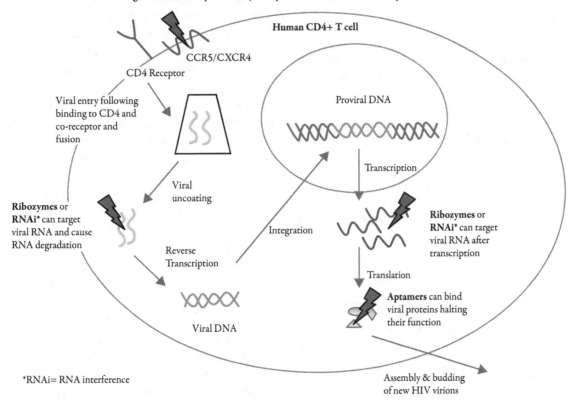

Zinc finger nucleases can permanently disrupt CCR5 and even CXCR4 expression

Human CD4+ T cell

CCR5/CXCR4

CD4 Receptor

Viral entry following binding to CD4 and co-receptor and fusion

Proviral DNA

Transcription

Viral uncoating

Ribozymes or **RNAi*** can target viral RNA and cause RNA degradation

Integration

Ribozymes or **RNAi*** can target viral RNA after transcription

Reverse Transcription

Translation

Aptamers can bind viral proteins halting their function

Viral DNA

*RNAi= RNA interference

Assembly & budding of new HIV virions

Figure 23.1 Schematic diagram of the HIV viral life cycle in host cell and gene therapy targets. SOURCE: Adapted from Zeller et al. (2011).

and to be associated with lower HIV viral loads after HIV challenge (Holt, 2010).

SB-728T, an infusion of ZFN-modified autologous CD4 T cells with the ability to knock out CCR5 expression, has been shown to increase CD4 cell over time, decrease proviral DNA, and restore the CD4-depleted population of the gut mucosa in chronically infected patients with CD4 counts >200 cells/μl (June, 2012; Lalezari, 2012). One subject with the highest level of CCR5 modification had an undetectable viral load when HAART treatment interruption occurred. In a well-publicized clinical trial, SB-728T was demonstrated to be safe in 12 patients who received the treatment, with one serious infusion reaction noted (Tebas, 2014). These subjects had significantly increased CD4+ T cell counts, and the gene-modified CD4 T cells persisted at low levels during long-term follow-up. Six of these patients underwent 12-week ART interruption, but in only 1 patient (heterozygous for the CCR5-delta 32 mutation) did the viral load decline to an undetectable level prior to ART reinitiation.

Additional studies of SB-728T are underway, with one examining CCR5-delta 32 heterozygotes and another examining the use of cytoxan prior to CD4+ T cell infusion to decrease the number of existing CD4+ T cells. Early data from the latter trial have demonstrated that cytoxan

treatment is well-tolerated with a dose-related increase in total CD4+ T cell count and engraftment of CCR5-modified cells (Blick, 2014).

One novel gene therapy approach currently in phase I trials is the use of MazF-T, autologous CD4+ T cells modified with the MAZF endoribonuclease gene, which can render T cells resistant to HIV replication (Saito, 2014). Additional trials using modified stem cells are also in early clinical stages for AIDS patients with hematologic malignancies. Although promising, it will be difficult to develop the previously discussed gene strategies for widespread use. Cost of the agents/technology, the development of an infrastructure for delivery, lack of availability of this technology in areas most affected by HIV-1, and patient insurance limitations all pose significant barriers to implementation.

Recommended Reading

Ahlensteil, C.L., Suzuki, K., Marks, K., et al. Controlling HIV-1: Non-coding RNA gene therapy approaches a functional cure. *Front Immunol.* 2015; 6:474.

Barouch, D.H., Deeks, S.G. Immunologic strategies for HIV-1 remission and eradication. *Science.* 2014; 345(6193):169–174.

Chomont, N., El-Far, M., Ancuta, P., et al. HIV reservoir size and persistence are driven by T cell survival and homeostatic proliferation. *Nat Med.* 2009; 15(8):893–900.

Frater, J. New approaches in HIV eradication research. *Curr Opin Infect Dis.* 2011; 24(6):593–598.

Kitchen, S.G., Shimizu, S., An, D.S. Stem cell-based anti-HIV gene therapy. *Virology.* 2011; 411:260–272.

Levy, J. Not an HIV cure, but encouraging new directions. *N Engl J Med.* 2009; 360:724–725.

Lewin, S., Rouzioux, C. HIV cure and eradication: How will we get from the laboratory to effective clinical trials? *AIDS.* 2011; 25:885–897.

Pett, S.L., Kelleher, A.D., Emery, S. Role of interleukin-2 in patients with HIV infection. *Drugs.* 2010; 70(9):1115–1130.

THERAPEUTIC VACCINES

LEARNING OBJECTIVE

Discuss the progression and current status of research in HIV therapeutic vaccines.

WHAT'S NEW?

HIV therapeutic vaccine research has seen a resurgence in recent years with different classes of vaccines showing promise in clinical trials.

KEY POINTS

- Therapeutic immunization is a strategy for boosting anti-HIV-1 immunity in chronically infected patients.

- Recent studies of therapeutic vaccines have provided more durable and diverse immune responses and lowering of viral load set points.

- Many different types of vaccines have progressed to phase II trials, including DNA, subunit, and dendritic cell vaccines.

Therapeutic immunization aims to induce a cellular immune response through vaccination with components of HIV-1 that will help contain viral replication through reconstitution of anti-HIV-1 immune responses. Data support the observation that the cellular immune response is critical in controlling HIV-1 replication, as reported in patients with primary HIV-1 infection and long-term nonprogressors (Borrow, 1994; Cao, 1995; Kroup, 1994; Rosenberg, 1997). Therapeutic vaccines can potentially be of benefit to ART-naive patients by potentially delaying progression to AIDS and time to initiation of ART. Among patients on ART, development of a durable vaccine can potentially intensify the effects of ART (accelerate response time to therapy, decrease risk of transmission, and potentiate the immune effects of ART including reduction of proviral DNA), simplify ART regimens, and support regimens with treatment interruption (Ensoli, 2014).

Clinical therapeutic vaccine research for HIV started prior to the introduction of HAART, first with a gp120-depleted inactivated HIV-1 preparation and then vectors expressing viral proteins (e.g., gag p17 and p24). Clinical trials of these agents largely failed to show efficacy and a sustained HIV-1-specific response (Hardy, 2007). Subsequent vaccines with recombinant HIV-1 glycoproteins (e.g., gp120 and gp160) also fared poorly, not altering the decline in CD4 count or halting disease progression in HIV-1-infected individuals in phase II trials (Eron, 1996; Pontesilli, 1998; Sandstrom, 1999; Tsoukas, 1998). In one of the largest of these trials, 608 HIV-1-infected individuals with CD4$^+$ T cell counts >400 cells/mm^3 were repeatedly immunized with a recombinant gp160 vaccine (VaxSyn HIV-1) or placebo and followed for 3–5 years. Although the vaccine had excellent immunogenicity (~70%), it failed to show a difference in reaching the primary clinical end points: a 50% decline in CD4$^+$ T cell count or disease progression to Walter Reed stages 4, 5, and 6 (Birx, 2000).

ANRS 093, a study of 70 HIV-1-infected patients, compared HAART to immunization with recombinant canary pox vector expressing several HIV genes (env, gag, pol, and nef) and lipo-6T (HIV-1 lipopepides) followed by SQ IL-2. The vaccine elicited a statistically significant interferon-γ (INF-γ)-producing CD8$^+$ T cell response that correlated with virologic control (Levy, 2005). The vaccine group was able to have a lower viral set point and, therefore, a significantly greater number of days off HAART (Levy, 2006), but the results of this study await validation in larger trials. In ACTG 5197, administration of a replication-defective adenovirus type 5 HIV-1 gag vaccine to HIV-infected patients with CD4$^+$ T cell counts >500 cells/mm^3 failed to be sufficiently immunogenic and lacked statistically significant efficacy (Schooley, 2010). The finding that the plasma viral load was 0.5 log$_{10}$ lower in the vaccine arm at 16 weeks post-HAART interruption prompted further analysis of the HLA class I alleles in all 110 participants because HLA classes have previously been shown to influence viral evolution and disease progression. Vaccinated patients with neutral HLA alleles in this cohort had a lower plasma viral load than those of both patients vaccinated with protective alleles and placebo participants with neutral alleles (Li, 2011).

One novel therapeutic vaccine strategy with promising results has targeted Tat, a transactivator of HIV gene expression essential for viral replication that is relatively conserved among HIV-1 subtypes. This vaccine is aimed at patients on ART with the hope of decreasing viral reservoirs

Table 23.2 SELECT THERAPEUTIC VACCINE TRIALS

VACCINE	DESCRIPTION	STAGE OF DEVELOPMENT	RESULTS
		DNA Vaccines	
Dermavir	Topically applied DNA vaccine	Phase II	Safe and immunogenic in ART-treated patients with GAG-specific T cell responses (Rodriguez, 2013)
GTU-multiHIV B	DNA plasmid vaccine	Phase II	Statistically significant decrease in log pHIV RNA in ART-naive patients compared to placebo; currently being studied with LIPO-5 as a prime boost strategy for patients on ART
		Subunit Vaccines	
Tat protein vaccine	Recombinant biologically active HIV-1 B Clade Tat protein	Phase II	Induction of anti-Tat antibodies in most patients on ART restoring T, B, and NK cells and CD4$^+$ and CD8$^+$ central memory subsets (Ensoli, 2015); significant reduction in proviral DNA seen at week 72
Vac-3S	Peptide-based vaccine aimed at eliciting a humoral response against the highly conserved region of gp41	Phase II	Trial ongoing
Vacc-4x	Peptide-based vaccine with four synthetic peptides based on the HIV-1 p24 protein	Phase II	Statistically significant lower HIV viral set point at week 48 compared to placebo in patients on ART; no change to time in treatment interruption and Cd4 count (primary endpoints)
HIV-v	T cell epitope HIV vaccine with synthetic peptides from conserved regions of Vpr, Vif, Rev, and Nef	Phase Ib/II	Safe, IgG responses in up to 75% of volunteers with 1 log reduction in viral load in ART-naive males with this response compared to placebo and non-responders (Boffito, 2013)
		Dendritic Cell Vaccines	
AGS-004	Patient-derived dendritic cells and loaded ex vivo with RNA encoding four (Gag, Nef, Rev, and Vpr) antigens plus CD40L	Phase II	Delay in continuous ART resumption in 24 treated subjects, but no improvement in CD4$^+$ T cell counts (DeBenedette, 2014)

ART, antiretroviral therapy; NK, natural killer.

and restoring immune homeostasis. In phase II trials, 168 patients controlled on ART and anti-Tat antibody negative at baseline administered the vaccine three or five times monthly showed specific and durable immune responses when followed for up to 144 weeks (Ensoli, 2015). Most patients (79%) developed anti-Tat antibodies, which was associated with significant reduction of proviral DNA seen after week 72. The vaccine was also associated with a restoration of T, B, and NK cells and CD4$^+$ and CD8$^+$ central memory subsets.

A multinational phase II trial examined the safety and immunogenicity of Vacc-4x, a peptide-based HIV-1 therapeutic vaccine targeting the conserved domains of p24Gag (Pollard, 2014). In chronically infected HIV-1 patients who were virologically suppressed on ART, the Vacc-4x vaccine did not alter time to ART resumption and did not lead to significant changes in CD4 count at week 28 during treatment interruption. However, there was a statistically significant

difference in HIV viral load at both week 48 (23,000 vs. 71,800 copies/ml) and week 52 (19,500 vs. 51,000 copies/ml).

The DNA plasmid vaccine GTU-multiHIV B, aimed at inducing immune responses to HIV-1 regulatory genes, has shown efficacy in HIV-1 subtype C chronically infected patients not on ART. In a population of 63 patients, the vaccine was deemed safe and was associated with a statistically significant decline in log pHIV-RNA with an increase in CD4$^+$ T cell counts nearing significance compared to placebo, especially after intramuscular injections (Vardas, 2012). The efficacy of GTU-multiHIV B DNA vaccine and LIPO-5 vaccine in a prime-boost strategy for lowering viral set point after treatment interruption for patients virologically suppressed on ART is currently being studied in phase II trials.

Significant attention has also focused on dendritic cells as cellular adjuvants for therapeutic HIV-1 vaccines because they have been shown to elicit strong CD4 and CD8 T cell responses in vivo. One uncontrolled study of immunization of 18 HIV-1-infected treatment-naive patients with dendritic cells pulsed with inactivated autologous virus reported a 90% decrease in viral load during the course of a year (Lu, 2004). A subsequent randomized control trial of 24 treatment-naive subjects with a similar vaccine, however, showed a weak HIV-1-specific response and a modest decrease in viral load compared to placebo (Garcia, 2011). In a trial of chronically infected patients on ART with CD4[+] T cell counts >450 cells/mm[3], the use of a monocyte-derived dendritic cell pulse with heat-inactivated whole HIV helped lower plasma viral load set point after treatment interruption, with an associated increased in HIV-1-specific T cell responses compared to placebo (Garcia, 2013). Recent trials have continued to demonstrate better vaccine responses and control of viral replication (Levy, 2014). Dendritic cells expressing the HIV proteins Gag, Tat, Rev, and Nef administered as a vaccine have been shown to elicit potent antiviral T cell responses in HIV-1 patients on HAART, including a Gag-specific IFN-γ response that correlated with HIV-1 inhibitory activity (van Gulck, 2012).

Although no therapeutic vaccine is currently FDA approved, the future of therapeutic vaccine research for both naive and ART-treated patients remains promising. Some of the key vaccines in development are highlighted in Table 23.2.

Recent data have been encouraging, but the results of therapeutic vaccine trials have not yielded a therapeutic vaccine strategy that can be implemented. In addition to further clinical trials of the vaccines discussed previously, additional studies investigating the heterogeneity of response to vaccines (e.g., genetic determinants) and the immunologic correlates of vaccine efficacy are needed for the field to advance.

Recommended Reading

Ensoli, B., Cafaro, A., Monini, P., et al. Challenges in HIV vaccine research for treatment and prevention. *Front Immunol.* 2014; 5:417.

Gilliam, B.L., Redfield, R.R. Therapeutic HIV vaccines. *Curr Top Med Chem.* 2003; 3(13):2536–1553.

Gotch, F.M., Imami, N., Hardy, G. Candidate vaccines for immunotherapy in HIV. *HIV Med.* 2001; 2:260–265.

Levy, Y. Therapeutic HIV vaccines: An update. *Curr HIV/AIDS Rep.* 2005; 2(1):5–9.

Van Gulck, E., Van Tendeloo, V.F., Berneman, Z.N., et al. Role of dendritic cells in HIV immunotherapy. *Curr HIV Res.* 2010; 8(4):310–322.

References

Abrams, D., Levy, Y., Losso, M.H., et al.; INSIGHT-ESPRIT Study Group; SILCAAT Scientific Committee. Interleukin 2 therapy in patients with HIV infection. *N Engl J Med.* 2009; 361(16):1548–1559.

ART Collaboration Cohort. Life expectancy of individuals on combination antiretroviral therapy in high-income countries: A collaborative analysis of 14 cohort studies. *Lancet.* 2008; 372:293–299.

Barouch, D.H., Whitney, J.B., Moldt, B., et al. Therapeutic efficacy of potent neutralizing HIV-1-specific monoclonal antibodies in SHIV-infected rhesus monkeys. *Nature.* 2013; 503:224–229.

Birx, D., Loomis-Price, L.D., Aronson, N., et al. Efficacy of recombinant human immunodeficiency virus (HIV) gp160 as a therapeutic vaccine in early-stage HIV-1-infected volunteers. *J Infect Dis.* 2000; 181:881–889.

Blick, G., Lalezari, J., Hsu, R., et al. Cyclophosphamide enhances SB-728T engraftment to levels associated with HIV-RNA control. Paper presented at the 21st Conference on Retroviruses and Opportunistic Infections, March 2014. Boston, MA. Abstract 141.

Boffito, M., Folx, J., Bowman, C., et al. Safety, immunogenicity and efficacy assessment of HIV immunotherapy in a multi-centre, double blind randomized placebo-controlled phase Ib human trial. *Vaccine.* 2013; 31(48):5680–5686.

Borrow, P., Lewicki, H., Hahn, B.H., et al. Virus specific CD8 cytotoxic T-lymphocyte activity associated with control of viremia in primary human immunodeficiency virus type 1 infection. *J Virol.* 1994; 68:6103–6110.

Bruno, J.B., Jacobson, J.M. Ibalizumab: An anti-CD4 monoclonal antibody for the treatment of HIV-1 infection. *J Antimicrob Chemother.* 2010; 65:1839–1841.

Bullen, C.K., Laird, G.M., Durand, C.M., et al. New ex vivo approached distinguish effective and ineffective single agents for reversing HIV-1 latency in vivo. *Nat Med.* 2014; 20(4):425–429.

Cao, Y., Qin, L., Zhang, L., et al. Virologic and immunologic characterization of long-term survivors of human immunodeficiency virus type 1 infection. *N Engl J Med.* 1995; 332:201–208.

Callebaut, C., Stepan, G., Tian, Y., et al. In vitro virology profile of tenofovir alafenamide, a novel oral prodrug of tenofovir with improves antiviral activity compared to that of tenofovir disoproxil fumarate. *Antimicrob Agents Chemother.* 2015; 59 (10):5909–5916.

Campos, N., Myburgh, R., Garcel, A., et al. Long lasting control of viral rebound with a new drug ABX 464 targeting Rev-mediated viral RNA biogenesis. *Retrovirology.* 2015; 12:64–66.

Caskey, M., Klein, F., Lorenzi, J.C., et al. Viraemia suppressed in HIV-1 infected humans by broadly neutralizing antibody 3BNC117. *Nature.* 2015; 522:487–493.

Centlivre, M., Legrand, N., Klamer, S., et al. Preclinical in vivo evaluation of the safety of a multi-shRNA-based gene therapy against HIV-1. *Mol Ther Nucleic Acids.* 2013; 2:e120.

Chen, W., Dmitrov, D. Monoclonal antibody-based candidate therapeutics against HIV type 1. *AIDS Res Hum Retroviruses.* 2012 May; 28(5):425–434.

DeBenedette, M., Tcherepanova, I., Gamble, A., et al. Immune function and viral load post AGS-004 administration to chronic HIV subjects undergoing STI. Paper presented at the 21st Conferences on Retroviruses and Opportunistic Infections (CROI), March 2014, Boston, MA. Abstract 343.

Emsig, F.N., Zangerle, R., Katsarou, O., et al. Long-term mortality in HIV-positive individuals virally suppressed for >3 years with incomplete CD4 recovery. *Clin Infect Dis.* 2014; 58(9):1312–1321.

Ensoli, B., Cafaro, A., Monini, P., et al. Challenges in HIV vaccine research for treatment and prevention. *Front Immunol.* 2014; 5:417.

Ensoli, F., Cafaro, A., Casabianco, A., et al. HIV-1 Tat immunization restores immune homeostasis and attacks the HAART-resistant blood HIV DNA: Results of a randomized plase II clinical exploratory clinical trial. *Retrovirology.* 2015; 12:33.

Eron, J.J., Jr., Ashby, M.A., Giordano, M.F., et al. Randomized trial of MNrgp120 HIV-1 vaccine in symptomless HIV-1 infection. *Lancet.* 1996; 348:1547–1551.

Forcina, G., d'Ettorre, G., Mastroianni, C., et al. Interleukin-15 modulated interferon-γ and β-chemokine production in patients with HIV infection: Implications for immune-based therapy. *Cytokine*. 2004; 25:283–290.

Garcia, F., Climent, N., Assoumou, L., et al. A therapeutic dendritic cell-based vaccine for HIV-1 infection. *J Infect Dis*. 2011; 203:473–478.

Garcia, F., Climent, N., Guardo, A.C., et al. A dendritic cell-based vaccine elicits T cell responses associated with control of HIV-1 replication. *Sci Transl Med*. 2013; 5:166ra62.

Gatell, J., Raffi, F., Plettenber, A., et al. Efficacy and safety of doravirine 100 mg QD vs. efavirenz 600 mg QD with TDF/FTC in ART-naïve HIV-infected patients: Week 24 results. Paper presented at the 8th International AIDS Society Conference on HIV Pathogenesis, Treatment and Prevention, July 2015, Vancouver, British Columbia, Canada. Abstract TUAB0104.

Gatell, J.M., Morales-Ramirex, J.O., Hagens, D. P., et al. Forty-eight week efficacy and safety and early CNS tolerability of doravirine (MK-1439), a novel NNRTI, with TDF/FTC in ART-naïve HIV-posiitve patients. *J Int AIDS Soc*. 2014; 17(4 Suppl 3):19532.

Heredia, A., Le, N., Gartenhaus, R.B., et al. Targeting of mTOR catalytic site inhibits multiple steps of the HIV-1 lifecycle and suppresses HIV-1 viremia in humanized mice. *Proc Natl Acad Sci USA*. 2015; 112 (30):9412–9417.

Hardy, G.A., Imami, N., Nelson, M.R. A phase I, randomized study of combined IL-2 and therapeutic immunization with antiretroviral therapy. *J Immune Based Therapies Vaccines*. 2007; 5:6.

Holt, N., Wang, J., Kim, K., et al. Human hematopoietic stem/progenitor cells modified by zinc-finger nucleases targeted to CCR5 control HIV-1 in vivo. *Nat Biotechnol*. 2010; 28(8);839–847.

Hutter, G., Nowak, D., Mossner, M., et al. Long-term control of HIV by CCR5 delta 32/delta 32 stem cell transplantation. *N Engl J Med*. 2009; 360:692–698.

Hwang, C., Schurmann, D., Sobotha, C., et al. Second generation HIV-1 maturation inhibitor BMS-955176: Overall antiviral activity and safety results from the phase IIa proof-of-concept study. Paper presented at the 15th European AIDS Conference, October 2015, Barcelona, Spain. Abstract AI468002.

Jacobson, J.M., Saag, M.S., Thompson, M.A., et al. Antiviral activity of a single dose PRO 140, a CCR5 monoclonal antibody in HIV-infected adults. *J Infect Dis*. 2008; 198:1345–1352.

Jacobson, J.M., Thompson, M., Lalezari, J., et al. Anti-HIV-1 activity of weekly or biweekly treatment with subcutaneous PRO 140, a CCR5 monoclonal antibody. *J Infect Dis*. 2010; 201(10):1481–1487.

June, C., Tebas, P., Stein, D., et al. Induction of acquired CCR5 deficiency with zinc finger nuclease-modified autologous CD4 T cells (SB-728-T) correlates with increases in CD4 count and effects on viral load in HIV-infected subjects. Paper presented at the 19th Conference on Retroviruses and Opportunistic Infection, February 2012, Seattle, WA. Abstract 155.

Khanlou, H., Devente, J., Fessel, J., et al. Durable efficacy and continued safety of ibalizumab in treatment-experienced patients. Abstracts of the IDSA Annual Meeting, Boston, MA, 2011. Abstract LB9.

Kroup, R.A., Safrit, J.T., Cao, Y., et al. Temporal association of cellular immune responses with the initial control of viremia in primary human immunodeficiency virus type 1 syndrome. *J Virol*. 1994; 68:4650–4655.

Laird, G.M., Bullen, C.K., Rosenbloom, D.I., et al. Ex vivo analysis identifies effective HIV-1 latency reversing drug combinations. *J Clin Invest*. 2015; 125(5):1901–1902.

Lalezari, J., Mitsuyasu, R., Wang, S., et al. A single infusion of zinc finger nuclease CCR5 modified autologous CD4 T cells (SB-728T) increased CD4 counts and leads to decrease in HIV proviral load in an aviremic HIV-infect subject. Paper presented at the 19th Conference on Retroviruses and Opportunistic Infection, February 2012, Seattle, WA. Abstract 433.

Lalezari, J.P., Latiff, G.H., Brinson, C., et al. Safety and efficacy of the HIV-1 attachment inhibitor prodrug BMS-663068 in treatment-experienced individuals: 24 week results of AI438011, a phase 2b randomized controlled trial. *Lancet HIV*. 2015; 2(10):e427–e437.

Levy, Y., Durier, C., Lascauz, A.S., et al. Sustained control of viremia following therapeutic immunization in chronically HIV-1 infected individuals. *AIDS*. 2006; 20:405–413.

Levy, Y., Gahery-Segard, H., Durier, C., et al. Immunologic and virologic efficacy of therapeutic immunization combined with interleukin-2 in chronically HIV-1 infected patients. *AIDS*. 2005; 19:279–286.

Levy, Y., Lacabaratz, C., Weiss, L., et al. Enhanced T cell recovery in HIV-1 infected adults through IL-7 treatment. *J Clin Invest*. 2009; 119(4):997–1007.

Levy, Y., Sereti, I., Tambussi, G., et al. Effects of recombinant human interleukin 7 on T-cell recovery and thymic output in HIV-infected patients receiving antiretroviral therapy: Results of a phase I/IIa randomized, placebo-controlled multicenter study. *Clin Infect Dis*. 2012; 55(2):291–300.

Levy, Y., Thiebaut, R., Montes, M., et al. Dendritic cell-based therapeutic vaccine elicits polyfunctional HIV-specific T-cell immunity associated with control of viral load. *Eur J Immunol*. 2014; 44:2802–2810.

Lewden, C., Chene, G., Morlat, P., et al. HIV-infected adults with a CD4 cell count greater than 500 cells/µl on long-term combination antiretroviral therapy reach same mortality rates as the general population. *J Acquir Immune Defic Syndr*. 2007; 46(1):72–77.

Li, J., Brumme, Z., Brumme, C., et al. Factors associated with viral rebound in HIV-1 infected individuals enrolled in a therapeutic HIV-1 gag vaccine trial. *J Infect Dis*. 2011; 203:976–983.

Lu, W., Arraes, C., Ferreira, W.T., et al. Therapeutic dendritic cell vaccination for chronic HIV-1 infection. *Nat Med*. 2004; 10:1359–1365.

Margolis, D.A., Brinson, C.C., Smith, G., et al. Cabotegravir plus rilpivirine, once a day, after induction with cabotegravir plus nucleoside reverse transcriptase inhibitors in antiretroviral-naïve adults with HIV-1 infection (LATTE): A randomised, phase 2b, dose-ranging trial. *Lancet Infect Dis*. 2015; 15:1145–1155.

Martin, A.R., Siciliano, R.F. Immune modulation with rapamycin as a potential strategy for HIV-1 eradication. Paper presented at the 22nd Conference on Retroviruses and Opportunistic Infections, February 2015, Seattle, WA. Abstract 415.

Mason, S.W., Sanisetty, S., Osuna Gutierrez, C., et al. Viral suppression was induced by anti-PD-L1 following ARV-interruption in SIV-infected monkeys. Paper presented at the 21st Conference on Retroviruses and Opportunistic Infections, March 2014, Boston, MA. Abstract 318LB.

Mitsuyasu, R.T., Merigan, T.C., Carr, A., et al. Phase 2 gene therapy trial of anti-HIV ribozyme in autologous CD34+ cells. *Nat Med*. 2009; 15(3):285–292.

Murga, J.D., Franti, M., Pevear, D.C., et al. Potent antiviral synergy between monoclonal antibody and small molecule CCR5 antagonists of human immunodeficiency virus type 1. *Antimicrob Agents Chemother*. 2006; 50(10):3289–3296.

Nettles, R., Schurmann, D., Zhu, L., et al. Pharmacodynamics, safety, and pharmacokinetics of BMS-663068: An oral HIV attachment inhibitor in HIV-1-infected patients. *J Infect Dis*. 2012; 206 (7):1002–1011.

Nowicka-Sans, B., Protack, T., Lin, Z., et al. Characterization of a second-generation HIV-1 maturation inhibitor. Presented at the 8th International AIDS Society Conference on HIV Pathogenesis, Treatment and Prevention, July 2015, Vancouver, British Columbia, Canada. Poster TUPEAO78.

Pallikkuth, S., Micci, L., Ende, Z.S., et al. Maintenance of intestinal Th17 cells and reduced microbial translocation in SIV-infected rhesus macaques treated with interleukin (IL)-21. *PLoS Pathog*. 2013; 9:e1003471.

Pallikkuth, S., Rogers, K., Villinger, F., et al. Interleukin-21 administration to rhesus macaques chronically infected with simian immunodeficiency viruses increases cytotoxic effector molecules in T cells and NK cells and enhances B cell function without increasing immune activation or viral replication. *Vaccine*. 2011; 29:9929–9938.

Palmer, C.S., Ostrowski, M., Zhou, J., et al. The mTORC1 inhibitors, temsirolimus and everolimus, suppress HIV-patient-derived CD4+

T-cell death and activation in vitro. Paper presented at the 22nd Conference on Retroviruses and Opportunistic Infections, February 2015, Seattle, WA. Abstract 320.

Pett, S.L., Carey, C., Lin, E., et al. Predictors of bacterial pneumonia in Evaluation of Subcutaneous Interleukin-2 in Randomized International TRIAL (ESPRIT). *HIV Med.* 2011; 12(4):219–227.

Pett, S.L., Kelleher, A.D., Emery, S. Role of interleukin-2 in patients with HIV infection. *Drugs.* 2010; 70(9):1115–1130.

Pollard, R.B., Rockstroh, J.K., Pantaleo, G., et al. Safety and efficacy of the peptide-based therapeutic vaccine for HIV-1, Vacc-4x: A phase 2 randomised double-blind, placebo-controlled trial. *Lancet Infect Dis.* 2014; 14(4):291–300.

Pontesilli, I., Guerra, E.S., Ammassari, A., et al. Phase II controlled trial of post-exposure immunization with recombinant gp160 versus antiretroviral therapy in asymptomatic HIV-1 infected adults. *AIDS.* 1998; 12:473–480.

Porichis, F., Kaufmann, D.E. Role of PD-1 in HIV pathogenesis and as a target for therapy. *Curr HIV/AID Rep.* 2012; 9(1):81–90.

Rodriguez, B., Asmuth, D.M., Matining, R.M., et al. Safety, tolerability and immunogenicity of repeated doses of dermavir, a candidate therapeutic HIV vaccine, in HIV-infected patients receiving combination antiretroviral therapy. *J Acquir Immune Defic Syndr.* 2013; 64(4):351–359.

Rosenberg, E.S., Billingsley, J.M., Caliendo, A.M., et al. Vigorous HIV-1-specific CD4R T cell responses associated with control of viremia. *Science.* 1997; 278:1447–1450.

Safarian, D., Carnec, X., Tsamis, F., et al. An anti-CCR5 monoclonal antibody and small molecular CCR5 antagonists synergize by inhibiting different stages of human immunodeficiency virus type 1 entry. *Virology.* 2006; 352(2)477–484.

Saito, N., Chono, H., Shibata, H., et al. CD4⁺ T cells modified by endoribonuclease MazF are safe and can persist in SHIV-infected rhesus macaques. *Mol Ther Nucleic Acids.* 2014; 3(6):e168.

Sandstrom, E., Wahren, B.; Nordic Vac-04 Study Group. Therapeutic immunization with recombinant gp160 in HIV-1 infection: A randomized double blind placebo-controlled trial. *Lancet.* 1999; 353:1735–1742.

Sax, P.E., Saag, M.S., Yin, M.T., et al. Renal and bone safety tenofovir alafenamide vs. tenofovir disoproxil fumarate. Paper presented at the 22nd Conference on Retroviruses and Opportunistic Infection, February 2015, Seattle, WA. Abstract 143LB.

Schooley, R.T., Spritzler, J., Wang, H., et al.; AIDS Clinical Trials Group 5197. A placebo-controlled trial of immunization of HIV-1-infected persons with a replication-deficient adenovirus type 5 vaccine expressing the HIV-1 core protein. *J Infect Dis.* 2010; 202(5):705–716.

Sereti, I., Dunham, R.M., Spritzler, J., et al. IL-7 administration drives T cell entry and expansion in HIV-1 infection. *Blood.* 2009; 113(25):6304–6314.

Shingai, M., Nishumura, Y., Klein, F., et al. Antibody-mediated immunotherapy of macaques chronically infected with SHIV suppresses viraemia. *Nature.* 2013; 503:277–281.

Singh, A., Palanichamy, J.K., Ramalingam, P., et al. Long-term suppression of HIV-1 C virus production in human peripheral blood mononuclear cells by LTR heterochromatization with a short double-stranded RNA. *J Anitmicrob Chemother.* 2014; 69:405–415.

Sogaard, O.S., Graversen, M.E., Leth, S., et al. The depsipeptide romdiepsin reverses HIV-1 latency in vivo. *PLoS Pathog.* 2015; 11(9):e1005142.

Stellbrink, H.J., van Lundzen, J., Westby, M., et al. Effects of interleukin-2 plus highly active antiretroviral therapy on HIV-1 replication and proviral DNA (COSMIC trial). *AIDS.* 2002; 16:1479–1487.

Tavel, J.A.; INSIGHT STALWART Study Group. Effect of intermittent IL-2 alone or with peri-cycle antiretroviral therapy in early HIV-1 infection: The STALWART study. *PloS One.* 2010; 5(2):e9334.

Tebas, P., Stein, D., Binder-Scholl, G., et al. Antiviral effects of autologous CD4 T cells genetically modified with a conditionally replicating lentiviral vector expressing long antisense to HIV. *Blood.* 2013; 121(9):1524–1533.

Tebas, P., Stein, D., Tang, W.W., et al. Gene editing of CCR5 in autologous CD4 T cells of persons infected with HIV. *N Engl J Med.* 2014; 370(10):901–910.

ter Brake, O., t Hooft, K., Liu, Y.P., et al. Lentiviral vector design for multiple shRNA expression and durable HIV-1 inhibition. *Mol Ther.* 2008; 16:557–564.

Tsoukas, C.M., Raboud, J., Bernard, N.F., et al. Active immunization of patients with HIV infection: A study of VaxSyn, a recombinant HIV envelope subunit vaccine, on progression of immunodeficiency. *AIDS Res Hum Retroviruses.* 1998; 14:483–490.

Van Gulck, E., Vlieghe, E., Vekemans, M., et al. mRNA-based dendritic cell vaccination induced potent antiviral responses in HIV-1 infected patients. *AIDS.* 2012; 26:F1–F12.

Van Lundzen, J., Glausinger, T., Stahmer, I., et al. Transfer of autologous gene-modified T cells in HIV-infected patients with advanced immunodeficiency and drug-resistant virus. *Mol Ther.* 2007; 15:1024–1033.

Vardas, E., Stanescu, I., Leinonen, M., et al. Indicators of a therapeutic effect in FIT-06, a phase II trial of a DNA vaccine, GTU-Multi-HIVB, in untreated HIV-1 infected subjects. *Vaccine.* 2012; 30(27):4046–4054.

Wei, D.G., Chaiang, V., Fyne, E., et al. Histone deacetylase inhibitor romidepsin induces HIV expression in CD4 T cells from patients on suppressive antiretroviral therapy at concentrations induced by clinical dosing. *PLoS Pathog.* 2014; 10(4):e1004071.

Wohl, D., Pozniack, D. A., Thompson, M., et al. Tenofovir alafenamide (TAF) in a single tablet regimen in initial HIV-therapy. Paper presented at the 22nd Conference on Retroviruses and Opportunistic Infection, February 2015, Seattle, WA. Abstract 113LB.

Wolstein, O., Boyd, M., Millington, M., et al. Preclinical safety and efficacy of an anti-HIV-1 lentiviral vector containing a short hairpin RNA to CCR5 and the C46 fusion inhibitor. *Mol Ther Methods Clin Dev.* 2014; 1:11.

Zeller, S., Kumar, P. RNA-based gene therapy for the treatment and prevention of HIV: From bench to bedside. *Yale J Biol Med.* 2011; 84(3):301–309.

Zhou, J., Rossi, J.J. Current progress in the development of RNAi based therapeutics for HIV-1. *Gene Ther.* 2011; 18:1134–1138.

24.

THE PHARMACIST'S ROLE IN CARING FOR HIV-POSITIVE INDIVIDUALS

Jennifer Cocohoba

LEARNING OBJECTIVES

- Describe common settings in which HIV pharmacists practice.

- List three potential ways in which pharmacists can contribute to the care of HIV-positive individuals.

KEY POINTS

- HIV pharmacists are a diverse group of providers that work to improve the health of HIV-positive individuals via medication therapy management, quality assurance practices, research, and other avenues.

- HIV pharmacists may be particularly skilled at managing complex antiretroviral drug–drug interactions, recommending therapies for resistant HIV virus, and providing education and support with regard to adherence.

- If practicing with a physician under a collaborative drug therapy management agreement, an HIV pharmacist may be able to provide more direct management (e.g., prescribing and ordering lab tests) for HIV and its associated conditions.

RISE OF THE HIV CLINICAL PHARMACIST

Medications for HIV have become more convenient but not less complex. For this reason, having a clinical pharmacist as a part of the health care team can greatly enhance the care of HIV-positive patients. HIV-specialized clinical pharmacists typically receive advanced training in HIV during postdoctorate residencies, infectious diseases fellowship programs, or HIV-specific fellowship programs, although some acquire their HIV knowledge through experience and intense self-study. Certification programs such as the American Academy of HIV Medicine's HIV Pharmacist (AAHIVP) certification program and the Introductory HIV Pharmaceutical Care Certificate Program offered through the University of Buffalo can help distinguish pharmacists who are well-versed in aspects of HIV pharmacotherapy.

SETTINGS IN WHICH HIV PHARMACISTS PROVIDE PATIENT CARE

People living with HIV/AIDS encounter many different pharmacists who may contribute to their care across the spectrum of their disease and medical visits. For patients who are acutely ill, the first setting in which they may interact with an HIV-specialized pharmacist is in the hospital. In many health systems, the infectious diseases (ID) team oversees consultative care for HIV-infected patients. HIV/ID pharmacists on these multidisciplinary teams may contribute their skills and knowledge to enhance care for HIV-positive patients. The paradigm of test and treat has increased the number of patients initiated on antiretroviral therapy (ART) during a hospital stay, but HIV pharmacotherapy is riddled with complex drug–drug interactions and requires close monitoring to dose adjust for renal insufficiency or hepatic dysfunction. HIV pharmacists on inpatient clinical services assist the team in selecting ART and appropriate opportunistic infection regimens, screen for complex drug–drug interactions, assist in ordering and interpreting resistance testing or therapeutic drug monitoring assays, provide discharge counseling for patients initiating new antiretroviral therapies, and can help coordinate benefit coverage for any antiretrovirals prescribed during an inpatient hospital stay.

HIV-specialized pharmacists play an important role in preventing and ameliorating medication errors. Published literature suggests that hospitalized HIV-positive patients are at high risk of incurring medication errors and that these errors—including incorrect antiretroviral regimens, incorrect dosing strategies, incorrect scheduling, or drug–drug interactions—may be initiated at various points during their hospital stay (Li, 2014).

A 3-year retrospective database study of 248 HIV-positive patients on ART identified a total of 551 medication errors in 381 hospital admissions (Merchen, 2011). Most medication errors occurred during the first 24 hours of admission, and an average of 23 hours passed before they were corrected. Mistakes in dosing or administration were the most common errors, comprising 66.9% of the total. Many errors had the potential to cause harm if they had not been corrected (as graded by National Coordinating Council for Medication Error Prevention criteria). Interventions by an HIV-specialized pharmacist resulted in an estimated cost avoidance of $24,273 per year for less serious medication errors and $124,080 per year for more serious medication errors. Pharmacy-led interventions such as antimicrobial stewardship programs, electronic medical record review, and pharmacy technician optimization programs have also been shown to be beneficial in reducing medication errors.

Patients in a clinic may interact with HIV-specialized pharmacists who work as part of an interdisciplinary ambulatory care team. These HIV clinical pharmacists have a wide range of duties commensurate with their experience and level of expertise. Responsibilities can include dispensing medications in a clinic-associated pharmacy; reviewing patient charts to ensure optimal pharmacotherapy; providing one-on-one patient education; consulting with patients and medical providers regarding medication-related problems, adherence, or resistance testing results; initiating and managing ART; ordering lab tests; and initiating, adjusting, or discontinuing medications for concomitant disease states.

Clinic-based HIV-specialized pharmacists can have an important impact on patient medication adherence and clinical outcomes. A study of 10,801 HIV-positive individuals conducted at Kaiser Permanente in California compared different clinic team structures to determine the optimal combination of clinicians that would increase adherence (Horberg, 2012). For patients starting a new ART regimen, the largest adherence increases at 12 months

were attributable to multidisciplinary teams composed of a clinical pharmacist, a social worker/benefits coordinator, and a non-HIV-specialized primary care provider (8.1% increase in mean adherence; 95% confidence interval (CI), 2.7–13.5%). Kaiser Permanente also conducted an ecological study to assess the effects of its HIV clinical pharmacists on adherence, health care utilization, and HIV outcomes (Horberg, 2007). Refill adherence at 24 months was statistically significantly higher for patients seen by an HIV clinical pharmacist (76.7% vs. 68.9%, $p = 0.02$). Odds of having a suppressed viral load or increase in CD4$^+$ cell count were modestly better for patients seen by HIV pharmacists. However, these point estimates did not achieve statistical significance and varied based on other factors such as provider panel size and patient factors such as length of time infected with HIV. The study did find that patients who worked with HIV pharmacists and whose providers had a smaller patient panel had a lower risk for medical office visits (relative risk = 0.81, $p < 0.001$). Rathbun et al. (2005) conducted a small, randomized, controlled clinical trial testing the effect of a pharmacist-run clinic adherence program on adherence and viral load. The intervention consisted of patient education, monitoring, and provision of adherence reminder devices. Patients were counseled at a clinic visit prior to starting ART. After initiation, they were contacted via telephone within 1 week and seen at a clinic visit after 2 weeks. Patients could be followed in additional clinic visits as necessary for the 12-week duration of the study. At week 28, adherence, as recorded by electronic drug monitors (74% vs. 51%), proportion of patients with viral suppression <50 copies/ml (63% vs. 53%), and median CD4$^+$ T cell count increases (142 vs. 97 cells) were all higher in the clinic pharmacist intervention group, although the point estimates did not achieve statistical significance. A number of studies on pharmacist-run adherence programs situated within community clinics, hospital clinics, and academic medical center clinics have found improvements in CD4$^+$ T cell counts, increased rates of viral suppression, fewer acute medical visits, and increased adherence for patients who interact with an HIV clinical pharmacist (Saberi, 2012).

ART is typically dispensed by a community pharmacist. Nearly all HIV-positive patients will interact with one at some point; the community pharmacist may be the health care provider with whom a healthy HIV-positive patient interacts most frequently. In larger metropolitan areas, pharmacists and staff who are knowledgeable about HIV disease may frequently be found at pharmacies that specialize in HIV care. These HIV-focused pharmacies may belong to large retail chains or can be independent pharmacies. Patient education and counseling, provision of reminder devices and adherence aids, managing the practical aspects of synchronizing and coordinating medication refills, and facilitating the procurement of antiretrovirals are just a few of the activities conducted by HIV community pharmacists.

Clinical researchers are beginning to study the impact of HIV-focused community pharmacies on patient-related outcomes. The major challenge of conducting this type of research is that pharmacy records typically do not link to medical and laboratory records, such that pharmacists may more easily evaluate the clinical impact of their interventions. The US Department of Health and Human Services funded a pilot program to support 10 California community pharmacies in providing medication therapy management (MTM) services for 1353 HIV-positive patients receiving Medicaid (Hirsch, 2009, 2011). Types of services offered in these HIV-focused pharmacies varied greatly; they included adherence enhancements such as automatic refill reminders, reminder packaging, and patient counseling when underuse or overuse of ART was detected (Rosenquist, 2010). After the first year of the program, patients using the pilot pharmacies were more adherent to their ART regimens (defined as having a medication possession ratio between 80% and 120%) compared to patients using nonpilot pharmacies (56.3% vs. 38.1%, $p < 0.001$). This trend continued at 3 years, at which time HIV-positive patients filling their ART at the pilot pharmacies ($n = 2234$) demonstrated higher medication possession ratios (69.4% vs. 47.3%, $p < 0.001$) and a higher odds of having optimal adherence (odds ratio, 2.74; 95% CI, 2.44–3.10) compared to those filling their ART at traditional pharmacies, after controlling for age, gender, and ethnicity (Hirsch, 2009, 2011). Costs at the end of the first year of the program were approximately $1,014 per pilot pharmacy patient. Although the funding for this program has since concluded, it demonstrates the potential for improvement in pharmacotherapy and adherence associated with patients using HIV-knowledgeable community pharmacies.

A SAMPLE
OF PHARMACIST SKILLS

Pharmacists make ideal treatment facilitators due to their extensive training in MTM. The goal of MTM is for a pharmacist to optimize a patient's treatment through identification, resolution, and prevention of medication-related problems (American Pharmacists Association and the National Association of Chain Drug Stores Foundation, 2008). This definition of MTM is intentionally broad so that it may accommodate the wide variety in activities that a pharmacist may perform to optimize a patient's therapy. For example, during a medication therapy review, a pharmacist may discover dangerous drug–drug interactions and poor patient adherence behaviors. The pharmacist may work closely with the patient and medical provider to create an action plan that addresses these issues. This section presents a sample of some of the skills that an HIV pharmacist may exercise when caring for an HIV-positive patient.

IDENTIFICATION AND
MANAGEMENT OF DRUG–DRUG
INTERACTIONS

Many antiretroviral agents strongly induce or inhibit the cytochrome P450 system, particularly the 3A4 isoform. Because approximately 60% of the most commonly prescribed drugs are also metabolized via cytochrome P450 3A4, pharmacists are trained to carefully review an HIV-positive patient's medication list to identify adverse drug interactions that may result in excess toxicity or subtherapeutic levels of the object drug or that may result in alterations in the HIV drug concentrations. Pharmacists provide management strategies for known interactions. For important theoretical interactions, pharmacists may suggest using therapeutic drug monitoring and can help interpret the levels garnered from these tests.

SUPPORTING ADHERENCE AND
PROVIDING PATIENT EDUCATION

In every setting, HIV pharmacists strive to support patients to adhere to their antiretroviral regimens. One very basic barrier is that patients may have difficulty adhering to medications that they cannot afford. Pharmacists can provide patients with information and resources regarding pharmaceutical company-run patient assistance programs and state-run AIDS drug assistance programs to help them afford their regimens. Hospital and clinic pharmacists may be knowledgeable regarding the local pharmacies that keep a consistent stock of antiretrovirals. Last, in the era of utilization management, pharmacists and their technicians play a critical role in selecting antiretroviral regimens that adhere to insurance formulary guidelines, providing clinical justification for prior authorizations, and managing those submissions so that patients do not have lapses in therapy.

Pharmacists have access to a wealth of reminder devices that may help improve adherence (Mahtani, 2011; Saberi,

2011). Some pharmacies offer specialized unit-dose packaging in plastic "bubble packs" or on medication cards ("blister packs") to help patients remember to take their doses. Pharmacists may train patients to use weekly medication boxes. Some community and clinic pharmacists may offer text messaging or may work with patients to set up cell phone alarms to serve as automated medication reminders. Pharmacies may offer a variety of other adherence-enhancing services, such as online management of medications, automatic prescription refills, telephone refill reminders, and home mailing or courier medication delivery.

Pharmacist services include patient counseling to enhance adherence. HIV clinical pharmacists make ideal treatment advocates because they are knowledgeable about ART and may help bridge the gap between patients and their providers. They offer personalized patient education regarding HIV disease, HIV treatment and opportunistic infection prophylaxis, and management of adverse effects. Using popular counseling techniques such as motivational interviewing, pharmacists may assess a patient's readiness to initiate ART and may help motivate the patient toward that goal (D'Antonio, 2010; Krummenacher, 2011). Although these items may be discussed during the treating clinician's visit rather than during a pharmacist visit, this type of education often takes up more time than allowed in a brief visit focused on acute medical problems. A visit with a pharmacist provides complementary education and serves as an extension of the provider's care. In clinic and community pharmacy settings, pharmacists may package all of these services into structured adherence programs that span the range of patient assessment, education, and counseling, offering reminder devices, dispensing medications, and providing continuity in the refill process. Although no two pharmacist-run adherence programs are exactly alike, many studies have illustrated their benefits with regard to patient outcomes (Krummenacher, 2011; March, 2007).

TESTING FOR HIV INFECTION

HIV testing is a service that is emerging predominantly in community pharmacies. These models of care typically encompass the use of point-of-care rapid HIV tests, counseling, and linkage to confirmatory testing and/or care. In preliminary studies, pharmacy-based testing appears to be acceptable to both patients and pharmacists. In one study, 939 HIV tests were provided by 22 pharmacy staff members at six different sites during a 12-month period (Lecher, 2015). Pre- and post-test counseling required an average of 4–12 minutes, and the average cost per person tested ranged from $32.17 to $47.21.

PROVIDING PATIENT CARE VIA COLLABORATIVE PRACTICE AGREEMENTS

In the United States, most states have legislation that allows for pharmacists to engage in collaborative practice; however, the requirements and regulations vary from state to state. In some states, pharmacists may enhance the care of HIV-positive patients via collaborative drug therapy management (CDTM) agreements. The specifics of any CDTM agreement depend on the collaborating physician and the qualifications and experience of the pharmacist.

The American College of Clinical Pharmacy defines a CDTM agreement as

> a collaborative practice agreement between one or more physicians and pharmacists wherein qualified pharmacists working within the context of a defined protocol are permitted to assume professional responsibility for performing patient assessments; ordering drug therapy-related laboratory tests; administering drugs; and selecting, initiating, monitoring, continuing, and adjusting drug regimens. (Hammond, 2003, p 1210)

The American Society of Health Systems Pharmacists recently published an updated statement on pharmacist involvement in HIV care that attempts to summarize the scope of practice for an HIV pharmacist (American Society of Health Systems Pharmacists, 2015). Collaborative protocols with physicians may allow pharmacists to select and initiate ART or opportunistic infection prophylaxis, draw and interpret pertinent labs that monitor efficacy or toxicity of the regimen, simplify regimens using fixed-dose combination tablets, and manage common antiretroviral-related side effects such as nausea and diarrhea. Knowledgeable pharmacists may order, interpret, and change a patient's ART based on resistance tests. Ma et al. (2010) conducted a before-and-after comparison of clinical outcomes for patients consulting with an HIV clinical pharmacist in a drug optimization clinic. Pharmacists reviewed patient medication histories and resistance tests, simplified or adjusted their ART regimens, and provided adherence training and education. After the pharmacist intervention, refill adherence was improved (89% vs. 81%, $p = 0.003$), a higher proportion of patients achieved undetectable viral loads (96% vs. 63%, $p < 0.001$), and a higher proportion of patients had increased absolute CD4[+] T cell counts (491 vs. 423 cells/mm^3 at visit, $p < 0.001$).

In addition to managing ART, some protocols allow pharmacists to assess and adjust medication therapy for HIV-related comorbidities such as depression, diabetes, hypertension, hepatitis C, or dyslipidemia. A retrospective cohort study found that an interdisciplinary primary care team that included an HIV pharmacist produced significantly improved outcomes in lipid management and smoking cessation for patients with HIV and diabetes, hypertension, or hyperlipidemia ($n = 96$) compared to a control group ($n = 50$) that was managed by an individual health care provider (Cope, 2015). The interdisciplinary team achieved a cost savings of approximately $3,000 per patient. This particular study examined pharmacist management of primary care conditions, and there are also emerging opportunities for pharmacists to practice collaboratively in the provision of pre-exposure prophylaxis and post-exposure prophylaxis for HIV.

A collaborative, interdisciplinary practice coupled with good communication between providers can serve as an excellent model for enhancing the care of HIV-positive patients and extending the provider's ability to reach the greatest number of patients. The roles, responsibilities, and impact of HIV pharmacists in clinical practice are likely to expand in the future as the profession of pharmacy lobbies for HIV pharmacists to be recognized as health care providers under US federal law.

PHARMACISTS: UNLIMITED POTENTIAL

The benefit of having an HIV clinical pharmacist extends beyond direct patient services. Pharmacists are becoming increasingly essential members of HIV hospital or clinic quality improvement teams. Performance measures, such as those for HIVQUAL, often involve chart abstraction to benchmark rates of ART, viral suppression, opportunistic infection prophylaxis, and adherence assessment. HIV clinical pharmacists have the clinical background and skills to assess these items (and others) quickly, accurately, and thoroughly. Pharmacists can also offer valuable insight for plan–do–study–act projects designed to improve any below-target performance measures.

Finally, an increasing number of trained HIV clinical pharmacist scientists are making a strong impact on HIV-related research. Their understanding of study design, drug therapy monitoring, and pharmacotherapy makes HIV clinical pharmacists ideal study coordinators or project managers for research studies being conducted within clinical settings. Advanced training through master's degree programs and complementary PhD programs also places HIV clinical pharmacists in an optimal position to serve as principal investigators on research studies regarding pharmacokinetics, pharmacodynamics, investigational drugs, adherence, drug resistance, or provision of health services. As pharmacists become further trained in clinical research methods, they will continue to contribute valuable information to the body of HIV knowledge.

CONCLUSION

HIV clinical pharmacists are a diverse group of health care practitioners with specialized skills and knowledge. Whether they are engaged in patient care, quality assurance, research, or a combination of these, they strive to benefit HIV-positive patients through their efforts. Although not all clinics or hospitals have available resources or grants to house an HIV specialized pharmacist, collaborations with HIV-focused community pharmacists can ensure that patients have access to this valuable health care team member and that they receive the highest quality medication care possible.

Recommended Reading

American Pharmacists Association and National Association of Chain Drug Stores Foundation. Medication therapy management in pharmacy practice: Core elements of an MTM service model (version 2.0). *J Am Pharm Assoc (2003)*. 2008; 48(3):341–353.

American Society of Health-Systems Pharmacists. ASHP guidelines on pharmacist involvement in HIV care. Available at http://www.ashp.org/DocLibrary/BestPractices/Guidelines-Pharmacist-Involvement-HIV-Care.aspx.

Scott, J. D., Abernathy, K. A., Diaz-Linares, M., et al. HIV clinical pharmacists—The US perspective. *Farm Hosp* 2010; 34(6):303–308.

References

American Society of Health Systems Pharmacists. ASHP guidelines on pharmacist involvement in HIV care. In: *ASHP Best Practices: Position & Guidance Documents of ASHP 2015–2016*. Bethesda, MD: American Society of Health Systems Pharmacists; 2015.

Cope, R., Berkowitz, L., Arcebido, R., et al. Evaluating the effects of an interdisciplinary practice model with pharmacist collaboration on HIV patient co-morbidities. *AIDS Patient Care STDS*. 2015; 29(8):445–453.

D'Antonio, N. Including motivational interviewing skills in the PharmD curriculum. *Am J Pharm Educ*. 2010; 74(8):152d.

Hammond, R. W., Schwartz, A. H., Campbell, M. J., et al. Collaborative drug therapy management by pharmacists—2003. *Pharmacotherapy*. 2003; 23(9):1210–1225.

Hirsch, J. D., Gonzales, M., Rosenquist, A., et al. Antiretroviral therapy adherence, medication use, and health care costs during 3 years of a community pharmacy medication therapy management program for Medi-Cal beneficiaries with HIV/AIDS. *J Manag Care Pharm*. 2011; 17(3):213–223.

Hirsch, J. D., Rosenquist, A., Best, B., et al. Evaluation of the first year of a pilot program in community pharmacy: HIV/AIDS medication therapy management for Medi-Cal beneficiaries. *J Manag Care Pharm*. 2009; 15(1):32–41.

Horberg, M. A., Bartemeier Hurley, L., James Towner, W., et al. Determination of optimized multidisciplinary care team for maximal antiretroviral therapy adherence. *J Acquir Immune Defic Syndr*. 2012; 60(2):183–190.

Horberg, M. A., Hurley, L. B., Silverberg, M. J., et al. Effect of clinical pharmacists on utilization of and clinical response to antiretroviral therapy. *J Acquir Immune Defic Syndr*. 2007; 44(5):531–539.

Krummenacher, I., Cavassini, M., Bugnon, O., et al. An interdisciplinary HIV-adherence program combining motivational interviewing and electronic antiretroviral drug monitoring. *AIDS Care*. 2011; 23(5):550–561.

Lecher, S. L., Shrestha, R. K., Botts, L. W., et al. Cost analysis of a novel HIV testing strategy in community pharmacies and retail clinics. *J Am Pharm Assoc* (2003). 2015; 55(5):488–492.

Li, E. H., and Foisy, M. M. Antiretroviral and medication errors in hospitalized HIV-positive patients. *Ann Pharmacother*. 2014 May 8; 48(8):998–1010.

Ma, A., Chen, D. M., Chau, F. M., et al. Improving adherence and clinical outcomes through an HIV pharmacist's interventions. *AIDS Care*. 2010; 22(10):1189–1194.

Mahtani, K. R., Heneghan, C. J., Glasziou, P. P., et al. Reminder packaging for improving adherence to self-administered long-term medications. *Cochrane Database System Rev*. 2011; 9:CD005025.

March, K., Mak, M., and Louie, S. G. Effects of pharmacists' interventions on patient outcomes in an HIV primary care clinic. *Am J Health Syst Pharm*. 2007; 64(24):2574–2578.

Merchen, A., Gerzenshtein, L., Scarsi, K., et al. HIV-specialized pharmacists' impact on prescribing errors in hospitalized patients on antiretroviral therapy. Paper presented at the 51st Interscience Conference on Antimicrobial Agents and Chemotherapy, Chicago, IL, September 17–20, 2011.

Rathbun, R. C., Farmer, K. C., Stephens, J. R., et al. Impact of an adherence clinic on behavioral outcomes and virologic response in the treatment of HIV infection: A prospective, randomized, controlled pilot study. *Clin Ther*. 2005; 27(2):199–209.

Rosenquist, A., Best, B. M., Miller, T. A., et al. Medication therapy management services in community pharmacy: A pilot programme in HIV specialty pharmacies. *J Eval Clin Pract*. 2010; 16(6):1142–1146.

Saberi, P., Dong, B. J., Johnson, M. O., et al. The impact of HIV clinical pharmacists on HIV treatment outcomes: A systematic review. *Patient Prefer Adherence*. 2012; 6:297–322.

Saberi, P., and Johnson, M. O. Technology-based self-care methods of improving antiretroviral adherence: A systematic review. *PLoS One*. 2011; 6(11):e27533.

25.

SOLID ORGAN TRANSPLANTATION IN HIV-INFECTED INDIVIDUALS

Eurides Lopes and Jennifer Husson

LEARNING OBJECTIVE

Discuss the indications and management of, and outcomes for HIV-infected solid organ transplant recipients.

WHAT'S NEW?

- Studies have found that patient and graft survival rates in HIV-infected transplant recipients can be as good as those in non-infected recipients.

- The HIV Organ Policy Equity (HOPE) Act, which was signed into law in the United States in November 2013, allows the use of HIV-infected donor organs for transplantation into HIV-infected recipients under research protocols.

KEY POINTS

- End-organ disease has become a major cause of morbidity and mortality in HIV-infected patients due to increased life expectancy, thus increasing the demand for organ transplantation in these patients.

- The care of HIV-infected transplant recipients warrants a multidisciplinary team approach, including the transplant team, pharmacists, infectious disease specialists, nurses, and patients and their families.

- The immunosuppression of HIV-infected recipients post-transplant does not appear to further advance HIV disease.

- The post-transplant risk of opportunistic infections for HIV-infected recipients does not appear to be increased by immunosuppression. However, the overall rate of infections is high, and it is even higher in hepatitis C virus (HCV) co-infected transplant recipients.

- HIV/HCV co-infected recipients have worse outcomes than both liver and kidney HIV-infected recipients.

INTRODUCTION

The arrival of antiretroviral (ARV) therapy in 1996 resulted in increased life expectancy of HIV-infected patients. Consequently, end-organ disease has become a major cause of morbidity and mortality in this population. Up to 30% of HIV-infected individuals have end-stage renal disease (ESRD) as a direct consequence of HIV infection (HIV-associated nephropathy), drug toxicities, or other comorbidities (Ahuja, 2002), accounting for 12.2% of HIV-related deaths (Locke, 2014). Because HIV-infected individuals with ESRD have a 5-year survival of only 65% compared to 94% for HIV-uninfected individuals with ESRD, and given the fact that co-infection with HCV is prevalent in this population, there is a growing need for renal and liver transplantation in these patients (Rodriguez, 2003).

PRETRANSPLANT EVALUATION

CRITERIA FOR TRANSPLANTATION

- Any opportunistic infections (OIs) or malignancies should be completely treated prior to transplant. A history of OIs or malignancies with suboptimal therapies (progressive multifocal leukoencephalopathy, visceral Kaposi's sarcoma, chronic cryptosporidiosis, or primary central nervous system lymphoma) should be excluded (Stock, 2010).

- Recipients must meet standard criteria for transplantation.

Renal Transplant

- CD4$^+$ cell counts should be ≥200 cells/μl prior to transplantation.

- Recipients must be on a stable ARV therapy.

- The HIV RNA should be below the limit of detection for *at least* 6 months prior to transplantation (Harbell, 2013; Stock, 2010).

Liver Transplant

- CD4$^+$ T cell counts must be ≥100 cells/μl, or they must be ≥200 cell/μl for recipients who have a history of previous OIs or malignancy. The CD4$^+$ T cell count threshold is lower for liver transplant recipients due to presumed splenic sequestration secondary to portal hypertension.

- Recipients must be on a stable ARV regimen.

- Ideally, HIV RNA should be suppressed at the time of transplant.

- For recipients who are not able to tolerate ARVs or who have recently started ARVs, an infectious diseases (ID) physician must be able to predict full HIV suppression on an acceptable ARV regimen (Harbell, 2013).

PRETRANSPLANT INFECTION SCREENING AND VACCINATIONS

Tuberculin Skin Test or Quantiferon Gold

- All candidates must be screened for latent tuberculosis (TB) prior to transplantation. Patients should be treated if they have a positive Quantiferon TB test, a tuberculin skin test >5 mm, or contact with a case of active TB. The preferred regimen is isoniazid (INH) + vitamin B$_6$ for 9 months, completing at least 6 of the 9 months prior to transplantation. For liver transplant when treatment cannot be completed prior or the risk of toxicity is too high, treatment should be completed after transplant.

Syphilis

- Test for and treat syphilis prior to transplant.

Serologies

- Test for cytomegalovirus (CMV), Epstein–Barr virus, herpes simplex virus, varicella zoster virus, and viral hepatitis serologies in all candidates. In addition, coccidioides and strongyloides serologies should be tested if the recipient has prolonged exposure to endemic areas.

Hepatitis A and B

- All candidates should be vaccinated against hepatitis A and B if not immune.

- Inactivated influenza vaccine should be given yearly.

- Pneumococcal/Prevnar vaccine should be given if not given in the past 5 years.

- Tdap vaccine should be given if not given in the past 10 years.

Human Papillomavirus Vaccine

- Vaccine should be given from ages 15 to 26 years.

Meningococcal Vaccine

- Vaccine should be given in appropriate context.

Varicella or Zoster, Measles, Mumps and Rubella (MMR)

- Vaccines are contraindicated if CD4$^+$ cell count <300 cells/μl (Miro, 2014).

WHEN TO REFER
Renal Transplant

- All HIV-infected patients on hemodialysis or with glomerular filtration rate ≤25 ml/min should be referred to a renal transplant center as long they meet the HIV inclusion criteria.

Liver Transplant

- All HIV-infected patients with decompensated cirrhosis, symptomatic disease, or hepatocellular carcinoma who meet the inclusion criteria should be referred for liver transplant evaluation. Patients with an albumin <3 g/dL, a prolonged prothrombin time, or a modified

Child–Turcotte–Pugh score ≥7 should also be considered.

POST-TRANSPLANT MANAGEMENT AND CARE

All pre-, peri-, and post-transplant care should be coordinated among a multidisciplinary team consisting of the transplant surgeon, an ID or HIV specialist, a nephrologist or hepatologist, a primary care provider, a transplant coordinator, a transplant pharmacist, a social worker, and nursing staff.

IMMUNOSUPPRESSION THERAPY

Induction

The multicenter HIVTR study suggested that the use of anti-thymocyte globulin (ATG) was associated with a higher risk of graft loss (Stock, 2010). However, subsequent studies found a 2.6-fold lower risk of acute rejection with ATG induction, with graft survival rates equivalent to those of a non-HIV-infected cohort (Locke, 2014). The choice of induction therapy should be patient-specific, accounting for the individual's risk of rejection, although recent evidence suggests ATG is generally safe in this population.

Maintenance

Maintenance immunosuppression generally consists of triple therapy including calcineurin inhibitors (CNIs) (e.g., cyclosporine and tacrolimus) with an antimetabolite (e.g., mycophenolate mofetil) and corticosteroids. An mTOR inhibitor (e.g., sirolimus and everolimus) may be substituted if patients are not able to tolerate CNIs or antimetabolites. The HIVTR study found an increased risk of rejection with the use of cyclosporine compared to tacrolimus (Stock, 2010), and sirolimus was found to be associated with a higher rate of rejection (Locke, 2014). However, given the uncertainty with drug interactions and small numbers of patients, the optimal regimen remains unclear.

ANTIRETROVIRAL THERAPY

Antiretroviral therapy should be reinitiated post-transplant as soon as oral medications can be tolerated (Roland, 2006). The regimen varies based on the individual patient's resistance pattern and prior drug exposure. There are also drug–drug interactions between CNIs, mTOR inhibitors, protease inhibitors (PIs), and non-nucleoside reverse transcriptase inhibitors (NNRTIs) due to effects on cytochrome P450 (CYP) 3A4 drug metabolism and P-glycoprotein (Frasetto, 2007; Trullas, 2011). This is significant because changes in antiretroviral medications (as well as other medications) can lead to altered metabolism of the immunosuppressants, thus leading to organ rejection or drug toxicity (van Maarseveen, 2012). However, there are no absolute contraindications because dosing modifications can compensate for the altered metabolism of these drugs.

Nucleoside Reverse Transcriptase Inhibitors

- When possible, nucleoside reverse transcriptase inhibitors (NRTIs) with significant mitochondrial toxicity should not be used with mycophenolate. Zidovudine and stavudine may have some antagonism when used with mycophenolate, and zidovudine may exacerbate bone marrow suppression. Abacavir, on the other hand, may have synergistic activity against HIV when used with mycophenolate (Chapuis, 2000; Margolis, 1999). Tenofovir should be avoided when possible due to the associated increase in creatinine.

NNRTIs

- These are strong CYP3A4 inducers, thus increasing the metabolism of CNIs and decreasing their serum levels. The dose of these immunosuppressive agents must be increased with close monitoring of drug levels.

Protease Inhibitors

- These are strong CYP3A4 inhibitors, which decrease the metabolism of CNIs and mTOR inhibitors resulting in higher levels of these agents. Thus, it is imperative that the dosages of both CNIs and mTOR inhibitors be decreased and the dosing interval increased with close monitoring of drug levels. PIs also decrease the clearance of glucocorticoids, which may cause a Cushing-like syndrome. In addition, they may exacerbate hyperlipidemia post-transplant and potentiate CNI-induced impaired glucose tolerance.

Integrase Inhibitors

- These do not interfere with CYP3A metabolism; thus, there are few potential drug interactions with immunosuppressants.

CCR5 Antagonists

- Sirolimus reduces the expression of CCR5 receptors and may enhance the antiviral activity of CCR5 antagonists such as Maraviroc (Gilliam, 2007; Heredia, 2008).

POST-TRANSPLANT INFECTION PROPHYLAXIS

In addition to standard post-transplant CMV prophylaxis, HIV solid-organ transplant (SOT) recipients should receive the following prophylaxis:

- *Pneumocystis jiroveci*
  - Lifelong prophylaxis with trimethoprim/sulfamethoxazole (TMP/SMX) or Dapsone (if sulfa allergic or bone marrow suppression is an issue) as long as glucose-6-phosphate dehydrogenase levels are normal.
- *Mycobacterium avium* complex
  - Azithromycin should be used if $CD4^+$ T cell count <75 cells/μl.
- Toxoplasmosis
  - TMP/SMX should be used if $CD4^+$ T cell count 200 cells/μl and if either the recipient or the donor carries IgG antibodies against *Toxoplasma gondii*.
- Prior OIs
  - Continue primary and secondary prophylaxis for OIs such as cryptococcus until $CD4^+$ T cell counts are above the threshold (i.e., $CD4^+$ >200 cells/μl) for approximately 3–6 months, although many may prefer lifelong secondary prophylaxis (Harbell, 2013).

OUTCOMES

PATIENT AND GRAFT SURVIVAL AND REJECTION

Renal Transplant

The overall patient and graft survival rates of HIV-infected renal transplant recipients in the HIVTR study were between the rates observed in HIV-uninfected, older recipients and all recipients, with rates of 94.6% ± 2% and 90.4% at 1 year and 88.2% ± 3.8% and 73.7% at 3 years,

respectively. Living donor grafts were also found to be protective, and the use of ATG, HCV co-infection, and older age were associated with decreased survival (Stock, 2010). Subsequently, the use of ATG induction was found to be associated with patient and graft survival rates equivalent to those of an HIV-uninfected cohort (Locke, 2014).

In the HIVTR study, the rate of acute rejection was found to be 2- to 3-fold higher and acute rejection was more aggressive, with a rate of 31% at 1 year and 41% at 3 years in HIV-infected recipients compared to the national rates (Stock, 2010). Further studies have also found higher rates of rejection, with a rate of 55% at 12 months and notably 28% at 1 month (Malat, 2012). ATG induction was associated with a 2.6-fold decrease in the rate of acute rejection compared to that of patients who did not receive any induction (Locke, 2014).

Liver Transplant

Studies have shown that dual organ transplantation, a lower pretransplant body mass index, older age, and HCV co-infection were associated with decreased survival, although there was a survival benefit for liver recipients with a pretransplant Model for End-Stage Liver Disease (MELD) score ≥15 (Stock, 2010). Recent data suggest that outcomes for mono-infected HIV-positive recipients have improved, with outcomes superior to those for HCV mono-infected or HIV/HCV co-infected recipients (Sawinski, 2015). However, there remains a 1.68-fold increased risk for death and 1.70-fold increased risk for graft loss compared to those risks for HIV non-infected recipients independent of HCV status (Locke, 2016). In addition, the 3-year rejection rate was 1.6-fold higher in HIV/HCV co-infected liver recipients compared to HCV mono-infected recipients (Terrault, 2012).

HIV/HCV CO-INFECTION

Renal Transplant

HIV/HCV co-infected renal transplant recipients have the lowest 3-year patient survival and graft survival rates (73% and 60%, respectively) compared to non-co-infected recipients (90% and 86%, respectively), HIV mono-infected recipients (89% and 81%, respectively), and HCV mono-infected recipients (84% and 78%, respectively) (Sawinski, 2015). This finding is consistent with those of other studies, suggesting that HCV co-infection has a negative impact on renal transplantation outcomes and emphasizing the need to treat HCV infection either pre- or post-transplant (Sawinski, 2015).

Liver Transplant

In general, HIV/HCV co-infected recipients tend to have poorer outcomes. Initial studies of liver transplantation in HIV-infected recipients showed that the 3-year patient and graft survival rates for the HIV/HCV co-infected patients were lower (53% and 74%, respectively) than those for HCV mono-infected recipients (60% and 79%, respectively) (Terrault, 2012). One explanation is that many of these patients will have recurrent HCV infection that can be very aggressive, leading to graft loss and death. Previously reported 5-year survival of approximately 50–55% may increase to 80% in co-infected liver recipients in whom the HCV viral infection has been cleared (Miro, 2015).

HIV/HEPATITIS B VIRUS CO-INFECTION

Renal Transplant

Kidney recipients with hepatitis B virus (HBV) infection have overall lower survival rates compared to non-infected recipients. The 10-year patient survival rate was 51.4% in HBV-infected recipients compared to 82.8% in non-infected recipients, and graft survival rates were 44% for HBV-infected recipients compared to 74.2% for non-infected recipients (Lee, 2001).

Liver Transplant

The overall outcomes for HIV/HBV co-infected recipients appear to be equivalent to those of HBV mono-infected recipients. A small study found that no patients developed clinical evidence of HBV recurrence despite low-grade viremia in 54% of co-infected recipients when treated with HBV immunoglobulin (HBIg) with or without anti-HBV antiviral therapy (Coffin, 2010). The recommended management for HBV-infected liver recipients includes two NRTIs with anti-HBV activity (lamivudine, tenofovir, and entecavir) and HBIg, with HBV DNA monitoring every 6 months (Harbell, 2013); this should be incorporated into or added to HIV/HBV co-infected recipients' ARV therapy.

PROGRESSION OF HIV DISEASE

The HIVTR study reported five cases of new opportunistic infections, including two cases of cutaneous Kaposi's sarcoma, one case of cryptosporidiosis, one presumed case of *P. jiroveci*, and one case of candidal esophagitis. Despite an initial decline in CD4+ T cell count post-transplant, which was more pronounced with ATG induction, there was no increase in complications associated with HIV disease or progression of HIV (Stock, 2010).

RISK OF INFECTION AND MALIGNANCY

Overall, 38% of kidney recipients had infections post-transplant in the HIVTR study, consisting of predominantly genitourinary infections (26%), respiratory tract infections (20%), and bacteremia (19%). This study also found that HCV co-infected recipients had a higher rate of serious infections compared to HCV-uninfected recipients (Stock, 2010).

Based on available data, the incidence of recurrent or new malignancy after SOT in HIV-infected patients is low and not significantly different from that of HIV-uninfected patients. In the HIVTR study, 9% of patients (11.2% of liver recipients and 8.7% of kidney recipients) developed post-transplant malignancies (including skin cancer, cutaneous Kaposi's sarcoma, penile squamous cell cancer, head and neck cancer, renal cell cancer, lymphoma, recurrence of pretransplant hepatocellular carcinoma, and cholangiocarcinoma), and 3% of patients died from a cancer-related cause (Stock, 2010). The same study showed an increased risk of developing high-grade squamous intraepithelial lesions after transplantation in 89 patients followed for anal cytology, which requires further study (Nissen, 2012).

FUTURE DIRECTIONS

With the increasing numbers of HIV-infected patients with ESRD and end-stage liver disease and the increased mortality associated with these conditions, the demand for organ transplantation is increasing. However, the organ pool does not currently meet demand. The use of HIV-infected donor organs may help to narrow this gap. Until recently, HIV-infected individuals were not allowed to be included in the transplant donor pool. There are still many concerns regarding the use of HIV-infected donor organs—namely the risk of superinfection with a new, possibly resistant HIV strain; the risk of transmitting donor-derived opportunistic infections; and the increased risk of acute rejection. Despite these concerns, in 2013, the HOPE Act, which allows the use of HIV-infected donor organs for transplantation into HIV-infected recipients, was signed into law in the United States. In addition, preliminary data from South Africa show patient survival rates among HIV-positive recipients of HIV-positive donor kidneys to be 84% at 1 year, 84% at

3 years, and 74% at 5 years, with graft survival rates of 93% at 1 year and 84% at both 3 and 5 years and rejection rates of 8% at 1 year and 22% at 3 years (Muller, 2015). As these organs becomes available, further research will be needed in an effort to optimize outcomes using HIV-infected donor organs, and issues such as the use of HIV-infected living donor organs and the use of HIV-infected donor organs for HIV non-infected recipients will need to be further debated.

CONCLUSION

HIV-infected patients have good survival benefit from transplantation, especially renal transplantation and some selected liver transplantation. Post-transplant immuno-suppression does not appear to further advance HIV disease or have an increased risk of opportunistic infection. HIV/HCV co-infected recipients continue to appear to have worse outcomes, partially due to a more aggressive post-transplant HCV recurrence, which emphasizes the importance of HCV treatment prior to or immediately post-transplant now that newer, less toxic therapies are available. The management of drug–drug interactions remains a crucial part of this process that cannot be ignored. This is a task that should include a large, integrated group of providers, including the transplant team, pharmacists, infectious disease specialists, and nurses, in addition to the patients.

References

Ahuja TS, Grady J, Khan S. Changing trends in the survival of dialysis patients with human immunodeficiency virus in the United States. *J Am Soc Nephrol*. 2002; 13(7):1889–1893.

Chapuis AG, Paolo Rizzardi G, D'Agostino C, et al. Effects of mycophenolic acid on human immunodeficiency virus infection in vitro and in vivo. *Nat Med*. 2000; 6:762–768.

Coffin CS, Stock PG, Dove LM, et al. Virologic and clinical outcomes of hepatitis B virus infection in HIV–HBV co-infected transplant recipients. *Am J Transp*. 2010; 10:1268–1275.

Frasetto LA, Browne M, Cheng A, et al. HYPERLINK "https://www.ncbi.nlm.nih.gov/pubmed/17949460" Immunosuppressant pharmacokinetics and dosing modifications in HIV-1 infected liver and kidney transplant recipients. *Am J. Transplant*. 2007 Dec; 7(12):2816–2820.

Gilliam B, Heredia A, Devico A, et al. Rapamycin reduces CCR5 mRNA levels in macaques: Potential applications in HIV-1 prevention and treatment. *AIDS*. 2007; 21(15):2108–2110.

Harbell J, Terrault NA, Stock P. Solid organ transplants in HIV-infected patients. *Curr HIV/AIDS Rep*. 2013; 10:217–225.

Heredia A, Latinovic O, Gallo RC, et al. Reduction of CCR5 with low-dose rapamycin enhances the antiviral activity of vicriviroc against both sensitive and drug-resistant HIV-1. *Proc Natl Acad Sci USA*. 2008; 105(51):20476–20481.

Lee WC, Shu KH, Cheng CH, et al. Long-term impact of hepatitis B, C virus infection on renal transplantation. *Am J Nephrol*. 2001; 21:300–306.

Locke JE, Durand C, Reed RD, et al. Long-term outcomes after liver transplantation among human immunodeficiency virus-infected recipients. *Transplantation*. 2016; 100(1):141–146.

Locke JE, James NT, Mannon RB, et al. Immunosuppression regimen and the risk of acute rejection in HIV-infected kidney transplant recipients. *Transplantation*. 2014; 97(4):446–450.

Malat GE, Ranganna KM, Sikalas N, et al. High frequency of rejections in HIV-positive recipients of kidney transplantation: A single center prospective trial. *Transplantation*. 2012; 94:1020–1024.

Margolis D, Heredia A, Gaywee J, et al. Abacavir and mycophenolic acid, an inhibitor of inosine monophosphate dehydrogenase, have profound and synergistic anti-HIV activity. *J AIDS*. 1999; 21:362–370.

Miro JM, Agüero F, Duclos-Vallée JC, et al. Infections in solid organ transplant HIV-infected patients. *Clin Microbiol Infect*. 2014; 20:119–130.

Miro JM, Stock P, Teicher E, et al. Outcome and management of HCV/HIV coinfection pre- and post-liver transplantation: A 2015 update. *J. Hepatol*. 2015; 62:701–711.

Muller E, Barday Z, Kahn D. HIV-positive-to-HIV-positive kidney transplantation: Results at 3 and 5 years. *N Engl J Med*. 2015; 372:613–620.

Nissen NN, Barin B, Stock PG. Malignancy in the HIV-infected patients undergoing liver and kidney transplantation. *Curr Opin Oncol*. 2012; 24:517–521.

Richterman A, Blumberg E. The challenges and promise of HIV-infected donors for solid organ transplantation. *Curr Infect Dis Rep*. 2015; 17:17.

Rodriguez RA, Mendelson M, O'Hare AM, et al. Determinants of survival among HIV-infected chronic dialysis patients. *J Am Soc Nephrol*. 2003; 14(5):1307–1313.

Roland ME, Stock PG. Liver transplantation in HIV-infected recipients. *Semin Liver Dis*. 2006; 26(3):273–284.

Sawinski D, Forde KA, Eddinger K, et al. Superior outcomes in HIV-positive kidney transplant patients compared with HCV-infected or HIV/HCV co-infected recipients. *Kidney Int*. 2015; 88:341–349.

Sawinski D, Goldberg DS, Blumberg E, et al. Beyond the NIH multicenter HIV transplant trial experience: Outcomes of HIV+ liver transplant recipients compared to HCV+ or HIV+/HCV+ co-infected recipients in the United States. *Clin Infect Dis*. 2015; 61(7):1054–1062.

Stock P, Barin B, Murphy B, et al. Outcomes of kidney transplantation in HIV-infected recipients. *N Engl J Med*. 2010; 363:2001–2014.

Terrault N, Roland ME, Schiano T, et al. Outcomes of liver transplant recipients with hepatitis C and human immunodeficiency virus coinfection. *Liver Transpl*. 2012; 18(6):716–726.

Trullas JC, Cofan F, Tuset M, et al. HYPERLINK "https://www.ncbi.nlm.nih.gov/pubmed/21248716" Renal transplantation in HIV-infected patients: 2010 update. *Kidney Int*. 2011 Apr; 79(8):825–842.

van Maarseveen EM, Rogers CC, Trofe-Clark J, et al. Drug–drug interactions between antiretroviral and immunosuppressive agents in HIV-infected patients after solid organ transplantation: A review. *AIDS Patient Care STDs*. 2012; 26(10):568–581.

26.

ANTIRETROVIRAL THERAPY IN PREGNANT WOMEN

William R. Short and Jason J. Schafer

LEARNING OBJECTIVE

Review the clinical management of HIV-infected pregnant women, including recommendations for the use of antiretrovirals (ARVs) and drug disposition.

WHAT'S NEW?

Darunavir/ritonavir is now a preferred protease inhibitor regimen, and lopinavir/ritonavir is an alternative regimen. Raltegravir is now a preferred integrase inhibitor regimen.

KEY POINTS

- ARVs should be initiated in all HIV-infected pregnant women regardless of CD4$^+$ T cell count or HIV-1 RNA level. ARVs should be given in combination therapy, similar to nonpregnant patients, with the goal of complete virologic suppression.

- Treatment changes during pregnancy have been associated with the loss of virologic control and independently associated with mother-to-child transmission.

- All cases of prenatal ARV exposure should be reported to the Antiretroviral Pregnancy Registry (www.apregistry.com).

BACKGROUND

Over time, research has demonstrated that proper prevention strategies and interventions during pregnancy, labor, and delivery can significantly reduce the rate of mother-to-child transmission (MTCT) of HIV. In 1994, a pivotal study in the field of HIV medicine, the Pediatric AIDS Clinical Trials Group (PACTG) 076, demonstrated that the use of zidovudine (ZDV) monotherapy during pregnancy substantially reduced the risk of HIV transmission to infants by 67% (Connor, 1994). The protocol is summarized in Table 26.1. It consisted of oral administration of ZDV initiated between 14 and 34 weeks of gestation and continued throughout pregnancy, followed by intrapartum administration of intravenous ZDV and then oral administration of ZDV to the newborn for 6 weeks after delivery. Additional studies have demonstrated the effectiveness of the use of combination antiretroviral therapy (ART), further decreasing the risk of HIV transmission to ≤2% (Cooper, 2002). Based on recent data, there have been modifications to the original protocol, including a more selective use of intravenous ZDV based on maternal viral load.

PHYSIOLOGIC CHANGES DURING PREGNANCY

There are physiologic changes that occur during pregnancy which may alter drug disposition and lead to decreased drug exposure. These changes may be associated with incomplete virologic suppression, virologic failure, and/or the development of drug resistance (Mirochnick, 2004). An understanding of the pharmacokinetic changes that can occur with ARVs during pregnancy is essential for making proper dose modifications to maintain efficacy and minimize toxicity. Box 26.1) summarizes some of the physiologic changes that occur during pregnancy which could affect drug disposition.

Table 26.1 THREE-PART ZIDOVUDINE (ZDV) CHEMOPROPHYLAXIS REGIMEN BASED ON PACTG 076

TIME OF ZDV ADMINISTRATION	REGIMEN
Antepartum	Oral administration of 100 mg ZDV five times daily,[a] initiated at 14–34 weeks of gestation and continued throughout pregnancy
Intrapartum	During labor, intravenous administration of ZDV in a 1-hour initial dose of 2 mg/kg body weight, followed by a continuous infusion of 1 mg/kg body weight/hour until delivery
Postpartum	Oral administration of ZDV to the newborn (ZDV syrup at 2 mg/kg body weight/dose every 6 hours) for the first 6 weeks of life, beginning 8–12 hours after birth[b]

[a]Oral ZDV administered as 200 mg three times daily or 300 mg twice daily is currently used in general clinical practice and is an acceptable alternative regimen to 100 mg five times daily.

[b]Intravenous dosage for full-term infants who can tolerate oral intake is 1.5 mg/kg body weight intravenously every 6 hours. ZDV dosing for infants less than 35 weeks of gestation at birth is 1.5 mg/kg/dose intravenously, or 2.0 mg/kg/dose orally, every 12 hours, advancing to every 8 hours at 2 weeks of age if more than 30 weeks of gestation at birth or at 4 weeks of age if less than 30 weeks of gestation at birth.

Box 26.1 EFFECT OF PREGNANCY ON DRUG DISPOSITION

Components of Drug Disposition

Absorption

- Decrease in intestinal motility resulting in increased gastric emptying

- Reduced gastric acid secretion with gastric pH increase affecting absorption of weak acids and bases

- Nausea and vomiting

Distribution

- Total body water increases

- Protein binding to albumin and α_1 acid glycoprotein decreases

Metabolism

- Induction of hepatic metabolic pathways

- Estrogen and progesterone may compete for metabolic binding sites

Excretion

- Increased clearance of drugs eliminated by renal clearance

TRANSPLACENTAL TRANSFER OF ANTIRETROVIRAL DRUGS

The placenta functions to transfer nutrients and oxygen to the fetus and assist in the removal of waste products (Syme, 2004). In general, nucleoside reverse transcriptase inhibitors (NRTIs), non-nucleoside reverse transcriptase inhibitors (NNRTIs), and integrase inhibitors readily cross the placenta. Protease inhibitors, such as lopinavir/ritonavir, are highly protein bound; therefore, only the small percentage of drug that is unbound is free to transfer (US Department of Health and Human Services (DHHS), 2016).

BASIC PRINCIPLES OF USE OF ANTIRETROVIRALS IN PREGNANCY

- Antiretrovirals should be initiated in *all* HIV-infected pregnant women regardless of CD4+ cell count or HIV-1 viral load.

- The regimen should have good efficacy and should be safe and well tolerated.

- The regimen should have one or more NRTIs with good placental passage.

- The provider should consider multiple factors when selecting a regimen, including baseline ARV resistance (determined by HIV genotype and treatment history), comorbidities, convenience, adverse effects, drug interactions, pharmacokinetics, and experience in pregnancy.

- Women entering pregnancy on ARVs should continue on their regimen if it is effective, well tolerated, and does not contain agents that are teratogenic.

RECOMMENDATIONS

ARV-NAIVE PATIENTS

All HIV-infected women should receive a potent ARV regimen to reduce the risk of perinatal transmission. Table 26.2

Table 26.2 RECOMMENDATIONS FOR USE OF ANTIRETROVIRAL DRUGS IN PREGNANT WOMEN

DRUG	COMMENT
	Preferred Regimens

Regimens with clinical trial data in adults demonstrating optimal efficacy and durability with acceptable toxicity and ease of use, PK data available in pregnancy, and no evidence to date of teratogenic effects or established adverse outcomes for mother/fetus/newborn. To minimize the risk of resistance, a PI regimen is preferred for women who may stop ART during the postpartum period.

Preferred Two-NRTI backbone Regimens

DRUG	COMMENT
ABC/3TC	Available as FDC. Can be administered once daily. ABC *should not be used* in patients who test positive for HLA-B*5701 because of the risk of hypersensitivity reaction. ABC/3TC with ATV/r or with EFV is not recommended if pretreatment HIV RNA >100,000 copies/ml.
TDF/FTC or 3TC	TDF/FTC available as FDC. Either TDF/FTC or TDF and 3TC can be administered once daily. TDF has potential renal toxicity; thus, TDF-based dual NRTI combinations should be used with caution in patients with renal insufficiency.
ZDV/3TC	Available as FDC. NRTI combination with most experience for use in pregnancy but has disadvantages of requirement for twice-daily administration and increased potential for hematologic toxicity.

Preferred PI Regimens

DRUG	COMMENT
ATV/r + a preferred two-NRTI backbone	Once-daily administration. Extensive experience in pregnancy. Maternal hyperbilirubinemia.
DRV/r + a preferred two-NRTI backbone	Better tolerated than LPV/r. PK data available. Increasing experience with use in pregnancy. Must be used twice daily in pregnancy.

Preferred NNRTI Regimen

DRUG	COMMENT
EFV + a preferred two-NRTI backbone *Note*: May be initiated after the first 8 weeks of pregnancy	Concern because of birth defects seen in primate study; risk in humans is unclear. Postpartum contraception must be ensured. Preferred regimen in women who require coadministration of drugs with significant interactions with PIs or the convenience of co-formulated, single-tablet, once-daily regimen.

Preferred Integrase Inhibitor Regimen

DRUG	COMMENT
RAL plus a preferred two-NRTI backbone	PK data available and increasing experience in pregnancy. Rapid viral load reduction. Useful when drug interactions with PI regimens are a concern. Twice-daily dosing required.
	Alternate Regimens

Regimens with clinical trial data demonstrating efficacy in adults but one or more of the following apply: Experience in pregnancy is limited; data are lacking or incomplete on teratogenicity; or regimen is associated with dosing, formulation, toxicity, or interaction issue.

PI Regimen

DRUG	COMMENT
LPV/r + a preferred two-NRTI backbone	Abundant experience and established PK in pregnancy. More nausea than preferred agents. Twice-daily administration. Once-daily LPV/r is not recommended for use in pregnant women.

NNRTI Regimen

DRUG	COMMENT
RPV/TDF/FTC (or RPV plus a preferred two-NRTI backbone)	RPV not recommended with pretreatment HIV RNA >100,000 copies/ml or CD4$^+$ cell count<200 cells/mm^3. Do not use with PPIs. PK data available in pregnancy but relatively little experience with use in pregnancy. Available in co-formulated single-pill, once-daily regimen.

Insufficient Data in Pregnancy to Recommend Routine Use in ART-Naive Women

Drugs that are approved for use in adults but lack adequate pregnancy-specific PK or safety data

DRUG	COMMENT
DTG	No data on use of DTG in pregnancy.
EVG/COBI/TDF/ FTC fixed drug combination	No data on use of EVG/COBI component in pregnancy.
FPV	Limited data on use in pregnancy.
MVC	MVC requires tropism testing before use. Few case reports of use in pregnancy.

Table 26.2 CONTINUED

DRUG	COMMENT
COBI	No data on use of COBI (including co-formulations with ATV or DRV) in pregnancy.

Not Recommended

Drugs whose use is not recommended because of toxicity, lower rate of viral suppression, or because not recommended in ART-naive populations

ABC/3TC/ZDV	Generally not recommended due to inferior virologic efficacy.
D4T	Not recommended due to toxicity.
DDI	Not recommended due to toxicity.
IDV/r	Nephrolithiasis, maternal hyperbilirubinemia.
NFV	Lower rate of viral suppression with NFV compared to LPV/r or EFV in adult trials.
RTV	RTV as a single PI is not recommended because of inferior efficacy and increased toxicity.
SQV/r	Not recommended based on potential toxicity and dosing disadvantages. Baseline ECG is recommended before initiation of SQV/r because of potential PR and QT prolongation; contraindicated with pre-existing cardiac conduction system disease. Limited data in pregnancy. Large pill burden. Twice-daily dosing required.
ETR	Not recommended in ART-naive populations.
T20	Not recommended in ART-naive populations.
TPV	Not recommended in ART-naive populations.

3TC, lamivudine; ABC, abacavir; ART, antiretroviral therapy; ARV, antiretroviral; ATV/r, atazanavir/ritonavir; CD4⁺, CD4⁺ T lymphocyte; COBI, cobicistat; d4T, stavudine; ddI, didanosine; DTG, dolutegravir; DRV/r, darunavir/ritonavir; ECG, electrocardiogram; EFV, efavirenz; ETR, etravirine; EVG, elvitegravir; FDC, fixed drug combination; FPV/r, fosamprenavir/ritonavir; FTC, emtricitabine; HSR, hypersensitivity reaction; IDV/r, indinavir/ritonavir; LPV/r, lopinavir/ritonavir; MVC, maraviroc; NFV, nelfinavir; NRTI, nucleoside reverse transcriptase inhibitor; NNRTI, non-nucleoside reverse transcriptase inhibitor; NVP, nevirapine; PI, protease inhibitor; PK, pharmacokinetic; RAL, raltegravir; RPV, rilpivirine; RTV, ritonavir; SQV/r, saquinavir/ritonavir; T20, enfuvirtide; TDF, tenofovir disoproxil fumarate; TPV, tipranavir; ZDV, zidovudine.

SOURCE: Adapted from the US Department of Health and Human Services, Panel on Treatment of HIV-Infected Pregnant Women and Prevention of Perinatal Transmission. Recommendations for use of antiretroviral drugs in pregnant HIV-1-infected women for maternal health and interventions to reduce perinatal HIV transmission in the United States. August 6, 2015. Available at https://aidsinfo.nih.gov/contentfiles/PerinatalGL.pdf. Accessed January 4, 2016.

lists the updated current DHHS preferred and alternate regimens for women who have never received ART and are pregnant. There is also a section on drug regimens that are no longer recommended and the rationale for the discontinuation of their use.

HIV-INFECTED PREGNANT WOMEN ON ANTIRETROVIRAL THERAPY

HIV-infected pregnant women who present for care in the first trimester should be counseled about the risks and benefits of ART. If possible, they should be maintained on their current ART regimen because discontinuations may lead to the loss of virologic control. This could adversely affect the health of the fetus, including HIV infection. In a prospective cohort of 937 mother–infant pairs, interruption of ART during the first and third trimesters was independently associated with MTCT of HIV. The overall rate of MTCT for all mother–infant pairs in the cohort was 1.3%, whereas the rates associated with first- and third-trimester interruptions of ART were 4.9% and 18.2%, respectively (Galli, 2009).

In the past, there has been concern regarding the teratogenic effects of efavirenz use in the first trimester of pregnancy. Preclinical primate data and retrospective reports raised concern about an increased risk of neural tube defects with efavirenz use in pregnancy. It is important to note that the neural tube closes at 36–39 days after the last menstrual period. Thus, the risk of neural tube defects is restricted to the first 5 or 6 weeks of pregnancy. Finally, a meta-analysis that included data on 1437 first-trimester efavirenz exposures showed no overall increased risk of birth defects compared to the risk for women on other ARV drugs. There was one neural tube defect, giving an incidence of 0.07% (Ford, 2011). The Panel on Treatment of HIV-Infected Pregnant Women and Prevention of Perinatal Transmission has recently changed its recommendation, noting that efavirenz can be continued in pregnant women who present for antenatal care in the first trimester, but are at least 8 weeks after conception, if they have achieved virologic suppression (DHHS, 2016).

HIV-INFECTED PREGNANT WOMEN WITH DETECTABLE VIREMIA

Raltegravir has been suggested for use in late pregnancy in women who have high viral loads because of its ability to rapidly suppress viral load (~2-log copies/ml decrease by week 2 of therapy). Two recent case series have reported the effect of adding raltegravir to ART regimens. In one case series, four women diagnosed with HIV infection in the third trimester experienced a mean viral load decline per week of 1.12 log after raltegravir was added to a standard ART regimen. In the second publication, raltegravir was either initiated as part of a combination ARV regimen in nine ARV-naive women or added to an existing ARV regimen in five women who conceived on ART but had persistent viremia. Raltegravir was initiated at a gestational age of 34 weeks or later. The median exposure time to raltegravir was 17 days, and the mean viral load decline was 2.6 log. Although no raltegravir-related side effects were noted in these reports, marked elevations in hepatic transaminases were reported in a single HIV-infected pregnant woman when raltegravir was added to an ART regimen. Because the efficacy and safety of this approach have only been described in anecdotal reports, it cannot be routinely recommended at this time for women who are ARV-naive (DHHS, 2016).

INTRAPARTUM ZIDOVUDINE DURING LABOR

HIV-infected women with HIV-1 RNA >1000 copies/ml or an unknown viral load near delivery should receive intravenous ZDV (DHHS, 2016). In the past, all HIV-infected women were given intravenous ZDV during pregnancy, regardless of viral load, because this was part of the PACTG 076 protocol noted previously (see Table 26.1).

The French Perinatal Cohort evaluated perinatal transmission in more than 11,000 HIV-infected pregnant women receiving ARV. Among women with HIV RNA <1000 copies/ml at delivery, zero transmissions occurred among 369 women who did not receive intravenous ZDV compared to 0.6% of those who received intravenous ZDV. Among women with HIV-1 RNA >1000 copies/ml, the risk of transmission was increased without intravenous ZDV (10.2%) compared to that with intravenous ZDV (2.5%) (Briand, 2013).

ANTIRETROVIRAL PREGNANCY REGISTRY

Established in 1989, the Antiretroviral Pregnancy Registry (APR) collects data on HIV-infected pregnant women taking ARVs with the goal of detecting any major teratogenic effects. Registration is voluntary and confidential; however, providers are strongly encouraged to enroll pregnant patients in the registry at the time of the initial evaluation of the pregnant woman. The study is an observational, exposure-registration and follow-up study. The APR is an international registry that has received reports from 67 countries, with the reports predominantly coming from the United States. More information can be obtained by visiting the registry website at www.apregistry.com.

References

Briand N, Warszawski J, Mandelbrot L, et al. Is intrapartum intravenous zidovudine for prevention of mother-to-child HIV-1 transmission still useful in the combination antiretroviral therapy era? *Clin Infect Dis.* 2013; 57(6):903–914.

Connor EM, Sperling RS, Gelber R, et al. Reduction of maternal-infant transmission of human immunodeficiency virus type 1 with zidovudine treatment. *N Engl J Med.* 1994; 331(18):1173–1180.

Cooper ER, Charurat M, Mofenson L, et al. Women and Infants' Transmission Study Group. *J AIDS.* 2002; 29(5):489–494.

Ford N, Calmy A, Mofenson L. Safety of efavirenz in the first trimester of pregnancy: An updated systematic review and meta-analysis. *AIDS.* 2011; 25(18):2301–2304.

Galli L, Puliti D, Chiappini E, et al. Is the interruption of antiretroviral treatment during pregnancy an additional major risk factor for mother-to-child transmission of HIV type 1? *Clin Infect Dis.* 2009; 48:1310–1317.

Mirochnick M, Capparelli E. Pharmacokinetics of antiretrovirals in pregnant women. *Clin Pharmacokinet.* 2004; 43(15):1071–1087.

Syme MR, Paxton JW, Keelan JA. Drug transfer and metabolism by the human placenta. *Clin Pharmacokinet.* 2004; 43(8):487–514.

US Department of Health and Human Services, Panel on Treatment of HIV-Infected Pregnant Women and Prevention of Perinatal Transmission. Recommendations for use of antiretroviral drugs in pregnant HIV-1-infected women for maternal United States. August 6, 2015. Available at https://aidsinfo.nih.gov/contentfiles/PerinatalGL.pdf. Accessed January 4, 2016.

27.

ANTIRETROVIRAL THERAPY IN CHILDREN AND NEWBORNS

Karin Nielsen-Saines

LEARNING OBJECTIVES

- Discuss advances in antiretroviral therapy for the prevention of mother-to child HIV transmission, particularly for post-exposure infant prophylaxis.

- Review pediatric-specific issues of early HIV diagnosis, timing and pathogenesis of HIV disease, and use of surrogate markers of HIV infection in this population.

- Discuss current guidelines for management of antiretrovirals in children within the context of what drugs to use, when to start them, and when to change antiretroviral therapy.

WHAT'S NEW?

- The US Department of Health and Human Services' (DHHS) antiretroviral treatment guidelines for children have been updated and now recommend that definitive exclusion or confirmation of HIV infection in children between the ages of 18 and 24 months who are HIV antibody-positive should be based on a nucleic acid test rather than on maternal antibody results because there could be residual maternal antibody in this age group.

- Early diagnosis of HIV infection in the United States was largely made through the use of DNA polymerase chain reaction (PCR) testing via the Amplicor HIV-1 DNA test, which is no longer commercially available. It is important to note that the sensitivity and specificity of noncommercial HIV-1 DNA tests that are currently being used may differ from the sensitivity and specificity of the previously US Food and Drug Administration (FDA)-approved Amplicor HIV-1 DNA test.

- Studies have continued to demonstrate a significant benefit of early antiretroviral treatment for infants younger than 12 months of age in the prevention of HIV mortality and morbidity. Treatment is recommended for all HIV-infected infants in this age group in all geographic settings, regardless of clinical findings, CD4$^+$ T cell counts, or virus load. The updated recommendation is that treatment of infants younger than 12 months of age who are diagnosed with HIV should be expedited and characterizes an urgent situation.

- Infant post-exposure prophylaxis with two or three antiretroviral agents initiated within 48 hours of life is preferred to standard zidovudine prophylaxis in situations in which mothers did not receive antiretrovirals during pregnancy until the time of labor and delivery. This strategy has been shown to further reduce the risk of intrapartum HIV acquisition in non-breast-feeding populations.

- Existing pharmacokinetic and safety data for HIV-infected preterm infants and term infants younger than 15 days of age are insufficient for the recommendation of a complete combination antiretroviral therapy (cART) regimen for this age group. DHHS guidelines recommend that neonatal care providers who are considering a three-drug antiretroviral (ARV) treatment regimen for term infants younger than 2 weeks or premature infants contact a pediatric HIV expert for guidance and individual case assessment of the risk:benefit ratio of treatment and for the latest information on neonatal drug doses. The National Perinatal HIV Hotline (1-888-448-8765) provides free clinical consultation on perinatal HIV care.

- World Health Organization (WHO) guidelines for resource-limited settings recommend cART for all pregnant women with HIV infection, regardless of CD4$^+$ T cell count or virus load, throughout pregnancy and for the duration of breast-feeding (WHO Option B). Many clinics have instituted cART for life for all women who are pregnant and living with HIV (WHO Option B+).

- Initial combination therapy for ART-naive children includes the use of integrase strand transfer inhibitor-based regimens as agents to be used in combination with two nucleoside analogue reverse transcriptase inhibitors (NRTIs). Raltegravir can be used in children aged 2 years or older and dolutegravir in children aged 12 years or older. Raltegravir is also licensed for infants as young as 4 weeks of age. The protease inhibitor (PI) atazanavir boosted with ritonavir is now considered an alternative PI in children aged 3 months through 5 years and remains a preferred drug for children aged 6 years or older. The two-NRTI combination of zidovudine and lamivudine or emtricitabine is now considered an alternative combination for adolescents older than age 13 years.

- Despite initial reports of a "functional" cure in an HIV-infected infant treated very early on with aggressive cART (the "Mississippi baby"), subsequent reports demonstrated that this approach has not been able to eradicate HIV but does appear to significantly limit seeding of viral reservoirs. The term "functional cure" has been replaced by the concept of HIV remission. Studies are underway to determine the extent and duration of HIV remission following prompt initiation of cART in HIV-infected infants who are treated soon after birth (i.e., during the acute infection process).

KEY POINTS

- HIV-infected infants and children have a different, more progressive disease course compared to adults given that early infection leads to sustained, high-magnitude viremia with significant seeding of reservoirs in the first months of life, prior to full maturation of the immune system.

- Early diagnosis of HIV infection is pivotal in the management of infants and the prevention of HIV-associated morbidity and mortality.

- The availability of potent pediatric antiretroviral formulations encompassing different classes of drugs for infected infants and young children is limited, and these need further development.

- Significant advancements have been achieved in the area of infant post-exposure prophylaxis, with new recommendations for in high-risk scenarios.

- Early antiretroviral treatment is still the mainstay for pediatric HIV infection, particularly for infants younger than 12 months of age, but it is also highly recommended for older children.

- Early treatment of young infants diagnosed soon after birth appears to be the best approach to reducing the seeding of viral reservoirs and potentially attaining prolonged periods of HIV remission off antiretrovirals—a strategy that is being evaluated in prospective clinical trials.

In the absence of interventions to curtail mother-to-child HIV-1 transmission, HIV-1 infection in children parallels that of women of childbearing age. Perinatal transmission of HIV-1 accounts for nearly all worldwide cases of pediatric HIV-1 infection today, with the exception of adolescent acquisition of HIV-1 via adult risk behaviors. HIV-1 transmission from mother to child occurs in 25–30% of cases when there is no maternal antiretroviral treatment (Newell, 1991; Scott, 1989), and if breast-feeding until 12 months of age is included, transmission risk can be as high as 40%. Infection may be transmitted during pregnancy, at the time of labor and delivery, and via breast-feeding. Worldwide, approximately 2000 HIV-infected infants are born daily, with 90% of cases occurring in sub-Saharan Africa (Marston, 2011). Breast-feeding transmission contributes another 300,000 infant infections per year (Marston, 2011). Although cART can reduce mother-to-child transmission to less than 1% in developed countries (Dorenbaum, 2002), failure to recognize HIV-1 infection in women and/or unavailability of treatment still contribute to continuing mother-to-child HIV transmission worldwide. Management of HIV-1 infection in children must consider the following factors: early diagnosis of infection, the natural history of HIV-1 infection in children and surrogate markers of disease, suitable pediatric drug formulations for children, drug metabolism and pharmacokinetics of antiretrovirals in children, and the general paucity of pediatric treatment data compared to data for adults.

DIAGNOSIS

Early diagnosis of HIV-1 infection is crucial for identification of at-risk infants and consequent initiation of treatment. All HIV-1-exposed infants carry maternal HIV-1 antibodies until approximately 15–18 months of age. Thus, early pediatric diagnosis relies on identification of the virus usually via HIV-1 DNA or RNA PCR techniques. The former measures integrated virus in the host genome, and the latter measures circulating plasma virus. Although it is also a reliable diagnostic method, HIV-1 co-culture is not routinely performed due to its high cost and time requirement. Infants infected in utero usually have positive PCR results within the first 48 hours of birth, whereas infants infected at the time of labor and delivery may have a negative HIV DNA or RNA PCR result at birth, followed by a positive result 1 week to 2 months following birth (Bryson, 1992). Breast-fed infants have continuing HIV-1 exposure and thus can develop a positive HIV DNA or RNA PCR result at any time. The risk of breast-feeding transmission by an HIV-1-positive mother is approximately 16% (Fowler, 2002). Therefore, repeat PCR testing in the first few months of life is critical for determination of the timing of infection, with sensitivity of a PCR result reaching 96% by 4 weeks of life in the absence of breast-feeding (Dunn, 1992; Nielsen, 2000).

TIMING OF INFECTION

The timing of HIV-1 infection (in utero vs. intrapartum) is somewhat predictive of the patient's subsequent clinical course (Dickover, 1994). Early onset of AIDS-defining conditions is more frequently observed in in utero-infected infants who sustain early, prolonged elevated HIV RNA levels (Figure 27.1).

As in adults, prolonged periods of elevated HIV RNA levels are predictive of disease progression. HIV-1-infected infants undergo primary infection, either in utero or soon after birth. Therefore, they tend to have very elevated virus loads in the first months of life (Figure 27.2).

EARLY TREATMENT INITIATION AND HIV REMISSION IN HIV-EXPOSED INFANTS

cART for infants and children suppresses viremia, reduces the high infant mortality rate, and improves clinical outcome; however, children must continue antiretroviral treatment lifelong. The major barrier to achieving HIV remission in children, as in adults, is the early establishment of long-lived latent cellular reservoirs in CD4+ T cells and other sites, with continued low-level replication and rebound viremia once taken off ART (Persaud, 2012). It is postulated that by treatment of very early HIV infection, the establishment, quantity, or even elimination of latent reservoirs could be achieved by reducing viral spread into memory CD4+ T cell reservoirs. This would potentially allow patients to thrive off of ART without viral rebound, as evidenced by the "Mississippi baby," who remained in ARV-free viral remission for 27 months post early cART (Luzuriaga, 2015; Persaud, 2013; Siliciano, 2014). Importantly, there are emerging data that very early therapy during acute HIV infection in both adults and children quantitatively modifies HIV persistence and may influence the rate of reservoir decay. This approach is being evaluated in ongoing clinical trials.

DISEASE COURSE

The natural history of pediatric HIV-1 infection is bimodal (Scott, 1991). Studies conducted in developed countries prior to the availability of antiretrovirals demonstrated that approximately 20% of children exhibit very rapid disease progression with rapid decline in CD4+ cell counts and

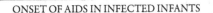

ONSET OF AIDS IN INFECTED INFANTS

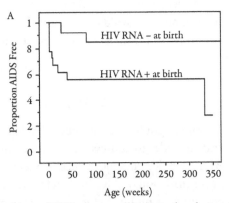
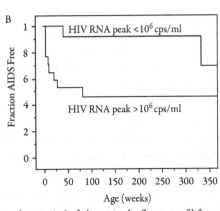

Figure 27.1 In utero acquisition of HIV infection and sustained peak viremia >10^6 copies/ml of plasma in the first year of life are predictive of HIV disease progression. SOURCE: Adapted from Dickover, 1996.

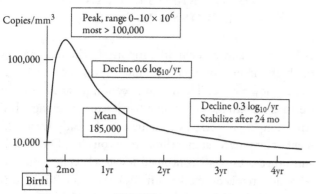

Dynamics of HIV-RNA in Infants

Peak, range $0-10 \times 10^6$ most > 100,000

Decline $0.6 \log_{10}/yr$

Decline $0.3 \log_{10}/yr$ Stabilize after 24 mo

Mean 185,000

Copies/mm³

100,000

10,000

2mo · 1yr · 2yr · 3yr · 4yr

Birth

Figure 27.2 Natural course of HIV RNA viremia in children. SOURCE: Adapted from Palumbo, 1998.

development of AIDS-defining conditions before 2 years of age (Nielsen, 1997). However, the majority of HIV-infected children (~60–65%) will have intermediate disease progression, with the presence of AIDS-defining events by age 7 or 8 years. Similar to adults, there is a small subset of children (~15–20% of patients) who have very slow or no disease progression by age 8 years, and there is an even smaller set of elite controllers (<5%). These children enter adolescence with minimal or no symptoms of HIV disease. Studies conducted in Africa have demonstrated an even faster pace of disease progression, with the majority of pediatric patients having AIDS-defining conditions by age 5 years (Newell, 2004). This might be due to the higher overall burden of disease and the presence of multiple co-infections. cART makes it possible to alter the natural history of HIV disease and transform disease progressors into nonprogressors. This results in improvement in the quality of life and reductions in HIV-associated disease morbidity and mortality.

SURROGATE MARKERS OF DISEASE

The goal of ART is to reduce the HIV-1 virus load as much as possible while restoring or preserving the immune function. Virus load is generally measured via plasma HIV-1 RNA reverse transcriptase PCR (Roche Molecular Systems), HIV RNA quantitation by branched (b) DNA (Chiron Corporation), or nucleic acid sequence-based amplification HIV-1 RNA quantitative assay (Organon Teknika). All three methods reliably measure free virus in plasma, with new-generation assays being able to identify virus isolates of different subtypes. Immune function in HIV disease is measured primarily by evaluating T cell subsets, particularly CD4+ cell absolute numbers and percentiles. Three-color

flow cytometry is generally the methodology employed for this purpose. Declining counts parallel disease progression, with declines in CD4+ cells usually following peak HIV RNA viremia. One important caveat in the management of HIV-infected children is that CD4+ cell numbers, particularly in infants, differ significantly from those of adults and do not achieve similar levels until after age 5 years. Therefore, an infant with a CD4+ cell count of 750 cells/mm³ or less is at significant risk for development of AIDS-defining conditions because normal values are generally in the range of 2000 cells/mm³.

ANTIRETROVIRAL THERAPY IN CHILDREN

One general principle in the use of ART is that continued viral replication in the presence of ARV drugs promotes development of drug resistance. Resistance to one specific ARV agent may in turn confer resistance to other drugs within the same class. Current standard of practice is that once therapy is started, long-term or lifelong treatment is warranted. In children, the efficacy of ART is often extrapolated from data obtained from adult clinical trials because of a lack of pediatric data. However, there are significant age-related differences between children and adults. These encompass body composition, renal excretion, liver metabolism, and gastrointestinal function. This leads to differences in drug distribution and metabolism, drug clearance, drug dosing, and toxicities between children and adults. In addition, protein binding and drug clearance of some specific ARVs may differ by race due to the presence of genetic polymorphisms. Nevertheless, often, therapeutic doses for infants and children are not available. Liquid or palatable formulations for children do not exist for many ARVs, and adherence depends on adult caretakers. It is crucial when initiating ARV therapy to take into consideration the presence of comorbidities and concomitant medications in order to avoid overlapping drug toxicities. It is also important to consider cross-resistance and later therapeutic options.

GUIDELINES

Treatment guidelines have been developed throughout the years in order to address critical concerns about the use of ART in children. Major concerns include the optimal timing of initiation of ART, the preferred choice of ARVs, the best ways to monitor efficacy and toxicities, and when to change therapy. There are variations in guidelines between developed and developing countries. In the United States, traditionally most children have been treated when identified as having HIV-1 infection, regardless of symptomatology. Given multiple therapeutic options and the general availability of virus load monitoring, guidelines in developed countries have relied on virus load measures for predicting early switches in therapy (DHHS, 2011, 2015). Randomized clinical trials such as the Cher trial in South Africa have demonstrated that early ARV treatment to infants diagnosed before 12 months of age is clearly beneficial in reducing morbidity and mortality (Violari, 2008). Current US pediatric ARV treatment guidelines recommend treatment of all infants younger than age 12 months, regardless of clinical findings, virus load, or CD4+ cell subsets (DHHS, 2015). For children between the ages of 1 and 5 years, guidelines recommend treatment initiation for those with AIDS or significant HIV-related symptoms, those with virus load >100,000 copies/ml of plasma, or those with a CD4+ cell percentage <25%. Treatment should be considered in this age group for children who are asymptomatic or who have a CD4+ percentage >25% or virus load <100,000 copies/ml plasma. Likewise, in children older than age 5 years, DHHS guidelines recommend treatment of all those with significant HIV-related symptoms, CD4+ cell count <500 cells/ mm³, or virus load >100,000 copies/ ml. For children who do not fulfill these criteria, guidelines recommend that treatment be considered. WHO treatment guidelines, however, recommend treatment for all children younger than age 12 months, regardless of clinical findings, and otherwise for children who have WHO clinical stage 3 or 4 (i.e., more symptomatic patients). WHO guidelines also use T cell subset measures as the main laboratory surrogate markers of disease (when available), as opposed to virus load measures for dictating initiation or switches in ART (Violari, 2008). Regardless of the specific guidelines in use, however, the decision to initiate therapy is based on disease severity and the risk of disease progression.

ANTIRETROVIRALS TO THE HIV-EXPOSED INFANT

The provision of antiretrovirals to infants born to HIV-infected mothers as prophylaxis has been standard of care in the Unites States since 1994, when results of Pediatric AIDS Clinical Trials Group study 076 were published (Connor, 1994). The study demonstrated that zidovudine to the mother started at 16 weeks of gestation, accompanied by an intravenous zidovudine infusion during labor and delivery followed by four-times daily dosing of zidovudine to the infant from birth to 6 weeks of age, was highly efficacious in preventing mother-to-child HIV transmission compared to placebo (8% vs. 25%, respectively; $p < 0.001$). In the developed country setting, 4–6 weeks of zidovudine (ZDV) to the infant initiated at birth, given at 2 mg/kg per dose four times a day or 4 mg/kg/dose twice a day, is standard of care (DHHS, 2015). The major toxicities of ZDV infant prophylaxis include anemia and neutropenia; however, these are dose-dependent and self-limiting, tend to occur toward the end of the course of treatment, and rarely require interruption of prophylaxis (Lahoz, 2010). In resource-limited settings, single-dose nevirapine to the infant (2 mg/kg) soon after birth is standard of care, and it has been implemented in multiple studies following publication of HIVNET 012 (Guay, 1999), which documented the efficacy of this approach in reducing mother-to-child transmission when associated with single-dose nevirapine to the mother at the time of labor. Among HIV-infected infants whose mothers were not treated with antiretrovirals throughout the course of pregnancy and are therefore at higher risk of HIV acquisition, double antiretroviral prophylaxis initiated within 48 hours of birth with three doses of nevirapine in the first week of life concurrently with 6 weeks of ZDV has been shown to be more efficacious for the prevention of HIV intrapartum infection than ZDV alone (Nielsen-Saines, 2011). An alternative regimen equally efficacious is the use of lamivudine and nelfinavir in the first 2 weeks of life concurrent with 6 weeks of ZDV (Nielsen-Saines, 2011). Due to the lack of availability of pediatric formulations of nelfinavir, however, the nevirapine/ZDV combination is preferable and therefore recommended (DHHS, 2011). Lopinavir/ritonavir suspension is currently not recommended by the FDA for use in infants younger than 2 weeks of age. In resource-limited settings, the use of daily nevirapine prophylaxis to the HIV-exposed infant for prevention of mother-to-child transmission has been evaluated up to 6 months of age and has been shown to be effective and safe in the prevention of postpartum HIV acquisition (Coovadia, 2012). Currently, however, most settings in sub-Saharan Africa have transitioned to WHO Options B or B+, which recommend treatment with cART to all HIV-infected women during pregnancy and lactation or from pregnancy onward with no further treatment interruption (WHO, 2014).

TIMING OF INITIATION OF THERAPY

Early versus deferred initiation of ARV treatment in HIV-infected children is a controversial matter. Clinical trials are ongoing in order to address this issue. Starting therapy early in asymptomatic children may control viral replication before genetic mutations develop, leading to fewer circulating viral strains. It also may prevent immune system destruction, which would avoid disease progression. With this strategy, viral seeding of latent cells or CD4$^+$ cell reservoirs may be circumvented. On the contrary, deferred treatment could be beneficial because there is no selective pressure for development of drug resistance, and it could also curtail potential toxicities. In addition, this could support greater adherence because patients improve with therapy. This strategy would also delay development of adverse effects from prolonged ARV exposure. Regardless of when therapy is started, the best predictor of treatment efficacy will be patient adherence to the ARV regimen.

CHANGE IN THERAPY

The decision to change antiretrovirals varies slightly according to the pediatric guidelines employed. The variability is mostly due to the surrogate markers used. Nevertheless, most experts agree that indicators of treatment failure include progression of HIV disease, growth failure, development of opportunistic infections while on established therapy, decline in CD4 percentiles, development or worsening of HIV encephalopathy, and significant increases in virus load.

SPECIFIC ANTIRETROVIRALS

Antiretrovirals currently available for use in the United States are listed in Table 27.1. Optimal ARV combinations for children may differ slightly from those of adults. In infants, particularly those younger than age 1 year, there is often a need to use very potent ARV regimens for reduction of persistently elevated virus loads (Luzuriaga, 2004; Palumbo, 2010). Therefore, in this scenario, four drug combinations including a protease inhibitor, two nucleoside analogs, and a non-nucleoside analog such as nevirapine may be indicated. The use of many ARVs is also limited in younger children (especially those younger than age 4 years) because of the lack of liquid formulations, as depicted in Table 27.1. Prevalent highly active antiretroviral therapy (HAART) regimens in pediatrics include one PI drug such as ritonavir/lopinavir, or atazanavir or darunavir (in older children), in combination with a double NRTI backbone, such as ZDV + lamivudine (3TC), stavudine (D4T) + 3TC, ZDV + didanosin (ddI), D4T + abacavir (ABC), ABC + 3TC, or emtricitabine/3TC (in older children). The PIs may be substituted by non-nucleoside reverse transcriptase inhibitors (NNRTI) drugs such as nevirapine

or efavirenz (the latter in older children). In special circumstances, it may be necessary to boost the main PI with additional PIs, such as ritonavir or saquinavir, in order to achieve higher blood concentrations. For instance, when atazanavir is used with tenofovir, additional boosting with 100 mg of ritonavir in the treatment of older children is often warranted. Triple NRTI regimens may have a role in specific case scenarios; however, they constitute less potent ARV regimens. Specific ARV regimens to be avoided include any type of mono- or dual therapy; efavirenz during pregnancy; atazanavir with tenofovir without ritonavir boosting; and combinations of of the following in pregnant patients: ZDV + D4T; zalcitabine (ddC) with 3TC, D4T, or ddI; or D4T and ddI. Clinical trials in the United States are currently evaluating the pharmacokinetics of integrase inhibitors in children, as well as the pharmacokinetics of R-5 receptor blockers. Newer-generation NNRTI drugs, such as etravirine and rilpivirine, have not yet been evaluated in children, nor are there dosing recommendations for multiple antiretrovirals in children younger than age 4 years. In resource-limited settings, treatment studies have demonstrated greater durability of virus load suppression in children treated with ritonavir/lopinavir regimens as opposed

Table 27.1 ANTIRETROVIRALS AVAILABLE FOR PEDIATRIC USE IN THE UNITED STATES

Nucleoside reverse transcriptase inhibitors	Protease inhibitors
Zidovudine (ZDV/AZT)[a]	Saquinavir soft gel
Lamivudine (3TC)[a]	Ritonavir[a]
Didanosine (ddI)[a]	Nelfinavir
Zalcitabine (ddC)	Indinavir
Stavudine (D4T)[a]	Fosamprenavir
Abacavir (ABC)[a]	Lopinavir/ritonavir[a]
Tenofovir (TDF)	Atazanavir
Emtricitabine (FTC)	Tipranavir
	Darunavir
Non-nucleoside reverse transcriptase inhibitors	**Fusion inhibitor**
Nevirapine[a]	Enfuvirtide (T-20)
Efavirenz	
Etravirine	
Rilpivirine	
Combination antiretrovirals[b]	**Other classes**
AZT/3TC	R-5 receptor inhibitor
AZT/3TC/ABC	Maraviroc
TDF/FTC	**Integrase inhibitors**
ABC/3TC	Raltegravir
EFV/TDF/FTC	Dolutegravir
FTC/RIL/TDF	

[a]Pediatric formulations available.

[b]Additional formulations, such as NVP/ZDV/3TC and NVP/D4T/3TC, are available to children in pediatric formulations as generic drugs in resource-limited settings.

to nevirapine-based regimens, although nevirapine has been shown to be associated with improved growth in this population (Chadwick, 2011).

TOXICITIES AND ADVERSE EFFECTS

There are multiple complications and side effects of specific ARVs. The most frequent toxicities of ZDV are hematologic, particularly anemia and neutropenia. These may resolve with dose reduction. All NRTIs may cause some degree of mitochondrial toxicity. ZDV may cause myopathy, and peripheral neuropathy is seen with this drug as well as with ddI, ddC, D4T, and, rarely, 3TC. ddI is associated with pancreatitis. D4T is associated with lipoatrophy and in combination with ddI may induce liver fatty acid syndrome, particularly during pregnancy. Abacavir is known to cause a fatal hypersensitivity reaction, which occurs in 1% of pediatric patients. It presents as flu-like symptoms with or without a rash, abdominal pain, sore throat, and myalgias. If the drug has been interrupted in this scenario, shock will ensue when restarted. The NNRTIs most commonly cause skin rashes (~40%) and have been associated with Steven–Johnsons syndrome. Efavirenz is teratogenic, and central nervous system findings such as dizziness, insomnia, and nightmares have been reported soon after initiation of treatment with this drug. There is some concern about the prolonged use of nevirapine during pregnancy in patients with higher CD4$^+$ cell counts who developed hepatic failure (Hitti, 2004), but there is controversy on the subject because additional studies have failed to demonstrate an association (DeLazzari, 2008).

Protease inhibitors have multiple drug–drug interactions because of their cytochrome P450 metabolism in the liver. Their most common side effects are gastrointestinal symptoms. Hepatitis and hyperbilirubinemia are not uncommon. In adults, they have been shown to induce lipodystrophy, diabetes, and increased atherosclerosis because of lipid abnormalities. These findings are beginning to be recognized in children, although complications occur to a lesser extent. Indinavir may induce renal stones by precipitation of the drug in the kidneys or tubules. There are also recent concerns about the potential for osteopenia and osteoporosis in children, induced either by HAART or by HIV disease (Mora, 2004).

Immune Reconstitution Syndrome

One recognized complication of potent ART is the immune reconstitution syndrome. It is most frequently observed in patients who initiate HAART with lower CD4$^+$ cell counts. It is attributed to a wide range of pathogens, with tuberculosis being a common underlying condition. The pathogenesis appears to be the colonization with opportunistic pathogens when patients have moderate to severe immunosuppression. With the initiation of HAART and subsequent recovery of immunity to the organism, there is a paradoxical clinical deterioration due to a dysregulated immune response. This syndrome usually presents in the first 6 weeks of HAART and may resolve either with the use of steroids or with temporary discontinuation of HAART. It is infrequently seen in pediatric HIV practiced in developed countries, particularly because children are generally treated earlier. However, it is very prevalent in the developing world and may carry high morbidity and mortality.

BENEFITS OF THERAPY

Despite the complications and controversies, the benefits of HAART in children with HIV are overwhelming. In the United States, the annual mortality in pediatric HIV patients decreased to less than 1% in 1999 due to the availability of treatment (Gortmaker, 2001; Jeremy, 2005). HAART decreases the virus load, preserves and restores the immune function, decreases the risk of comorbidities, decreases hospitalizations, improves survival, improves quality of life, and restores hope to children and their families. As illustrated in the clinical cases, some children in treatment are now young adults attending college and preparing for adult life. HAART has also changed the AIDS paradigm. As one patient noted, HIV is no longer a disease you die from but a disease you live with.

References

Bryson YJ, Luzuriaga K, Sullivan JL, et al. Proposed definitions for in utero versus intrapartum transmission of HIV-1. *N Engl J Med.* 1992; 327:1246–1247.

Chadwick EG, Yogev R, Alvero CG, et al.; International Pediatric Adolescent Clinical Trials Group (IMPAACT) P1030 Team. Long-term outcomes for HIV-infected infants less than 6 months of age at initiation of lopinavir/ritonavir combination antiretroviral therapy. *AIDS.* 2011; 25:643–649.

Connor EM, Sperling RS, Gelber R, et al.; Pediatric AIDS Clinical Trials Group Protocol 076 Study Group. Reduction of maternal–infant transmission of human immunodeficiency virus type 1 with zidovudine treatment. *N Engl J Med.* 1994; 331:1173–1180.

Coovadia HM, Brown ER, Fowler MG, et al.; HPTN 046 protocol team. Efficacy and safety of an extended nevirapine regimen in infant children of breastfeeding mothers with HIV-1 infection for prevention of postnatal HIV-1 transmission (HPTN 046): A randomised, double-blind, placebo-controlled trial. *Lancet.* 2012; 379(9812):221–228.

De Lazzari E, León A, Arnaiz JA, et al. Hepatotoxicity of nevirapine in virologically suppressed patients according to gender and CD4$^+$ cell counts. *HIV Med.* 2008; 9:221–226.

Dickover RE, Dillon M, Gillette SG, et al. Rapid increases in load of human immunodeficiency virus correlate with early disease progression and loss of CD4[+] cells in vertically infected infants. *J Infect Dis*. 1994; 170:1279–1284.

Dickover RE, Dillon M, Leung KM, et al. Early prognostic indicators in primary perinatal human immunodeficiency virus type 1 infection: Importance of viral RNA and the timing of transmission on long-term outcome. *J Infect Dis*. 1998; 178:375–387.

Dorenbaum A, Cunningham CK, Gelber RD, et al. Two-dose intrapartum/newborn nevirapine and standard antiretroviral therapy to reduce perinatal HIV transmission: A randomized trial. *JAMA*. 2002; 288:189–198.

Dunn DT, Newell ML, Ades AE, et al. Risk of human immunodeficiency virus type 1 transmission through breastfeeding. *Lancet*.1992; 340:585–588.

Fowler MG, Newell ML. Breastfeeding and HIV-1 transmission in resource-limited settings. *J AIDS*. 2002; 30:230–239.

Gortmaker SL, Hughes M, Cervia J, et al.; Pediatric AIDS Clinical Trials Group Protocol 219 Team. Effect of combination therapy including protease inhibitors on mortality among children and adolescents infected with HIV-1. *N Engl J Med*. 2001; 345(21):1522–1528.

Guay LA, Musoke P, Fleming T, et al. Intrapartum and neonatal single-dose nevirapine compared with zidovudine for prevention of mother-to-child transmission of HIV-1 in Kampala, Uganda: HIVNET 012 randomised trial. *Lancet*. 1999; 354:795–802.

Hitti J, Frenkel LM, Stek AM, et al.; PACTG 1022 Study Team. Maternal toxicity with continuous nevirapine in pregnancy: Results from PACTG 1022. *J Acquir Immune Defic Syndr*. 2004; 36:772–776.

Jeremy RJ, Kim S, Nozyce M, et al.; Pediatric AIDS Clinical Trials Group (PACTG) 338 & 377 Study Teams. Neuropsychological functioning and viral load in stable antiretroviral therapy-experienced HIV-infected children. *Pediatrics*. 2005; 115:380–387.

Lahoz R, Noguera A, Rovira N, et al. Antiretroviral-related hematologic short-term toxicity in healthy infants: Implications of the new neonatal 4-week zidovudine regimen. *Pediatr Infect Dis J*. 2010; 29:376–379.

Luzuriaga K, Gay H, Ziemniak C, et al. Viremic relapse after HIV-1 remission in a perinatally infected child. *N Engl J Med*. 2015; 372:786–788.

Luzuriaga K, McManus M, Mofenson L, et al.; PACTG 356 Investigators. A trial of three antiretroviral regimens in HIV-1-infected children. *N Engl J Med*. 2004; 350(24):2471–2480.

Marston M, Becquet R, Zaba B, et al. Net survival of perinatally and postnatally HIV-infected children: A pooled analysis of individual data from sub-Saharan Africa. *Int J Epidemiol*. 2011; 40:385–396.

Mora S, Zamproni I, Beccio S, et al. Longitudinal changes of bone mineral density and metabolism in antiretroviral-treated human immunodeficiency virus-infected children. *J Clin Endocrinol Metab*. 2004; 89:24–28.

Newell ML. The natural history of vertically acquired HIV infection: The European Collaborative Study. *J Perinat Med*. 1991; 19(Suppl 1):257–262.

Newell ML, Coovadia H, Cortina-Borja M, et al.; Ghent International AIDS Society (IAS) Working Group on HIV Infection in Women and Children. Mortality of infected and uninfected infants born to HIV-infected mothers in Africa: A pooled analysis. *Lancet*. 2004; 364:1236–1243.

Nielsen K, Bryson YJ. Diagnosis of HIV infection in children. *Pediatr Clin North Am*. 2000; 47:39–63.

Nielsen K, McSherry G, Petru A, et al. A descriptive survey of pediatric human immunodeficiency virus-infected long term survivors. *Pediatrics*. 1997; 99:pe4.

Nielsen-Saines K, Watts DH, Veloso VG, et al; for the NICHD HPTN 040/ PACTG 1043 Protocol Team. Phase III randomized trial of the safety and efficacy of three neonatal antiretroviral regimens for prevention of intrapartum HIV-1 transmission (NICHD HPTN 040/ PACTG 1043). Late Breaker Abstract 124LB. Paper presented at the 18th Conference on Retroviruses and Opportunistic Infections, Boston, MA, February 27–March 2, 2011.

Palumbo P, Lindsey JC, Hughes MD, et al. Antiretroviral treatment for children with peripartum nevirapine exposure. *N Engl J Med*. 2010; 363:1510–1520.

Palumbo PE, Raskino C, Fiscus S, et al. Predictive value of quantitative plasma HIV RNA and CD4[+] lymphocyte count in HIV-infected infants and children. *JAMA*. 1998; 279:756–761.

Persaud D, Gay G, Ziemniak C, et al. Absence of detectable HIV-1 viremia after treatment cessation in an infant. *N Engl J Med*. 2013; 369:1828–1835.

Persaud D, Palumbo PE, Ziemniak C, et al. Dynamics of the resting CD4[+] T cell latent HIV reservoir in infants initiating highly active antiretroviral therapy less than six months of age. *AIDS*. 2012 Jul 31; 26(12):1483–1490.

Scott GB. HIV infection in children: Clinical features and management. *J Acquir Immune Defic Syndr*. 1991; 4:109–115.

Scott GB, Hutto C, Makuch RW, et al. Survival in children with perinatally acquired human immunodeficiency virus type 1 infection. *N Engl J Med*. 1989; 321:1791–1796.

Siliciano JD, Siliciano RF. Recent developments in the search for a cure for HIV-1 infections: Targeting the latent reservoir for HIV-1. *J Allergy Clin Immunol*. 2014 Jul; 134:12–19.

US Department of Health and Human Services, Panel on Antiretroviral Therapy and Medical Management of HIV-Infected Children. Guidelines for the use of antiretroviral agents in pediatric HIV infection. August 11, 2011. Available at https://aidsinfo.nih.gov/content-files/lvguidelines/pediatricguidelines.pdf. Accessed March 25, 2011.

US Department of Health and Human Services, Panel on Antiretroviral Therapy and Medical Management of HIV-Infected Children. Guidelines for the use of antiretroviral agents in pediatric HIV infection. March 5, 2015. Available at https://aidsinfo.nih.gov/ guidelines/html/2/pediatric-arv-guidelines/45/whats-new-in-the-guidelines. Accessed December 23, 2015.

Violari A, Cotton MF, Gibb DM, et al.; CHER Study Team. Early antiretroviral therapy and mortality among HIV-infected infants. *N Engl J Med*. 2008; 359:2233–2244.

World Health Organization. March 2014 supplement to the 2013 consolidated guidelines on the use of antiretroviral drugs for treating and preventing HIV infection recommendations for a public health approach. March 2014. Available at http://apps.who.int/ iris/bitstream/10665/104264/1/9789241506830_eng.pdf?ua=1. Accessed December 29, 2015.

28.

IMMUNOSUPPRESSANTS AND ANTIRETROVIRAL THERAPY IN HIV-POSITIVE TRANSPLANT PATIENTS

Carolyn Kramer and Emily Blumberg

LEARNING OBJECTIVE

Explain how to assess and manage key drug-drug interactions between immunosuppressive agents and antiretroviral therapy in HIV-positive organ transplant recipients.

WHAT'S NEW?

With the increase in number of available integrase inhibitors, clinicians and patients can more frequently choose an antiretroviral regimen that minimizes the risk of drug–drug interactions with immunosuppressive agents. Dolutegravir in particular provides an option that minimizes drug interactions while maintaining a high barrier to resistance.

KEY POINTS

- Protease inhibitors (PIs), especially ritonavir, are inhibitors of CYP3A4 and P-gp1, and they can significantly increase levels of calcineurin inhibitors (e.g., tacrolimus or cyclosporine) and mammalian target of rapamycin (mTOR) inhibitors (e.g., sirolimus or everolimus).

- Although data and clinical experience are limited, cobicistat is an inhibitor of CYP3A4, and its effect on levels of calcineurin inhibitors and mTOR inhibitors is likely to be similar to that of ritonavir.

- Many non-nucleoside reverse transcriptase inhibitors (NNRTIs) are inducers of CYP3A4. Efavirenz in particular may result in lower concentrations of calcineurin inhibitors and mTOR inhibitors.

- Dose reduction and careful attention to monitoring drug levels are critical to avoid toxicity and maintain therapeutic immunosuppressive concentrations when PIs or cobicistat are coadministered with calcineurin inhibitors or mTOR inhibitors. If NNRTIs are used, calcineurin inhibitor and mTOR inhibitor doses will need to be increased; careful monitoring is required.

- Nucleoside reverse transcriptase inhibitors (NRTIs) and integrase inhibitors are not metabolized by CYP3A4, nor are they inducers or inhibitors of CYP3A4. These classes are not expected to significantly alter dosing or levels of immunosuppressants.

- Mycophenolate mofetil is not a substrate for CYP3A4 or P-gp1 and has no expected or documented interactions with antiretroviral therapy.

- Although there is no formalized recommendation for the ideal antiretroviral therapy regimen in HIV-positive transplant recipients, a regimen consisting of two NRTIs and an integrase inhibitor minimizes the risk of drug–drug interactions and simplifies dosing of immunosuppressive agents while maintaining a high barrier to resistance.

BACKGROUND

As survival for HIV-positive individuals improves and advances in antiretroviral therapy allow more patients to remain suppressed on more tolerable combination therapies, the focus of HIV care has shifted to management of chronic comorbidities. End-stage renal disease and cirrhosis occur frequently among this population due to shared comorbidities, and solid organ transplant, once considered contraindicated among HIV-positive individuals, has been increasingly successful. Recent data suggest that in the absence of HCV co-infection, HIV-positive liver transplant recipients have a risk of death and graft loss similar to that of uninfected recipients (Sawinski, 2015). Renal transplant data demonstrate comparable patient and graft survival in the absence of HCV co-infection, at least compared with older recipients, and there may be a survival advantage compared with remaining on dialysis (Gathogo, 2014; Kumar, 2008; Landin, 2010; Sawinski, 2015; Stock, 2010). Managing interactions between immunosuppressive agents and antiretroviral therapy can be a particularly challenging aspect of caring for the HIV-positive transplant recipient. In the outpatient setting, clinicians will most frequently encounter maintenance immunosuppressive regimens consisting of a combination of a calcineurin inhibitor (e.g., tacrolimus or cyclosporine), corticosteroids, and potentially an antiproliferative agent (mycophenolate mofetil or, less frequently, azathioprine). In some cases, mTOR inhibitors will be used in place of one of these agents or as adjunctive therapy. Understanding the pharmacokinetics of each of these drug classes is crucial to safely managing antiretroviral therapy. Calcineurin inhibitors are substrates and inhibitors of cytochrome P450 3A4 (CYP3A4) and P-glycoprotein 1 (P-gp1) and therefore have potential for significant interaction with antiretroviral agents that are substrates, inhibitors, or inducers of CYP3A4 or P-gp1. Overexposure to tacrolimus can result in nephrotoxicity and neurotoxicity, and administration of tacrolimus requires careful monitoring of trough levels in all patients. mTOR inhibitors are substrates of both CYP3A4 and P-gp1, and dosing must be adjusted in the presence of inhibitors or inducers of CYP3A4. The antimetabolites mycophenolate mofetil and azathioprine are not substrates for CYP3A4 or P-gp1, and they have no expected or documented interactions with antiretroviral therapy.

KEY DRUG–DRUG INTERACTIONS

PROTEASE INHIBITORS

Protease inhibitors are both substrates and inhibitors of CYP3A4 and P-gp1. Both boosted (i.e., coadministered with ritonavir or cobicistat) and unboosted PIs can significantly alter metabolism and transport of calcineurin inhibitors and mTOR inhibitors, resulting in increased levels of these immunosuppressive agents. Case reports of coadministration of calcineurin inhibitors and PIs suggest that significant dose reductions in tacrolimus or cyclosporine and frequent monitoring of drug levels are critical to minimize

toxicity related to overexposure and to avoid subtherapeutic trough levels. An observational study of patients undergoing orthotopic liver transplantation found that those who initiated therapy with lopinavir/ritonavir required a dose reduction of tacrolimus of 99% to maintain therapeutic levels (Teicher, 2007). A similar dose reduction is necessary to maintain appropriate trough levels of cyclosporine when coadministered with PIs. Liver transplant recipients receiving a ritonavir-boosted PI showed an increase in half-life of cyclosporine of up to 38 hours, requiring reductions to 5–20% of standard doses (Vogel, 2004). Modeling pharmacokinetic curves of pretransplant test doses of tacrolimus in patients on a ritonavir-boosted regimen may allow for more targeted post-transplant dosing (van Maarseveen, 2013). Sirolimus has shown similar pharmacokinetic alterations when coadministered with PIs. A case study of an HIV-positive liver transplant recipient who initiated nelfinavir showed that the 24-hour trough level of sirolimus was increased by fivefold, peak concentration was increased by 3.2 times, and half-life was extended by 60% (Jain, 2002). Drug levels of tacrolimus, cyclosporine, sirolimus, and everolimus must be monitored carefully for patients taking concomitant protease inhibitors, particularly ritonavir. Although data and clinical experience are limited, cobicistat (structurally very similar to ritonavir) is a known potent inhibitor of CYP3A4, and similar caution should be used.

NNRTIS

The most commonly administered NNRTIs are substrates of CYP3A4. In addition, efavirenz, nevirapine, and etravirine are inducers of CYP3A4. Although published data are sparse, the effect of NNRTIs on immunosuppressant metabolism may be greatest for efavirenz. In a study of 35 liver or kidney transplant patients, those taking efavirenz required significantly increased doses of cyclosporine (Frassetto, 2007). In a relatively recent case report, a heart transplant recipient on efavirenz required an increased dose of everolimus to maintain therapeutic levels (Durante-Mangoni, 2014). Transplant recipients on an antiretroviral regimen that includes an NNRTI, particularly efavirenz, should have immunosuppressant levels monitored closely, and it should be anticipated that they will require higher doses of calcineurin and mTOR inhibitors than typically administered.

NRTIS

NRTIs are not metabolized via the CYP pathway, and there is no expected interaction between immunosuppressive agents and NRTIs. A pharmacokinetic study of tacrolimus coadministered with tenofovir/emtricitabine to healthy volunteers demonstrated no clinically relevant interaction between these drugs (Chittick, 2008). Case reports among HIV-positive transplant recipients are consistent with this expectation. A 2007 study of tacrolimus pharmacokinetics in HIV-positive liver transplant recipients reported little change in the tacrolimus dose required to maintain therapeutic levels in a patient who initiated therapy with an NRTI-based regimen (Teicher, 2007). The current standard dual-NRTI backbone of antiretroviral therapy appears to be appropriate and safe in transplant recipients and does not require alterations to standard doses of immunosuppressive agents.

INTEGRASE INHIBITORS

Integrase inhibitors, which are metabolized chiefly by glucuronidation rather than via CYP3A4, have been shown to have negligible interaction with calcineurin inhibitors and mTOR inhibitors. Although experience is greatest with raltegravir, the absence of interaction and stability of dosing are likely to be similar for dolutegravir. A pharmacokinetic study among four HIV-positive liver transplant recipients showed no interaction between raltegravir and cyclosporine (Barau, 2014), and case reports have demonstrated successful coadministration of these agents (Di Biagio, 2009). Case reports have shown similar stability without dose adjustment of tacrolimus when administered with raltegravir (Cirioni, 2013; Miro, 2010). An observational study of 13 HIV-positive liver and kidney transplant recipients maintained on a combination of two NRTIs and raltegravir found that target levels of tacrolimus and cyclosporine were stable and easily achieved with no adjustment to standard immunosuppressant doses. Among these 13 patients, HIV remained well controlled, and there were no cases of acute rejection (Tricot, 2009). Data for sirolimus, although limited, suggest a similar safety profile without need for dose adjustment. A case report of a liver transplant recipient with tacrolimus-induced renal toxicity in the setting of PI coadministration demonstrated safety of raltegravir and sirolimus with no adjustment to standard dosing of sirolimus (Moreno, 2008). Integrase inhibitors provide a safe option for antiretroviral therapy that, when combined with dual NRTIs, avoids clinically relevant drug interactions with immunosuppressive agents.

SUMMARY

Understanding interactions between immunosuppressive agents and antiretroviral therapy and the effects that changes in highly active antiretroviral therapy (HAART) can have on metabolism of immunosuppressive agents—and ultimately the longevity of the transplant organ—is critical to caring for HIV-positive transplant recipients. PIs, as inhibitors of CYP3A4, can drastically increase levels of calcineurin inhibitors and mTOR inhibitors, resulting in overexposure and potential toxicity if doses are not adjusted and monitored carefully. Many NNRTIs are inducers of CYP3A4 and can decrease levels of calcineurin inhibitors and mTOR inhibitors, resulting in subtherapeutic trough levels and ultimately increasing the risk of rejection. The ideal antiretroviral therapy regimen, although not formally defined, may be a combination of NRTIs and an integrase inhibitor because neither of these classes has significant interactions with calcineurin inhibitors or mTOR inhibitors. Clinicians caring for HIV-positive transplant recipients should be aware of the key interactions between antiretroviral therapy and immunosuppressive agents and take these interactions into consideration when making changes to HAART.

ACKNOWLEDGMENTS

This chapter is an extension of the work by the authors of previous editions of this chapter, Ian R. McNicholl and Joan J. McNicholl.

Recommended Reading

Blumberg EA, Rogers CC; AST Infectious Diseases Community of Practice. Human immunodeficiency virus in solid organ transplantation. *Am J Transplant*. 2013; 13(Suppl 4):169–178.

Conte AH, Kittleson, MM, Dilibero D, et al. Successful orthotopic heart transplantation and immunosuppressive management in 2 human immunodeficiency virus-seropositive patients. *Tex Heart Inst J*. 2016; 43(1):69–74.

Locke JE, James NT, Mannon RB, et al. Immunosuppression regimen and the risk of acute rejection in HIV-infected kidney transplant recipients. *Transplantation*. 2014; 97(4):446–450.

Roland ME, Barin B, Huprikar S, et al; HIVTR Study Team. Survival in HIV-positive transplant recipients compared with transplant candidates and with HIV-negative controls. *AIDS*. 2016 Jan 28; 30(3):435–444.

References

Barau C, Braun J, Vincent C, et al. Pharmacokinetic study of raltegravir in HIV-infected patients with end-stage liver disease: The LIVERAL-ANRS 148 study. *Clin Infect Dis*. 2014; 59(8):1177–1184.

Chittick GE, Zong J, Begley JA, et al. Pharmacokinetics of emtricitabine/tenofovir disoproxil fumarate and tacrolimus at steady state when administered alone or in combination. *Int J Clin Pharmacol Ther*. 2008; 46(12):627–636.

Cirioni O, Weimer LE, Fragola V, et al. A simplified HAART regimen with raltegravir and lamivudine, and pharmacokinetic interactions with a combined immunosuppressive therapy with tacrolimus and everolimus in an HIV/HCV/HBV/HDV patient after liver transplantation. *West Indian Med J*. 2014; 63(7):779–784.

Di Biagio A, Rosso R, Siccardi M, et al. Lack of interaction between raltegravir and cyclosporine in an HIV-infected liver transplant recipient. *J Antimicrob Chemother*. 2009; 64(4):874–875.

Durante-Mangoni E, Maiello C, Limongelli G, et al. Management of immunosuppression and antiretroviral treatment before and after heart transplant for HIV-associated dilated cardiomyopathy. *Int J Immunopathol Pharmacol*. 2014; 27(1):113–120.

Frassetto LA, Browne M, Cheng A, et al. Immunosuppressant pharmacokinetics and dosing modifications in HIV-1 infected liver and kidney transplant recipients. *Am J Transplant*. 2007; 7(12):2816–2820.

Gathogo EN, Hamzah L, Hilton R, et al. Kidney transplantation in HIV-positive adults: The UK experience. *Int J STD AIDS*. 2014; 25(1):57–66.

Jain AK, Venkataramanan R, Fridell JA, et al. Nelfinavir, a protease inhibitor, increases sirolimus levels in a liver transplantation patient: A case report. *Liver Transpl*. 2002; 8(9):838–840.

Kumar MSA, Ranganna K, Malat GE, et al. In HIV+ patients with end stage renal disease (ESRD) kidney transplantation significantly prolongs long-term patient survival compared to chronic dialysis treatment. *Am J Transplant*. 2008; 8:S179.

Landin L, Rodriguez-Perez JC, Garcia-Bello MA, et al. Kidney transplants in HIV-positive recipients under HAART: A comprehensive review and meta-analysis of 12 series. *Nephrol Dial Transplant*. 2010; 25(9):3106–3115.

Miro JM, Ricart MJ, Trullas JC, et al. Simultaneous pancreas–kidney transplantation in HIV-infected patients: A case report and literature review. *Transplant Proc*. 2010; 42(9):3887–3891.

Moreno A, Barcena R, Quereda C, et al. Safe use of raltegravir and sirolimus in an HIV-infected patient with renal impairment after orthotropic liver transplantation. *AIDS*. 2008; 22(4):547–548.

Sawinski D, Forde KA, Eddinger K, et al. Superior outcomes in HIV-positive kidney transplant patients compared with HCV-infected or HIV/HCV coinfected recipients. *Kidney Int*. 2015; 88:341–349.

Sawinski D, Goldberg DS, Blumberg E, et al. Beyond the NIH multicenter HIV transplant trial experience: Outcomes of HIV+ liver transplant recipients compared to HCV+ or HIV+/HCV+ coinfected recipients in the United States. *Clin Infect Dis*. 2015; 61(7):1054–1062.

Stock PG, Barin B, Murphy B, et al. Outcomes of kidney transplantation in HIV-infected recipients. *N Engl J Med*. 2010; 363(21):2004–2014.

Teicher E, Vincent I, Bonhomme-Faivre L, et al. Effect of highly active antiretroviral therapy on tacrolimus pharmacokinetics in hepatitis C and HIV co-infected liver transplant recipients in the ANRS HC-80 study. *Clin Pharmacokinet*. 2007; 46(11):941–952.

Tricot L, Teicher E, Peytavin G, et al. Safety and efficacy of raltegravir in HIV-infected transplant patients cotreated with immunosuppressive drugs. *Am J Transplant*. 2009; 9(8):1946–1952.

van Maarseveen EM, Crommelin HA, Mudrikova T, et al. Pretransplant pharmacokinetic curves of tacrolimus in HIV-infected patients on ritonavir-containing cART: A pilot study. *Transplantation*. 2013; 95(2):397–402.

Vogel M, Voigt E, Michaelis HC, et al. Management of drug-to-drug interactions between cyclosporine A and the protease-inhibitor lopinavir/ritonavir in liver-transplanted HIV-infected patients. *Liver Transpl*. 2004; 10(7):939–944.

29.

UNDERSTANDING AND MANAGING ANTINEOPLASTIC AND ANTIRETROVIRAL THERAPY

Jason J. Schafer, Elizabeth M. Sherman, Taylor K. Gill, and Jatandra Birney

CHAPTER GOAL

To identify contemporary challenges and describe strategies in managing antineoplastic and antiretroviral therapy in patients with cancer and HIV infection.

LEARNING OBJECTIVE

To review both general and specific concepts regarding the safe and effective use of antineoplastic and antiretroviral therapy in patients with HIV and cancer.

WHAT'S NEW?

To address the challenges of complicated interactions and toxicities associated with antiretroviral and antineoplastic therapies, HIV-infected patients with cancer should receive multidisciplinary care that includes primary care providers, infectious disease clinicians, hematologists/oncologists, and clinical pharmacists.

KEY POINTS

- The use of combination antiretroviral therapy in patients with malignancies is associated with improved HIV and cancer-related outcomes.

- Combining antiretroviral and antineoplastic therapy is often complicated by significant drug–drug interactions, drug–disease state monitoring interactions, and overlapping toxicities.

- Definitive pharmacokinetic studies evaluating drug interactions between antineoplastics and antiretrovirals are uncommon, and clinical judgment must often be used to determine the potential for significant interactions.

- Adjusting antiretroviral therapy in response to significant drug interactions or overlapping toxicities is often more feasible than modifying antineoplastic protocols.

INTRODUCTION TO CANCER IN HIV

Before the widespread use of antiretroviral therapy (ART), AIDS-defining malignancies (ADMs) such as Kaposi's sarcoma, non-Hodgkin's lymphoma, and invasive cervical cancer accounted for the largest burden of cancer in patients with HIV infection (Rubinstein, 2014). These malignancies occur most commonly in patients with severe immune suppression characterized by advanced HIV, and all are associated with oncogenic viruses.

Following the widespread use of combination ART in the mid-1990s, a substantial decline in the number of new AIDS diagnoses and AIDS-related deaths was observed (Rubinstein, 2014). The ability to reconstitute the immune system with ART also led to a decrease in ADMs. During the same time period, however, the occurrence of non-AIDS-defining malignancies (NADMs) increased. These malignancies include Hodgkin's lymphoma; leukemia; and cancers of the head, neck, lung, kidney, liver, gastrointestinal tract, anus, and skin. Currently, NADMs cause more cancer-related morbidity and mortality than ADMs in patients with HIV.

Although ADMs most commonly occur in patients with severe immune suppression, low CD4 cell counts (<500 cells/mm³) have been identified as a risk factor for both ADMs and NADMs (Torres, 2014). This suggests that initiating ART to suppress HIV replication and reconstituting CD4 cell counts may reduce the overall risk of malignancies in patients living with HIV. Furthermore, in patients with a cancer diagnosis, the use of ART alongside chemotherapy is now routinely recommended as a means to improve overall survival.

The administration of chemotherapy and ART concurrently is complicated by a number of factors (Rudek, 2011), including limited data regarding safe and effective therapy combinations; significant drug–drug interactions among ART, antineoplastics, and supportive care medications; drug–disease state monitoring interactions; and overlapping drug toxicities (Table 29.1). This chapter reviews contemporary information regarding the use of chemotherapy and ART in combination, including strategies for managing potential and established drug–drug interactions and considerations for preventing and/or monitoring for toxicity.

GENERAL CONSIDERATIONS FOR COMBINING ANTINEOPLASTIC AND ANTIRETROVIRAL THERAPY

Drug interactions between ART and antineoplastic agents may occur via several different mechanisms. The first and most common are the interactions that occur during metabolism of medications from active to inactive substances via the hepatic cytochrome P450 system (CYP450). Medications may be substrates of the CYP450 system, meaning that they use this system for metabolism and their concentrations may be altered by concurrent administration with other agents. In addition, medications may be inducers or inhibitors of individual CYP450 isoenzymes, such as 3A4. CYP450 inducers will increase the metabolism of CYP450 substrates, thus decreasing the concentration of medication, which may lead to subtherapeutic medication levels. Conversely, CYP450 inhibitors will decrease the metabolism of CYP450 substrates, thus increasing the medication concentration, which may lead to toxicity. The timing of the CYP450 interactions may also be variable because enzyme inhibition occurs rapidly, with maximum effect occurring when a medication is at steady state and enzyme induction occurring more slowly due to the need for enzyme synthesis (Di Francia, 2014). Many antiretroviral, antineoplastic, and supportive care medications utilize the CYP450 system for metabolism, and drug interactions are expected to be a challenge in this setting.

To add to the complications of the interactions that occur with medication metabolism, there may also be absorption interactions with the p-glycoprotein efflux pump in the gastrointestinal tract. Similar to the CYP450 interactions, medications may be p-glycoprotein substrates, inducers, or inhibitors. P-glycoprotein inducers will stimulate the efflux of medications back into the gastrointestinal lumen and will thus decrease the absorption and plasma concentrations of these medications. Likewise, p-glycoprotein inhibitors will increase the absorption of medication and increase plasma concentrations of substrates, which could lead to toxicities. The literature has shown that p-glycoprotein is highly expressed in HIV-associated malignancies such as non-Hodgkin's lymphoma and can play a significant role in the effectiveness of both antiretroviral and antineoplastic therapy (Klibanov, 2007). Clinicians should be aware of antiretroviral, antineoplastic, and supportive care agents that affect p-glycoprotein and should realize the potential for drug interactions with medications that influence, or are influenced by, this mechanism.

In addition to drug interactions, clinicians will also need to consider overlapping toxicities of the medication classes. Some antiretroviral therapy and antineoplastic agents are known for causing severe adverse effects that may become additive when used in combination. It is vitally important when devising medication regimens that serious adverse effects of all agents be identified and overlapping toxicities minimized when possible.

Last, the presence of drug–disease interactions will need to be recognized when combining antiretroviral and antineoplastic agents. Disease monitoring interactions are a concern because there are certain antiretroviral medications that increase oncologic disease markers such as bilirubin. Conversely, there are also concerns that antineoplastic agents may affect the level of CD4 cells, rendering the monitoring parameters of both disease states inaccurate (Klibanov, 2007). To supplement the monitoring parameter concerns, there may also be medication absorption concerns due to the presence of disease complications such as gastrointestinal tumors, mucositis, and graft-versus-host disease (Torres, 2014). Clinicians may need to be creative in these situations, such as selecting medication regimens available in liquid formulations or alternative routes of administration.

The key concepts of drug interactions, overlapping toxicities, and drug–disease interactions are just a few examples of the complexity in utilizing combination antiretroviral and antineoplastic therapy. Specific literature and guideline

Table 29.1 POTENTIAL DRUG INTERACTIONS AND OVERLAPPING TOXICITIES IN A SAMPLE OF COMMONLY USED ANTINEOPLASTIC AND ANTIRETROVIRAL AGENTS

ANTINEOPLASTIC	SOME CANCERS TREATED	INFLUENCES OR INFLUENCED BY CYP450	OTHER METABOLISM	INFLUENCES OR INFLUENCED BY P-GLYCOPROTEIN	DOCUMENTATION OF INTERACTIONS WITH ANTIRETROVIRAL THERAPY	OVERLAPPING TOXICITY	COMMENT
Folate Antagonists							
Methotrexate	Most cancers	No	Renal (80% unchanged drug)	No	No	Renal, BMS	Caution when used with sulfamethoxazole–trimethoprim
Pyrimidine/Purine Antagonists							
5-Fluorouracil	A, C, Br, L, Pan, H&N	Yes	DPD metabolism	No	No	Mucositis, diarrhea, rash	
Cytarabine	Leuk, HD, NHL	Yes	Cytidine deaminase	No	No	Renal, BMS	
Gemcitabine	Br, HD, NHL, L, Pan, S	No	Cytidine deaminase	No	No	BMS, hepatic	
Platinums							
Cisplatin	Most solid tumors	No	Possibly spontaneous degradation	Yes	No	Renal, PN	May need to renal adjust ART due to cisplatin toxicity
Carboplatin	B, Br, H&N, L	No	Spontaneous hydrolysis	No	No data available	N	Active study pending results with ART and carboplatin
Oxaliplatin	C, HD, NHL, Br, Pan	No	Extensive biotransformation in blood	No	No	N	
Alkylating Agents							
Cyclophosphamide/ ifosphamide	Most cancers	Yes	Renal excretion	No	No	BMS, renal	
Dacarbazine	B, HD, Pan, S	Yes	Hepatic activation	No	Yes	Hepatic	Regimen ABVD with ritonavir-boosted regimen had documented increased toxicities
Procarbazine	B, HD, L, MM, NHL	Yes	Renal excretion	No	No	BMS, rash	

(continued)

Table 29.1 CONTINUED

ANTINEOPLASTIC	SOME CANCERS TREATED	INFLUENCES OR INFLUENCED BY CYP450	OTHER METABOLISM	INFLUENCES OR INFLUENCED BY P-GLYCOPROTEIN	DOCUMENTATION OF INTERACTIONS WITH ANTIRETROVIRAL THERAPY	OVERLAPPING TOXICITY	COMMENT
Antitumor Antibiotics							
Dactinomycin	Leuk, Br, KS, S	Unknown	Hepatic	Yes	No data available	BMS, hepatic, rash	
Doxorubicin	Leuk, Br, H&N, KS, HD, NHL, L, MM, S	Yes	Hepatic	Yes	No	BMS, hepatic	Regimen ABVD with ritonavir-boosted regimen had documented increased toxicities
Idarubicin	Leuk	Yes	Plasma	No	No	BMS	
Bleomycin	H&D, HD, NHL, KS, S	Unknown	Intracellular hydrolysis	No	Yes	Renal, rash	Regimen ABVD with ritonavir-boosted regimen had documented increased toxicities
Mitomycin	A, C, L, Pan, H&N	Unknown	Hepatic	Yes	No data available	BMS	No data published about interactions with ART in anal cancer studies
Microtubules							
Vinblastine	Br, Leuk, H&N, HD, NHL, KS, L	Yes	Hepatic	Yes	Yes	N	Caution when used with ritonavir-boosted regimens
Vincrisitine	Leuk, B, Br, CRC, S, H&N, KS, L, MM, P, HD, NHL	Yes	Hepatic	Yes	No	N	
Taxanes							
Docetaxel	L, H&N, Br, KS, Pan, S	Yes	Hepatic	Yes	Yes	N, BMS	Caution when used with ritonavir-boosted regimens
Paclitaxel	Br, H&N, L, KS	Yes	Hepatic	Yes	Yes	BMS, mucositis	Conflicting reports of interactions in published data

A, anal; ART, antiretroviral therapy; ABVD, doxorubicin, bleomycin, vinblastine, dacarbazine; B, brain; BMS, bone marrow suppression; Br, breast; C, : CRC, colorectal; DPD, dihydropyrimidine dehydrogenase; G, gastric; HD, Hodgkin's lymphoma; H&N, head and neck; KS, Kaposi's sarcoma; L, lung; Leuk, leukemia; MM, Multiple myeloma; N, neck; NHL, non-Hodgkin lymphoma; Pan, pancreas; S, sarcoma; UGT, uridine 5'-diphosphoglucronosyltransferase.

SOURCE: Gold Standard, Inc. Clinical pharmacology [database online]. Available at http://www.clinicalpharmacology.com. Accessed December 3, 2015.

recommendations to guide the selection, dosing, and monitoring of these agents when used in combination are scarce. Thus, these concepts should be considered on a case-by-case basis and explored when crafting a medication regimen in the treatment of both HIV and oncologic diseases.

SPECIFIC CONSIDERATIONS FOR COMBINING ANTINEOPLASTIC AND ANTIRETROVIRAL THERAPIES BY ANTIRETROVIRAL DRUG CLASS

ENTRY/FUSION INHIBITORS

There are limited data on the use of HIV entry/fusion inhibitors, maraviroc and enfuvirtide, with chemotherapy agents. Maraviroc, a CCR5 antagonist, is a substrate of CYP3A4 but does not induce or inhibit this enzyme. It is also a substrate of p-glycoprotein. Therefore, maraviroc is unlikely to affect levels of antineoplastic drugs, although it may be susceptible to drug interactions with antineoplastic and supportive care medications. The prescribing information for maraviroc contains a warning of hepatotoxicity associated with allergic features including rash and fever approximately 4 weeks after starting treatment (Selzentry package insert, GlaxoSmithKline). Such an adverse effect should be considered when combining maraviroc with chemotherapy agents with a high risk of hepatotoxicity due to the potential for overlapping toxicity.

Enfuvirtide, an HIV fusion inhibitor, is not metabolized by nor an inhibitor or inducer of CYP450 enzymes. Rather, it undergoes catabolism to its constituent amino acids. Enfuvirtide is not expected to have drug interactions with any antineoplastic agent or supportive therapy agent. However, the use of enfuvirtide is limited by its tolerability, which includes injection site reactions.

NUCLEOSIDE/NUCLEOTIDE REVERSE TRANSCRIPTASE INHIBITORS

The nucleoside/nucleotide reverse transcriptase inhibitors (NRTIs) were the first available class of antiretrovirals and are still commonly used today. The class consists of seven individual agents and is the backbone of many current HIV treatment regimens. Therefore, it should be expected that at least one and probably two agents in this class will be used concurrently with antineoplastic agents.

In analyzing the concurrent usage of this class and oncologic treatments, fewer drug interactions are expected but concern regarding additive and overlapping adverse effects remains.

Regarding drug interactions, NRTIs are excreted unchanged in the urine or metabolized outside of the hepatic CYP450 system. In addition, NRTIs do not induce or inhibit any of the CYP450 enzymes. The majority of NRTIs are also completely absorbed without involvement of the p-glycoprotein system, with the exception of tenofovir, which is a p-glycoprotein substrate (Torres, 2014). Due to these pharmacokinetic properties, the NRTIs have minimal drug interactions with other medications. When devising complex antineoplastic medication regimens, the NRTIs will be easy to utilize concurrently, and drug interactions should not be a major concern.

Although NRTIs have the benefits of being efficacious and easily utilized in combination regimens due to lack of drug interactions, their tolerability and adverse effects have historically been limitations. The older NRTIs have severe adverse effect profiles; however, the tolerability has greatly improved with the advancement of the newer agents. There are specific overlapping toxicities that should be considered when NRTIs and antineoplastic agents are utilized in combination:

- Neutropenia: The most severe and troublesome is the occurrence of neutropenia when zidovudine is used with any cytotoxic class of chemotherapy. Due to both medications causing a decrease in the white blood cell count (WBC), it is recommended to avoid the use of zidovudine if possible and use other NRTI agents. If this is not possible, then it is recommended to use less toxic chemotherapy (Rudek, 2011).

- Peripheral neuropathy: Two specific NRTI agents, didanosine and stavudine, may cause severe and potentially nonreversible peripheral neuropathy. There are also certain classes of chemotherapy agents, such as taxanes, platinums, vinca alkaloids, and the individual agent bortezomib, that may cause peripheral neuropathy. The development of peripheral neuropathy is often dose related and cumulative with ongoing therapy. Also, peripheral neuropathy may be expected when utilizing these agents in combination. The literature suggests using different NRTI medications, changing to an alternative chemotherapy regimen, or temporarily discontinuing antiretroviral therapy when antineoplastic agents causing peripheral neuropathy are administered (Rudek, 2011).

- Hepatotoxicity: Many medications have the potential to cause hepatoxicity, but some NRTIs have a higher propensity than others. As previously mentioned, the older NRTIs of zidovudine, didanosine, and stavudine have more adverse effects and also have the potential for hepatotoxicity. Therefore, it is recommended that these agents not be used in combination with cytotoxic chemotherapy agents that undergo hepatic metabolism. The newer NRTIs, such as abacavir, lamivudine, emtricitabine, and tenofovir, may be preferred in combination with such chemotherapy, or a reduced antineoplastic dose may be considered (Rudek, 2011).

- Nephrotoxicity: Tenofovir disoproxil fumarate, a commonly used NRTI, has been associated with the occurrence of nephrotoxicity. When used in combination with nephrotoxic chemotherapy such as cisplatin or carboplatin, an additive toxic effect may occur, and rigorous monitoring of serum creatinine is recommended (Rubinstein, 2014).

NON-NUCLEOSIDE REVERSE TRANSCRIPTASE INHIBITORS

There are four commonly used non-nucleoside reverse transcriptase inhibitors (NNRTIs): efavirenz, nevirapine, etravirine, and rilpivirine. The potential for drug interactions with these agents is high because they are extensively metabolized by and induce or inhibit the CYP450 system. In addition, NNRTI-mediated modulation of p-glycoprotein may provide another mechanism whereby the pharmacokinetics of antineoplastic drugs may be altered.

Both efavirenz and nevirapine are metabolized by CYP3A4 and CYP2B6 enzymes and induce CYP3A4. In addition, efavirenz inhibits CYP2B6, CYP3A4, and CYP2C9/19, whereas nevirapine induces CYP3A4, CYP2B6, and p-glycoprotein. The use of these NNRTIs in combination with chemotherapy agents is limited by their drug interactions and prolonged half-life. Theoretically, either efavirenz or nevirapine could lower therapeutic levels of chemotherapeutic agents that are metabolized by CYP3A4 due to strong enzyme induction. Interacting agents include vinblastine, vincristine, paclitaxel, docetaxol, ifosfamide, cyclophosphamide, tyrosine kinase inhibitors, and corticosteroids that are metabolized by CYP3A4 (Rubinstein, 2014).

Etravirine is a substrate of CYP3A4, CYP2C9, and CYP2C19, and it can both induce and inhibit P450 enzymes. Etravirine acts as an inhibitor of CYP2C9/19 and an inducer of CYP3A4 and p-glycoprotein. Limited experience exists with regard to treating cancer patients with this newer NNRTI, which has unpredictable drug interactions with both chemotherapeutic agents and immunosuppressants (Torres, 2014).

Rilpivirine is a substrate of CYP450 3A4 but does not induce or inhibit the CYP450 system and theoretically should not affect chemotherapeutic or immunosuppressant drug levels. Rilpivirine may cause benign increases in serum creatinine due to inhibition of tubular creatinine secretion without effects on actual glomerular filtration. This elevation normally occurs in the first few weeks of treatment and then stabilizes. Patients receiving rilpivirine-containing ART regimens should have serum creatinine monitored routinely. If serum creatinine elevations above 0.1–0.4 mg/dl occur, particularly outside of this time window, other causes should be considered.

Various NNRTI-based regimens are associated with rash and hepatic transaminase elevations, and overlapping toxicities with antineoplastic agents should be considered. Hepatotoxicity is also common with most chemotherapeutic classes. The literature supports chemotherapeutic agents that can be administered without any dose reductions in the setting of liver toxicity, including cisplatin, gemcitabine, and bleomycin (Rubinstein, 2014).

INTEGRASE INHIBITORS

The integrase inhibitor class of antiretroviral medications is the newest and perhaps most diverse HIV medication class. This class includes raltegravir, elvitegravir, and dolutegravir, and although all have the same mechanism of action, the agents differ dramatically in terms of their pharmacokinetic profiles. Therefore, it is important to assess each agent individually in terms of drug interactions and additive adverse effect potential.

Regarding to drug interactions, the first-generation integrase inhibitor, raltegravir, is metabolized by uridine 5-diphosphate–glucuronosyltransferase (UGT) 1A1 and is unlikely to have any major drug interactions with antineoplastic therapy (Beumer, 2014). Conversely, elvitegravir is a CYP450 3A4 substrate and modest 2C9 inducer and must be boosted by the potent CYP3A4 and 2D6 inhibitor cobicistat. Therefore, when given individually boosted or in the once-daily single-tablet regimen of Stribild or Genvoya, elvitegravir can be expected to cause drug interaction concerns. Antineoplastic therapy that utilizes or influences CYP450 3A4, 2D6, or 2C9 will need to be monitored closely when used with elvitegravir boosted with cobicistat because this agent may lead to heightened chemotherapy concentrations. The second-generation integrase inhibitor dolutegravir is primarily metabolized by UGT and, to a lesser extent, CYP450 3A4. Specifically, dolutegravir is a substrate but not an inducer or inhibitor of the CYP450 3A4 isoenzyme. Caution should be used when dolutegravir is used with chemotherapy agents that are inhibitors or inducers of CYP450 3A4 because alterations in dolutegravir concentrations may occur.

In addition to CYP450 interactions, p-glycoprotein effects are also agent specific. Raltegravir has no p-glycoprotein involvement and is not expected to cause drug interactions via this mechanism. When boosted with cobicistat, elvitegravir is a p-glycoprotein inducer and may decrease the concentration of antineoplastic agents that utilize p-glycoprotein for absorption. Dolutegravir is a p-glycoprotein substrate, and its absorption may be altered by antineoplastic therapies that are p-glycoprotein inhibitors or inducers. Thus, within the integrase inhibitor class, raltegravir is considered the cleanest agent in terms of drug interactions and has been specifically studied in combination with chemotherapy. The literature has shown that raltegravir-based ART is safe and effective when combined with antineoplastic chemotherapy, regardless of the tumor type and the type and duration of chemotherapy (Banon, 2014).

Although the metabolism of the individual integrase inhibitors differs, a benefit of the class as a whole is that these inhibitors have minimal adverse effects. Integrase inhibitors are well tolerated, and overlapping toxicities with antineoplastic agents are not projected to be a major concern. Therefore, due to the lack of drug interactions and minimal adverse effects, the integrase inhibitor raltegravir is an attractive option within a complete ART regimen when antiretroviral and antineoplastic therapy must be given concurrently.

PROTEASE INHIBITORS

The HIV protease inhibitors (PIs) remain among the most commonly used antiretroviral drug classes. They are potent antiretrovirals that are often effective in both treatment-naive and -experienced patients, and they have a high barrier to HIV resistance. In addition, newer PIs have a more favorable dosing schedule than previous agents as a result of pharmacologic boosting. All PIs (aside from nelfinavir) can be pharmacologically boosted when coadministered with cobicistat or low-dose ritonavir.

The boosting process begins in the gastrointestinal tract, where low doses of ritonavir or cobicistat inhibit intestinal p-glycoprotein and CYP3A4. Because nearly all PIs are substrates of both p-glycoprotein and CYP3A4, the inhibition of these proteins allows the companion PI to achieve better bioavailability. The process continues in the liver, where ritonavir and cobicistat inhibit CYP3A4-mediated PI metabolism. This step prolongs therapeutic PI concentrations, reducing the need for frequent dosing.

Boosting improves the administration of PIs but also results in a higher likelihood of significant drug–drug interactions with other medications. Several antineoplastic agents are substrates, inducers, or inhibitors of CYP3A4 and/or p-glycoprotein (Rubinstein, 2014). For example, alkylating agents, taxanes, tyrosine kinase inhibitors, and vinca alkaloids can be substrates and inhibitors or inducers of CYP isoenzymes. The result is complex bidirectional interactions with ART (Rudek, 2011). Furthermore, although pharmacologic boosting improves the pharmacokinetic profile of PIs through CYP3A4 inhibition, both ritonavir and cobicistat can cause collateral drug interactions with other metabolic and drug elimination pathways. For example, ritonavir and cobicistat also inhibit CYP2D6, whereas ritonavir can induce CYP2B6, CYP2C9, and certain enzymes involved in glucuronidation. Again, the result is complex interactions with antineoplastic agents that could limit efficacy or introduce the possibility of toxicity.

With regard to toxicity, PIs have been found to potentiate the myelosuppressive effects of certain chemotherapy (Torres, 2014). They may also lead to greater gastrointestinal upset, including nausea, vomiting, and diarrhea. Specific PIs, such as atazanavir and lopinavir/ritonavir, have been associated with QT prolongation (Rudek, 2014). Because of the potential for arrhythmias and sudden death, these PIs should be avoided when antineoplastic agents also known to cause QT prolongation are administered. These include anthracyclines, arsenic trioxide, dasatanib, lapatinib, and tamoxifen.

In addition to some overlapping toxicities, some PIs may also complicate the dosing and monitoring of certain chemotherapy (Beumer, 2014). For example, bilirubin is often used as a means for determining dosage adjustments for a number of chemotherapeutic agents, such as docetaxel, paclitaxel, doxorubicin, etoposide, ironotecan, imatinib, and vincristine. Atazanavir and indininivir may cause unconjugated hyperbilirubinemia secondary to UGT1A1 inhibition, leading to possible inaccuracies in chemotherapy dosage calculations.

STRATEGIES FOR CLINICAL MANAGEMENT OF PATIENTS WITH CANCER AND HIV

Treatment of patients with HIV-related malignancies is complex. The administration of ART with chemotherapy improves clinical response and prolongs survival, but concerns often arise regarding pharmacokinetic drug interactions and additive toxicity. The data regarding pharmacokinetic and pharmacodynamic interactions between antiretrovirals and chemotherapy agents are limited. To address the challenges of these complicated interactions and toxicities, HIV-infected patients with cancer should be treated using a multidisciplinary approach including primary care providers, infectious disease clinicians, hematologists/oncologists, and clinical pharmacists. Communication among these professions is essential.

In combining ART and anticancer drug therapy, overlapping toxicity profiles can be avoided by altering either the ART regimen or the chemotherapy regimen. Interruption of ART is not recommended because it has been associated with an increase in mortality. In many instances, one or more components of a patient's ART regimen may be substituted in order to avoid risk of drug interactions or additive toxicity. ART regimen changes should always be carried out in conjunction with an HIV specialist utilizing the patient's complete antiretroviral treatment history, past adverse events, and resistance test results. More intensive monitoring of tolerability, viral suppression, adherence, and laboratory changes is recommended during the first 3 months after a regimen switch. In addition, modifications to the drugs in an antineoplastic regimen may also be considered due to concerns regarding drug interactions and/or overlapping toxicities. Dose adjustments of anticancer therapy, based on patient tolerance and response, can also be considered. Regardless, both ART and chemotherapy should be individualized according to patient characteristics.

For the majority of antiretroviral drugs that are CYP450 substrates, inducers, or inhibitors, coadministration with other metabolized drugs could result in drug accumulation and possible toxicity, or it could result in decreased efficacy of one or both drugs. Because standardized dosing algorithms do not exist for managing such interactions, increased monitoring for efficacy and toxicity is recommended when coadministering any ART regimen with chemotherapy. When determining interaction potential, drug interaction resources such as the following should be consulted: the Toronto General Hospital Immunodeficiency Clinic (http://hivclinic.ca/drug-information/antiretroviral-interactions-with-chemotherapy-regimens) and the University of Liverpool HIV drug interaction website (http://www.hivdruginteractions.org). Due to the paucity of available literature and the variability in the quality of evidence, clinical management should be assessed individually for each patient.

Last, in HIV-infected patients with cancer, opportunistic infection prophylaxis should be tailored and expanded with antimicrobials required for specific chemotherapy regimens or hematopoietic stem cell transplantation. The need for opportunistic infection prophylaxis should be re-evaluated on a regular basis and adjusted as needed via coordination among both the infectious disease team and the oncology team. Prophylaxis may need to be modified as the patient's CD4$^+$ T cell count decreases with some chemotherapy regimens or increases after completion of therapy.

FUTURE DIRECTIONS

As patients with HIV infection live longer and develop ADMs or NADMs, more information on how to treat patients with anticancer treatment and supportive therapies will be needed. The AIDS Malignancy Consortium, a National Cancer Institute clinical trials group, aims to meet these needs by conducting prospective clinical trials with molecularly targeted agents in HIV-infected patients receiving ART. As anticancer therapy moves from cytotoxics to molecularly targeted agents, there may be fewer concerns about drug interactions and overlapping toxicities with ART. Due to the rapidly evolving nature of both HIV and cancer treatments, clinicians should be cognizant of the potential for interactions and toxicities and remain current on the latest clinical information. (Richterman A, Blumberg E. 2015)

Recommended Reading

Beumer JH, Venkataramanan R, Rudek MA. Pharmacotherapy in cancer patients with HIV/AIDS. *Clin Pharmcol Ther*. 2014 April; 95(4):370–372.

Rubinstein PG, Aboulafia DM, Zloza A. Malignancies in HIV/AIDS: From epidemiology to therapeutic challenges. *AIDS*. 2014 February 20; 28(4):453–465.

Rudek MA, Flexner C, Ambinder RF. Use of antineoplastic agents in patients with cancer who have HIV/AIDS. *Lancet Oncol*. 2011; 12:905–912.

References

Banon S, Machuca I, Araujo S, et al. Efficacy, safety and lack of interactions with the use of raltegravir in HIV-infected patients undergoing antineoplastic chemotherapy. *J Intern AIDS*. 2014; 17(Suppl 3):19590.

Beumer JH, Venkataramanan R, Rudek MA. Pharmacotherapy in cancer patients with HIV/AIDS. *Clin Pharmcol Ther*. 2014; 95(4):370–372.

Di Francia R, Di Paolo M, Valente D, et al. Pharmacogenetic based drug–drug interactions between highly active antiretroviral therapy (HAART) and antiblastic chemotherapy. *WCRJ*. 2014; 1(2):e386.

Gold Standard, Inc. Clinical pharmacology [database online]. Available at http://www.clinicalpharmacology.com. Accessed December 3, 2015.

Klibanov OM, Clark-Vetril R. Oncologic complications of human immunodeficiency virus infection: Changing epidemiology, treatments, and special considerations in the era of highly active antiretroviral therapy. *Pharmacotherapy*. 2007; 27(1):122–136.

Rubinstein PG, Aboulafia DM, Zloza A. Malignancies in HIV/AIDS: From epidemiology to therapeutic challenges. *AIDS*. 2014; 28(4):453–465.

Rudek MA, Chang CY, Steadman K, et al. *Cancer Chemother Pharmacol.* 2014 Apr; 73(4):729–736.

Rudek MA, Flexner C, Ambinder RF. Use of antineoplastic agents in patients with cancer who have HIV/AIDS. *Lancet Oncol.* 2011; 12(9):905–912.

Selzentry package insert. Available at https://www.gsksource.com/pharma/content/dam/GlaxoSmithKline/US/en/Prescribing_Information/Selzentry/pdf/SELZENTRY-PI-MG.PDF. Accessed December 1, 2015.

Torres HA, Mulanovich V. Management of HIV infection in patients with cancer receiving chemotherapy. *Clin Infect Dis.* 2014; 59(1):106–114.

30.

SUBSTANCE ABUSE IN HIV POPULATIONS

Elizabeth David and John P. Casas

CHAPTER GOAL

This chapter discusses issues, implications, diagnosis, and treatment of substance abuse in HIV-infected individuals.

LEARNING OBJECTIVES

- Describe the bidirectional interactions between HIV and substance abuse.

- Recognize substance abuse in their patients.

- Provide an initial outline of potential approaches to the treatment of substance use disorders in this population.

WHAT'S NEW?

The chapter has been updated to reflect the terminology of the fifth edition of the *Diagnostic and Statistical Manual of Mental Disorders* (American Psychiatric Association, 2013). More thorough and specific treatment modalities and recommendations are included.

INTRODUCTION

The prevalence of substance use in HIV-infected individuals is high, with rates of abuse/dependence much greater than those in the normal population. These substances include alcohol, opioids, cocaine/crack, methamphetamine, MDMA ("ecstasy" or "molly"), benzodiazepines, marijuana, ketamine, GHB, anabolic steroids, nitrite inhalants, barbiturates, nicotine, and newer synthetic compounds ("bath salts," "kush," etc.)—all of which can have long- and short-term physiological, psychological, social, and neurocognitive effects when used in excess.

The relationship between substance use and HIV illness, illness progression, and treatment is complex. Whereas early in the course of the epidemic it was theorized that substance abuse was a causative factor or cofactor in HIV disease (Friedman, 1988; Goedert, 1984; Newell, 1985), it has become increasingly obvious that the interaction is behavioral as much as biological. Many behaviors associated with substance use result in increased risk of exposure to the virus, both directly through routes such as needle sharing and more indirectly through mechanisms relating to impaired judgment (unprotected sex, sex with multiple partners, trading sex for drugs, and "adventurous" sex including anal penetration) (Hillfors, 2007; Mackesy-Amiti, 2010; Semples, 2009) and sociocultural issues (homelessness and being embedded in a community with a high incidence of HIV disease) (Millett, 2007). In addition, low adherence to HIV treatment in this population with poor impulse control, unstructured and unhealthy lifestyles, multiple barriers to treatment (including fear of legal reprisals), and patterns of immediate wish gratification lead to increased morbidity and mortality (Cofrancesco, 2008; DeLorenze, 2011). Mental illness and substance abuse are separate and additive risk factors for HIV infection. One study of HIV-positive patients revealed that those who have the dual diagnosis of mental illness and substance use have an HIV prevalence of 4.7% as opposed to 2.4% for those with substance use disorder diagnosis alone—almost double the rate. This highlights the importance of a comprehensive approach in the treatment of those with dual diagnoses, which inherently place them at a higher risk of contracting or transmitting sexually transmitted diseases (STDs) including HIV. Problems with adherence to medical treatment seem to be additive in this group (Moore, 2008; Sullivan, 2011). Finally, substance abuse is associated with a host of medical sequelae (liver disease, infection, diabetes, cardiovascular disease, and neurocognitive changes), complicating treatment of the virus in a population already at risk for these problems and leading to increased disease progression. Despite this known connection between substance abuse and HIV, and despite the knowledge that successful treatment of substance abuse can increase adherence to combination antiretroviral therapy regimens to levels comparable to those of non-substance abusers (Catz, 2000; Palepu, 2011; Vallecillo, 2010), a study revealed that fewer than half of all US substance abuse treatment facilities conduct on-site infectious disease screening (Substance Abuse and Mental Health Services Administration, 2010).

DIAGNOSIS AND GENERAL ISSUES IN THE TREATMENT OF SUBSTANCE USE DISORDERS

Although there are precise criteria for the diagnosis of abuse and dependence (American Psychiatric Association, 2013), delineating the degree of severity of use is difficult and may ultimately be relatively insignificant. Some drugs are extremely destructive with almost any use, whereas some people manage to adapt and function despite ongoing and heavy abuse. Practically speaking, substance use disorders represent maladaptive patterns of substance use that interfere with a person's ability to function on a day-to-day basis. Generally when use reaches these levels, there is disturbance of employment, disruption of relationships, possible medical consequences, and the substance use becomes central to the person's daily life, with requirement for increasingly more of the substance to feel "normal" or get the same high/ sense of relief as previously experienced. Despite these obvious costs, the patient frequently does not view his or her use as a problem ("denial") or, perceiving a problem, cannot cut down. Despite traditional views of this as a condition of character weakness or poor choice, addiction is recognized as a disease process by the medical community.

These patients are often difficult to treat. Their frequent relapses—the norm rather than an exception—tend to demoralize them and those treating them. In addition, their patterns of denial and of using and abusing often extend to the people and systems around them, leaving treaters (as well as family, friends, and sometimes strangers) feeling angry, drained, frustrated, manipulated, and overwhelmed. When possible, the use of a treatment team (primary care physician, substance abuse counselor, psychiatrist when necessary, nursing staff, and social services/case manager) and a very clear treatment contract can mitigate these difficulties.

Screening for substance abuse can be done quickly and easily. Numerous specific screening questionnaires are available through the National Institute on Alcohol Abuse and Alcoholism, the Center for Substance Abuse Treatment, and other governmental agencies. However, the validity of simple one-question ("How often in the past year have you had 4 (for women)/5 (for men) or more drinks?" (Smith, 2009)), two-question ("Have you ever had a substance use problem? When was your last use of that substance?" (Cyr, 1988)), or CAGE/CAGE-AID (cut down, annoyed, guilty, eye-opener) (Brown, 1995; Willenbring, 2009) is well established, including the modifications made for various other substances. Even for those not currently using, ongoing monitoring of substance use is important in this population known for frequent relapse, and questions at each visit as well as periodic urine drug screens, liver function tests, and complete blood count (to check mean corpuscular volume) can be helpful.

There are several stages in the treatment of substance abuse. When denial and continued use are unquestioned by the abuser, he or she is said to be in a "precontemplative" phase—a term suggesting that everyone has a hope for treatment. Prior to initiation of treatment ("contemplative" phase), there must be acknowledgment by the individual that there is a problem and the beginnings of readiness to consider stopping use. This is followed by detoxification— abstaining from active use of the drug until it is no longer present in the body and the immediate effects of intoxication are gone, usually within 4–10 days, depending on the drug of abuse. Only at this point is the individual physically and cognitively prepared to move on to the tasks of sobriety. Rehabilitation, the next phase, usually lasts approximately 30 days and involves reorganizing one's life patterns to exclude abuse and finding more healthy and adaptive ways of coping. For those with a lengthy history of substance use and/or early onset of use, the rehabilitation portion of treatment is likely to be longer and much more complex. This process may be augmented by participation in a therapeutic community, which is a less structured but still supportive transitional living arrangement, typically lasting 6 months to 1 year. During the rehabilitation phase, active and aggressive treatment of any comorbid psychiatric illness should be initiated (see Chapter 37). The fifth phase is relapse prevention. Finally, because relapse is very common in this population, rapid response to relapse must be considered as yet another part of treatment.

Traditional outpatient treatment involves the use of frequent diagnosis-specific psychosocial groups—12-step programs such as Alcoholics Anonymous, Narcotics Anonymous, and Cocaine Anonymous—accompanied by more individualized interaction with a personal sponsor. These groups are readily available to patients in almost every community, and they are organized and led by individuals with similar problems who have achieved some period of sobriety. Individuals utilizing this approach ("working the program") have access to a strong support network but remain within their own community (family, employment, and neighborhood). Thus, they often encounter problems when habit patterns have formed around the circumstances and stressors that exist within their home environment—potentially a positive situation if they continue to utilize the resources and skills they are building in the treatment process. These programs often incorporate strong spiritual beliefs into their techniques, and in Western culture, that frequently involves a very Judeo-Christian outlook, which some might find problematic. There are other treatment approaches that rely on totally different mechanisms. Acupuncture is a less traditional outpatient adjunct to reduce cravings and is recognized by the National Institutes of Health (1997), although questions about efficacy have been raised (Margolin, 2002). Cognitive–behavioral therapy (group or individual) has also been used with some success (Roll, 2006). Use of various medications to reduce cravings, block effects of intoxication, and negatively reinforce use is discussed later.

Individuals with long-standing abuse, with physiological dependence (particularly on benzodiazepines, barbiturates, or alcohol, withdrawal from which can be life threatening), with a history of frequent relapses, or with other significant risk factors (including medical illness and pregnancy) may require an inpatient rehab program. Both medical and nonmedical programs are available, with the nonmedical facilities traditionally prohibiting all psychoactive substances, including medications for mental health issues and pain management as well as those to assist in detox. These medications include tapered doses of benzodiazepines, usually long-acting, to safely withdraw from benzodiazepines or alcohol, sometimes with the addition of carbamazepine or gabapentin to prevent seizures; tapering doses of long-acting narcotics along with symptomatic treatment with clonidine and nonsteroidal anti-inflammatory drugs for comfortable detox from narcotic drugs; and antidepressants or clonidine for comfortable withdrawal from cocaine or methamphetamine.

Traditionally, the goal of treatment is sustained abstinence from all drugs of abuse. This involves strategies for relapse prevention, including avoiding prescribing medications that could lead to increased cravings (e.g., judicious use of benzodiazepines), appropriate treatment of pain (a frequent trigger for relapse), careful observation during periods of increased stress, and prompt treatment of mental health issues (New York State Department of Health AIDS Institute, 2009). Even short-term abstinence, however, can

be helpful in stabilizing the individual's life and support network, allowing the body a chance to heal what it can and decreasing the degree of physiological tolerance to a given agent. Psychopharmacological strategies to assist in maintenance of sobriety and relapse prevention include aversive therapy (disulfiram for alcohol abuse), blockade of reinforcement (naltrexone for opioid abuse), drive suppression (bupropion, varenicline, or naltrexone for tobacco abuse; buprenorphine for opiate abuse; and bupropion, modafinil, or baclofen for methamphetamine abuse), substituted addiction (methadone, levo-α-acetylmethadol (LAAM), or buprenorphine for opioid abuse), and tapered addiction (nicotine patch/spray/gum/inhaler for smoking cessation). The treatment regimens for withdrawal and sustained sobriety for specific drugs of abuse are discussed later.

An alternative approach to substance abuse treatment involves establishing a hierarchy of harm reduction. The highest level of harm reduction is, of course, abstinence. In the case of intravenous (IV) drug use, if the patient is not yet ready for total cessation of use, will he or she consider stopping injection use? If not stopping injection, will the patient use new needles and syringes? Will the patient clean needles/syringes with bleach? Will he or she avoid sharing injection equipment with others? Will the patient inject in social environments in which consequences of intoxication are lower (i.e., less risk of unsafe sex while intoxicated)?

SPECIFIC DRUGS OF ABUSE

ALCOHOL

As previously noted, alcohol use/misuse is closely linked to risk behaviors exposing individuals to HIV and other STDs. These risk factors have been shown to increase proportionally with higher consumption of alcohol and decrease with abstinence. The impact of alcohol on these risk factors has been shown to be independent of other drug use (Ruiz, 2007). Treatment strategies for alcohol abuse relate to achievement of sobriety/abstinence.

Medications for achieving and maintaining abstinence have utilized two mechanisms of action, one through blocking the reinforcing effects of intoxication by interfering with reward systems and the other focusing on stabilizing systems that have become deregulated by chronic alcohol use.

Disulfiram (Antabuse)

Originally studied as a possible antiparasitic treatment, this medication was discovered to have aversive effects when used with alcohol. In 1954, the US Food and Drug

Administration (FDA) approved disulfiram for the treatment of alcohol dependence in the United States. Disulfiram causes irreversible inhibition of acetaldehyde dehydrogenase, a key enzyme in the metabolism of alcohol that leads to buildup of acetaldehyde, resulting in very unpleasant symptoms, including nausea, vomiting, tachycardia, headaches, hypertension/hypotension, diaphoresis, flushing, vertigo, dysphoria, and dyspnea—thus the aversive reaction. Disulfiram works best in individuals who are motivated or where abstinence is strictly supervised. Adherence to disulfiram increases with behavioral couples therapy (BCT), which provides contingency for sobriety and increased psychosocial support for positive change. In BCT, couples provide a caring and supportive positive nonjudgmental environment. Meta-analysis of randomized studies of BCT has shown superior results in reducing alcohol use, consequence of use, and integrity relationships with others (O'Farrell, 2000). Disulfiram should be avoided in patients with a history of cardiovascular disease, myocardial infarction (MI), congestive heart failure, and end-stage liver disease. Caution should also be used in patients with a history of psychosis (inhibition of dopamine dehydroxylase results in increased dopamine levels, potentially increasing psychotic symptoms), those with peripheral neuropathy (can be exacerbated), and those taking metronidazole (will trigger aversive side effects). Aversive reactions can occur up to 2 weeks after last dose and can be precipitated by alcohol-containing foods, alcohol over-the-counter medicines, and toiletries. Patients must wait at least 12 hours after last drink before starting disulfiram.

Naltrexone

Naltrexone is a μ-opioid receptor antagonist originally marketed for opioid dependence. In1994, it was approved by the FDA for prevention of heavy alcohol bingeing in those with alcohol dependence. It acts through blockade of naturally occurring opiates (i.e., endorphins and encephalins) released during alcohol consumption, minimizing release of dopamine in the nucleus accumbens and thus blocking the effects of pleasure and reinforcement. This results in decreased craving as well as disruption of the euphoric feelings associated with alcohol intoxication. Naltrexone use is contraindicated in patients with significant liver disease (hepatitis and liver failure), and all patients should have liver function tested prior to initiation of this drug because it may cause liver damage, especially in HIV patients, in whom certain antiviral medications can also impair liver function. Naltrexone should also be avoided in those who are currently going through acute opioid withdrawal.

Patients should be opioid free for a minimum of 7–10 days prior to starting naltrexone because it can precipitate severe opioid withdrawal. Patients should be started first on the short-acting oral formulation, and if able to tolerate it, they may be switched to monthly injections. The medication may initially cause symptoms of dysphoria, which patients often describe as "feeling weird, odd, not right." These symptoms are due to naltrexone's indirect effect on dopamine levels in the nucleus accumbens. Symptoms will eventually subside as neurochemical systems stabilize. Some patients may try to overcome naltrexone μ-receptor blockade by taking large amounts of exogenous opioids, which may lead to life-threatening opioid intoxication.

Acamprosate (Campral)

Acamprosate is an NMDA receptor antagonist that modulates GABA and glutamate activity, resulting in alleviation of negative dysphoric symptoms associated with alcohol abstinence while also decreasing cravings. It is recommended that it be started as soon as possible after alcohol withdrawal and establishment of sobriety and that it should be continued even when relapse occurs. Common side effects include nausea, vomiting, diarrhea, gas, stomach pain, loss of appetite, headache, drowsiness, dizziness, constipation, fatigue, weight gain/loss, muscle/joint pain, change in sexual desire, and decreased sexual ability. Acamprosate carries a warning for possible increase in suicidal behavior. Although many of these events occurred in the context of alcohol relapse, no consistent pattern of relationship between the clinical course of recovery from alcoholism and the emergence of suicidality was identified (Campral/acamprosate product information, Forest Pharmaceuticals). The interrelationship between alcohol dependence, depression, and suicidality is well recognized and complex. All alcohol-dependent patients, including those being treated with this medication, should be monitored for the development of symptoms of depression or suicidal thinking. Families and caregivers of patients being treated with acamprosate should be advised to monitor patients for the emergence of symptoms of depression. This drug is eliminated by kidney and is contraindicated in patients with severe renal impairment. Dosage must be adjusted for patients with less severe renal impairment.

OPIOIDS

Use of opioid-based drugs, particularly IV drug abuse, has long been associated with HIV infection and transmission. The risk has been shown to be even higher in those who also have psychiatric illness. Depression in IV drug users has been linked to increased rates of sharing of needles and other paraphernalia, resulting in a greater risk for HIV infection. It is therefore crucial to treat both the psychological disorders and the behavioral risk factors in IV drug use (Ruiz, 2007).

The degree to which opioids are abused depends on the interaction between each opioid and its receptor (full agonist, partial agonist, or antagonist). Drugs that act as a full agonist (heroin, morphine, codeine, oxycodone, hydrocodone, meperidine, methadone, propoxyphene, fentanyl, and LAAM) have a high likelihood of being abused. They produce positive mood effects (euphoria) as well as physical signs such as myosis, nausea, vomiting, constipation, mental clouding, and decreased libido. Abrupt cessation after sustained use results in withdrawal, with specific symptoms depending on when opioids were last used: Early symptoms (24 hours to 2 weeks) include rhinorrhea, lacrimation, gastrointestinal disturbance, piloerection, insomnia, irritability; late symptoms (2 weeks to 2 years—"late abstinence syndrome") include depressed mood, anhedonia, decreased libido, bone pain, and muscle aches. Overdoses and death are common with IV opioid use because the purity of street drugs is notoriously uneven. Overdoses result in respiratory depression, pinpoint pupils, coma, hypotension, bradycardia, and pulmonary edema.

Initial treatment of opioid dependence consists of a period of detoxification, which can be assisted by use of methadone, buprenorphine, clonidine, and lofexidine, as well as supportive/symptomatic treatments for specific complaints. If rapid detox is necessary, clonidine and naltrexone are generally used. There is also the possibility for "ultra-detoxification," which would involve inpatient care and sedation/anesthesia. Because partial agonist and antagonist agents cause less euphoria, are generally less rewarding, and are generally less abused, they have become a staple of longer term medication treatment for opiate abuse. With the exception of methadone, most of the medications used to treat opioid dependence are from these classes of receptor action.

Methadone

Developed in the 1960s, methadone is a μ-receptor agonist as well as a weak NMDA receptor antagonist, and it has proved to be a very effective treatment for opiate addiction. The use of methadone has been shown to decrease the use of IV opioid drugs and the spread of communicable diseases such as HIV, hepatitis B virus, and hepatitis C virus by modifying behaviors such as IV drug use (Lollis, 2000).

Methadone treatment for opioid dependence is provided in specialized opioid treatment programs (OTPs), which require federal licensing and certification. In addition to supplying methadone to its patients, OTP clinics also give counseling, drug testing, and vocational training/assistance. It is illegal for noncertified health care entities to provide methadone maintenance treatment. Doses are carefully titrated to the needs of the patient. Studies have shown that methadone doses in the range of 20–40 mg/day are effective in suppressing symptoms of withdrawal, but they may not be effective in reducing or stopping symptoms of craving (Strain, 1993a, 1993b).

Unfortunately, there are many issues with the use of methadone in HIV-infected individuals because this medication has many side effects and drug–drug interactions. Methadone prolongs QT/QTc intervals; therefore, close monitoring is required in patients who are taking other QT interval-prolonging drugs. Antiretrovirals known to significantly interfere with methadone serum levels include lopinavir/ritonavir, efavirenz, and nevirapine. Other medications that have been shown to have drug–drug interaction with methadone include the anticonvulsants carbamazepine and phenytoin as well as some antibiotics, such as rifampin. In general, use of these medications should be avoided in patients who are being treated or plan to be treated with methadone. If such medication combinations are required, then methadone doses should be titrated upward to avoid withdrawal symptoms and continue maximized treatment. Methadone has been shown to be safe during pregnancy (especially relative to opioid use or withdrawal) and safe with breast-feeding. Some newborns may experience neonatal abstinence syndrome, which consists of blotchy skin coloring (mottling), diarrhea, high-pitched crying, excessive sucking, fever, hyperactive reflexes, increased muscle tone, irritability, poor feeding, and, in rare cases, seizures.

Buprenorphine (Subutex) and Buprenorphine Plus Naloxone (Suboxone)

Buprenorphine is a partial agonist to the μ-opioid receptor and antagonist at the κ-opioid receptor. When patients are not taking opioids, buprenorphine acts as an agonist, whereas it acts as an antagonist when patients attempt to take opioids. Naloxone is added to reduce the abuse potential of the drug. These medications require special certification for prescription, but they can be prescribed in an office setting. Initial doses are low (regardless of the patient's wish to start at higher dose) to avoid potential side effects—2 or 4 mg is standard, and ideally patients should be in some form of opioid withdrawal. If well tolerated and there are still signs of withdrawal, this dosage can be repeated 1 or 2 hours later. Titration to the target dose (generally 8–16 mg/day, although up to 24 mg/day can be used) is done quickly to minimize patient dropout and withdrawal symptoms. If a patient requires doses greater than 24 mg/day, issues of diversion or misuse must be considered. Suboxone has ceiling effects: Unlike other opioid treatment drugs, it plateaus at a certain dose (32 mg/day), and a higher dose has no therapeutic benefit. Overdose can still occur, resulting in respiratory distress that may require airway management. Other potential side effects include central nervous system depression and hepatitis. Those with a history of traumatic brain injury should be monitored for increased intracranial pressure because all potent opioids may elevate cerebrospinal fluid pressure. Buprenorphine is metabolized by CYP450 3A4 enzyme, and there are several clinically significant drug–drug interactions. Those taking CYP450 3A4 inhibitors such as nefazodone, fluvoxamine, fluoxetine, ketoconazole, intraconazole, erythromycin, clarithromycin, grapefruit juice, and most protease inhibitors (especially ritonavir) should take reduced doses of buprenorphine.

Naltrexone

See the section on alcohol.

COCAINE/CRACK

In addition to the increased incidence of risk behaviors in cocaine abusers, recent studies have shown that cocaine abuse may have broad-ranging effects on human immunity. With regard to HIV infection, in vitro studies have shown that cocaine enhances infection of stimulated lymphocytes. Moreover, cohort studies in the pre- and post-highly active antiretroviral therapy (HAART) era have linked stimulant abuse with increased HIV pathogenesis (Baum, 2009). It is therefore crucial to treat HIV-infected patients with cocaine dependence.

Cocaine blocks dopamine (DA) reuptake at the presynaptic site, thus increasing levels of DA at the nucleus accumbens, resulting in its addictive properties. Cocaine effects depend on the mode of use, with smoked (crack) and IV administration having the quickest effects (seconds to 30 minutes; peak, 15–30 minutes), and intranasal administration having slightly more delayed effects (5–90 minutes; peak, 30 minutes). Mild to moderate intoxication gives sympathomimetic symptoms—generally increased heart rate and blood pressure, decreased appetite, insomnia, euphoria,

hyperalertness, and irritability. With severe intoxication, there is dilation of the pupils, and severe hypertension, hyperthermia, cardiac arrhythmias/MIs, stroke, seizures, coma, and death may occur. At any level of intoxication, there may also be psychiatric symptoms—auditory/visual/tactile hallucinations, delusions, paranoia, and aggression/violence. For patients with severe cocaine intoxication (i.e., malignant HTN, hyperthermia, and seizure), the goal is stabilization of vital signs and the elimination of seizure activities. Patients should be given phentolamine, cooling, and other supportive measures for HTN crisis and hyperthermia; benzodiazepine should be given to prevent seizures and agitation. Antipsychotics may be useful for severe agitation/aggression/psychosis but should be avoid in patient with seizures because neuroleptics may further decrease the seizure threshold.

Research into medications for treating cocaine addiction has failed to show conclusive evidence of effectiveness, but efforts are ongoing. Recent ongoing research has been focused on creating a cocaine vaccine that uses modified cold virus attached to cocaine-like molecules to trigger the body to produce cocaine antibodies. Other promising agents include modafanil, topiramate, and desipramine, which may decrease cocaine craving.

METHAMPHETAMINE

Unlike many of the other drugs of abuse, which tend to be predominate in urban areas, methamphetamine use has grown exponentially in both rural and urban areas during the past few decades. It is an extremely addictive drug that heightens sexual arousal with reduced inhibition and judgment, placing its users at risk of contracting STDs such as HIV. It can be smoked, snorted, injected, or rectally inserted. It is a fairly inexpensive drug with rapid onset and long-lasting high (half-life of 11 or 12 hours). Use increases the release of newly synthesized dopamine, norepinephrine, and serotonin. It is also an indirect catecholamine and 5-HT agonist. Like cocaine, methamphetamine can deplete dopamine stores and lead to significant symptoms of depression and, in some cases, suicide. Other symptoms that may be experienced include psychosis (that may last weeks to months), aggression, thought disorders, and gum disease with long-term use. Acute intoxication of methamphetamine is treated similar to cocaine with phentolamine, cooling, and other supportive measure for hypertension crisis and hyperthermia; benzodiazepine is used to prevent seizures and agitation. Antipsychotics may also be required to control severe aggression/agitation. Addiction is more difficult to treat because there are no current approved FDA medications. Some medications have shown promise, including naltrexone, mirtazapine, and topiramate. Unlike other drugs of its kind, methamphetamine may induce sensitization, which results in enhanced response to the drug because of prior exposure and thus a higher likelihood of overdosing.

ECSTASY OR MOLLY (MDMA)

Dubbed the "intimacy drug," Ecstasy use has been shown to produce profound feelings of closeness, which may lead to high-risk sexual behavior and HIV exposure. Some studies have shown that those using Ecstasy may perceive less danger of contracting HIV and other STDs compared to non-Ecstasy users (Theall, 2006). It is therefore critical that those with HIV and those at higher risk of contracting HIV be educated about the dangers of Ecstasy use in addition to the other known heath issues that may result from Ecstasy use. Currently, there is no FDA-approved medication for treatment of Ecstasy abuse, and acute management is geared toward treating life-threatening conditions such as serotonin syndrome and hyperthermia that are commonly seen in rave parties.

SPECIAL CONSIDERATIONS IN HIV POPULATIONS

Interactions between substances of abuse and antiretroviral (ARV) agents have been reported. The toxicity of amphetamines, MDMA, meperidine, and GHB is dangerously increased by ritonavir, even in boosting doses. Barbiturates induce the cytochrome systems responsible for metabolism of protease inhibitors (PI), non-nucleoside reverse transcriptase inhibitors (NNRTIs), maraviroc, and raltegravir, significantly decreasing their effectiveness. Oral midazolam and triazolam are contraindicated with PIs, NNRTIs, efavirenz, and delavirdine. The toxicity of ketamine and PCP is dangerously increased by PIs, delavirdine, and etravirine.

All the agents listed for use in detox and maintenance of sobriety have utility in the HIV population, but there are special considerations:

- Buprenorphine administration is office based but requires special training and certification. Also, clinically significant interactions occur with ARVs, including delavirdine, amprenavir, atazanavir, darunavir, fosamprenavir, indinavir, ritonavir, and saquinavir (increased buprenorphine activity and sedation—especially with atazanavir), and etravirine, nevirapine, and tipranavir (decreased buprenorphine activity, with tipranavir levels also significantly decreased). Fluconazole can increase the activity of buprenorphine, whereas phenobarbital, phenytoin, rifabutin, and rifampin decrease the effective amounts, sometimes causing withdrawal symptoms.

- Bupropion (used for smoking cessation) decreases the seizure threshold, particularly in patients with weight loss or electrolyte instability.

- Disulfiram (Antabuse) has a high risk of hepatotoxicity and cannot be used with tipranavir/ritonavir capsules (they contain alcohol) or with amprenavir oral solution (decreases metabolism of amprenavir and increases central nervous system and metabolic toxicity). Use in individuals with heart disease is also problematic.

- Methadone maintenance cannot be done outside a registered clinic, and this agent has several clinically significant adverse interactions with ARVs (blood levels of abacavir, didanosine, stavudine, and amprenavir are all decreased; blood level of zidovudine is increased; abacavir and delavirdine increase blood levels of methadone, and dose adjustment may be required to avoid sedation; efavirenz, nevirapine, amprenavir, darunavir, fosamprenavir, lopinavir, ritonavir (even in boosting doses), saquinavir, and tipranavir all decrease methadone availability, with withdrawal symptoms reported in some cases). Drug interactions with other medications frequently used in the HIV population are also reported (carbamazepine, phenobarbital, phenytoin, and rifampin sharply decrease methadone levels, and fluconazole significantly increases methadone blood levels).

- Naltrexone cannot be used in individuals requiring narcotic pain control but does not seem to interact with ARVs.

SUMMARY

Substance use or misuse is common in the HIV population and requires early and aggressive diagnosis and treatment, both to minimize further spread of the disease through ungoverned risk behaviors and to maximize the ability of the individual to fully participate in HIV treatment. Both of these will obviously decrease morbidity and mortality from both conditions. Adequate treatment with decreased substance use can improve adherence to HIV regimens (clinic visits and ARV use) to levels comparable to those seen in non-addicted HIV populations. These principles apply even more stringently in those with "triple diagnosis"—substance abuse, mental illness, and HIV. As with any treatment process, success involves establishing a collaborative alliance—a therapeutic relationship between treatment staff and patient. This sets the stage for honest communication, mutual respect of boundaries, and continued participation in treatment (on both sides) despite temporary setbacks and failures. Integrated treatment of substance abuse and HIV (or substance abuse, HIV, and mental illness in the case of triple diagnosis) offers distinct advantages for these complex cases with multiple barriers to participation. Factors in a decision to start antiretroviral treatment in individuals with active substance abuse are obviously complex, but substance use alone should not be an absolute contraindication to HAART.

Recommended Reading

Ruiz P, Strain EC. Alcohol abstinence pharmacotherapy treatment. In *The Substance Abuse Handbook*. Philadelphia: Lippincott Williams & Wilkins; 2014.

Ruiz P, Strain EC. Amphetamines and other stimulants. In: *The Substance Abuse Handbook*. Philadelphia: Lippincott Williams & Wilkins; 2014.

Ruiz P, Strain EC. Buprenorphine treatment. In: *The Substance Abuse Handbook*. Philadelphia: Lippincott Williams & Wilkins; 2014.

Ruiz P, Strain EC. Cocaine and crack. In: *The Substance Abuse Handbook*. Philadelphia: Lippincott Williams & Wilkins; 2014.

Ruiz P, Strain EC. Methadone maintenance treatment. In: *The Substance Abuse Handbook*. Philadelphia: Lippincott Williams & Wilkins; 2014.

Ruiz P, Strain EC. Naltrexone and other pharmacotherapies for opioid dependence. In: *The Substance Abuse Handbook*. Philadelphia: Lippincott Williams & Wilkins; 2014.

References

American Psychiatric Association. *Diagnostic and Statistical Manual of Mental Disorders*, 5th ed. Washington, DC: APA Press; 2013.

Baum MK, Rafie C, Lai S, et al. Crack-cocaine use accelerates HIV disease progression in a cohort of HIV-positive drug users. *J Acquir Immune Defici Syndr*. 2009; 50(1):93–99.

Brown RL, Rounds LA. Conjoint screening questionnaires for alcohol and other drug abuse: Criterion validity in primary practice. *Wis Med J*. 1995; 94:135–140.

Campral (Acamprosate calcium) delayed release tablets [product information]. Forest Pharmaceuticals, St. Louis, MO, 2004.

Catz SL, Kelly JA, Bogart LM, et al. Patterns, correlates, and barriers to medication adherence among persons prescribed new treatments for HIV disease. *Health Psychol*. 2000; 19:124–133.

Cofrancesco J Jr, Scherzer R, Tien PC, et al. Illicit drug use and HIV treatment outcomes in a US cohort. *AIDS*. 2008; 22:237–245.

Cyr MG, Wartman SA. The effectiveness of routine screening in the detection of alcoholism. *JAMA*. 1988; 259:51–54.

DeLorenze GN, Weisner C, Tsai AL, et al. Excess mortality among HIV-infected patients diagnosed with substance use dependence or abuse receiving care in a fully-integrated medical care program. *Alcohol Clin Exp Res*. 2011; 35:203–210.

Friedman H, Klein T, Sperter S, et al. Drugs of abuse and virus susceptibility. *Adv Biochem Psychopharmacol*. 1988; 44:125–137.

Goedert JJ. Recreational drugs: Relationship to AIDS. *Ann N Y Acad Sci*. 1984; 437:192–199.

Hillfors DD, Iritani BJ, Miller WC, et al. Sexual and drug behavior patterns and HIV and STD racial disparities: The need for new directions. *Am J Public Health*. 2007; 97(1):125–132.

Lollis CM, Strothers HS, et al. Sex, drugs and HIV: Does methadone maintenance reduce drug use and risky sexual behavior? *J Behav Med*. 2000, 23; 6:545–557.

Mackesy-Amiti ME, Fendrich M, Johnson TP. Symptoms of substance dependence and risky sexual behavior in a probability sample of HIV negative men who have sex with men in Chicago. *Drug Alcohol Dependence*. 2010; 110(1–2):38–43.

Margolin A, Avants SK, Holford TR. Interpreting conflicting findings from clinical trials of auricular acupuncture for cocaine addiction: Does treatment context influence outcome? *J Altern Complement Med*. 2002; 8:111–121.

Millett GA, Flores SA, Bakeman R. Explaining disparities in HIV infection among Black and White men who have sex with men: A meta-analysis of HIV risk behaviors. *AIDS*. 2007; 21(15):2083–2091.

Moore RM, Gebo KA, Lucas GM, et al. Rate of co-morbidities not related to HIV infection or AIDS among HIV-infected patients by CD4 count and HAART use status. *Clin Infect Dis*. 2008; 47(8):1102–1104.

National Institutes of Health. Acupuncture. *NIH Consensus Statement*. 1997; 15:1–34.

New York State Department of Health AIDS Institute. *Substance Use in Patients with HIV/AIDS*. Albany, NY: New York State Department of Health; 2009.

Newell GR, Mansell PW, Spitz MR, et al. Volatile nitrites: Use and adverse effects related to the current epidemic of the acquired immune deficiency syndrome. *Am J Med*. 1985; 78(5):811–816.

O'Farrell TJ, William-Fals S. Behavioral couples therapy for alcoholism and drug abuse. *J Substance Abuse Treatment* 2000; 18:51–54.

Palepu A, Milloy MJ, Derr T, et al. Homelessness and adherence to antiretroviral therapy among a cohort of HIV-infected injection drug users. *J Urban Health*. 2011; 88(3):545–555.

Roll JM, Petry NM, Stitzer ML, et al. Contingency management for the treatment of methamphetamine use disorders. *Am J Psychiatry*. 2006; 163:1993–1999.

Ruiz P, Strain EC. Psychiatric complications of HIV-1 infection and drug abuse. In: *The Substance Abuse Handbook*. Philadelphia: Lippincott Williams & Wilkins; 2014.

Semples SJ, Strathdee SA, Zians J, et al. Sexual risk behavior associated with co-administration of methamphetamine and other drugs in a sample of HIV-positive men who have sex with men. *Am J Addict*. 2009; 18:65–72.

Smith PC, Schmidt SM, Allensworth-Davies D, et al. Primary care validation of a single-question alcohol screening test. *J Gen Intern Med*. 2009; 24:783–788.

Strain EC, Stitzer ML, Lisbon IA, et al. Dose–response effects of methadone in the treatment of opioid dependence. *Ann Intern Med*. 1993a; 119:23–27.

Strain EC, Stitzer ML, Lisbon IA, et al. Methadone dose and treatment outcome. *Drug Alcohol Depend* 1993b; 33:105–117.

Substance Abuse and Mental Health Services Administration. National Survey of Substance Abuse Treatment Services: The N-SSATS report. February 25, 2010.

Sullivan LE, Goulet JL, Justice AC, et al. Alcohol consumption and depressive symptoms over time: A longitudinal study of patients with and without HIV infection. *Drug Alcohol Depend.* 2011; 117:158–163.

Theall KP, Elifson KW, Sterk CE. Sex, touch, and HIV risk among Ecstasy users. *AIDS Behav.* 2006; 10(2):169–178.

Vallecillo G, Sanvisens A, Martinez E, et al. Use of highly active antiretroviral therapy is increasing in HIV-positive severe drug users. *Curr HIV Res.* 2010; 8(8):641–648.

Willenbring ML, Gardner MB. Helping patients who drink too much: An evidence-based guide for primary care clinicians. *Am Fam Phys.* 2009; 80:44–50.

31.

UNDERSTANDING THE USE OF ANTIRETROVIRAL DRUGS IN THE AGING PATIENT

Brandon H. Samson and James D. Scott

CHAPTER GOAL

Identify the growing relevance of long-term antiretroviral use in geriatric populations and be able to apply treatment strategies involving antiretroviral use for this population.

CHAPTER OBJECTIVES

After reading the chapter, the reader will be able to

- discuss the course of HIV disease in people older than age 50 years;

- list treatment issues that are of greater concern in older people with HIV;

- discuss the outcomes of clinical trials focused on older people with HIV; and

- discuss the factors that make drug–drug interactions more complicated in older people with HIV.

WHAT'S NEW?

In addition to a brief discussion on pharmacokinetic and pharmacodynamic considerations for the aging patient, this chapter includes discussion and recommendations based on the availability of treatment considerations from the HIV and Aging Consensus Project and the US Department of Health and Human Services (DHHS). Recent HIV studies pertaining to the geriatric population are also included, as well as information on a recent US Food and Drug Administration (FDA)-approved drug therapy.

KEY POINTS

- Treatment of HIV in aging patients is based on the consideration of adverse effects associated by antiretroviral therapy (ART) with regard to renal, hepatic, cardiovascular, metabolic, and bone health as well as the potential for increased drug–drug interactions.

- The effect of ART on cardiovascular disease (CVD) risk is mediated by the underlying cardiovascular risk associated with HIV infection; hence, ART is not guaranteed to reduce the risk of CVD.

- Certain antiretroviral agents (notably tenofovir disoproxil fumarate) are associated with nephrotoxicity, so monitoring of renal function is crucial, especially in patients also receiving additional nephrotoxic agents.

- Multiple classes of antiretroviral agents are associated with hepatotoxicity, and certain agents have such a severe degree of liver injury that they are no longer recommended as preferred agents by guidelines.

- ART is associated with decreased bone mineral density, with a variable amount of bone loss being a consistent feature of all agents used for initial treatment.

- Health care providers should routinely review patients' medication lists to search for significant drug–drug interactions (DDIs) and perform drug interaction checks using available resources.

INTRODUCTION

In 2012, people aged 55 years old or older represented roughly 25% of the estimated 1.2 million people living with

HIV infection in the United States at the time, with this population more likely to be diagnosed with HIV later in the course of their disease (Centers for Disease Control and Prevention (CDC), 2015). Often, health care providers and older people mistake the presence/progression of HIV with the normal aging process, especially because both involve chronic inflammation and activation of the immune system (Nasi, 2014). This presents a unique challenge to health care providers because they must balance optimal ART selection with additional noncommunicable diseases/comorbidities, DDIs, renal and/or hepatic function, and the increased likelihood of ART-associated events. There is currently a paucity of clinical trials, systematic reviews, and guidelines available to assist health care providers in safe and appropriate decision-making for the geriatric HIV population. Nevertheless, the significance of patients living longer while on ART cannot be ignored.

Although the association between long-term antiretroviral exposure and increased toxicity is less apparent, there is evidence that older age is significantly associated with higher viral load at diagnosis and, consequently, faster CD4 cell count decline (Grabar, 2004; Winston, 2015). Because ART is associated with both beneficial and deleterious effects, health care providers should weigh the negative effects against the positive effects of viral suppression (Guaraldi, 2014). Unfortunately, there is a lack of data on the long-term safety of specific antiretroviral (ARV) drugs in older patients, with recommendations for older patients based on the adverse effects of therapy based on renal, hepatic, cardiovascular, metabolic, and bone health (DHHS, 2012). In the absence of information about the pharmacokinetic effects of long-term antiretroviral use in HIV-infected individuals older than age 60 years, the following section presents important practice-related considerations regarding antiretroviral use in geriatric populations (Schoen, 2013).

METABOLIC COMPLICATIONS ASSOCIATED WITH ANTIRETROVIRAL THERAPY

Prior to ART that was FDA approved after 2009, ARVs associated with lipodystrophy were predictive of atherosclerotic lesions in HIV patients. Although newer drugs have a more lipid-friendly profile from a metabolic standpoint, this benefit does not necessarily translate into a guaranteed CVD risk reduction in HIV-infected patients because the effect of ART on CVD risk is mediated by the underlying cardiovascular risk associated with HIV infection. As an additional consideration, an initial ritonavir-boosted protease inhibitor-based regimen should be avoided in individuals with diabetes mellitus or hyperinsulinemia if possible (Abrass, 2012). For further information on these topics, see Chapter 41 (cardiovascular disease), Chapter 46 (lipodystrophy and lipoatrophy), and Chapter 47 (dyslipidemia).

RENAL COMPLICATIONS ASSOCIATED WITH ANTIRETROVIRAL THERAPY

Based on studies showing preservation of renal function associated with ART, possible improvement in renal function, and declining renal function during treatment interruption, optimal ART can prevent the development or stop the progression of HIV-associated nephropathy. However, certain antiretroviral agents (notably tenofovir disoproxyl fumarate) are associated with nephrotoxicity, so monitoring of renal function is crucial, especially in patients also receiving additional nephrotoxic agents (Hall, 2011). For additional information on effective renal dosing, the DHHS guidelines provide a valuable reference for medication dosing in settings involving renal or hepatic dysfunction. Clinical data for a newer formulation of tenofovir (tenofovir alafenamide, currently approved in single-tablet co-formulated combination with elvitegravir, cobicistat, and emtricitabine as Genvoya (Gilead Sciences, Redwood City, CA)) show smaller increases in serum creatinine and decreases in estimated glomerular filtration rate compared to those with tenofovir disoproxyl fumarate and, accordingly, lower creatinine clearance cut-offs for treatment initiation (Zolopa, 2013; Sax, 2015). For further information on this topic, see Chapter 42.

HEPATOTOXICITY ASSOCIATED WITH ANTIRETROVIRAL THERAPY

Multiple classes of antiretroviral agents are associated with hepatotoxicity, and certain agents have such a severe degree of liver injury that they are no longer recommended as preferred agents by guidelines (e.g., didanosine associated with noncirrhotic portal hypertension and stavudine associated with increased frequency of acute liver injury) (Chang, 2012; Clark, 2002). The 2012 World Health Organization (WHO) guidelines on the use of antiretroviral drugs for treating and preventing HIV infection included recommendations to progressively reduce the use of stavudine due to well-recognized toxicities, including lipoatrophy, peripheral neuropathy, and lactic acidosis (WHO, 2012).

With regard to currently relevant antiretroviral agents in use (most notably protease inhibitors), hepatotoxicity may occur some months after commencing treatment. Further hepatic deterioration may also result in impaired drug elimination and drug accumulation. For further information on this topic, see Chapter 39.

EFFECTS ON BONE AND VITAMIN D ASSOCIATED WITH ANTIRETROVIRAL THERAPY

ART is associated with decreased bone mineral density, with a variable amount of bone loss a consistent feature of all agents used for initial treatment. This is believed to be caused by a decrease in bone turnover as ART reduces viral load and increases inflammatory cytokines. In addition, certain agents (efavirenz and zidovudine) can also affect vitamin D levels. For patients with known risk factors for osteoporosis, long-term concurrent use of proton pump inhibitors or corticosteroids should be avoided if possible. For further information on this topic, see Chapter 45.

CENTRAL NERVOUS SYSTEM/NERVOUS SYSTEM TOXICITY ASSOCIATED WITH ANTIRETROVIRAL THERAPY

Antiretroviral therapy, most notably efavirenz, may be associated with neurocognitive/psychiatric complications. Peripheral neuropathy can also be associated with combination ART but less so with current regimens. In the absence of further available recommendations, caution should be exercised in individual clinical situations. For further information on this topic, see Chapter 38.

DRUG–DRUG INTERACTIONS/ MEDICATION FATIGUE ASSOCIATED WITH ANTIRETROVIRAL THERAPY

Although health care providers should communicate the critical need for adherence to ART, they must also be aware of common DDIs among older patients. There are many drug interaction studies documenting significant DDIs between antiretroviral drugs and medications that are commonly prescribed in older patients, but the majority of these pharmacokinetic studies were conducted in young, healthy volunteers who were not HIV-infected. As a result, these studies may not be generalizable to older HIV-infected patients. Health care providers should routinely review patients' medication lists to search for significant DDIs

and perform drug interaction checks using available online resources (e.g., http://www.hiv-druginteractions.org), the DHHS guidelines for the use of antiretroviral agents, or the CDC/National Institutes of Health guidelines for the prevention and treatment of opportunistic infections (Nachega, 2012).

STUDIES INVESTIGATING ANTIRETROVIRAL MEDICATION RESPONSE IN OLDER HIV-POSITIVE PATIENTS

- A post-hoc analysis evaluating potential differences in efficacy and safety in older (≥50 years) versus younger (<50 years) patients from the ECHO and THRIVE trials revealed similar virologic response rates between older (77%) and younger (76%) patients on rilpivirine and numerically higher response rates in older (84%) versus younger (76%) patients on efavirenz (EFV) (Ryan, 2013). No clinically relevant age-related differences were observed in immunologic responses. Minor differences were noted in older versus younger patients with regard to adverse events (higher rates of depression, insomnia, and rash in older EFV-treated patients), laboratory abnormalities (increased low-density lipoprotein cholesterol and hyperglycemia in older EFV-treated patients and increased amylase in older patients across treatments), bone mineral density (larger decreases in older patients across treatments), and progression to severe vitamin D deficiency (greater in older vs. younger EFV-treated patients).

- In a national, retrospective cohort analysis of 161 patients ≥50 years old when they first began combination ART (112 starting with emtricitabine (FTC)/tenofovir disoproxil fumarate (TDF) and 49 with other nucleotide reverse transcriptase inhibitors), use of FTC/TDF was generally safe and effective without any statistically significant differences between FTC/TDF and non-FTC/TDF users for any output except persistence (log rank 0.001; adjusted hazard ratio, 2.10; 95% confidence interval, 1.34–3.29) (Blanco, 2013). In this study, the authors defined persistence as the duration during which a patient remains on a prescribed therapy.

- In a study that enrolled 12,196 eligible patients, immunologic response decreased with increasing age (age groups: 18 to <30 years: reference; 30 to

<40 years: adjusted hazard odds ratio (aHOR), 0.92 (0.85, 1.00); 40 to <50 years: aHOR, 0.85 (0.78, 0.92); 50 to <60 years: aHOR, 0.82 (0.74, 0.90); and >60 years: aHOR, 0.74 (0.65, 0.85)), and this relationship was independent of the antiretroviral regimen (Althoff, 2010).

- The COHERE study enrolled 49,921 antiretroviral-naive patients who started ART from 1998 to 2006 with the objective of measuring virological and immunological response by age (COHERE Study Group, 2008). The probability of virologic response was higher in those aged 50–54 years (adjusted hazard ratio, 1.24), 55–59 years (1.24), and 60 years or older (1.18), but the probability of immunologic response in subjects aged 60 years or older was 7% less (0.93 (0.87–0.98)). After adjusting for the latest $CD4^+$ T cell count as a time-updated covariate, the risk of AIDS remained higher in those aged 55–59 years and 60 years or older (55–59 years: 1.18 (1.05–1.34); 60 years or older: 1.32 (1.17–1.48)).

- Additional supporting data are available from a retrospective cohort analysis of HIV-positive patients being treated throughout Kaiser Permanente California in which virologic and immunologic outcomes were measured and stratified by age group in a retrospective analysis of 5090 patients (Silverberg, 2007). Patients older than 50 years were more likely to achieve an undetectable viral load compared to younger patients, but this age effect disappeared when antiretroviral adherence was controlled for. In contrast, younger patients had a higher probability of achieving a greater increase in $CD4^+$ cells (131.8 cells/µl/year) than patients older than 50 years (111.8 cells/µl/year; $p = 0.046$). This effect was most pronounced during the first year of ART. A greater risk for increased serum creatinine and lower hemoglobin concentrations was also noted for patients older than 50 years.

- The mean time to undetectable viral loads was shorter in older patients (>50 years) compared to younger patients (<40 years), with a mean time to undetectable of 3.2 months versus 4.4 months, respectively ($p = 0.001$) (Greenbaum, 2008). In this study, no differences were noted in either age group with regard to immunologic response. Unfortunately, older patients also had a shorter

survival time and an overall higher mortality compared to younger patients, with both of these outcomes being statistically significant.

ACKNOWLEDGMENT

The authors of this chapter acknowledge the author of this chapter in the 2012 edition, Dr. Ian McNicholl, for the portions of his work that have endured in this version.

Recommended Reading

Abrass CK, Appelbaum JS, Boyd CM, et al. Summary report from the Human Immunodeficiency Virus and Aging Consensus Project: Treatment strategies for clinicians managing older individuals with the human immunodeficiency virus. *J Am Geriatr Soc.* 2012 May; 60(5):974–979.

Nachega JB, Hsu AJ, Uthman OA, et al. Antiretroviral therapy adherence and drug–drug interactions in the aging HIV population. *AIDS.* 2012 Jul 31; 26(Suppl 1):S39–S53.

US Department of Health and Human Services. HIV and the older patient. January 28, 2016. Available at https://aidsinfo.nih.gov/guidelines/html/1/adult-and-adolescent-arv-guidelines/277/hiv-and-the-older-patient.

References

Abrass CK, Appelbaum JS, Boyd CM, et al. Summary report from the Human Immunodeficiency Virus and Aging Consensus Project: Treatment strategies for clinicians managing older individuals with the human immunodeficiency virus. *J Am Geriatr Soc.* 2012 May; 60(5):974–979.

Althoff KN, Gebo KA, Gange SJ, et al. HYPERLINK "https://www.ncbi.nlm.nih.gov/pubmed/21159161" CD4 count at presentation for HIV care in the United States and Canada: are those over 50 years more likely to have a delayed presentation? *AIDS Res Ther.* 2010 Dec 15; 7:45.

Blanco JR, Caro-Murillo AM, Castaño MA, et al. HYPERLINK "https://www.ncbi.nlm.nih.gov/pubmed/24144897" Safety, efficacy, and persistence of emtricitabine/tenofovir versus other nucleoside analogues in naive subjects aged 50 years or older in Spain: the TRIP study. *HIV Clin Trials.* 2013 Sep–Oct; 14(5):204–215.

Centers for Disease Control and Prevention. HIV among people aged 50 and over. October 2015. Available at http://www.cdc.gov/hiv/group/age/olderamericans/index.html.

Chang HM, Tsai HC, Lee SS, et al. Noncirrhotic portal hypertension associated with didanosine: A case report and literature review. *Jpn J Infect Dis.* 2012; 65(1):61–65.

Clark SJ, Creighton S, Portmann B, et al. Acute liver failure associated with antiretroviral treatment for HIV: A report of six cases. *J Hepatol.* 2002 Feb; 36(2):295–301.

Grabar S, Kousignian I, Sobel A, et al. Immunologic and clinical responses to highly active antiretroviral therapy over 50 years of age: Results from the French Hospital Database on HIV. *AIDS.* 2004; 18(15):2029–2038.

Greenbaum AH, Wilson LE, Keruly JC, et al. HYPERLINK "https://www.ncbi.nlm.nih.gov/pubmed/18981772" Effect of age and

HAART regimen on clinical response in an urban cohort of HIV-infected individuals. *AIDS*. 2008 Nov 12; 22(17):2331–2339.

Guaraldi G, Prakash M, Moecklinghoff C, et al. Morbidity in older HIV-infected patients: Impact of long-term antiretroviral use. *AIDS Rev*. 2014 Apr–Jun; 16(2):75–89.

Hall A, Hendry B, Nitsch D, et al. Tenofovir-associated kidney toxicity in HIV-infected patients: A review of the evidence. *Am J Kidney Dis*. 2011; 57:773–780.

Nachega JB, Hsu AJ, Uthman OA, et al. Antiretroviral therapy adherence and drug–drug interactions in the aging HIV population. *AIDS*. 2012 Jul 31; 26(Suppl 1):S39–S53.

Nasi M, Pinti M, De Biasi S, et al. Aging with HIV infection: A journey to the center of inflammAIDS, immunosenescence and neuroHIV. *Immunol Lett*. 2014 Nov; 162(1 Pt B):329–333.

Ryan R, Dayaram YK, Schaible D, et al. HYPERLINK "https://www.ncbi.nlm.nih.gov/pubmed/24467642" Outcomes in older versus younger patients over 96 weeks in HIV-1-infected patients treated with rilpivirine or efavirenz in ECHO and THRIVE. *Curr HIV Res*. 2013 Oct; 11(7):570–575.

Sax PE, Wohl D, Yin MT, et al. Tenofovir alafenamide versus tenofovir disoproxil fumarate, coformulated with elvitegravir, cobicistat, and emtricitabine, for initial treatment of HIV-1 infection: Two randomised, double-blind, phase 3, non-inferiority trials. *Lancet*. 2015 Jun 27; 385(9987):2606–2615.

Schoen JC, Erlandson KM, Anderson PL. Clinical pharmacokinetics of antiretroviral drugs in older persons. *Expert Opin Drug Metab Toxicol*. 2013 May; 9(5):573–588.

Silverberg MJ, Leyden W, Horberg MA, et al. Ol HYPERLINK "https://www.ncbi.nlm.nih.gov/pubmed/17420427" der age and the response to and tolerability of antiretroviral therapy. *Arch Intern Med*. 2007 Apr 9; 167(7):684–691.

US Department of Health and Human Services. HIV and the older patient. March 2012. Available at https://aidsinfo.nih.gov/guidelines/html/1/adult-and-adolescent-arv-guidelines/277/hiv-and-the-older-patient.

Winston A, Underwood J. Emerging concepts on the use of antiretroviral therapy in older adults living with HIV infection. *Curr Opin Infect Dis*. 2015 Feb; 28(1):17–22.

World Health Organization. Phasing out stavudine: Progress and challenges. Available at http://www.who.int/hiv/pub/guidelines/arv2013/arv2013supplement_to_chapter09.pdf.

Zolopa A, Sax PE, DeJesus E, et al. HYPERLINK "https://www.ncbi.nlm.nih.gov/pubmed/23392460" A randomized double-blind comparison of coformulated elvitegravir/cobicistat/emtricitabine/tenofovir disoproxil fumarate versus efavirenz/emtricitabine/tenofovir disoproxil fumarate for initial treatment of HIV-1 infection: analysis of week 96 results. *J Acquir Immune Defic Syndr*. 2013 May 1; 63(1):96–100.

32.

OPPORTUNISTIC INFECTIONS

Ben J. Barnett, Lisa Armitige, and Karen J. Vigil

TIMING OF ANTIRETROVIRAL THERAPY INITIATION AND IMPACT ON OPPORTUNISTIC INFECTIONS

LEARNING OBJECTIVES

- Describe the issues concerning starting antiretroviral therapy (ART) in the setting of an opportunistic infection.

- Summarize the recommendations for starting antiretroviral therapy (ART) in the setting of an opportunistic infection.

WHAT'S NEW?

Data and guidelines on starting ART in patients with cryptococcal meningitis.

KEY POINTS

- Early initiation of ART was associated with a decrease in AIDS progression or death in the ACTG A5164 trial.

- Early initiation of ART near the time of starting treatment for an opportunistic infection should be considered for most patients, with the possible exception of patients with cryptococcal meningitis.

INTRODUCTION

The question of when to initiate ART in the setting of an acute or ongoing opportunistic infection (OI) has been controversial. On the one hand, the immediate initiation of ART in the presence of an OI may provide better clinical outcomes as the immune system improves. On the other hand, rapidly decreasing HIV viral load has been associated

with the immune reconstitution inflammatory syndrome (IRIS), which may lead to further complications in the setting of an OI. There are also questions of increasing pill burden, potential drug–drug interactions, additive toxicity and adverse events, and the more practical problem of continuity of care if ART is started in a hospital setting for a newly diagnosed patient with HIV, without established outpatient care already in place. This problem could be particularly troublesome for patients who do not have health insurance or otherwise do not have affordable access to ART in the outpatient setting.

Some conditions associated with severe immunosuppression, such as HIV encephalopathy or HIV-associated nephropathy, do not have adequate treatment other than ART. For these patients, the only way to improve the condition is by starting ART, so it makes sense to start ART immediately. However, for OIs such as *Pneumocystis jirovecii* pneumonia (PCP) or *Cryptococcus neoformans* meningitis, targeted antimicrobial treatment is available to stabilize the condition, and the patient can improve in the absence of ART. It is for these patients that controversy has existed about the optimal time to start ART.

CLINICAL TRIAL RESULTS

AIDS Clinical Trials Group (ACTG) study A5164 was designed to address the question of the optimal timing of ART initiation for individuals presenting with AIDS-defining OIs or serious bacterial infections (BIs) for which effective antimicrobial therapies were available. This was a randomized, open-label strategy trial to evaluate early (defined as within 14 days of starting acute OI treatment) versus deferred (given after OI treatment is completed) initiation of ART in patients starting treatment of acute OIs or BIs, using clinical and virologic end points at 48 weeks. Results of this study were published in 2009 (Zolopa, 2009). A total of 282 patients were evaluable, with 141 in each arm. Most study participants were from racial/ethnic minority groups (73%) and male (85%), with a median age of 38 years, median CD4+ cell count of 29 cells/ml, and a median HIV RNA of 5.07 log₁₀ copies/ml. The most common entry OIs included PCP (63%), cryptococcal meningitis (12%), and BIs (12%). ART was initiated a mean of 12 days after starting OI treatment in the "early" arm and a mean of 45 days after OI treatment in the "deferred" arm.

The study found a decrease in the number of study patients with AIDS progression or death in the early treatment arm (14.2%) compared to the deferred arm (24.1%), which was a statistically significant result (odds ratio, 0.51; 95% confidence interval, 0.27–0.94). The time to AIDS progression or death was also longer in the early treatment arm, again a statistically significant result. The impact of these differences was seen most prominently in the first 6 months after the OI. The number of adverse events was not different in the two arms, and IRIS was reported in 8 subjects in the early arm and 12 subjects in the deferred arm. Based on these data, it appears that early initiation of ART during treatment for an acute OI or serious bacterial infection is beneficial if there are no major contraindications to doing so. A cost-effectiveness analysis, supportive of this early treatment strategy, has also been published (Sax, 2010).

The overall rates of IRIS in A5164 were lower than some rates observed in previous retrospective trials. This was possibly because of the types of the OIs in this study (largely PCP) and because patients with *Mycobacterium tuberculosis* infection were excluded from entry due to the fact that it was the subject of a separate trial. Factors that were found to be associated with IRIS in A5164 were the presence of fungal infections (*Cryptococcus* or *Histoplasma*), lower baseline CD4+ cell counts, and higher baseline HIV RNA levels. IRIS was also associated with higher CD4+ cell counts and lower HIV RNA levels while on ART. Early initiation of ART did not increase the incidence of IRIS in this study.

However, recommendations regarding the timing of starting ART specifically in the setting of meningitis due to *C. neoformans* have been more complex. A study on IRIS related to meningitis caused by *C. neoformans* was published in 2009 (Sungkanuparph, 2009). Although this study of 101 patients employed a different methodology than ACTG 5164, it also found no association between the timing of ART initiation and the diagnosis of IRIS. Rather, it found that an increased baseline serum cryptococcal antigen titer was a risk factor for IRIS. In contrast, a study of 54 patients in Zimbabwe showed early initiation of ART (within 72 hours of diagnosis) in patients with cryptococcal meningitis versus delayed initiation (after 10 weeks of treatment with fluconazole alone) was associated with increased mortality in that setting, in which the

optimal management of increased intracranial pressure may not be available (Makadzange, 2010). Furthermore, a 2014 study of 177 patients from Uganda and South Africa who had cryptococcal meningitis reported increased mortality (hazard ratio, 1.73) at 26 weeks for patients who started ART within 1 or 2 weeks compared to those who had deferral of ART for 5 weeks (Boulware, 2014). Patients in the early group started ART a median of 8 days after antifungal therapy, and patients in the deferred group started ART at a median of 36 days. Most of the increase in mortality was observed within the first 8–30 days of the study. The differences in mortality were especially pronounced in patients who had cerebrospinal fluid (CSF) white blood cell (WBC) counts of <5 cells/μl. Although it was unclear if the increase in mortality in this study was due to progression of cryptococcal disease or IRIS, recommendations regarding the timing of ART in the presence of cryptococcal meningitis have been recently revised (discussed later).

Implementation of the findings of A5164 and similar studies may prove difficult in practice, particularly in settings in which patients may not have existing linkage to primary care and limited access to ongoing treatment with ART after the resolution of the acute OI. However, effective implementation of early ART was accomplished and published by an academic medical center, and this may be a model for bringing early ART to a "real-world" population (Geng, 2011).

RECOMMENDATIONS OF GUIDELINES

The guidelines for prevention and treatment of OIs in HIV-infected adults and adolescents were updated from 2013 to 2015 and are available in the latest form online (US Department of Health and Human Services (DHHS), 2015). These guidelines provide recommendations regarding the timing of initiation of ART in the setting of specific opportunistic conditions, and they should be referenced for guidance in the treatment of patients with those conditions. These guidelines generally reiterate the findings of A5164 suggesting that unless contraindications are present, early initiation of ART near the time of treatment of an OI should be considered for most patients with an acute OI. Other elements that should be considered are degree of immunosuppression, availability of treatment for the OI, drug–drug interactions and overlapping toxicities, and the risk and potential consequences of IRIS.

In many instances, it is recommended that ART should be started as soon as possible. These conditions include progressive multifocal leukoencephalopathy (caused by the John Cunningham (JC) virus), cryptosporidiosis, microsporidiosis, and fungal infections other than meningitis caused by *C. neoformans*. For PCP and invasive BIs, the guidelines recommend starting ART within 2 weeks of diagnosis, although the panel notes that no patients with respiratory failure requiring mechanical ventilation were enrolled in study A5164. For *Toxoplasma gondii* encephalitis, the panel cites expert opinion to start ART within 2 or 3 weeks. For disseminated *Mycobacterium avium* complex, the panel cites expert opinion to consider starting ART after the first 2 weeks of antimycobacterial therapy in order to decrease the overall initial pill burden and also decrease the possibility for IRIS. For cytomegalovirus (CMV) retinitis, the panel notes that many experts would not delay ART for more than 2 weeks after the start of CMV-specific treatment.

Last, regarding cryptococcal meningitis, the panel notes that it would be prudent to defer ART at least until the initial 2-week antifungal induction is complete and possibly until the completion of the consolidation phase at 10 weeks, especially if the patient has increased intracranial pressure or a low CSF WBC count. The panel also notes that if ART is started prior to 10 weeks of antifungal treatment, then the clinician should be prepared to promptly investigate and treat manifestations of IRIS, including increased intracranial pressure.

CONCLUSION

Although substantial barriers to early initiation of ART in the setting of an acute OI exist, the weight of the available evidence falls on the side of starting ART as soon as possible for most patients with acute OIs and invasive BIs, with the notable exception of meningitis due to *C. neoformans*.

Recommended Reading

Boulware DR, Meya DB, Muzoora C, et al. Timing of antiretroviral therapy after diagnosis of cryptococcal meningitis. *N Engl J Med* 2014 Jun 26; 370(26):2487–2498.

Zolopa A, Andersen J, Powderly W, et al. Early antiretroviral therapy reduces AIDS progression/death in individuals with acute opportunistic infections: A multicenter randomized strategy trial. *PLoS One.* 2009; 4(5):e5575.

MYCOBACTERIAL INFECTIONS

LEARNING OBJECTIVE

Discuss the available tests and treatment modalities to appropriately manage patients with HIV and infection with *M. tuberculosis, M. avium* complex, and *Mycobacterium kansasii*, the most common mycobacterial diseases associated with HIV infection.

KEY POINTS

- HIV infection markedly increases the likelihood of a patient progressing from latent tuberculosis infection (LTBI) to active TB disease.

- Interferon-γ release assays (IGRAs) increase specificity but not sensitivity over tuberculin skin testing in the diagnosis of TB in HIV-infected patients.

- Rifamycins are a critical component of effective TB therapy in HIV patients but have many drug–drug interactions.

- *Mycobacterium avium* complex (MAC) disease most commonly presents as disseminated disease with fever, night sweats, weight loss, and gastrointestinal symptoms.

- Optimal treatment of MAC disease should include medications for both MAC and HIV (to reconstitute the immune system).

- MAC should be treated with multidrug therapy, including clarithromycin and ethambutol optimally.

- Individuals with a CD4 count <50 cells/mm³ should receive chemoprophylaxis for MAC with azithromycin or clarithromycin once they have been ruled out for active disease.

- *Mycobacterium kansasii* infection closely resembles TB with more frequent pulmonary presentation than MAC.

- First-line antituberculosis drugs (except for pyrazinamide) are highly effective against *M. kansasii*.

- Diagnosis and treatment of *M. kansasii* as outlined in the American Thoracic Society guidelines are the same for HIV-infected and -uninfected individuals.

MYCOBACTERIUM TUBERCULOSIS

Epidemiology

There were 9.6 million cases of TB worldwide in 2014; 1.2 million of these cases (~12%) were in HIV-positive individuals (World Health Organization, 2015). Recognition of the vulnerability of the HIV population to TB and increased awareness of the need to rapidly diagnose and treat TB/HIV-co-infected individuals have led to a steady decrease in HIV-associated TB deaths since the numbers peaked globally in 2004. Deaths from TB in HIV-infected individuals declined from 540,000 in 2004 to 360,000 in 2013. Despite these gains, TB still kills an estimated 1 in

5 persons with AIDS annually worldwide (World Health Organization, 2015 factsheet).

The total number of TB cases in the United States peaked in 1992 and has been steadily declining since. The American Thoracic Society, Infectious Diseases Society of America, and Centers for Disease Control and Prevention (CDC) have recommended testing for HIV in all active cases of TB (American Thoracic Society, 2000). HIV testing has increased to 89% of reported TB cases in the United States, with 6% of cases reported as HIV-positive in 2014. This is down significantly from the peak in 1992, when nearly two-thirds of TB cases in 25- to 44-year-olds were HIV-positive. Attention to screening and treatment in the HIV population in the United States has resulted in a decrease in HIV-associated TB cases and a faster decline than in the general population (CDC, 2014).

Unlike other HIV-related opportunistic infections, CD4 count does not predict risk of TB infection. Rates of TB in HIV-infected patients are higher than those in non-HIV-infected individuals at all CD4 counts.

Clinical Presentation

Infection with *M. tuberculosis* generally occurs after inhalation of infectious particles coughed into the air by a person with active pulmonary TB disease. A less common route of infection involves ingestion of unpasteurized dairy products produced from the milk of *Mycobacterium bovis*-infected cows (bovine TB). Once infected, individuals will either progress to active disease (progressive primary disease) or their immune system will contain growth of the organism but not kill it (LTBI). Host immune factors play a major role in which route initial infection will take. Host factors also play a role in whether patients with LTBI will progress to active TB disease (post-primary or reactivation disease).

Tuberculosis in individuals who are not infected with HIV typically presents as pulmonary disease. Often, the upper lobes of the lung are involved, and cavitary lesions are characteristic. Pulmonary disease is frequently accompanied by constitutional symptoms such as fever, night sweats, and weight loss. These findings are more typical of reactivation disease rather than progressive primary infection found when there is poor containment of the infecting organism by the immune system.

CD4$^+$ cells play a pivotal role in the containment of *M. tuberculosis*. As HIV infection progresses and there is a decline in the number of these cells, there is less containment of infecting organisms. The clinical presentation of TB in HIV-infected individuals differs based on the CD4$^+$ count. Patients with CD4$^+$ counts >350 cells/mm^3 often present with the classic pulmonary presentation described. As the CD4$^+$ count decreases, the clinical presentation can look more like progressive primary disease. In patients with CD4$^+$ counts <200 cells/mm^3, pulmonary lesions may involve any lobe of the lungs and range from infiltrates to pneumonia. Cavitary lesions become less common with advanced HIV disease, and HIV–TB co-infected patients may have no abnormalities on chest X-ray.

Another feature of HIV-associated TB is extrapulmonary disease. Extrapulmonary disease is found in up to 50% of individuals in some series. Lymph node disease is the most common extrapulmonary site. Disseminated (military) disease and mycobacteremia are far more common in patients with low CD4$^+$ counts.

Diagnosis

Diagnosis of TB infection in an HIV-infected patient requires a high index of suspicion. Recent advances in diagnostic tests for TB, such as IGRAs, have not translated into a major improvement in the diagnosis of TB in patients with HIV. Diagnosis requires the HIV physician to remain vigilant.

Traditionally, screening for TB infection has been via the tuberculin skin test (TST). The assay involves injection of 0.1 ml (comprising 5 tuberculin units) of purified protein derivative subcutaneously into the volar surface of the forearm. Individuals who have been previously infected with *M. tuberculosis* develop a delayed-type hypersensitivity reaction to the injected proteins. Induration caused by this reaction is measured after 48–72 hours. A TST measurement of 5 mm of induration or greater is considered positive in a person infected with HIV. Sensitivity of this test has always been poor in HIV-infected individuals, and it can be as low as 30% in TB patients with CD4$^+$ counts <200 cells/mm^3. It is also important to note that the TST will not distinguish between patients with latent TB infection and those with active TB, and it may be falsely positive in patients vaccinated with Bacillus Calmette–Guérin (BCG) due to cross-reaction with the antigens found in the BCG vaccine.

IGRAS are newer diagnostic tests developed in the past 10 years for detection of *M. tuberculosis* infection. These tests are based on immune responses to antigens unique to *M. tuberculosis*. IGRAs have the benefits of negating the false positives seen with BCG vaccination and offering a blood draw that requires a single visit. There are two commercially available US Food and Drug Administration-approved IGRAs—the QuantiFERON-TB Gold In-Tube (QFT-GIT) and the T.SPOT.*TB* (T-spot). Meta-analyses (Cattamanchin, 2011; Santin, 2012) show the sensitivity of these tests to be approximately 60% for the QFT-GIT and 70% for the T-spot. Although this appears to be an improvement over the TST, there was not a significant difference in head-to-head sensitivity with either test compared to the TST. The T-spot seems to be less affected by the level of immunosuppression than either the QFT-GIT or TST in HIV-infected patients. The studies highlight the fact that there are still a large number of cases of LTBI or active disease that may be missed by these tests, and a high index of suspicion is still warranted. As highlighted in the recommendations on IGRAs outlined by the CDC (CDC, 2010), these tests are most useful in BCG-vaccinated populations (adding greater specificity) and in populations with poor rates of return (negating the need for a return visit for reading). These same guidelines state clearly that routine testing with both the TST and an IGRA is not recommended.

HIV-infected individuals should be screened for TB infection by a TST or IGRA at the time of HIV diagnosis and regularly thereafter. Individuals who travel to countries with a high TB burden or who reside in areas with high rates of TB should be tested annually. All others should be tested when there is suspicion of exposure to an active case after their initial testing. Individuals with CD4+ counts <200 cells/mm^3 at HIV diagnosis should have a repeat diagnostic test after CD4+ count recovery to >200 cells/mm^3.

An individual with a positive diagnostic test (TST or IGRA) without evidence of active TB disease should be given a diagnosis of LTBI. HIV patients with LTBI are at very high risk for advancing to active TB. Individuals with LTBI without HIV have a 5–10% lifetime risk of developing active TB, whereas individuals with HIV and LTBI have a 10% annual risk. Generally, persons with HIV and LTBI are 29.6 (27.1–32.1) times more likely to progress to active disease than persons without HIV (World Health Organization, 2015 factsheet). LTBI treatment in this population is paramount and has formed the cornerstone of progress in reducing global TB cases.

Diagnosis of active TB disease requires utilization of many pieces of data. A thorough history is useful in most cases. Important information to note includes exposure to an active TB case, residence in high-risk settings such as jail or homeless shelters, and prior diagnosis of untreated LTBI. Signs and symptoms of active disease may include cough lasting longer than 3 weeks, unexplained weight loss, fevers, and/or night sweats. There are no physical exam findings specific for TB, but a thorough physical exam may reveal suspicious lymphadenopathy, draining fistulas, respiratory sounds, or signs of meningitis.

Diagnostic tests such as the TST and IGRA can add to available data but cannot be relied on entirely. One may also consider performing more than one of these tests to increase sensitivity, especially when the patient has a low CD4 count. In general, a positive TST or IGRA result should be taken as evidence of infection.

All patients suspected of having active TB should receive a chest X-ray because the lungs are the most common entry point and a frequent site of infection. As previously noted, the chest X-ray can be normal in patients with culture-positive pulmonary TB. Any patient with respiratory symptoms, regardless of chest X-ray findings, should have sputum (three specimens) collected 8–24 hours apart with at least one sputum being an early morning specimen.

Patients with lower CD4+ counts are more likely to have extrapulmonary TB with infection in tissues that are more difficult to access and that have fewer organisms. It may be necessary to obtain biopsy specimens such as lymph nodes, bone marrow, or lung tissue to make the diagnosis. CSF, ascitic, or abscess fluid may also be diagnostic. All tissue from suspected sites of infection should be submitted for smear and culture analysis for acid-fast bacilli and, if indicated, histopathologic analysis searching for characteristic granulomas on pathology.

Treatment

Treatment of latent TB in HIV-infected patients is essentially the same as that in patients without HIV. The preferred regimen for treatment of LTBI in HIV-infected patients is 9 months of isoniazid (INH) dosed daily or intermittently (twice weekly) by directly observed therapy (DOT). In individuals without HIV, 6 months of INH is an acceptable alternative, but this regimen has a lower rating for HIV-infected individuals.

Rifampin taken for 4 months is an acceptable LTBI treatment in patients who are intolerant of INH or who are exposed to an INH-resistant case. Rifampin interacts with all antiretrovirals except the nucleoside analogues (excluding zidovudine) and enfuvirtide. In many cases, rifabutin can be substituted for rifampin. When a rifamycin is used in the treatment of a patient on ART, drug–drug interactions must be carefully considered. Guidance is available in a regularly updated document at https://aidsinfo.nih.gov.

The most recently approved treatment regimen for LTBI is INH–rifapentine dosed weekly for 12 weeks by DOT. Although this regimen is appropriate for patients with HIV, it is contraindicated in patients receiving any form of antiretroviral treatment.

Treatment of active TB in HIV-infected patients is also essentially the same as that for HIV-negative patients. All patients diagnosed in the United States with active TB should be started on a four-drug regimen consisting of isoniazid, rifampin, ethambutol, and pyrazinamide unless there is known resistance or baseline severe impairment of hepatic or renal function. After 2 months of this four-drug therapy (initial phase) and if the patient's organism is not resistant, the regimen can be reduced to INH and rifampin for the duration of treatment (continuation phase). Length of treatment will depend on the site and extent of disease. Most cases can be treated with 6–9 months of total therapy, whereas infections involving the bones or meninges should be treated for a total of 9–12 months. Infections of the pericardium or meninges should be treated with steroids in addition to anti-TB medications.

The most significant differences between treatment of HIV-positive patients and that of HIV-negative patients involve use of the rifamycins and frequency of dosing. As previously noted, there is significant interaction between rifampin and most antiretrovirals, so care must be taken in introducing this class of medications into the regimen. Treatment regimens for active TB that do not contain a rifamycin require up to 18 months of therapy and have very high rates of relapse. Every effort should be made to include a rifamycin in the treatment of patients co-infected with HIV and TB. Regularly updated guidance on how to manage drug interactions can be found at https://aidsinfo.nih.gov.

DOT is highly recommended for all cases of active TB treated in the United States. Patients can receive intermittent dosing but only if receiving DOT. Highly intermittent dosing of TB therapy (once- or twice-weekly dosing) is associated with an increased risk of relapse with rifampin-resistant disease and should be avoided in patients infected with HIV (CDC, 2003). This is especially noted in patients with $CD4^+$ counts <100 cells/mm^3.

The question of when to initiate antiretroviral treatment in a patient co-infected with HIV and TB is not a trivial one. Treatment for both diseases simultaneously can result in a large pill burden, potential for multiple drug interactions, and potential for multiple drug toxicities. Although it is clear that patients who are diagnosed with TB should be started immediately on anti-TB medications, until recently the timing of adding ART was less clear. Several studies (Blanc, 2011; Karim, 2011; Martinson, 2011) conducted at multiple sites have shown a survival benefit (reduced mortality) when starting ART within 2 weeks of starting TB medications in patients with $CD4^+$ counts <50 cells/mm^3. At CD4 counts >50 cells/mm^3, the incidence of IRIS events increased. In patients with severe disease who have $CD4^+$ counts ≥50 cells/mm^3, the current recommendation is to start treatment for HIV within 2–4 weeks of starting

TB therapy and within 8–12 weeks in patients with $CD4^+$ counts ≥50 cells/mm^3 who do not have severe disease.

If IRIS does occur in the course of treatment, it is important that both antiretroviral and TB treatment be continued. Mild cases of IRIS can be observed or treated with nonsteroidal anti-inflammatory agents or, if more severe, a short course of steroids may be necessary.

Special consideration should be given to patients with HIV and TB meningitis. IRIS involving central nervous system disease leads to worse outcomes. Patients with HIV and TB meningitis must be monitored carefully and treated with steroid therapy to reduce the inflammatory effects associated with disease. Treatment with antiretroviral medication should be added with careful monitoring of the patient for any evidence of IRIS.

Drug-resistant disease in an HIV-infected patient requires individualized therapy and should be approached with an expert in drug-resistant TB. Patients with multidrug-resistant or extensively drug-resistant TB should have ART initiated within 2–4 weeks after initiation of second-line TB drug therapy.

Prevention

Individuals with HIV should be screened for TB by a TST or IGRA at the time of diagnosis and periodically thereafter. Individuals with HIV who are found to have a positive TST or IGRA without evidence of active disease should be treated for LTBI to prevent progression to active disease.

HIV-positive individuals who are contacts to an infectious pulmonary case of TB and have no evidence of active disease should be treated with a full course of therapy for LTBI, even with a negative diagnostic test. As outlined previously, available diagnostic tests are not sensitive enough to rule out TB infection, and patients exposed to an infectious case are highly susceptible. Active disease should be ruled out in all patients prior to initiation of treatment for LTBI.

Patients who have a history of untreated or inadequately treated TB who do not have evidence of currently active disease should receive treatment for LTBI. This may be manifest as old fibrotic lesions on chest X-ray noted during routine screening.

MYCOBACTERIUM AVIUM COMPLEX

Epidemiology

MAC, also known as MAI, consists of *M. avium* and *M. intracellulare*, two organisms so similar that they can only be differentiated using DNA probes. MAC infections are the most common nontuberculous mycobacteria (NTM) infections in both HIV-positive and HIV-negative patients (Griffith, 2007).

These organisms are ubiquitous and are found environmentally in water, soil, and animal sources. Despite the many places from which the organisms can be isolated, the actual route of infection in HIV-infected patients is unclear. There is no evidence for human-to-human or animal-to-human transmission.

Disseminated disease is the most common presentation of MAC infection associated with HIV and occurs almost exclusively in patients with profound immunosuppression who are not yet receiving ART. Disseminated disease is most commonly found in patient with CD4$^+$ counts <50 cells/mm^3. Having a high HIV viral load (>100,000 copies/mm^3) has also been identified as a risk factor. The incidence of disseminated MAC has declined steadily since the introduction of effective antiretroviral treatment, with most cases occurring in individuals who have not accessed care.

Clinical Presentation

As stated previously, the most common presentation of MAC infection in HIV patients is disseminated disease. Symptoms tend to be nonspecific and typically include fever; night sweats; anorexia weight loss; and gastrointestinal symptoms such as nausea, vomiting, diarrhea, and abdominal pain. It is important to remember that these same symptoms can be associated with other opportunistic infections, such as TB and fungal disease.

Disseminated MAC infection tends to involve the reticuloendothelial system and, subsequently, physical exam findings may include hepatomegaly, splenomegaly, and lymphadenopathy. Pulmonary disease is rare, even with disseminated disease, but occasionally can manifest as nodules, infiltrates, cavities, or mediastinal/hilar adenopathy. Pulmonary findings are more likely to be associated with infection due to *M. tuberculosis* or *M. kansasii*.

Immune reconstitution in patients newly started on ART may "unmask" preexisting, previously undetected disease. The presentation in this case may manifest as disseminated disease or perhaps localized disease.

Diagnosis

Isolation of MAC from a normally sterile site, such as the blood, should be considered diagnostic for disseminated disease. In the absence of a positive blood culture, other more invasive approaches, such as lymph node, liver, or bone marrow biopsy, may be necessary to obtain an adequate specimen for diagnosis.

Isolation of MAC from nonsterile sites such as the respiratory or gastrointestinal tracts may represent true pathology but can also represent colonization. In these cases, it is important to make an effort to determine if other pathogens may be at play.

Treatment

Optimally, the approach to treatment of disseminated MAC disease should include treatment of both MAC and HIV. Like treatment of TB and other NTM infections, treatment of MAC infection should include multidrug therapy.

Clarithromycin should be the first drug added to a MAC treatment regimen. In the event of clarithromycin intolerance or unacceptable drug interaction with other medications, azithromycin may be substituted. Studies have shown treatment with clarithromycin to be associated with faster clearance of bacteremia than treatment with azithromycin (CDC, 2015).

The second drug added should be ethambutol. Addition of ethambutol to a macrolide is associated with decreased relapse in the treatment of MAC. Rifabutin can also be added to the MAC treatment regimen but has not been shown to improve outcomes over the combination of a macrolide and ethambutol alone. Addition of rifabutin also adds the potential for significant interaction with many antiretrovirals and can lower serum drug levels of clarithromycin when used in combination. Prior to addition of rifabutin to the treatment of a mycobacterial infection, TB must be ruled out to prevent the emergence of rifampin-resistant TB disease.

Based on data from non-HIV-infected patients, agents such as amikacin and streptomycin can be utilized if there is a need for additional medication options due to resistance or toxicity.

IRIS has been documented with treatment of MAC disease, as it has with TB. The presentation generally manifests as a return of fever and worsening lymphadenitis with negative blood cultures. Mild cases can be simply monitored or treated with a nonsteroidal anti-inflammatory agent or, in severe cases, a short course of steroids. Treatment for both MAC and HIV should be continued during management of IRIS reactions.

Treatment of disseminated disease should continue until there is a response to ART. Patients who complete a 12-month course of therapy, who remain free of signs or symptoms of disease, and who show a sustained increase in CD4$^+$ count to >100 cells/mm^3 for at least 6 months have a low risk of relapse. If a previously treated patient experiences a decrease in CD4$^+$ count <100 cells/mm^3, the patient should be placed back on preventive prophylaxis treatment.

Prevention/Prophylaxis

No direct route for infection with MAC has been identified and, thus, there is no specific action known to prevent exposure to MAC. Patients with a CD4$^+$ count <50 cells/mm^3 are at high risk for disseminated MAC and should receive chemoprophylaxis to prevent development of disease.

Azithromycin dosed at 1200 mg weekly is the preferred prophylactic regimen. Clarithromycin dosed at 500 mg twice daily is effective, but due to the increased pill burden, it is considered an alternative to azithromycin. Before starting prophylaxis, disseminated MAC should be ruled out.

Rifabutin is an alternative when there is evidence of macrolide-resistant disease or macrolide intolerance, but rifabutin is less effective in this capacity and adds increased risk of drug interactions with many of the antiretrovirals. Before use of rifabutin, every effort should be made to rule out active TB.

MYCOBACTERIUM KANSASII

Epidemiology

Mycobacterium kansasii infection is the second most common NTM infection in HIV-infected patients (after MAC infection). Tap water appears to be the most likely environmental reservoir for strains causing human disease (Griffith, 2002; Jones, 2002). Lung disease caused by *M. kansasii* closely resembles disease caused by *M. tuberculosis* in both HIV-infected and non-HIV-infected patients. Despite its similarities to TB, there is no evidence of human-to-human transmission of *M. kansasii*. Similar to MAC, infection with *M. kansasii* is most commonly found in patients with CD4$^+$ counts <50 cells/mm^3.

Clinical Presentation

Unlike MAC disease, which is most commonly disseminated and rarely pulmonary, *M. kansasii* can be disseminated but is more commonly pulmonary. Radiographically, *M. kansasii* infection closely resembles infection with *M. tuberculosis*, with symptoms that include cough, fever, night sweats, weight loss, and hemoptysis.

Diagnosis

Diagnosis requires isolation of the organism from a sterile site or meeting the criterion outlined in the guidelines set forth by the American Thoracic Society (ATS). Briefly, the ATS criteria for both HIV-infected and non-infected individuals require that the individual in question have pulmonary symptoms with suggestive radiography, exclusion of other diagnoses, positive culture results from two separate expectorated sputa, or at least one bronchoalveolar lavage specimen or bronchial biopsy with suggestive histopathology.

Mycobacterium kansasii isolated from the sputum of a patient with pulmonary lesions can trigger an unnecessary public health investigation for TB. Testing with a nucleic acid amplification test can rule out TB in these cases.

Treatment

Mycobacterium kansasii responds well to anti-TB medications with the exception that the organism is widely resistant to pyrazinamide. Treatment with isoniazid, ethambutol and rifampin or rifabutin is recommended for 18 months, with at least 12 months of culture-negative sputum. Rifamycins in the treatment regimen of *M. kansasii* patients (unlike those with MAC disease) provide clear benefit and prevent relapse. The choice and dose of rifamycin should be guided by the patient's antiretroviral treatment, with special attention to potential drug interactions.

As with infections caused by other mycobacteria, IRIS has been documented with treatment of *M. kansasii*. Mild cases can be simply monitored or treated with a nonsteroidal anti-inflammatory agent or, in severe cases, a short course of steroids. It is important that treatment for both *M. kansasii* and HIV be continued during management of IRIS reactions.

Recommended Reading

Centers for Disease Control and Prevention. Targeted tuberculin testing and treatment of latent tuberculosis infection. *MMWR*. 2000; 49(RR-6).

Centers for Disease Control and Prevention. Treatment of tuberculosis. *MMWR*. 2003; 52(RR-11).

Centers for Disease Control and Prevention. Guidelines for prevention and treatment of opportunistic infections in HIV-infected adults and adolescents. *MMWR*. 2009; 58(RR-4).

Griffith DE. Management of disease due to *Mycobacterium kansasii. Clin Chest Med*. 2002; 23:613–621.

Griffith DE, Aksamit T, Brown-Elliott BA, et al. An official ATS/IDSA statement: Diagnosis, treatment, and prevention of nontuberculous mycobacterial diseases. *Am J Respir Crit Care Med*. 2007; 175:367–416.

US Department of Health and Human Services, Panel on Antiretroviral Guidelines for Adults and Adolescents. Guidelines for the use of antiretroviral agents in HIV-1-infected adults and adolescents. Available at https://www.aidsinfo.nih.gov/ContentFiles/AdultandAdolescentGL.pdf.

OPPORTUNISTIC INFECTIONS: VIRAL INFECTIONS

LEARNING OBJECTIVE

Discuss the established and evolving science regarding diagnosis, treatment, and prophylaxis of opportunistic viral infections associated with HIV infection in order to improve quality of life and length of survival.

WHAT'S NEW?

Suppressive acyclovir therapy is recommended in HIV-infected patients with CD4$^+$ cell count <250 cells/mm^3 who are starting highly active antiretroviral therapy (HAART) to reduce the risk of genital ulcer disease.

KEY POINTS

Herpes Simplex Virus

- Herpes simplex virus (HSV) is a very common disease in HIV-infected patients, typically presenting with orolabial, genital, and/or anorectal ulcers that may be very severe in the setting of advance immunosuppression. HSV could also manifest as proctitis (particularly in men who have sex with men), esophagitis, keratitis, meningitis, encephalitis, radiculitis, and retinitis (presenting as acute retinal necrosis).

- Treatment is generally with acyclovir or one of its derivatives. Acyclovir resistance is more common among HIV-infected individuals. HSV suppression should be considered for individuals with frequent or severe recurrent episodes.

Varicella Zoster Virus

- Varicella zoster reactivation disease in HIV-infected patients is often more severe, multidermatomal, or disseminated. Severe complications such as progressive outer retinal necrosis must be treated quickly to prevent permanent sequelae. For mild disease, oral therapy with acyclovir or one of its derivatives is appropriate; in severe cases, however, intravenous therapy is required.

Cytomegalovirus

- Cytomegalovirus may cause a variety of clinical manifestations in HIV-infected patients with CD4$^+$ cell counts <50 cells/mm^3. Retinitis and colitis are the most common manifestations. Ganciclovir (or the oral prodrug valganciclovir) or foscarnet are the most common

therapies, but they carry significant risk of toxicity. Primary prophylaxis is not recommended.

JC Virus

- JC virus causes progressive multifocal leukoencephalopathy, a progressive, demyelinating disease of the central nervous system that leads to relatively rapid accumulation of neurologic deficits with dementia, coma, and death. Diagnosis is generally made clinically with the support of typical magnetic resonance imaging (MRI) findings and polymerase chain reaction (PCR) testing for JC virus in the CSF. Definitive diagnosis is made by brain biopsy. No specific antiviral therapy exists for JC virus. ART often results in stabilization or regression of disease.

HERPESVIRUS

Herpes Simplex Virus

Herpes simplex virus types 1 and 2 (HSV-1 and HSV-2) are highly prevalent in HIV-infected patients. Classically, HSV-1 caused oral ulcers, whereas HSV-2 caused genital ulcers; currently, however, both are recognized as a cause of genital infection, especially in young women and men who have sex with men.

HSV-2 is one of the most common sexually transmitted infections worldwide and the primary cause of genital ulcer disease. The overall national HSV-2 prevalence was reported as 16.2% in 2010 (Xu, 2006); however, in HIV-infected patients, seroprevalence rates near 70% have been reported (Corey, 2004). The primary mode of transmission is through direct contact with oral secretions or genital secretions. Clinical HSV disease is common in the absence of HIV infection, but manifestations are more common, more severe, or atypical in the setting of HIV infection.

Clinical Presentation

The classical presentation of herpes infection is large, painful, grouped vesicles with an erythematous base typically in the orolabial, genital, and anorectal regions; however, they may involve any areas of the body. In patients with advanced HIV-associated immunosuppression, anogenital lesions may be severe, and they may be refractory to treatment or secondary to acyclovir-resistant virus (Safrin, 1994). Dissemination is possible, but it is rarely seen in HIV-infected patients. Proctitis (particularly in men who have sex with men), keratitis, meningitis, encephalitis, radiculitis, and retinitis (presenting as acute retinal necrosis) are possible complications. HSV esophagitis may occur in people with CD4+ cell counts <50 cells/mm³ and typically presents with retrosternal chest pain and odynophagia.

Reactivation of HSV is more common in HIV-infected patients. Recurrent lesions are often more frequent, more extensive, and of longer duration in this population. In addition, there is prolonged shedding of the virus even in the absence of lesions, especially in patients with lower CD4+ cell counts and higher plasma HIV-1 RNA levels.

Diagnosis

Diagnosis is made clinically. However, laboratory confirmation should be done, when possible, with viral culture, examination of lesion scrapings using immunofluorescent staining, Tzanck preparation (multinucleated giant cells), or PCR amplification techniques. Culture specimens can also be tested for antiviral drug susceptibility.

Treatment

Table 32.1 shows the current treatment recommendations from the 2009/2015 "Guidelines for the Prevention and Treatment of Opportunistic Infections" published by the Centers for Disease Control and Prevention, the National Institutes of Health, and the HIV Medicine Association of the Infectious Diseases Society of America (DHHS, 2015). Oral acyclovir, valacyclovir, and famciclovir are comparable alternatives. In patients with extensive mucocutaneous lesions, it is recommended to use intravenous acyclovir. Resistance to acyclovir has been reported in up to 5% of HIV-infected patients with HSV-2 infection and is more frequent in patients with prolonged acyclovir use. In these cases, foscarnet or cidofovir are alternate options.

Prophylaxis

The "Guidelines for the Prevention and Treatment of Opportunistic Infections" (DHHS, 2015) recommends the use of condoms to prevent transmission of HSV-2. The use of 1% tenofovir vaginal gel has been shown to be associated with a 50% risk reduction of HSV-2 acquisition in women at high risk of HIV infection. However, this has not been confirmed in other studies. In addition, in patients taking oral tenofovir, the rates of vaginal shedding of HSV-1 and HSV-2 are similar. Suppressive therapy with oral acyclovir, valacyclovir, or famciclovir is effective in preventing genital herpes recurrences, and it should be discussed with all HSV-2-infected patient (Table 32.2). Immune reconstitution improves the frequency and severity of clinical episodes of genital herpes, but it does not decrease shedding.

In individuals with CD4+ cell count <250 cells/mm³ who will start ART, there is an increased risk of HSV-2 shedding and genital ulcer diseases in the first 6 months. It is recommended to give suppressive antiviral therapy because it decreases the risk of genital ulcer diseases by 60%.

VARICELLA ZOSTER VIRUS

Varicella zoster virus (VZV), the third herpesvirus, causes initial infection in childhood (chickenpox) and later reactivates, causing herpes zoster. The prevalence of herpes zoster is 3–5% in the general population, but it is 15–25 times higher in HIV-infected patients (Buchbinder, 1992). Lower CD4+ cell counts have been associated with more atypical presentations of the disease but not with increased incidence.

Clinical Presentation

The initial clinical presentation is similar to that of immunocompetent patients. It manifests as a prodrome of cutaneous burning or pain, followed by a cutaneous eruption of grouped vesicles on an erythematous base along a dermatome. However, HIV-infected patients are at increased risk for multidermatomal or disseminated zoster, including neurologic and ophthalmologic complications. Approximately 20–30% of HIV-infected patients will experience subsequent episodes of herpes zoster, either in the same or in different dermatomes. The probability of a recurrence of herpes zoster within 1 year of the index episode is 10% (Gebo, 2005). Post-herpetic neuralgia is reported in 10–15% of HIV-infected patients (Gebo, 2005; Harrison, 1999).

Atypical VZV presentations such as chronic hyperkeratotic lesions or chronic disseminated ecthyma have also been reported. Meningitis, multifocal leukoencephalitis, ventriculitis, myelitis, cranial nerve palsies, and focal brainstem lesions are possible neurological complications.

Involvement of the ophthalmic division of the trigeminal nerve causes anterior uveitis, corneal scarring, and vision loss. Ocular involvement with acute retinal necrosis and progressive outer retinal necrosis are syndromes similar to CMV retinitis but of faster progression that typically occurs at CD4+ cell counts <100 cells/mm³ and may result in retinal blindness (Engstromm, 1994).

Diagnosis

The diagnosis is made clinically. Laboratory confirmation could be done by viral culture, direct immunofluorescence testing, and the PCR assay, which is the most sensitive test.

Table 32.1 HERPES SIMPLEX VIRUS TREATMENT RECOMMENDATIONS

CONDITION	FIRST CHOICE TREATMENT	ALTERNATIVE TREATMENT
Orolabial lesions	Valacyclovir 1 g PO BID or Famciclovir 500 mg PO BID or Acyclovir 400 mg PO TID for 5–10 days	
Initial or recurrent genital lesions	Valacyclovir 1 g PO BID or Famciclovir 500 mg PO BID or Acyclovir 400 mg PO TID for 5–10 days	
Severe mucocutaneous lesions	Acyclovir 5 mg/kg IV every 8 hours until lesions regress, then switch to acyclovir 400 mg PO TID until lesions are healed	
Esophagitis	Valacyclovir 1 g PO TID or Famciclovir 500 mg PO TID or Acyclovir 400 mg PO five times daily for 14–21 days	
Encephalitis and hepatitis	Acyclovir 10–15 mg/kg IV every 8 hours for 21 days	
Acyclovir-resistant herpes	Foscarnet 80–120 mg/kg/day IV 2–3 times daily until clinical response	Topical trifluridine, or Cidofovir 1% gel, or Topical imiquimod 5% three times weekly for 21–28 days or longer based on clinical response

Treatment

VZV treatment is summarized in Table 32.3.

CYTOMEGALOVIRUS

CMV is a DNA herpesvirus and the largest virus that infects humans. It is typically acquired from close contact during youth or adolescence. In the general population, the percentage of people with evidence of previous CMV infection ranges from 40% to 100% and varies with ethnicity and country. Active disease associated with HIV typically results from reactivation of latent infection in the setting of advanced immunosuppression with CD4$^+$ counts <50 cells/mm^3 (Dieterich, 1991). Other risk factors for CMV disease include plasma HIV RNA levels >100,000 copies/ml and the presence of other opportunistic infections.

Table 32.2 HERPES SIMPLEX VIRUS SUPPRESSIVE THERAPY RECOMMENDATIONS

CONDITION	FIRST CHOICE TREATMENT
Genital lesions	Valacyclovir 500mg PO BID or Famciclovir 500 mg PO BID or Acyclovir 400–800 mg PO BID or TID

Before the use of ART, CMV retinitis was the most common intraocular infection in patients with AIDS, occurring in up to 40% of patients (Whitcup, 2000). Currently, the incidence of new cases of CMV end-organ disease has declined to <6 cases/100 person-years (Jabs, 2007).

Clinical Presentation and Diagnosis

CMV can infect different organs of the body. Retinitis accounts for 85% of CMV manifestations and is the leading cause of vision loss among HIV-infected individuals. Other CMV clinical syndromes include esophagitis, colitis, polyradiculopathy, ventriculoencephalitis, pneumonitis, adrenalitis, and pancreatitis. In addition, CMV infections can present in patients with IRIS.

Chorioretinitis

CMV chorioretinitis presents with painless progressive loss of vision, floaters, and/or visual field cut defects. Symptoms are unilateral at first, but without treatment they can become bilateral. The diagnosis is exclusively made by recognition of typical retinal changes during a fundoscopic examination: creamy or yellow-white granular areas with perivascular exudates and hemorrhage. These lesions initially are

Table 32.3 VARICELLA ZOSTER VIRUS TREATMENT RECOMMENDATIONS

CONDITION	FIRST CHOICE TREATMENT
Varicella zoster virus infection, immunocompromised patients	Acyclovir 10–15 mg/kg IV every 8 hours for 7–10 days May switch to PO if no evidence of visceral involvement
Herpes zoster, acute localized dermatomal	Valacyclovir 1 g TID or Famciclovir 500 mg TID or Acyclovir 800 mg PO 5 times daily Each administered for 7–10 days Consider longer duration if lesions slow to resolve

Herpes zoster, extensive cutaneous lesion or visceral involvement	Acyclovir 10–15 mg/kg IV every 8 hours
	
	After clinical improvement is evident, switch to oral therapy:
	
	    Valacyclovir 1 g TID or
	
	    Famciclovir 500 mg TID or
	
	    Acyclovir 800 mg 5 times daily
	
	    Each administered for 10–14 days

Acute retinal necrosis	Acyclovir 10 mg/kg IV every 8 hours for 10–14 days Followed by oral valacyclovir 1 g TID for 6 weeks
Progressive outer retinal necrosis	Ganciclovir 5 mg/kg IV plus Foscarnet 90 mg/kg IV every 12 hours plus Ganciclovir 2 mg/0.05 ml intravitreal twice weekly and/or Foscarnet 1.2 mg/0.05 ml intravitreal twice weekly
Acyclovir-resistant varicella zoster virus infection	Foscarnet 90 mg/kg IV every 12 hours

found in the periphery of the fundus but can later involve the macula and the optic disc, resulting in blindness.

Colitis

CMV colitis is the second most common manifestation of CMV infection in HIV-infected patients. Patients present with severe diarrhea, abdominal pain and cramping, anorexia, weight loss, and fever. The diagnosis is achieved via detection of mucosal ulcerations on endoscopic examination combined with colonoscopic or rectal biopsy. Pathology will reveal intracytoplasmatic or intranuclear inclusions. A positive culture itself does not confirm the diagnosis. Mucosal hemorrhage and perforation rarely occur, but they are life threatening.

Esophagitis

CMV esophagitis causes odynophagia, nausea, fever, and retrosternal pain. Diagnosis is made by endoscopic examination that reveals diffuse inflammation of the esophagus and/or esophageal ulcers. Biopsy specimens also reveal intranuclear inclusions. A positive culture itself does not make the diagnosis.

CMV Polyradiculopathy

CMV polyradiculopathy presents with sacrolumbar radicular pain and lower limb paresthesia that may develop into progressive flaccid paralysis of the legs with decreasing and ultimately absent tendon reflexes. Urinary retention and stool incontinence may occur. If untreated, the condition rapidly advances up the spine, causing ascending sensory loss and growing flaccidity in the upper limbs, similar to Guillain–Barré-like paralysis. The CSF may have a pleocytosis with a predominance of polymorphonuclear cells, elevated protein, and moderately low glucose. Diagnosis is made by viral culture of the CSF. Lumbar MRI reveals gadolinium enhancement of the cauda equina in 33% of patients. CMV antigen assays and detection of CMV deoxyribonucleic acid via PCR may also be useful.

Ventriculoencephalitis

CMV ventriculoencephalitis is a late manifestation of CMV disease. It presents with fever, lethargy, confusion, and an acute course consisting of cranial nerve palsies, nystagmus, and other focal neurologic deficits that rapidly leads to death. MRI with gadolinium may reveal a characteristic periventricular ring-like enhancement. Viral culture of the CSF is not always positive, although CMV deoxyribonucleic acid can often be detected in CSF using PCR. Computed tomography (CT) and MRI scans show white matter enhancement.

Dementia

CMV dementia can present with fever, lethargy, and confusion, and it may be clinically similar to dementia caused directly by HIV. Central nervous system fluid (CSF) reveals pleocytosis that may be polymorphonuclear, low to normal glucose, and normal to high protein. CT and MRI scans may show cerebral atrophy.

Pneumonia

CMV pneumonitis is uncommon in AIDS patients. Symptoms include shortness of breath, dyspnea, dry nonproductive cough, and hypoxia. Imaging studies show diffuse interstitial infiltrates. A definitive diagnosis is made when multiple CMV inclusion bodies are seen in lung tissue.

CMV may be isolated in bronchial washings and lavage fluid from approximately 50% of HIV-infected patients undergoing bronchoscopy secondary to viral shedding.

CMV viremia is common in asymptomatic persons with low CD4+ counts (<100 cells/mm³). Viremia is typically present in active disease but may also be present in the absence of end-organ disease, so the tests are of limited value. The absence of CMV antibody may be helpful in excluding CMV disease; however, rarely, active disease can present during primary CMV infection with negative antibodies, and immunoglobin G antibody tests may revert to negative in individuals with advanced immunosuppression.

Treatment

Table 32.4 shows the current treatment recommendations from the "Guidelines for the Prevention and Treatment of Opportunistic Infections" (DHHS, 2015).

For CMV chorioretinitis, treatment consists of an induction phase of high-dose drug given for at least 2 weeks. Once retinitis is stable, patients are placed on chronic maintenance therapy until there is evidence of immune recovery (sustained CD4+ cell counts >100 cells/mm³ for ≥6 months). In the absence of antiretroviral-mediated immune reconstitution, most patients will have a reactivation of CMV infection despite suppressive therapy and will require reinduction therapy. Intraocular therapy may be useful in salvage therapy for patients who cannot tolerate systemic therapy. Any local therapy should be accompanied by systemic anti-CMV therapy. Systemic therapy has been shown to decrease CMV involvement of the contralateral eye, to reduce the risk of CMV disease in other organs, and to increase survival rates. Intraocular therapy alone has been associated with progression of CMV to the contralateral eye, as well as with systemic disease (Martin, 1994).

Table 32.4 CYTOMEGALOVIRUS TREATMENT RECOMMENDATIONS

CONDITION	FIRST CHOICE TREATMENT	ALTERNATIVE TREATMENT
CMV retinitis	*Sight-threatening lesions* Intravitreal injections Ganciclovir or foscarnet plus Valganciclovir 900 mg PO BID for 14–21 days, then once daily *For small peripheral lesions* Valganciclovir 900 mg PO bid for 14–21 days, then 900 mg once daily Or any of the alternative treatments	Intravitreal injections Ganciclovir or foscarnet plus Ganciclovir 5 mg/kg IV every 12 hours for 14–21 days, then 5 mg/kg IV daily or Ganciclovir 5 mg/kg IV every 12 hours for 14–21 days, then valganciclovir 900 mg PO daily Foscarnet 60 mg/kg IV every 8 hours or Foscarnet 90 mg/kg IV every 12 hours for 14–21 days, then 90–120 mg/kg IV every 24 hours or Cidofovir 5 mg/kg/week IV for 2 weeks, then 5 mg/kg every other week with saline hydration and probenecid 2 g PO 3 hours before the dose followed by 1 g 2 hours and 8 hours after the dose (total of 4 g)
Secondary prophylaxis (previously called maintenance therapy) for CMV retinitis	Valganciclovir 900 mg PO daily or Ganciclovir implant (replaced every 6–8 months if CD4+ count remains <100 cells/mm³) plus Valganciclovir 900 mg PO daily until immune recovery	Ganciclovir 5 mg/kg IV 5–7 times weekly or Foscarnet 90–120 mg/kg body weight IV once daily or Cidofovir 5 mg/kg body weight IV every other week as above
CMV colitis or esophagitis	Ganciclovir IV or Foscarnet IV for 21–28 days	
CMV neurological disease	Ganciclovir IV plus Foscarnet IV Until symptomatic improvement	

BID, twice daily; CMV, cytomegalovirus; IV, intravenous; PO, orally.

Ganciclovir and valganciclovir, foscarnet, and cidofovir carry significant risk for toxicity. Ganciclovir and valganciclovir can cause neutropenia, thrombocytopenia, nausea, diarrhea, renal dysfunction, and central venous catheter infection. Foscarnet more commonly causes nephrotoxicity, electrolyte abnormalities seizures, genital ulcers, and central venous catheter infection. Cidofovir, when used, is associated with nephrotoxicity and intraocular hypotony.

Prevention/Prophylaxis

In patients with $CD4^+$ cell count <100 cells/mm³, early recognition of the manifestations of end-organ CMV disease is the primary method of prevention. Primary prophylaxis against CMV is not recommended. Patients with $CD4^+$ cell counts <100 cells/mm³ should have annual ophthalmology exam. Secondary prophylaxis is done with valganciclovir until $CD4^+$ cell count has been >100 cells/mm³ for 3–6 months and the lesions are not life threatening. If $CD4^+$ cell count decreases to <100 cells/mm³, secondary prophylaxis should be reinstituted.

HUMAN HERPESVIRUS-8

The prevalence of human herpesvirus-8 (HHV-8) ranges between 1% and 5% in the general population, but it is between 20% and 77% in men who have sex with men (Pauk, 2000). HHV-8 is associated with all forms of Kaposi's sarcoma, primary effusion lymphoma, and lymphoproliferative disorders such as multicentric Castleman's disease (see Chapter 33).

JC VIRUS

JC virus causes progressive multifocal leukoencephalopathy (PML), a disease characterized by focal demyelination. Approximately 85% of adults are seropositive for JC virus worldwide. The incidence of PML has decreased significantly since the widespread use of ART. However, PML has also been reported in HIV-infected patients with $CD4^+$ cell counts >300 cells/mm³ and as a complication of IRIS (Berger, 1998; Cinque, 2003).

Clinical Presentation

The clinical presentation of PML depends on the localization of brain lesions, and the specific deficits vary from patient to patient. Patients present with symptoms of diffuse encephalopathy to focal deficits such as ataxia, hemiparesis, or speech difficulties. Symptoms tend to progress rapidly over several weeks to months. Fever and headache may be present; seizures are seen in 20% of cases.

Diagnosis

Brain biopsy will reveal the typical findings of focal myelin loss with peculiar astrocytes and lipid-laden macrophages, and it is used to make a definitive diagnosis. MRI of the brain demonstrates distinct white matter lesions in areas of the brain corresponding to the clinical deficits. The lesions are usually white on T2 images, and they are also characteristically dark on T1 images. PCR detection of the JC virus in CSF has a diagnostic sensitivity of 70–80% and specificity of 100%.

Treatment

Initiation of effective ART is the treatment of choice. It prolongs survival and improves neurologic deficits when immune reconstitution is achieved. The early use of a five-drug antiretroviral regimen after PML diagnosis appears to improve survival (Gasnault, 2011). Other treatments have been attempted with no improvement in survival.

References

American Thoracic Society. Targeted tuberculin testing and treatment of latent tuberculosis infection. 2000. Available at http://www.cdc.gov/mmwr/preview/mmwrhtml/rr4906a1.htm.

Berger JR, Levy RM, Flomenhoft D. Predictive factors for prolonged survival in acquired immunodeficiency syndrome-associated progressive multifocal leukoencephalopathy. *Ann Neurol*. 1998; 44:341–349.

Blanc FX, Sok T, Laureillard, D, et al. 2011. Earlier versus later start of antiretroviral therapy in HIV-infected adults with tuberculosis. *N Engl J Med*. 2011; 365(16):1471–1481.

Boulware DR, Meya DB, Muzoora C, et al. Timing of antiretroviral therapy after diagnosis of cryptococcal meningitis. *N Engl J Med*. 2014 Jun 26; 370(26):2487–2498.

Buchbinder SP, Katz MH, Hessol NA, et al. Herpes zoster and human immunodeficiency virus infection. *J Infect Dis*. 1992; 166:1153–1156.

Cattamanchi A, Smith R, Steingart KR, et al. Interferon-gamma release assays for the diagnosis of latent tuberculosis infection in HIV-infected individuals: A systematic review and meta-analysis. *J Acquir Immune Defic Syndr*. 2011; 56:230–238.

Centers for Disease Control and Prevention. Treatment of tuberculosis. *MMWR* 2003; 52(RR-11).

Centers for Disease Control and Prevention. Updated guidelines for using interferon gamma release assays to detect *Mycobacterium tuberculosis* infection—United States, 2010. Available at http://www.cdc.gov/mmwr/preview/mmwrhtml/rr5905a1.htm?s_cid=rr5905a1_e.

Centers for Disease Control and Prevention. Reported tuberculosis in the United States, 2014. Atlanta, GA: US Department of Health and Human Services; October 2011.

Centers for Disease Control and Prevention. Guidelines for prevention and treatment of opportunistic infections in HIV-infected adults and adolescents. 2015. Available at https://aidsinfo.nih.gov/guidelines/html/4/adult-and-adolescent-oi-prevention-and-treatment-guidelines/0.

Cinque P, Bossolasco S, Brambilla AM, et al. The effect of highly active antiretroviral therapy-induced immune reconstitution on development and outcome of progressive multifocal leukoencephalopathy: Study of 43 cases with review of the literature. *J Neurovirol.* 2003; 9:73–80.

Corey L, Wald A, Celum CL, et al. The effects of herpes simplex virus-2 on HIV-1 acquisition and transmission: A review of two overlapping epidemics. *J Acquir Immune Defic Syndr.* 2004; 35:435–445.

Dieterich DT, Rahmin M. Cytomegalovirus colitis in AIDS: Presentation in 44 patients and a review of the literature. *J Acquir Immune Defic Syndr.* 1991; 4:s29–s35.

Engstrom RE Jr, Holland GN, Margolis TP, et al. The progressive outer retinal necrosis syndrome: A variant of necrotizing herpetic retinopathy in patients with AIDS. *Ophthalmology.* 1994; 101:1488–1502.

Fenner L, Gagneux S, Janssens JP, et al. Tuberculosis in HIV-negative and HIV-infected patients in a low-incidence country: Clinical characteristics and treatment outcomes. *PLoS One.* 2012; 7(3):e34186.

Gasnault J, Costagliola D, Hendel-Chavez H, et al. Improved survival of HIV-1-infected patients with progressive multifocal leukoencephalopathy receiving early 5-drug combination antiretroviral therapy. *PLoS One.* 2011; 6:e20967.

Gebo KA, Kalyani R, Moore RD, et al. The incidence of, risk factors for, and sequelae of herpes zoster among HIV patients in the highly active antiretroviral therapy era. *J Acquir Immune Defic Syndr.* 2005; 40:169–174.

Geng EH, Kahn JS, Chang OC, et al. The effect of AIDS Clinical Trials Group Protocol 5164 on the time from *Pneumocystis jirovecii* pneumonia diagnosis to antiretroviral initiation in routine clinical practice: A case study of diffusion, dissemination, and implementation. *Clin Infect Dis.* 2011 Nov; 53(10):1008–1014.

Griffith DE. Management of disease due to *Mycobacterium kansasii. Clin Chest Med.* 2002; 23:613–621.

Griffith DE, Aksamit T, Brown-Elliott BA, et al. An official ATS/IDSA statement: Diagnosis, treatment, and prevention of nontuberculous mycobacterial diseases. *Am J Respir Crit Care Med.* 2007; 175:367–416.

Harrison RA, Soong S, Weiss HL, et al. A mixed model for factors predictive of pain in AIDS patients with herpes zoster. *J Pain Symptom Manage.* 1999; 17:410–417.

Jabs DA, Van Natta ML, Holbrook JT, et al. Longitudinal study of the ocular complications of AIDS: 1. Ocular diagnoses at enrollment. *Ophthalmology.* 2007; 114:780–786.

Jones D, Havlir DV. Nontuberculous mycobacteria in the HIV infected patient. *Clin Chest Med.* 2002; 23:665–674.

Karim SSA, Naidoo K, Grobler A, et al. Integration of antiretroviral therapy with tuberculosis treatment. *N Engl J Med.* 2011; 365(16):1492–1501.

Makadzange AT, Ndhlovu CE, Takarinda K, et al. Early versus delayed initiation of antiretroviral therapy for concurrent HIV infection and cryptococcal meningitis in sub-Saharan Africa. *Clin Infect Dis.* 2010 Jun 1; 50(11):1532–1538.

Martin DF, Parks DJ, Mellow SD, et al. Treatment of cytomegalovirus retinitis with an intraocular sustained-release ganciclovir implant: A randomized controlled clinical trial. *Arch Ophthalmol.* 1994; 112:1531–1539.

Martinson NA, Hoffmann CJ, RE Chaisson. Epidemiology of tuberculosis and HIV. *Proc Am Thorac Soc.* 2011; 8:288–293.

Pauk J, Huang ML, Brodie SJ, et al. Mucosal shedding of human herpesvirus 8 in men. *N Engl J Med.* 2000; 343:1369–1377.

Safrin S, Elbeik T, Phan L, et al. Correlation between response to acyclovir and foscarnet therapy and in vitro susceptibility result for isolates of herpes simplex virus from human immunodeficiency virus-infected patients. *Antimicrob Agents Chemother.* 1994; 38:1246–1250.

Santin M, Munoz L, Rigau D. Interferon-c release assays for the diagnosis of tuberculosis and tuberculosis infection in HIV-infected adults: A systematic review and meta-analysis. *PLoS One.* 2012 March; 7(3):e32482.

Sax PE, Sloan CE, Schackman BR, et al. Early antiretroviral therapy for patients with acute AIDS-related opportunistic infections: A cost-effectiveness analysis of ACTG A5164. *HIV Clinical Trials.* 2010; 11(5):248–259.

Sungkanuparph S, Filler SG, Chetchotisakd P, et al. Cryptococcal immune reconstitution inflammatory syndrome after antiretroviral therapy in AIDS patients with cryptococcal meningitis: A prospective multicenter study. *Clin Infect Dis.* 2009 Sep 15; 49(6):931–934.

US Department of Health and Human Services, Panel on Opportunistic Infections in HIV-Infected Adults and Adolescents. Guidelines for the prevention and treatment of opportunistic infections in HIV-infected adults and adolescents: Recommendations from the Centers for Disease Control and Prevention, the National Institutes of Health, and the HIV Medicine Association of the Infectious Diseases Society of America. Available at https://aidsinfo.nih.gov/content-files/lvguidelines/adult_oi.pdf. Accessed December 17, 2015.

Whitcup S. Cytomegalovirus retinitis in the era of highly active antiretroviral therapy. *JAMA.* 2000; 283:653–657.

World Health Organization. Global tuberculosis report 2015, 20th ed. Available at http://apps.who.int/iris/bitstream/10665/191102/1/9789241565059_eng.pdf?ua=1.

World Health Organization. TB/HIV factsheet 2015. Available at http://www.who.int/tb/challenges/hiv/tbhiv_factsheet_2015.pdf?ua=1.

Xu F, Sternberg MR, Kottiri BJ, et al. Trends in herpes simplex virus type 1 and type 2 seroprevalence in the United States. *JAMA.* 2006; 296:964–973.

Zolopa A, Andersen J, Powderly W, et al. Early antiretroviral therapy reduces AIDS progression/death in individuals with acute opportunistic infections: A multicenter randomized strategy trial. *PLoS One.* 2009; 4(5):e5575.

33.

MALIGNANT DISEASES IN HIV

Nora Oliver and Elizabeth Chiao

CHAPTER GOALS

- Review the epidemiology and role of antiretroviral therapy (ART) on the impact of AIDS-defining malignancies, which remain common among individuals with HIV.

- Discuss the role of human herpes virus-8 (HHV-8) in the development of Kaposi's sarcoma (KS), which remains the most common tumor associated with HIV infection.

- Discuss the role Epstein–Barr virus (EBV) in primary central nervous system lymphoma and other HIV-associated lymphomas.

- Review the role of human papillomavirus (HPV) vaccination in virally mediated anogenital squamous cell cancers in both men and women.

- Discuss non-AIDS-defining malignancies, including lung, prostate, oropharyngeal, liver, breast, and pancreatic cancer.

- Emphasize that ART initiation is of utmost importance for all AIDS-defining malignancies and non-AIDS-defining malignancies.

INTRODUCTION

LEARNING OBJECTIVE

Discuss AIDS-associated and non-AIDS-associated malignancies.

WHAT'S NEW?

Use of integrase inhibitors, the newest class of antiretrovirals, makes concurrent chemotherapeutic options safer and more feasible for many patients.

KEY POINTS

- Malignancies in HIV-positive patients remain a major health concern.

- ART continues to influence the epidemiology of malignancies, with decreasing rates overall.

Malignancies were one of the earliest recognized manifestations that led to the eventual description of the AIDS epidemic. Kaposi's sarcoma (KS) became one of the first entities described in association with AIDS (Ziegler, 1984). Subsequently, intermediate-grade and high-grade non-Hodgkin's lymphoma (NHL), invasive cervical cancer, and primary central nervous system lymphoma (PCNSL) were defined by the Centers for Disease Control and Prevention (CDC) as "AIDS-defining conditions" (CDC, 2008). Since the advent of combination ART, several other cancers that are not AIDS-defining have been found to have an increased incidence in patients with HIV. These include, but are not limited to, Hodgkin's disease and anal, liver, lung, oropharyngeal, colorectal, and renal cancers (Patel, 2008). They are generally referred to as "non-AIDS-defining cancers" (NADCs). The increasing longevity of persons living with HIV as well as concurrent modifiable risk factors such as tobacco use may also influence epidemiology of these malignancies.

The introduction of combination ART in the mid-1990s has significantly impacted the clinical history and outcomes of HIV infection. In addition to changing the natural history of HIV disease, in terms of survival and incidence of opportunistic diseases, it has also dramatically decreased the incidence of virally mediated HIV-associated malignancies, such as Kaposi's sarcoma, and PCNSL (Silverberg, 2015). The impact of ART on the overall incidence and natural history of HPV-mediated cancers, such as cervical and anogenital squamous cell cancer, remains uncertain.

Management of malignancies in patients with HIV infection presents the clinician with many challenges, including the risk of further compromise to the immune system of these patients receiving chemotherapy, toxicities of treatment, pharmacologic interaction between ART and chemotherapy drugs, and the risk of intercurrent opportunistic infections (Mandell, 2010). The safety profile and feasibility of ART administration with concurrent chemotherapy have also improved with the introduction and increased use of integrase inhibitors during the past several years.

This chapter reviews the malignancies most commonly associated with HIV, with brief mention of other cancers in the setting of HIV infection.

Recommended Reading

Patel P, Hanson DL, Sullivan PS, et al. Incidence of types of cancer among HIV-infected persons compared with the general population in the United States, 1992–2003. *Ann Intern Med.* 2008; 148(10):728–736.

Silverberg MJ, Lau B, Achenbach CJ, et al. Cumulative incidence of cancer among persons with HIV in North America. *Ann Intern Med.* 2015; 163(7):507–518.

KAPOSI'S SARCOMA

LEARNING OBJECTIVES

- Discuss the epidemiology of KS.

- Discuss the pathogenesis and clinical manifestations.

- Review the treatments for KS, including local and systemic therapies.

WHAT'S NEW?

The incidence of KS continues to decline with the use of ART, but it remains significantly elevated in areas with endemic disease, such as Sub-Saharan Africa.

KEY POINTS

- The presence of HHV-8 and advanced immunosuppression are both associated with risk of KS development and other lymphoproliferative states, such as multicentric Castleman's disease and primary body cavity lymphoma.

- Treatment for KS includes ART, local therapy, and systemic therapy.

- The goals of treatment are suppressive and generally noncurative.

Chemotherapy and radiotherapy are palliative treatments for KS. In general, treatment decisions and referrals to oncology should be based on evidence of symptomatic or systemic disease. Radiotherapy should be avoided in the pelvis and lower extremities because of damage to the lymphatics and the potential for lymphedema and skin breakdown.

EPIDEMIOLOGY

Kaposi's sarcoma was first described in 1872 by Moritz Kaposi, a Hungarian dermatologist. Four types of KS have been described: classic, endemic, transplant-associated, and AIDS-associated or epidemic KS. Classic KS is typically seen in elderly men of Mediterranean or Eastern European descent and is characterized by cutaneous lesions of the lower extremities (Iscovich, 2000). The endemic form, found primarily in sub-Saharan Africa, often is more aggressive and morbid with visceral involvement (Friedman-Kien, 1990). Transplant-associated KS was first described in the 1970s and is seen in immunosuppressed allograft recipients. Both cutaneous disease and visceral disease are common (Penn, 1979).

AIDS-associated KS was first described in gay men in the early 1980s, at the advent of the HIV epidemic (Friedman-Kien, 1981), and is the most common neoplasm occurring in HIV-infected individuals (Frisch, 2001). AIDS-associated KS disproportionately affects gay men with HIV, who are estimated to have a 20-fold higher risk of developing KS in comparison with other HIV transmission risk groups (Beral, 1990; Hoover, 1993). KS is rarely reported in intravenous (IV) drug users or other HIV risk groups (Mitsuyasu, 1984; Safai, 1987).

The incidence of KS in resource-abundant countries has declined markedly since the early 1990s with the widespread use of ART. Of the 85,922 cases of KS in the United States, the proportion of KS in persons with AIDS declined from 89% in 1990–1995 to 67% in 2001–2007 ($p < 0.001$) (Shiels, 2011). Cumulative incidence of KS by age 75 years was among the highest compared to other cancers (lung, anal, colorectal, Hodgkin's lymphoma, liver, and oropharyngeal) from 1995 to 2009 at 4.1%. However, there were significant decreases in incidence of KS by 4% per year from 2005 to 2009 compared to 1996–1999 rates ($p < 0.01$) (Silverberg, 2015). Similarly, the Swiss HIV Cohort Study showed that the KS incidence was 33.3 per 1000 patient-years in 1984–1986 and did not change significantly in the subsequent periods until 1996–1998, when it declined to 5.1 per 1000 patient-years (95% confidence interval (CI), 3.9–6.5) and then further decreased to 1.4 per 1000 patient-years in 1999–2001 and remained constant thereafter (Franceschi, 2008). A Brazilian retrospective cohort also described a decreased incidence of KS from 1998 to 2010, with an incidence rate ratio per year of 0.89 (95% CI, 0.83–0.97) (Castilho, 2015).

In areas of southern Africa where KS is endemic, this cancer has reached epidemic proportions due to lack of ART. For instance, in Zimbabwe, KS is reported to represent 40% of all cancers in men (Chokunonga, 2000). A prospective cohort from 2004–2010 found that the incidence in Zimbabwe, Botswana, South Africa, and Zambia reached 413/100,000 patient-years (95% CI, 342–497), with higher rates among age groups older than age 60 years (Rohner, 2014). Despite the increased availability of ART in these countries, estimates of KS have minimally decreased in the HIV population on ART, with the incidence of KS remaining high at 164/100,000 patient-years (95% CI, 151–178) (Rohner, 2014). Individuals with KS in this geographic region have high tumor burdens and aggressive disease progression, and survival from time of diagnosis is often less than 6 months (Campbell, 2003).

PATHOGENESIS

In 1994, Chang and Moore (Chang, 1994) discovered a new herpesvirus, human herpesvirus type 8 (HHV-8) or KS herpes virus (KSHV), in more than 90% of AIDS-KS tissue samples. Although the KS types vary in epidemiology and clinical presentation, all are associated with HHV-8. In 2003, Engels et al. demonstrated HHV-8 viremia to be an early marker of KS, and Newton found that the risk of developing disease increased with HHV-8 antibody titers (Engels 2003; Newton, 2003). HHV-8 also is associated with rare lymphoproliferative diseases most often seen in individuals with HIV, including multicentric Castleman's disease and a rare form of NHL called primary effusion or body cavity lymphoma. Although infection with KSHV is necessary for the development of KSHV-associated disease, it is not sufficient. Among individuals with HIV, immunosuppression confers the greatest risk and is most predictive of development of KS (Jacobson, 2000; Renwick, 1998).

The pathogenesis of KS is complex and involves viral processes and dysregulation of cytokine pathways. The HHV-8 genome encodes many homologues of human cellular gene products that are involved in inflammation, cell cycle regulation, and angiogenesis, such as viral cyclin-D1, vascular endothelial growth factor, basic fibroblast growth factor, and interleukin-6 (Cannon, 2000). Cytokines released from spindle cells and inflammatory cells stimulate the growth of tumors. A regulatory transactivating (Tat) protein of HIV is released by infected cells and guards KS

cells from apoptosis (Deregibus, 2002), stimulates growth and angiogenesis (Barillari, 2002; Ensoli, 1990), and also increases the production and release of matrix metalloproteinases (MMPs) from endothelial and inflammatory cells. MMPs contribute to the angiogenesis found in KS lesions (Impola, 2003; Lafrenie, 1996).

The mechanism of HHV-8 transmissibility remains unclear. HHV-8 has been detected in semen, prostate tissue (Monini, 1996), and breast milk (Dedicoat, 2004). The virus is often shed from the oropharynx of both immunocompetent and immunocompromised men and women in areas where KSHV is endemic (Casper, 2004, 2007). Behaviors associated with exposure to saliva are correlated with a higher risk of KSHV infection, implicating both sexual and horizontal transmission (Casper, 2006; Plancoulaine, 2000). A relatively high KSHV seroprevalence has been described among injection drug users, and an increased incidence of KSHV infection has been noted among transfusion recipients in areas where KSHV is endemic, suggesting that parenteral transmission may be possible (Cannon, 2001; Hladik, 2006). Finally, transmission of KSHV from donors of solid organs has been described (Barozzi, 2003; Luppi, 2000).

CLINICAL MANIFESTATIONS

KS is an angioproliferative disease varying from an indolent to fulminant disease with potential for significant morbidity and mortality. The disease can occur in patients with a wide range of CD4+ cell counts but becomes increasingly common as immune function declines. The progression of disease may be rapid or slow. Patients with limited disease and controlled HIV infection usually do reasonably well. However, in the setting of uncontrolled HIV viral replication and low CD4+ counts, KS progresses rapidly.

The skin is the most common site of presentation. Visceral involvement is quite common, and as the disease progresses, KS frequently involves the gastrointestinal (GI) tract. At autopsy, almost every organ system can show involvement. Visceral disease is uncommon in the absence of extensive cutaneous disease.

The cutaneous presentation of KS occurs in 95% of cases. Lesions may occur anywhere on the skin. Common sites include the face (particularly the periorbital area and tip of the nose), external ear, mouth, torso, and lower extremities. They can evolve from macules or nodular tumors to large plaque-like tumor masses that involve extensive cutaneous surfaces and eventually evolve into ulcerating tumors. Their color may vary from violaceous in light-skinned individuals to brownish-black in dark-skinned individuals. These lesions are generally nonblanching, nonpruritic, and painless. Lesions of KS may become painful in the setting of immune reconstitution inflammatory syndrome (IRIS).

Lymphedema associated with KS usually appears in patients with visible cutaneous lesions, and edema may be out of proportion to the extent of visible lesions. Lymphedema also may occur in patients with no visible skin lesions. Common sites include the face, neck, external genitals, and lower extremities. A contiguous area of skin usually is involved as well.

Oral cavity involvement is seen in approximately one-third of KS patients and is the initial site of diagnosis 15% of the time (Dezube, 2004). These lesions may be flat or nodular and are red or purplish. They usually appear on the hard palate, but they may develop on the soft palate, gingival areas, and tongue. Oral lesions, if extensive, may cause tooth loss, pain, and ulceration. Involvement of the oral cavity correlates with KS in the GI tract.

Gastrointestinal KS has been reported in 40% of cases at initial diagnosis (Dezube, 2004) with any segment of the GI tract involved. Visceral spread of KS that involves the GI tract is rarely symptomatic. However, with disease progression, patients may have symptoms of abdominal pain, nausea, vomiting, or GI bleeding (Danzig, 1991). Rare cases of obstruction, perforation, or protein-losing enteropathy have been reported (Friedman, 1988). In those with advanced immunosuppression (CD4$^+$ cell count <100 cells/mm^3), GI KS may be more severe with complications. Some believe that screening endoscopy to detect occult disease may be warranted in these patients (Nagata, 2012).

Pulmonary KS is also common; however, in contrast to KS at other visceral sites, lung involvement is generally symptomatic. Common symptoms include cough, bronchospasm, dyspnea, and hemoptysis. This complication tends to occur in the setting of advanced AIDS, with most individuals having CD4$^+$ cell counts <100 cells/mm^3 (Gill, 1989), and in patients with more extensive cutaneous disease (e.g., with >50 lesions). Of note, it can occur in patients with minimal and absent cutaneous KS. The disease is often rapidly progressive when it involves the lungs, with a median survival time of only 2–6 months in the pre-ART era (Kaplan, 1988). Respiratory failure is often the cause of death. The radiographic appearance is variable, with the characteristic reticulonodular pattern seen in approximately one-third of patients (Kaplan, 1988). Otherwise, diffuse interstitial infiltrates, pleural effusions, and hilar adenopathy may be seen (Levine, 2001).

Once KS is clinically suspected, diagnosis is made by biopsy and histologic examination or by presumptive diagnosis based on the endoscopic appearance of a visceral lesion (Aboulafia, 2001). A histologic confirmation is essential to exclude other conditions that can mimic KS. Endoscopically, the classic appearance of small submucosal vascular nodules establishes the diagnosis of GI KS. It may be difficult to establish a diagnosis of GI KS by biopsy because many of the lesions are submucosal (Hengge, 2002). In patients with suspected pulmonary KS, violaceous endobronchial lesions typically are observed on bronchoscopic examination. A presumptive diagnosis of pulmonary KS can be made based on characteristic radiographic and endobronchial findings in patients who have had KS at other sites (Kaplan, 1988). Endobronchial biopsy is discouraged because of the risk of hemorrhage. Gallium scanning may be helpful in differentiating KS from pulmonary infection because KS is not gallium avid (Kaplan, 1988).

In the pre-ART era, the AIDS Clinical Trials Group (ACTG) developed a staging system based on tumor extent (T), severity of immunosuppression (I), and the presence of systemic illness (S) (Krown, 1997). Two different risk categories were noted based on this staging system: a good risk defined as T0I0S0 and a poor risk defined as T1I1S1 (Table 33.1).

Based on epidemiological, clinical, staging, and survival data of patients in two Italian prospective cohort studies ($N = 211$), Nasti et al. concluded that in the era of ART, a refinement of the ACTG staging system is needed (Nasti, 2003). Patient CD4$^+$ cell counts in this study did not provide prognostic information, and only the combination of T1S1 identified patients with unfavorable prognosis. The 3-year survival rate for patients with T1S1 was 53%, which was significantly lower compared to the 3-year survival rates of patients with T0S0, T1S0, and T0S1, which were 88%, 80%, and 81%, respectively. Several studies have found other prognostic markers for KS. Stebbing et al. developed a prognostic index predicting poor survival. The index included the following variables: not having Kaposi's sarcoma as the AIDS-defining illness, decreasing CD4$^+$ cell count, age 50 years or older, and having another AIDS-associated illness at the same time (Stebbing, 2006). Other variables, including CD8$^+$ cell count (Stebbing, 2007) and detectable HHV-8 DNA in plasma at the time of diagnosis (El Amari, 2008), have also been associated with poor KS prognosis.

TREATMENT

Treatment of KS is generally not considered curative and was not shown to have a significant impact on survival in the pre-ART era. An older retrospective review of 194 cases of KS (Volberding, 1989) showed no significant difference in survival time between patients treated with chemotherapy

Table 33.1 ACTG TUMOR STAGING SYSTEM

CHARACTERISTIC	GOOD RISK (0)	POOR RISK (1)
	All of the following:	Any of the following:
Tumor (T)	Tumor confined to skin and/or lymph nodes and/or minimal oral disease[a]	Tumor-associated edema or ulceration; extensive oral KS; GI KS; other visceral KS
Immune system (I)	CD4 count ≥150 cells/mm^3	CD4 count <150 cells/mm^3
Systemic illness (S)	No history of OI or thrush; no systemic symptoms; Karnofsky performance status ≥70	History of OI and/or thrush; systemic symptoms; Karnofsky performance status <70; other HIV-related illnesses

[a]Nonnodular KS confined to the palate.

GI, gastrointestinal; KS, Kaposi's sarcoma; OI, opportunistic infection.

SOURCE: Adapted from Krown (1989) and incorporating revision by Krown (1997), with permission from the American Society of Clinical Oncology.

or interferon-α and patients not treated. In a recent randomized trial done in South Africa of ART alone versus ART plus chemotherapy for KS, there was a significant difference in KS response but no difference in survival between the two arms (Mosam, 2012). In the United States, the primary goals of treatment for patients with KS are palliation of symptoms and improved cosmesis. Consultation with a KS-experienced oncologist or dermatologist should be considered for most patients diagnosed with this malignancy.

Impact of Antiretroviral Therapy

ART is a key component in the treatment of KS and should be initiated or optimized to achieve complete HIV RNA suppression in all patients with AIDS-associated KS. The inhibition of HIV replication, decreased production of the Tat protein, restored immunity to HHV-8, and the direct antiangiogenic activity of some protease inhibitors are among the many benefits of ART (Noy, 2003). Some older data suggested that protease inhibitors (PIs) have an anti-KS effect (Sgadari, 2003); however, non-PI-containing ART regimens also lead to KS regression.

Combination ART has been associated with a lengthening of time to treatment failure with either local or systemic therapy for KS. A retrospective study found a median time of 20.4 months from the initiation of ART plus chemotherapy versus 6 months with just chemotherapy to detect treatment failure among HIV-infected individuals with KS (Bower, 1999). It has also been demonstrated that HIV-infected individuals who were receiving ART at KS diagnosis had a less aggressive presentation versus individuals who were ART naive at the time of KS diagnosis (Nasti, 2003). Another retrospective analysis from 1990 to 1999 found an 81% reduction in the risk of death among HIV-infected individuals with KS after the initiation of ART (Tam, 2002).

KS-associated IRIS has been well described. Some patients may experience painful enlarged lesions or progression of KS lesions during the first months of ART. In a prospective study of 69 patients with HIV and KSHV co-infection, approximately 12% of patients experienced IRIS-KS after initiation of ART (Letang, 2010).

Local Treatment

Local treatment should be reserved for patients with minimal or locally symptomatic disease. These patients should concurrently receive ART. Current options for local treatment include the following:

- Radiotherapy has been the mainstay of local therapy for KS. It is best suited for patients with single or a few locally symptomatic areas or for symptomatic disease that requires rapid tumor reduction. Electron beam radiation applied to the entire face is highly effective in relief of facial edema. Radiotherapy also can be useful for treatment of dysphagia caused by pharyngeal lesions and tumor masses of the eye or the extremities (Hill, 1987). Radiotherapy, whether given as whole-body electron beam therapy, fractionated focal radiation therapy, or single treatments, has produced complete remissions in 50–80% of patients (Cooper, 1991; Pluda, 1992). Complications such as severe mucositis, radiotherapy fibrosis, loss of skin compliance, and chronic lymphedema may occur with these treatments.

- With intralesional chemotherapy, vinblastine has been most commonly used, with a reported response rate of 70% in older studies (Boudreaux, 1993). Small cutaneous lesions can be treated with intralesional chemotherapy for cosmetic purposes. Repeated treatments may be necessary. Intralesional chemotherapy can cause significant pain and also areas of hyperpigmentation after treatment.

- Alitretinoin gel (Panretin) is a topical treatment that may be used for relatively asymptomatic patients with KS lesions that do not respond to ART alone and for whom the KS is predominantly an issue of cosmesis. A response rate of 49% ($N = 184$) in a phase III study was reported (Walmsley, 1999). Adverse effects include dry skin and light hypersensitivity.

- Cryotherapy with liquid nitrogen and laser therapy has been used successfully for the treatment of isolated small KS lesions. Given the significant mucosal toxicity associated with radiotherapy in the treatment of oral lesions, laser surgery may be substituted for radiation.

Systemic Treatment

Systemic chemotherapy is used for more severe disease, including symptomatic visceral disease, extensive skin involvement, significant edema, or rapidly progressive KS. As described previously, the goal of systemic chemotherapy is mainly palliation of symptoms.

Large randomized studies have established liposomal anthracyclines (doxorubicin and daunorubicin) as first-line single-agent chemotherapy agents with promising results compared to combination chemotherapy treatment (Gill, 1996; Northfelt, 1998; Stewart, 1998). These studies found that liposomal anthracyclines alone can achieve response rates equal to or better than those of combination chemotherapy with a lower incidence of toxicity such as nausea, fatigue, alopecia, and neuropathy. Neutropenia, however, occurred as frequently with the liposomal agent as with the standard combination regimen.

Paclitaxel is a highly active agent that is often used as second-line therapy. It has significant antitumor activity in patients with previously untreated (Gill, 1995) and refractory KS (Saville, 1995). The most significant side effects are hypersensitivity, myelosuppression, peripheral neuropathy, alopecia, and drug interactions with ART. This agent is the treatment of choice for refractory KS or if there are contraindications to the use of anthracyclines.

Combination regimens with adriamycin, bleomycin, and vincristine have produced overall response rates of 24–60% in patients with pulmonary KS (Gill, 1996; Ireland-Gill, 1992). The use of these agents has declined dramatically since the introduction of the single agents mentioned previously. Imatinib, a platelet-derived growth factor receptor/c-kit inhibitor, induced responses in 10 of 30 patients

with KS when given up to 1 year in a multicenter phase II trial (Koon, 2014). The vascular endothelial growth factor-A inhibitor, bevacizumab, was shown in another phase II trial to produce complete and partial responses in 3 and 2 of 16 patients, respectively (Uldrik, 2012). Inhibition of the KS-activated mammalian target of rapamycin (mTOR) signaling pathway has also been examined in an AIDS Malignancy Consortium (AMC) study and has shown promising therapeutic results (Krown, 2012).

Recommended Reading

Gill PS, Wernz J, Scadden DT, et al. Randomized phase III trial of liposomal daunorubicin versus doxorubicin, bleomycin, and vincristine in AIDS-related Kaposi's sarcoma. *J Clin Oncol.* 1996; 14(8):2353–2364.

Shiels MS, Pfeiffer RM, Hall HI, et al. Proportions of Kaposi sarcoma, selected non-Hodgkin lymphomas, and cervical cancer in the United States occurring in persons with AIDS, 1980–2007. *JAMA.* 2011; 305(14):1450–1459.

HIV-RELATED PRIMARY CENTRAL NERVOUS SYSTEM LYMPHOMA

LEARNING OBJECTIVES

- Review the epidemiology of PCNSL in HIV patients.
- Review the pathophysiology and clinical presentation.
- Review chemotherapeutic strategies for treatment.
- Discuss survival among these patients.

WHAT'S NEW?

Fluorodeoxyglucose–positron emission tomography (FDG-PET) and magnetic resonance spectroscopy provide less invasive strategies to characterize invasiveness of disease and distinguish from other pathologies.

KEY POINTS

- EBV-mediated oncogenesis in the setting of advanced immunosuppression is largely responsible for PCNSL.
- Treatment with ART should be initiated and maintained for all HIV patients with PCNSL.
- Despite improved survival in the ART era, overall survivability remains poor.

Primary CNS lymphoma is a rare type of NHL, accounting for 1% or 2% of all NHLs and <5% of all primary brain tumors (Lister, 2002). PCNSL has been diagnosed in 1.6–9.0% of patients with AIDS and represents the second most common intracranial mass lesion in this population (Rosenblum, 1988; Welch, 1984). The vast majority of PCNSL has been linked to EBV-infected B cells that reach the CNS during advanced immunodeficiency (Cingolani, 2005). MacMahon and colleagues noted that EBV genes important for oncogenesis are abundant in patients with primary CNS lymphoma, suggesting a pathogenic role of EBV in this setting (MacMahon, 1991). This association suggests that the pathogenesis of PCNSL might differ from systemic NHL, which has a 40–50% association with EBV (Ballerini, 1993; Hamilton-Dutoit, 1989).

EPIDEMIOLOGY

In the era before effective ART, the relative risk of PCNSL was approximately 1000-fold and as high as 3600-fold in individuals with AIDS compared to the general population (Cote, 1996).

The age-adjusted incidence of PCNSL in the United States has increased substantially since the 1970s, from 0.16 per 100,000 in 1973–1984 to 0.48 per 100,000 in 1985–1997 (Olson, 2002). However, with the introduction of ART in the mid to late 1990s, the incidence of PCNSL in AIDS has significantly decreased (Hoffman, 2001; Wolf, 2005). In the Multicenter AIDS Cohort Study, the incidence rate in 2734 HIV-infected men declined from 4.3 to 0.4 per 100,000 (Sacktor, 2001). Despite this dramatic decrease in incidence, survival rates have not significantly improved, especially compared to those of HIV-negative counterparts (Bayraktar, 2011; Conti, 2000).

CLINICAL PRESENTATION

The clinical presentation of CNS lymphoma is similar irrespective of HIV status. Symptoms may include headaches, confusion, lethargy, memory loss, personality changes, and seizures. On examination, patients may present with hemiparesis, aphasia, and cranial nerve palsies. Lesions are most common in the cerebrum, basal ganglia, and brainstem. More diffuse and multifocal involvement is seen in HIV-related PCNSL (Gage, 2000). These lesions are contrast enhancing on computed tomography (CT) and MRI. Before ART, the median CD4 cell count at presentation was <50/mm³ (Levine, 1991).

PCR to detect EBV DNA in the cerebrospinal fluid is useful for diagnosing AIDS-associated CNS lymphoma.

Identification of EBV by PCR can detect most cases of AIDS-related PCNSL with a sensitivity of 80–100% and specificity for lymphoma of 93–100% (Bossolasco, 2002). Cerebrospinal fluid cytology alone has limited utility due to poor sensitivity and specificity (Ekstein, 2006).

Single photon emission computed tomography has been suggested as a less invasive technique for diagnosis. However, due to conflicting results in terms of sensitivity and specificity, its role in the diagnosis of PCNSL remains limited (Licho, 2002; Ruiz, 1994). FDG-PET and magnetic resonance spectroscopy are two other imaging modalities that can aid in the diagnosis of cerebral PCNSL lesions apart from other infectious CNS pathologies such as toxoplasmosis. Magnetic resonance spectroscopy typically shows decreased N-acetylaspartate and increased choline, which reflects neoplastic cell proliferation (Westwood, 2013). FDG-PET can also help identify extracerebral systemic disease involvement (Lewitschnig, 2013). Currently, the gold standard for diagnosis of PCNSL is stereotactic brain biopsy. In patients in whom a brain biopsy is unobtainable, the combination of imaging, negative toxoplasma serology, previous toxoplasmosis prophylaxis, and positive EBV cerebrospinal fluid by PCR may be sufficient to make a presumptive diagnosis.

TREATMENT AND SURVIVAL

The relative rarity of PCNSL precludes large-scale randomized trials; therefore, the optimal treatment for PCNSL has not been determined. Norden et al. showed that HIV/AIDS significantly reduced median overall survival to 2 months versus 12 months in non-HIV patients (Norden, 2011). Despite good initial response rates to treatment, median survival times with treatment remain only 2–5.5 months (Baumgartner, 1990). The previous standard treatment of patients with AIDS-related CNS lymphoma was palliative corticosteroids and whole-brain radiation that achieved a complete response in 20–50% of patients (Cote, 1996). Radiation alone can improve symptoms and extend median survival, but this is likely affected by a patient's baseline functional status and not the dose of radiation received (Goldstein, 1991).

Regarding AIDS-related PCNSL, an uncontrolled pilot study published in 1997 used high-dose IV methotrexate in 15 patients, including 10 with histologically confirmed lymphoma. The median time since clinical onset was 27 days (range, 7–69 days), and the mean CD4⁺ cell count was 30 cells/mm³. Complete responses, defined as clinical improvement and disappearance of contrast-enhancing brain abnormalities on CT or MRI, was obtained in 7 of

15 patients (3 of 10 patients with histological diagnosis and 4 of 5 patients without histological confirmation). One patient relapsed at 6 months. Six patients failed to respond, and 2 patients died of severe sepsis. The median survival time was 290 days for the 10 patients with histological diagnosis and 347 days for the 5 patients without histological confirmation. In addition, steroids were also administered, and individuals ultimately received ART including a protease inhibitor (Jacomet, 1997). In HIV-negative individuals with primary CNS lymphoma, high-dose IV methotrexate remains the standard of care for those who can tolerate the therapy. Whole-brain radiation is reserved for those with poor performance status (National Comprehensive Cancer Network (NCCN) PSCNL version 1.2015). Further investigation of other treatment strategies, including use of anti-CD20 monoclonal antibodies and hematopoietic stem cell transplantation, is needed (Gabarre, 2004; Wolf, 2014).

ROLE OF ANTIRETROVIRAL THERAPY

Combination ART should be initiated in all individuals with AIDS-related PCNSL who are undertaking treatment because it is associated with significant improvement in survival. In the pre-ART era, radiotherapy prolonged survival for 2–5.5 months compared to palliative care (Donahue, 1995). McGowan and Shah (McGowan, 1998) were the first to describe a case of remission maintained for more than 2 years after treatment with ART alone in an individual who had PCNSL. Other case reports have also reported similar PCNSL response to ART (Aboulafia, 2007; Corales, 2000; Travi, 2012). In a retrospective analysis, Hoffman and colleagues (Hoffman, 2001) showed that survival times of patients receiving ART in addition to radiotherapy differed significantly from those of patients receiving radiotherapy or palliative care alone. Four of the six patients receiving ART survived for more than 1.5 years. In another retrospective analysis, Skiest and Crosby (Skiest, 2003) demonstrated a prolonged median survival of 667 days in individuals who received ART. These findings strongly suggest that immune recovery contributes to recovery and longer remission in HIV patients with PCNSL.

Recommended Reading

Cingolani A, Fratino L, Scoppettuolo G, et al. Changing pattern of primary cerebral lymphoma in the highly active antiretroviral therapy era. *J Neurovirol.* 2005; 11(Suppl 3):38–44.
Westwood TD, Hogan C, Julyan PJ, et al. Utility of FDG-PETCT and magnetic resonance spectroscopy in differentiating between cerebral lymphoma and non-malignant CNS lesions in HIV-infected patients. *Eur J Radiol.* 2013; 82(8):e374–e379.

SYSTEMIC NON-HODGKIN'S LYMPHOMA

LEARNING OBJECTIVES

- Review the epidemiology of NHL.
- Review the pathophysiology and clinical manifestations of NHL
- Review the treatment of NHL and survival outcomes.

WHAT'S NEW?

- Survival for NHL continues to improve in the ART era; however, incidence continues to be significantly higher compared to that for HIV-negative persons.
- Intensive chemotherapy and autologous hematopoietic cell transplantation (HCT) are safe in patients with HIV and are associated with improved outcomes.

KEY POINTS

- NHL development is likely a multifactorial interplay among host immune factors as well as the presence of viral mediators including EBV and HHV-8. Disease can occur in a variety of nodal and extranodal sites, and some forms of NHL are more aggressive than others, such as primary effusion lymphoma (PEL).
- Prognostic factors include host immunity, the presence of injection drug use, performance status, and the degree of tumor burden.
- Treatment with ART and intensive chemotherapy with consideration of HCT are cornerstones of NHL treatment.

The first cases of AIDS-related NHL were described in 1982 (Ziegle, 1982). In 1985, NHL was added to the list of AIDS-defining malignancies. Before the ART era, it was estimated to occur in approximately 8% of all HIV cases (Kaplan, 1989), and it is currently the second most common neoplasm occurring among HIV-infected individuals (Knowles, 2001).

The World Health Organization has divided AIDS-related lymphomas (ARLs) into three categories (Table 33.2):

Table 33.2 AIDS-RELATED LYMPHOMAS: WORLD HEALTH ORGANIZATION CLASSIFICATION

Lymphomas also occurring in immunocompetent patient
  Burkitt's lymphoma
  Diffuse large B cell lymphoma: Centroblastic, immunoblastic, and anaplastic variants
Lymphomas occurring specifically in HIV-infected patients
  Primary effusion lymphoma
  Plasmablastic lymphoma
Lymphomas also occurring in other immunodeficiency states
  Polymorphic or post-transplant lymphoproliferative disorder-like B cell lymphoma

SOURCE: Adapted from Raphael (2008).

1. Lymphomas also occurring in immunocompetent patients, such as Burkett's lymphoma and diffuse large B cell lymphoma

2. Lymphomas occurring specifically in HIV-infected patients, such as PEL and plasmablastic lymphoma

3. Lymphomas also occurring in other immunodeficiency states, such as polymorphic or post-transplant lymphoproliferative disorder-like B cell lymphoma

Diffuse large B cell lymphoma (DLBCL) and Burkitt's lymphoma are the most common ARLs, representing approximately 90% of these malignancies (Besson, 2001). Only intermediate-grade or high-grade lymphomas are considered AIDS-defining.

EPIDEMIOLOGY

Individuals with impaired cell-mediated immunity show a marked increase in the incidence of NHL. This has been best described in immunosuppressed allograft recipients. Similar trends were seen in HIV-infected individuals in the pre-ART era. The CDC examined data of 2824 NHL cases occurring in 97,258 HIV-infected individuals between 1981 and 1989 in the United States. The risk was 60 times greater in HIV-infected individuals (Beral, 1991). The risk also varies by histologic subtype, with up to 600-fold excess risk for immunoblastic lymphoma (IBL) (Cote, 1997). In a recent study evaluating the cumulative incidence of NHL in persons with HIV living in the United States and Canada ($n = 86,620$), the incidence of NHL from 1996 to 2009 was 4.5% by age 75 years compared to only 0.7% in HIV-negative persons ($n = 196,987$) (Silverberg, 2015).

PATHOGENESIS

The pathogenesis of HIV NHL is most likely multifactorial, involving HIV; immune dysfunction; cytokine dysregulation; and other viral antigens, including EBV and HHV-8 (Gates, 2003). EBV is present in approximately 40–50% of cases of AIDS-related systemic NHL (Hamilton-Dutoit, 1989). This contrasts with a report by Ballerini and colleagues, who reported 100% EBV co-infection in the IBL variant of DLBCL (Ballerini, 1993). The expression of the latent EBV transforming proteins EBNA-2 and LMP-1 is known to play a central role in the initiation and maintenance of EBV-induced B cell growth and proliferation (Liebowitz, 1989). Both EBNA-2 and LMP-1 can serve as targets for cytotoxic T cells; thus, their expression induces T cell immune surveillance and regulates lymphomagenesis in individuals who are immunocompetent. With immunodeficiency states such as late-stage HIV, EBNA-2 and LMP-1 expression may become unregulated and subsequently lead to uncontrolled proliferation of EBV-infected cells (Gaidano, 1995). Genetic alterations involving oncogenes and tumor suppressor genes may also occur, and often *MYC* and *BCL6* translocations are implicated in neoplastic development (Chadburn, 2013).

Expression of HHV-8 has also been associated with PEL, which often presents as malignant effusions in both the chest and the abdomen with a paucity of nodal masses. It is aggressive and often refractory to chemotherapy. HHV-8 has been universally found in malignant cells, often in conjunction with EBV (Komanduri, 1996).

CLINICAL CHARACTERISTICS

Approximately two-thirds of ARLs are classified as DLBCL (Navarro, 2006). AIDS-related systemic NHL usually presented as widespread disease involving extranodal sites in the pre-ART era (Knowles, 1988). The most common sites of extranodal disease are the gastrointestinal tract, CNS, bone marrow, and liver. Ziegler et al. reported that 95% of patients from several institutions had evidence of extranodal disease, including 42% with CNS involvement and 33% with bone marrow involvement (Ziegler, 1984). Of note, GI NHL occurs in approximately 30% of HIV-infected patients with NHL. Most of these cases involve the stomach, but virtually any site in the GI tract or hepatobiliary tree can be involved (Burkes, 1986). Interestingly, plasmablastic lymphomas are associated with characteristic development of oral cavity lesions in the majority of cases and predominate in mucosal sites (Chadburn, 2013).

In the ART era, among patients with undetectable plasma HIV RNA levels, Gerard et al. found that NHL occurred at a median CD4 cell count of 297. In addition, they found that 65% of the cases occurred within 18 months of initiating HIV treatment with ART (Gerard, 2009). Other studies have shown that PEL and immunoblastic NHL are seen in patients with lower CD4 cell counts, of older age, and with a prior diagnosis of AIDS, whereas Burkitt's NHL tends to occur in patients with more preserved immune function (Knowles, 1996).

PROGNOSTIC FEATURES

Historically, poor prognostic factors for patients with HIV-related NHL have included age older than 35 years, CD4$^+$ T cell count <100 cells/mm^3, history of injection drug use, history of AIDS-defining condition, poor performance status, elevated lactate dehydrogenase, tumor bulk or stage of disease, and International Prognostic Index (IPI) (Straus, 1998). The IPI includes clinical features that reflect the growth and invasive potential of the tumor (tumor stage, serum lactate dehydrogenase (LDH) level, and number of extranodal disease sites), the patient's response to the tumor (performance status), and the patient's ability to tolerate intensive therapy (age and performance status). The simplified model for younger patients (the age-adjusted IPI) uses a subgroup of these clinical features (tumor stage, LDH level, and performance status).

Lim and colleagues compared the prognostic factors for survival and the use of the IPI in pre- and post-ART HIV-infected individuals with diffuse large-cell lymphoma (Lim, 2005) In groups with low-, low-intermediate-, and high-intermediate-risk IPI disease, 3-year overall survival rates were 20%, 22%, and 5% in the pre-ART era and improved to 64%, 64%, and 50% in the post-ART era, respectively. Of note, PEL and extracavity PEL are known to be aggressive malignancies, with median survival time of 6 months and fewer survivors beyond 12 months. Poor performance status and lack of ART portend poorer prognosis (Boulanger, 2005).

TREATMENT

The treatment for AIDS-related lymphoma is similar to that of non-HIV-infected individuals, with some exceptions. Intrathecal chemotherapy prophylaxis is necessary because patients with HIV are at an increased risk for CNS involvement. Those cases include lymphomas with aggressive pathologic features, including Burkitt's lymphoma, plasmablastic lymphoma, and presentations consistent with possible CNS involvement (Chari, 2005). The use of hematopoietic stimulants such as granulocyte colony-stimulating factor (G-CSF) may aid in reducing chemotherapy-induced cytopenic complications. *Pneumocystis jirovecii* pneumonia prophylaxis is administered with standard-dose chemotherapy, irrespective of CD4 cell count.

Chemotherapy in the Pre-ART Era

In the pre-ART era, HIV-infected individuals with NHL had a poor prognosis, were managed on low-dose chemotherapy regimens because of concern for toxicity, and had a median survival of 5–8 months (Kaplan, 1997; Sandler, 1996). In addition to persistent neoplasia contributing to death, many patients in this era died due to the infectious complications of opportunistic diseases (Lowenthal, 1988).

Chemotherapy in the ART Era

In the ART era, more recent standard chemotherapy regimens have been reported without excessive toxicity due to restored immunity. The AMC reported on 65 patients who were given reduced doses of cyclophosphamide and doxorubicin combined with vincristine and prednisone (modified CHOP) or full doses of CHOP combined with G-CSF with concomitant ART. Complete response rates were 30% and 48% in the reduced- and full-dose groups, respectively (Ratner, 2001). No long-term outcomes were reported in this study. Other studies of CHOP-based chemotherapy and concurrent ART have reported median survival of 2 years. In patients with Burkitt's lymphoma, a particularly aggressive form of NHL, intensive chemotherapy with cyclophosphamide, doxorubicin, high-dose methotrexate/ifosfamide, etoposide, and high-dose cytarabine (CODOX-M/IVAC) resulted in similar rates of event-free survival and remission as those of their HIV-negative counterparts (Wang, 2003).

Risk-adaptive chemotherapy has also been studied comparing the post- to pre-ART era. A total of 485 HIV-infected individuals were assigned randomly to chemotherapy after risk stratification based on an HIV score (comprising performance status, prior AIDS, and CD4$^+$ cell counts <100 cells/mm^3). Of these patients, there were 218 good risk patients (HIV score 0), who received doxorubicin, cyclophosphamide, vindesine, bleomycin, and prednisone (ACVBP) or CHOP; 177 intermediate risk patients (HIV score 1), who received CHOP or low-dose CHP; and 90 poor risk patients (HIV score 2 or 3), who received low-dose CHOP or vincristine and steroid. Five-year overall survival in the good risk group was 51%

for ACVBP versus 47% for CHOP ($p = 0.85$), that in the intermediate risk group was 28% for CHOP versus 24% for low-dose CHOP ($p = 0.19$), and that in the poor risk group was 11% for low-dose CHOP versus 3% for vincristine and steroid ($p = 0.14$). The significant factors in this study for overall survival were ART (relative risk (RR), 1.6; $p = 0.0002$), HIV score (RR, 1.7; $p = 0.0001$), and IPI score (RR, 1.5; $p = 0.0012$), but not the intensity of chemotherapy (Mounier, 2006).

An infusional regimen of cyclophosphamide, doxorubicin, and etoposide with or without ART (only didanosine) resulted in a complete response rate of 45% and median overall survival of 12.8 months. At the time of the analysis, 30% in the pre-ART group were alive, compared with 47% in the ART group. Furthermore, patients in the ART group experienced less nonhematologic toxicity (22% vs. 42%), thrombocytopenia (31% vs. 52%), and anemia (9% vs. 27%) (Sparano, 2004).

Chemotherapy ART Interactions

Cyclophosphamide and vincristine are metabolized via the CYP3A4 isoenzyme. PIs and non-nucleoside reverse transcriptase inhibitors both inhibit and induce CYP3A4, with the potential for altered chemotherapeutic and cytotoxic effects. Thus, chemotherapy without antiretroviral drugs has been studied due to concerns of drug interactions with chemotherapy and noncompliance with ART resulting in increased resistance (Powles, 2000). Furthermore, PIs (in ART regimens) have been associated with increased incidence of neutropenia with concomitant chemotherapy (Bower, 2004). The National Cancer Institute used a dose-adjusted regimen of etoposide, vincristine, and doxorubicin (4 days) and daily oral prednisone (5 days), followed by cyclophosphamide. The study consisted of 39 patients, and antiretrovirals were not given until after the final cycle of chemotherapy. A complete remission rate of 74% was achieved (Little, 2003).

Recently, raltegravir, an integrase inhibitor that is eliminated via glucuronidation, has been utilized during CHOP administration, resulting in minimal drug–drug interactions. It has also been used in the presence of other antimetabolites such as gemcitabine and methotrexate, as well as monoclonal antibodies rituximab and trastuzumab, with good tolerability and durable viral suppression (Bañon, 2014). Raltegravir improves virologic and immunologic responses in antiretroviral treatment-naive patients and is considered in the US Department of Health and Human Services (DHHS) ART guidelines for HIV disease as an acceptable first-line therapy; thus, it could be a suitable alternative for preventing chemotherapeutic–ART interactions (Fulco, 2010).

Rituximab

Kaplan and colleagues reported a randomized trial in the ART era using CHOP versus CHOP and rituximab (anti-CD20 antibody) given with each cycle and with an additional three monthly doses after complete response was attained (Kaplan, 2003). Median event-free survival at approximately 1 year was similar for both groups. The group treated with rituximab and CHOP, however, had an increased risk of death from infection (14% vs. 2%; $p = 0.027$). Up to 60% of deaths occurred in patients with a CD4 count <50 cells/mm³, and 40% occurred during the maintenance phase of rituximab. In non-HIV-infected individuals, rituximab benefit is limited to lymphomas that overexpress blc-2, and this overexpression is found less commonly in ARL, which may explain the decreased response to immunotherapy in this study (Avivi, 2003).

Sparano et al. examined rituximab plus infusional etoposide, vincristine, doxorubicin, cyclophosphamide, and prednisone (EPOCH) given either concurrently or sequentially. In the concurrent arm, 35 of 48 evaluable patients (73%; 95% CI, 58–85%) had a complete response, whereas 29 of 53 evaluable patients (55%; 95% CI, 41–68%) had a complete response. Toxicity was comparable in the two arms, although patients with a baseline CD4 count <50 cells/mm³ had a high infectious death rate in the concurrent arm (Sparano, 2010).

Regarding Burkitt's lymphoma, a 2012 study examined CODOX-M, followed by IVAC with or without rituximab. The majority of patients were on ART and had a median CD4 count of 375 cells/mm³. Ten of the 14 patients who received ART, intensive chemo, and rituximab survived to the follow-up period of nearly 12 months. Complications included late neutropenia, which responded well to G-CSF. Due to predilection of herpesvirus reactivation with rituximab, prophylaxis for herpes simplex and varicella zoster and preemptive monitoring of cytomegalovirus were also undertaken (Rodrigo, 2012).

Hematopoietic-Cell Transplantation for AIDS-Related NHL

Poor outcomes were observed using allogeneic or syngeneic bone marrow transplantation in the setting of HIV disease in the 1980s (Hassett, 1983; Holland, 1989). Several authors have reported on small series of patients treated at individual institutions for high first risk remission, relapsed, or refractory AIDS-related lymphoma. No definitive conclusions regarding efficacy can be made due to the small and varied group of patients. Although autologous HCT has long remained the optimal therapy for high-risk and refractory NHL in non-HIV patients, a sufficient number of HIV-infected individuals have now undergone autologous HCT to determine that it is a safe and feasible approach for ARL patients who meet criteria for transplantation (Navarro, 2006). Uninterrupted ART should be continued in these patients during the peritransplant period, when feasible, to maintain virological suppression and avoid untoward effects of acute virological rebound, including acute retroviral syndrome and opportunistic infections (Woolfrey, 2008). Administration of ART is generally considered safe with minimal effect on the transplantation course, including adverse drug–drug interactions or other significant adverse events (Johnston, 2016).

One study showed that low CD4 cell count, marrow involvement, and poor performance status independently affected survival with HCT (Re, 2009). Overall survival has been reported to be 50% at 9 months (Gabarre, e2000), 85% at 32 months (Krishnan, 2005), 55% at 9 months (Re, 2003), and 71% at 21 months (Diez-Martin, 2003). A few opportunistic infections were reported in patients receiving transplants, and success rates have ranged from 80% to 100%.

All studies except the French series by and colleagues (Diez-Martin, 2003) have required HIV disease to be under control for HCT, either by low to undetectable HIV RNA levels or by CD4 cell counts >100 cells/mm³. In another study, Diez-Martin et al. showed similar incidence of relapse, overall survival, and progression-free survival in cohorts of HIV-positive and HIV-negative lymphoma patients who received HCT (Diez-Martin, 2009). Long-term survival of autologous HCT for relapsed/refractory lymphoma has been examined in a 2015 retrospective review of HIV-positive survivors. This study found a survival of 65% at 5 years for 37 patients. Among 26 patients who achieved complete remission, overall survival at 10 years was 91% and event-free survival was 36%. Nine patients developed opportunistic infections at a median of 0.4 years post HCT (Zanet, 2015).

Impact of ART

Most studies have shown that the incidence of HIV NHL, like that for most other AIDS-defining cancers (ADCs), has declined throughout the years. In a meta-analysis by Appleby et al. (Appleby, 2000) that included 47,936 HIV-infected individuals with NHL (inclusive of PCNSL), the incidence declined from 6.2 cases/1000 person-years (py) in the pre-ART era to 3.6 cases/1000 py in the post-ART era ($p < 0.0001$).

In a population-based, record-linkage study of cancer in 472,378 individuals with AIDS from 1980 to 2006, the cumulative incidence of NHL declined from 3.8% during 1990–1995 to 2.2% during 1996–2006. Of note, NHL was the most common ADC during the ART era (53%) (Simard, 2011). In addition, the Swiss Cohort study examined 429 NHL cases of 12,959 HIV-infected individuals from 1993 to 2006. NHL incidence reached 13.6 per 1000 py in 1993–1995 and declined to 1.8 in 2002–2006. Combination ART use was associated with a decline in NHL incidence (hazard ratio (HR), 0.26; 95% CI, 0.20–0.33) (Polesel, 2008).

A recent retrospective study using US and Canadian data from 1996–2009 showed a significant decline in the annual hazard rate of NHL (–8%) in HIV-infected persons compared to that of uninfected persons, signifying a narrowing of the gap of NHL burden between HIV-infected and -uninfected groups (Silverberg, 2015). This reduction also represents the benefit of immunological recovery and viral control.

Recommended Reading

Bañon S, Machuca I, Araujo S, et al. Efficacy, safety, and lack of interactions with the use of raltegravir in HIV-infected patients undergoing antineoplastic chemotherapy. *J Intern AIDS Soc.* 2014; 17(4 Suppl 3):19590.

Zanet E, Taborelli M, Rupolo M, et al. Postautologous stem cell transplantation long-term outcomes in 26 HIV-positive patients affected by relapsed/refractory lymphoma. *AIDS.* 2015; 29(17):2303–2308.

NON-AIDS-DEFINING CANCERS

LEARNING OBJECTIVES

- Review the risk factors and epidemiology of NADCs.
- Review the impact of anogenital neoplasias and squamous cell cancer of the anus (SCCA) in men and women.
- Discuss treatment of anogenital neoplasias and SCCA, including the role of ART.

WHAT'S NEW?

- Women are more recognized as a high-risk group for SCCA, and pre-disposing factors include positivity for high-risk HPV serotypes.

KEY POINTS

- Due to the aging HIV population, NADCs are responsible for an increasing number of deaths. Immunologic control with ART, however, has decreased the incidence of some cancers, including anogenital cancers.

- Screening with cervical Papanicolaou (Pap) smear in women is a key surveillance measure for detecting precancerous lesions. Screening with anal Pap smear in men and women with risk factors is also recommended, although uptake of this practice may be contingent on the availability of high-resolution anoscopy.

- HPV vaccination for HIV-positive men and women is safe and efficacious.

Since the advent of widely available ART in the United States, individuals with HIV infection have had significantly improved survival and decreased mortality from AIDS-related infections and ADCs. However, with longer survival, it has become evident that individuals with HIV disease are now at increased risk for NADCs. Multiple risk factors for NADCs include degree and duration of viremia, low CD4$^+$ nadir, co-infection with oncogenic viruses (e.g., HPV and HBV), and personal carcinogenic exposure, which also should be considered when implementing risk mitigation strategies (Kowalkowski, 2014; Reidel, 2015; Vallet-Prichard, 2004).

Simard et al. confirmed the benefits of immunological control in a population-based, record-linkage study examining cancers in 472,378 individuals with AIDS from 1980 to 2006 (Simard 2011). The cumulative incidence of ADCs declined sharply across three AIDS calendar periods (from 18% in 1980–1989 to 11% in 1990–1995 and 4.2% in 1996–2006). The cumulative incidence of NADC increased from 1.1% to 1.5%, with no change thereafter (1% in 1996–2006). However, the cumulative incidence increased steadily over time for specific NADCs (anal cancer, Hodgkin's lymphoma, and liver cancer) (Simard, 2011). Another study (Simard, 2010) showed an elevated incidence for the following NADCs in patients 3–10 years after the onset of AIDS: Hodgkin's lymphoma and cancers of the oral cavity and/or pharynx, tongue, anus, liver, larynx, lung and/or bronchus, and penis. These data demonstrate that having previously diagnosed advanced immunosuppression appears to increase the risk for NADCs as well as ADCs.

The increased risk of NADCs among HIV-infected individuals has been reported by Patel et al. (Patel, 2008). The incidences of the following cancers were significantly higher: anal (standardized rate ratio (SRR), 42.9; 95% CI, 34.1–53.3), vaginal (SRR, 21.0; CI, 11.2–35.9), Hodgkin's lymphoma (SRR, 14.7; CI, 11.6–18.2), liver (SRR, 7.7; CI, 5.7–10.1), lung (SRR, 3.3; CI, 2.8–3.9), melanoma (SRR, 2.6; CI, 1.9–3.6), oropharyngeal (SRR, 2.6; CI, 1.9–3.4), leukemia (SRR, 2.5; CI, 1.6–3.8), colorectal (SRR, 2.3; CI, 1.8–2.9), and renal (SRR, 1.8; CI, 1.1–2.7). The incidence of prostate cancer was significantly lower among HIV-infected persons compared to the general population (SRR, 0.6; CI, 0.4–0.8). Only the relative incidence of anal cancer increased over time (Patel, 2008). Of particular note, none of the AIDS–cancer match studies found an increased risk of breast, colon, or prostate cancer. It is unclear if there is a definite link between the level of immunodeficiency and certain NADCs. Some studies have failed to show such a relationship (Burgi, 2005). Conversely, Reekie et al. utilized data from 4453 patients in the prospective, multinational EuroSIDA cohort (Reekie 2010). The incidence of NADCs in this cohort from 1994 to 2007 was 4.3 per 1000 py of follow-up. After adjustment, a higher current CD4$^+$ cell count was independently associated with a decreased incidence of NADCs. In addition, an increased rate of virus-related cancers and non-virus-related epithelial cancers was found in immunodeficient patients. Hodgkin's lymphoma, anal cancer, and lung cancer were all found at a higher rate in patients with lower current CD4$^+$ cell counts after adjustment for other demographic and traditional risk factors (Reekie, 2010).

It has also been previously hypothesized that individuals with HIV are at higher risk for malignancies at younger age. Shiels et al. (Shiels, 2010) used the national US AIDS Cancer Registry Match to demonstrate that individuals with HIV are not at increased risk for colon, prostate, or breast cancer at younger ages, but they were younger at the time of diagnosis for lung and anal cancers. They also found that the age of diagnosis of Hodgkin's lymphoma was significantly older than that of the general population. A recent study using data from the HIV/AIDS Cancer Match study found that HIV-infected patients with cancer tended to be younger than age 50 years compared to their uninfected counterparts, whose cancer occurred more often after age 60 years. This study also found that those with HIV presented with more advanced stage cancers with distant disease (32.2%) compared to uninfected patients (17.7%), and they experienced higher cancer-specific mortality (Coghill, 2015).

NADCs are responsible for an increasingly large proportion of deaths in patients with HIV disease in the ART era, which is likely due to longer survival among individuals with HIV. A study conducted by the Data Collection on Adverse Events of Anti-HIV Drugs (D:A:D) evaluated factors associated with mortality due to NADCs and ADCs (Monforte, 2008). The study included 23,437 patients under active follow-up from December 1999 through April 2001. It was found that the overall mortality rate due to NADCs was higher than that due to ADCs. The death rate from NADCs was 1.8 per 1000 py of follow-up (95% CI, 1.5–2.1) compared to 1.1 per 1000 py of follow-up (95% CI, 0.9–1.2) for ADCs. In addition, based on multivariable analysis, it was found that most recent CD4 cell count and increasing age were associated with an increased risk of death from ADCs and NADCs. Other factors, such as ART utilization, increased the risk of death for NADMs only. It is unlikely that HIV treatment itself increases the risk for NADMs. Rather, it underscores the complex relationship between prolonged survival with HIV disease, immunosuppression, and the diagnosis of and survival from NADCs.

The Mortalite study in France captured the changing patterns of AIDS-related deaths in that country (Bonnet, 2005; Lewden, 2005). Lewden reported on cancer deaths among HIV-infected individuals in the original study and found that in 2000, NADCs were the third leading cause of death. It was also found that as the patient population increased above age 45 years, deaths due to malignant disease eclipsed those due to infectious etiologies. The study was subsequently updated in 2005, and it was found that the rate of death from non-AIDS/hepatitis-related cancers increased from 38% in 2000 to 50% in 2005. A subsequent follow-up study found that the combination of ADCs and NADCs has become the leading cause of death in France (Morlat, 2014).

A retrospective study from the United States found that cancer-related mortality among HIV-infected individuals compared to HIV-uninfected patients (1996–2010) was significantly elevated for colorectal (HR, 1.49; 95% CI, 1.2–1.8), pancreatic (HR, 1.7; CI, 1.35–2.18), lung (HR, 1.28; CI, 1.17–1.3), melanoma (HR, 1.72; CI, 1.09–2.7), breast (HR, 2.61; CI, 2.06–3.3), and prostate cancer (HR, 1.57; CI, 1.02–2.41) (Coghill, 2015).

Regardless of etiology, as the HIV-infected population ages, the risk of NADCs will also undoubtedly increase. Some evidence suggests that treatment of these individuals

may be more difficult than that of the general population, that HIV-infected patients may present with more advanced disease, and that HIV-infected patients may not tolerate cancer therapies as well as HIV-negative patients (Bower, 2003). Screening for early signs of malignancy may be an important method for earlier diagnosis. However, no studies of screening approaches have been performed, and no specific recommendations for alternative screening practices different from what is recommended for the general population exist for HIV-infected adults for the majority of cancers.

Most studies of treatment outcomes for NADCs in the ART era demonstrate that HIV-infected individuals have similar outcomes as HIV-uninfected individuals. Simard and Engels evaluated cause of death in the pre-ART and ART eras and showed that death from NADCs (lung, Hodgkin's lymphoma, anal cancers, and other unspecified cancers) decreased steadily from 1980 to 2006 (Simard, 2010). For all NADCs, the number of deaths/1000 py from 1980–1989 to 1996–2006 significantly declined from 2.21 to 0.84 (Simard, 2010). Due to the benefit of ART on cancer outcomes in HIV-infected individuals, it is recommended that most patients be treated similarly to those without HIV infection and that ART should be administered concurrently with chemotherapy or radiotherapy (Chiao, 2010).

ANOGENITAL NEOPLASIA

Anogenital neoplasia refers to anal and cervical carcinomas and their precursor lesions. One of the most important risk factors associated with anogenital neoplasia is HPV infection. Human papillomavirus is a DNA virus and generally infects stratified squamous epithelium. More than 100 HPV serotypes have been identified to date, and at least 30 of these have a high predilection for the anogenital tract. HPV serotypes 6 and 11 have been associated with benign disease, whereas serotypes 16, 18, and 31 are associated with high-grade cervical or anal squamous intraepithelial lesions (SILs) or cervical and anal carcinomas.

In HIV, HPV infection has a well-established relationship with the increased risk of developing anogenital neoplasia (Bjorge, 2002; Palefsky, 1991). Frisch reported an increase in both invasive and in situ forms of not only cervical and anal cancer but also vulvar/vaginal and penile cancers among HIV-infected individuals (Frisch, 2000).

Pathogenesis of HPV in HIV Infection

The increased prevalence of HPV disease associated with HIV infection may be mediated by impaired T cell and antigen-presenting cell function. However, local effects of HIV infection may also upregulate HPV replication and oncogenesis. The HPV viral oncogenes E6 and E7 are able to immortalize primary keratinocytes and can transform cells in culture (Barbosa, 1989; Munger, 1989). In an animal model of estrogen-stimulated HPV-induced cervical cancer, expression of E7 alone resulted in precancers and cancer, whereas the expression of E6 and E7 together resulted in larger cancers (Riley, 2003). Although the exact mechanisms of HIV-related immunosuppression and HPV co-infection have not been determined, several in vitro studies have shown that the HIV tat protein can drive the replication of HPV-16 and HPV-18 through the overexpression of E7 and other genes in the early region (Tornesello, 1993; Vernone, 1993).

Epidemiology of HIV-Associated Cervical Carcinoma

Since 1993, invasive cervical cancer has been listed by the CDC as an "AIDS-defining" condition. However, quantifying the contribution of HIV infection to the development of cervical cancer among HIV-infected women remains unclear. A 1996 study that evaluated the relationship between HIV and cervical cancer found no conclusive evidence that HIV per se increased the risk of cervical cancer among HIV-infected women (International Agency for Research on Cancer, 1996). Subsequent studies continue to yield conflicting results. In developed countries with access to ART, several studies have shown an increased risk of cervical cancer. Using a national AIDS–cancer linked registry database of cases through 1998, Frisch et al. found a relative risk of 5.4 for invasive cervical cancer among HIV-positive women compared to the general population (Frisch, 2001). However, no increased risk in cervical cancer has been noted in case–control studies from multiple sub-Saharan African countries, where endemic rates of cervical cancer are higher and women have shorter survival (Gichangi, 2002; La Ruche, 1998; Patil, 1995).

As noted previously, with the use of ART since the mid-1990s, there have been definite declines in the incidence of AIDS-related cancers. This has been attributed to the improved immune function and control of oncogenic viruses seen with ART. This declining trend has not been consistently seen in AIDS-related cervical cancer. Shiels et al. showed an increasing proportion of cervical cancers in persons with AIDS from 0.11% in 1980–1989 (95% CI, 0.08–0.13) to 0.69% in 2001–2007 (95% CI, 0.49–0.89) (Shiels, 2011). A 2016 study from the Kaiser group found that HIV-positive women had twofold higher odds

of cervical intraepithelial neoplasia grade 2$^+$ (CIN2$^+$) and CIN3$^+$, but this was only in women with a recent CD4 count <500 cells/mm^3 (Silverberg, 2016).

Epidemiology of HIV-Associated Cervical Intraepithelial Neoplasia

The relationship between HIV infection and increased prevalence of CIN has been shown in many studies. Mandelblatt et al. performed a meta-analysis of 15 cross-sectional studies published between 1986 and 1998 that evaluated prevalence of cervical neoplasia, HPV infection, and HIV infection among women (Mandelblatt, 1999). They found that among women infected with HPV, HIV-infected women were significantly more likely to develop cervical neoplasia, and this effect was related to the degree of immunodeficiency. Several other studies have also shown that HIV-infected women are at higher risk for CIN, including that by Ahdieh et al., who found that 13% of HIV-positive women versus 2% of HIV-negative women had abnormal cytological findings (Ahdieh, 2000). They also found that HIV-positive women had a much lower rate of HPV clearance on follow-up exams, and that in a multivariate model, the increased rate of CIN among HIV-positive women was fully accounted for by HPV persistence (Ahdieh, 2000).

Effect of ART on HIV-Associated Cervical Dysplasia

Although ART has significantly improved the survival of HIV-infected individuals through immune reconstitution and has decreased the incidence of opportunistic infections, the effects of ART on HPV infection and CIN among HIV-infected women remain unclear. Whereas three older studies did not find a significant reduction in risk of cervical dysplasia among women on ART (Lillo, 2001; Moore, 2002; Orlando, 1999), a recent prospective study did find a reduction in cervical dysplasia risk related to ART (Minkoff, 2010).

The largest retrospective analysis performed by the Women's Interagency HIV Study (WIHS) group found that among 741 HIV-positive women, those on ART were 40% (95% CI, 4–81) more likely to exhibit a regression of cervical lesions and were also significantly less likely to have progression of CIN (odds ratio (OR), 0.68). Minkoff prospectively evaluated 286 HIV-positive women who initiated ART (Minkoff, 2010). They were assessed semiannually for HPV infection (by PCR) and SILs. Combination ART initiation among adherent women was associated with a significant reduction in HPV prevalence, incident detection of oncogenic HPV infection, and decreased prevalence and more rapid clearance of oncogenic HPV-positive SILs. Effects were smaller among nonadherent women (Minkoff, 2010). Conflicting observations regarding the effect of ART on cervical SIL or CIN from these reports are likely in part due to differences in study design, inclusion criteria, clinical end points, and statistical methodologies. Collectively, the data suggest that treating HIV infection with ART has a modest beneficial effect on progression of HPV-related cervical disease.

Treatment and Prevention of HIV-Associated Cervical Dysplasia

Invasive cervical cancer diagnosed in women with HIV infection is treated using the same criteria and protocols as those for women without HIV infection, as long as no other contraindications for treatment exist. In addition, close post-treatment surveillance is also recommended. Current US Public Health Service and Infectious Diseases Society of America guidelines recommend that HIV-positive women undergo a complete history and physical that includes a pelvic exam and Pap test at the time of initial evaluation. The Pap test is the primary mode for cervical cancer screening for HIV-infected women. Screening for these women should commence within 1 year of the onset of sexual activity regardless of mode of HIV transmission (e.g., sexual activity and perinatal exposure) but no later than age 21 years. Women ages 21–29 years should have a Pap test at the time of initial diagnosis with HIV. If the initial Pap test for young (or newly diagnosed) HIV-infected women is normal, the next Pap test should be performed in 12 months (although some experts still recommend a repeat Pap test at 6 months after baseline testing). If the results of the three consecutive Pap tests are normal, follow-up Pap tests can be done every 3 years. Co-testing (Pap test with HPV testing) is no longer recommended for HIV-infected women younger than age 30 years. Either Pap testing only or Pap testing and HPV co-testing is acceptable for screening. If screening is done with Pap tests alone, the HIV-infected woman should have a Pap test at the time of HIV diagnosis (baseline) and then every 12 months. If the results of the three consecutive Pap tests are normal, follow-up Pap tests may be done every 3 years. For women age 30 years or older, Pap and HPV testing should be done at the time of HIV diagnosis (or starting at age 30 years). If the Pap is normal and the HPV screening test is negative HPV, repeat cervical cancer screening can be done in 3 years. Any HIV-infected woman with an abnormal Pap smear, including atypical squamous

cell of undetermined significance–high grade, high-grade squamous intraepithelial lesions, or atypical glandular cells, should undergo colposcopy (CDC, 2015). Cervical cancer screening in HIV-infected women should continue throughout their lifetime (and not end at age 65 years, as in the general population).

Prevention

There are currently three US Food and Drug Administration (FDA)-approved HPV vaccines: bivalent, quadrivalent, and 9-valent. All three prevent HPV-16 and HPV-18 infections and also prevent precancers (and likely cancers) caused by HPV-16 and HPV-18. In addition, the quadrivalent and 9-valent HPV vaccines prevent HPV-6 and HPV-11 infections and genital warts due to these types. The 9-valent vaccine also prevents infection and precancers due to five additional types (31, 33, 45, 52, and 58). The CDC currently recommends HPV vaccine for HIV-infected women through age 26 years that is given in three doses (0, 2, and 6 months) (CDC, HPV Fact Sheet, 2015).

The HPV vaccine has been tested in several groups of older women with HIV and has been found to be safe and effective but is not yet FDA approved for this population. The AIDS Clinical Trials Group Protocol A5240 was a phase II, international, multicenter trial that enrolled 319 HIV-positive women with a median age of 36 years. Rates of seroconversion were significantly more robust in those with $CD4^+$ cell counts >200 cells/mm^3 and virological suppression (HIV RNA <400 copies/ml) (Kojic, 2014). Similar results of safety and efficacy were seen using the bivalent vaccine containing anti-HPV-16/18 antibodies in both HIV-positive and HIV-negative women in South Africa (Denny, 2013).

EPIDEMIOLOGY OF HIV-ASSOCIATED SQUAMOUS CELL CANCER OF THE ANUS

Even before the HIV epidemic, anal cancer incidence among men who have sex with men (MSM) was estimated to be as high as approximately 35 cases per 100,000 py. This rate is comparable to the incidence of cervical cancer in the United States before the advent of routine cervical cytology (Daling, 1987; Melbye, 1994). In the 1960s, the annual incidence of SCCA among men in the United States was relatively low and stable, with approximately 0.5 cases per 100,000 persons. Since then, studies have shown a steady increase. A US population-based analysis of the

Surveillance, Epidemiology and End Results (SEER) program data found that the incidence of SCCA in the United States among men increased from 1.06 per 100,000 persons from 1973 to 1979 to 2.04 per 100,000 persons from 1996 to 2004 (Johnson, 2004).

Many studies have shown that the incidence of SCCA is higher in HIV-positive persons. In a meta-analysis, Machalek examined nine studies published before November 2011 reporting anal cancer incidence in MSM (Machalek, 2012). Six were linkage studies based on data obtained from HIV/AIDS and cancer registries, and three were observational cohort studies. The incidence of anal cancer was significantly higher in HIV-positive men than in HIV-negative men ($p = 0.011$). This result has been mirrored in several studies in the United States and Europe, which show that the incidence of anal cancer among HIV-positive individuals ranges from 42 to 137 cases per 100,000 py, a rate 30–100 times higher than that of the general population (D'Souza, 2008; Patel, 2008; Piketty, 2008).

Squamous cell cancers of the anus may be overlooked in the female population; however, the rate of HPV-related anal cancers among women appears to be higher than that in men (1.8 vs. 1.2 per 100,000 population) (CDC, April 20, 2012). Other publications have found incidence rates as high as 18–30 per 100,000 persons (Piketty, 2012; Silverberg, 2012). Like the effects of HPV on cervical endothelium, the virus can lead to high-grade precancerous lesions and anal cancer. A recent systematic review of SCCA in women revealed higher prevalence of HPV in the anus versus cervix in the majority of studies reviewed (16–85% vs. 17–70%, respectively) and that concordant HPV genotypes were found in 9–16% of women. Risk factors for anal HPV included cervical HPV, low CD4 cell count, smoking, and perianal warts (Stier, 2015). Furthermore, Machalek et al. found that the incidence of anal cancer was actually higher in the ART era. For example, from 1996 onward, the incidence of SCCA was 78 per 100,000 population per year compared to 22 per 100,000 population per year prior to this time. The reason for this increase is unclear. Improved survival associated with ART may allow for sufficient time for men with chronic HPV infection to develop anal cancer. Increases in screening are unlikely to explain this trend because routine screening is not yet currently recommended or routinely implemented in most clinical practice settings (Machalet, 2012). However, risk factors associated with SCCA have been shown to be associated with greater immunosuppression, including nadir CD4 cell count and median HIV RNA levels >500,000 copies/ml (Guiguet, 2009).

EPIDEMIOLOGY OF HIV-ASSOCIATED ANAL INTRAEPITHELIAL NEOPLASIA

Unlike cervical HPV infection, which peaks in the third decade in women, anal HPV infection is highly prevalent throughout adult life among MSM well into the sixth decade (Chin-Hong, 2004; Schiffman, 2003). Several studies have reported the prevalence of anal intraepithelial neoplasia (AIN) among HIV-infected men and women. Palefsky found that the relative risk of developing high-grade squamous intraepithelial lesions (HSIL) was 3.7 for HIV-positive compared to HIV-negative MSM (Palefsky, 2001). Sixteen studies demonstrated that between 41% and 97% of HIV-infected men are found to have anal dysplasia on anal Pap smear screening (Kiviat, 2002; Palefsky, 2001; Piketty, 2008). In a meta-analysis of 31 studies, Machalek showed that the pooled prevalence of anal HPV detected by PCR was 89% in HIV-infected compared to 53.6% in HIV-negative men ($p = 0.047$) (Machalek 2012). In addition, the prevalence of HPV-16 and HPV-18, associated with high-grade neoplasia and malignancy, was also significantly higher in HIV-positive men compared to HIV-negative men.

TREATMENT AND PREVENTION OF HIV-ASSOCIATED ANAL DYSPLASIA

Treatment outcomes for anal dysplasia have only been reported from small case series. Current treatment options are similar for HIV-positive and HIV-negative individuals. These include topical trichloroacetic acid, liquid nitrogen, imiquimod, infrared coagulation, electrocautery, CO_2 laser, and surgical excision.

As discussed previously, HIV-infected individuals are at an increased risk for SCCA and AIN. In addition, SCCA shares many biologic similarities with cervical cancer, including detectable dysplastic precursor lesions and high-risk HPV infection. Consequently, many have recommended annual anal Pap screening for HIV-infected patients (Bosch, 1995). Anal Pap smears are acquired by randomly obtaining squamous cells from the anal canal using a Dacron swab. They are then fixed in liquid cytology media. Similar to cervical cytology protocols, abnormal anal cytologic findings are confirmed by high-resolution anoscopy directed biopsy of visualized lesions (Figure 33.1). Anal cytology is categorized according to the Bethesda system for cervical cytology: atypical squamous cells of unknown significance (ASCUS), low-grade squamous intraepithelial lesion (LSIL), and high-grade squamous intraepithelial lesion (HSIL). Anal Pap smears have a similar sensitivity and specificity as cervical Pap smears. Note that there are no definitive clinical studies showing that anal Pap smears decrease SCCA-related morbidity and mortality among HIV-infected individuals. Furthermore, anal cytology should not be performed if evaluation with high-resolution anoscopy is not available for the patient.

There is a lack of consensus and rigorous evidence regarding recommendations for performing annual digital rectal exam (DRE) in patients at risk for SCCA, such as MSM. The 2015 European AIDS Clinical Society (EACS) guidelines recommend DRE with or without an anal Pap smear every 1–3 years in MSM (EACS, 2015). The 2015 "Guidelines for Prevention and Treatment of Opportunistic Infections in HIV-Infected Adults and Adolescents" suggest that annual DRE is only a class B, grade III recommendation (DHHS, 2015).

Similar to females, routine vaccination with quadrivalent HPV or the 9-valent HPV vaccine is recommended for males aged 11–26 years in the general population. Vaccination is also recommended for MSM and HIV-positive men through age 26 years to prevent genital warts and the development of precancerous and cancerous HPV-mediated lesions (Advisory Committee on Immunization Practices, 2013). Vaccination for those older than age 26 years is not established. However, a growing body of evidence suggests that vaccination may be beneficial and cost-effective in the prevention of high-grade AIN and anal cancer (Cranston, 2014; Deshmukh, 2015; Swedish, 2014). Definitive studies on efficacy in older men and women are ongoing.

Figure 33.1 demonstrates the protocol for screening of AIN.

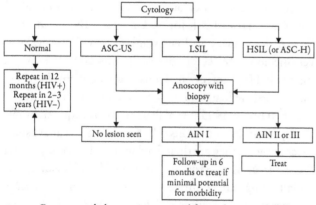

Figure 33.1 Recommended screening protocol for anal intraepithelial neoplasia. ASC-H, atypical squamous cells, cannot rule out HSIL; ASC-US, atypical squamous cells of undetermined significance; HSIL, high-grade squamous intraepithelial lesion; LSIL, low-grade squamous intraepithelial lesion SOURCE: *Curr Infect Dis Rep.* 2010 March; 12(2): 126–133.

EFFECT OF ART ON ANAL DYSPLASIA

Similar to studies evaluating the effect of ART on cervical dysplasia, studies evaluating the effect of HIV therapy on anal dysplasia have found conflicting results. This may be related to the significant design and methodological differences among these studies. There are two small case series (*n* = 4 and 26 patients, respectively) describing outcomes of HIV-associated SCCA, with 5-year survival rates of 47–60% (Jephcott, 2004; Myerson, 2001). In studies that specifically compared survival among patients with SCCA in the pre-ART versus ART eras, there was a nonsignificant trend toward improved survival, better tolerability of chemoradiotherapy, and improved local tumor control in the ART era (Bower, 2004; Cleator, 2000; Stadler, 2004).

A study linking the New York State cancer registry with the New York City HIV/AIDS registry found that in the early ART era (1990–1996), the 24-month survival was 76% for patients with AIDS compared to 78% for patients without AIDS, suggesting that at least during this time period, HIV-infected patients with SCCA have equivalent survival with HIV-negative patients.

Palefsky and colleagues compared the rates of progression and regression of anal dysplasia after 6 months of ART (Palefsky, 2001). They found that the likelihood of lesion progression or regression was not affected by ART initiation, but they noted that among the patients starting ART at higher CD4 cell counts, ART demonstrated a nonsignificant benefit on anal dysplasia lesions. In contrast, Wilkin et al. conducted a cross-sectional study evaluating anal HPV infection and anal dysplasia in 98 HIV-positive men (Wilkin, 2004). In a multivariate analysis, they found that ART and higher nadir CD4 cell count were significantly protective for anal dysplasia by histology but were not protective of anal HPV infection. A recent study from Canada retrospectively evaluated 1691 HIV-positive MSM and found that immunosuppression with nadir CD4 cell count <100 cells/mm^3 was a risk factor for anal cancer (OR, 3.08; *p* = 0.01). They also found that men treated during the pre-ART era had a higher incidence (370 vs. 93/100,000 py) and shorter lead time to development of anal cancer compared to those in the post-ART era (Duncan, 2015). Therefore, it remains unclear if ART initiation influences the natural history of AIN in HIV-infected individuals. However, ART is beneficial for men undergoing treatment for HPV-related disease.

Recommended Reading

Kojic EM, Kang M, Cespedes MS, et al. Immunogenicity and safety of the quadrivalent human papillomavirus vaccine in HIV-1-infected women. *Clin Infect Dis.* 2014; 59(1): 127–135.

Piketty C, Selinger-Leneman H, Grabar S, et al. Marked increase in the incidence of invasive anal cancer among HIV-infected patients despite treatment with combination antiretroviral therapy. *AIDS (London)*. 2008; 22(10):1203–1211.

Stier EA, Sebring MC, Mendez AE, et al. Prevalence of anal human papillomavirus infection and anal HPV-related disorders in women: A systematic review. *Am J Ob Gyn*. 2015; 213(3):278–309.

LUNG CANCER

LEARNING OBJECTIVES

- Review the epidemiology and risks of lung cancer in those with HIV.

- Review the pathogenesis of lung cancer.

- Discuss the treatment of lung cancer.

- Discuss the treatment outcomes and mortality associated with lung cancer in HIV-infected persons.

WHAT'S NEW?

- HIV-positive patients have an increasing incidence of lung cancer during the ART era.

- Surgery, chemotherapy, and radiation are mainstays of standard treatment for patients with HIV.

- Treatment disparities between HIV and non-HIV patients may contribute to poor survivability of those with lung cancer.

KEY POINTS

- Tobacco cessation is of utmost importance in preventing lung cancers in patients with HIV.

- People with HIV have a higher incidence of lung cancer than the general population, although predominant histology of non-small cell lung cancer is common in both groups.

- HIV-positive patients have worse survival, which may be due to frequent presentation with advanced disease.

- No specific guidelines for treating HIV patients with lung cancer exist, and more rigorous studies evaluating standards of care are needed.

Lung cancer is the leading cause of death due to cancer in the general US population, and it also represents the most common non-AIDS cancer in people with HIV (Frisch, 2001). Lung cancers in HIV are primarily non-small cell cancer (NSCLC) types, including adenocarcinoma and squamous cell carcinoma. This largely reflects the trend of histology types among the general population in Western settings (Cadranel, 2006). Mortality from lung cancer remains high in HIV-infected individual compared to the general population, especially for patients presenting at advanced stages (Coghill, 2015, Shiels, 2010).

The incidence of lung cancer, like that of other NADCs, has increased for several reasons, including increased life expectancy in the era of ART and longer cumulative exposure to carcinogens known to be associated with lung cancer development, namely tobacco smoke. Notably, tobacco exposure in the HIV population remains a significant health problem, with disproportionate use compared to the general population (Clifford, 2012; Rahmanian, 2011). Due to this increased risk, smoking cessation is of utmost importance in this patient population. Immunosuppression may also be a contributing factor; however, this relationship is not clearly understood.

EPIDEMIOLOGY OF LUNG CANCER IN HIV

Engels et al. examined data from large HIV and cancer registries in the United States to estimate the incidence of lung cancer. They found the incidence in the HIV population to be 59 per 100,000 py during a period from 1991 to 2002 (Engels, 2008). This same study found that the incidence of lung cancer increased from 51/100,000 py to 126/100,000 py between those with HIV compared to those with an AIDS diagnosis (Engels, 2008). In a recent study of US and Canadian data, researchers found that from 1996 to 2009, the incidence of lung cancer in HIV persons was 129/100,000 py compared to 45.4/100,000 py in uninfected persons. The incidence of lung cancer was higher for persons aged 75 years than for those aged 65 years (3.4% vs. 2.2%), which supports the increased risk of cancer development as the population ages (Silverberg, 2015).

A Ugandan study evaluating overall cancer incidence (ADC and NADCs) in HIV-infected persons from 1988 to 2002 found the incidence over time to be increased, with a standardized incidence ratio (SIR) of 5 (Mbulaiteye, 2006). Another study using the Swiss HIV Cohort Study and Swiss cancer registries found that cancers of the trachea, lung, and bronchus were significantly elevated compared to those of the general population, with an SIR of 3.2 (Clifford, 2005).

The impact of ART on the incidence and risk of lung cancer remains unclear. Studies attempting to evaluate the incidence of lung cancer during the pre-ART and ART eras have found mixed results, with increased incidence in both eras. The previously cited study by Silverberg et al. showed that cumulative incidence of lung cancer in North America continues to increase in the ART era (Silverberg, 2015). They found a cumulative incidence of 3.7% from 2005 to 2009 compared to 1.8% from 1996 to 2009 (Silverberg, 2015). Another study that examined data from 34 states showed similar results, with a steady increase in the number of lung cancers (35 to 283 cases) from 1991 to 2005, which largely occurred in persons older than 50 years (Shiels, 2011). This phenomenon speaks to the increasing longevity of the HIV population and accumulation of malignant comorbidities.

RISK FACTORS ASSOCIATED WITH LUNG CANCER IN HIV

Risk factors for lung cancer are multiple and include tobacco exposure, injection drug use, and possibly HIV infection itself. Other comorbid pulmonary diseases, such as chronic obstructive pulmonary disease and bacterial pneumonia, are more common in HIV-infected people than in uninfected people and may place HIV-infected people at higher risk for cancer due to persistent states of inflammation (Crothers, 2011; Shebl, 2010). Inflammatory markers circulating in the blood have been associated with theoretical risk of lung cancer; these include C-reactive protein, serum amyloid, soluble tumor necrosis factor receptor-2, lymphoid differentiation cytokine interleukin-7, and various leukocyte-derived chemokines (Shiels, 2013). However, it remains to be determined exactly how these inflammatory states that are not confounded by smoking or other traditional risks factors impact the risk of lung cancer.

Cigarette smoking has repeatedly been implicated as a major risk factor for lung cancer in the general population as well as the HIV population. Prevalence of cigarette smoking among HIV-positive persons is estimated to be between 42% and 59%, and it greatly exceeds that in the general population by two- to threefold (Mdodo, 2015; Tesoriero, 2010). In the Swiss study, Clifford and others reported that all persons with cancer of the respiratory tract were smokers, and there was a threefold higher excess risk of these cancers (Clifford, 2005). A similar finding was demonstrated in a US study that showed patients with HIV and lung cancer were 1.3 times more likely to be current or former smokers and to have greater pack-year tobacco consumption history compared to those with HIV but without

cancer (D'Jaen, 2010). Shiels et al. also examined the role of cigarette smoking in the development of lung cancer in HIV. They found that those with HIV who smoked more than 1.43 packs per day had twice the risk of lung cancer compared to those with HIV who smoked less. Compared to HIV-negative patients who smoked less than 1.43 packs per day, those with HIV and who smoked more than 1.43 packs per day had 7.2 times higher risk of developing lung cancer (Shiels, 2010).

Other studies have not found the same association with smoking. Engels et al. studied 5238 HIV-infected patients and found that the overall smoking-adjusted standardized incidence ratio for lung cancer was 2.5 times higher than that of the general population (95% CI, 1.6–3.5) (Engels, 2006). However, in an analysis assuming all subjects smoked, the smoking-adjusted standardized incidence ratio was only 1.7. This suggests that smoking did not account for all excess risk of lung cancer in HIV (Engels, 2006). In the mortality analysis by Shiels et al., it was found that after adjusting for smoking and other patient characteristics, the risk of death was 3.8 times higher for HIV-positive versus HIV-negative patients (Shiels, 2010). A large Veterans Administration study found that the incidence rate ratio (1.7) of lung cancer in HIV patients remained significantly elevated after multivariable adjustment for confounders including smoking compared to persons without HIV (Sigel, 2012). These studies suggest that independent of smoking, HIV positivity portends a higher incidence and mortality risk for lung cancer.

Injection drug use (IDU) among HIV-infected patients has also been associated with an increased risk of lung cancer compared with that for non-users in several studies. One study in particular, from southern Europe, demonstrated that those with IDU, with or without HIV, had an increased risk of lung cancer, with a standardized incidence ratio of 14.3 and 6.2, respectively (Serraino, 2000). Other studies have found little evidence to support this risk factor, however. In a study by Kirk et al. that included 2086 participants (the AIDS Link to the Intravenous Experience Study), IDU was not associated with increased risk of lung cancer (Kirk, 2007).

HIV itself may also be associated with the development of lung cancer due to directly acting oncogenic effects. HIV-1 replication depends on Tat protein expression, which has the ability to upregulate expression of protooncogenes c-myc, c-fos, and c-jun to enhance cellular proliferation, including human adenocarcinoma cell lines (El-Solh, 1997). Allelic loss and changes in microsatellites, which are short tandem repeat DNA sequences, have also been described in other malignancies, such as KS, NHL, and SCCA, and have been found in lung cancers of HIV-positive patients (Wistuba, 1998). These genetic alterations may lead to activation of oncogenes and loss of tumor suppressor genes. However, the lack of HIV viral integration into cellular DNA of somatic neoplastic cells challenges this hypothesis of oncogenesis because cancer cells can have background genetic alterations and immunosuppression can also be associated with microsatellite changes (Bedi, 1995).

Although men historically have been considered at higher risk for lung cancer, women also share a significant proportion of lung cancer diagnoses. This may be due to the increase in women tobacco smokers in the population or the increase in the number of HIV-positive women. The WIHS compared data from the National Health and Nutritional Examination (NHANES) II and SEER. Researchers found that HIV-infected women have higher lifetime cigarette consumption as well as an elevated SIR of 3 (95% CI, 1.7–5.1) compared to the general population with a SIR of 2.11 (95% CI, 0.25–7.61). Furthermore, these data did not vary by pre-ART era versus ART era (Levine, 2010). A French study evaluating cancer in HIV-infected patients in the pre-ART and ART eras found that the SIR of women was three times higher than that of men in the ART era (6.28 vs. 2.12) (Herida, 2003). Several additional studies have shown greater incidence in women with SIR ranging from 1.6 to 16.7 (Calabresi, 2013; Clifford, 2005; Ramirez-Marrero, 2010).

DIAGNOSIS AND CLINICAL PRESENTATION OF LUNG CANCER IN HIV

Despite the increased risk of cancer with aging, HIV-infected persons with lung cancer tend to be younger. In several studies, age at presentation ranged from 38 to 57 years. This is far below the age of presentation among the general population, which is closer to the seventh decade of life (Winstone, 2013). Stage at presentation also tends to be advanced in HIV-positive patients, with a majority presenting with stages III or IV. This likely contributes to the poor survivability of these patients (Sigel, 2012; Winstone, 2013).

The majority of histological types mirror those of the general population, with greater than 50% consisting of NSCLC. Adenocarcinoma is the predominant non-small cell cancer (36%), followed by squamous cell carcinoma (30%) (Sigel, 2012). Many patients present with advanced disease and have symptoms of persistent cough and chest pain (Karp, 1993). Early diagnosis of lung cancer improves prognosis; however, screening with plain chest radiography at any interval has not been shown to be effective and is not recommended. Use of low-dose chest CT may be beneficial in these patients. Recent recommendations by the US Preventive Services Task Force to screen high-risk patients for lung cancer with low-dose chest CT were based on the findings from the National Lung Screening Trial (National Lung Screening Trial Research Team, 2011). This was a large randomized trial that found a 20% reduction in lung cancer mortality after implementing annual screening by low-dose CT in patients aged 55–74 years and at least a 30 pack-year smoking history. The benefit and cost-effectiveness of low-dose CT in patients infected with HIV remain unknown, but following these general guidelines is reasonable after discussing risks (e.g., false positives and radiation exposure) and benefits (e.g., early detection and better prognosis) with patients. Currently, a French multicenter, prospective pilot study (ANRS EP48 HIV-CHEST cohort) is evaluating the utility of low-dose CT in HIV-positive individuals (NCT01207986; Makinson, 2015).

TREATMENT OF LUNG CANCER

There are no alternative or specific treatment guidelines for lung cancer in the HIV population. Most randomized trials for lung cancer have historically excluded HIV-positive patients due to concerns regarding immune suppression, toxicity, and drug interactions with ART (Persad, 2008). Current treatment strategies are mainly with protocols for patients without HIV and depend on tumor histology, stage of disease, and underlying host factors such as comorbidities and pulmonary function. Patients with NSCLC are staged (I–IV) based on the tumor node metastasis system, with stage I disease confined to localized tumor without invasion into the chest wall, diaphragm, mediastinum, or surrounding structures and stage IV to metastatic disease (Shepherd, 2007). MRI of the brain should also be pursued for stage II or higher to identify intracranial metastasis. For localized, nonmetastatic disease, surgical resection is the preferred strategy with intent to cure for those patients able to undergo surgery. Surgery (lobectomy, sublobular resection, and video-assisted thoracoscopy) may be followed by adjuvant chemotherapy or radiation for those with more advanced stages or invasion (NCCN, 2.2016). For nonsurgical candidates, ablation with radiotherapy can be considered. Studies evaluating surgery in HIV-infected patients have been described in mainly small case–control series and case reports. Patients undergoing surgery for localized disease (stage I or stage II) tolerated surgery well with minimal complications (Cadranel, 2006).

For patients with advanced NSCLC or recurrence after initial definitive therapy, goals of therapy are largely palliative. For patients with solitary metastasis or recurrence, curative intention with additional surgery or radiotherapy may be indicated and beneficial to help prolong survival. However, risks and benefits must be weighed in advanced disease to avoid undue adverse events and toxicities. Systemic therapy with combination chemotherapy with platinum-based regimen is the mainstay agent with or without additional agents, such as the vascular endothelial growth factor inhibitor bevacizumab (NCCN, 2.2016). Additional molecular, genetic mutation analysis for potential genetic-directed therapy targets has been explored. These should be performed when possible in patients with advanced stage NSCLC, namely for the presence of epidermal growth factor receptor (EGFR) and anaplasmic lymphoma kinase (NCCN, 2.2016). Other targets include RAS family oncogenes, the mTOR signaling pathway, and the MEK signaling pathway. Treatment with EGFR tyrosine kinase inhibitors such as erlotinib may also be considered for patients with this specific EGFR mutation in the tumor. However, long-term survival has yet to be established with use of these agents (Okuma, 2014).

Use of chemotherapy in HIV-positive patients is feasible, and it has been used in patients to treat metastatic disease as well as an adjuvant therapy and in combination with radiation for locally advanced disease. One large retrospective study found similar rates of treatment modality between HIV and non-HIV patients (Sigel, 2013). Limited data from case series have provided heterogeneous results regarding use of chemotherapeutic agents, efficacy, and drug toxicities in HIV patients with lung cancer (Bower, 2003; Powles, 2003; Spano, 2004). Additional studies to evaluate efficacy, tolerability, and safety of chemotherapy in HIV patients are needed.

SURVIVAL OF LUNG CANCER IN HIV

Survival among patients with HIV and lung cancer is worse compared to that of their uninfected counterparts. Coghill et al. analyzed data from 1996–2010 and found that in 1058 HIV-positive patients, all-cause mortality and cancer-specific mortality risk were respectively 85% and 28% higher for HIV patients with lung cancer compared to HIV-negative patients (Coghill, 2015). For patients with local-stage NSCLC receiving standard cancer therapy, those with HIV continued to have greater cancer-related deaths compared to HIV-uninfected patients (HR, 1.8; 95% CI, 1.21–2.7) (Coghill, 2015). Another large study utilizing SEER registry data compared 267 HIV-infected to 1428 non-infected patients with similar cancer stage and histology of NSCLC (Sigel, 2013). Both groups with stage I–IIIA disease received surgery, chemotherapy, and radiotherapy at similar rates.

Among the HIV-infected group, 82% died during follow-up compared to 66% of of the uninfected group ($p < 0.001$). Median overall survival for HIV patients was only 6 months compared to 20 months for the uninfected cohort. Overall 5-year survival was also poor for HIV-infected patients at 9% compared to 23% for the non-infected group. Patients with HIV and advanced disease (stage IIIB–IV) had the worst survival, with 9–20 times greater risk of death compared to HIV patients with only localized disease. Moreover, a major proportion of those with HIV also died from non-cancer-related causes (31% vs. 9%; $p < 0.001$).

Such disparity in outcomes in the previously discussed studies may be explained by several hypotheses, including the fact that patients with HIV experience overall greater mortality than the general population. It may be that tumors behave more aggressively in patients with HIV due to tumor effect or poor immunological surveillance due to lack of fully intact cellular immunity. Poor tolerability of surgery and chemotherapy may also contribute to worse outcomes. More studies are needed to clarify these issues.

Last, health disparities in treatment between HIV-positive and non-HIV populations may contribute to poor survivability. Data from the Texas Cancer registry from 1995–2009 showed that patients with HIV and NSCLC less frequently received any cancer treatments despite greater numbers presenting at younger ages and with distant-stage disease (Suneja, 2013). Patients with HIV and local-stage NSCLC were less likely to receive surgery (45.5% vs. 62.5%; $p = 0.04$) than uninfected patients. Those with regional disease and HIV were less likely to receive systemic chemotherapy. For distant disease, HIV-positive patients received less chemotherapy or radiation (31.1% vs. 45.5%; $p = 0.0009$) (Suneja, 2013).

Recommended Reading

Coghill AE, Shiels MS, Suneja G, et al. Elevated cancer-specific mortality among HIV-infected patients in the United States. *J Clin Oncol.* 2015; 33(21):2376–2383.

Sigel K, Crothers K, Dubrow R, et al. Prognosis in HIV-infected patients with non-small cell lung cancer. *Br J Cancer.* 2013; 109:1974–1980.

Suneja G, Shiels MS, Melville SK. Disparities in the treatment and outcomes of lung cancer among HIV-infected Individuals. *AIDS.* 2013; 27(3):459–468.

PROSTATE CANCER

LEARNING OBJECTIVES

- Review the epidemiology and risk factors for prostate cancer in men with HIV.

- Review the current screening recommendations for prostate cancer.

- Discuss the treatment options for prostate cancer in men with HIV.

Prostate cancer remains the leading cancer diagnosis among men in the United States and other industrialized countries. It is the second leading cause of cancer deaths after lung cancer. Increased screening efforts in the United States led to increased incidence after the PSA test became widely available in 1992. However, screening and treatment among HIV-negative and HIV-positive patients have been controversial due to the occult and often indolent nature of untreated prostate cancer, especially in older men with limited life expectancy. The mortality benefit of diagnosis and treatment of early stage prostate cancer remains unproven; thus, emphasis on screening and early detection has waned in recent years. Compared to other NADCs such as lung or anal cancer, some studies have demonstrated HIV infection

to be associated with a reduced risk of prostate cancer. Regardless, diagnosis of prostate cancer carries a significant clinical impact on patients' sexual, genitourinary, and overall health.

EPIDEMIOLOGY OF PROSTATE CANCER IN HIV

HIV-positive men experienced an increased incidence of prostate cancer in the United States after 1990 compared to the preceding decade from 0.2% to 2.2% of all cancers in a retrospective study of population-based registry data (Engels, 2006). In the same study, the incidence increased during the pre-ART and post-ART eras, which may be explained by the introduction of the PSA screening test. Another study that was a large retrospective review also found that prostate cancer in HIV-positive men increased during the time from 1992 to 2003, similar to the aforementioned study (Patel, 2008). However, the HIV-positive group had statistically significantly lower rates of cancer compared to the general population in the pre-ART era (15 vs. 47 per 100,000 py) and the ART era (38 vs. 61 per 100,000 py) (Patel, 2008). Another study that examined the PSA testing era (1992–2007) found an incidence of 28 per 100,000 py in HIV-positive men. However, the incidence in HIV-positive men compared to the expected rate in the general population during this same time period was significantly reduced, with a standardized incidence ratio of only 0.5 (95% CI, 0.44–0.57) (Shiels, 2010).

RISK FACTORS FOR PROSTATE CANCER

Postulated risk factors that promote development of prostate cancer in HIV-positive men include exposure to carcinogens and use of androgen supplementation to treat hypogonadism. Co-infection with oncogenic viruses may also promote neoplasia (Montgomery, 2006). Chronic inflammatory states promoted by HIV systemically and localized to the prostate as well as chronic prostatitis may contribute to cancer development (Leport, 1989; Smith, 2004).

Prostate cancer and risk of death have been associated with tobacco exposure in several studies. However, other studies have demonstrated conflicting data. Two large meta-analyses examined this issue and found similar results (Huncharek, 2010; Islami, 2014). Huncharek found a dose-dependent relationship with incidence of prostate cancer in non-HIV patients. The heaviest smokers had a 13% increased risk of cancer. These data derived from 7 prospected cohort studies. Based on 19 prospective studies, Islami found smoking to be associated with an increased risk of death (RR, 1.24) from prostate cancer, which was dose dependent. The incidence of prostate cancer, however, was not statistically significant overall. In fact, baseline cigarette smoking was inversely associated with incidence of prostate cancer (Islami 2014).

Unlike other malignancies in HIV, immunological control with increasing $CD4^+$ cell count has been associated with increased risk of prostate cancer, with a relative risk that is three times greater in the ART era (Shiels, 2010). In several studies, HIV-positive men with prostate cancer had robust $CD4^+$ cell counts >300 cells/mm^3 (Hsiao, 2009; Marcus, 2014; Pantanowitz, 2008). Overall, data from numerous studies suggest that variations in prostate cancer deficits in HIV-infected men are due to differential PSA screening in this population and not to immunologic status.

PROSTATE CANCER SCREENING

The primary tools for diagnosis of prostate cancer include serum PSA measurement, DRE, and ultimately prostate biopsy for definitive histologic diagnosis. Both European and US guidelines have recommended against routine screening with PSA in both HIV-negative and HIV-positive men (Heidenreich, 2013; Moyer, 2012). Rather, whether to perform individual screening with PSA for early detection should be a well-informed, mutual decision between physician and patient based on possible benefits and harms of a positive PSA test. Optimal interval of PSA screening has also not been established. DRE alone has limited sensitivity (6–8%) of detecting prostate cancer (Gosselaar, 2009; Okotie, 2007). The combination of an abnormal DRE versus normal DRE with PSA level >3 ng/ml may enhance positive predictive value of cancer detection at 48% versus 22% (Gosselaar, 2008).

CLINICAL PRESENTATION

Prostate cancer diagnosis in HIV often occurs in the fifth and sixth decades of life, and patients often have a positive family history of prostate cancer (Hsiao, 2009; Ong, 2015; Shiels, 2010). Men with HIV may present more often with late-stage disease compared to the general population, although this is supported by limited data (Shiels, 2015). A large California cohort found more localized cancer compared to regional or distant disease among HIV-positive men (88% vs. 7%), which was similar to the pattern found in HIV-negative men (Marcus, 2014). Other studies have found no difference in presentation with early or advanced disease (Hsiao, 2009; Riedel, 2015). HIV-negative African Americans have a greater likelihood of presenting with advanced-stage prostate cancer in the general population (Siegel, 2012). Within the HIV population, African Americans may represent a higher risk group for prostate cancer because they comprise a large proportion of HIV prevalence and annual HIV diagnoses in the United States.

TREATMENT AND TREATMENT OUTCOMES OF PROSTATE CANCER

Treatment of prostate cancer in HIV-positive men is similar to that of HIV-negative men and is based on stage and grade of disease with use of the Gleason score (ranging from 2 to 10). For localized disease (stage I and stage II) not spread to lymph nodes or distant sites, strategies include active surveillance (PSA monitoring and/or repeat biopsy), radical prostatectomy, or radiation therapy (external beam radiation and/or brachytherapy) with or without androgen deprivation. For locally advanced disease (stage III) that has spread outside the prostate gland, surgery or radiation with androgen deprivation therapy are alternatives. A Gleason score greater than 8 represents high-risk neoplasia, even if disease is localized. The optimal choice between surgical intervention and radiation is unclear for these patients, and careful consideration of individual risks and benefits should be discussed on a case-by-case basis (Grimm, 2012).

Treatment of disseminated disease, which often involves osteoblastic lesions, typically involves androgen deprivation therapy, castration (medical or surgical), and systemic chemotherapy. Two recent phase III trials examining the use of abiraterone and enzalutamide for treatment of metastatic, castration-resistant prostate cancer have shown clinical benefit with these agents, which target the androgen-synthesis pathway (Loriot, 2015; Ryan, 2015). Chemotherapy with taxane-based regimens has also shown success in prolonging survival in men with castration-resistant prostate cancer. Docetaxel plus prednisone is currently the standard, initial cytotoxic chemotherapy used in metastatic, castration-resistant disease (Berthold, 2008).

Few studies have evaluated the safety, tolerability, and efficacy of treatments for prostate cancer in men with HIV. Most studies have been small and limited to evaluation of external beam radiation therapy (EBRT) with heterogeneity of dosing. One Veterans Administration study reported 15 patients who received an EBRT dose-escalation approach (75.6 Gy to 79.2 Gy) for localized disease. Of the 15 patients, 13 were treated with concomitant ART, and the 5-year event-free survival was 92.3% (Schreiber, 2014).

Toxicities included urinary frequency and rectal bleeding. Eight patients on ART had a transient decline in CD4$^+$ cell count, which returned to near or above baseline in the follow-up period. Another study evaluating EBRT (72 Gy to 81 Gy) for localized prostate cancer in HIV-positive compared to HIV-negative men found that 26% of men with HIV had biochemical failure compared to 12% of matched HIV-negative controls. At a mean of 36 months, there were no deaths in the HIV group. Genitourinary and anal adverse events were overall mild (Kahn, 2012).

The risk of death from prostate cancer is associated with advanced disease compared to local or regional prostate cancer (Shiels, 2010). In a large retrospective study of HIV and cancer registries from 1996 to 2010, mortality of prostate cancer was significantly higher compared to that of HIV-uninfected patients (HR, 1.57; 95% CI, 1.02–2.41) even after adjusting for patient characteristics and cancer stage (Coghill, 2015). Cancer deaths were also greater in HIV-infected men after adjusting for treatment but not significantly so (HR, 1.64; 95% CI, 0.93–2.89). A recently published study that used data from 1996 to 2002 found a 2.1-fold increased risk of death from prostate cancer in HIV-positive compared to HIV-negative men. Interestingly, in this study, HIV-infected men had more localized disease (Marcus, 2014).

Recommended Reading

Coghill AE, Shiels MS, Suneja G, et al. Elevated cancer-specific mortality among HIV-infected patients in the United States. *J Clin Oncol.* 2015; 33(21):2376–2383.

Marcus JL, Chao CR, Leyden WA, et al. Prostate cancer incidence and prostate-specific antigen testing among HIV-positive and HIV-negative men. *J Acquir Immune Defic Syndr.* 2014; 66:495–502.

Moyer VA. Screening for prostate cancer: U.S. Preventive Services Task Force recommendation statement. *Ann Intern Med.* 2012; 157(2):120–135.

Shiels MS, Goedert JJ, Moore RD, et al. Risk of prostate cancer in U.S. men with AIDS. *Cancer Epidemiol Biomarkers Prev.* 2010; 19(11):2910–2915.

COLORECTAL ADENOCARCINOMA

LEARNING OBJECTIVES

- Review the epidemiology of colorectal cancer in the HIV population.

- Discuss the screening methods for colorectal cancer.

- Review treatment modalities and outcomes in HIV patients with colorectal cancer.

WHAT'S NEW?

- The incidence of colon cancer has increased in the HIV population compared to the general population in the ART era, and mortality remains high compared to that of the HIV-negative population.

- Patients with HIV disproportionately receive less colorectal cancer screening than the general population.

- Standard chemoradiation and surgical approaches for treating colorectal cancer appear to be well tolerated in patients with HIV, although more research is needed in this area.

KEY POINTS

- Colorectal cancer presents a major health and mortality burden in the HIV population.

- Colorectal cancer presentation occurs often in younger patients and with more advanced disease compared to the general population.

- Significant disparities exist in screening HIV patients for colorectal cancer compared to HIV-negative patients.

- Standard treatment includes surgery and neoadjuvant and/or adjuvant chemoradiation.

- Survival is significantly worse compared to that of non-HIV=infected patients with colorectal cancer.

In the United States, colorectal cancer (CRC) is the third leading cause of cancer death in the general population for both men and women. It has been the focus of large-scale primary prevention screening efforts to identify patients with early disease (Siegel, 2014). Non-AIDS cancers such as colorectal adenocarcinoma in the HIV population have become increasingly recognized as a significant health problem as patients are living longer and may accrue greater risk factors for cancer development. Vigilance for neoplastic processes such as colorectal cancer must be maintained in HIV patients because they are often diagnosed at advanced stages and can be overlooked due to presentation at a younger age and lack of traditional risk factors such as family history (Chapman, 2009; Yegüez, 2003). This phenomenon was characterized by early case reports of colorectal adenocarcinoma in HIV. Patients were often males, aged 20s–40s, and with advanced immunosuppression (Cappell, 1988; Klugman, 1994; Ravalli, 1989).

HIV patients who are considered "average" risk are offered screening less frequently than the general population (Nayudu, 2012). Furthermore, disparities in cancer treatment between HIV-positive and HIV-negative patients are also prevalent. Persons with HIV are less likely to receive treatment for colon cancer than their HIV-negative counterparts (Suneja, 2013). The lack of screening and treatment is likely to contribute to poorer outcomes and excess mortality in the HIV population.

EPIDEMIOLOGY OF COLON CANCER IN HIV

Patients with HIV have incurred a higher incidence of CRC than the general population. A large US study that examined cancer incidence in HIV patients compared to the general population from 1992 to 2003 found an increased standardized incidence rate during the early time period of 1992–1995 (39.9 per 100,000 py) compared to the later time period of 2000–2003 (66.2 per 100,000 py). During both time periods, the rates were greater than those of the general population (20.4 and 21.1 per 100,000 py, respectively) (Patel, 2008).

In a recent study using US and Canadian data from 2006 to 2009, the incidence rate of CRC in HIV was 36.4 per 100,000 py compared to 27.7 per 100,000 py in uninfected patients. During this study period, the cumulative incidence declined by 6% per year for HIV-negative patients but increased in those with HIV by 5% per year. This may be a reflection of the declining death rate among persons with HIV (Silverberg, 2015).

A large Taiwanese study that used the National Health Insurance Research Database from 1998 to 2009 found that among 1282 persons with HIV and cancer, the incidence of CRC, excluding anal cancer, was 51 per 100,000 py with a SIR of 5.9 (95% CI, 4.15–8.37). Interestingly, colon cancer was the most common NADC in females, with an incidence of 156 per 100,000 py (Chen, 2014). In the US surveillance study using the HIV/AIDS Cancer Match Study registry data from 1991 to 2002, the incidence of CRC, excluding anal cancer, was 15 per 100,000 py (Engels, 2008).

Immunosuppression likely plays a role in the epidemiology of CRC, as demonstrated in the previously discussed case reports from the pre-ART era. A study by Silverberg et al. stratified groups of $CD4^+$ cell count and found that those with HIV and <200 cells/mm³ had an 80% higher relative risk compared to a protective effect of higher $CD4^+$ cell counts (Silverberg, 2011). Another study that used flexible sigmoidoscopy for CRC screening in HIV patients found that patients with duration of HIV >10 years and

$CD4^+$ cell count <200 cells/mm³ had greater odds of having distal colon neoplastic lesions compared to those with higher $CD4^+$ cell counts (Bini, 2006). On the contrary, many other studies have not shown significant differences in rates among AIDS patients or reduction of CRC in the ART era. Several studies support increases in CRC in the ART era. The lack of reporting of CRC in advanced immunosuppression coupled with the increase in CRC in the ART era may be explained by increased longevity of the HIV population as well as an increase in screening measures allowing for more diagnoses.

An Australian study that used national HIV and cancer registry data in the pre-ART era evaluated the incidence of cancer among those with HIV. It did not find significantly increased incidence rates among AIDS patients before and after developing advanced immunosuppression (Gulrich, 2002). A US study examined cancer data of patients with an AIDS diagnoses from 1978 to 1996 (Frisch, 2001). It found the relative risk of colon cancer in patients with newly diagnosed AIDS to be no different in the period prior to AIDS or in the 5 years thereafter (RR, 0.9) (Frisch, 2001). A prospective study at the University of Alabama at Birmingham followed HIV patients from 1989 to 2002. It demonstrated an incidence during that period of 60 cases of NADC, with an increase in annual incidence of 0.65 cases per 1000 py in the pre-ART era and 2.34 cases per 1000 py in the ART era. Although the study found an increase in the incidence of the relative risk in the ART era of 3.6 (95% CI, 0.8–16.3), this difference was not statistically significant (Bedimo, 2004). These findings can likely be attributed to improved longevity and screening methods in the ART era. However, a lack of information on screening efforts reported in many of these studies is a major limitation in accurately measuring the true incidence of colorectal cancer in the HIV population.

COLORECTAL CANCER SCREENING IN THE HIV POPULATION

Screening for CRC in HIV patients reflects that recommended for the general population with normal cancer risk. This is defined as no personal history of CRC, adenomatous polyps, or inflammatory bowel disease and no first-degree relative with a history of CRC. The US Preventive Services Task Force recommends that for adults with an average risk of CRC, screening with fecal occult blood testing, flexible sigmoidoscopy, or colonoscopy should begin at age 50 years and continue until age 75 years. The current screening interval for colonoscopy is 10 years. These recommendations have been effective for reducing the incidence and mortality of CRC. For those with increased risk, such as an immediate family member with a history of CRC, screening should begin at age 40 years or 10 years prior to the relative's age at onset of CRC, whichever occurs first (Whitlock, 2008). Interestingly, even in the general population, screening is underutilized. The CDC found that only 64.5% of screening-eligible people aged 50–75 years surveyed in the Behavioral Risk Factor Surveillance System reported having one of the recommended tests (Joseph, 2012).

Screening the HIV population based on standard guidelines has been more challenging, with significant disparity compared to the general population. A retrospective study in New York identified 565 screening-eligible HIV patients with average risk and found that only 25% underwent screening colonoscopy within 10 years of the review. The median age was 58 years, and the majority of these patients had well-controlled HIV compared to those who did not have colonoscopy. Among those who had colonoscopy and biopsy, 32% of biopsies were of tubular adenomas, which exceeds the detection rate of tubular adenomas in the general population for men (34%) and women (27%) (Nayudu, 2012). A prospective study performed among New York veterans from 1998 to 2003 sought to describe the prevalence of adenomas or CRC in the distal colon with flexible sigmoidoscopy (Bini, 2006). The study included 2217 HIV-negative controls and 165 HIV-positive patients (85.5% on ART and 45.5% with undetectable HIV viral load). Among the HIV-positive group eligible for CRC screening, 91.9% underwent flexible sigmoidoscopy, which was similar to the percentage who underwent it in the HIV-negative cohort. More polyps were identified in the HIV group compared to the control group (30.9% vs. 23%; $p = 0.2$), and polyps in the HIV group were more likely to have neoplastic features compared to those of the controls (25.5% vs. 13.1%; $p < 0.001$; OR, 2.27; 95% CI, 1.57–3.29). The study found that duration of HIV more than 10 years and lower $CD4^+$ cell count were significantly associated with having distal neoplasias. Those with positive sigmoidoscopy went on to have full colonoscopy, which showed a higher prevalence of proximal colon neoplastic lesions in the HIV group compared to the HIV-negative controls (61.2% vs. 47.8%; $p = 0.07$) (Bini, 2006). Although not statistically significant, it appears that HIV-infected patients are at high risker for malignant potential compared to their HIV-negative counterparts. Another study comparing CRC screening in HIV patients and controls demonstrated similar results as those obtained in the New York veterans study. This study compared 302 HIV-positive and 302 HIV-negative patients and found that those with HIV were significantly less likely to have any type of screening modality (55.6% compared to 77.8%; $p < 0.0001$). Undetectable HIV RNA levels, older age, and a family history were variables associated with having at least one CRC screening (Reinhold, 2005).

Appropriate use of screening for eligible persons is of utmost importance for the HIV population because polyps may have more high-risk features than those of the general population. Barriers to colonoscopy referral and screening should be identified and managed. Increased provider and patient education may also be beneficial. One pilot study that randomizing screening-eligible HIV patients to receive educational material and in-person decision-making support showed increased screening colonoscopy uptake (Ferron, 2015). Based on this evidence, efforts to increase on-time screening in eligible HIV-positive patients should be undertaken.

CLINICAL PRESENTATION

At the time of diagnosis in HIV patients, CRC is often advanced and occurs in younger patients compared to the general population. Researchers from the Italian Cooperative Group AIDS and Tumors evaluated 27 HIV-positive and 54 matched, HIV-negative patients who were diagnosed with CRC between 1985 and 2003 (Berretta, 2009). The majority were diagnosed in the ART era, with a median age of 48 years in both groups. However, the majority of patients in the HIV cohort were younger than age 45 years. Median $CD4^+$ cell count at the time of diagnosis was 325 cells/mm^3. In the HIV-positive group, the stage was predominantly Dukes' stage D (distant metastasis) compared to those without HIV (74% vs. 35%; $p = 0.002$). Histopathology showed poorly differentiated adenocarcinoma in 66% of the HIV cohort compared to 26% in the HIV-negative matched controls (Berretta, 2009).

A case–control study from Southern California also found that CRC of HIV-positive patients occurred mainly in those younger than age 50 years (72%) and with advanced disease (stages III and IV). HIV patients had a younger to older age ratio of 3:1 compared to the population controls, whose ratio was 1.33. In the majority of patients, biopsy findings revealed poorly differentiated adenocarcinoma (64%). Of note, the mean $CD4^+$ cell count at time of diagnosis was robust at 467 cells/mm^3 (Wasserberg, 2007).

One multicenter retrospective study of 17 HIV patients with confirmed CRC from 1988 to 2003 reported that patients had a mean age of 43 years and a majority had a $CD4^+$ cell count <500 cells/mm^3 (not specified further) (Chapman, 2009). The majority of tumors arose in the right side of the colon (57%) and with advanced stage IV disease (47%) and histopathology with grade 2 or 3 adenocarcinomas (79%). The majority of metastatic sites were to the liver but also included lung, peritoneum, and subcutaneous sites (Chapman, 2009). Given the presence of right-sided colonic tumors, colonoscopy in HIV patients may have a greater diagnostic yield compared to flexible sigmoidoscopy. Further prospective studies should be performed to evaluate the various screening techniques in the HIV-positive population.

TREATMENT FOR COLORECTAL CANCER IN HIV

Treatment for CRC in HIV-positive patients is the same as that for those without HIV and primarily depends on clinical staging of the malignancy, which is determined by physical exam and radiographic imaging. CT is mandatory for determining regional extension, nodal involvement, or distant metastasis in the tumor, nodal, and metastatic staging system. Stages range from stage I to stage IV as the disease advances from confined disease to the colonic mucosa, regional lymph node involvement, and involvement of one or more distant organs including peritoneal seeding. For patients with stage II–IV disease, imaging with CT scan of the chest, abdomen, and pelvis is recommended (NCCN Colon Cancer, 2.2016). Further imaging with MRI may be useful for better characterization of the liver for metastatic disease, especially in the setting of background steatosis (Shahani, 2014). Testing with the tumor marker carcinoembryonic antigen (CEA) should be performed prior to treatment to help serve as a guide in the post-treatment follow-up. This test has not been validated for use specifically in the HIV population, nor has there been robust evidence supporting survival benefit in the general population, but CEA remains a standard pre- and post-treatment test for its prognostic utility (Locker, 2006).

Role of Surgery in Treatment of CRC

Treatment for localized disease can be curative with endoscopic resection of a carcinomatous polyp or surgical resection with simple colectomy and anastomosis. Surgery remains the cornerstone of therapy for localized disease, and margins should be free of cancer. Locally advanced disease or poorly differentiated polypoid lesions may warrant more invasive or radical surgery. If invasion involves surrounding structures, larger resection of contiguous, multivisceral structures is indicated to ensure negative margins in the affected noncolonic organs (NCCN Colon Cancer, 2.2016). This approach has yielded improved prognosis and outcomes in patients with locally advanced disease

(Govindarajan, 2006; Lehnert, 2002). Tumor location is also an important aspect in consideration of surgical approach because management of CRC involving the rectum (especially the lower rectum) may compromise anal sphincter tone and genitourinary function. If the anus is involved, sphincter-sparing surgery may be considered with adjuvant or neoadjuvant chemotherapy and radiation (NCCN, 1.2016; Sauer, 2012).

Colorectal adenocarcinoma typically metastasizes to the liver, lung, lymph nodes, and peritoneum. With limited metastatic disease, curative surgery still remains an option to improve survival; however, recurrence of disease is a reality for some patients (Neef, 2009; Shah, 2006).

Chemoradiotherapy CRC

Neoadjuvant and adjuvant chemotherapies are generally considered for patients with advanced or metastatic disease when the expectation of noncurative surgery is present. Neoadjuvant chemoradiotherapy is a standard approach to therapy in locally advanced rectal cancer (T3 or N1-2) prior to surgery or rectal cancer that is unresectable or medically inoperable. This consists of fractionated radiation therapy usually with a 5-fluorouracil (5-FU)-based regimen in combination with other agents, such as capecitabine or oxaliplatin and leucovorin (NCCN, 1.2016; Sauer, 2012). Adjuvant chemoradiotherapy following resection to eliminate microscopic foci of tumors and promote recurrence-free survival has been most beneficial in patients with nodal involvement (stage III), which has been shown in randomized controlled trials (Smith, 2004). Typical regimens include 5-FU/leucovorin- or capecitabine-based regimens (NCCN Colon Cancer, 2.2016). Other adjuvant therapies in metastatic disease include the vascular endothelial and epidermal growth factor inhibitor bevacizumab and cetuximab, respectively. Overall survival benefit of these agents remains controversial, and they may cause excess adverse events (da Gramont, 2012; Taieb, 2014).

TREATMENT OUTCOMES AND SURVIVAL OF PATIENTS WITH HIV AND CRC

There is a paucity of data on the efficacy, tolerability, and treatment outcomes of CRC for patients with HIV infection. Case series have provided much of the data on this population. As previously discussed, patients with HIV tend to present with more advanced disease, which may require both surgery and chemoradiation. In one case series, 10 HIV-positive patients with stage III or IV disease underwent segmental colon or rectal resection. One of these patients underwent complete pelvic exenteration (Wasserberg, 2007). All patients also received first-line adjuvant chemotherapy with 5-FU/leucovorin. Four of the patients received additional CPT-11 or irinotecan for metastatic disease. Of the patients with rectal involvement, 1 patient received neoadjuvant 5-FU/leucovorin-based chemoradiation, and 3 patients received adjuvant radiation. Overall, chemotherapy was tolerated well, but some patients did experience grade 3 adverse events with neutropenia and anemia (Wasserberg, 2007).

Another case series from Italy reported on 27 HIV-positive patients, the majority with metastatic CRC (Berretta, 2009). Of those with metastatic disease, 3 received neoadjuvant oxaliplatin-based chemotherapy for liver metastasis, 7 underwent palliative chemotherapy, and 2 were treated with 5-FU chemoradiation. The remaining patients with metastatic disease underwent palliation. One patient who received radiation incurred hemorrhagic proctitis, which prompted treatment cessation (Berretta, 2009). Overall, chemotherapy was tolerated well in the group, with few grade 3 neutropenic events.

Surgical resection provides the best curative treatment for localized colon cancer, and this has been demonstrated with SEER data (2005–2011) showing 5-year survival rates of 90% for localized disease. However, survival declines steeply with regional or nodal involvement (70%) and with distant metastasis (13%) (Howlader, 2015). Patients with HIV may not receive surgery when indicated, giving them a survival disadvantage. This disparity was highlighted in a follow-up study by the previously mentioned Italian group. In the following year, the group released a brief report on its experience treating HIV patients with liver metastasis (Berretta, 2010). The group reported on 14 patients in its center who had HIV and CRC-related liver metastasis. Only 3 patients initially had unresectable liver metastasis as determined by a multidisciplinary team; however, the other 11 patients underwent FOLFOX-4 treatment. Three patients in the group of those who were able to undergo surgical approach received neoadjuvant chemotherapy with FOLFOX-4 or FOLFIRI, followed by liver segmentectomy (2 patients) and liver segmentectomy plus radiofrequency ablation (1 patient). These 3 patients tolerated the treatments well, remained on ART without any grade 3 or 4 toxicities, and 2 of the 3 patients remained disease-free at 21-month follow-up. Although the number of patients was small, these researchers demonstrated that an aggressive surgical approach for metastatic CRC can be successfully performed in patients with HIV. Narrowing the treatment gap between the HIV population and the general population remains an important goal in the care of malignancies in HIV that may help improve survival outcomes for this group.

Mortality for HIV patients with CRC remains high compared to that for the general population. A large retrospective study estimated that those with HIV and CRC have a 50% higher risk of mortality compared to uninfected patients (Coghill, 2015). Smaller case–control studies have shown markedly poorer survivability for HIV patients compared to negative controls, with 4-year survival of 15% and 49%, respectively (Berretta, 2009). Although the smaller aforementioned studies have demonstrated tolerability of chemotherapy and surgery in HIV patients with ability to continue with ART, larger population-based studies have demonstrated that a survival disparity remains. It has been hypothesized that HIV-infected individuals are less likely to receive therapy and therefore, on a population level, will have poorer survival. HIV positivity should not preclude delivery of the standard of care, and further studies are needed to rigorously evaluate the standard of care delivered to these patients. Disparities in screening and treatment of HIV patients with CRC are likely to perpetuate their less than optimal survival outcomes relative to those of HIV-negative patients.

Recommended Reading

Berretta M, Cappellani A, Di Benedetto F, et al. Clinical presentation and outcome of colorectal cancer in HIV-positive patients: A clinical case–control study. *Onkologie.* 2009; 32:319–324.

Bini EJ, Park J, Francois F. Use of flexible sigmoidoscopy to screen for colorectal cancer in HIV-infected patients 50 years of age or older. *JAMA Intern Med.* 2006; 166(15):1626–1631.

References

Aboulafia DM. Kaposi's sarcoma. *Clinics Derm.* 2001; 19(3):269–283.

Aboulafia DM, Puswella AL. Highly active antiretroviral therapy as the sole treatment for AIDS-related primary central nervous system lymphoma: A case report with implications for treatment. *AIDS Patient Care STDS.* 2007; 21(12):900–907.

Advisory Committee on Immunization Practices. Recommended adult immunization schedule: United States, 2013. *Ann Intern Med.* 2013; 158:191–199.

Ahdieh L, Munoz A, Vlahov D, et al. Cervical neoplasia and repeated positivity of human papillomavirus infection in human immunodeficiency virus-seropositive and -seronegative women. *Am J Epidemiol.* 2000; 151(12):1148–1157.

Appleby P, Beral V, Newton R, et al. Highly active antiretroviral therapy and incidence of cancer in human immunodeficiency virus-infected adults. *Cancer Inst.* 2000; 92:1823–1830.

Avivi I, Robinson S, Goldstone A. Clinical use of rituximab in haematological malignancies. *Br J Cancer.* 2003; 89(8):1389–1394.

Ballerini P, Gaidano G, Gong JZ, et al. Multiple genetic lesions in acquired immunodeficiency syndrome-related non-Hodgkin's lymphoma. *Blood.* 1993; 81(1):166–176.

Barillari G, Ensoli B. Angiogenic effects of extracellular human immunodeficiency virus type 1 Tat protein and its role in the pathogenesis of AIDS-associated Kaposi's sarcoma. *Clin Microbiol Rev.* 2002; 15(2):310–326.

Bañon S, Machuca I, Araujo S, et al. Efficacy, safety, and lack of interactions with the use of raltegravir in HIV-infected patients undergoing antineoplastic chemotherapy. *J Intern AIDS Soc.* 2014; 17(4 Suppl 3):19590.

Barbosa MS, Schlegel R. The E6 and E7 genes of HPV-18 are sufficient for inducing two-stage in vitro transformation of human keratinocytes. *Oncogene.* 1989; 4(12):1529–1532.

Barozzi P, Luppi M, Facchetti F, et al. Post-transplant Kaposi sarcoma originates from the seeding of donor-derived progenitors. *Nature Med.* 2003; 9(5):554–561.

Baumgartner JE, Rachlin JR, Beckstead JH, et al. Primary central nervous system lymphomas: Natural history and response to radiation therapy in 55 patients with acquired immunodeficiency syndrome. *J Neurosurg.* 1990; 73(2):206–211.

Bayraktar S, Bayraktar UD, Ramos JC, et al. Primary CNS lymphoma in HIV positive and negative patients: Comparison of clinical characteristics, outcome and prognostic factors. *J Neurooncol.* 2011; 101:257–265.

Bedi GC, Westra WH, Farzedegan H, et al. Microsatellite instability in primary neoplasms from HIV+ patients. *Nature Med.* 1995; 1(1):65–68.

Bedimo R, Chen RY, Accortt NA, et al. Trends in AIDS-defining and non-AIDS defining malignancies among HIV-infected patients: 1989–2002. *Clin Infect Dis.* 2004; 39(9):1380–1384.

Beral V, Peterman TA, Berkelman RL, et al. Kaposi's sarcoma among persons with AIDS: A sexually transmitted infection? *Lancet.* 1990; 335(8682):123–128.

Beral V, Peterman T, Berkelman R, et al. AIDS-associated non-Hodgkin lymphoma. *Lancet.* 1991; 337(8745):805–809.

Berretta M, Cappellani A, Di Benedetto F, et al. Clinical presentation and outcome of colorectal cancer in HIV-positive patients: A clinical case–control study. *Onkologie.* 2009; 32:319–324.

Berretta M, Zanet E, Basile F, et al. HIV positive patients with liver metastasis from colorectal cancer deserve the same therapeutic approach as the general population. *Onkkologie.* 2010; 33:203–204.

Berthold DR, Pond GR, Soban F, et al. Docetaxel plus prednisone or mitoxantrone plus prednisone for advanced prostate cancer: Updated survival in the TAX 327 study. *J Clin Oncol.* 2008; 26(2):242–245.

Besson C, Goubar A, Gabarre J, et al. Changes in AIDS-related lymphoma since the era of highly active antiretroviral therapy. *Blood.* 2001; 98(8):2339–2344.

Bini EJ, Park J, Francois F. Use of flexible sigmoidoscopy to screen for colorectal cancer in HIV-infected patients 50 years of age or older. *JAMA Intern Med.* 2006; 166(15):1626–1631.

Bjorge T, Engeland A, Luostarinen T, et al. Human papillomavirus infection as a risk factor for anal and perianal skin cancer in a prospective study. *Br J Cancer.* 2002; 87(1):61–64.

Bonnet F, Burty C, Lewden C, et al. Changes in cancer mortality among HIV-infected patients: The Mortalite 2005 Survey. *Clin Infect Dis.* 2009; 48(5):633–639.

Bosch FX, Manos MM, Munoz N, et al. Prevalence of human papillomavirus in cervical cancer: A worldwide perspective. *J Natl Cancer Inst.* 1995; 87(11):796–802.

Bossolasco S, Cinque P, Ponzoni M, et al. Epstein–Barr virus DNA load in cerebrospinal fluid and plasma of patients with AIDS-related lymphoma. *J Neurovirol.* 2002; 8(5):432–438.

Boudreaux AA, Smith LL, Cosby CD, et al. Intralesional vinblastine for cutaneous Kaposi's sarcoma associated with acquired immunodeficiency syndrome: A clinical trial to evaluate efficacy and discomfort associated with infection. *J Am Acad Derm.* 1993; 28(1):61–65.

Boulanger E, Gerard L, Gabarre J, et al. Prognostic factors and outcome of human herpesvirus 8-associated primary effusion lymphoma in patients with AIDS. *J Clin Oncol.* 2005; 23(19):4372–4380.

Bower M, Fox P, Fife K, Gill J, Nelson M, Gazzard B. Highly active anti-retroviral therapy (HAART) prolongs time to treatment failure in Kaposi's sarcoma. *AIDS (London, England).* 1999;13(15):2105–2111.

Bower M, McCall-Peat N, Ryan N, et al. Protease inhibitors potentiate chemotherapy-induced neutropenia. *Blood.* 2004; 104(9):2943–2946.

Bower M, Powles T, Nelson M, et al. HIV-related lung cancer in the era of highly active antiretroviral therapy. *AIDS (London).* 2003; 17(3):371–375.

Bower M, Powles T, Newsom-Davis T, et al. HIV-associated anal cancer: Has highly active antiretroviral therapy reduced the incidence or improved the outcome? *J Acquir Immune Defic Syndr.* 2004; 37(5):1563–1565.

Burgi A, Brodine S, Wegner S, et al. Incidence and risk factors for the occurrence of non-AIDS-defining cancers among human immunodeficiency virus-infected individuals. *Cancer.* 2005; 104(7):1505–1511.

Burkes RL, Meyer PR, Gill PS, et al. Rectal lymphoma in homosexual men. *Arch Intern Med.* 1986; 146(5):913–915.

Cadranel J, Garfield D, Lavole A, et al. Lung cancer in HIV infected patients: Facts, questions, and challenges. *Thorax.* 2006; 61:1000–1008.

Calabresi A, Ferraresi A, Festa A, et al. Incidence of AIDS-defining cancers and virus-related and non-virus-related non-AIDS-defining cancers among HIV-infected patients compared with the general population in a large health district of northern Italy, 1999–2000. *HIV Med.* 2013; 14(8):481–490.

Campbell TB, Borok M, White IE, et al. Relationship of Kaposi sarcoma (KS)-associated herpesvirus viremia and KS disease in Zimbabwe. *Clin Infect Dis.* 2003; 36(9):1144–1151.

Cannon MJ. Kaposi's sarcoma-associated herpesvirus and acquired immunodeficiency syndrome-related malignancy. *Semin Oncol.* 2000; 27:408–419.

Cannon MJ, Dollard SC, Smith DK, et al. Blood-borne and sexual transmission of human herpesvirus 8 in women with or at risk for human immunodeficiency virus infection. *N Engl J Med.* 2001; 344(9):637–643.

Cappell MS, Yao F, Cho KC. Colonic adenocarcinoma associated with the acquired immune deficiency syndrome. *Cancer.* 1988: 62:616–619.

Casper C, Carrell D, Miller KG, et al. HIV serodiscordant sex partners and the prevalence of human herpesvirus 8 infection among HIV negative men who have sex with men: Baseline data from the EXPLORE Study. *Sex Transm Infect.* 2006; 82(3):229–235.

Casper C, Krantz E, Selke S, et al. Frequent and asymptomatic oropharyngeal shedding of human herpesvirus 8 among immunocompetent men. *J Infect Dis.* 2007; 195(1):30–36.

Casper C, Redman M, Huang ML, et al. HIV infection and human herpesvirus-8 oral shedding among men who have sex with men. *J Acquir Immune Defic Syndr.* 2004; 35(3):233–238.

Castilho JL, Luz PM, Shepherd BE, et al. HIV and cancer: A comparative retrospective study of Brazilian and U.S. clinical cohorts. *Infect Agent Cancer.* 2015; 10(4):1–10.

Centers for Disease Control and Prevention. AIDS-defining conditions. 2008. Available at https://www.cdc.gov/mmwr/preview/mmwrhtml/rr5710a2.htm.

Centers for Disease Control and Prevention. Human papillomavirus-associated cancers—United States, 2004–2008. *Morbid Mortal Wkly Rep.* 2012 April 20; 61(15):258–261.

Centers for Disease Control and Prevention. Estimated HIV incidence in the United States, 2007–2010. *HIV Surveill Suppl Rep* 2012; 17(4).

Centers for Disease Control and Prevention. Human papilloma virus (HPV) fact sheet. Available at www.cdc.gov/std/hpv. Accessed May 11, 2016.

Chadburn A, Abdul-Nabi AM, Teruya BS, et al. Lymphoid proliferations associated with human immunodeficiency virus infection. *Arch Path Lab Med.* 2013; 137(3):360–370.

Chang Y, Cesarman E, Pessin MS, et al. Identification of herpesvirus-like DNA sequences in AIDS-associated Kaposi's sarcoma. *Science.* 1994; 266(5192):1865–1869.

Chapman C, Aboulafia DM, Dezube BJ, et al. Human immunodeficiency virus-associated adenocarcinoma of the colon: Clinicopathologic findings and outcome. *Clin Colorectal Cancer*. 2009; 8(4):215–219.

Chari A, Kaplan L, Volberding PA, et al. Diagnosis and management of non-Hodgkin's lymphoma and Hodgkin's lymphoma. 2005.

Chen YH, Lin MW, Bhatia K, et al. Cancer incidence in a nationwide HIV/AIDS patient cohort in Taiwan in 1998–2000. *J Acquir Immune Defic Syndr*. 2014; 65(4):463–472.

Chiao EY, Dezube BJ, Krown SE, et al. Time for oncologists to opt in for routine opt-out HIV testing? *JAMA*. 2010; 304(3):334–339.

Chin-Hong PV, Vittinghoff E, Cranston RD, et al. Age-specific prevalence of anal human papillomavirus infection in HIV-negative sexually active men who have sex with men: The EXPLORE study. *J Infect Dis*. 2004; 190(12):2070–2076.

Chokunonga E, Levy LM, Bassett MT, et al. Cancer incidence in the African population of Harare, Zimbabwe: Second results from the cancer registry 1993–1995. *Int J Cancer*. 2000; 85(1):54–59.

Cingolani A, Fratino L, Scoppettuolo G, et al. Changing pattern of primary cerebral lymphoma in the highly active antiretroviral therapy era. *J Neurovirol*. 2005; 11(Suppl 3):38–44.

Cleator S, Fife K, Nelson M, et al. Treatment of HIV-associated invasive anal cancer with combined chemoradiation. *Eur J Cancer (Oxford: 1990)*. 2000; 36(6):754–758.

Clifford GM, Lise M, Franceschi S, et al. Lung cancer in the Swiss HIV Cohort Study: Role of smoking, immunodeficiency, and pulmonary infection. *Br J Cancer*. 2012; 106:448–452.

Clifford GM, Polesel J, Richenbach M, et al. Cancer risk in the Swiss HIV Cohort Study: Associations with immunodeficiency, smoking, and highly active antiretroviral therapy. *J Natl. Cancer Inst*. 2005; 97(6):425–432.

Coghill AE, Shiels MS, Suneja G, et al. Elevated cancer-specific mortality among HIV-infected patients in the United States. *J Clin Oncol*. 2015; 33(21):2376–2383.

Conti S, Masocco M, Pezzotti P, et al. Differential impact of combined antiretroviral therapy on the survival of Italian patients with specific AIDS-defining illnesses. *J Acquir Immune Defic Syndr (1999)*. 2000; 25(5):451–458.

Cooper JS, Steinfeld AD, Lerch I. Intentions and outcomes in the radiotherapeutic management of epidemic Kaposi's sarcoma. *Int J Radiat Oncol Biol Phys*. 1991; 20(3):419–422.

Corales R, Taege A, Rehm S, et al. Regression of AIDS-related CNS lymphoma with HAART. Proceedings of the XIII International AIDS Conference, Durban, South Africa, 2000. [Abstract MoPpB1086]

Cote TR, Biggar RJ, Rosenberg PS, et al. Non-Hodgkin's lymphoma among people with AIDS: Incidence, presentation and public health burden. *Int J Cancer*. 1997; 73(5):645–650.

Cote TR, Manns A, Hardy CR, et al.; AIDS/Cancer Study Group. Epidemiology of brain lymphoma among people with or without acquired immunodeficiency syndrome. *J Natl Cancer Inst*. 1996; 88(10):675–679.

Cranston R, Yang M, Paczuski P, et al. Baseline data of a phase 3 trial of the quadrivalent HPV vaccine in HIV+ males and females: ACTG 5298. Paper presented at the 21st Conference on Retroviruses and Opportunistic Infections; Boston, MA, March 3–6, 2014.

Crothers K, Huang, L, Goulet JL, et al. HIV infection and risk for incident pulmonary diseases in the combination antiretroviral therapy era. *Am J Respir Crit Care Med*. 2011; 183(3):388–395.

Da Gramont A, Van Cutsem E, Schmoll HJ, et al. Bevacizumab plus oxaliplatin-based chemotherapy as adjuvant treatment for colon cancer (AVANT): A phase 3 randomised controlled trial. *Lancet Oncol*. 2012; 13(12):1225–1233.

Daling JR, Weiss NS, Hislop TG, et al. Sexual practices, sexually transmitted diseases, and the incidence of anal cancer. *N Engl J Med*. 1987; 317(16):973–977.

Danzig JB, Brandt LJ, Reinus JF, et al. Gastrointestinal malignancy in patients with AIDS. *Am J Gastroenterol*. 1991; 86(6):715–718.

Dedicoat M, Newton R, Alkharsah KR, et al. Mother-to-child transmission of human herpesvirus-8 in South Africa. *J Infect Dis*. 2004; 190(6):1068–1075.

Denny L, Hendricks B, Gordon C, et al. Safety and immunogenicity of the HPV-16/18 AS04-adjuvanted vaccine in HIV-positive women in South Africa: A partially-blind randomised placebo-controlled study. *Vaccine*. 2013; 31(48):5743–5753.

Deregibus M, Cantalupp IV, Doublier S, et al. HIV-1-Tat protein activates phosphatidylinositol 3-kinase/AKT-dependent survival pathways in Kaposi's sarcoma cells. *J Biol Chem*. 2002; 277(28):25195–25202.

Deshmukh AA, Chhatwal J, Chiao EY, et al. Long-term outcomes of adding HPV vaccine to the anal intraepithelial neoplasia treatment regimen in HIV-positive men who have sex with men. *Clin Infect Dis*. 2015; 61(10):1527–1535.

Dezube BJ, Pantanowitz L, Aboulafia DM. Management of AIDS-related Kaposi sarcoma: Advances in target discovery and treatment. *AIDS Reader*. 2004; 14(5):236–238, 243.

Diez-Martin J, Balsalobre P, Carrion R. et al. Long term survival after autologous stem cell transplant (ASCT) in AIDS related lymphoma patients [Abstract 868]. *Blood*. 2003; 247a:102.

Diez-Martin JL, Balsalobre P, Re A, et al. Comparable survival between HIV+ and HIV– non-Hodgkin and Hodgkin lymphoma patients undergoing autologous peripheral blood stem cell transplantation. *Blood*. 2009; 113(23):6011–6014.

D'Jaen GA, Pantanowitz L, Bower M, et al. Human immunodeficiency virus-associated primary lung cancer in the era of highly active antiretroviral therapy: A multi-institutional collaboration. *Clin Lung Cancer*. 2010; 11(6):396–404.

Donahue BR, Sullivan JW, Cooper JS. Additional experience with empiric radiotherapy for presumed human immunodeficiency virus-associated primary central nervous system lymphoma. *Cancer*. 1995; 76(2):328–332.

D'Souza G, Wiley D, Li X, et al. Incidence and epidemiology of anal cancer in the multicenter AIDS cohort study. *J Acquir Immune Defic Syndr*. 2008; 48:491–499.

Duncan KC, Chan KJ, Chiu CG, et al. HAART slows progression to anal cancer in HIV-infected MSM. *AIDS*. 2015; 29:305–311.

Ekstein D, Ben-Yehuda D, Slyusarevsky E, et al. CSF analysis of IgH gene rearrangement in CNS lymphoma: Relationship to the disease course. *J Neurol Sci*. 2006; 247:39–46.

El Amari EB, Toutous-Trellu L, Gayet-Ageron A, et al. Predicting the evolution of Kaposi sarcoma in the highly active antiretroviral therapy era. *AIDS*. 2008; 22(9):1019–1028.

El-Solh A, Kumar NM, Nair MP, et al. An RDG-containing peptide from HIV-1 TAT-(65–80) modulates protooncogene expression in human bronchoalveolar carcinoma cell line, A549. *Immunol Invest*. 1997; 26(3):351–370.

Engels EA, Biggar RJ, Hall I, et al. Cancer risk in people infected with human immunodeficiency virus in the United States. *Intern J Cancer*. 2008; 123:187–194.

Engels EA, Biggar RJ, Marshall VA, et al. Detection and quantification of Kaposi's sarcoma-associated herpesvirus to predict AIDS-associated Kaposi's sarcoma. *AIDS (London)*. 2003; 17(12):1847–1851.

Ensoli B, Barillari G, Salahuddin S, et al. Tat protein of HIV-1 stimulates growth of cells derived from Kaposi's sarcoma lesions of AIDS patients. *Nature*. 1990; 345(6270):84–86.

European AIDS Clinical Society. Guidelines version 8.0. October 2015. Available at http://www.eacsociety.org/files/2015_eacsguidelines_8.0-english_revised-20151104.pdf. Accessed May 13, 2016.

Ferron P, Asfour SS, Metsch LR, et al. Impact of a multifaceted intervention on promoting adherence to screening colonoscopy among persons in HIV primary care: A pilot study. *Clin Transl Sci*. 2015; 8(4):290–297.

Franceschi S, Dal Maso L, Rickenbach M, et al. Kaposi sarcoma incidence in the Swiss HIV Cohort Study before and after highly active antiretroviral therapy. *Br J Cancer*. 2008; 99(5):800–804.

Friedman SL. Gastrointestinal and hepatobiliary neoplasms in AIDS. *Gastroenterol Clin North Am.* 1988; 17(3):465–486.

Friedman-Kien AE. Disseminated Kaposi's sarcoma syndrome in young homosexual men. *J Am Acad Dermatol.* 1981; 5(4):468–471.

Friedman-Kien AE, Saltzman BR. Clinical manifestations of classical, endemic African, and epidemic AIDS-associated Kaposi's sarcoma. *J Am Acad Dermatol.* 1990; 22(6 Pt 2):1237–1250.

Frisch M, Biggar RJ, Engels EA, et al.; AIDS–Cancer Match Registry Study Group. Association of cancer with AIDS-related immunosuppression in adults. *JAMA.* 2001; 285(13):1736–1745.

Frisch M, Biggar RJ, Goedert JJ. Human papillomavirus-associated cancers in patients with human immunodeficiency virus infection and acquired immunodeficiency syndrome. *J Nat Cancer Institute.* 2000; 92(18):1500–1510.

Frisch M, Goodman MT. Human papillomavirus-associated carcinomas in Hawaii and the mainland U.S. *Cancer.* 2000; 88(6):1464–1469.

Fulco PP, Hynicka L, Rackley D. Raltegravir-based HAART regimen in a patient with large B-cell lymphoma. *Ann Pharmacother.* 2010; 44(2):377–382.

Gabarre J, Azar N, Autran B, et al. High-dose therapy and autologous haematopoietic stem-cell transplantation for HIV-1-associated lymphoma. *Lancet.* 2000; 355(9209):1071–1072.

Gabarre J, Marcelin AG, Azar N, et al. High-dose therapy plus autologous hematopoietic stem cell transplantation for human immunodeficiency virus (HIV)-related lymphoma: Results and impact on HIV disease. *Haematologica.* 2004; 89(9):1100–1108.

Gage JT, Vance EA, Hildenbrand PG, et al. Brain lesion and AIDS. *Proc Baylor Univ Medical Center.* 2000; 13(4):424–429.

Gaidano G, Dalla-Favera R. Molecular pathogenesis of AIDS-related lymphomas. *Adv Cancer Res.* 1995; 67:113–153.

Gates AE, Kaplan LD. Biology and management of AIDS-associated non-Hodgkin's lymphoma. *Hematol Oncol Clin North Am.* 2003; 17(3):821–841.

Gerard L, Meignin V, Galicier L, et al. Characteristics of non-Hodgkin lymphoma arising in HIV-infected patients with suppressed HIV replication. *AIDS.* 2009; 23(17):2301–2308.

Gichangi P, De Vuyst H, Estambale B, et al. HIV and cervical cancer in Kenya. *Intern J Gynaecol Obst.* 2002; 76(1):55–63.

Gill ON, Weinberg JR, Fisher IS, et al. Meta-surveillance—Safer cyber-surveillance. *Lancet.* 1995; 346(8977):776.

Gill PS, Akil B, Colletti P, et al. Pulmonary Kaposi's sarcoma: Clinical findings and results of therapy. *Am J Med.* 1989; 87(1):57–61.

Gill PS, Wernz J, Scadden DT, et al. Randomized phase III trial of liposomal daunorubicin versus doxorubicin, bleomycin, and vincristine in AIDS-related Kaposi's sarcoma. *J Clin Oncol.* 1996; 14(8):2353–2364.

Goldstein JD, Dickson DW, Moser FG, et al. Primary central nervous system lymphoma in acquired immune deficiency syndrome: A clinical and pathologic study with results of treatment with radiation. *Cancer.* 1991; 67(11):2756–2765.

Gosselaar C, Roobol MJ, van den Bergh RC, et al. Digital rectal examination and the diagnosis of prostate cancer—A study based on 8 years and three screenings within the European Randomized Study of Screening for Prostate Cancer (ERSPC), Rotterdam. *Eur Urol.* 2009; 55(1):139–146.

Gosselaar C, Roobol MJ, Roemeling S, et al. The role of the digital rectal examination in subsequent screening visits in the European Randomized Study of Screening for Prostate Cancer (ERSPC), Rotterdam. *Eur Urol.* 2008; 54:581–588.

Govindarajan A, Coburn NH, Kiss A, et al. Population-based assessment of the surgical management of locally advanced colorectal cancer. *J Natl Cancer Inst.* 2006; 98(20):1474–1481.

Grimm P, Billiet I, Bostwick D, et al. Comparative analysis of prostate specific antigen free survival outcomes for patients with low, intermediate, and high risk prostate cancer treatment by radical therapy: Results from the Prostate Cancer Results Study Group. *Br J Urol Int.* 2012; 109(Suppl 1):22–29.

Guiguet M, Boue F, Cadranel J, et al. Effect of immunodeficiency, HIV viral load, and antiretroviral therapy on the risk of individual malignancies (FHDH-ANRS CO4): A prospective cohort study. *Lancet Oncol.* 2009; 10(12):1152–1159.

Gulrich AE, Yueming L, McDonald A, et al. Rates of non-AIDS defining cancers in people with HIV infection before and after AIDS diagnoses. *AIDS.* 2002; 16:1155–1161.

Hamilton-Dutoit SJ, Pallesen G, Karkov J, et al. Identification of EBV-DNA in tumour cells of AIDS-related lymphomas by in-situ hybridisation. *Lancet.* 1989; 1(8637):554–552.

Hassett JM, Zaroulis CG, Greenberg ML, et al. Bone marrow transplantation in AIDS. *N Engl J Med.* 1983; 309(11):665.

Heidenreich A, Bastian PJ, Bellmunt J, et al. European Association of Urology (EAU) guidelines on prostate cancer: Part 1. Screening, diagnosis, and local treatment with curative intent—Update 2013. *Eur Urol.* 2014; 65(1):124–137.

Hengge UR, Ruzicka T, Tyring SK, et al. Update on Kaposi's sarcoma and other HHV8 associated diseases: Part 1. Epidemiology, environmental predispositions, clinical manifestations, and therapy. *Lancet Infect Dis.* 2002; 2(5):281–292.

Herida M, Mary-Krause M, Kaphan R, et al. Incidence of non-AIDS defining cancers before and during the highly active antiretroviral therapy era in a cohort of human immunodeficiency virus-infected patients. *J Clin Oncol* 2003; 21;3447–3453.

Hill DR. The role of radiotherapy for epidemic Kaposi's sarcoma. *Semin Oncol.* 1987; 14:1207.

Hladik W, Dollard SC, Mermin J, et al. Transmission of human herpesvirus 8 by blood transfusion. *N Engl J Med.* 2006; 355(13):1331–1338.

Hoffmann C, Tabrizian S, Wolf E, et al. Survival of AIDS patients with primary central nervous system lymphoma is dramatically improved by HAART-induced immune recovery. *AIDS (London).* 2001; 15(16):2119–2127.

Holland HK, Saral R, Rossi JJ, et al. Allogeneic bone marrow transplantation, zidovudine, and human immunodeficiency virus type 1 (HIV-1) infection: Studies in a patient with non-Hodgkin lymphoma. *Ann Intern Med.* 1989; 111(12):973–981.

Hoover DR, Black C, Jacobson LP, et al. Epidemiologic analysis of Kaposi's sarcoma as an early and later AIDS outcome in homosexual men. *Am J Epidemiol.* 1993; 138(4):266–278.

Howlader N, Noone AM, Krapcho M, et al. SEER statistics review, 1975–2012. Bethesda, MD: National Cancer Institute. 2015. Available at http://seer.cancer.gov/archive/csr/1975_2012. Accessed May 13, 2016

Hsiao W, Anastasia K, Hall J, et al. Association between HIV status and positive prostate biopsy in a study of U.S. veterans. *ScientificWorldJournal.* 2009; 9:102–108.

Huncharek M, Haddock KS, Reid R, et al. Smoking as a risk factor for prostate cancer: A meta-analysis of 24 prospective cohort studies. *Am J Pub Health.* 2010; 100(4):693–701.

Impola U, Cuccuru MA, Masala MV, et al. Preliminary communication: Matrix metalloproteinases in Kaposi's sarcoma. *Br J Dermatol.* 2003; 149(4):905–907.

International Agency for Research on Cancer. *Human Immunodeficiency Viruses and Human T-Cell Lymphotropic Viruses.* Geneva: World Health Organization; 1996.

International Collaboration on HIV and Cancer. Highly active antiretroviral therapy and incidence of cancer in human immunodeficiency virus-infected adults. *J Natl Cancer Institute.* 2000; 92(22):1823–1830.

Ireland-Gill A, Espina BM, Akil B, et al. Treatment of acquired immunodeficiency syndrome-related Kaposi's sarcoma using bleomycin-containing combination chemotherapy regimens. *Semin Oncol.* 1992; 19(2 Suppl 5):32–36.

Iscovich J, Boffetta P, Franceschi S, et al. Classic Kaposi sarcoma: Epidemiology and risk factors. *Cancer.* 2000; 88(3):500–517.

Islami F, Moreira DM, Boffetta P, et al. A systematic review and meta-analysis of tobacco use and prostate cancer mortality and incidence in prospective cohort-studies. *Eur Urol.* 2014; 66(6):1054–1064.

Jacobson LP, Jenkins FJ, Springer G, et al. Interaction of human immunodeficiency virus type 1 and human herpesvirus type 8 infections on the incidence of Kaposi's sarcoma. *J Infect Dis.* 2000; 181(6):1940–1949.

Jacomet C, Girard PM, Lebrette MG, et al. Intravenous methotrexate for primary central nervous system non-Hodgkin's lymphoma in AIDS. *AIDS (London).* 1997; 11(14):1725–1730.

Jephcott CR, Paltiel C, Hay J. Quality of life after non-surgical treatment of anal carcinoma: A case–control study of long-term survivors. *Clin Oncol.* 2004; 16(8):530–535.

Johnson LG, Madeleine MM, Newcomer LM, et al. Anal cancer incidence and survival: The surveillance, epidemiology, and end results experience, 1973–2000. *Cancer.* 2004; 101(2):281–288.

Johnston C, Harrington R, Jain R, et al. Safety and efficacy of combination antiretroviral therapy in human immunodeficiency virus-infected adults undergoing autologous or allogeneic hematopoietic cell transplantation for hematologic malignancies. *Biol Blood Marrow Transplant.* 2016; 22:149–156.

Joseph DA, King JB, Miller JW, et al. Prevalence of colorectal cancer screening among adults—Behavioral risk factor surveillance system, United States, 2010. *Morbid Mortal Wkly Rep.* 2012; 61(2):51–56.

Kahn S, Jani A, Edelman S, et al. Matched cohort analysis of outcomes of definitive radiotherapy for prostate cancer in human immunodeficiency virus-positive patients. *Int Radiat Oncol Biol Physics.* 2012; 83(1):16–21.

Kaplan LD, Abrams DI, Feigal E, et al. AIDS-associated non-Hodgkin's lymphoma in San Francisco. *JAMA.* 1989; 261(5):719–724.

Kaplan LD, Hopewell PC, Jaffe H, et al. Kaposi's sarcoma involving the lung in patients with the acquired immunodeficiency syndrome. *J Acquir Immune Defic Syndr.* 1988; 1(1):23–30.

Kaplan LD, Straus DJ, Testa MA, et al. Low-dose compared with standard-dose m-BACOD chemotherapy for non-Hodgkin's lymphoma associated with human immunodeficiency virus infection. National Institute of Allergy and Infectious Diseases AIDS Clinical Trials Group. *N Engl J Med.* 1997; 336(23):1641–1648.

Karp J, Profeta G, Marantz PR, et al. Lung cancer in patients with immunodeficiency syndrome. *Chest.* 1993; 103(2):410–413.

Kirk GD, Merlo C, O'Driscoll P, et al. HIV infection is associated with an increased risk for lung cancer, independent of smoking. *Clin Infect Dis.* 2007; 45(1):103–110.

Kiviat NB, Hawes S, Lampinen T, et al. The effect of HAART on detection of anal HPV and squamous intraepithelial lesions among HIV infected homosexual men. Paper presented at the 6th International Conference on Malignancies in AIDS and Other Immunodeficiencies, Bethesda, MD, 2002.

Klugman AD, Schaffner J. Colon adenocarcinoma in HIV infection: A case report and review. *Am J Gastroenterol.* 1994; 89(2):254–256.

Knowles DM. Etiology and pathogenesis of AIDS-related non-Hodgkin's lymphoma. *Hematol Oncol Clin North Am.* 1996; 10(5):1081–1109.

Knowles DM. *Neoplastic Hematopathology.* Philadelphia: Lippincott Williams & Wilkins; 2001.

Knowles DM, Chamulak GA, Subar M, et al. Lymphoid neoplasia associated with the acquired immunodeficiency syndrome (AIDS): The New York University Medical Center experience with 105 patients (1981–1986). *Ann Intern Med.* 1988; 108(5):744–753.

Kojic EM, Kang M, Cespedes MS, et al. Immunogenicity and safety of the quadrivalent human papillomavirus vaccine in HIV-1-infected women. *Clin Infect Dis.* 2014; 59(1):127–135.

Komanduri KV, Luce JA, McGrath MS, et al. The natural history and molecular heterogeneity of HIV-associated primary malignant lymphomatous effusions. *J Acquired Immune Defic Syndr.* 1996; 13(3):215–226.

Koon HB, Krown SE, Lee JY, et al. Phase II trial of imatinib in AIDS-associated Kaposi's sarcoma: AIDS Malignancy Consortium Protocol 042. *J Clin Oncol.* 2014; 32(5):402–408.

Kowalkowski MA, Day RS, Chan W, et al. Cumulative HIV viremia and non-AIDs-defining malignancies among a sample of HIV-infected male veterans. *J Acquir Immune Defic Syndr* 2014; 62(2):204–211.

Krishnan A, Molina A, Zaia J, et al. Durable remissions with autologous stem cell transplantation for high-risk HIV-associated lymphomas. *Blood.* 2005; 105(2):874–878.

Krown SE, Metroka C, Wernz JC. Kaposi's sarcoma in the acquired immune deficiency syndrome: a proposal for uniform evaluation, response, and staging criteria. AIDS Clinical Trials Group Oncology Committee. *J Clin Oncol.* 1989 Sep; 7(9):1201–1207.

Krown SE, Testa MA, Huang J. AIDS-related Kaposi's sarcoma: Prospective validation of the AIDS Clinical Trials Group staging classification. AIDS Clinical Trials Group Oncology Committee. *J Clin Oncol.* 1997; 15(9):3085–3092.

Krown WE, Roy D, Lee JY, et al. Rapamycin with antiretroviral therapy in AIDS-associated Kaposi sarcoma: An AIDS Malignancy Consortium Study. *J Acquir Immune Defic Syndr.* 2012; 59(5):447–454.

La Ruche G, You B, Mensah-Ado I, et al. Human papillomavirus and human immunodeficiency virus infections: Relation with cervical dysplasia–neoplasia in African women. *Int J Cancer.* 1998; 76(4):480–486.

Lafrenie RM, Wahl LM, Epstein JS, et al. HIV-1-Tat modulates the function of monocytes and alters their interactions with microvessel endothelial cells: A mechanism of HIV pathogenesis. *J Immunol (Baltimore, 1950).* 1996; 156(4):1638–1645.

Lehnert T, Methner M, Pollok A, et al. Multivisceral resection for locally advanced primary colon and rectal cancer: An analysis of prognostic factors in 201 patients. *Ann Surg.* 2002: 235(2):217–225.

Leport C, Rousseau F, Perronne C, et al. Bacterial prostatitis in patients infected with the human immunodeficiency virus. *J Urol.* 1989; 141(2):334–336.

Letang E, Almeida J, Miró J, et al. Predictors of immune reconstitution inflammatory syndrome-associated with Kaposi sarcoma in Mozambique: A prospective study. *J Acquir Immune Defic Syndr.* 2010; 53(5):589–597.

Levine AM, Seaberg EC, Hessol NA, et al. HIV as a risk factor for lung cancer in women: Data from the Women's Interagency HIV Study. *J Clin Oncol.* 2010; 28(9):1514–1519.

Levine AM, Sullivan-Halley J, Pike MC, et al. Human immunodeficiency virus-related lymphoma: Prognostic factors predictive of survival. *Cancer.* 1991; 68(11):2466–2472.

Levine AM, Tulpule A. Clinical aspects and management of AIDS-related Kaposi's sarcoma. *Eur J Cancer (Oxford: 1990).* 2001; 37(10):1288–1295.

Lewden C, Salmon D, Morlat P, et al. Causes of death among human immunodeficiency virus (HIV)-infected adults in the era of potent antiretroviral therapy: Emerging role of hepatitis and cancers, persistent role of AIDS. *Int J Epidemiol.* 2005; 34(1):121–130.

Lewitschnig S, Gedela K, Toby M, et al. 18F-FDG PET/CT in HIV-related central nervous system pathology. *Eur J Nucl Mol Imaging.* 2013; 40(9):1420–1427.

Licho R, Litofsky NS, Senitko M, et al. Inaccuracy of Tl-201 brain SPECT in distinguishing cerebral infections from lymphoma in patients with AIDS. *Clin Nuclear Med.* 2002; 27(2):81–86.

Liebowitz D, Kieff E. Epstein–Barr virus latent membrane protein: Induction of B-cell activation antigens and membrane patch formation does not require vimentin. *J Virol.* 1989; 63(9):4051–4054.

Lillo FB, Ferrari D, Veglia F, et al. Human papillomavirus infection and associated cervical disease in human immunodeficiency virus-infected women: Effect of highly active antiretroviral therapy. *J Infect Dis.* 2001; 184(5):547–551.

Lim S-T, Karim R, Tulpule A, et al. Prognostic factors in HIV-related diffuse large-cell lymphoma: Before versus after highly active antiretroviral therapy. *J Clin Oncol.* 2005; 23(33):8477–8482.

Lister A, Abrey LE, Sandlund JT. Central nervous system lymphoma. *Am Soc Hematol. Educ Prog.* 2002; 283–296.

Little RF, Pittaluga S, Grant N, et al. Highly effective treatment of acquired immunodeficiency syndrome-related lymphoma with dose-adjusted EPOCH: Impact of antiretroviral therapy suspension and tumor biology. *Blood.* 2003; 101(12):4653–4659.

Locker GY, Hamilton S, Harris J, et al. ASCO 2006 update of recommendations for the use of tumor markers in gastrointestinal cancer. *J Clin Oncol.* 2006: 24(33):5313.

Loriot Y, Miler K, Sternberg CN, et al. Effect of enzalutamide on health-related quality of life, pain, and skeletal-related events in asymptomatic and minimally symptomatic, chemotherapy-naïve patients with metastatic castration-resistant prostate cancer (PREVAIL): Results from a randomised, phase 3 trial. *Lancet Oncol.* 2015; 16(5):509–521.

Lowenthal DA, Straus DJ, Wise Campbell S, et al. AIDS-related lymphoid neoplasia: The Memorial Hospital experience. *Cancer.* 1988; 61(11):2325–2337.

Luppi M, Barozzi P, Santagostino G, et al. Molecular evidence of organ-related transmission of Kaposi sarcoma-associated herpesvirus or human herpesvirus-8 in transplant patients. *Blood.* 2000; 96(9):3279–3281.

Machalek DA, Poynten M, Jin F, et al. Anal human papillomavirus infection and associated neoplastic lesions in men who have sex with men: A systematic review and meta-analysis. *Lancet Oncol.* 2012; 13(5):487–500.

MacMahon EM, et al. Epstein–Barr virus in AIDS-related primary central nervous system lymphoma. *Lancet.* 1991; 338(8773):969–973.

Makinson A, Cheret A, Abgrall S, et al. Early lung cancer diagnosis in HIV infected population with an important smoking history with low-dose Ct: A pilot study (EP48 HIV CHEST). Bethesda, MD: National Library of Medicine. 2015. Available at https://www.clinicaltrials.gov/ct2/show/NCT01207986?term=NCT01207986&rank=1. NLM Identifier: NCT 01207986.

Mandelblatt JS, Kanetsky P, Eggert L, et al. Is HIV infection a cofactor for cervical squamous cell neoplasia? *Cancer Epidemiol.* 1999; 8(1):97–106.

Mandell SP, Mack CD, Bulger EM. Motor vehicle mismatch: A national perspective. *Injury Prev.* 2010; 16(5):309–314.

Marcus JL, Chao CR, Leyden WA, et al. Prostate cancer incidence and prostate-specific antigen testing among HIV-positive and HIV-negative men. *J Acquir Immune Defic Syndr.* 2014; 66:495–502.

Mbulaiteye SM, Katabira ET, Wabinga H, et al. Spectrum of cancers among HIV-infected persons in Africa: The Uganda AIDS-Center Registry Match Study. *Int J Cancer.* 2006; 118(4):985–990.

McGowan JP, Shah S. Long-term remission of AIDS-related primary central nervous system lymphoma associated with highly active antiretroviral therapy. *AIDS (London).* 1998; 12(8):952–954.

Mdodo R, Frazier EL, Dube SR, et al. Cigarette smoking prevalence among adults with HIV compared with the general adult population in the United States: Cross-sectional surveys. *Ann Intern Med.* 2015; 162(5):335–344.

Melbye M, Rabkin C, Frisch M, et al. Changing patterns of anal cancer incidence in the United States, 1940–1989. *Am J Epidemiol.* 1994; 139(8):772–780.

Minkoff H, Zhong Y, Burk RD, et al. Influence of adherent and effective antiretroviral therapy use on human papillomavirus infection and squamous intraepithelial lesions in human immunodeficiency virus-positive women. *J Infect Dis.* 2010; 201(5):681–690.

Mitsuyasu RT, Groopman JE. Biology and therapy of Kaposi's sarcoma. *Semin Oncol.* 1984; 11(1):53–59.

Monforte A, Abrams D, Pradier C, et al. HIV-induced immunodeficiency and mortality from AIDS-defining and non-AIDS-defining malignancies. *AIDS (London).* 2008; 22(16):2143–2153.

Monini P, de Lellis L, Fabris M, et al. Kaposi's sarcoma-associated herpesvirus DNA sequences in prostate tissue and human semen. *N Engl J Med.* 1996; 334(18):1168–1172.

Moore AL, Sabin CA, Madge S, et al. Highly active antiretroviral therapy and cervical intraepithelial neoplasia. *AIDS (London).* 2002; 16(6):927–929.

Morlat P, Roussillon C, Henard S, et al. Causes of death among HIV-infected patients in France in 2010 (national survey): Trends since 2000. *AIDS.* 2014; 28(8):1181–1191.

Mosam A, Shaik F, Uldrick TS, et al. A randomized controlled trial of HAART versus HAART and chemotherapy in therapy-naive patients with HIV-associated Kaposi sarcoma in South Africa. *J Acquir Immune Defic Syndr.* 2012; 60(2):150.

Mounier N, Spina M, Gabarre J, et al. AIDS-related non-Hodgkin lymphoma: Final analysis of 485 patients treated with risk-adapted intensive chemotherapy. *Blood.* 2006; 107(10):3832–3840.

Moyer VA. Screening for prostate cancer: U.S. Preventive Services Task Force recommendation statement. *Ann Intern Med.* 2012; 157(2):120–135.

Munger K, Phelps WC, Bubb V, et al. The E6 and E7 genes of the human papillomavirus type 16 together are necessary and sufficient for transformation of primary human keratinocytes. *J Virol.* 1989; 63(10):4417–4421.

Myerson RJ, Kong F, Birnbaum EH, et al. Radiation therapy for epidermoid carcinoma of the anal canal: Clinical and treatment factors associated with outcome. *Radiother Oncol.* 2001; 61(1):15–22.

Nagata N, Shimbo T, Yazaki H, et al. Predictive clinical factors in the diagnosis of gastrointestinal Kaposi's sarcoma and its endoscopic severity. *PLoS One.* 2012; 7(11):1–7.

Nasti G, Martellotta F, Berretta M, et al. Impact of highly active antiretroviral therapy on the presenting features and outcome of patients with acquired immunodeficiency syndrome-related Kaposi sarcoma. *Cancer.* 2003; 98(11):2440–2446.

Nasti G, Talamini R, Antinori A, et al. AIDS-related Kaposi's sarcoma: Evaluation of potential new prognostic factors and assessment of the AIDS Clinical Trial Group Staging System in the HAART Era—The Italian Cooperative Group on AIDS and Tumors and the Italian Cohort of Patients Naive From Antiretrovirals. *J Clin Oncol.* 2003; 21(15):2876–2882.

National Comprehensive Cancer Network. NCCN clinical practice guidelines in oncology. Primary CNS lymphoma version 1.2015. May 1, 2015. Available at https://www.nccn.org/professionals/physician_gls/pdf/cns.pdf. Accessed December 13, 2015.

National Comprehensive Cancer Network. NCCN clinical practice guidelines in oncology. Rectal cancer version 1.2016. November 4, 2015. Available at https://www.nccn.org/professionals/physician_gls/pdf/rectal.pdf. Accessed May 13, 2016.

National Comprehensive Cancer Network. NCCN clinical practice guidelines in oncology. Non-small cell lung cancer version 2.2016. November 23, 2015. Available at https://www.nccn.org/professionals/physician_gls/pdf/nscl.pdf. Accessed December 8, 2015.

National Comprehensive Cancer Network. NCCN clinical practice guidelines in oncology. Colon cancer version 2.2016. November 23, 2015. Available at https://www.nccn.org/professionals/physician_gls/pdf/colon.pdf. Accessed May 13, 2016.

National Lung Screening Trial Research Team. Reduced lung-cancer mortality with low-dose computed tomographic screening. *N Engl J Med.* 2011; 365(5):395–409.

Navarro WH, Kaplan LD. AIDS-related lymphoproliferative disease. *Blood.* 2006; 107(1):13–20.

Naydu SK, Balar B. Colorectal cancer screening in human immunodeficiency virus populations: Are they at average risk? *World J Gastrointestinal Oncol.* 2012; 4(12):259–264.

Neef H, Horth W, Makowiec F, et al. Outcome after resection of hepatic and pulmonary metastasis of colorectal cancer. *J Gastrointest Surg.* 2009; 13(10):1813–1820.

Newton R, Ziegler J, Bourboulia D, et al. Infection with Kaposi's sarcoma-associated herpesvirus (KSHV) and human immunodeficiency virus

(HIV) in relation to the risk and clinical presentation of Kaposi's sarcoma in Uganda. *Br J Cancer*. 2003; 89(3):502–504.

Norden AD, Drappatz J, Wen PY, et al. Survival among patients with primary central nervous system lymphoma, 1973–2004. *J Neuro-Oncol*. 2011; 101(3):487–493.

Northfelt DW, Dezube BJ, Thommes JA, et al. Pegylated-liposomal doxorubicin versus doxorubicin, bleomycin, and vincristine in the treatment of AIDS-related Kaposi's sarcoma: Results of a randomized phase III clinical trial. *J Clin Oncol*. 1998; 16(7):2445–2451.

Noy A. Update in Kaposi sarcoma. *Curr Opin Oncol*. 2003; 15(5):379–381.

Okotie OT, Roehl KA, Han M, et al. Characteristics of prostate cancer detected by digital rectal examination only. *Urology*. 2007; 70(6):1117–1120.

Okuma Y, Hosomi Y, Imamura A. Lung cancer patients harboring epidermal growth factor receptor mutation among those infected by human immunodeficiency virus. *Onco Targets Ther*. 2014; 31:111–115.

Olson JE, Janney CA, Rao RD, et al. The continuing increase in the incidence of primary central nervous system non-Hodgkin lymphoma: A surveillance, epidemiology, and end results analysis. *Cancer*. 2002; 95(7):1504–1510.

Ong WL, Manohar P, Millar J, et al. Clinicopathological characteristics and management of prostate cancer in the human immunodeficiency virus (HIV)-positive population: Experience in an Australian major HIV center. *Br J Urol Int*. 2015: 116(Suppl 3):5–10.

Orlando G, Fasolo MM, Schiavini M, et al. Role of highly active antiretroviral therapy in human papillomavirus-induced genital dysplasia in HIV-1-infected patients. *AIDS (London)*. 1999; 13(3):424–425.

Palefsky JM, Holly EA, Gonzales J, et al. Detection of human papillomavirus DNA in anal intraepithelial neoplasia and anal cancer. *Cancer Res*. 1991; 51(3):1014–1019.

Palefsky JM, Holly EA, Ralston ML, et al. Effect of highly active antiretroviral therapy on the natural history of anal squamous intraepithelial lesions and anal human papillomavirus infection. *J Acquir Immun Defic Syndr (1999)*. 2001; 28(5):422–428.

Pantanowitz L, Bohac G, Cooley T, et al. Human immunodeficiency virus-associated prostate cancer: Clinicopathological findings and outcome in a multi-institutional study. *Br J Urol Int*. 2008; 101:1519–1523.

Park IU, Palefsky JM. Evaluation and Management of Anal Intraepithelial Neoplasia in HIV-Negative and HIV-Positive Men Who Have Sex with Men. *Curr Infect Dis Rep*. 2010 Mar; 12(2):126–133.

Patel P, Hanson DL, Sullivan PS, et al. Incidence of types of cancer among HIV-infected persons compared with the general population in the United States, 1992–2003. *Ann Intern Med*. 2008; 148(10):728–736.

Patil P, Elem B, Zumla A. Pattern of adult malignancies in Zambia (1980–1989) in light of the human immunodeficiency virus type 1 epidemic. *J Tropical Med Hygiene*. 1995; 98(4):281–284.

Penn I. Kaposi's sarcoma in organ transplant recipients: Report of 20 cases. *Transplantation*. 1979; 27(1):8–11.

Persad GC, Little RF, Grady C. Including persons with HIV infection in cancer clinical trials. *J Clin Oncol*. 2008; 26(7):1027–1032.

Piketty C, Seliger-Leneman H, Bouvier AM. Incidence of HIV-related anal cancer remains increased despite long-term combined antiretroviral treatment: Results from the French Hospital Database on HIV. *J Clin Oncol*. 2012; 30(35):4360–4366.

Piketty C, Selinger-Leneman H, Grabar S, et al. Marked increase in the incidence of invasive anal cancer among HIV-infected patients despite treatment with combination antiretroviral therapy. *AIDS (London)*. 2008; 22(10):1203–1211.

Plancoulaine S, Abel L, van Beveren M, et al. Human herpesvirus 8 transmission from mother to child and between siblings in an endemic population. *Lancet*. 2000; 356(9235):1062–1065.

Pluda J, Broder S, Yarchoan R. Therapy of AIDS and AIDS-associated neoplasms. *Cancer Chemother Biol Response Modif*. 1992; 13:404–439.

Polesel J, Clifford GM, Rickenbach M, et al. Non-Hodgkin lymphoma incidence in the Swiss HIV Cohort Study before and after highly active antiretroviral therapy. *AIDS (London)*. 2008; 22(2):301–306.

Powles T, Matthews G, Bower M. AIDS related systemic non-Hodgkin's lymphoma. *Sex Transm Infect*. 2000; 76(5):335–341.

Powles T, Thirwell C, Newsom-Davis T, et al. Does HIV adversely influence the outcome in advanced non-small-cell lung cancer in the era of HAART? *Br J Cancer*. 2003; 89:457–459.

Rahmanian S, Wewers ME, Koletar S, et al. Cigarette smoking in the HIV-infected population. *Proc Am Thorac Soc*. 2011; 8(3):313–319.

Ramirez-Marrero FA, Smit E, de la Torre-Feliciano T, et al. Risk of cancer among Hispanics with AIDS compared with the general population in Puerto Rico: 1987–2003. *Puerto Rico Health Sci J*. 2010; 29(3):256–264.

Raphael M, Said J, Dorisch B, et al. Lymphomas associated with HIV infection. In: Swerdlow SH, Campo E, Harris NL, et al. (Eds.), *World Health Organization Classification of Tumours of Haematopoietic and Lymphoid Tissue*, 4th ed. Lyon, France: IARC Press; 2008:340–342.

Ratner L, Lee J, Tang S, et al. Chemotherapy for human immunodeficiency virus-associated non-Hodgkin's lymphoma in combination with highly active antiretroviral therapy. *J Clin Oncol*. 2001; 19(8):2171–2178.

Ravalli S, Chabon A, Khan A. Gastrointestinal neoplasia in young HIV antibody-positive patients. *Am J Clin Pathol*. 1989: 91:458–461.

Re A, Cattaneo C, Michieli M, et al. High-dose therapy and autologous peripheral-blood stem-cell transplantation as salvage treatment for HIV-associated lymphoma in patients receiving highly active antiretroviral therapy. *J Clin Oncol*. 2003; 21(23):4423–4427.

Re A, Michieli M, Casari S, et al. High-dose therapy and autologous peripheral blood stem cell transplantation as salvage treatment for AIDS-related lymphoma: Long-term results of the Italian Cooperative Group on AIDS and Tumors (GICAT) study with analysis of prognostic factors. *Blood*. 2009; 114(7):1306–1313.

Reekie J, Kosa C, Engsig F, et al. Relationship between current level of immunodeficiency and non-acquired immunodeficiency syndrome-defining malignancies. *Cancer*. 2010 Nov 15;116(22): 5306–5315.

Reinhold JP, Moon M, Tenner CT, et al. Colorectal cancer screening in HIV-infected patients 50 years of age and older: Missed opportunities for prevention. *Am J Gastroenterol*. 2005; 100:1805–1812.

Renwick N, Halaby T, Weverling GJ, et al. Seroconversion for human herpesvirus 8 during HIV infection is highly predictive of Kaposi's sarcoma. *AIDS (London)*. 1998; 12(18):2481–2488.

Riedel DJ, Cox ER, Stafford KA, et al. Clinical presentation and outcomes of prostate cancer in an urban cohort of predominantly African American, human immunodeficiency virus-infected patients. *Urology*. 2015; 85(2):415–421.

Riedel DJ, Rositch AF, Redfield RR. Patterns of HIV viremia and viral suppression before diagnosis of non-AIDS-defining cancers in HIV-infected individuals. *Infect Agent Cancer*. 2015; 38(10):1–7.

Riley RR, Duensing S, Brake T, et al. Dissection of human papillomavirus E6 and E7 function in transgenic mouse models of cervical carcinogenesis. *Cancer Res*. 2003; 63(16):4862–4871.

Rodrigo JA, Hicks LK, Cheung MC, et al. HIV-associated Burkitt lymphoma: Good efficacy and tolerance of intensive chemotherapy including CODOX-M/IVAC with or without rituximab in the HAART era. *Adv Hematol*. 2012; 2012:1–9.

Rohner E, Valeri F, Maskew M, et al. Incidence rate of Kaposi sarcoma in HIV-infected patients on antiretroviral therapy in southern Africa: A prospective multicohort study. *J Acquir Immune Defic Syndr*. 2014; 67(5):547–554.

Rosenblum ML, Levy RM, Bredesen DE, et al. Primary central nervous system lymphomas in patients with AIDS. *Ann Neurol*. 1988; 23(Suppl):S13–S16.

Ruiz A, Ganz WI, Post MJ, et al. Use of thallium-201 brain SPECT to differentiate cerebral lymphoma from toxoplasma encephalitis in AIDS patients. *Am J Neuroradiol*. 1994; 15(10):1885–1894.

Ryan CJ, Smith MR, Fizazi K, et al. Abiraterone acetate plus prednisone versus placebo plus prednisone in chemotherapy-naïve men with metastatic castration-resistant prostate cancer (COU-AA-302): Final overall survival analysis of a randomised, double-blind, placebo-controlled phase 3 study. *Lancet Oncol.* 2015; 16(2):152–160.

Sacktor N, Lyles RH, Skolasky R, et al. HIV-associated neurologic disease incidence changes: Multicenter AIDS Cohort Study, 1990–1998. *Neurology.* 2001; 56(2):257–260.

Safai B. Pathophysiology and epidemiology of epidemic Kaposi's sarcoma. *Semin Oncol.* 1987; 2:7–12.

Sandler AS, Kaplan LD. Diagnosis and management of systemic non-Hodgkin's lymphoma in HIV disease. *Hematol Oncol Clin North Am.* 1996; 10(5):1111–1124.

Sauer R, Liersch T, Merkel S, et al. Preoperative versus postoperative chemoradiotherapy for locally advanced rectal cancer: Results of the German CAO/ARO/AIO-94 randomized phase III trial after a median follow-up of 11 years. *J Clin Oncol.* 2012; 20(16):1926–1933.

Saville M, Lietzau J, Pluda J, et al. Activity of placlitaxel (Taxol) as therapy for HIV-associated Kaposi's sarcoma. *Lancet.* 1995; 346:26–28.

Schiffman M, Kjaer SK. Natural history of anogenital human papillomavirus infection and neoplasia. *JNCI Monographs.* 2003; 2003(31):14–19.

Schreiber D, Chhabra A, Rineer J, et al. Outcomes and tolerance of human immunodeficiency virus-positive veterans undergoing dose-escalated external beam radiotherapy for localized prostate cancer. *Clin Genitourinary Cancer.* 2014; 12(2):94–99.

Serraino D, Boschini A, Carrieri P, et al. Cancer risk among men with, or at risk of, HIV infection in southern Europe. *AIDS.* 2000; 14(5):553–559.

Sgadari C, Monini P, Barillari G, et al. Use of HIV protease inhibitors to block Kaposi's sarcoma and tumour growth. *Lancet Oncol.* 2003; 4(9):537–547.

Shah R, Al-Sukhni W, Kim RD, et al. Resection of hepatic and pulmonary metastasis from colorectal carcinoma. *JACS.* 2006; 202(3):468–475.

Shebl FM, Engels EA, Goedert JJ, et al. Pulmonary infections and risk of lung cancer among persons with AIDS. *J Acquir Immune Defic Syndr.* 2010; 55:375–379.

Shepherd FA, Crowley J, van Houtte P, et al.; the IASLC Lung Cancer Staging Project. Clinical staging of small cell lung cancer in the forthcoming (seventh) edition of the Tumor, Node, Metastasis Classification for Lung Cancer. *J Thoracic Oncol.* 2007; 2(12):1067–1077.

Shiels, MS, Cole SR, Mehta SH, et al. Lung cancer incidence and mortality among HIV-infected and HIV-uninfected injection drug users. *J Acquir Immune Defic Syndr.* 2010; 55(4):510–515.

Shiels MS, Copeland G, Goodman M, et al. Cancer stage at diagnosis in patients infected with the human immunodeficiency virus and transplant recipients. *Cancer.* 2015; 121(12):1063–2071.

Shiels MS, Goedert JJ, Moore RD, et al. Reduced risk of prostate cancer in U.S. men with AIDS. *Cancer Epidemiol Biomarkers Prev.* 2010; 19(11):2910–2915.

Shiels MS, Pfeiffer RM, Engels EA. Age at cancer diagnosis among persons with AIDS in the United States. *Ann Intern Med.* 2010; 153(7):452–460.

Shiels MS, Pfeiffer RM, Gail MH, et al. Cancer burden in the HIV-infected population in the United States. *J Nat Cancer Institute.* 2011; 103:753–762.

Shiels MS, Pfeiffer RM, Hall HI, et al. Proportions of Kaposi sarcoma, selected non-Hodgkin lymphomas, and cervical cancer in the United States occurring in persons with AIDS, 1980–2007. *JAMA.* 2011; 305(14):1450–1459.

Shiels MS, Pfeiffer RM, Hildesheim A, et al. Circulating inflammation markers and prospective risk for lung cancer. *J Nat Cancer Inst.* 2013; 105(24):1871–1880.

Siegel R, DeSantis C, Jemal A. Colorectal cancer statistics, 2014. *CA Cancer J Clinicians.* 2014; 64(2):104–117.

Siegel R, Naishadham D, Jemal A. Cancer statistics, 2012. *CA Cancer J Clinicians.* 2012; 62(1):10–29.

Sigel K, Crothers K, Dubrow R, et al. Prognosis in HIV-infected patients with non-small cell lung cancer. *Br J Cancer.* 2013; 109:1974–1980.

Sigel K, Wisnevesky J, Gordon K, et al. HIV as an independent risk factor for incident lung cancer. *AIDS.* 2012; 26:1017–1025.

Silverberg MJ, Chao C, Leyden WA, et al. HIV infection, immunology, viral replication, and the risk of colon cancer. *Cancer Epidemiol Biomarkers Prev.* 2011; 20(12):2551–2559.

Silverberg MJ, Lau B, Achenbach CJ, et al. Cumulative incidence of cancer among persons with HIV in North America. *Ann Intern Med.* 2015; 163(7):507–518.

Silverberg MJ, Lau B, Justic AC, et al. Risk of anal cancer in HIV-infected and HIV-uninfected individuals in North America. *Clin Infect Dis.* 2012; 54(17):1026–1034.

Silverberg MJ, Leyden W, Steven Gregorich S, et al. Is intensive cervical cancer screening justified in immunosuppressed women? Paper presented at the Conference on Retroviruses and Opportunistic Infections (CROI), February 22–25, 2016, Boston. [Abstract 162]

Simard EP, Engels EA. Cancer as a cause of death among people with AIDS in the United States. *Clin Infect Dis.* 2010; 51(8):957–962.

Simard EP, Pfeiffer RM, Engels EA. Spectrum of cancer risk late after AIDS onset in the United States. *Arch Intern Med.* 2010; 170(15):1337–1345.

Simard EP, Pfeiffer RM, Engels EA. Cumulative incidence of cancer among individuals with acquired immunodeficiency syndrome in the United States. *Cancer.* 2011; 117(5):1089–1096.

Skiest DJ, Crosby C. Survival is prolonged by highly active antiretroviral therapy in AIDS patients with primary central nervous system lymphoma. *AIDS.* 2003; 17(12):1787–1793.

Smith DM, Kingery JD, Wong JK, et al. The prostate as a reservoir for HIV-1. *AIDS.* 2004; 18(11):1600–1602.

Smith RE, Colangelo L, Wieand HS, et al. Randomized trial of adjuvant therapy in colon carcinoma: 10-Year results of NSABP Protocol C-01. *J Natl Cancer Inst.* 2004; 96(15):1128–1132.

Spano JP, Massiani MA, Bentata M, et al. Lung cancer in patients with HIV infection and review of the literature. *Med Oncol.* 2004; 21:109–115.

Sparano JA, Lee S, Chen MG, et al. Phase II trial of infusional cyclophosphamide, doxorubicin, and etoposide in patients with HIV-associated non-Hodgkin's lymphoma: An Eastern Cooperative Oncology Group Trial (E1494). *J Clin Oncol.* 2004; 22(8):1491–1500.

Sparano JA, Lee JY, Kaplan LD, et al. Rituximab plus concurrent infusional EPOCH chemotherapy is highly effective in HIV-associated B-cell non-Hodgkin lymphoma. *Blood.* 2010; 115(15):3008–3016.

Stadler RF, Gregorcyk SG, Euhus DM, et al. Outcome of HIV-infected patients with invasive squamous-cell carcinoma of the anal canal in the era of highly active antiretroviral therapy. *Dis Colon Rectum.* 2004; 47(8):1305–1309.

Stebbing J, Sanitt A, Nelson M, et al. A prognostic index for AIDS-associated Kaposi's sarcoma in the era of highly active antiretroviral therapy. *Lancet.* 2006; 367(9521):1495–1502.

Stebbing J, Sanitt A, Teague A, et al. Prognostic significance of immune subset measurement in individuals with AIDS-associated Kaposi's sarcoma. *J Clin Oncol.* 2007; 25(16):2230–2235.

Stewart S, Jablonowski H, Goebel FD, et al. Randomized comparative trial of pegylated liposomal doxorubicin versus bleomycin and vincristine in the treatment of AIDS-related Kaposi's sarcoma: International Pegylated Liposomal Doxorubicin Study Group. *J Clin Oncol.* 1998; 16(2):683–691.

Stier EA, Sebring MC, Mendez AE, et al. Prevalence of anal human papillomavirus infection and anal HPV-related disorders in women: A systematic review. *Am J Ob Gyn.* 2015; 213(3):278–309.

Straus DJ, Huang J, Testa MA, et al. Prognostic factors in the treatment of human immunodeficiency virus-associated non-Hodgkin's lymphoma: Analysis of AIDS Clinical Trials Group protocol 142—Low-dose versus standard-dose m-BACOD plus granulocyte-macrophage colony-stimulating factor; National Institute of Allergy and Infectious Diseases. *J Clin Oncol.* 1998; 16(11):3601–3606.

Suneja G, Shiels MS, Melville SK. Disparities in the treatment and outcomes of lung cancer among HIV-infected individuals. *AIDS.* 2013; 27(3):459–468.

Swedish KA, Goldstone SE. Prevention of anal condyloma with quadrivalent human papillomavirus vaccination of older men who have sex with men. *PLoS One.* 2014; 9(4):e93393.

Taieb J, Tabernero J, Mini E, et al. Oxaliplatin, fluorouracil, and leucovorin with or without cetuximab in patients with resected stage III colon cancer (PETACC-8): An open-label, randomised phase III trial. *Lancet Oncol.* 2014; 15(8):862–873.

Tam HK, Zhang Z-F, Jacobson LP, et al. Effect of highly active antiretroviral therapy on survival among HIV-infected men with Kaposi sarcoma or non-Hodgkin lymphoma. *Int J Cancer.* 2002; 98(6):916–922.

Tesoiero JM, Gieryic SM, Carrascal A, et al. Smoking among HIV-positive New Yorkers: Prevalence, frequency, and opportunities for cessation. *AIDS Behav.* 2010; 14(4):824–835.

Tornesello ML, Buonaguro FM, Beth-Giraldo E, et al. Human immunodeficiency virus type 1 tat gene enhances human papillomavirus early gene expression. *Intervirology.* 1993; 36(2):57–64.

Travi G, Ferreri A, Cinque P, et al. Long term remission of HIV-associated primary CNS lymphoma achieved with highly active antiretroviral therapy alone. *J Clin Oncol.* 2012; 30(10):e119–e121.

Uldrick TS, Wyvill KM, Kumar P, et al. Phase II trial of bevacizumab in patients with HIV-associated Kaposi's sarcoma receiving antiretroviral therapy. *J Clin Oncol.* 2012; 30(13):1476–1483.

US Department of Health and Human Services, Panel on Opportunistic Infections in HIV-Infected Adults and Adolescents. Guidelines for the prevention and treatment of opportunistic infections in HIV-infected adults and adolescents: Recommendations from the Centers for Disease Control and Prevention, the National Institutes of Health, and the HIV Medicine Association of the Infectious Diseases Society of America. Updated September 24, 2015. Available at https://aidsinfo.nih.gov/contentfiles/lvguidelines/Adult_OI.pdf. Accessed May 13, 2016.

Vallet-Pichard A, Pol S. Hepatitis viruses and human immunodeficiency virus co-infection: Pathogenesis and treatment. *J Hepatol.* 2004; 41(1):156–166.

Vernon SD, Hart CE, Reeves WC, et al. The HIV-1 tat protein enhances E2-dependent human papillomavirus 16 transcription. *Virus Res.* 1993; 27(2):133–145.

Volberding P, Kusick P, Feigal D. Effects of chemotherapy for HIV-associated Kaposi's sarcoma on long-term survival. *Proc Am Soc Clin Oncol.* 1989; 3(9): Abstract 11.

Walmsley S, Northfelt DW, Melosky B, et al. Treatment of AIDS-related cutaneous Kaposi's sarcoma with topical alitretinoin (9-cis-retinoic acid) gel: Panretin Gel North American Study Group. *J Acquir Immune Defic Syndr.* 1999; 22(3):235–246.

Wang ES, Straus DJ, Teruya-Felstein J, et al. Intensive chemotherapy with cyclophosphamide, doxorubicine, high-dose methotrexate/ifosfamide, etoposide, and high-dose cytarabine (CODOX-M/IVAC) for human immunodeficiency virus-associated Burkett lymphoma. *Cancer.* 2003; 98(3):1196–1205.

Wasserberg N, Nunoo-Mensah JW, Gonzalez Ruiz C, et al. Colorectal cancer in HIV-infected patients: A case–control study. *Colorectal Dis.* 2007; 22(10):1217–1221.

Welch K, Finkbeiner W, Alpers CE, et al. Autopsy findings in the acquired immune deficiency syndrome. *JAMA.* 1984; 252(9): 1152–1159.

Westwood TD, Hogan C, Julyan PJ, et al. Utility of FDG-PETCT and magnetic resonance spectroscopy in differentiating between cerebral lymphoma and non-malignant CNS lesions in HIV-infected patients. *Eur J Radiol.* 2013; 82(8):e374–e379.

Whitlock EP, Lin JS, Liles E, et al. Screening for colorectal cancer: A targeted, updated systematic review for the U.S. Preventive Services Task Force. *Ann Intern Med.* 2008; 149(9):638–658.

Wilkin TJ, Palmer S, Brudney KF, et al. Anal intraepithelial neoplasia in heterosexual and homosexual HIV-positive men with access to antiretroviral therapy. *J Infect Dis.* 2004; 190(9):1685–1691.

Winstone, TA, Man SF, Hull M, et al. Epidemic of lung cancer in patients with HIV infection. *Chest.* 2013; 143(2):305–314.

Wistuba IL, Behrens C, Milchgrub S, et al. Comparison of molecular changes in lung cancers in HIV-positive and HIV-indeterminate subjects. *JAMA.* 1998; 279(19):1554–1559.

Wolf T, Brodt H-R, Fichtlscherer S, et al. Changing incidence and prognostic factors of survival in AIDS-related non-Hodgkin's lymphoma in the era of highly active antiretroviral therapy (HAART). *Leuk Lymphoma.* 2005; 46(2):207–215.

Wolf T, Kiderlen T, Atta J, et al. Successful treatment of AIDS-associated, primary CNS lymphoma with rituximab- and methotrexate-based chemotherapy and autologous stem cell transplantation. *Infection.* 2014; 42:445–447.

Woolfrey AE, Malhotra U, Harrington RD, et al. Generation of HIV-1-specific CD8+ cell responses following allogeneic hematopoietic cell transplantation. *Blood.* 2008; 112(8):3484–3487.

Yegüez JF, Martinez SA, Sands DR, et al. Colorectal malignancies in HIV-positive patients. *Am Surg.* 2003; 69(11):981–987.

Zanet E, Taborelli M, Rupolo M, et al. Postautologous stem cell transplantation long-term outcomes in 26 HIV-positive patients affected by relapsed/refractory lymphoma. *AIDS.* 2015; 29(17):2303–2308.

Ziegler JL, Drew WL, Miner RC, et al. Outbreak of Burkitt's-like lymphoma in homosexual men. *Lancet.* 1982; 2(8299):631–633.

Ziegler JL, Templeton AC, Vogel CL. Kaposi's sarcoma: A comparison of classical, endemic, and epidemic forms. *Semin Oncol.* 1984; 11(1):47–52.

34.

DERMATOLOGIC COMPLICATIONS

Kudakwashe Mutyambizi

CHAPTER GOAL

This chapter reviews dermatologic complications of HIV infection and treatment.

OVERVIEW OF CUTANEOUS FINDINGS IN HIV INFECTION

LEARNING OBJECTIVE

Review the approach to skin findings in the context of HIV.

WHAT'S NEW?

Multiple biopsies increase diagnostic yield for identification of cutaneous complications of HIV.

KEY POINTS

- Dermatoses that are rare in the general population but common in HIV populations should prompt testing for HIV when there is no preexisting diagnosis.

- Correct diagnosis and management of skin complaints can improve the quality of life of HIV-infected patients who have increased longevity in the highly active antiretroviral therapy (HAART) era.

- The appearance of AIDS-defining cutaneous illnesses in previously immune reconstituted patients on HAART should prompt a reassessment of CD4$^+$ T cell count and HIV RNA levels.

- In patients who have been on HAART for less than 24 weeks, the appearance or worsening of dermatoses may be due to the immune reconstitution inflammatory syndrome (IRIS).

The hallmark of HIV infection is immune dysregulation and immunosuppression. As the immune system deteriorates, inflammatory dermatoses, metabolic dysregulation, adverse drug reactions, opportunistic infections, and cutaneous malignancies become more common, atypical in presentation, and recalcitrant to therapy. Both acute and chronic skin complaints contribute significantly to reduced quality of life for HIV patients (Mirmirani, 2002).

The Centers for Disease Control and Prevention (CDC) recommends that individuals between ages 13 and 64 years be tested for HIV at least once in their lifetime, with increased screening of high-risk individuals and testing based on symptoms. The presence of dermatoses uncommon in the general population but concentrated in the HIV population, or dermatoses strikingly recalcitrant to therapy, should warrant suspicion and testing for HIV. In patients with known HIV/AIDS, there is a correlation between CD4$^+$ T cell count and the occurrence of characteristic dermatoses (Goldstein, 1997; Rigopoulos, 2004). Direct CD4$^+$ T cell testing is the gold standard assessment of immune function; however, the World Health Organization's (WHO) clinical staging provides guidelines regarding skin findings that should raise suspicion for immune deterioration, prompting CD4$^+$ T cell testing, and have significance in international settings in which CD4$^+$ T cell testing is of limited availability (Baveewo, 2011; Weinberg, 2010). The occurrence of AIDS-defining illnesses such as Kaposi's sarcoma or acute systemic illnesses and infections in patients previously immunocompetent by CD4$^+$ T cell count, or previously well controlled on HAART, should prompt an assessment of CD4$^+$ T cell count and HIV RNA levels to evaluate for immune deterioration. In patients who have been on HAART for less than 24 weeks, acute systemic illnesses may be due to IRIS or treatment toxicity and during this period do not closely parallel the WHO clinical staging guidelines (Ratnam, 2006). With these caveats, the dermatoses discussed in this chapter are presented along with the corresponding CD4$^+$ T cell count at which they typically occur (Zancanaro, 2006).

HIV practitioners can competently diagnose many of the dermatological conditions discussed in this chapter, as well as perform diagnostic biopsies and minor cosmetic procedures. Busy HIV practices sometimes maintain a supply of liquid nitrogen to treat warts and an electrocautery machine known as a hyfrecator to electrodessicate lesions such as molluscum contagiosum. Referral to a dermatologist is recommended when presented with diagnostic or management uncertainty, particularly in the acutely ill patient, common or chronic dermatoses recalcitrant to therapies familiar to the HIV practitioner, and for optimal tissue procurement when the clinician is uncertain of appropriate biopsy site or method.

It is important for HIV practitioners to be aware that a number of serious disseminated opportunistic infections, some of which may be fatal, may first manifest as an acute cutaneous eruption. Therefore, it is important for a skin biopsy to be performed in an acutely febrile HIV/AIDS patient with a newly developed skin eruption. The biopsy should be accompanied with a request for urgent processing with special stains for bacteria, atypical mycobacteria, fungi, and viruses as appropriate. Tissue is placed in 10% formalin for routine processing, but a portion should be placed in normal saline so that cultures for microorganisms can be performed for definitive diagnosis.

In general, when sampling a lesion, especially one that is papular or pustular, an early, new lesion that is not excoriated is most likely to yield tissue with changes that afford the dermatopathologist the best opportunity to make an accurate diagnosis (Altman, 2015). A pertinent exception in this population is biopsy of suspected Kaposi's sarcoma because early lesions can present a confusing picture histologically. An older, more mature lesion, if present, will have greater diagnostic yield (Maurer, 2005). When in doubt, one should consider taking multiple biopsies from the lesion in different stages of evolution and from different cutaneous sites. If the practitioner is not comfortable performing a good skin biopsy, dermatological referral for evaluation and biopsy determination should be made. Table 34.1 provides guidelines for referral.

Recommended Reading

Altman, K., Vanness, E., & Westergaard, R. P. (2015). Cutaneous manifestations of human immunodeficiency virus: A clinical update. *Curr Infect Dis Rep*, 17(3), 464.

Mirmirani, P., Maurer, T. A., Berger, T. G., et al. (2002). Skin-related quality of life in HIV-infected patients on highly active antiretroviral therapy. *J Cutan Med Surg*, 6(1), 10–15.

INFLAMMATORY DERMATOSES AND HIV

LEARNING OBJECTIVE

Discuss the incidence, presentation, and management of inflammatory dermatoses in HIV.

WHAT'S NEW?

Traditional immunosuppressants and biologic therapies have been used safely in controlled settings and for short courses in HIV patients with refractory psoriasis and debilitating psoriatic arthritis who are on concurrent HAART.

KEY POINTS

- Initiation of HAART, ultraviolet B (UVB), and oral retinoids are good initial therapies for patients with psoriatic arthritis.

- Topical tacrolimus inhibitors and UV light have both been used safely in HIV patients.

- Patients receiving systemic biologics for debilitating psoriatic arthritis should be carefully selected and closely monitored.

- Papular pruritic eruption of AIDS and HIV-associated eosinophilic pustular folliculitis are HIV/AIDS-associated dermatologic illnesses and should prompt testing for HIV in a previously undiagnosed patient.

Table 34.1 INDICATIONS FOR REFERRAL TO A DERMATOLOGIST

Diagnostic uncertainty

Management uncertainty

Life-threatening differential diagnoses

Rapid progression

Persistence or recurrence despite therapy

Requires specialized medications

Requires specialized procedures

Suspected skin cancer

Indications for skin cancer screening

Pigmented lesions

Improve compliance

Patient request

SEBORRHEIC DERMATITIS

Seborrheic dermatitis is a common skin disorder, with a prevalence of approximately 5% in the general population. It was noted to be the most common dermatosis in HIV-infected individuals, with a prevalence of greater than 83% in HIV/AIDS populations in the pre-HAART era (Sadick, 1990). Seborrheic dermatitis is seen at all clinical stages of disease. *Malassezia* species are the causative organisms. The typical presentation is of episodic variably pruritic thin erythematous plaques with branny or greasy yellow-white scale involving the scalp and central face, particularly the eyebrows and nasolabial folds. Scalp involvement ranges from light "dandruff" to crusted plaques. Involvement of the anterior chest and groin areas is common. HIV should be considered in rapid and exaggerated presentations with thick extensive plaques and also in cases recalcitrant to advanced treatment regimens. The clinical differential for facial seborrheic dermatitis includes rosacea, an overlap presentation with psoriasis called sebopsoriasis that is often more difficult to treat than standard seborrheic dermatitis, contact dermatitis, tinea faciei, and connective tissue disease. In tinea faciei, a potassium hydroxide (KOH) preparation can identify dermatophytes exhibiting characteristic hyphae. In contrast, seborrheic dermatitis is thought to be an inflammatory response to the commensal yeast *Malassezia* species (thus, KOH evaluation has no role), with the increased presentation in HIV/AIDS patients thought to be due to a more vigorous inflammatory response as the yeast proliferate in the setting of $CD4^+$ T cell lymphopenia (Oble, 2005; Pedrosa, 2014). Seborrheic dermatitis is a clinical diagnosis; thus, biopsy is infrequently performed. Histology reveals psoriasiform hyperplasia, neutrophilic spongiosis, perifollicular mound parakeratosis with necrotic keratinocytes, and plasma cells occasionally present in HIV-associated seborrheic dermatitis (Soeprono, 1986). First-line therapy is with topical antifungals and low-potency topical steroids. HAART therapy improves seborrheic dermatitis occurring in the setting of HIV/AIDS; however, patients typically continue to experience episodic flares.

PSORIASIS

Psoriasis also presents at all clinical stages of HIV, more frequently at $CD4^+$ T cell counts <350 cells/ mm^3 (Bartlett, 2007). Psoriasis has a prevalence of approximately 2% or 3% in the general population, with various series suggesting a similar or higher incidence in HIV populations (Mallon, 2000; Obuch, 1992). The prevalence of psoriatic arthritis in the general population has previously been underestimated and is now thought to be approximately 11% in the US psoriasis population, and it is concentrated in the HIV-positive psoriasis population (Dover, 1991; Gelfand, 2005). Psoriasis characteristically presents as variably pruritic, episodic, well -demarcated plaques with silvery white scale anywhere on the body but with a predilection for the scalp, elbows, lower back, gluteal folds, external genitalia, and acral sites. Preexisting psoriasis can worsen with HIV infection and immune deterioration, and psoriasis can develop de novo with HIV infection. De novo psoriasis in HIV often involves palmar plantar locations with pustules, nail dystrophy, and psoriatic arthritis that can be debilitating. Inverse psoriasis (involving intertriginous areas), generalized pustular psoriasis, and erythrodermic psoriasis also occur more frequently in HIV (Obuch, 1992). Erythrodermic psoriasis can be difficult to distinguish from other causes of erythroderma, including atopic dermatitis, drug-induced erythroderma, pityriasis rubra pilaris, Sezary syndrome, and a paraneoplastic presentation or HIV presentation; thus, it typically warrants a biopsy. Histology reveals parakeratosis, collections of neutrophils in the stratum corneum and epidermis, and a diminished granular layer. Whereas increased defensins and canthelicidins in the skin of psoriatics in the general population have been associated with their relatively low frequency of bacterial superinfection compared to other chronic dermatoses that also result in a compromised skin barrier such as atopic dermatitis, there is an increased frequency of bacterial superinfection in HIV psoriatics (Mallon, 2000; Zheng, 2007). Theories regarding the increased incidence and severity of psoriasis in HIV include the fact that overexpression of tumor necrosis factor (TNF) occurs in both psoriasis and HIV. Furthermore, $CD4^+$ T cell depletion in HIV skews the T cell population to CD8 cells, the effector cells in psoriasis, whereas the HIV tat gene directly induces epidermal proliferation (Duvic, 1990; Kim, 1992).

In treating psoriasis, exacerbating medications should be discontinued. Of note, systemic steroids exacerbate psoriasis. Topical treatments including topical steroids, vitamin D analogues, and topical calcineurin inhibitors such as tacrolimus are first-line therapies for mild to moderate plaque psoriasis. A black box warning on tacrolimus and malignancy risk has not identified a causal relationship, and studies have shown that topical calcineurin inhibitors can be safely used in the immunosuppressed HIV population (de Moraes, 2007; Toutous-Trellu, 2005). Randomized controlled studies have not been conducted to evaluate the efficacy and safety of systemic treatments for psoriasis in the HIV setting; thus, much of the following data are derived from case reports and case series. Systemic therapies can be used in combination with each other and with topical treatments to optimized efficacy. HAART can effectively treat both moderate to severe psoriasis and psoriatic arthritis, and it is a first-line treatment, as is UV light, for this severity category (Duvic, 1994; Menon, 2010; Meola, 1993). UVB is preferentially used over psoralens plus UVA (PUVA) given its more favorable side effect profile. Although in vitro studies have shown that UVB light can activate latent HIV in chronically infected monocytes, it has not been associated with short-term changes in immune function in vivo or changes in HIV RNA levels in patients receiving concomitant suppressive HAART therapy (Breuer-McHam, 1999; Meola, 1993; Stanley, 1989). Oral retinoids, particularly acitretin, are an attractive second-line therapy because they are non-immunosuppressants with efficacy for moderate to severe psoriasis and also psoriatic arthritis. Acitretin use is limited by hypertriglyceridemia, liver function test (LFT) elevation particularly in combination with some antiretroviral medications, and an extended 3-year teratogenicity period in women of childbearing age due to reesterification to etretinate (Dogra, 2014). Patients with refractory psoriasis or debilitating psoriatic arthritis are candidates for immunosuppressant therapies that have shown efficacy in this patient population, including low-dose methotrexate and brief courses of cyclosporine and TNF-α inhibitors. In a case report, dramatic improvement of HIV-associated psoriatic arthritis was achieved but frequent polymicrobial infections were experienced on etanercept (Aboulafia, 2000). In summary, concomitant HAART therapy, strict prophylaxis against opportunistic infections, CD4$^+$ T cell counts, monitoring of HIV RNA levels, and close clinical monitoring of rigorously selected patients are advised when treating HIV-associated psoriasis with immunosuppressant therapy.

ATOPIC DERMATITIS AND XEROSIS

The prevalence of eczema in the US adult population is estimated at 10.7%, with approximately 17% of the population experiencing at least one of four eczematous symptoms (Hanifin, 2007). An atopic dermatitis-like condition occurs frequently in HIV populations, often despite never having had a history of atopic dermatitis in childhood. One series reported that 29% of HIV/AIDS patients who attended an urban HIV clinic in the pre-HAART era had this condition (Lin, 1995). This atopic dermatitis-like condition is characterized by pruritus and a spectrum of generalized scaling from xerosis to ichthyosis, with variable plaques and lichenification involving extremities and flexural areas (Singh, 2003). Often, this xerotic condition initially presents when the CD4$^+$ T cell count is still >400

cells/mm^3 and is thus an early clinical sign of HIV/AIDS, typically preceding the other papulosquamous disorders. The generalized icthyotic form typically occurs with CD4$^+$ T cell counts <50 cells/mm^3 (Sadick, 1990). Decreased cellular immunity and a switch to the TH2-like cytokine profile resulting in polyclonal activation of B cells with increased IgE production are thought to contribute to the increase in atopic conditions in HIV (Nissen, 1999). In addition, nutritional deficits and autonomic nervous dysfunction causing alterations in sweating, sebaceous gland secretion, and reduction in natural moisturizing factor secretion are thought to contribute to xerosis and ichthyosis (Cockerell, 2013). Biopsy, which is not regularly performed for this diagnosis, shows variable hyperkeratosis and parakeratosis, spongiosis, and superficial perivascular lymphocytic infiltrate. The clinical differential diagnosis includes scabies, psoriasis, and contact dermatitis. For erythematous plaques, topical steroid preparations, preferably ointments, and topical calcineurin inhibitors are appropriate first-line therapies. Topical keratolytics such as urea and lactic acid formulations are useful for areas of lichenification. Widespread flares may require short courses of systemic steroids, bridging to phototherapy for sustained flares. Oral antihistamines and a dry skin care regimen of short lukewarm showers, frequent use of non-allergic emollients, and avoidance of allergens should be used in conjunction. Bacterial superinfection is common and should be managed with antibiotics.

PAPULAR PRURITIC ERUPTION
OF AIDS

Papular pruritic eruption (PPE) is a markedly pruritic papulosquamous eruption characterized by symmetric crops of nonfollicular, often urticarial erythematous papules involving the extensor extremities. Excoriations and prurigo nodularis are frequently associated secondary changes due to marked pruritus in this condition. PPE is uncommon in the general adult population but has a prevalence in the HIV population of 11–46%, thus the designation papular pruritic eruption of AIDS (Eisman, 2006). It has a greater prevalence in HIV/AIDS cohorts in sub-Saharan Africa than in the United States. Among other theories, PPE is hypothesized to be due to an exaggerated response to arthropod antigens that occurs in the setting of immune dysregulation (Resneck, 2004). PPE can develop well before other symptoms and serologic diagnosis of HIV is made; however, its occurrence also correlates with lower CD4$^+$ T cell counts, and it is common in patients with CD4$^+$ T cell counts <100 cells/mm^3 (Boonchai, 1999;

Cockerell, 2013). The clinical differential includes eosinophilic folliculitis, which in contrast affects the face and upper trunk, and differentiation of active lesions of PPE from lesions of prurigo nodularis that may also be pruritic. The diagnosis is typically made clinically based on the distribution of lesions. Early lesions without secondary changes carry the highest histologic diagnostic yield, and they may show a dense perivascular and interstitial infiltrate of lymphocytes and some eosinophils and neutrophils, which may extend deeply around adnexa and vessels, although nonspecific findings occur (Calonje, 2012). The disease has a chronic waxing and waning course and is associated with decreased quality of life due to pruritus (Hevia, 1991; Liu, 2013). Given its association with low CD4+ T cell counts, initiation of HAART may improve the disease, although it can also flare with immune reconstitution. UVB has been shown to decrease both papules and pruritus, and it may have greater efficacy in regimens combining other modalities including oral antihistamines, pentoxifylline, topical steroids, topical tacrolimus, and topical anti-itch preparations (Bellavista, 2013). Reducing exposure to bites by wearing clothing that covers skin and application of insect repellant is also recommended.

HIV-ASSOCIATED EOSINOPHILIC PUSTULAR FOLLICULITIS

Eosinophilic pustular folliculitis (Ofugi's disease) is rare in the general adult population but common in the HIV/AIDS population, particularly once the CD4+ T cell count declines below 250 cells/mm³. HIV-associated eosinophilic folliculitis is characterized by persistent markedly pruritic erythematous, mostly follicular papules and occasional pustules on the face, trunk, and upper extremities. Urticarial plaques and nonfollicular erythematous papules are also described. Peripheral eosinophilia can also be common along with elevated IgE levels (Rosenthal, 1991). It is thought to be an exaggerated cutaneous reaction to *Malassezia* yeast or other microorganisms colonizing the follicular infundibulum and reflects TH1/2 immune dysregulation. Recently, CD163+ macrophages have been implicated in the pathogenesis (Okada, 2013). Additional theories include autoimmune activation against antigens in sebocytes in HIV-positive individuals (Fearfield, 1999). The clinical differential includes PPE as well as acne, molluscum, and drug reactions. Biopsy may be useful, with erythematous nonexcoriated follicular lesions carrying the highest diagnostic yield. Spongiosis involving the follicular epithelium and intra- and perifollicular mixed infiltrate is typically seen, with eosinophilic

abscess formation in long-standing lesions. Treatment is often difficult, with pruritus contributing to reduced quality of life. Phototherapy (UVB or UVA), oral antihistamines, itraconazole, isotretinoin, and metronidazole are all reported treatments; however, no controlled clinical trials have been performed. First-line therapy with UVB phototherapy, topical steroids, and oral antihistamines is suggested.

Recommended Reading

Cockerell, C. C., & Calame, A. (2013). *Cutaneous Manifestations of HIV Disease*. London, UK: Manson.

Toutous-Trellu, L., Abraham, S., Pechere, M., et al. (2005). Topical tacrolimus for effective treatment of eosinophilic folliculitis associated with human immunodeficiency virus infection. *Arch Dermatol, 141*(10), 1203–1208.

HIV DRUG REACTIONS AND INTERACTIONS

LEARNING OBJECTIVE

Describe common or important cutaneous adverse drug reactions, and pertinent factors in their management, in the HIV population.

WHAT'S NEW?

In recent years, several adverse drug reactions to HAART medications have been identified that were not observed or were underrepresented in preapproval trials.

KEY POINTS

- Non-nucleoside reverse transcriptase inhibitors are the most common antiretroviral drugs that cause morbilliform skin eruptions.

- Abacavir hypersensitivity reaction can be fatal, and predisposed patients can be identified by testing for the HLA-B5701 allele prior to commencing abacavir therapy.

- The injectable fillers poly-L-lactic acid and calcium hydroxyapatite are approved for facial fat loss treatment in HIV.

- Ritonavir, a CYP34A inhibitor often used to booster other antiretroviral drugs, increases the levels of corticosteroids, which can result in hypothalamic–pituitary–adrenal (HPA) axis dysfunction and Cushing's syndrome.

The incidence of medication-related skin rashes in the HIV-positive population is approximately 50% (Davis, 2008). Drug hypersensitivity reactions are classified into two categories: those secondary to HAART regimens and those secondary to other medications taken by HIV-positive patients. Since its inception, HAART has revolutionized the management of HIV/AIDS, with new drug classes and single-tablet combination formulations designed to decrease pill burden now available. However, antiretroviral drugs have been complicated by adverse drug reactions, including reactions that may not have been recognized or underrepresented in preapproval clinical trials (Introcaso, 2010). Thus, recognition of known and identification of previously unreported drug reactions are extremely important in the management of antiretroviral-related drug hypersensitivity reactions. It can be a particular challenge to differentiate between drug hypersensitivity reactions, IRIS, and worsening HIV infection when patients are commencing antiretroviral therapy. Some of the adverse drug reactions are mediated through genetic and immunologic factors via the major histocompatibility complex (Chaponda, 2011). IgE levels increase with progression of HIV, and altered cytokine profiles are also believed to play a role (Davis, 2008). Immune dysregulation in HIV is also thought to make HIV patients more susceptible to non-HAART medications. In addition, antiretroviral drugs can result in alterations in metabolism of other medications, particularly through the cytochrome P450 pathway, thus increasing their toxicity.

NON-NUCLEASE REVERSE TRANSCRIPTASE INHIBITORS

Non-nucleoside reverse transcriptase inhibitors are the most common antiretroviral agents to cause morbilliform skin eruptions, which are usually distributed over the face, trunk, and extremities. In particular, nevirapine is well known for its ability to cause rash, particularly within the first 6 weeks of use. According to the manufacturer, 13% of patients taking nevirapine develop some degree of morbilliform eruption during early treatment; this has been reported to be as high as 28% in some populations in practice (Introcaso, 2010). Many patients with mild or moderate rash can continue therapy with close monitoring, and the rash will spontaneously resolve. Severe rash is seen in at least 8% of patients, and development of concomitant hepatitis in the drug hypersensitivity syndrome is an indication for immediate discontinuation of nevirapine given the potential for fatal hepatitis. Risk factors for the development of morbilliform eruption with the use of nevirapine include higher CD4+ T cell count (>250

cells/mm^3 in women and >400 cells/mm^3 in men), lower HIV-1 RNA levels, Chinese ethnicity, and female gender (Davis, 2008). In addition, nevirapine can cause the mucocutaneous Stevens–Johnson syndrome at a rate of 0.5–1%, although patients with CD4+ T cell counts <200 cells/mm^3 (i.e., with AIDS) have a 1000-fold higher risk (Warren, 1998). The incidence may be higher in sub-Saharan Africa, where nevirapine is more commonly used in antiretroviral regimens. Steven–Johnson syndrome is characterized by flat, atypical targets or pruritic papules that are widespread or distributed on the trunk first and then spread to the neck, face, and proximal upper extremities. The palms and soles may be an early site of involvement. Bullae developing on the conjunctivae and mucous membranes of the nares, mouth, anorectal junction, vulvovaginal region, and urethral meatus are characteristic, with toxic epidermal necrolysis diagnosed when there is more than 30% body surface area skin detachment (Bolognia, 2012). In several studies, the use of prednisone and/or a 2-week lead-in dose of nevirapine 200 mg once daily failed to decrease the occurrence of the nevirapine-associated rash (Knobel, 2001). A dose escalation protocol is now recommended starting with nevirapine 200 mg daily for 2 weeks, followed by an increase to the standard 400-mg daily dose only if there is no rash or no worsening rash after the trial 2-week period (Anton, 1999).

NUCLEOSIDE REVERSE TRANSCRIPTASE INHIBITOR

Abacavir, a nucleoside reverse transcriptase inhibitor, can cause a well-documented, multiorgan, potentially life-threatening hypersensitivity reaction. This abacavir hypersensitivity reaction (AHR) is seen in 5–8% of HIV-positive patients on treatment. Symptoms consist of fever, rash, malaise, fatigue, tachypnea, pharyngitis, cough, wheezing, nausea, vomiting, and diarrhea that commence 9–11 days after initiating therapy. Symptoms that become worse with each subsequent dose are a classic characteristic of AHR. Symptoms of AHR recur within 24 hours of rechallenge and can be fatal. Therefore, the use of abacavir in any person suspected to have AHR is contraindicated. Pre-ART genetic testing has shown that the absence of the HLA-B5701 allele dramatically decreases (by 99.9%) the likelihood of developing abacavir hypersensitivity (Mallal, 2008). For this reason, the ART guidelines of both the US Department of Health and Human Services and the International Antiviral Society–USA recommend obtaining this test prior to initiation of any abacavir-containing regimen.

PROTEASE INHIBITORS

The protease inhibitors are generally associated with lipodystrophy, abnormal fat distribution, and central adiposity, which can be an indication for discontinuation. The injectable fillers poly-L-lactic acid and calcium hydroxyapatite are approved for facial fat loss treatment in HIV (Jagdeo, 2015). Indinavir has the greatest variety of cutaneous side effects among protease inhibitors, including acute porphyria, Stevens–Johnson syndrome, hypersensitivity syndrome, morbilliform drug eruptions, gynecomastia, alopecia, pyogenic granuloma-like lesions, and paronychia (Ward, 2002). Ritonavir is a CYP34A inhibitor, and through this mechanism, it decreases clearance of corticosteroids, thus increasing their levels and the risk of HPA axis dysfunction and Cushing's syndrome (Hyle, 2013). This should be considered when prescribing topical steroids for application to a large body surface area and systemic steroids for longer courses.

OTHER ANTIRETROVIRAL THERAPIES

Few other antiretroviral drugs have a strong association with severe adverse drug reactions. Approximately 6% of persons taking atazanavir, a protease inhibitor, have reported typically mild rash not requiring treatment cessation. A hypersensitivity to the fusion inhibitor enfuvirtide has been seen in less than 1% of persons taking it. However, 98% of users experience injection site reactions, which are frequently symptomatic (Ball, 2003). The enfuvirtide injection site reaction is characterized by tender erythema, induration, and nodule or cyst formation. On histology, a palisaded granulomatous response may be seen, with multinucleated cells aggregated around altered collagen, and surrounding eosinophils, histiocytes, lymphocytes, plasma cells, and variable fibrosis. Recently, the package insert for raltegravir, an integrase inhibitor, was updated to include dermatological side effects including Stevens–Johnson syndrome and toxic epidermal necrolysis.

ANTIBIOTICS

Antibiotic drug reactions appear at a higher rate in HIV-positive patients than in the general population. Trimethoprim–sulfamethoxazole is a commonly used antibiotic in HIV, especially for the prophylaxis of *Pneumocystis jirovecii* pneumonia (PCP). Given its importance in the prevention of PCP pneumonia, a desensitization schedule has been developed for those patients who have had reactions in the past and would benefit from its use. Desensitization has been successful using the following dosing schedule: an initial dose of trimethoprim 0.4 mg and sulfamethoxazole 2 mg, followed by doubling the dose daily over days 2–9 and at 10 days administering the full-strength dose (trimethoprim 160 mg/sulfamethoxazole 800 mg) (Gompels, 1999).

Recommended Reading

Hyle, E. P., Wood, B. R., Backman, E. S., et al. (2013). High frequency of hypothalamic–pituitary–adrenal axis dysfunction after local corticosteroid injection in HIV-infected patients on protease inhibitor therapy. *J Acquir Immune Defic Syndr*, 63(5), 602–608.

Introcaso, C. E., Hines, J. M., & Kovarik, C. L. (2010). Cutaneous toxicities of antiretroviral therapy for HIV: Part II. Nonnucleoside reverse transcriptase inhibitors, entry and fusion inhibitors, integrase inhibitors, and immune reconstitution syndrome. *J Am Acad Dermatol*, 63(4), 563–569; quiz 569–570.

CUTANEOUS OPPORTUNISTIC INFECTIONS

LEARNING OBJECTIVE

Discuss the diagnosis and management of viral, fungal, bacterial, and parasitic opportunistic infections occurring in HIV patients.

WHAT'S NEW?

In 2014, the US Food and Drug Administration (FDA) approved the topical agents efinaconazole and tavoraole, which show some efficacy for the treatment of onychomycosis.

KEY POINTS

- Cutaneous *Cryptococcus* may manifest before systemic symptoms; therefore, prompt diagnosis and management can prevent fatal outcomes.

- Molluscum, histoplasmosis, and *Cryptococcus* may all present with umbilicated papulonodules; however, there is a central white core to the molluscum lesion, and patients are well as opposed to systemically ill with cryptococcal infection.

- Postherpetic neuralgia is very common in HIV patients who develop herpes zoster, and initiation of neurontin along with antiviral therapy at diagnosis may mitigate neuralgia.

- The prozone effect may result in a false-negative syphilis test in HIV patients, and dilution of the assay should be requested when syphilis is suspected.

- The CDC now recommends an intensive regimen for the management of crusted scabies as follows: ivermectin dosed at 200 μg/kg taken on days 1, 2, 8, 9, and 15 and, for severe disease, also days 22 and 29, in combination with topical permethrin daily for 7 days and then twice a week until cure.

ONYCHOMYCOSIS

Onychomycosis is reported to affect approximately 2–13% of the general population (Rosen, 2015) and is very common in the HIV-positive population. Dermatophytes *Trichophyton mentagrophytes* and *Trichophyton rubrum* are responsible for most infections. Proximal subungual onychomycosis is a pattern seen commonly in HIV-positive patients, especially those with a CD4+ T cell count <450 cells/mm³, and although it is not considered an AIDS-defining condition, it should prompt testing for HIV infection if not already determined. *Trichophyton rubrum* is usually the causative dermatophyte for this pattern, although it can also be caused by *Trichophyton megninii*. Superficial white onychomycosis, for example, is typically caused by *T. mentagrophytes* in the general population, whereas it is typically caused by *T. rubrum* in the HIV population. The clinical differential includes psoriasis, lichen planus, trauma, and periungual squamous cell carcinoma. Most topical antifungals do not penetrate the thick nail keratin and thus are ineffective. Efinaconazole is a topical triazole solution recently released on the market for the treatment of onychomycosis; it is applied daily for 48 weeks to affected nails. Localized dermatitis is a potential side effect. In preapproval trials, 15.2–17.8% of patients achieved complete cure of onychomycosis. Tavorabole, a boron-based agent that was FDA approved for onychomycosis in 2014, had even lower efficacy, with 6.5–9.1% of patients achieving clearance (Zeichner, 2015). Terbinafine is considered first-line systemic therapy, dosed at 250 mg daily for 3 or 4 months for toenails and 6 weeks for fingernails (~50% cure rate). Itraconazole may also be effective at 200 mg daily for 3 months for toenails and 6 weeks for fingernails or at 200 mg twice daily for 1 week per month for 3 months for toenails and 2 months for fingernails. The efficacy of fluconazole is lower than that of terbinafine and itraconazole. Patients with active liver disease should not receive terbinafine, and testing of LFTs at baseline and every 4–6 weeks is recommended given the risk of hepatotoxicity. Congestive heart disease is a contraindication to itraconazole use. In addition, itraconazole interacts with more medications compared to terbinafine (de Berker, 2009). Finally, the causative agent may differ between the general population and HIV-infected populations, which is relevant when selecting therapy. For example, nondermatophyte molds, such as *Scytalidium*, *Aspergillus*, and *Fusarium*, and yeast such as *Candida* are implicated in onychomycosis in HIV patients more often than in the general public. Much higher cure rates are achieved with itraconazole than with terbinafine for these organisms, whereas the reverse is true for dermatophytes (Cambuim, 2011; Warshaw, 2005). For these reasons, and given the potential side effects of systemic therapies, culture of nail clippings involved with onychomycosis is recommended before initiation of therapy by some dermatologists.

CANDIDIASIS

Angular cheilitis is typically caused by *Candida albicans* and presents as fissured white plaques at the angles of the lips. It occurs with some frequency in the elderly, but it may suggest HIV infection in young adults and may warrant testing if there is no other known reason for immunosuppression. Topical antifungal creams are effective and avoid systemic circulation for this focal disease. Associated burning and dysphagia suggest oral candidiasis, with atrophic or removable yellow white pseudomembranous or hyperplastic plaques typically seen on the tongue or dorsal palate. Oral candidiasis is often a harbinger of immunologic failure in patients on antiretroviral therapy, although it can also be caused by steroids and antibiotics (Cockerell, 2013). Nystatin or clotrimazole troches, and oral antifungals such as fluconazole or ketoconazole when there is associated odynophagia, are effective. Ketoconazole should be taken with food and should be avoided in the setting of malabsorption given the risk of treatment failure.

Candida intertrigo is common in HIV-infected populations, and it can appear as eroded glistening erythematous plaques or as pustules with scale over a macerated erythematous surface within and extending from skin folds. Treatment with oral fluconazole or ketoconazole for larger or extensive plaques is suggested over topical antifungals.

CUTANEOUS CRYPTOCOCCOSIS

Cryptococcus neoformans causes a systemic infection in which there is skin involvement in 10% of cases. It is an AIDS-defining illness, with skin involvement preceding the more common central nervous system and pulmonary involvement in 10% of cases. The patient is typically febrile and very ill. Skin lesions can present as papules that may be umbilicated, nodules, pustules, ulcers, and plaques. A skin biopsy is necessary for diagnosis, revealing round yeast with narrow-based budding and a slimy capsule in a granulomatous or gelatinous background, highlighted by fungal stains. Culture is definitively diagnostic, and treatment is with amphotericin B or fluconazole; adjunctive flucytosine can also be used (Cockerell, 2013). Antiretroviral therapy has decreased the incidence of cryptococcal infection; however, institution of HAART in patients with cryptococcal infection can result in fatal IRIS (Lortholary, 2005). Relapses are not uncommon, and secondary prophylaxis with fluconazole 200–400 mg daily for patients with CD4+ T cell counts <200 cells/mm³ is recommended.

CUTANEOUS HISTOPLASMOSIS

Histoplasmosis manifests with cutaneous lesion secondary to pulmonary or disseminated disease; primary manifestation is rare. The rash is nonspecific, characterized by diffuse erythematous macules, papules that may be umbilicated, pustules, crusted ulcers, or psoriasisform papules. The face is most often involved, followed by truncal and extremity involvement (Cockerell, 2013). The clinical differential diagnosis includes molluscum contagiosum and cryptococcosis. HIV patients with cutaneous histoplasmosis may be well appearing on initial presentation; however, prompt diagnosis is important because they can rapidly and fatally decompensate with systemic involvement (Wheat, 1990). Diagnosis of cutaneous histoplasmosis requires tissue biopsy, which reveals spores with a pseudo-capsule (the fungal wall) parasitizing macrophages. Culture confirms the diagnosis. Mild infection in the general public is self-limiting and may not require treatment; however, treatment is indicated in HIV patients. Treating systemic disease also treats skin involvement and is typically done with itraconazole; amphotericin is reserved for meningitis or other disseminated infection (Hage, 2015). Similar to cryptococcosis, relapses can occur, and secondary prophylaxis with itraconazole in AIDS patients is advised.

MOLLUSCUM CONTAGIOSUM

Molluscum is a common viral infection in children and their caregivers, but it warrants testing for HIV in adults with limited exposure to children. Skin-colored discrete umbilicated papules are typical, although giant facial molluscum and extensive beard involvement occur with advanced immunosuppression. Giant molluscum can persist even after immune reconstitution; it is extremely difficult to treat and is stigmatizing. Molluscum is differentiated from cryptococcosis and histoplasmosis, which can also have umbilicated papules by the presence of a central core in molluscum lesions. Also, patients appear well with molluscum infection, whereas they are systemically ill with cryptococcal infection. Treatment options include cryotherapy for smaller lesions and curettage and excision for larger lesions. Topical imiquimod, cidofivir, and photodynamic therapy with 5-aminolevulinic acid have all shown efficacy in case reports (Drain, 2014; Foissac, 2014).

CONDYLOMA ACCUMINATUM

Condyloma accuminatum (anogenital warts), which is caused by the human papillomavirus (HPV), is the most common sexually transmitted infection in the United States. Warts appear as flesh-colored to gray, rounded to pointy papules, frequently on a short peduncle. Podophyllin, trichloroacetic acid, and cryotherapy are three of the most commonly used treatments for genital warts. Cryotherapy and trichloroacetic acid yield a treatment success rate of 75%, whereas that of podophyllin is reported to be 20–50% (Murray, 2015). Therapies for recalcitrant anogenital warts include topical 5-fluoracil, cidofovir, intralesional interferon-α, and surgical excision (Nambudiri, 2013). Approximately 5% of men who have sex with men (MSM) and 15% of HIV-positive MSM have a history of perianal warts. Anogenital warts are more common in women, and HIV-infected women are five times more likely than their counterparts to have these warts (Hagensee, 2004). In addition, squamous epithelial lesions occur in 79% of HIV-positive women with anal HPV infection compared to 43% of HIV-negative women. The frequency of intraepithelial neoplasia within anogenital warts is higher than previously realized, warranting aggressive surveillance and treatment (McCloskey, 2007).

HERPES SIMPLEX

Herpes simplex virus (HSV) infection is caused by either HSV-1 or HSV-2 and is a common viral infection in the general population. It presents as grouped vesicles on an erythematous base. In HIV-positive patients, the infections occur more frequently and are less likely to self-resolve. When CD4+ T cells decrease below 100 cells/mm³, the incidence of HSV outbreaks reaches 27% (Severson, 1999). Recommended treatment for an HIV-positive patient with recurrent herpes infection is valacyclovir 1 g twice daily for 5–10 days or acyclovir 200 mg five times a day for the same period. Acyclovir-resistant HSV has become a problem in patients with AIDS. Reported acyclovir resistance in HIV-positive patients is 10-fold higher than that in immunocompetent counterparts—0.6% and 6%, respectively

(Lolis, 2008). Resistance to acyclovir also implies resistance to valacyclovir, and in many cases famciclovir is also not an effective treatment. Treatment of choice for acyclovir-resistant HSV is intravenous foscarnet or cidofovir. Topical cidofovir and foscarnet have been used as successful treatments as well (Strick, 2006).

HERPES ZOSTER

Herpes zoster, also known as shingles, is caused by the reactivation of varicella zoster virus (VZV), which also causes chickenpox. Ten to twenty percent of adults are affected by shingles. As T cell immunity wanes, with age or immunosuppression, the incidence of infection increases. Therefore, herpes zoster is very common with HIV infection, and it may be the presenting manifestation. In immunocompetent patients, the infection is usually limited to one dermatome. Pain, constitutional symptoms of fever, malaise, and headache may precede the eruptive phase, which consists of clusters of vesicles on an erythematous base within a dermatome. Involvement of multiple dermatomes is common in HIV-positive individuals, and disseminated infection is frequent. Treatment is with acyclovir 800 mg daily for 7–10 days, valacyclovir 1 g three times a day, or acyclovir 10 mg/kg when intravenous treatment is warranted. Foscarnet 40 mg/kg three times a day is used for treatment of acyclovir-resistant VZV (Cockerell, 2013). Continual pain, referred to as postherpetic neuralgia (PHN), can occur and can last months to years. Immunocompromised patients are at a higher risk of developing PHN, and initiation of gabapentin at presentation along with antivirals should be considered. Varicella vaccine is recommended in adults without varicella immunity and CD4$^+$ T cell counts >200 cells/mm^3. Zoster vaccine should be avoided in HIV-infected patients with AIDS or manifestations of HIV and CD4$^+$ T cell counts <200 cells/mm^3 or CD4$^+$ T cell T lymphocytes ≤15% (CDC, Advisory Committee on Immunization Practices).

METHICILLIN-RESISTANT STAPHYLOCOCCUS AUREUS

Staphylococcus aureus has acquired the mecA gene, which makes it less sensitive to many of the antibiotics typically used to treat skin and soft tissue infections. Methicillin-resistant *Staphylococcus aureus* (MRSA) has grown to epidemic proportions during approximately the past decade. There is a higher rate of MRSA infection in the HIV-positive population. One study reported that the prevalence was 18 times higher in the HIV population compared to the general population (Crum-Cianflone, 2007).

Incision and drainage is the most important component of treatment for localized skin infections. Many cutaneous MRSA infections are generally sensitive to the antibiotics trimethoprim–sulfamethoxazole, doxycycline, clindamycin, and linezolid. These antibiotics are generally effective against MRSA, and culture and sensitivity data are helpful in guiding treatment.

Both skin and nasal colonization are potential reservoirs for reinfection. Studies have indicated that mupirocin can be used to eradicate nasal colonization, whereas chlorhexidine can be used for the skin (Kuehnert, 2006).

BACILLARY ANGIOMATOSIS

This infectious disease occurs rarely in HIV-infected patients, but awareness of bacillary angiomastosis (BA) is important because it is a clinical mimicker of Kaposi's sarcoma (KS) that can be treated effectively with erythromycin 500 mg four times a day; it is potentially systemic and fatal if untreated. Clinically, purple "grape-like" papules to nodules are seen in a focal or widespread distribution. In contrast to KS, they only rarely manifest as patches or plaques. BA can be distinguished from KS on histology, with a lobular capillary proliferation with an edematous stroma and clusters of neutrophils seen throughout the lesion (Cockerell, 2013). There is often an amorphous material that represents colonies of bacteria, and culture for *Bartonella* speciation has relevance given that *Bartonella quintana* is more frequently associated with neurologic sequelae compared to *Bartonella henselae* (Gasquet, 1998).

SYPHILIS

Primary syphilis typically presents with an asymptomatic orogenital ulcer, whereas secondary syphilis is typically papulosquamous to psoriasiform but can mimic many other dermatoses. The color is characteristic, resembling a "clean-cut ham" or having a coppery tint. Palms and soles may present with classic coppery-colored scaly plaques. Temporal irregular, "moth-eaten" alopecia of the beard, scalp, and eyebrows may occur. Of concern, syphilis has an accelerated rate of progression in HIV, with potential development of neurosyphilis, and can have atypical presentations including multiple chancres and syphilitic vasculitis. Diagnosis can be complicated by the prozone effect, in which a false-negative rapid plasma reagin or Venereal Disease Research Laboratory test is achieved due to overwhelming antibody titers interfering with formation of antigen antibody lattice network in the test. Dilution of the assay overcomes this false-negative result, and this should be requested when syphilis is suspected and there is a negative result (Smith, 2004). Treatment is with penicillin formulations, and better response with decreased progression to neurosyphilis has been noted in HIV patients on antiretroviral therapy (Ghanem, 2007).

SCABIES

Scabies is caused by an infestation of the skin by the *Sarcoptes scabiei* mite. The first symptom of scabies is usually pruritus, especially at night. Scabies is a very common infection, with an approximate prevalence of 300 million annual cases (CDC, 2006). Scabies mites cannot jump or fly and therefore require skin-to-skin contact for infection to occur. Scabies mites have not demonstrated the ability to transmit HIV. Diagnosis is made through clinical examination. Burrow scrapings can be examined under a microscope for scabies mites, eggs, and feces; however, the absence of these on microscopic evaluated does not eliminate the possibility of infection. Recently, dermoscopy has been shown to be a valuable tool in the diagnosis of scabies, with a characteristic "delta wing jet" appearance of burrows identified on dermoscopy (Suh, 2014).

"Norwegian" or "crusted" scabies is a more florid infection leading to crusted burrows. These crusted lesions typically occur in the web spaces of the hands and feet, over the elbows, and on the ears or temples. This typically occurs in immunocompromised patients, including HIV-infected patients with low CD4+ T cell counts. Norwegian scabies are much more infectious and can be easily spread to health care workers by skin-to-skin contact.

Per CDC guidelines, first-line treatment of scabies is either topical permethrin cream or oral ivermectin (Workowski, 2015). Permethrin cream is applied below the neck (and above the neck if lesions are evident) and washed off after 8–14 hours on days 1 and 14, or ivermectin 200 µg/kg is given on days 1 and 14. The updated CDC recommendation for treatment of crusted scabies to avoid treatment failure is an intensive regimen of ivermectin dosed at 200 µg/kg taken on days 1, 2, 8, 9, and 15, and, for severe disease, also days 22 and 29, in combination with topical permethrin daily for 7 days and then twice a week until cure (Ortega-Loayza, 2013). Compliance may be a challenge.

AMOEBA

Naegleria fowleri, *Balamuthia mandrillaris*, and *Acanthamoeba* are free-living protozoa that cause a rapidly progressive fatal infection in the immunocompromised.

Acanthamoeba is a recognized pathogen in immunocompromised patients and has been cultured from the cornea, nasal and sinus cavities, ears, throat, lungs, and skin. *Acanthamoeba* can infect the skin directly or can spread to the skin by hematogenous dissemination from primary foci in the lungs or sinuses (Chandrasekar, 1997). More frequent sites of cutaneous involvement include the face, trunk, and extremities. The lesions typically present as nonspecific necrotic ulcers or nodules that may be quite tender or asymptomatic. Evaluations should include biopsy with histology showing trophozoites and culture for speciation. The survival rate is poor. Optimal treatment has not been determined; thus, combination therapy is recommended with miltefosine, fluconazole, and pentamadine. Trimethoprim–sulfamethoxazole, metronidazole, and a macrolide can be added to this regime in patients failing therapy (Mayer, 2011).

Recommended Reading

Drain, P. K., Mosam, A., Gounder, L., et al. (2014). Recurrent giant molluscum contagiosum immune reconstitution inflammatory syndrome (IRIS) after initiation of antiretroviral therapy in an HIV-infected man. *Int J STD AIDS*, 25(3), 235–238.

McCloskey, J. C., Metcalf, C., French, M. A., et al. (2007). The frequency of high-grade intraepithelial neoplasia in anal/perianal warts is higher than previously recognized. *Int J STD AIDS*, 18(8), 538–542.

Smith, G., & Holman, R. P. (2004). The prozone phenomenon with syphilis and HIV-1 co-infection. *South Med J*, 97(4), 379–382.

CUTANEOUS MALIGNANCIES IN HIV

LEARNING OBJECTIVE

Review the status of cutaneous malignancies in HIV patients.

WHAT'S NEW?

As life expectancy of HIV-positive patients has increased, cancers have become a more prevalent cause of morbidity and mortality.

KEY POINTS

- In the United States, first-line treatment for HIV-associated KS remains antiretroviral therapy, with chemotherapy indicated for progressive cutaneous disease or visceral involvement and radiation therapy for bulky obstructive tumors.

- There is an increased risk of metastatic disease in HIV patients with invasive melanoma, with worse outcomes associated with lower CD4$^+$ T cell counts.

- There is a three- to fivefold increased risk of developing nonmelanoma skin cancer in HIV, and basal and squamous cell cancers are more aggressive in HIV patients.

KAPOSI'S SARCOMA

Prior to the HIV epidemic, KS was rare in the United States. It was seen mostly in elderly men from the Mediterranean or recipients of solid organ transplants. The increasing prevalence of KS in the early HIV years led to the discovery of human herpesvirus-8 (HHV-8), the causative agent of KS. Mucocutaneous violaceous patches, plaques, or nodules may be seen, with biopsy revealing a vascular proliferation on histology with confirmatory HHV-8 immunostaining. First-line treatment for HIV-associated KS is antiretroviral therapy. IRIS can result in KS progression during the initiation of antiretroviral therapy, and patients on antiretroviral therapy can still develop KS (Krown, 2008). Chemotherapy is indicated for rapidly progressive cutaneous KS, when there is visceral involvement, and radiation may be helpful when bulky plaques cause pain or lymphatic blockage (Murphy, 1997). There have been reports of HHV-8 reactivation and development of KS in patients exposed to topical and systemic steroids (Boudhir, 2013).

MELANOMA AND NONMELANOMA SKIN CANCERS

The non-AIDS-defining skin cancers in HIV include basal cell cancers, squamous cell cancers, and melanomas. Case reports suggest an increased incidence of melanoma in HIV patients (Wilkins, 2006). In addition, HIV patients are more likely to develop metastases with invasive melanoma, and lower CD4$^+$ T cell count is predictive of worse prognosis (Rodrigues, 2002). Screening guidelines are the same as those for the general population. In addition, there is a three- to fivefold increased risk of developing nonmelanoma skin cancer in HIV. Basal cell carcinomas are more common than squamous cell carcinomas (SCCs), as is the case in the general population but in contrast to immunocompromised transplant patients, in whom SCCs are more common. Both basal cell carcinomas and SCCs are more aggressive in the HIV population (Wilkins, 2006).

ACKNOWLEDGMENT

The author acknowledges John M. Curtain, PA-C, MPH, the author of this chapter in the previous edition.

Recommended Reading

Wilkins, K., Turner, R., Dolev, J. C., et al. (2006). Cutaneous malignancy and human immunodeficiency virus disease. *J Am Acad Dermatol*, *54*(2), 189–206; quiz 207–110.

References

Aboulafia, D. M., Bundow, D., Wilske, K., & Ochs, U. I. (2000). Etanercept for the treatment of human immunodeficiency virus-associated psoriatic arthritis. *Mayo Clin Proc*, *75*(10), 1093–1098.

Altman, K., Vanness, E., & Westergaard, R. P. (2015). Cutaneous manifestations of human immunodeficiency virus: A clinical update. *Curr Infect Dis Rep*, *17*(3), 464.

Anton, P., Soriano, V., Jimenez-Nacher, I., et al. (1999). Incidence of rash and discontinuation of nevirapine using two different escalating initial doses. *AIDS*, *13*(4), 524–525.

Ball, R. A., Kinchelow, T., & Group, I. S. R. S. (2003). Injection site reactions with the HIV-1 fusion inhibitor enfuvirtide. *J Am Acad Dermatol*, *49*(5), 826–831.

Bartlett, B. L., Khambaty, M., Mendoza, N., et al. (2007). Dermatological management of human immunodeficiency virus (HIV). *Skin Therapy Lett*, *12*(8), 1–3.

Baveewo, S., Ssali, F., Karamagi, C., et al. (2011). Validation of World Health Organisation HIV/AIDS clinical staging in predicting initiation of antiretroviral therapy and clinical predictors of low CD4$^+$ T cell cell count in Uganda. *PLoS One*, *6*(5), e19089.

Bellavista, S., D'Antuono A., Infusino, S. D., Trimarco, R., & Patrizi, A. (2013). Pruritic papular eruption in HIV: A case successfully treated with NB-UVB. *Dermatol Ther*, *26*(2), 173–175.

Bolognia, J. L., Jorizzo J. L., & Schaffer, J. (2012). *Dermatology* (3rd ed.). New York, NY: Elsevier.

Boonchai, W., Laohasrisakul, R., Manonukul, J., & Kulthanan, K. (1999). Pruritic papular eruption in HIV seropositive patients: A cutaneous marker for immunosuppression. *Int J Dermatol*, *38*(5), 348–350.

Boudhir, H., Mael-Ainin, M., Senouci, K., et al. (2013). [Kaposi's disease: An unusual side-effect of topical corticosteroids]. *Ann Dermatol Venereol*, *140*(6–7), 459–461.

Breuer-McHam, J., Marshall, G., Adu-Oppong, A., et al. (1999). Alterations in HIV expression in AIDS patients with psoriasis or pruritus treated with phototherapy. *J Am Acad Dermatol*, *40*(1), 48–60.

Calonje, E., Brenn, T., Lazar, A., & Mckee, P. (2012). *McKee's Pathology of the Skin* (4th ed.), p. 901. St. Louis, MO: Saunders.

Cambuim, II, Macedo, D. P., Delgado, M., et al. (2011). [Clinical and mycological evaluation of onychomycosis among Brazilian HIV/AIDS patients]. *Rev Soc Bras Med Trop*, *44*(1), 40–42.

Chandrasekar, P. H., Nandi, P. S., Fairfax, M. R., & Crane, L. R. (1997). Cutaneous infections due to *Acanthamoeba* in patients with acquired immunodeficiency syndrome. *Arch Intern Med*, *157*(5), 569–572.

Chaponda, M., & Pirmohamed, M. (2011). Hypersensitivity reactions to HIV therapy. *Br J Clin Pharmacol*, *71*(5), 659–671.

Cockerell, C., & Calame, A. (2013). *Cutaneous Manifestations of HIV Disease*. London, UK: Manson.

Crum-Cianflone, N. F., Burgi, A. A., & Hale, B. R. (2007). Increasing rates of community-acquired methicillin-resistant *Staphylococcus aureus* infections among HIV-infected persons. *Int J STD AIDS*, *18*(8), 521–526.

Davis, C. M., & Shearer, W. T. (2008). Diagnosis and management of HIV drug hypersensitivity. *J Allergy Clin Immunol*, *121*(4), 826–832, e825.

de Berker, D. (2009). Clinical practice: Fungal nail disease. *N Engl J Med, 360*(20), 2108–2116.

de Moraes, A. P., de Arruda, E. A., Vitoriano, M. A., et al. (2007). An open-label efficacy pilot study with pimecrolimus cream 1% in adults with facial seborrhoeic dermatitis infected with HIV. *J Eur Acad Dermatol Venereol, 21*(5), 596–601.

Dogra, S., & Yadav, S. (2014). Acitretin in psoriasis: An evolving scenario. *Int J Dermatol, 53*(5), 525–538.

Dover, J. S., & Johnson, R. A. (1991). Cutaneous manifestations of human immunodeficiency virus infection: Part II. *Arch Dermatol, 127*(10), 1549–1558.

Drain, P. K., Mosam, A., Gounder, L., et al. (2014). Recurrent giant molluscum contagiosum immune reconstitution inflammatory syndrome (IRIS) after initiation of antiretroviral therapy in an HIV-infected man. *Int J STD AIDS, 25*(3), 235–238.

Duvic, M. (1990). Immunology of AIDS related to psoriasis. *J Invest Dermatol, 95*(5), 38S–40S.

Duvic, M., Crane, M. M., Conant, M., et al. (1994). Zidovudine improves psoriasis in human immunodeficiency virus-positive males. *Arch Dermatol, 130*(4), 447–451.

Eisman, S. (2006). Pruritic papular eruption in HIV. *Dermatol Clin, 24*(4), 449–457, vi.

Fearfield, L. A., Rowe, A., Francis, N., Bunker, C. B., & Staughton, R. C. (1999). Itchy folliculitis and human immunodeficiency virus infection: Clinicopathological and immunological features, pathogenesis and treatment. *Br J Dermatol, 141*(1), 3–11.

Foissac, M., Goehringer, F., Ranaivo, I. M., et al. (2014). [Efficacy and safety of intravenous cidofovir in the treatment of giant molluscum contagiosum in an immunosuppressed patient]. *Ann Dermatol Venereol, 141*(10), 620–622.

Gasquet, S., Maurin, M., Brouqui, P., Lepidi, H., & Raoult, D. (1998). Bacillary angiomatosis in immunocompromised patients. *AIDS, 12*(14), 1793–1803.

Gelfand, J. M., Gladman, D. D., Mease, P. J., et al. (2005). Epidemiology of psoriatic arthritis in the population of the United States. *J Am Acad Dermatol, 53*(4), 573.

Ghanem, K. G., Erbelding, E. J., Wiener, Z. S., & Rompalo, A. M. (2007). Serological response to syphilis treatment in HIV-positive and HIV-negative patients attending sexually transmitted diseases clinics. *Sex Transm Infect, 83*(2), 97–101.

Goldstein, B., Berman, B., Sukenik, E., & Frankel, S. J. (1997). Correlation of skin disorders with CD4+ T cell lymphocyte counts in patients with HIV/AIDS. *J Am Acad Dermatol, 36*(2 Pt 1), 262–264.

Gompels, M. M., Simpson, N., Snow, M., et al. (1999). Desensitization to co-trimoxazole (trimethoprim-sulphamethoxazole) in HIV-infected patients: is patch testing a useful predictor of reaction? *J Infect, 38*, 111–115.

Hage, C. A., Azar, M. M., Bahr, N., Loyd, J., & Wheat, L. J. (2015). Histoplasmosis: Up-to-date evidence-based approach to diagnosis and management. *Semin Respir Crit Care Med, 36*(5), 729–745.

Hagensee, M. E., Cameron, J. E., Leigh, J. E., & Clark, R. A. (2004). Human papillomavirus infection and disease in HIV-infected individuals. *Am J Med Sci, 328*(1), 57–63.

Hanifin, J. M., Reed, M. L., Eczema, P., et al.; Impact Working Group (2007). A population-based survey of eczema prevalence in the United States. *Dermatitis, 18*(2), 82–91.

Hevia, O., Jimenez-Acosta, F., Ceballos, P. I., et al. (1991). Pruritic papular eruption of the acquired immunodeficiency syndrome: A clinico-pathologic study. *J Am Acad Dermatol, 24*(2 Pt 1), 231–235.

Hyle, E. P., Wood, B. R., Backman, E. S., et al. (2013). High frequency of hypothalamic–pituitary–adrenal axis dysfunction after local corticosteroid injection in HIV-infected patients on protease inhibitor therapy. *J Acquir Immune Defic Syndr, 63*(5), 602–608.

Introcaso, C. E., Hines, J. M., & Kovarik, C. L. (2010). Cutaneous toxicities of antiretroviral therapy for HIV: Part II. Nonnucleoside reverse transcriptase inhibitors, entry and fusion inhibitors, integrase inhibitors, and immune reconstitution syndrome. *J Am Acad Dermatol, 63*(4), 563–569; quiz 569–570.

Jagdeo, J., Ho, D., Lo, A., & Carruthers, A. (2015). A systematic review of filler agents for aesthetic treatment of HIV facial lipoatrophy (FLA). *J Am Acad Dermatol, 73*(6), 1040–1054, e1014.

Kim, C. M., Vogel, J., Jay, G., & Rhim, J. S. (1992). The HIV tat gene transforms human keratinocytes. *Oncogene, 7*(8), 1525–1529.

Knobel, H., Miro, J. M., Domingo, P., et al. (2001). Failure of a short-term prednisone regimen to prevent nevirapine-associated rash: A double-blind placebo-controlled trial: the GESIDA 09/99 study. *J Acquir Immune Defic Syndr, 28*(1), 14–18.

Krown, S. E., Lee, J. Y., Dittmer, D. P., & Consortium, A. M. (2008). More on HIV-associated Kaposi's sarcoma. *N Engl J Med, 358*(5), 535–536; author reply 536.

Kuehnert, M. J., Kruszon-Moran, D., Hill, H. A., et al. (2006). Prevalence of *Staphylococcus aureus* nasal colonization in the United States, 2001–2002. *J Infect Dis, 193*(2), 172–179.

Lin, R. Y., & Lazarus, T. S. (1995). Asthma and related atopic disorders in outpatients attending an urban HIV clinic. *Ann Allergy Asthma Immunol, 74*(6), 510–515.

Liu, Z., Xie, Z., Zhang, L., et al. (2013). Reliability and validity of dermatology life quality index: Assessment of quality of life in human immunodeficiency virus/acquired immunodeficiency syndrome patients with pruritic papular eruption. *J Tradit Chin Med, 33*(5), 580–583.

Lolis, M. S., Gonzalez, L., Cohen, P. J., & Schwartz, R. A. (2008). Drug-resistant herpes simplex virus in HIV infected patients. *Acta Dermatovenerol Croat, 16*(4), 204–208.

Lortholary, O., Fontanet, A., Memain, N., et al.; Cryptococcosis Study Group (2005). Incidence and risk factors of immune reconstitution inflammatory syndrome complicating HIV-associated cryptococcosis in France. *AIDS, 19*(10), 1043–1049.

Mallal, S., Phillips, E., Carosi, G., et al. (2008). HLA-B*5701 screening for hypersensitivity to abacavir. *N Engl J Med, 358*(6), 568–579.

Mallon, E., & Bunker, C. B. (2000). HIV-associated psoriasis. *AIDS Patient Care STDS, 14*(5), 239–246.

Maurer, T. A. (2005). Dermatologic manifestations of HIV infection. *Top HIV Med, 13*(5), 149–154.

Mayer, P. L., Larkin, J. A., & Hennessy, J. M. (2011). Amebic encephalitis. *Surg Neurol Int, 2*, 50.

McCloskey, J. C., Metcalf, C., French, M. A., et al. (2007). The frequency of high-grade intraepithelial neoplasia in anal/perianal warts is higher than previously recognized. *Int J STD AIDS, 18*(8), 538–542.

Menon, K., Van Voorhees, A. S., Bebo, B. F., et al. (2010). Psoriasis in patients with HIV infection: From the medical board of the National Psoriasis Foundation. *J Am Acad Dermatol, 62*(2), 291–299.

Meola, T., Soter, N. A., Ostreicher, R., Sanchez, M., & Moy, J. A. (1993). The safety of UVB phototherapy in patients with HIV infection. *J Am Acad Dermatol, 29*(2 Pt 1), 216–220.

Mirmirani, P., Maurer, T. A., Berger, T. G., et al. (2002). Skin-related quality of life in HIV-infected patients on highly active antiretroviral therapy. *J Cutan Med Surg, 6*(1), 10–15.

Murphy, M., Armstrong, D., Sepkowitz, K. A., et al. (1997). Regression of AIDS-related Kaposi's sarcoma following treatment with an HIV-1 protease inhibitor. *AIDS, 11*(2), 261–262.

Murray, H., Barber, C. J., Foreman, R. M., et al.; GBD 2013 DALYs and HALE Collaborators (2015). Global, regional, and national disability-adjusted life years (DALYs) for 306 diseases and injuries and healthy life expectancy (HALE) for 188 countries, 1990–2013: Quantifying the epidemiological transition. *Lancet, 386*, 2145–2191.

Nambudiri, V. E., Mutyambizi, K., Walls, A. C., et al. (2013). Successful treatment of perianal giant condyloma acuminatum in an immuno-compromised host with systemic interleukin 2 and topical cidofovir. *JAMA Dermatol, 149*(9), 1068–1070.

Nissen, D., Nolte, H., Permin, H., et al. (1999). Evaluation of IgE-sensitization to fungi in HIV-positive patients with eczematous skin reactions. *Ann Allergy Asthma Immunol, 83*(2), 153–159.

Oble, D. A., Collett, E., Hsieh, M., et al. (2005). A novel T cell receptor transgenic animal model of seborrheic dermatitis-like skin disease. *J Invest Dermatol, 124*(1), 151–159.

Obuch, M. L., Maurer, T. A., Becker, B., & Berger, T. G. (1992). Psoriasis and human immunodeficiency virus infection. *J Am Acad Dermatol, 27*(5 Pt 1), 667–673.

Okada, S., Fujimura, T., Furudate, S., et al. (2013). Immunosuppression-associated eosinophilic pustular folliculitis (IS-EPF) developing after highly active anti-retroviral therapy (HAART): The possible mechanisms through CD163+ M2 macrophages. *Eur J Dermatol, 23*(5), 713–714.

Ortega-Loayza, A. G., McCall, C. O., & Nunley, J. R. (2013). Crusted scabies and multiple dosages of ivermectin. *J Drugs Dermatol, 12*(5), 584–585.

Pedrosa, A. F., Lisboa, C., & Goncalves Rodrigues, A. (2014). Malassezia infections: A medical conundrum. *J Am Acad Dermatol, 71*(1), 170–176.

Ratnam, I., Chiu, C., Kandala, N. B., & Easterbrook, P. J. (2006). Incidence and risk factors for immune reconstitution inflammatory syndrome in an ethnically diverse HIV type 1-infected cohort. *Clin Infect Dis, 42*(3), 418–427.

Resneck, J. S., Jr., Van Beek, M., Furmanski, L., et al. (2004). Etiology of pruritic papular eruption with HIV infection in Uganda. *JAMA, 292*(21), 2614–2621.

Rigopoulos, D., Paparizos, V., & Katsambas, A. (2004). Cutaneous markers of HIV infection. *Clin Dermatol, 22*(6), 487–498.

Rodrigues, L. K., Klencke, B. J., Vin-Christian, K., et al. (2002). Altered clinical course of malignant melanoma in HIV-positive patients. *Arch Dermatol, 138*(6), 765–770.

Rosen, T., Friedlander, S. F., & Kircik, L. (2015). Onychomycosis: epidemiology, diagnosis, and treatment in a changing landscape. *J Drugs Dermatol, 14*(3), 223–233.

Rosenthal, D., LeBoit, P. E., Klumpp, L., & Berger, T. G. (1991). Human immunodeficiency virus-associated eosinophilic folliculitis. A unique dermatosis associated with advanced human immunodeficiency virus infection. *Arch Dermatol, 127*(2), 206–209.

Sadick, N. S., McNutt, N. S., & Kaplan, M. H. (1990). Papulosquamous dermatoses of AIDS. *J Am Acad Dermatol, 22*(6 Pt 2), 1270–1277.

Severson, J. L., & Tyring, S. K. (1999). Relation between herpes simplex viruses and human immunodeficiency virus infections. *Arch Dermatol, 135*(11), 1393–1397.

Singh, F., & Rudikoff, D. (2003). HIV-associated pruritus: Etiology and management. *Am J Clin Dermatol, 4*(3), 177–188.

Smith, G., & Holman, R. P. (2004). The prozone phenomenon with syphilis and HIV-1 co-infection. *South Med J, 97*(4), 379–382.

Soeprono, F. F., Schinella, R. A., Cockerell, C. J., & Comite, S. L. (1986). Seborrheic-like dermatitis of acquired immunodeficiency syndrome: A clinicopathologic study. *J Am Acad Dermatol, 14*(2 Pt 1), 242–248.

Stanley, S. K., Folks, T. M., & Fauci, A. S. (1989). Induction of expression of human immunodeficiency virus in a chronically infected promonocytic cell line by ultraviolet irradiation. *AIDS Res Hum Retroviruses, 5*(4), 375–384.

Strick, L. B., Wald, A., & Celum, C. (2006). Management of herpes simplex virus type 2 infection in HIV type 1-infected persons. *Clin Infect Dis, 43*(3), 347–356.

Suh, K. S., Han, S. H., Lee, K. H., et al. (2014). Mites and burrows are frequently found in nodular scabies by dermoscopy and histopathology. *J Am Acad Dermatol, 71*(5), 1022–1023.

Toutous-Trellu, L., Abraham, S., Pechere, M., et al. (2005). Topical tacrolimus for effective treatment of eosinophilic folliculitis associated with human immunodeficiency virus infection. *Arch Dermatol, 141*(10), 1203–1208.

Ward, H. A., Russo, G. G., & Shrum, J. (2002). Cutaneous manifestations of antiretroviral therapy. *J Am Acad Dermatol, 46*(2), 284–293.

Warren, K. J., Boxwell, D. E., Kim, N. Y., & Drolet, B. A. (1998). Nevirapine-associated Stevens–Johnson syndrome. *Lancet, 351*(9102), 567.

Warshaw, E. M., Nelson, D., Carver, S. M., et al. (2005). A pilot evaluation of pulse itraconazole vs. terbinafine for treatment of *Candida* toenail onychomycosis. *Int J Dermatol, 44*(9), 785–788.

Weinberg, J. L., & Kovarik, C. L. (2010). The WHO clinical staging system for HIV/AIDS. *Virtual Mentor, 12*(3), 202–206.

Wheat, L. J., Connolly-Stringfield, P. A., Baker, R. L., et al. (1990). Disseminated histoplasmosis in the acquired immune deficiency syndrome: Clinical findings, diagnosis and treatment, and review of the literature. *Medicine (Baltimore), 69*(6), 361–374.

Wilkins, K., Turner, R., Dolev, J. C., et al. (2006). Cutaneous malignancy and human immunodeficiency virus disease. *J Am Acad Dermatol, 54*(2), 189–206; quiz 207–110.

Workowski, K. A., & Bolan, G. A. (2015). Sexually transmitted diseases treatment guidelines, 2015. *MMWR Recomm Rep, 64*(RR-03), 1–137.

Zancanaro, P. C., McGirt, L. Y., Mamelak, A. J., et al. (2006). Cutaneous manifestations of HIV in the era of highly active antiretroviral therapy: An institutional urban clinic experience. *J Am Acad Dermatol, 54*(4), 581–588.

Zeichner, J. A. (2015). New topical therapeutic options in the management of superficial fungal infections. *J Drugs Dermatol, 14*(10), s35–s41.

Zheng, Y., Niyonsaba, F., Ushio, H., et al. (2007). Cathelicidin LL-37 induces the generation of reactive oxygen species and release of human alpha-defensins from neutrophils. *Br J Dermatol, 157*(6), 1124–1131.

35.

ENDOCRINE DISORDERS

Rajagopal V. Sekhar

LEARNING OBJECTIVE

After reading this chapter, the reader should be able to describe the mechanism and clinical management of endocrine disease in HIV-infected patients.

WHAT'S NEW?

- The prevalence of diabetes mellitus (DM) is increasing in HIV-infected patients worldwide.

- Recent data suggest that middle-aged HIV-infected women have a higher adjusted fracture rate compared to that of HIV-uninfected women.

- Zoledronic acid, administered annually by the intravenous route, has been shown to improve bone mineral density (BMD) in HIV-infected patients.

KEY POINTS

- Abnormalities in glucose and lipids are common in HIV.

- HIV patients have a higher prevalence of metabolic syndrome.

- HIV infection, antiretroviral drugs (ARVs), and other factors play a role in the development of endocrine disease.

- For endocrine disorders in HIV, early referral to an endocrinologist is suggested.

HIV infection is now a chronic disease, and it is associated with an increasing prevalence of metabolic and endocrine abnormalities. The underlying etiology of these disorders can be attributed to multiple factors, including, but not limited to, the effects of HIV itself, ARVs, the effects of immune dysfunction, and other opportunistic infections.

Any endocrine glandular system can be involved; hence, appropriate clinical suspicion, endocrinological dynamic testing for accurate diagnosis, and effective therapy are important in the identification and management of these disorders.

MECHANISMS OF ENDOCRINE DISEASE IN HIV

The mechanisms through which HIV infection affects the endocrine system are complex and involve abnormalities in hormonal secretion, transport, metabolism, and resistance. However, the underlying mechanisms for many of these disorders are still not completely understood, such as in the case of HIV-associated lipodystrophy or accelerated aging in HIV.

One important contributing factor is immune dysfunction in the context of HIV, with abnormalities in cytokine, chemokine, and other immune phenomena that affect endocrine function (Merrill, 1989; Salin, 1988; Tracey, 1990). For example, interleukin-1 (IL-1) has been shown to increase adrenocorticotropic hormone (ACTH) in cultured pituitary cells (Meyer, 1987; Szebeni, 1991). Other pituitary hormones may also be affected; effects include prolactin elevations (Parra, 2004) and deficient growth hormone secretion (Koutkia, 2004). HIV-infected mononuclear cells can increase interferon-α (Grunfeld, 1992) and impair glucocorticoid receptor activity (Norbiato, 1996), and abnormalities in IL-1 and tumor necrosis factor can affect gonadal function by inhibiting gonadal steroidogenesis (Calkins, 1988; Hales, 1992; Xiong, 1993).

Another contributor to HIV-related endocrine disease is opportunistic infections. For example, cytomegalovirus (CMV) infection predisposes to an increased risk of developing adrenalitis (Glasgow, 1985). Infections caused by mycobacterial pathogens may also affect adrenal function, whereas CMV, cryptococcal, and toxoplasma infections can affect central nervous system function and cause retinitis, meningitis, and pituitary disease (Giampalmo, 1982). CMV infection has been reported in one instance to cause hypernatremia, likely through a reset osmostat (Keuneke, 1999). Thyroid function can be affected by opportunistic pathogens in HIV, including pneumocystis, which is a rare cause of thyroiditis (Drucker, 1990).

The development and clinical use of antiretroviral therapy (ART) have led to significant benefits for HIV patients, including decreased early mortality, decreased opportunistic infection, and improved nutritional status. However, these benefits are associated with increases in the incidence and prevalence of endocrine and metabolic complications, most notably dyslipidemia, and changes in body morphology ranging from lipodystrophy (Carr, 1998) to central obesity in the context of metabolic syndrome.

PROTEASE INHIBITORS

The initial use of these drugs led to observations of varying abnormalities in total body fat distribution, most notably an increase in abdominal fat that was initially described by colorful names such as the "protease paunch" (Mishriki, 1998) or "Crixivan belly" (Huff, 1998). Since then, the protease inhibitor (PI) class of drugs has been linked to the development of abdominal obesity and biochemical abnormalities comprising severe hypertriglyceridemia, dyslipidemia, insulin resistance, and diabetes. Many PI drugs, including Kaletra (lopinavir/ritonavir), nelfinavir, amprenavir, and saquinavir, are metabolized by the hepatic cytochrome 450 CYP3A4 isoenzyme pathway. PI drugs have been shown to directly impact insulin resistance. For example, indinavir can inhibit GLUT4 activity and thus impair insulin-stimulated glucose uptake and predispose to hyperglycemia (Caron, 2001; Murata, 2000). In addition to their permissive role in metabolic and glycemic abnormalities, PI drugs have also been implicated in the development of prolactin abnormalities (Hutchinson, 2000) and in osteomalacia (Cozzolino, 2003).

NUCLEOSIDE REVERSE TRANSCRIPTASE INHIBITORS

Nucleoside reverse transcriptase inhibitors have also been described to induce changes in body morphology. For example, stavudine has been linked to the development of lipoatrophy in HIV (Saint-Marc, 1999). These drugs have also been linked to the development of mitochondrial dysfunction (Mallon, 2005), which could result in abnormalities of glucose and lipid metabolism (Sekhar, 2002; Shikuma, 2001).

NON-NUCLEOSIDE REVERSE TRANSCRIPTASE INHIBITORS

Non-nucleoside reverse transcriptase inhibitors have been linked to dyslipidemia (Padmapriyadarsini, 2011) and fat depletion in 3T3-L1 cells (Minami, 2011).

ENDOCRINE DISORDERS IN HIV

HIV infection is associated with an increased risk of diabetes and the metabolic syndrome, but it can also affect adrenal, thyroid, pituitary, and gonadal function, in addition to bone, electrolytes, and dyslipidemia.

DIABETES AND METABOLIC SYNDROME IN HIV

The prevalence of DM is increasing in HIV-infected patients worldwide (Tzur, 2015) and ranges from 1.5–2.6% in ART-naive patients (El-Sadr, 2005; Tien, 2007) to 5.9% when co-infected with hepatitis C (Visnegarwala, 2004). As reported in the Multicenter AIDS Cohort Study, exposure to ART results in a 14% incidence of DM in HIV-infected men, which is fourfold higher than that for HIV-seronegative controls (Brown, 2005). HIV-infected individuals with lipodystrophy have up to 35% prevalence of impaired glucose tolerance and 7% prevalence of diabetes (Hadigan, 2001).

HIV-infected individuals also have a higher risk of developing metabolic syndrome (MS). Whereas the prevalence of MS in non-HIV-infected individuals is 3%, HIV-infected patients taking ART have a prevalence of 1618% (Samaras, 2007). HIV-infected women appear to have an even higher burden of MS, with a 33% prevalence compared to 22% for HIV-seronegative women (Sobieszczyk, 2008).

Clinically, the previously discussed data translate to patients having an increased incidence and prevalence of abdominal obesity, insulin resistance, dyslipidemia, and hypertension, all of which contribute to elevated cardiometabolic risk in HIV-infected patients. Treatment of these disorders involves a combination of patient education; adherence to dietary control; encouragement of physical activity and exercise, where possible; and appropriate pharmacotherapy targeting glycemic control, blood pressure, and lipids. Details of dyslipidemia in HIV patients are provided in Chapter 47.

ADRENAL DISORDERS

HIV infection can be associated with adrenal dysfunction. The incidence of hypoadrenalism has been reported to be 20% in HIV-infected patients (González- González, 2001), and postmortem studies have shown that up to two-thirds of patients with AIDS may have adrenal involvement (Bricaire, 1988). Presentation of adrenal dysfunction may be subtle, and it is relatively common in hospitalized patients with HIV (Membreno, 1987). Adrenal hypofunction can range from primary hypoadrenalism with elevations in ACTH levels (Villette, 1990) to secondary hypoadrenalism due to pituitary suppression possibly caused by exogenous steroid use (Danaher, 2009; Kaviani, 2011). HIV-infected patients have also been described to develop hyperadrenalism with iatrogenic Cushing's syndrome when administered steroids via oral, inhaled, and parenteral routes (Gray, 2010; Johnson, 2006; Samaras, 2005; Yombi, 2008).

HIV-infected patients may also have abnormalities in the mineralocorticoid axis (Stricker, 1999). HIV-infected women with the wasting syndrome may have significant shunting of adrenal steroid metabolism away from androgenic pathways and toward cortisol production (Grinspoon, 2001).

THYROID ABNORMALITIES

The clinical presentation of thyroid abnormalities in HIV infection ranges from asymptomatic hypo- or hyperthyroidism to clinically overt disease. The prevalence of thyroid dysfunction in HIV patients is generally similar to that seen in non HIV-infected populations (Hoffman, 2007), but there may be an increased risk of hypothyroidism (Beltran, 2003). Factors contributing to thyroid disorders in HIV infection include, but are not limited to, ARVs, infection, and immune factors.

ARVs could play a role in the development of thyroid abnormalities in HIV-infected patients. For example, HIV-related non-autoimmune primary hypothyroidism and subclinical hypothyroidism have been linked to stavudine, decreased $CD4^+$ T cell counts, and male gender (Calza, 2002; Quirino, 2004).

HIV-related immune and other factors are also linked to the development of abnormal thyroid function tests. For example, $CD4^+$ T cell counts have been inversely correlated with thyroid binding globulin (Bourdoux, 1991), and diminished levels of triiodothyronine (T3) and reverse T3 with increased thyroid binding globulin may be associated with HIV progression. Hyperthyroidism can also occur in HIV-infected patients. Autoimmune Graves' disease is an anti-thyroid-stimulating hormone receptor antibody after the initiation of ART and after an increase in $CD4^+$ T cell count (Jubault, 2000).

Infection as an etiological factor for thyroid disease was much more prevalent in the pre-ART era and was caused by a wide variety of infectious microorganisms. However, these can still be seen in patients not on ART, those with ART drug resistance, or those who are noncompliant with medications.

Although the clinical presentation of thyroid abnormalities ranges from asymptomatic hypo- or hyperthyroidism to clinically overt disease, the diagnostic workup is similar to that in HIV-negative patients.

GONADAL DYSFUNCTION

Gonadal dysfunction is common in HIV-infected patients (Crum, 2005; Rietschel, 2000). In male patients, decreased levels of testosterone may be associated with fatigue, muscle wasting and sarcopenia, decreased bone density, low libido, weight loss, decreased strength (Grinspoon, 1996; Wanke, 2000), and impotence (Mylonakis, 2001). In a study of 300 HIV patients, 17% were found to be hypogonadal, and all patients with low testosterone had secondary hypogonadism. Interestingly, there was no correlation between hypogonadism and erectile dysfunction, but increasing age and a higher body mass index were positively correlated with hypogonadism, whereas smoking was negatively correlated (Crum-Cianflone, 2007). Although underlying causes are not fully understood, elevated levels of prolactin have been implicated in the development of male hypogonadism (Collazos, 2009). Treatment of patients with AIDS wasting syndrome with testosterone or placebo was associated with a sustained increase in lean mass only with testosterone after a 6-month period (Grinspoon, 1999). Testosterone therapy, especially in older patients, should involve careful monitoring of prostate-specific antigen levels, liver profiles, and hematocrit levels.

HIV-infected women have increased rates of oligomenorrhea and amenorrhea. HIV has been shown to infect the cervix, uterus, and fallopian tubes (Howell, 1997). In one study, 8% of women with HIV had evidence of early menopause and 48% had anovulatory cycles, whereas women who ovulated had higher $CD4^+$ T cell counts (Chirgwin, 1996).

Gynecomastia

Male patients with HIV have a 2.9% incidence of developing gynecomastia, which is not linked to progression of HIV disease (Biglia, 2004) but is linked to hypogonadism, lipoatrophy, and hepatitis C (Manfredi, 2001) and also lipodystrophy (Biglia, 2004). The role of ARVs in the development of gynecomastia is controversial, with no correlation found in some studies (Manfredi, 2001), whereas other studies have linked gynecomastia with PI-based antiretroviral regimens (Manfredi, 2004; Peyriere, 1999; Toma, 1998). When associated with PI therapy, gynecomastia does not resolve after cessation of ART, and underlying mechanisms are not clear. Treatment of gynecomastia includes removal of any identifiable cause and, in extreme cases, surgical removal.

Pituitary Disease

The pituitary gland is located in the sella turcica and comprises the anterior pituitary (adenohypophysis) and posterior pituitary (neurohypophysis). The adenohypophyseal hormones are intimately involved in controlling thyroid, adrenal, and gonadal function, growth, and milk secretion; the neurohypophysis controls water balance, acting via antidiuretic hormone.

Growth Hormone Disorders

Disorders of growth hormone (GH) are reported in HIV infection. Adult patients with HIV-associated lipodystrophy are described to have GH deficiency with reduced pulse and amplitude of GH secretion, which may be related to an increased somatostatin tone, decreased ghrelin, and increased circulatory free fatty acid concentrations (Koutkia, 2004). HIV-infected children and adults with AIDS wasting syndrome have low levels of insulin-like growth factor-1 (IGF-1) and IGF binding protein 3 and increased concentrations of GH, suggesting resistance to GH (Frost, 1996; Pinto, 2000; Ratner, 1997; Rondanelli, 2002).

Pituitary Adrenal Disorders

Iatrogenic Cushing's syndrome, together with secondary hypoadrenalism, has been reported in HIV patients receiving steroid therapy (Danaher, 2009; Gray, 2010; Johnson, 2006; Kaviani, 2011; Samaras, 2005; Yombi, 2008). This is likely caused by the effect of several antiretroviral agents (almost entirely ritonavir or cobicistat boosting) on the hepatic cytochrome P450 system, which prolongs the half-life of steroids. This results in elevated levels of exogenously administered steroids and suppression of ACTH and thereby of endogenous cortisol production, resulting in iatrogenic Cushing's syndrome together with endogenous adrenal insufficiency. Because sudden withdrawal of exogenous steroids in this situation could precipitate a catastrophic adrenal crisis, caution must be exercised while discontinuing steroids, and a gentle taper is recommended.

Prolactin Disorders

Patients with HIV have been reported to have disturbances in basal and rhythmic prolactin secretions associated with CD4[+] T lymphocytes (Parra, 2004). Elevation in serum prolactin is described in HIV-infected patients (Collazos, 2002), and hyperprolactinemia in HIV-infected men has been linked to hypogonadism and gynecomastia (Collazos, 2009). Although the etiology of the hyperprolactinemia is unclear, use of PIs has been linked to elevations in prolactin (Ram, 2004).

Posterior Pituitary Disorders

Posterior pituitary disorders are caused by excess secretion of antidiuretic hormone (ADH), resulting in hyponatremia, or a paucity of ADH, resulting in diabetes insipidus. In one report, one-third of AIDS patients were found to be hyponatremic primarily due to the syndrome of inappropriate ADH (Agarwal, 1989).

HIV AND BONE LOSS

Disorders of bone loss, such as osteoporosis and osteopenia, are occurring more frequently in HIV-infected patients, and the prevalence of osteoporosis and osteopenia is reported to be 15–23% and 48–55%, respectively (Bonjoch, 2010; Brown, 2006; Cazanave, 2008). Consequently, decreases in BMD on dual-energy X-ray absorptiometry scanning are being observed with increasing frequency. In one study, 73% of HIV-infected patients receiving ART had reduced BMD compared to 30% of HIV-negative patients of similar age (Tebas, 2000). Interestingly, HIV infection per se, but not ART, may be related to an age-adjusted bone loss in addition to other traditional risk factors, such as low body weight, smoking, and steroid use (Amiel, 2004). HIV-infected women have a higher prevalence of osteopenia compared to age-matched non-HIV women (Dolan, 2004), and a lower vertebral bone density was associated with increased visceral adiposity in HIV-infected patients (Koutkia, 2005). Not surprisingly, HIV-infected patients are reported to have an increased risk of fractures (Martin, 2004; McComsey, 2004; Prieto-Alhambra, 2014; Triant, 2008), and in the multicenter HIV Outpatient Study (HOPS), the age-adjusted fracture rate was higher in HIV-infected patients compared to the HIV-negative population (Young, 2011). A recent publication from the Women's Interagency HIV Study (WIHS) cohort noted that middle-aged HIV-infected women had a higher adjusted fracture rate compared to that of HIV-uninfected women (Sharma, 2015).

In addition to traditional risk factors contributing to bone loss—including advanced age, female gender, low body mass index, lack of physical activity, smoking and alcohol abuse, deficiency of vitamin D together with secondary hyperparathyroidism, subnormal calcium intake, and hypogonadism—the presence of HIV infection per se, co-infection with hepatitis C, and the use of certain antiretroviral medications such as tenofovir can also facilitate bone loss in HIV-infected patients (Cotter, 2014; Dao, 2011; Gibellini, 2008; Jacobson, 2008; Kooij, 2015; Muller, 2010; Sherwood, 2012; Womack, 2013). In addition, secondary causes of bone loss caused by hyperthyroidism, hypercortisolemia (endogenous or iatrogenic), hypogonadism, hyperparathyroidism, renal impairment, and hypovitaminosis D must be actively screened for and treated.

Treatment of osteoporosis in HIV patients is similar to that in the general population. Traditional risk factors discussed previously should be addressed, and any identified secondary causes should be treated. Vitamin D deficiency should be corrected and patients encouraged to increase calcium intake. Pharmacotherapy with oral weekly alendronate is effective, convenient, and simple (Rozenberg, 2012). Alendronate, vitamin D, and oral calcium have been successfully used to increase BMD in HIV patients with osteopenia and osteoporosis (Mondy, 2005). Zoledronic acid, another bisphosphonate, is administered annually by the intravenous route and has been shown to improve BMD in HIV-infected patients (Bolland, 2012; Negredo, 2015).

CONCLUSIONS

HIV-infected patients can be affected by endocrine abnormalities. Although the more common disorders are dyslipidemia, diabetes, metabolic syndrome, and insulin resistance, other disorders affecting bone, adrenal glands, pituitary, and thyroid function may also be present. For rapid diagnosis and treatment of endocrine disorders in HIV-infected patients, both early referral to and working together with an endocrinologist are recommended.

References

Agarwal A, Soni A, Ciechanowsky M, et al. Hyponatremia in patients with the acquired immunodeficiency syndrome. *Nephron.* 1989; 53:317–321.

Amiel C, Ostertag A, Slama L, et al. BMD is reduced in HIV-infected men irrespective of treatment. *J Bone Miner Res.* 2004; 19:402–409.

Beltran S, Lescure FX, Desailloud R, et al. Increased prevalence of hypothyroidism among human immunodeficiency virus-infected patients: A need for screening. *Clin Infect Dis.* 2003; 37:579–583.

Biglia A, Blanco JL, Martínez E, et al. Gynecomastia among HIV-infected patients is associated with hypogonadism: A case–control study. *Clin Infect Dis.* 2004 Nov 15; 39(10):1514–1519.

Bolland MJ, Grey A, Horne AM, et al. Effects of intravenous zoledronate on bone turnover and bone density persist for at least five years in HIV-infected men. *J Clin Endocrinol Metab.* 2012 Jun; 97(6):1922–1928.

Bonjoch A, Figueras M, Estany C, et al. High prevalence of and progression to low bone mineral density in HIV-infected patients: A longitudinal cohort study. *AIDS.* 2010; 24:2827.

Bourdoux PP, De Wit SA, Servais GM, et al. Biochemical thyroid profile in patients infected with human immunodeficiency virus. *Thyroid.* 1991; 1:147–149.

Bricaire F, Marche C, Zoubi D, et al. Adrenocortical lesions and AIDS. *Lancet.* 1988; 1:881.

Brown TT, Cole SR, Li X, et al. Antiretroviral therapy and the prevalence and incidence of diabetes mellitus in the multicenter AIDS cohort study. *Arch Intern Med.* 2005; 165:1179–1184.

Brown TT, Qaqish RB. Antiretroviral therapy and the prevalence of osteopenia and osteoporosis: A meta-analytic review. *AIDS.* 2006; 20:2165.

Calkins JH, Siegel MM, Nankin HR, et al. Interleukin-1 inhibits Leydig cell steroidogenesis in primary cell culture. *J Clin Endocrinol Metab.* 1988; 123:1605–1610.

Calza L, Manfredi R, Chiodo F. Subclinical hypothyroidism in HIV-infected patients receiving highly active antiretroviral therapy. *J Acquir Immune Defic Syndr.* 2002; 31:361–363.

Caron M, Auclair M, Vigouroux C, et al. The HIV protease inhibitor indinavir impairs sterol regulatory element-binding protein-1 intranuclear localization, inhibits preadipocyte differentiation, and induces insulin resistance. *Diabetes.* 2001; 50:1378–1388.

Carr A, Samaras K, Burton S, et al. A syndrome of peripheral lipodystrophy, hyperlipidaemia and insulin resistance in patients receiving HIV protease inhibitors. *AIDS.* 1998 May 7; 12(7):F51–F58.

Cazanave C, Dupon M, Lavignolle-Aurillac V, et al. Reduced bone mineral density in HIV-infected patients: Prevalence and associated factors. *AIDS.* 2008; 22:395.

Chirgwin KD, Feldman J, Muneyyirci-Delale O, et al. Menstrual function in human immunodeficiency virus-infected women without acquired immunodeficiency syndrome. *J Acquir Immune Defic Syndr Hum Retrovirol.* 1996. 12:489–494.

Collazos J, Esteban M. Has prolactin a role in the hypogonadal status of HIV-infected patients? *J Int Assoc Physicians AIDS Care (Chic).* 2009 Jan–Feb; 8(1):43–46.

Collazos J, Ibarra S, Martinez E, et al. Serum prolactin concentrations in patients infected with HIV. *HIV Clin Trials.* 2002; 3: 133–138.

Cotter AG, Sabin CA, Simelane S, et al. Relative contribution of HIV infection, demographics and body mass index to bone mineral density. *AIDS.* 2014; 28:2051.

Cozzolino M, Vidal M, Arcidiacono MV, et al. HIV-protease inhibitors impair vitamin D bioactivation to 1,25-dihydroxyvitamin D. *AIDS.* 2003; 17:513–520.

Crum NF, Furtek KJ, Olson PE, et al. A review of hypogonadism and erectile dysfunction among HIV-infected men during the pre- and post-HAART eras: Diagnosis, pathogenesis, and management. *AIDS Patient Care STDS.* 2005 Oct; 19(10):655–671.

Crum-Cianflone NF, Bavaro M, Hale B, et al. Erectile dysfunction and hypogonadism among men with HIV. *AIDS Patient Care STDS.* 2007; 21:9–19.

Danaher PJ, Salsbury TL, Delmar JA. Metabolic derangement after injection of triamcinolone into the hip of an HIV-infected patient receiving ritonavir. *Orthopedics.* 2009 Jun; 32(6):450.

Dao CN, Patel P, Overton ET, et al. Low vitamin D among HIV-infected adults: Prevalence of and risk factors for low vitamin D Levels in a cohort of HIV-infected adults and comparison to prevalence among adults in the US general population. *Clin Infect Dis.* 2011; 52:396.

Dolan SE, Huang JS, Killilea KM, et al. Reduced bone density in HIV-infected women. *AIDS*. 2004; 18:475–483.

Drucker DJ, Bailey D, Rotstein L. Thyroiditis as the presenting manifestation of disseminated extrapulmonary *Pneumocystis carinii* infection. *J Clin Endocrinol Metab*. 1990; 71:1663–1665.

El-Sadr WM. Effects of HIV disease on lipid, glucose and insulin levels: Results from a large antiretroviral-naive cohort. *HIV Med*. 2005; 6:114–121.

Frost RA, Fuhrer J, Steigbigel R. Wasting in the acquired immune deficiency syndrome is associated with multiple defects in the serum insulin-like growth factor system. *Clin Endocrinol (Oxf)*. 1996: 44:501.

Gallant JE, Staszewski S, Pozniak AL, et al. Efficacy and safety of tenofovir DF vs. stavudine in combination therapy in antiretroviral-naive patients: A 3-year randomized trial. *JAMA*. 2004; 292:191.

Giampalmo A, Buffa D, Quaglia AC. AIDS pathology: Various critical considerations (especially regarding the brain, the heart, the lungs, the hypophysis and the adrenal glands). *Pathologica*. 1990 Nov–Dec; 82(1982):663–677.

Gibellini D, De Crignis E, Ponti C, et al. HIV-1 triggers apoptosis in primary osteoblasts and HOBIT cells through TNFalpha activation. *J Med Virol*. 2008; 80:1507.

Glasgow BJ, Steinsapir KD, Anders K, et al. Adrenal pathology in the acquired immune deficiency syndrome. *Am J Clin Pathol*. 1985; 84:594–597.

González-González JG, de la Garza-Hernández NE, Garza-Morán RA, et al. Prevalence of abnormal adrenocortical function in human immunodeficiency virus infection by low-dose cosyntropin test. *Int J STD AIDS*. 2001 Dec; 12(12):804–810.

Gray D, Roux P, Carrihill M, et al. Adrenal suppression and Cushing's syndrome secondary to ritonavir and budesonide. *S Afr Med J*. 2010 May 4; 100(5):296–297.

Grinspoon S, Corcoran C, Anderson E, et al. Sustained anabolic effects of long-term androgen administration in men with AIDS and wasting. *Clin Infect Dis*. 1999; 28:634–636.

Grinspoon S, Corcoran C, Lee K, et al. Loss of lean body and muscle mass correlates with androgen levels in hypogonadal men with acquired immunodeficiency syndrome and wasting. *J Clin Endocrinol Metab*. 1996; 81:4051–4058.

Grinspoon S, Corcoran C, Stanley T, et al. Mechanisms of androgen deficiency in human immunodeficiency virus-infected women with the wasting syndrome. *J Clin Endocrinol Metab*. 2001; 86:4120–4126.

Grunfeld C, Pang M, Doerrler W, et al. Lipids, lipoproteins, triglyceride clearance, and cytokines in human immunodeficiency virus infection and the acquired immunodeficiency syndrome. *J Clin Endocrinol Metab*. 1992; 74:1045–1052.

Hadigan C, Meigs JB, Corcoran C, et al. Metabolic abnormalities and cardiovascular disease risk factors in adults with human immunodeficiency virus infection and lipodystrophy. *Clin Infect Dis*. 2001; 32:130–139.

Hales DB. Interleukin1 inhibits Leydig cell steroidogenesis primarily by decreasing 17αhydroxylase/C17–20 lyase cytochrome P450 expression. *Endocrinology*. 1992; 131:2165–2172.

Hoffman CJ, Brown TT. Thyroid function abnormalities in HIV infected patients. *Clin Infect Dis*. 2007; 45:488–494.

Howell AL, Edkins RD, Rier SE, et al. Human immunodeficiency virus type 1 infection of cells and tissues from the upper and lower human female reproductive tract. *J Virol*. 1997; 71:3498–3506.

Huff A. Protease inhibitor side effects take people by surprise. *GMHC Treat Issues*. 1997–1998 Winter; 12(1):25–27.

Hutchinson J, Murphy M, Harries R, et al. Galactorrhoea and hyperprolactinoma associated with protease inhibitors. *Lancet*. 2000; 356:1003–1004.

Jacobson DL, Spiegelman D, Knox TK, et al. Evolution and predictors of change in total bone mineral density over time in HIV-infected men and women in the nutrition for healthy living study. *J Acquir Immune Defic Syndr*. 2008; 49:298.

Johnson SR, Marion AA, Vrchoticky T, et al. Cushing syndrome with secondary adrenal insufficiency from concomitant therapy with ritonavir and fluticasone. *J Pediatr*. 2006 Mar; 148(3):386–388.

Jubault V, Penformin F, Schillo F, et al. Sequential occurrence of thyroid autoantibodies and Grave's disease after immune restoration in severely immunocompromised human immuno-deficiency virus-1 infected patients. *J Clin Endocrinol Metab*. 2000; 85:4254–4257.

Kaviani N, Bukberg P, Manessis A, et al. Iatrogenic osteoporosis, bilateral HIP osteonecrosis, and secondary adrenal suppression in an HIV-infected man receiving inhaled corticosteroids and ritonavir-boosted highly active antiretroviral therapy. *Endocr Pract*. 2011 Jan–Feb; 17(1):74–78.

Keuneke C, Anders HJ, Schlöndorff D. Adipsic hypernatremia in two patients with AIDS and cytomegalovirus encephalitis. *Am J Kidney Dis*. 1999 Feb; 33(2):379–382.

Kooij KW, Wit FW, Bisschop PH, et al. Low bone mineral density in patients with well-suppressed HIV infection: Association with body weight, smoking, and prior advanced HIV disease. *J Infect Dis*. 2015; 211:539.

Koutkia P, Canavan B, Breu J, et al. Effects of growth hormone-releasing hormone on bone turnover in human immunodeficiency virus-infected men with fat accumulation. *J Clin Endocrinol Metab*. 2005; 90:2154–2160.

Koutkia P, Meininger G, Canavan B, et al. Metabolic regulation of growth hormone by free fatty acids, somatostatin, and ghrelin in HIV-lipodystrophy. *Am J Physiol Endocrinol Metab*. 2004 Feb; 286(2):E296–E303.

Mallon PW, Unemori P, Sedwell R, et al. In vivo, nucleoside reverse-transcriptase inhibitors alter expression of both mitochondrial and lipid metabolism genes in the absence of depletion of mitochondrial DNA. *J Infect Dis*. 2005 May 15; 191(10):1686–1696.

Manfredi R, Calza L, Chiodo F. Gynecomastia associated with highly active antiretroviral therapy. *Ann Pharmacother*. 2001 Apr; 35(4):438–439.

Manfredi R, Calza L, Chiodo F. Another emerging event occurring during HIV infection treated with any antiretroviral therapy: Frequency and role of gynecomastia. *Infez Med*. 2004 Mar; 12(1):51–59.

Martin K, Lawson-Ayayi S, Miremont-Salamé G, et al. Symptomatic bone disorders in HIV-infected patients: Incidence in the Aquitaine cohort (1999–2002). *HIV Med*. 2004; 5:421.

McComsey GA, Huang JS, Woolley IJ, et al. Fragility fractures in HIV-infected patients: Need for better understanding of diagnosis and management. *J Int Assoc Physicians AIDS Care (Chic)*. 2004; 3:86.

Membreno L, Irony I, Dere W, et al. Adrenocortical function in acquired immunodeficiency syndrome. *J Clin Endocrinol Metab*. 1987; 65:482–487.

Merrill JE, Koyanagi Y, Chen ISY. Interleukin-1 and tumor necrosis factor α can be induced from mononuclear phagocytes by human immunodeficiency virus type 1 binding to the CD4 receptor. *J Virol*. 1989; 63:4404–4408.

Meyer WJ, Smith EM, Richards GE, et al. In vivo immunoreactive adrenocorticotropin (ACTH) production by human mononuclear leukocytes from normal and ACTH-deficient individuals. *J Clin Endocrinol Metab*. 1987; 64:98–105.

Minami R, Yamamoto M, Takahama S, et al. Comparison of the influence of four classes of HIV antiretrovirals on adipogenic differentiation: The minimal effect of raltegravir and atazanavir. *J Infect Chemother*. 2011 Apr; 17(2):183–188.

Mishriki YY. A baffling case of bulging belly: Protease paunch. *Postgrad Med*. 1998 Sep; 104(3):45–46.

Mondy K, Powerly WG, Claxton SA, et al. Alendronate, vitamin D, and calcium for the treatment of osteopenia/osteoporosis associated with HIV infection. *J Acquir Immune Defic Syndr*. 2005; 38:426–431.

Mueller NJ, Fux CA, Ledergerber B, et al. High prevalence of severe vitamin D deficiency in combined antiretroviral therapy-naive and successfully treated Swiss HIV patients. *AIDS*. 2010; 24:1127.

Murata H, Hruz PW, Mueckler M. The mechanism of insulin resistance caused by HIV protease inhibitor therapy. *J Biol Chem*. 2000; 275:20251–20254.

Mylonakis E, Koutkia P, Grinspoon S. Diagnosis and treatment of androgen deficiency in human immunodeficiency virus-infected men and women. *Clin Infect Dis.* 2001; 33:857–864.

Negredo E, Bonjoch A, Pérez-Álvarez N, et al. Comparison of two different strategies of treatment with zoledronate in HIV-infected patients with low bone mineral density: Single dose versus two doses in 2 years. *HIV Med.* 2015 Aug; 16(7):441–448.

Norbiato G, Bevilacqua M, Vago T, et al. Glucocorticoids and interferon-alpha in the acquired immunodeficiency syndrome. *J Clin Endocrinol Metab.* 1996; 81:2601–2606.

Padmapriyadarsini C, Ramesh Kumar S, et al. Dyslipidemia among HIV-infected patients with tuberculosis taking once-daily nonnucleoside reverse-transcriptase inhibitor-based antiretroviral therapy in India. *Clin Infect Dis.* 2011 Feb 15; 52(4):540–546.

Parra A, Reyes-Terán G, Ramírez-Peredo J, et al. Differences in nocturnal basal and rhythmic prolactin secretion in untreated compared to treated HIV-infected men are associated with CD4+ T-lymphocytes. *Immunol Cell Biol.* 2004 Feb; 82(1):24–31.

Peyriere H, Mauboussin JM, Rouanet I, et al. Report of gynecomastia in five male patients during antiretroviral therapy for HIV infection. *AIDS.* 1999. 13:2167–2169.

Pinto G, Blanche S, Thiriet I, et al. Growth hormone treatment of children with human immunodeficiency virus-associated growth failure. *Eur J Pediatr.* 2000; 159:937–938.

Prieto-Alhambra D, Güerri-Fernández R, De Vries F, et al. HIV infection and its association with an excess risk of clinical fractures: A nationwide case–control study. *J Acquir Immune Defic Syndr.* 2014; 66:90.

Quirino T, Bongiovanni M, Ricci E, et al. Hypothyroidism in HIV-infected patients who have or have not received HAART. *Clin Infect Dis.* 2004; 38:596–597.

Ram S, Acharya S, Fernando JJ, et al. Serum prolactin in HIV infection. *Clin Lab.* 2004; 50:617–620.

Ratner Kaufman F, Gertner JM, Sleeper LA, et al. Growth hormone secretion in HIV-positive versus HIV-negative hemophilic males with abnormal growth and pubertal development. The Hemophilia Growth and Development Study. *J Acquir Immune Defic Syndrome Hum Retrovirol.* 1997; 15:137–144.

Rietschel P, Corcoran C, Stanley T, et al. Prevalence of hypogonadism among men with weight loss related to human immunodeficiency virus infection who were receiving highly active antiretroviral therapy. *Clin Infect Dis.* 2000; 31:1240–1244.

Rondanelli M, Caselli D, Arico M, et al. Insulin-like growth factor 1 (IGF-1) and IGF-binding protein 3 response to growth hormone is impaired in HIV-infected children. *AIDS Res Hum Retroviruses.* 2002; 18:331–339.

Rozenberg S, Lanoy E, Bentata M, et al.; Fosivir Study Group. Effect of alendronate on HIV-associated osteoporosis: A randomized, double-blind, placebo-controlled, 96-week trial (ANRS 120). *AIDS Res Hum Retroviruses.* 2012 Sep; 28(9):972–980.

Saint-Marc T, Partisani M, Poizot-Martin I, et al. A syndrome of peripheral fat wasting (lipodystrophy) in patients receiving long-term nucleoside analogue therapy. *AIDS.* 1999 Sep 10; 13(13):1659–1667.

Salim YS, Faber V, Wiik A, et al. Anticorticosteroid antibodies in AIDS patients. *APMIS.* 1988; 96:889–894.

Samaras K, Pett S, Gowers A, et al. Iatrogenic Cushing's syndrome with osteoporosis and secondary adrenal failure in human immunodeficiency virus-infected patients receiving inhaled corticosteroids and ritonavir-boosted protease inhibitors: Six cases. *J Clin Endocrinol Metab.* 2005 Jul; 90(7):4394–4398.

Samaras K, Wand H, Law M, et al. Prevalence of metabolic syndrome in HIV infected using International Diabetes Foundation and Adult Treatment Panel III criteria: Associations with insulin resistance, disturbed body fat compartmentalization, elevated C-reactive protein, and hypoadiponectinemia. *Diabetes Care.* 2007; 30:113–119.

Sekhar RV, Jahoor F, White AC, et al. Metabolic basis of HIV-lipodystrophy syndrome. *Am J Physiol Endocrinol Metab.* 2002 Aug; 283(2):E332–E337.

Sharma A, Shi Q, Hoover DR, et al. Increased fracture incidence in middle-aged HIV-infected and HIV-uninfected women: Updated results from the Women's Interagency HIV Study. *J Acquir Immune Defic Syndr.* 2015 Sep 1; 70(1):54–61.

Sherwood JE, Mesner OC, Weintrob AC, et al. Vitamin D deficiency and its association with low bone mineral density, HIV-related factors, hospitalization, and death in a predominantly black HIV-infected cohort. *Clin Infect Dis.* 2012; 55:1727.

Shikuma CM, Hu N, Milne C, et al. Mitochondrial DNA decrease in subcutaneous adipose tissue of HIV-infected individuals with peripheral lipoatrophy. *AIDS.* 2001; 15:1801–1809.

Sobieszczyk ME, Hoover DR, Anastos K, et al. Prevalence and predictors of metabolic syndrome among HIV-infected and HIV-uninfected women in the Women's Interagency HIV Study. *J Acquir Immune Defic Syndr.* 2008; 48:272–280.

Stricker RB, Goldberg DA, Hu C, et al. A syndrome resembling primary aldosteronism (Conn syndrome) in untreated HIV disease. *AIDS.* 1999; 13:1791–1792.

Szebeni J, Dieffenbach C, Wahl SM, et al. Induction of alpha interferon by human immunodeficiency virus type 1 in human monocyte–macrophage cultures. *J Virol.* 1991; 65:6362–6364.

Tebas P, Powderly WG, Claxton S, et al. Accelerated bone mineral loss in HIV-infected patients receiving potent antiretroviral therapy. *AIDS.* 2000; 14:F63–F67.

Tien PC, et al. Antiretroviral therapy exposure and incidence of diabetes mellitus in the Women's Interagency HIV study. *AIDS.* 2007; 21:1739–1745.

Toma E, Therrien R. Gynecomastia during indinavir antiretroviral therapy in HIV infection. *AIDS.* 1998; 12:681–682.

Tracey KJ, Cerami A. Metabolic responses to cachectin/TNF: A brief review. *Ann N Y Acad Sci.* 1990; 587:325–331.

Triant VA, Brown TT, Lee H, et al. Fracture prevalence among human immunodeficiency virus (HIV)-infected versus non-HIV-infected patients in a large U.S. healthcare system. *J Clin Endocrinol Metab.* 2008; 93:3499.

Tzur F, Chowers M, Agmon-Levin N, et al. Increased prevalence of diabetes mellitus in a non-obese adult population: HIV-infected Ethiopians. *Isr Med Assoc J.* 2015 Oct; 17(10):620–623.

Villette JM, Bourin P, Doinel C, et al. Circadian variations in plasma levels of hypophyseal, adrenocortical and testicular hormones in men infected with human immunodeficiency virus. *J Clin Endocrinol Metab.* 1990; 70:572–577.

Visnegarwala F, Chen L, Raghavan S, et al. Prevalence of diabetes mellitus and dyslipidemia among antiretroviral naïve patients co-infected with hepatitis C virus (HCV) and HIV-1 compared to patients without co-infection. *J Infect.* 2005; 50:331–337.

Wanke CA, Silva M, Knox TA, et al. Weight loss and wasting remain common complications in individuals infected with human immunodeficiency virus in the era of highly active antiretroviral therapy. *Clin Infect Dis.* 2000; 31:803.

Womack JA, Goulet JL, Gibert C, et al. Physiologic frailty and fragility fracture in HIV-infected male veterans. *Clin Infect Dis.* 2013; 56:1498.

Xiong Y, Hales DB. The role of the tumor necrosis factor-alpha in the regulation of mouse Leydig cell steroidogenesis. *Endocrinology.* 1993; 132:2438–2444.

Yombi JC, Maiter D, Belkhir L, et al. Cushing's syndrome and secondary adrenal insufficiency after a single intra-articular administration of triamcinolone acetonide in HIV-infected patients treated with ritonavir. *Clin Rheumatol.* 2008 Dec; 27(Suppl 2):S79–S82.

Young B, Dao CN, Buchacz K, et al. Increased rates of bone fracture among HIV-infected persons in the HIV Outpatient Study (HOPS) compared with the US general population, 2000–2006. *Clin Infect Dis.* 2011; 52:1061.

36.

NON-OPPORTUNISTIC INFECTIONS

RESPIRATORY COMPLICATIONS

Karen J. Vigil

LEARNING OBJECTIVE

Discuss the established and evolving science regarding non-infectious respiratory complications related to HIV infection so that conditions will be accurately diagnosed and treated.

KEY POINTS

Lymphocytic Interstitial Pneumonitis

- Lymphocytic interstitial pneumonitis (LIP) is a common respiratory complication of HIV infection in children but a rare complication in HIV-infected adults.

- It presents with slowly progressive dyspnea, nonproductive cough, and fever. X-ray findings are nonspecific but characteristically show bilateral reticulonodular "interstitial" infiltrates with a lower lung zone predominance.

- The diagnosis requires histologic confirmation by biopsy. Antiretroviral therapy has been used with success for treatment.

Nonspecific Interstitial Pneumonitis

- Nonspecific interstitial pneumonitis (NSIP) presents with dyspnea, nonproductive cough, and fever in a patient with CD4$^+$ T cell counts >200 cells/mm^3. X-ray findings are nonspecific but characteristically show bilateral reticulonodular "interstitial" infiltrates.

- The diagnosis of NSIP requires histologic confirmation by biopsy. The optimum treatment remains unclear.

Pulmonary Arterial Hypertension

- The prevalence of pulmonary arterial hypertension (PAH) is higher in HIV-infected patients compared to the general population.

- The clinical presentation is similar to that in the general population, with progressive dyspnea, nonproductive cough, chest pain, and sometimes syncope or near syncope.

- The diagnosis is first suggested by chest radiograph revealing prominent pulmonary arteries or by electrocardiogram. Right heart catheterization is the standard of diagnosis. Patients have a mean pulmonary arterial pressure (mPAP) ≥25 mmHg, a mean pulmonary capillary wedge pressure ≤15 mmHg, and a normal or reduced cardiac output.

- Potential therapies for HIV-associated PAH include HIV antiretroviral therapy as well as supportive therapy, including oxygen, diuretics, and anticoagulation. Although there are no controlled clinical trials, prostanoids (epoprostenol, treprostinil, and iloprost), endothelin receptor antagonists (bosentan), and phosphodiesterase-5 inhibitors (sildenafil) have been used in patients with HIV-associated PAH.

HIV LYMPHOID INTERSTITIAL PNEUMONITIS

Lymphoid interstitial pneumonitis accounts for 40% of lung diseases in children with AIDS but only 1% or 2% of lung diseases in HIV-infected adults (Anderson, 1988; Stover, 1985).

Histologically, LIP is characterized by diffuse infiltration with predominantly small lymphocytes and plasma cells and histiocytes in the alveolar septae and along lymphatic vessels (Halprin, 1972). Although the etiology of LIP is not clear, it has been suggested that Epstein–Barr virus (EBV) may play a role. EBV DNA samples have been found in fragments of lung tissues taken from children with LIP (Reddy, 1988). In addition, Epstein–Barr-positive serology has been identified in HIV-infected children and adults with LIP (Barbera, 1992). HIV itself may play a role in the pathology of LIP. HIV RNA copies have been obtained in lung biopsy samples of patients with LIP, and HIV-specific IgG is frequently present in the bronchoalveolar lavage fluid (Resnick, 1987). Human T-lymphotropic virus type I (HTLV-I) has been linked to LIP in Japan (Setoguchi, 1991).

The clinical presentation of LIP is similar in adults and children. Patients complain of slowly progressive dyspnea, nonproductive cough, and fever. Chest pain, weight loss, and arthralgias have also been reported. Physical exam may be completely normal or may reveal crackles. Children may have clubbing, salivary gland enlargement, lymphadenopathy, and hepatosplenomegaly.

Chest X-rays are normal or show bilateral reticular or nodular opacities. Focal areas of confluent pulmonary opacifications have been described as well as pulmonary cysts and patchy consolidations, the latter being less common. Chest computed tomography shows diffuse ground-glass opacities with small nodules (2–3 mm) in a peribronchovascular distribution (Pitcher, 2010). Similar to other diffuse interstitial lung diseases, spirometry typically shows decreased total lung capacity and decreased diffusing capacity.

There is no consensus regarding the optimal treatment for LIP in HIV-infected patients. Corticosteroids at a dosage of 1 mg/kg/day are recommended. However, in several case reports, highly active antiretroviral therapy (HAART) has been demonstrated to be effective by itself (Garcia Lujan, 2004; Innes, 2004; Ripamonti, 2003).

NONSPECIFIC INTERSTITIAL PNEUMONITIS

The prevalence of NIP is unknown. It was found in 48% of asymptomatic patients with AIDS in the 1980s (Ognibene, 1988) and in 38% of patients with AIDS and pulmonary symptoms or abnormal imaging studies (Suffredini, 1987). Different from LIP, it has been characterized only in adults and not in children.

The etiology of NIP is unknown. Histologically, it is characterized by the presence of lymphoid aggregates with or without germinal centers, mainly peribronchiolar and perivascular; however, these are also found along the pleura and interlobar fibrous septate (Travis, 1992).

Clinical symptoms are minimal or nonexistent; dyspnea, nonproductive cough, and fever have been reported (Suffredini, 1987). Physical exam may reveal crackles. Imaging studies may be normal or may show diffuse interstitial infiltrates. Pleural effusions, alveolar infiltrates, and nodules may also be seen. Similar to LIP, spirometry typically shows decreased diffusing capacity. Definitive diagnosis is made by histologic confirmation. The treatment is unclear.

PULMONARY ARTERIAL HYPERTENSION

Pulmonary arterial hypertension has a higher prevalence among HIV-1-infected patients compared to the general population. It was reported to be 0.5% in 1991 (Speich, 1991) and remains the same in the HAART era (Opravil, 2008; Sitbon, 2008; Zuber, 2004).

The occurrence of PAH in HIV-infected patients is not related to the CD4[+] T cell count. No risk factors have been found. However, it is more frequent in intravenous drug users. In a series that compared PAH in HIV-infected patients and PAH in non-HIV-infected subjects, the HIV-infected patients were significantly younger and had milder disease (50% vs. 75% had New York Heart Association functional class III or IV) (Petipretz, 1994).

The clinical presentation of patients with HIV and PAH is similar to that of uninfected patients. Patients experience symptoms related to right heart dysfunction, such as progressive shortness of breath, pedal edema, nonproductive cough, fatigue, syncope, and chest pain. Physical exam may reveal increased intensity of the pulmonary second heart sound, third and fourth sound gallop, tricuspid and pulmonary regurgitation murmurs, elevated jugular venous pressure, and peripheral edema.

The diagnosis is usually made 6 months after the development of symptoms. Chest X-rays may show cardiomegaly, enlarged pulmonary artery, but clear lung fields. Transthoracic Doppler echocardiogram shows systolic flattening of the interventricular septum, enlargement of the right atrium and the right ventricle, and a reduction in both left ventricular systolic and left ventricular diastolic dimensions. It is important to note that a thorough evaluation should be done to exclude other causes of pulmonary hypertension.

Right heart catheterization is still the standard for diagnosing HIV PAH and for assessing its severity and response to treatment. PAH is defined by an mPAP ≥25 mmHg, a mean pulmonary capillary wedge pressure ≤15 mmHg, and a normal or reduced cardiac output (Galie, 2009).

Treatment of HIV-associated PAH is similar to that of PAH in non-HIV-infected patients. Supportive therapy includes oxygen administration, diuretics, digoxin, and oral anticoagulants. Oxygen is recommended if arterial blood oxygen pressure is ≤60 mmHg. Diuretics reduce the right ventricular preload and are recommended in patients with right ventricular failure. The role of digoxin is controversial; however, it has been shown to improve cardiac output in patients with acutely right ventricular dysfunction attributable to PAH. Due to evidence of thrombosis of the small arterioles on postmortem examination in patients with idiopathic PAH, long-term anticoagulation is recommended. Specific therapy for PAH has also been evaluated in patients with HIV-associated PAH. Although there are no controlled clinical trials, prostanoids (epoprostenol, treprostinil, and iloprost), endothelin receptor antagonists (bosentan), and phosphodiesterase-5 inhibitors (sildenafil) have been used in patients with HIV-associated PAH and have been shown to improve symptoms and hemodynamic parameters. Caution should be taken with the use of these medications due to possible severe drug interactions, particularly with protease inhibitors. Although there is no evidence of the effect of antiretrovirals on the progression of HIV-associated PAH, it is recommended to start HAART in all patients with PAH, regardless of the CD4+ cell count. HAART has been demonstrated to cause improvements in pressure gradient over time and to significantly reduce the risk of death in patients with HIV-associated PAH.

Prognosis is poor. The majority of patients with HIV and PAH die within 1 year of diagnosis mainly of complications of PAH rather than HIV infection.

References

Anderson V, Lee H. Lymphocytic interstitial pneumonitis in pediatric AIDS. *Pediatr Pathol.* 1988; 8:417–421.

Barbera J, Hayashi S, Hegele R, et al. Detection of Epstein–Barr virus in lymphocytic interstitial pneumonia by in situ hybridization. *Am Rev Respir Dis.* 1992; 145:940–946.

Galie N, Hoeper M, Humbert M. Guidelines for the diagnosis and treatment of pulmonary hypertension. *Eur Heart J.* 2009; 30:2493–2537.

Garcia Lujan R, Echave-Sustaeta J, Garcia Quero C, et al. Lymphoid interstitial pneumonia resolved through antiretroviral therapy in an adult infected by human immunodeficiency virus. *Arch Bronconeumol.* 2004; 40:537–539.

Halprin G, Ramirez J, Pratt O. Lymphoid interstitial pneumonia. *Chest.* 1972; 62:418–423.

Innes A, Huang L, Nishimura S. Resolution of lymphocytic interstitial pneumonitis in an HIV infected adult after treatment with HAART. *Sex Transm Infect.* 2004; 80:417–418.

Ognibene F, Masur H, Rogers P, et al. Nonspecific interstitial pneumonitis without evidence of *Pneumocysitis carinii* in asymptomatic patients infected with human immunodeficiency virus (HIV). *Ann Intern Med.* 1988; 109:874–879.

Opravil M, Sereni D. Natural history of HIV-associated pulmonary arterial hypertension: Trends in the HAART era. *AIDS.* 2008; 22:35–40.

Petipretz P, Brenot F, Azarian R. Pulmonary hypertension in patients with human immunodeficiency virus infection: Comparison with primary pulmonary hypertension. *Circulation.* 1994; 89:2722–2727.

Pitcher R, Beningfield S, Zar H. Chest radiographic features of lymphocytic pneumonitis in HIV-infected children. *Clin Radiol.* 2010; 65:150–154.

Reddy A, Lyall E, Crawford D. Epstein–Barr virus and lymphoid interstitial pneumonitis: An association revisited. *Pediatr Infect Dis J.* 1988; 17:82–83.

Resnick L, Pitchenik A, Fisher E, et al. Detection of HTLVIII/LAV specific IgG and antigen in bronchoalveolar lavage fluid from two patients with lymphocytic interstitial pneumonitis associated with AIDS related complex. *Am J Med.* 1987; 82:553–556.

Ripamonti D, Rizzi M, Maggiolo F, et al. Resolution of lymphocytic interstitial pneumonia in a human immunodeficiency virus infected adult following the start of highly antiretroviral therapy. *Scand J Infect Dis.* 2003; 35:348–351.

Setoguchi Y, Takahashi S, Nukiwa T, et al. Detection of human T-cell lymphotropic virus type I-related antibodies in patients with lymphocytic interstitial pneumonia. *Am Rev Respir Dis.* 1991; 144:1361.

Sitbon O, Lascoux-Combe C, Delfraissy JF, et al. Prevalence of HIV-related pulmonary arterial hypertension in the current antiretroviral therapy era. *Am J Respir Crit Care Med.* 2008; 177:108–113.

Speich R, Jenni R, Opravil M, et al. Primary pulmonary hypertension in HIV infection. *Chest.* 1991; 100:1268–1271.

Stover D, White D, Romano P, et al. Spectrum of pulmonary diseases associated with the acquired immune deficiency syndrome. *Am J Med.* 1985; 78:429–437.

Suffredini A, Ognibene F, Lack E, et al. Nonspecific interstitial pneumonitis: A common cause of pulmonary disease in the acquired immunodeficiency syndrome. *Ann Intern Med.* 1987; 107:7–13.

Travis W, Fox C, Devaney K. Lymphoid pneumonitis in 50 adult patients infected with the human immunodeficiency virus: Lymphocytic interstitial pneumonitis versus nonspecific interstitial pneumonitis. *Hum Pathol.* 1992; 23:529–541.

Zuber J, Calmy A, Evison J. Pulmonary arterial hypertension related to HIV infection improved hemodynamics and survival associated with antiretroviral therapy. *Clin Infect Dis.* 2004; 38:1178–1185.

37.

PSYCHIATRIC ILLNESS AND TREATMENT IN HIV POPULATIONS

Elizabeth David

CHAPTER GOAL

This chapter discusses the psychiatric concomitants of HIV illness and the role of psychiatric care in the overall treatment of HIV populations.

LEARNING OBJECTIVES

- Discuss the bidirectional causes of the close association between HIV infection and psychiatric illness/symptoms.

- Recognize symptoms suggesting the presence of a psychiatric component to the clinical picture.

- Describe general principles of treatment and when specifically intervention by mental health professionals is advised.

WHAT'S NEW?

This chapter has been updated to reflect terminology from the fifth edition of the *Diagnostic and Statistical Manual of Mental Disorders* (DSM-5; American Psychiatric Association, 2013), and additional recommendations regarding in- and outpatient psychiatric consultation have been added.

INTRODUCTION

From the earliest recognized AIDS deaths in 1981 to the commencement of highly active antiretroviral therapy (HAART) in the mid-90s and the simpler combination ART regimens now available, HIV has remained a disease and an epidemic in constant evolution. For many years

a near-certain death sentence, it has become a treatable chronic condition, with issues of HIV-associated dementia and rapid death by opportunistic infection generally replaced by treatment of "premature" aging and slow neurological decline and questions of maximizing adherence to treatment. Issues that have not changed include the tremendous psychosocial burden to the individual and family, the economic cost to the patient and society, as well as factors of stigmatization and marginalization of HIV populations. Many HIV-infected individuals were already stigmatized before contracting this illness. The prevalence of HIV infection is much higher in gay/bi/transsexual populations, in people of color, in substance abusers, in prison populations, in the homeless, in individuals with histories of physical and emotional trauma, and in people with mental illness (Whetten, 2008). HIV infection then adds to the burden through the psychological manifestations it causes (demoralization, depression, mania, anxiety, insomnia, and neurocognitive deficits), through disturbances in appearance (wasting, lipodystrophy, and Kaposi's sarcoma) and function (kidney disease, diabetes, and chronic pain), and through tremendous losses (people, independence, health, employment, and sense of control). From the earliest days of the epidemic, it has been recognized that mental illness and HIV infection are closely related (Hoffman, 1984), with some estimates of comorbidity as high as 50–70% (Blashill, 2011; Gaynes, 2008). Psychiatric illnesses are in and of themselves potentially lethal conditions, with increased rates of suicide and increased rates of illness and death from other conditions, including cancer, diabetes, and cardiovascular and cerebrovascular disease. They are associated with tremendous costs in terms of quality of life, lost productivity, and treatment. In combination with HIV-related illness, these issues are magnified.

Addressing these complex mental health issues is central to prevention, diagnosis, and treatment of HIV-related illness. Psychiatric illness is both a risk factor for disease and a barrier to adequate treatment. Substance abuse and "triple diagnosis" patients (HIV, substance abuse, and mental illness) have been particularly problematic (see Chapter 30). The chronically mentally ill are both overrepresented in this population and more difficult to reach and treat due to homelessness, distrust, and the unstructured nature of their lives. Survivors of physical and emotional trauma are a group increasingly recognized as both vulnerable to HIV infection and difficult to treat. They are prone to risk behaviors but slow to establish trusting relationships with treaters. In addition to these issues of primary mental illness is the factor of secondary mental health problems—those caused by the virus and/or its treatment.

MENTAL ILLNESS AND HIV INFECTION

The interaction between HIV and mental illness is complex. For many individuals, the psychiatric condition is a preexisting one, predisposing to HIV infection through behavioral factors and risk environment (Rhodes, 2002). The risk factors for HIV are well established and involve blood/bodily fluid contact with infected individuals through unprotected sexual behaviors, needle sharing, multiple sexual partners, and fetal/natal exposure. Individuals with preexisting psychiatric illness often engage in risky behaviors with little thought or fear of consequences. This relates to increased emotional immaturity and impulsivity (bipolar disorder, personality disorders, anxiety conditions, and post-traumatic stress disorder (PTSD)), poor contact with reality (schizophrenia and other psychotic conditions), denial and disinhibition (substance use disorders), cognitive dysfunction (major neurocognitive disorders and dementia), active thoughts of self-harm (depression), and victimization or impaired judgment (Kent, 2011; Owe-Larssom, 2009). Barriers to treatment, such as distrust of authority (including fear of legal consequences), poor communication skills, limited access (financial and transportation), lack of motivation, and unstructured lifestyle, all result in poor overall health care and delayed diagnosis of all health issues. Diagnosis of mental health issues is frequently challenging, and adherence to treatment is frequently impacted by these same factors.

Even for patients without psychiatric illness, the diagnosis of serious medical illness is a significant emotional blow. Freud stated that emotional health involves the ability to integrate and balance aspects of love, work, and play (Freud, 1910). What could more thoroughly disrupt this balance and integration than an illness such as HIV, with so many devastating consequences, such a complex regimen of treatment, and so many far-reaching biological, psychological, and social consequences? Every day, every pill, every medical visit, and every secret kept from family, friends, and coworkers is a reminder that one is compromised, vulnerable, damaged, not normal. In her landmark work, Kubler-Ross discussed this trauma and the individual's response to it through repetitive processes of denial, anger, bargaining, and depression before (ideally) reaching a degree of acceptance (Kubler-Ross, 1969). Treaters see the negative aspect of this emotional upheaval in its behavioral correlates: unrealistic anger at medical staff, equally unrealistic expectations of outcomes, guilt, fear, increased substance use, demoralization/hopelessness/amotivation, poor adherence to treatment, suicidal thoughts/suicide, and helplessness/neediness. We can help through building a positive and supportive treatment alliance that facilitates communication, acknowledges the huge cost to the patient, tolerates some of the stress behaviors, and does not take these behaviors personally but also sets limits of appropriateness. Timely referral to a psychiatrist or a psychotherapist is essential when stress becomes distress and behavior goes beyond those limits of appropriateness or when the patient becomes dangerous to him- or herself or others.

HIV enters the central nervous system (CNS) very early in the course of systemic infection, and the brain becomes an important site of damage in patients with HIV/AIDS (Ho, 1985). This causes many of those infected to develop neurological and psychological symptoms with etiology posited to relate to the presence of viral particles, neuro-immunological and neuroinflammatory responses, disruption of dopamine pathways and dopamine depletion (Kumar, 2011), and cytokine activation (Brafanca, 2011). Accelerated aging from HIV infection and HIV treatments, damage caused by opportunistic infections or comorbid medical conditions (e.g., hepatitis C virus), and concomitant use of drugs of abuse (Gannon, 2011) also play important roles. AIDS mania and a continuum of neurocognitive deficits from very subtle to frank and debilitating dementia are well-defined psychiatric syndromes directly related to the presence of virus, but depression, insomnia, and anxiety are also among the mental health symptoms that result from the infection itself. This part of disease progression seems to be less amenable to treatment with HAART compared to the more peripheral manifestations (Heaton, 2010), although antiretrovirals with higher levels of CNS penetration may promote improvement in some functions (Cysique, 2004). Unfortunately, those agents capable of crossing the blood–brain barrier are also the medications most likely to have psychiatric symptomatology as a side effect of use—a Pyrrhic victory in many ways.

Regardless of etiology, the presence of psychiatric symptoms and substance abuse is associated with poorer outcomes in HIV illness—lower levels of treatment adherence, slower virologic suppression, less subjective quality of life, increased morbidity and mortality, and increased utilization of medical services (Blashill, 2011; Carrico, 2011; Leserman, 2008; Nel, 2011; Pence, 2007). Adequate treatment of the psychiatric illness, however, improves outcome across all categories (Cook, 2006; Horberg, 2008; Mellins, 2009; Walkup, 2008). Although most of the literature cited in this chapter relates to HIV-infected adults, the diagnostic descriptions and treatments can, for the most part, be applied to adolescents and children (Benton, 2010; Rao, 2007).

PSYCHIATRIC DISORDERS AND TREATMENT

Careful diagnosis is essential given the complex interaction between psychiatric illness, HIV infection, substance abuse, comorbid medical conditions, and side effects of medications. Psychiatric illness cannot be diagnosed if these others medical factors play the primary role in causing symptoms (i.e., delirium), and psychiatric medications will seldom be of benefit in those cases. The following brief descriptions are based on the criteria from DSM-5 (American Psychiatric Association, 2013). The context of HIV infection results in no appreciable changes from the usual clinical manifestations of psychiatric disorders, with the possible exception of AIDS mania. Equally, pharmacological and nonpharmacological approaches to the treatment of psychiatric illness in the context of HIV illness are not radically different from those in HIV-negative populations. HIV-infected patients do seem to have some increased sensitivity to the side effects of the older "first-generation" antipsychotic drugs, even absent antiretroviral treatment (Kent, 2011). Because many psychopharmacologic agents are metabolized by the same elements of the cytochrome P450 isoenzyme system that metabolize protease inhibitors and non-nucleoside/nucleotide reverse transcriptase inhibitors, there were many fears early on that they could not be used concomitantly. In fact, however, there are surprisingly few clinically significant interactions except as specifically noted in the following sections. As in all clinical situations, however, a "start low and go slow" philosophy is warranted, and the relative risks and benefits of treatment must be carefully weighed.

Stress and Adjustment Disorders

There are multiple stressors associated with living with a serious and debilitating illness. Some kinds of emotional and behavioral reactions to this stress are normal, short-lived, and do not require treatment beyond support, reassurance, education, and therapeutic optimism. Assistance with access to resources and support networks or with informing family or significant others of the diagnosis can be "curative." Such reactions typically occur immediately after diagnosis and at periods of acute change in the illness (opportunistic infections, deteriorating CD4/viral load indices, initiation of antiretroviral therapy, and onset of other comorbid medical complications) or in social circumstances (loss and financial problems). Typically, patients with these acute stress reactions are able to attribute the onset and nature of their symptoms to specific life events. They can also be distracted from their emotions and symptoms and are capable of feeling pleasure and interest in other things. *Adjustment reactions* (normal responses to stressful circumstances) are typically treated with supportive counseling and psychotherapy. It is only when stress reactions—anger, worry, guilt, sadness, and insomnia—are sustained for months, reach a point that they interfere with normal life functioning, or actually threaten survival (substance abuse, high-risk activities, and self-destructive thoughts/behaviors) that they require intervention. *Adjustment disorders* may also respond to support and psychotherapy, but they may necessitate psychiatric medications and/or hospital admission. The specific medication used depends on the symptoms being manifested. A complex of sadness, guilt, and insomnia frequently responds to use of antidepressants, particularly the more sedating ones (sertraline and mirtazapine). Symptoms on the anxiety continuum may benefit from use of almost any medication with a sedating side effect. Low-dose trazodone or antihistamine (hydroxyzine or diphenhydramine are commonly used) can be helpful, although caution must be used because these agents tend to cause drying of mucous membranes, which can exacerbate oral thrush. The use of benzodiazepines is rarely indicated (see later discussion). Because of the known relationship between stress and compromised immune function, early appropriate intervention is important (Leserman, 2008).

Anxiety Disorders and PTSD

This group of illnesses includes generalized anxiety disorder (persistent feelings of anxiety), the phobias (irrational fear of a particular thing or behavior), panic disorder (spontaneous attacks of intense anxiety), and obsessive–compulsive disorder (intrusive anxiety-provoking thoughts that compel ritualized behaviors thought to alleviate that anxiety). PTSD (anxiety-related thoughts and behaviors connected to memories of past traumatic life experiences) was formerly included in this group, but it has been separated into its own category in DMS-5. All involve activation of the sympathetic nervous system (psychological and physiological fight–flight–freeze responses) in situationally inappropriate circumstances because there is no current emergency. Careful diagnosis requires that endocrine disorders (especially thyroid-related), substance use (including caffeine, steroids, and psychostimulants), agitated depression, dementia, and delirium be eliminated as primary etiological factors. HIV-infected individuals have rates of anxiety disorders greater than those of the general population (Gaynes, 2008; Klinkenberg, 2004; Martinez, 2002), as well as an increased incidence of past traumatic experiences (Pence, 2009). Treatment ideally consists of a combination of psychotherapy (supportive, interpersonal, mindfulness, cognitive–behavioral, biofeedback, exposure and response prevention, flooding, etc.) and psychopharmacotherapy with antidepressants and/or anti-anxiety agents. Because therapeutic benefit with antidepressant is delayed in onset, it may be useful to supplement early treatment with low-dose benzodiazepine—lorazepam or other short-acting agent for panic disorder or phobis (used prn onset of panic attack or exposure to phobic object, but no more than three or four times a day) and clonazepam or other long-acting medication for generalized anxiety. Benzodiazepines are rarely the regimen of choice for more than the first 2–4 weeks, however, and should be discontinued at the earliest time practical. Some alternative treatments have also been shown to be effective, including relaxation/meditation, breath training, acupuncture, and guided imagery. All of the antidepressants except bupropion have efficacy in anxiety disorders, and selection of a specific medication should be based on safety (the serotonin and serotonin/norepinephrine reuptake inhibitors (SNRIs) are overall much safer than tricyclics or monoamine oxidase inhibitors), side effect profile (relative sedation vs. excitation, potential for gastric symptoms, appetite stimulation vs. suppression, anticholinergic effects, concerns for liver function, assistance with pain control, etc.), and past response to medications in the patient or a family member. The selective serotonin reuptake inhibitors (SSRIs) can increase dream and flashback symptoms in patients with past traumatic experiences, although small doses of prazocin can mitigate this effect. As noted previously, anti-anxiety agents include benzodiazepines, antihistamines, buspirone, and small doses of antidepressants (e.g., trazodone) or atypical antipsychotics (e.g., seroquel—an

off-label use). All except buspirone work by sedating the patient, and they can be taken at the onset of anxiety symptoms. (Buspirone, like the antidepressants, must be taken on a regular basis to be effective.) The benzodiazepines also disinhibit behaviors, cause various degrees of cognitive impairment including amnesia and motor slowing/incoordination (a serious issue in a population already at risk for neurocognitive impairment), increase the risk of falls, and can trigger relapse or increased substance use in patients with substance abuse problems. They are meant for temporary use only and can usually be discontinued when the antidepressants have become effective (2–4 weeks). A consensus survey of psychiatrists treating HIV revealed clonazepam to be the most frequently used benzodiazepine, followed by lorazepam (Freudenreich, 2010). Alprazolam, midazolam, and triazolam should be avoided due to their high potential for addiction and their adverse interactions with antiretroviral drugs (ARVs). Again, the byword for concomitant use of any psychopharmacologic agent with ARV is "Start low. Go slow."

Affective Disorders

Disorders of mood, particularly depression, are the most common psychiatric manifestations of HIV disease, with rates much higher in HIV-infected individuals than in the general population (Berger-Greenstein, 2007; Gaynes, 2011; Treisman, 2007) and increasing frequency with advancing disease (Atkinson, 2008). Depression hinders treatment of HIV-infected individuals, increasing risk of disease progression and spread (Benton, 2008; Villes, 2007), and may have direct effects on immune responses (Alciati, 2007). Risk of suicidal ideation and attempts is significantly increased (Fermamdez, 2006), as is successful suicide (Carrico, 2010). Adequate treatment, however, reverses all these trends for both depression (Horberg, 2008; Mellins, 2009; Walkup, 2008) and bipolar disorder (Walkup, 2011).

Major depression consists of a constellation of symptoms related to persistent low mood (crying spells, guilt, low self-esteem, negative ruminations, social isolation, and loss of pleasure and interest), mental slowing (poor attention, concentration, memory, and energy; loss of libido; and motor retardation), and changes in behavior (increased or decreased sleep or appetite). Those with severe illness may also have psychotic symptoms—hallucinations and delusions—usually with depressive content. Careful diagnosis is essential because many of these symptoms might also be caused by serious medical illness, major neurocognitive impairment (dementia and delirium), side effects of medications, substance abuse, or grief and loss. Unlike adjustment disorders, patients with major depression generally cannot cite a precipitating event nor be distracted from their negative emotions. It is the relentless nature of the symptoms that results in a sense of hopelessness and despair with a progressive narrowing of emotional focus until it may seem that death (suicide) is the only way out. Treatment ideally consists of combined psychotherapy and psychopharmacology with antidepressant medications, sometimes adding augmenting agents (a second antidepressant from another class, lithium, testosterone, thyroid medications, psychostimulants, and mood stabilizers). Low doses of antipsychotics are indicated on a temporary basis if psychotic features are present. Ketamine in very low doses is being used in some centers, but it must be used with extreme caution in patients on antiretroviral treatment. Alternative treatments including exercise, meditation/relaxation, acupuncture, and herbal medications have been found to be helpful. Patients on St. John's wort should be cautioned, however, because this popular herbal antidepressant has significant adverse clinical interactions with multiple ARVs, anticancer drugs, anti-inflammatory agents, antibiotics, psychopharmacologic agents, cardiovascular drugs, antihypoglycemics, oral contraceptives, proton pump inhibitors, statins, and anti-asthmatic medications (Di, 2008). All of the normal antidepressant drugs show efficacy in the HIV-infected population, and choice of a particular medication should be based on safety (Watkins, 2011), side effect profile, and past response to medications in the patient or a family member. A consensus study revealed that the SSRIs are the most common first-line drugs, with citalopram the number one choice (Freudenreich, 2010), although this may be changing with newer US Food and Drug Administration warnings about QT prolongation caused by this medication in higher doses. The SSRIs do have an anticoagulant effect, and used long term, they can result in significant decreases in bone density. They can also cause bruxism and extrapyramidal side effects as well as sexual dysfunction. Switching drugs within a pharmacologic class is of benefit if patients find specific side effects intolerable. If a medication in any given class of antidepressants fails to show therapeutic benefit (8- to 12-week trial of adequate doses), a switch to another class of drugs is advised because agents within any given class have similar efficacy (Warden, 2007), so a switch to an SNRI (venlafaxine and duloxetine) and then to bupropion is a useful algorithm when there is treatment failure (Freudenreich, 2010). Particular caution is suggested in using bupropion (either as an antidepressant or in smoking cessation) in combination with the protease inhibitors (especially saquinavir or indinavir) or non-nucleoside reverse transcriptase inhibitors

(NNRTIs; especially efavirenz) because metabolism of bupropion can be inhibited, thus increasing the risk of seizures. Lopinavir/ritonavir, on the other hand, increases metabolism of bupropion, so bupropion doses must be increased when used with this antiretroviral combination (Hogeland, 2007). Currently, mirtazapine is considered to be a second-line choice, although it can be particularly useful for patients with chronic pain, weight loss, nausea, and vomiting (especially from chemotherapy regimens). Monoamine oxidase inhibitors (MAOIs) are not generally used in this population, and they are contraindicated for concomitant use with other antidepressants and most antipsychotics. (Remember that the antibiotic linezolid is also an MAOI.) All antidepressant regimens take several weeks to have therapeutic benefit, and the symptoms may not all resolve simultaneously. For this reason, particular caution and close observation are warranted in the early weeks of treatment: If energy, motivation, and a sense of agency return before suicidal thoughts and impulses disappear, a person who has had suicidal thoughts but insufficient energy to act on them may suddenly find the energy to act. The use of antidepressants in children and younger adolescents is particularly fraught with danger of suicide, and most antidepressant medications now carry a black box warning for this population. Inpatient psychiatric treatment is necessary if there are questions of safety, and this is obviously a situation in which it is best to err on the side of caution. Duration of treatment is a significant question. In the general population, an individual with a single episode of depression is generally treated for 4–6 months, whereas individuals with more than two episodes receive protracted therapy with antidepressants. Because of concurrent medical illnesses, stress, and the propensity for HIV virus to cause/exacerbate affective symptoms, long-term use of antidepressants is frequently necessary.

Bipolar disorder is defined by intermittent episodes of low (depressive) and high (hypomanic or manic) moods, each lasting days, weeks, or months and in a continuum of severity from mild to disabling. These mood swings are not a reaction to life events. The lows are identical to the depressive episodes described previously. The high episodes consist of persistent elevated mood tone (euphoric or irritable), increased energy (racing thoughts that bounce from topic to topic, little need for sleep, rapid speech, and increased libido), and an inflated sense of self-worth, and they often lead to engaging in risky behaviors. In mania, there is frank psychosis, with delusions (usually grandiose), disorganized thinking, and hallucinations, leading to severe impairment in functioning and judgment. Psychopharmacologic treatment consists of mood stabilizer medications (lithium, valproic acid, carbamazepine, lamotrigine, and "second-generation" antipsychotic medications), with antidepressants and antipsychotics added if these symptoms are prominent. Some clinicians believe that long-acting benzodiazepine can be helpful in the first days of treatment for active mania, but these agents can further disinhibit and should be used only on a short-term basis. All of these medications are effective and reasonably safe in HIV populations. Lithium has a very narrow window of safety, and it is eliminated by the kidney. Particular caution is necessary in patients with kidney dysfunction, diarrhea, electrolyte disturbances, or cognitive impairment, but there are no specific interactions with antiretrovirals. Lithium can cause or exacerbate thyroid dysfunction, tremor, acne, and psoriasis. Valproic acid appears to have few clinically significant drug interactions with the antiretrovirals. However, it is metabolized by the liver, and it can increase liver enzymes and cause ammonemia. In addition, there is risk of severe hepatitis, weight gain, thrombocytopenia, nystagmus, and tremor. The use of carbamazepine is more complicated: It is metabolized by the cytochrome P450 system, and it induces its own metabolism. There have been reports of clinically significant carbamazepine toxicity when used in combination with ritonavir and other potent CYP3A4 inhibitors and also of virologic failure caused by enzyme induction. In addition, carbamazepine causes a significant risk for bone marrow suppression. Lamotrigine is effective particularly for depressive symptoms and appears to be safe when used in combination with antiretroviral therapy. Initiation and discontinuation of this agent must be managed very carefully due to the risk of life-threatening rashes (Stevens–Johnson syndrome). It should be remembered that use of antidepressants without a mood stabilizer in a bipolar patient can trigger a manic episode.

AIDS mania is a specific manifestation of late-stage HIV infection. The mood is more likely to be irritable, sullen, and withdrawn than euphoric and hypertalkative, and there is frequently no prior personal or family history of psychiatric illness. Otherwise, the symptoms are typical of mania. Episodes, however, tend to be protracted, frequently with a prodrome of progressive cognitive decline. Symptoms do not usually respond to the usual psychopharmacological approaches, nor is there spontaneous remission if the condition is left untreated. The treatment of choice is initiation of aggressive antiretroviral therapy.

Psychotic Disorders

The psychotic disorders are defined by loss of contact with reality (hallucinations and delusions) as well as by varying degrees of disorganized thinking and behavior. Insight and judgment are compromised, and it is frequently difficult to communicate clearly with these individuals because they can seem lost in their own, sometimes quite bizarre, world. Symptoms can be present on a temporary/episodic basis (brief psychotic episode and schizophreniform disorder) or may be more chronic (schizophrenia). Although disruption of thinking and behavior are most typical, any psychotic illnesses may involve some affective symptoms, even if only because patients recognize that they are somehow damaged and different. When symptoms of an emotional nature (depression or excitation) are a prominent and invariate part of the psychosis, schizoaffective disorder must be considered. Differential diagnosis includes affective disorder with psychotic features, medical illness (psychosis secondary to a medical condition such as HIV), side effects of medications, delirium/dementia, and substance abuse. Initial medical workup of anyone with a new-onset psychosis should probably include a urine drug screen (although many of the newer synthetic substances do not appear on standard tests), serology, endocrine screen, liver function tests, and computed tomography and/or magnetic resonance imaging of the brain. Visual hallucinations are rare in primary psychiatric illness, and they should also prompt a more complete medical evaluation. The chronically mentally ill are at increased risk of exposure to HIV due to factors such as homelessness, poor insight/judgment, lack of knowledge, victimization, and increased rates of substance abuse and other high-risk behaviors. Without adequate psychiatric treatment, their psychosis is a serious barrier to medical treatment due to poor adherence, difficulties communicating with providers, and unstable lifestyle (Carrico, 2011). Treatment consists of control of symptoms with medications along with psychosocial support. All of the antipsychotic medications work in HIV-infected patients. As previously noted, HIV-positive individuals, even without antiretroviral treatment, seem to be somewhat more sensitive to the dopamine-mediated extrapyramidal side effects of these drugs. These side effects are most common with the high-potency first-generation antispychotics (i.e., haloperidol and fluphenazine). Both the first-generation and newer antipsychotics have significant risk for metabolic, cardiac (prolonged QT intervals), and endocrine side effects, and all are metabolized by the liver. They do not seem to have clinically significant interactions with antiretroviral treatments with the possible exception of lurasidone, but the issue of QT prolongation should be closely monitored because some of the antiretrovirals also have this side effect. In the consensus survey, quetiapine was the most commonly used agent for psychosis, perhaps because it is also useful in mood stabilization and sedation (Freudenreich, 2010). A recent meta-analysis also revealed that quetiapine is the safest of the antipsychotic drugs to use for psychosis and behavioral control in demented patients (Kales, 2012). Clozapine and the low-potency first-generation medications (chlorpromazine and thioridazine) are seldom used (Freudenreich, 2010), although certainly not contraindicated. Use of depo injections tends to result in fewer side effects than seen with daily oral formulations and can be particularly useful in individuals for whom compliance with antipsychotic medication is problematic. It is safest, however, to initiate treatment with oral medication and then switch to the long-acting forms later.

Personality Disorders and the Difficult-to-Treat Patient

Personality can be thought of as enduring patterns of behavior, and this is partly what we refer to when we say we "know" a person—he or she has somewhat predictable responses to given circumstances, a familiar emotional tone, consistent belief systems, and a well-formed sense of identity and agency. When these patterns are stable and healthy, one's responses to adversity (coping techniques) help to mitigate stress, and one can modulate emotional responses to fit the circumstances, thus maintaining a stable sense of self and other and control over one's world. In personality disorders, an individual is stuck in repetitive patterns that do not work: coping techniques that actually escalate stressful situations, relationship paradigms that result in little perceived support and an increasing sense of frustration by and with others, spiraling loss of emotional control, and ultimately the fearful recognition that one is out of control of both internal and external worlds. Borderline and antisocial personality disorders are common in HIV-infected populations because these individuals tend to engage in high-risk behaviors that expose them to contracting the virus. The presence of these character pathologies also complicates treatment adherence (Hansen, 2009). They tend to be easily frustrated, to expect immediate gratification, to want sure-fire/magical interventions, and to demand "special" treatment from everybody. They also challenge authority and have limited ability to adequately and consistently structure their own lives. As difficult and challenging as it can be to work with these individuals, it is important to remember that their behavior is not intentional—it is their best effort to adjust to and control their chaotic world (Groves, 1978). Frequently, the emotions they engender in others are only reflections of the emotional turmoil within themselves. These are patients for whom referral

to psychotherapy and the presence of a strong, consistent treatment team with a clearly delineated treatment contract are essential to preserve coherent participation in medical care. Because their psychological symptoms tend to be so reactive to events in the environment, switching rapidly and wildly, caution should be used in initiating medications. Although consistent use of an SSRI or a mood stabilizer may be useful, chasing symptoms with medications is contraindicated. It is generally much more useful to help these patients understand that their problems are related to their own patterns of response and poor behavioral choices than to teach them that some medication is going to provide them with internal peace or a sense of purpose, meaning, security, and attachment.

Substance Use Disorders

For a full discussion of this topic, see Chapter 30. Suffice it to say here that concurrent substance abuse complicates diagnosis and treatment of all other psychiatric conditions as well as HIV-related illnesses. These complications, as well as problems with adherence to treatment and overall morbidity and mortality, are additive in nature. It is essential to good treatment of HIV illness that clinicians screen for substance abuse and address it consistently and aggressively.

Major Neurocognitive Disorders (Delirium and Dementia)

HIV infection is associated with a number of CNS complications that may be temporary (delirium) or permanent (the continuum of neurocognitive deficits from asymptomatic to frank dementia). Dementia is a common manifestation of HIV illness, and it is discussed in Chapter 45. Delirium is a potentially life-threatening medical condition, generally of sudden and rapid onset and pursuing a waxing and waning course. Neurologists call this encephalopathy, and it is the most common neuropsychiatric diagnosis in hospitalized or critically ill HIV patients, with an estimated frequency of 40–65% (Gallago, 2011). It can manifest with any psychiatric symptom (anxiety, depression, mania, and psychosis) but most frequently includes disturbances in orientation, awareness/alertness, reality testing (hallucinations, including visual—which are very unusual in primary psychiatric conditions), communication (mumbled, incoherent speech), and motor behavior (lethargy, agitation, and picking at skin/clothing/intravenous lines). Several screening tools are used to diagnose delirium, of which the Cognitive Assessment Measurement Scale (CAMS and CAMS-ICU) is probably the most thoroughly researched. Definitive treatment involves correction of the underlying medical condition (infection, electrolyte disturbance, medication side effect, endocrine imbalance, intoxication, etc.). *Temporary* use of low-dose antipsychotic medications can be helpful, but they should be tapered and discontinued as the delirium resolves. Avoid the use of any anticholinergic agents and of antipsychotics with high anticholinergic side effects (thorazine and thioridazine). Olanzapine, a sedating antipsychotic, may help with agitation but has been reported to cause/exacerbate/prolong delirium in some cases. Use of benzodiazepines is also generally counterproductive with the obvious exception of delirium caused by alcohol or benzodiazepine withdrawal. Measures that improve the patient's connection with reality can be very helpful. These include constant soft lighting (patients tend to misperceive shadows), quiet and soothing background noise, a visible clock and/or calendar in the room, a written list of names of nursing staff and others, and repeated self-introduction of caregivers and visitors.

Sexual Dysfunction

Sexual dysfunctions are very common in HIV illness. Disorders of desire (hypoactive sexual desire disorder) may be almost universal in HIV-positive men and women, and erectile dysfunction is very common in men with AIDS (Shindel, 2011). Although certainly related to stress, depression, and uncertainties about spreading the disease to sexual partners, it also seems likely that the virus itself, the myriad comorbid conditions (including hypogonadism, diabetes, and peripheral neuropathy), and the multiple medications used to treat all these conditions play a role. Treatment, therefore, is obviously complex. To the degree that these disorders are due to secondary issues, efforts can be made to change those conditions. Depression, stress, and comorbid conditions can be treated, and sometimes medications can be changed or doses modified to minimize sexual side effects. Sexual counseling and therapy are helpful in teaching the patient that sexual behavior and loving are not always about intercourse. Medications for erectile dysfunction (sildenafil, vardenafil, and tadalafil) can be used in this population, but doses must be reduced when given in the context of antiretroviral therapy because metabolism is delayed. This obviously increases the probability of adverse side effects from the erectile dysfunction drugs, including visual changes, priapism, hypotension, and myocardial infarct. As with all medications, risks and benefits must be carefully weighed by the patient and the clinician.

SLEEP DISTURBANCE

Insomnia is defined as difficulty initiating and/or maintaining sleep or overall non-restful sleep. It tends to impair daytime function, and it is even more common in HIV-positive individuals than in the general population. This condition has been linked to poor quality of life and nonadherence to treatment (Saberi, 2011). Stress and depression play a role in etiology, and some antiretrovirals disrupt sleep continuity. Efavirez, a medication from the NNRTI class, is most consistently associated with sleep disturbances, including delayed sleep initiation, impaired sleep maintenance, and vivid nightmares. However, it appears that insomnia may be a primary symptom of viral presence, with changes in sleep architecture and decreased sleep efficiency noted even prior to onset of any symptoms of HIV/AIDS (Norman, 1992). Pharmacological treatment of insomnia includes the use of benzodiazepines, nonbenzodiazepine hypnotics, antihistamines, antidepressants, and antipsychotics. Of the benzodiazepines, clonazepam, lorazepam, oxazepam, and temazepam are relatively safe, although as previously noted, their use in patients with current or past substance abuse is problematic. Use of alprazolam, flurazepam, quazepam, and triazolam is contraindicated with antiretrovirals and ketoconazole and also in patients with kidney or hepatic disease. Sustained use of benzodiazepine medications is rarely, if ever, indicated. All of the nonbenzodiazepine hypnotics (eszopiclone, zaleplon, and zolpidem) are relatively safe in HIV populations, although dosages of zolpidem should be reduced if it used with protease inhibitors, even in boosting dosages. Dosages of all nonbenzodiazepine hypnotics should also be reduced in patients with hepatic disease. Antihistamines (especially diphenhydramine and hydroxyzine) are effective in many patients, and they are safe in HIV populations. However, it should be remembered that some patients have paradoxical excitatory responses to these medications. Sleep induction is an off-label use for any antidepressant or antipsychotic. Nonetheless, low-dose tricyclics (especially doxepin and amitriptyline) and mirtazapine can be very useful in this regard. They can also help with control of neuropathic pain, which can improve sleep quality. In higher doses, all are associated with weight gain, which can be beneficial in some cases. Trazodone is frequently used to induce and maintain sleep in normal populations, but its use in HIV-positive patients on antiretroviral therapy is problematic because final metabolism of the trazodone is slowed and untoward side effects (sleep disruption, vivid dreams, increased sedation, anxiety, and hypotension) occur. Of the antipsychotics, quetiapine and olanzapine are frequently used, although again, this is an off-label usage. As previously noted, HIV-infected individuals are much more sensitive to the extrapyramidal side effects of these medications. They also cause endocrine disturbances (prolactinemia) and metabolic side effects that may be cumulative with those of antiretroviral therapy, such as lipodystrophy, hyperlipidemia, and insulin resistance (Omonuwa, 2009).

PSYCHIATRIC EFFECTS OF ANTIRETROVIRAL THERAPY

Many of the antiretroviral agents have prominent psychiatric side effects that have been discussed previously. The most prominent of these psychiatric symptoms is vivid dreams and nightmares. Unfortunately, these issues seem to be more common, problematic, and sustained in individuals who are already vulnerable or experiencing psychiatric symptoms—that is, those with chronic mental illness. The vivid dreams and nightmares can be especially troubling for individuals with PTSD or past traumatic experiences. Although psychiatric diagnoses should not be a contraindication for use of these agents when indicated, special caution and close follow-up are certainly warranted. As with PTSD, low-dose prazocin can sometimes ameliorate the sleep disturbance experienced.

USE OF PSYCHIATRIC CONSULTATION

Mental health issues in HIV-infected individuals are very common. In an ideal world, mental health professionals would be integrated into every HIV treatment setting, and patients suspected of having significant illness or distress could be seen rapidly and frequently after referral. In reality, this is rarely the case, and even when psychiatrists and other mental health providers are on-site, visits are commonly delayed due to sheer numbers of patients. So when is referral most warranted and useful? First and foremost, the patient must be aware of and agree to mental health evaluation. Exceptions to this relate to those individuals who are incapable of understanding the need for assessment and treatment, who are imminently dangerous to self or other, or who are systematically destroying themselves and their treatment/treatment team by their behavior. Beyond that, the first part of a decision for referral rests on the primary problem and referring to the correct person. Certain individuals will benefit most from referral to support groups of like-minded people with similar problems, and many actually prefer this form of treatment. Although there are certainly exceptions, most psychiatrists are not the primary resource

for either substance abuse counseling or for individual/marital/group psychotherapy. The first task is handled, in general, by specific substance abuse counselors and by self-help groups (Alcoholics Anonymous, Narcotics Anonymous, etc.). Psychotherapy is also more frequently done by behavioral specialists other than psychiatrists—psychologists, social workers, licensed counselors, etc. Pain management and medical management of substance detox and sobriety are also frequently handled by other caregivers. In most settings, it is possible to refer directly to these providers, who can then screen for cases requiring specific psychiatric intervention. Psychologists are specifically trained in diagnostic processes (including psychological and neuropsychological testing and screening) and in psychotherapeutic interventions. Psychiatrists, although trained in behavioral interventions and therapy techniques, are medical doctors, and they are the first-line resource for evaluation of individuals with complex psychiatric/medical issues, those who will probably require psychotropic medications, and those who have not responded to conventional psychotropic medications. Although psychiatrists can be helpful in diagnosing delirium and can assist in behavioral management of symptoms, the presence of these major neurocognitive disorders (including acute intoxication) generally makes it impossible to ascertain if there is true psychiatric illness underlying the current medical process. The final caveat is this: When in doubt, consult. I know I would much rather be included when I am not needed than absent when I could be of help, and I think most psychiatrists feel the same.

CONCLUSIONS

From the earliest days of the AIDS epidemic, it has been apparent that large numbers of HIV-infected people also have psychiatric illness. This, of course, raises the question of the direction of relatedness: Is psychiatric illness a risk factor for HIV infection, or does the HIV virus cause or predispose to psychiatric symptoms? The answer seems to be "yes"—the association goes both ways. Individuals with psychiatric illness (depression, bipolar disorders, anxiety disorders, PTSD, schizophrenia, dementia, and substance use disorders) tend to engage in behaviors that place them at increased risk for exposure to the HIV virus. Contracting HIV infection results in numerous psychosocial stressors that trigger or exacerbate expression of psychological symptoms in vulnerable individuals. The virus itself precipitates changes in the CNS that cause psychiatric manifestations. Finally, treatment with certain of the current antiretroviral agents can result in psychiatric/behavioral symptoms. In turn, the presence of these psychiatric symptoms creates additional problems with diagnosis and treatment of HIV-related illnesses. All HIV-infected individuals should be screened for the presence of psychiatric illness. Fortunately, HIV-infected individuals respond well to traditional psychopharmacological and psychotherapeutic approaches to mental distress and illness, and with adequate psychiatric treatment, they have good adherence and response to HIV treatment. Psychiatric illness alone is no longer considered to be a contraindication to full treatment of HIV or AIDS.

References

Alciati A, Gallo L, Monforte AD, et al. Major depression-related immunological changes and combination antiretroviral therapy in HIV-seropositive patients. *Hum Psychopharmacol.* 2007; 22(1):33–40.

American Psychiatric Association. *Diagnostic and Statistical Manual of Mental Disorders* (5th ed.). Arlington, VA: American Psychiatric Publishing; 2013.

Atkinson JH, Heaeton RK, Patterson TL, et al. Two-year prospective study of major depressive disorder in HIV-infected men. *J Affect Disord.* 2008; 108:225–233.

Benton TD. Depression and HIV/AIDS. *Curr Psychiatry Rep.* 2008 Jun; 10(3):280–205.

Benton TD. Psychiatric considerations in children and adolescents with HIV/AIDS. *Child Adolesc Psychiatr Clin North Am.* 2010 Apr; 19(2):387–400.

Berger-Greenstein JA, Cuevas CA, Brady SM, et al. Major depression in patients with HIV/AIDS and substance abuse. *AIDS Patient Care STDS.* 2007; 21:942–949.

Blashill AJ, Perry N, Safren SA. Mental health: A focus on stress, coping, and mental illness as it relates to treatment retention, adherence, and other health outcomes. *Curr HIV/AIDS Rep.* 2011 Dec; 8(4):215–222.

Brafanca M, Palha A. HIV associated neurocognitive disorders. *Actas Esp Psiquiatr.* 2011; 39(6):374–383.

Carrico A. Elevated suicide rate among HIV-positive persons despite benefits of antiretroviral therapy: Implications for a stress and coping model of suicide. *Am J Psychiatry.* 2010; 167:117–119.

Carrico AW, Bangsberg DR, Weisner SD, et al. Psychiatric correlates of HAART utilization and viral load among HIV-positive impoverished persons. *AIDS.* 2011 May 15; 25(8):1113–1118.

Cook JA, Burke-Miller J, Anastos K, et al. Effects of treated and untreated depressive symptoms on highly active antiretroviral therapy use in a US multi-site cohort of HIV-positive women. *AIDS Care.* 2006 Feb; 18(2):3–100.

Cysique LA, Maruff P, Brew BJ. Prevalence and pattern of neuropsychological impairment in human immunodeficiency virus-infected/acquired immunodeficiency syndrome (HIV/AIDS) patients across pre- and post-highly active antiretroviral therapy eras: A combined study of two cohorts. *J Neurovirol.* 2004 Dec; 10(6):350–357.

Di YM, Li CG, Xue CC, et al. Clinical drugs that interact with St. John's wort and implication in drug development. *Curr Pharm Des.* 2008; 14(17):1723–1742.

Fernandez F, Ruiz P. *Psychiatric Aspects of HIV/AIDS.* Philadelphia: Lippincott Wilkins & Williams; 2006.

Freud S. Five lectures on psycho-analysis. *Am J Psychol.* 1910; 21.

Freudenreich O, Goforth HW, Cozza KL, et al. Psychiatric treatment of persons with HIV/AIDS: An HIV psychiatry consensus survey of current practices. *Psychosomatics.* 2010; 51:480–488.

Gallego L, Barreiro P, Lopez-Ibor JJ. Diagnosis and clinical features of major neuropsychiatric disorders in HIV infection. *AIDS Rev.* 2011; 13:171–179.

Gannon P, Khan MZ, Kolson DL. Current understanding of HIV-associated neurocognitive disorders pathogenesis. *Curr Opin Neurol.* 2011 Jun; 24(3):275–283.

Gaynes BN, Farley JF, Dusetzina SB, et al. Does the presence of accompanying symptom clusters differentiate the comparative effectiveness of second-line medication strategies for treating depression? *Depress Anxiety.* 2011 Nov; 28(11):989–998.

Gaynes BN, Pence BW, Eron JJ Jr, et al. Prevalence and comorbidity of psychiatric diagnoses based on reference standard in an HIV+ population. *Psychosom Med.* 2008; 70:505–511.

Groves, JE. Taking care of the hateful patient. *N Engl J Med.* 1978; 298:883–887.

Hansen N, Vaughan E, Cavanaugh C, et al. Health-related quality of life in bereaved HIV-positive adults: Relationships between HIV symptoms, grief, social support, and axis II indication. *Health Psychol.* 2009; 28:249–257.

Heaton RK, Clifford DB, Franklin DR, et al. HIV-associated neurocognitive disorders persist in the era of potent antiretroviral therapy: CHARTER study. *Neurology.* 2010 Dec 7; 75(23):2087–2096.

Ho D, Tota TR, Schooley RT, et al. Isolation of HTV-III from cerebrospinal fluid and neural tissues of patients with neurologic syndromes relate to the acquired immunodeficiency syndrome. *N Engl J Med.* 1985; 313(24):1493–1497.

Hoffman, RS. Neuropsychiatric complications of AIDS. *Psychosomatics.* 1984; 25:393–395.

Hogeland GW, Swindells S, McNabb JC, et al. Lopinavir/ritonavir reduces bupropion plasma concentrations in healthy subjects. *Clin Pharmacol Ther.* 2007 Jan; 81(1):69–75.

Horberg MA, Silverberg MJ, Hurley LB, et al. Effects of depression and selective serotonin reuptake inhibitor use on adherence to highly active antiretroviral therapy and on clinical outcomes in HIV-infected patients. *J Acquir Immune Defic Syndr.* 2008; 7(3):384–390.

Kales HC, Kim HM, Zivin K, et al. Risk of mortality among individual antipsychotics in patients with dementia. 2012 Jan 1; 169:71–79.

Kent LK, Blumenfield M. Psychodynamic psychiatry in the general medical setting. *J Am Acad Psychoanal Dyn Psychiatry.* 2011 Spring; 9(1):41–62.

Klinkenberg WD, Dacks SL; HIV/AIDS Treatment Adherence, Health Outcomes and Cost Study Group. Mental disorders and drug abuse in persons living with HIV/AIDS. *AIDS Care.* 2004; 16(Suppl 1):S22–S42.

Kubler-Ross E. *On Death and Dying.* New York, NY: Macmillan; 1969.

Kumar AM, Ownby RL, Waldrop-Valverde D, et al. Human immunodeficiency virus infection in the CNS and decreased dopamine availability: Relationship with neuropsychological performance. *J Neurovirol.* 2011; 17:26–40.

Leserman J. Role of depression, stress and trauma in HIV disease progression in HIV. *Psychosom Med.* 2008; 70:539–545.

Martinez A, Israelski BS, Walker C, et al. Posttraumatic stress disorder in women attending human immunodeficiency virus outpatient clinics. *AIDS Patient Care STDs.* 2002; 98:9–17.

Mellins CA, Havens JF, McDonnell C et al. Adherence to antiretroviral medications and medical care in HIV-infected adults diagnosed with mental and substance abuse disorders. *AIDS Care.* 2009 Feb; 21(2):168–177.

Nel A, Kagee A. Common mental health problems and antiretroviral therapy adherence. *AIDS Care.* 2011 Nov; 23(11):1360–1365.

Norman SE, Cheick AD, Freeman C, et al. Sleep disturbances in men with asymptomatic human immunodeficiency (HIV) infection. *Sleep.* 1992; 15:150–155.

Omonuwa TS, Goforth HW, Preud'homme X, et al. The pharmacologic management of insomnia in patients with HIV. *J Clin Sleep Med.* 2009 June 15; 5(3):251–262.

Owe-Larssom B, Sall, L, Allgulander C. HIV infection and psychiatric illness. *Afr J Psychiatry.* May 2009; 115–128.

Pence BW. The impact of mental health and traumatic life experiences on antiretroviral treatment outcomes for people living with HIV/AIDS. *J Antimicrob Chemother.* 2009 April; 63(4):636–640.

Pence BW, Miller WC, Gaynes BN, et al. Psychiatric illness and virologic response in patients initiating highly active antiretroviral therapy. *J Acquir Immune Defic Syndr.* 2007; 44(2):159–165.

Rao R, Sagar R, Kabra SK, et al. Psychiatric morbidity in HIV-infected children. *AIDS Care.* 2007 Jul; 19(6):828–833.

Rhodes T. The "risk environment": A framework for understanding and reducing drug-related harm. *Int J Drug Policy.* 2002; 13:85–94.

Saberi P, Neilands TB, Johnson MO. Quality of sleep: associations with antiretroviral nonadherence. *AIDS Patient Care STDS.* 20011 Sep; 26(9):517–524.

Shindel A, Horberg M Smith J, et al. Sexual dysfunction, HIV, and AIDS in men who have sex with men. *AIDS Patient Care STD.* 2011; 25:41–49.

Treisman G, Angelinno A. Interrelation between psychiatric disorders and the prevention and treatment of HIV infection. *Clin Infect Dis.* 2007; 45(Suppl 4):S313–S317.

Villes V, Spire B, Lewden C, et al. The effect of depressive symptoms at ART initiation on HIV clinical progression and mortality: Implications in clinical practice. *Antivir Ther.* 2007; 12:1067–1071.

Walkup J, Wei W, Sambamoorthi U, et al. Antidepressant treatment and adherence to combination antiretroviral therapy among patients with AIDS and diagnosed depression. *Psychiatr Q.* 2008; 79(1):43.

Walkup JT, Akincigil A, Chakravarty S, et al. Bipolar medication use and adherence to antiretroviral therapy among patients with HIV-AIDS and bipolar disorder. *Psychiatr Serv.* 2011 Mar; 62(3):313–316.

Warden D, Rush AJ. The STAR*D project results: A comprehensive review of findings. *Curr Psychiatry Rep.* 2007; 9(6):449–459.

Watkins CC, Pieper AA, Treisman GJ. Safety considerations in drug treatment of depression in HIV-positive patients: An updated review. *Drug Saf.* 2011 Aug 1; 34(8):623–639.

Whetten K, Reif S, Whetten R, et al. Trauma, mental health, distrust and stigma among HIV-positive persons: Implications for effective care. *Psychosom Med.* 2008; 70(5):531–538.

38.

HIV-ASSOCIATED NEUROCOGNITIVE DISORDERS

Rodrigo Hasbun, Richard Dunham, Joseph S. Kass, Rituparna Das,

Karen Nunez-Wallace, Lydia J. Sharp, and Doris Kung

LEARNING OBJECTIVE

Discuss the clinical features, differential diagnosis, and management of HIV-associated neurocognitive disorders.

WHAT'S NEW?

- CD8[+] T cell encephalitis has been described as a severe form of HIV-associated neurocognitive disorder (HAND).

- The central nervous system (CNS) penetration effectiveness score has been correlated with cerebrospinal fluid (CSF) viral escape.

- Recommendations in the diagnostic and therapeutic approach to HAND have been published by the Mind Exchange Group.

- Neurocognitive impairment has been associated with lack of retention in care in older adults.

- The impact of the CNS-targeted combination antiretroviral therapy (ART) on HAND is currently being explored.

KEY POINTS

- There is a high prevalence of HAND in antiretroviral treatment-naive patients and in patients treated with ART with virological suppression.

- Rapid screening tools such as the Montreal Cognitive Assessment test have been evaluated for their use in diagnosing HAND in the clinic.

- HAND is associated with significant cognitive, behavioral, and motor abnormalities that can impact ART compliance, retention in care in older individuals, and quality of life.

- CNS-targeted ART can be considered in patients with HAND, and corticosteroids can be considered in patients with CD8[+] T cell encephalitis.

Despite the use of combination ART, up to 39% of patients currently experience HAND (Robertson, 2007). It is unclear if inadequate CSF penetration by the majority of the antiretrovirals accounts for the high prevalence and whether CNS active ART improves cognitive impairment. However, higher CSF penetration scores have been correlated with a lower probability of detectable CSF HIV RNA levels.

HIV causes a chronic form of encephalitis (HIVE) that is clinically characterized by either dementia or mild neurocognitive impairment. Since the introduction of ART in 1996, the incidence of HIV dementia has decreased by 50% (McArthur, 2005), but the prevalence of mild neurocognitive disorder (MND) has increased up to 39% (Robertson, 2007). HIVE is the result of direct microglial infection, interruption of trophic factors, or caused by inflammatory cytokines (Boisse, 2008). HIV enters the brain primarily by the "Trojan horse mechanism": It is carried by monocytes and lymphocytes that cross the blood–brain barrier. HIV has a predilection for the basal ganglia, deep white matter, and hippocampus, resulting in a subcortical dementia. Brain computed tomography (CT) scanning or magnetic resonance imaging (MRI) typically show cerebral atrophy and symmetrical white matter lesions. HIV dementia is a diagnosis of exclusion; other co-infections (e.g., JC virus-associated progressive multifocal leukoencephalopathy, hepatitis C, neurosyphilis, and cryptococcal meningitis), cerebrovascular disease, malnutrition, and drug abuse should be ruled out before making the diagnosis. In patients receiving ART with immunological response, a novel condition called "CD8[+] T cell encephalitis" was recently described (Lescure, 2013). Patients can present

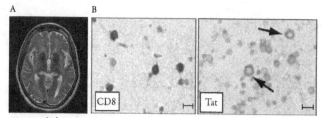

Figure 38.1 (A) Magnetic resonance imaging of an HIV-positive patient with virological suppression for 4 years with biopsy-proven CD8$^+$ T cell encephalitis. (B) The presence of CD8$^+$ T cells and HIV Tat antigens on brain biopsy. SOURCE: Adapted with permission from Johnson TP, Patel K, Johnson KR, et al. Induction of IL-17 and nonclassical T-cell activation by HIV-Tat protein. *Proc Natl Acad Sci USA.* 2013 Aug 13; 110:13588–13593.

with HAND, headache, focal neurological deficits, and seizures, with MRI of the brain showing bilateral white matter lesions. CSF usually shows a lymphocytic pleocytosis with CD8$^+$ T cells greater than 65%. A brain biopsy, if performed, shows pronounced CD8$^+$ T cell infiltration with the presence of scant HIV antigens (Figure 38.1) (Johnson, 2013). Patients improve dramatically with corticosteroids and with improved CNS penetration of their ART regimen. The optimal dose and duration of corticosteroids are currently unknown.

Neuropsychological impairment is a surrogate marker for the presence of HIVE on autopsy (Cherner, 2002). Cognitive impairment has also been associated with ART nonadherence (Maggiolog, 2007), lack of retention in care in older adults (Jacks, 2015), an negative impact on quality of life. In the pre-ART era, it was shown to be an independent predictor of death (Ellis, 1997). Furthermore, CSF HIV RNA levels are increased in HIV-1-infected individuals with neurocognitive impairment, as are several CSF biomarker levels, such as tumor necrosis-α, neurofilament light, neopterin, β_2 microglobulin, and monocyte chemotactic protein-1 (Boisse, 2008). A recent clinical model identified the following variables as associated with detectable CSF viral load: detectable serum HIV RNA on polymerase chain reaction (PCR), a CNS penetration score <9, non-Caucasian race, <95% ART adherence, depression, and <36 months of ART duration (Hammond, 2014).

CLINICAL MANIFESTATIONS OF HAND

The clinical features of HAND are related to the involvement of HIV in the subcortical structures. The following can occur: slowing of processing speed; motor and psychomotor abnormalities; and executive, planning, or multitasking dysfunction (Valcour, 2011a). HAND affects the following three areas:

- Cognitive: Memory, concentration, mental processing speed, and comprehension

- Behavioral: Apathy, depression, agitation, and sometimes mania

- Motor function: Unsteady gait, poor coordination, abnormal tone, and tremors

In addition, patients with CD8$^+$ T cell encephalitis can also manifest with new-onset seizures, status epilepticus, and altered mental status.

RISK FACTORS

Several studies have documented host genetic factors (polymorphisms in apolipoprotein E4, chemokine receptor CCR2, and monocyte chemoattractant protein-1), HIV-specific disease factors (history of AIDS-defining illness or low CD4$^+$ T cell nadir, particular HIV variants, HIV RNA levels in CSF, duration of HIV infection, and older age at conversion), and comorbidities (>50 years of age, anemia, vascular disease, metabolic abnormalities, and hepatitis C co-infection) associated with HAND (Alfahad, 2013).

SCREENING TOOLS FOR COGNITIVE IMPAIRMENT

Despite the high prevalence of HAND in HIV clinics, it has not become routine to screen patients for cognitive impairment or to consider more CNS-active ART for those affected, even though there are now recommendations from an international consortium to do so (Mind Exchange Working Group, 2013). Screening tools that have been evaluated in HAND include several versions of the HIV dementia scale, the Mini Mental Status Exam (MMSE), standardized questionnaires that assess symptoms such as the Medical Outcomes survey, and the Montreal Cognitive Assessment (MoCA). The dementia scales are reliable but only in severe cases of HAND, the MMSE is not sensitive enough to detect HAND, and the subjective reporting of cognitive symptoms will miss patients due to poor insight or due to mood disturbances (Valcour, 2011a,b). The MMSE is now proprietary. Recent studies have shown that the MoCA is a rapid, reliable, and sensitive test to detect cognitive impairment in HIV-1-infected individuals (Hasbun, 2012), and it is now the preferred screening test for HAND.

DEFINITIONS OF NEUROCOGNITIVE DISORDERS

In 2007, the diagnostic criteria for HIV-associated neurocognitive disorders were revised (Antinori, 2007). Three HANDs were defined in these new criteria: asymptomatic neurocognitive impairment (ANI), MND, and HIV-associated dementia (HAD). ANI was defined as having a combination of the following: (1) an acquired mild to moderate impairment in cognitive function documented by a score of at least 1 standard deviation (SD) below demographically corrected norms on tests on at least two different cognitive domains, (2) the functional impairment has been seen for more than 1 month, (3) the impairment does not meet criteria for delirium or dementia, and (4) the cognitive impairment is not fully explained by comorbid conditions. The definition of MND is identical to that of ANI, but it also includes interference with activities of daily living. The diagnosis of HAD includes a marked impairment of cognitive impairment.

CEREBROSPINAL FLUID ACTIVITY OF ANTIRETROVIRALS

There are currently more than 30 US Food and Drug Administration (FDA)-approved antiretrovirals or combinations in six mechanistic classes for treatment of HIV infection, but only some have adequate CSF penetration (US Department of Health and Human Services, 2016). The CNS penetration-effectiveness score has been designed to classify the different antiretrovirals with regard to their capability of lowering CSF RNA levels (Letendre, 2011). Antiretrovirals were assigned a score of from 1 to 4 based on their chemical properties, CSF penetration, and/or effectiveness in CNS studies (Table 38.1). A higher CNS penetration score was associated with higher virological suppression in the CSF (Letendre, 2010). Furthermore, a study showed that 10% of patients with virological suppression in the serum had viral escape (detectable CSF viral loads) (Eden, 2010). In addition, a higher CSF penetration score is associated with a lower rate of neurocognitive impairment (Carvalhal, 2016).

Very few randomized studies have evaluated the impact of CNS active antiretrovirals in HIV neurocognitive disorders. In the pre-ART era, zidovudine (AZT) demonstrated efficacy in the treatment of HIV-associated dementia in a randomized clinical trial. AIDS Clinical Trial Group Study 005 randomized HIV patients with dementia to 2000 mg of AZT per day, 1000 mg AZT per day, or placebo (Sidtis, 1993). The greatest neuropsychological improvement was seen in those patients treated with high-dose AZT. In the ART era, a trial involving 49 patients found no neurocognitive benefit of CNS-targeted ART (Ellis, 2014). Future HIV treatment guidelines are anticipated to change and

Table 38.1 CENTRAL NERVOUS SYSTEM PENETRATION-EFFECTIVENESS SCORE OF DIFFERENT ANTIRETROVIRALS (CPE SCORE)

	CPE SCORE			
DRUG CLASS	4	3	2	1
NRTIs	Zidovudine	Abacavir Emtricitabine	Didanosine Lamivudine Stavudine	Tenofovir Zalcitabine
NNRTIs	Nevirapine	Delavirdine Efavirenz	Etravirine	
Protease inhibitors	Indinavir	Darunavir/r Fosamprenavir/r Indinavir Lopinavir/r	Atazanavir Atazanavir/r Fosamprenavir	Nelfinavir Ritonavir Saquinavir Saquinavir/r Tipranavir/r
Entry/fusion inhibitors		Maraviroc		Enfuvirtide
Integrase inhibitors		Raltegravir Dolutegravir		

NNRTIs, non-nucleoside reverse transcriptase inhibitors; NRTIs, nucleoside reverse transcriptase inhibitors.

SOURCE: Adapted from Letendre (2011).

recommend cognitive screening and CNS ART as part of patients' evaluations.

Recommended Reading

Calcagno A, Di Perri G, Bonora S. Pharmacokinetics and pharmacodynamics of antiretrovirals in the central nervous system. *Clin Pharmacokinet*. 2014; 53(10):891–906. Available at https://www.ncbi.nlm.nih.gov/pubmed/25200312.

Letendre SL, Mills AM, Tashima KT, et al. ING116070: A study of the pharmacokinetics and antiviral activity of dolutegravir in cerebrospinal fluid in HIV-1-infected, antiretroviral therapy-naive subjects. *Clin Infect Dis*. 2014; 59(7):1032–1037. Available at https://www.ncbi.nlm.nih.gov/pubmed/24944232.

MYELOPATHY

LEARNING OBJECTIVE

Discuss the clinical presentation, differential diagnosis, and management of myelopathy in HIV-infected patients.

WHAT'S NEW?

The incidence of vacuolar myelopathy (VM) has been reduced significantly. It remains a cause of disability in end-stage HIV and has a poor prognosis.

KEY POINTS

- VM is an uncommon complication of HIV infection and tends to occur in the late stages of HIV infection.

- Acute transverse myelitis and inflammatory CSF are unlikely to be VM.

- Human T cell lymphotropic virus type 1 (HTLV-1) infection is another infectious cause of myelopathy, and it should be considered in endemic geographic areas and in cases of co-infection with HIV.

- HIV and HTLV-1 can both cause a chronic myelopathy involving dorsal and lateral columns.

- The workup for a myelopathic patient includes MRI of the spine with and without contrast and may include CSF analysis and investigations for nutritional deficiencies and toxic agents.

HIV-ASSOCIATED MYELOPATHY

Spinal cord injury, nonspecifically referred to as either myelopathy or myelitis, is a neurologic complication of HIV infection. Myelopathies in HIV-infected individuals can be due to either the direct effect of HIV invasion of the spinal cord, referred to as HIV-associated VM, or a secondary process such as an opportunistic infection or neoplasm that either invades or compresses the spinal cord.

VM is a chronic myelopathy seen in the late stages of HIV infection and affects 10–15% of untreated AIDS patients. Patients typically experience a slow, painless progression of neurologic symptoms over several months, most commonly lower extremity weakness and spasticity (Di Rocco, 1999). Patients also complain of progressive weakness or clumsiness in the lower extremities, as well as leg cramps and difficulty walking. Urinary symptoms such as frequency and urgency are also common, as is difficulty in achieving and maintaining an erection. Sensation in the legs, particularly proprioception and vibratory sense, is usually impaired, but a clear sensory level on the trunk is unusual. Arms are typically spared until advanced-stage disease. Localized back pain is not a common feature. Patients are also typically hyperreflexic in the lower extremities (hyperreflexia may spread to the upper extremities if the cervical cord is involved) and exhibit extensor plantar responses. VM patients present very similarly to patients with subacute combined degeneration due to vitamin B_{12} deficiency. Acute transverse myelitis, a prominent sensory level, or high numbers of inflammatory cells in the CSF should suggest another diagnosis. Although new HIV infections have been associated with acute myelopathy, this acute inflammatory process is a different entity from VM. Acute transverse myelitis associated with HIV seroconversion may respond well to steroids, intravenous immunoglobulin (IVIG), and ART (Hamada, 2011).

VM is the result of a chronic inflammatory degeneration with vacuolization and myelin pallor of the lateral and posterior tracts, typically affecting the thoracic cord most severely. On histologic examination, the lateral and dorsal columns demonstrate axonal injury and macrophage infiltration with lipid-laden macrophages and microglia infected with HIV (Dal Pan, 1997; Petito, 1994; Tyor, 1993). As many as 20–50% of AIDS patients may have pathological evidence of VM at autopsy (Dal Pan, 1994; Di Rocco, 1998; McArthur, 2005). However, it is relatively uncommon clinically, affecting only 6.5–10% of HIV-infected patients (Cho, 2012).

There is no effective treatment for VM. Patients with VM often have coexisting HIV-associated dementia and peripheral neuropathies. Rehabilitation is helpful to maximize physical capacity. ART does not appear to alter the natural history of the disease (Banks, 2002). Antispasmodic agents such as baclofen, tizanidine, and botulinum toxin can be used for symptomatic relief.

The differential diagnosis for myelopathy in an HIV patient is broad and includes the following categories: (1) infections including HTLV-1-associated myelopathy/tropical spastic paraparesis (HAM/TSP; discussed later), tuberculosis spondylitis or meningomyelitis, cytomegalovirus radiculomyelitis, varicella zoster myelitis, toxoplasma myelopathy, neurosyphilis with tabes dorsalis, and bacterial epidural abscess (particularly among intravenous drug users); (2) neoplastic diseases, especially lymphoma and spinal metastases from systemic neoplasms; (3) nutritional deficiencies such as B_{12}, folate, copper, thiamine (presenting as beriberi), and vitamin E; and (4) toxic etiologies such as lathyrism (Di Rocco, 1998). Thus, an MRI of the spinal cord with and without contrast, lumbar puncture with CSF analysis, and serum analysis for vitamin and mineral deficiencies will be needed to evaluate for these etiologies (Chong, 1999).

Clinicians should consider common infectious causes initially. One study from Cape Town, Africa—an area known for a high prevalence of tuberculosis (TB) and HIV—reviewed 216 cases of myelopathy and cauda equina syndrome in HIV-infected patients (median $CD4^+$ count 185 cell/mm^3). Investigators found that 68% of myelopathy cases were due to TB (Candy, 2014). This large number of TB-related myelopathy cases in HIV patients has also been seen in other small studies in Africa (Bhigjee, 2001; Modi, 2011). TB spondylitis could be diagnosed radiographically with a high degree of certainty using MRI, and the diagnosis was confirmed with either CSF analysis or open biopsy.

HTLV-1-ASSOCIATED MYELOPATHY/ TROPICAL SPASTIC PARAPARESIS

HTLV-1 is a retrovirus that is T cell-tropic and causes a proliferation of T cells (Manns, 1999). Although its full disease spectrum remains unknown, this virus is associated with adult T cell leukemia/lymphoma, uveitis, and HAM, which is also referred to as TSP. The prevalence of HTLV-1 infection increases with age, and it is more common in women than in men. It is also geographically clustered, with high rates in southern Japan, the Caribbean, areas of Africa, the Middle East, South America, the Pacific Melanesian Islands, and Papua New Guinea. Among low-risk groups in the United States and Europe, seroprevalence is approximately 1%. The majority of these patients remain asymptomatic during their lifetime. Approximately 1% of these patients develop a myelopathy (Pillat, 2011). Given the

overlapping risk factors for both HIV infection and HTLV-1 infection, it is important to consider HIV and HTLV-1 co-infection in HIV patients presenting with a slowly progressive myelopathy.

HAM patients present with progressive muscle weakness in the legs, hyperreflexia, clonus, extensor plantar responses, sensory disturbances, urinary incontinence, impotence, and lower back pain. HTLV-1 antibodies are present in both plasma and the CSF, as well as in brain and spinal cord tissue.

The diagnostic approach to HAM/TSP is similar to that outlined previously for VM, including MRI of the spine with and without contrast, lumbar puncture, and an investigation for nutritional deficiencies and toxic exposures. Definitive diagnosis requires an assay to detect HTLV-1 antibodies in plasma and CSF, including an assay capable of distinguishing between HTLV-1 and HTLV-2.

There is evidence that immune-modulating therapy, such as corticosteroids and IVIG, may be beneficial in the treatment of HTLV-1 myelopathy. Research is underway to develop new therapies in addition to preventive and therapeutic vaccines for HTLV-1 (Martin, 2011), but currently, prevention education, particularly regarding breast-feeding and sexual behavior, is the only known method of reducing incidence.

MRI IN HIV-ASSOCIATED VACUOLAR MYELOPATHY

MRI of the spinal cord in VM is nonspecific and thus lacks pathognomonic features to differentiate it from non-HIV-related spinal cord disease. The spinal cord may appear normal, but the most affected spinal cords appear atrophic with or without hyperintensities on T_2-weighted images (Chong, 1999; Yousem, 2010).

Recommended Reading

Di Rocco, A. Diseases of the spinal cord in human immunodeficiency virus infection. *Semin Neurol.* 1999; 19:151–155.

Manns A, Hisada M, La Grenade L. Human T-lymphotropic virus type I infection. *Lancet.* 1999; 353:1951–1958.

INTRACRANIAL LESIONS

LEARNING OBJECTIVE

Discuss the clinical presentation, differential diagnosis, and treatment of intracranial lesions in HIV-infected patients.

Intracranial mass lesions are common neurologic findings and account for as much as half of the neurologic disorders seen in HIV patients. Although intracranial mass lesions typically occur in patients with known HIV infections with advanced immunosuppression (CD4+ counts <200 cells/mm³), an intracranial lesion can occasionally be the initial presenting symptom of AIDS. Intracranial lesions in HIV-infected patients can be broadly categorized into three groups: opportunistic infections, neoplasms, and cerebrovascular disease (American Academy of Neurology, 1998).

The clinical presentation of intracranial lesions varies depending on the underlying etiology. Typical presenting clinical symptoms include alteration in level of awareness and consciousness as well as focal neurologic deficits. In developed countries such as the United States, the most common etiologies include toxoplasmosis, PCNSL, bacterial and fungal abscesses, and PML. Additional differential diagnosis includes primary brain tumor, brain metastasis

from systemic cancer, tuberculoma, and lesions of fungal origin. Differentiating among this large differential diagnosis of intracranial lesions can be challenging and controversial, especially with regard to use of biopsy for establishing the diagnosis. However, in patients with large lesions with mass effect and impending herniation, open biopsy with decompression is recommended. Nevertheless, making the correct diagnosis is paramount to effectively managing the causal pathogen in a timely manner. Achieving this goal requires a knowledge-based diagnostic algorithm that accounts for the relative frequency of various etiologies of intracranial lesions. Figure 38.2 provides a useful process of differential considerations based on level of immunosuppression, typical clinical and radiographic presentation, management options, and prognosis with or without empirical treatment (American Academy of Neurology, 1998).

Cerebral toxoplasmosis is the most common cause of space-occupying intracranial focal mass lesions in HIV/AIDS. It often results from reactivation of latent infection of *Toxoplasma gondii*, an obligate intracellular parasite (American Academy of Neurology, 2000a). In the United States, there has been a decline in the incidence of cerebral toxoplasmosis due to widespread use of prophylaxis agents such as trimethoprim–sulfamethoxazole and ART in HIV-infected patients (American Academy of Neurology, 1998).

Toxoplasmosis often presents with subacute changes in level of consciousness, fever, headaches, seizures, and focal neurologic deficit. It should be suspected in any HIV patient with an intracranial mass lesion, especially if the patient has a CD4+ count <100 cells/mm³, is not receiving toxoplasmosis prophylaxis, and has immunoglobulin G antibodies to *T. gondii* (American Academy of Neurology, 2000a). Investigative studies such as CSF analysis, toxoplasma serology, or imaging studies do not always provide a definitive diagnosis. In this patient population, obtaining lumbar puncture is often contraindicated due to the presence of lesions with mass effect and increased risk of herniation. In cases in which CSF is obtained, analysis frequently shows nonspecific mild mononuclear pleocytosis with elevated protein. PCR can increase utility of CSF analysis. PCR can detect *T. gondii* with high specificity (100%) but variable sensitivity (30–50%) (American Academy of Neurology, 2002). Consequently, whereas a positive PCR result is highly suggestive of the diagnosis, a negative result does not exclude it.

Imaging studies can also provide supportive information. MRI, with or without contrast, has greater sensitivity than contrast-enhanced CT, especially for detecting multiple lesions, subcortical lesions, and posterior fossa involvement. However, neither imaging modality alone is

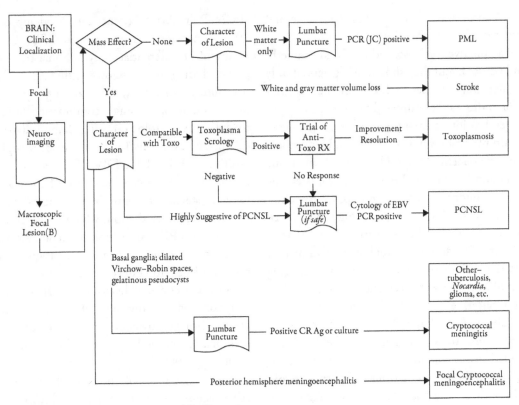

Figure 38.2 General algorithm for diagnostic evaluation of focal brain diseases.

sufficient enough to make a diagnosis because there is no pathognomonic radiographically distinguishing feature of toxoplasmosis compared to PCNSL. Toxoplasmosis typically presents as multiple, homogeneous, ring-enhancing lesions with cerebral edema and mass effect. It has a predilection for the basal ganglia and corticomedullary junction, with involvement of both white and gray matter (American Academy of Neurology, 2000a). Although a solitary mass lesion with edema is often observed in PCNSL, it can also be seen in toxoplasmosis (American Academy of Neurology, 2000a). Thallium single-photon emission computed tomography (SPECT) and positron emission tomography (PET) can be useful in distinguishing toxoplasmosis from lymphoma. Lymphoma has increased thallium uptake on SPECT and hypermetabolism of glucose and methionine on PET. Toxoplasma is hypometabolic on PET and does not show uptake of thallium (American Academy of Neurology, 2000a). As a result of the limitation of the investigative modalities mentioned previously, diagnosis of toxoplasmosis is often presumptive and based on clinical and radiographic findings, as well as clinical and radiographic response to empirical treatment within the first 2 weeks. Open or stereotactic brain biopsy can yield a definitive diagnosis; however, there is morbidity and even mortality associated with the procedure due to subsequent

intracranial hemorrhage. Biopsy is often pursued as a last resort in patients who do not improve with empirical management, have large mass effect with impending herniation, and require a definite diagnosis.

Empirical anti-toxoplasma therapy is usually started once toxoplasmosis is suspected. First-line treatment includes the use of sulfadiazine, pyrimethamine, and folinic acid (leucovorin) (American Academy of Neurology, 2000a). Folinic acid must be given to counteract myelosuppression from use of pyrimethamine. Treatment duration is at least 6 weeks before resuming secondary prophylaxis. Recrudescence occurs in up to 30% of patients, usually due to poor adherence to secondary prophylaxis; however, it can occur despite good adherence to the treatment plan (American Academy of Neurology, 2000a). In patients with sulfa allergy or intolerance, clindamycin is an alternative to sulfadiazine; however, use of clindamycin is associated with a slightly increased incidence of recrudescence. If the patient is intolerant to both sulfadiazine and clindamycin, alternatives include high-dosed trimethoprim–sulfamethoxazole, azithromycin, and atovaquone. Atovaquone is less tolerated due to gastrointestinal side effects. There is usually clinical improvement within the first 10–14 days of treatment. Clinical improvement occurs prior to radiographic evidence of improvement, which may be noted within 2 or 3 weeks. Lack of improvement within the first 2 weeks should raise suspicion for an alternative diagnosis.

The use of adjunctive corticosteroids, such as dexamethasone, should be brief, and they should implemented only in very particular circumstances, such as when there is clinical evidence of midline shift or impending herniation, signs of critically elevated intracranial pressure, or clinical deterioration within the first 48 hours of therapy. Under these circumstances, the benefits of steroids outweigh the many risks of steroid administration. The use of steroids can be a diagnostic confounder because it can improve the clinical presentation, making it difficult to distinguish between effects of steroid use and the therapeutic effectiveness of empiric treatment. In addition, steroid anti-inflammatory actions affect the radiographic presentation by decreasing the intensity of contrast enhancement and surrounding edema, thus interfering with reliable comparative interpretation of subsequent radiographic images. Steroids can also complicate the pathological diagnosis of PCNSL if a biopsy is needed, rendering the biopsy falsely negative for the presence of lymphoma. Aside from more acute steroid complications such as avascular necrosis, hyperglycemia, and psychiatric symptoms, the prolonged use of steroids can also make the patient susceptible to other opportunistic infections.

An important differential diagnosis is PCNSL. It is one of the four AIDS-defining neoplasms, which include systemic non-Hodgkin's lymphoma, Kaposi's sarcoma, and invasive cervical carcinoma. PCNSL is commonly seen in HIV patients with CD4$^+$ counts <50 cells/mm^3 and is rarely the initial presenting symptom of AIDS. The pathogenesis is also strongly related to reactivation of latent Epstein–Barr virus (EBV) infection. The clinical presentation is very similar to that of toxoplasmosis, with alteration of the level of consciousness, impaired cognitive function, seizures, and focal neurologic deficits such as aphasia and hemiparesis. Investigative studies such as CSF analysis and imaging are often utilized. Lumbar puncture should only be obtained if there are no contraindications, such as risk of herniation. CSF analysis, particularly cytology, can be helpful, but it has a very low sensitivity. PCR assay of CSF for EBV DNA can be diagnostic. PCR for EBV has a sensitivity greater than 80% and a specificity greater than 95%. As with toxoplasmosis, MRI often provides higher diagnostic yield than CT scan, but CT with contrast remains useful particularly in patients who have contraindication for getting an MRI. PCNSL can present with single or multiple well-defined, ring or patchy enhancing lesions with edema and mass effect. It often involves supratentorial regions such as the corpus callosum and periventricular or periependymal areas

(PCNSL in AIDS) (American Academy of Neurology, 2000b). As previously mentioned, SPECT and PET can be useful in differentiating lymphoma from other etiologies, including toxoplasmosis. Although PET and SPECT have limited sensitivity, they have high specificity. A diagnosis is often made using a combination of CSF cytology, toxoplasmosis serologic testing, failure of trial of empirical antibiotics usually for treatment of toxoplasmosis, and positive CSF PCR for EBV; if necessary, a brain biopsy is obtained (American Academy of Neurology, 2000b). Open or stereotactic brain biopsy is usually required prior to whole brain irradiation, which is the current mainstay treatment for PCNSL. Whole brain radiation appears to be able to prevent further neurologic progression or produce reversal of deficits. However, the treatment plan is based on the patient's overall health status. There can be spread of lymphoma with involvement of the eyes; therefore, a complete ophthalmologic examination including a slit-lamp examination should be performed (American Academy of Neurology, 2000b).

Other etiologies of intracranial mass lesions include other neoplasms, cerebrovascular disease, and opportunistic infections. Other neoplasms associated with HIV include glioma, Kaposi's sarcoma, and metastatic cancer.

Opportunistic infections can be classified based on the pathogen: parasitic, fungi, and bacteria. Most of these opportunistic infections present with meningitis and focal lesion. Common parasitic infections with intracranial lesion include neurocysticercosis. On imaging studies, the appearance of neurocysticercosis varies depending on the stage of infection. MRI is favored over CT scan, especially for evaluation of intraventricular and cisternal/subarachnoidal cysts as well as cystic degeneration and pericystic inflammatory reaction.

Common bacterial mass lesions include abscess from *Mycobacterium tuberculosis*, *Nocardia*, *Listeria monocytogenes*, and *Treponema pallidum*. In developing countries, particularly in highly endemic areas such as Southeast Asia and Africa, tuberculous meningitis is common. Due to its proclivity for the basal meninges, tuberculous meningitis often presents clinically with multiple cranial neuropathies and hydrocephalus (American Academy of Neurology, 2000a). Neuroimaging may show masses, which are often tuberculomas. Intracranial tuberculomas can be seen on MRI as hypointense or isointense due to varying amounts of caseous necrosis. This variable appearance of intracranial tuberculoma is attributed to the changing nature of the granulomatous lesion (Park, 2008). The diagnosis of tuberculous meningitis can be challenging and requires a combination of CSF analysis including culture for TB, acid-fast bacilli stain, and TB PCR along with a clinical evaluation for systemic tuberculosis.

Common etiologies of fungal abscesses include *Cryptococcus neoformans, Candida albicans,* aspergilliosis, mucomycosis, histoplasmosis, and coccidioidomycosis. Of these fungi, cryptococcosis is the most common opportunistic fungal infection in HIV-infected patients and arises from an acquired infection from *C. neoformans,* an encapsulated yeast. With widespread use of fluconazole as prophylaxis, there is a decreased incidence. Neuroimaging, usually a contrast-enhanced brain MRI, may show cryptococcomas—multiple enhancing lesions of various sizes most often seen within perivascular spaces. These lesions usually resolve with treatment. A definitive diagnosis is made by a positive CSF culture for *C. neoformans,* a positive CSF India ink stain, or a reactive CSF cryptococcal antigen test. For additional information, see Chapter 32.

PML is characterized by multifocal areas of demyelinating often in subcortical and periventricular areas. The pathogenesis is reactivation of JC virus infecting oligodendroglia in the setting of advanced immunosuppression. On imaging studies, the lesions are usually nonenhancing with contrast and do not produce any edema or mass effect. The subcortical U fibers are involved. However, in the setting of immune reconstitution inflammatory syndrome (IRIS), on MRI with contrast, PML can present with contrast enhancement, focal edema, and mass effect (Tan, 2009).

HIV-infected patients with intracranial lesions are at heightened risk for developing seizures. Antiepileptic drugs (AEDs) should not be given for routine prophylaxis to patients with a CNS mass lesion because not all patients with CNS lesions will develop seizures. However, once the patient experiences a seizure, chronic AED administration is appropriate. In 2012, the American Academy of Neurology issued an evidence-based guideline for clinicians about AED selection for people with HIV/AIDS (Birbeck, 2012). The guideline describes the strength of evidence for each of its recommendations based on the quality of evidence available from clinical investigations. The vast majority of the recommendations in this guideline were rated as having weak evidence.

The American Academy of Neurology guideline states that it may be important to avoid enzyme-inducing AEDS (EI-AEDs) in people on antiretroviral (ARV) regimens that include protease inhibitor (PI) or non-nucleotide reverse transcriptase inhibitors (NNRTIs) because pharmacokinetic interactions may result in virologic failure (Birbeck, 2012). Examples of EI-AEDs include phenobarbital, phenytoin, and carbamazepine. The guideline identifies circumstances in which specific dose adjustments to the ARV regimen of the AED are advised to maintain adequate serum levels of the mediations. For example, patients concurrently on phenytoin and lopinavir/ritonavir may need a 50% dosage increase in lopinavir/ritonavir to maintain adequate serum levels of the PI and virologic control. Patients coadministered atazanavir/ritonavir and lamotrigine may require a 50% increase in lamotrigine dose to maintain adequate serum levels of the AED and seizure control. Patients taking both zidovudine and the P450 inhibitor valproic acid may require a zidovudine dose reduction to maintain unchanged zidovudine levels (Birbeck, 2012). Although not specifically recommended in the guideline, renally excreted medications such as levetiracetam are often favored for patients on ARVs given their lack of drug–drug interactions. However, in the setting of status epilepticus, the use of intravenous phenytoin or fosphenytoin remains the recommended therapeutic intervention for cessation of clinical and subclinical seizures.

Using the approach discussed in this chapter, common etiologies of intracranial mass lesion can be systemically evaluated in order to make a diagnosis and institute therapy. In settings with limited resources such as sophisticated neuroimaging, CSF PCR, and biopsy, clinical findings on history and physical combined with the prevalence of infectious etiologies should guide the diagnosis and subsequent empiric therapeutic intervention.

MENINGITIS

LEARNING OBJECTIVE

Review the differential diagnosis and clinical management of meningitis in HIV-positive patients.

WHAT'S NEW?

- Timing of ART should be deferred in *Cryptococcus.*
- Meningococcal A vaccine has decreased the burden of meningitis in Africa.

KEY POINTS

- The differential diagnosis is broad.
- Meningitis in HIV-infected patients is usually treatable, and a cause should be investigated.

Table 38.2 CAUSES OF MENINGITIS IN HIV-POSITIVE PATIENTS

Viral	Acute HIV seroconversion, CD8[+] T cell encephalitis, enterovirus, herpes simplex virus, arboviruses (West Nile virus, St. Louis encephalitis), cytomegalovirus, varicella zoster virus, influenza virus, Epstein–Barr virus, lymphocytic choriomeningitis virus, mumps
Bacterial	Bacterial meningitis, endocarditis, parameningeal focus (e.g., epidural abscess and mastoiditis), syphilis, Lyme disease, *Mycoplasma pneumoniae*, *Bartonella henselae*, *Brucella* species, *Ehlichia*, *Rickettsia*, leptospirosis, *Mycobacterium tuberculosis*
Fungal	*Cryptococcus neoformans*, *Coccidiodes immitis*, *Histoplasma capsulatum*, *Aspergillus* species, zygomycosis
Parasitic	*Naegleria/Acanthamoeba*, *Taenia solium*, *Angiostrongylus cantonensis*, *Toxoplasma gondii*
Non-infectious	Medications (e.g., antibiotics and nonsteroidal anti-inflammatory drugs), meningeal carcinomatosis (lymphoma and leukemia), vasculitis, chemical meningitis (intrathecal injections and spinal anesthesia), seizures

A meta-analysis of studies of meningitis in HIV-infected patients in Africa documented that the three most common causes were *C. neoformans*, *M. tuberculosis*, and bacterial meningitis.

The differential diagnosis of meningitis in HIV-infected individuals is broad (viral, bacterial, fungal, mycobacterial, lymphomatous, etc.) (Table 38.2).

EARLY HIV STAGE

Acute HIV infection may manifest as an "aseptic meningitis" presentation (Hasbun, 2000). Patients with recent HIV exposure present with severe headache, stiff neck, diffuse macular rash, photophobia, and a lymphocytic pleocytosis in the CSF. Patients typically have positive HIV RNA levels and/or a positive HIV p24 antigen.

During the early stages of the HIV disease (CD4[+] T cell count >200 cells/mm³), patients can have the more typical viral causes of aseptic meningitis: enteroviruses, herpes simplex type 2, and arboviruses (West Nile and St. Louis encephalitis). Enteroviruses should be suspected in the late spring and summer in young patients with small children at home with recent illness (gastroenteritis or with flu-like syndromes). Herpes simplex type 2 can present with the initial genital outbreak of herpes or in patients with recurrent episodes of aseptic meningitis (Mollaret's meningitis). Arboviruses should be suspected in the summer and fall in patients with fever and recent mosquito bites. Unfortunately, viral PCR and arboviral serologies are obtained in the minority of patients with meningitis (Nesher, 2016).

Other less common causes of meningitis in the HIV-infected patient include varicella zoster virus (VZV), syphilis, and bacterial meningitis. VZV can present with a dermatomal vesicular rash and an aseptic meningitis presentation, and it should prompt screening for HIV. In more advance stages of HIV infection, it can present as

disseminated VZV. It can also present without a rash (*Zoster sine herpete*); with the Ramsay–Hunt syndrome; or with stroke, myelopathy, retinitis, or encephalitis. The diagnosis is made with a CSF VZV PCR or with culturing the virus from a vesicular lesion, and the treatment is intravenous acyclovir. Syphilis can also present as an aseptic meningitis syndrome in patients with a diffuse rash that involves the palms and soles. A serum rapid plasma reagin >1:32 and a CD4 T cell count <350 cells/mm³ are associated with neurosyphilis and should prompt the performance of a lumbar puncture (Marra, 2004). Bacterial meningitis represents a diagnostic consideration in all of the stages of HIV, but its incidence has decreased with the advent of the conjugate vaccines (Lopez, 2014). If bacterial meningitis is suspected, intravenous dexamethasone and antibiotic therapy with vancomycin, ceftriaxone, and ampicillin should be started to cover for *Streptococcus pneumoniae*, *Neisseria meningitides*, and *Listeria monocytogenes* until CSF cultures are negative (Tunkel, 2004). Furthermore, the introduction of the meningococcal A conjugate vaccine in 2010 in 26 countries in Africa has dramatically decreased the burden of disease (*Weekly Epidemiological Record*, 2015).

LATE HIV STAGES (CD4[+] T CELL COUNT <200 CELLS/MM³)

The most common cause of meningitis in patients with advance immunosuppression is *C. neoformans*. CSF examination typically shows a lymphocytic pleocytosis, but inflammation may be absent. CSF India ink examination is positive in up to 50% of cases, and the CSF cryptococcal antigen test is positive in approximately 90% of cases. An opening pressure should be documented because its elevation is associated with higher CSF fungal burden and also higher neurological morbidity and mortality (Gambarin, 2002). The preferred therapy for cryptococcal meningitis is a combination of intravenous amphotericin B deoxycholate at 0.7–1 mg/kg per day plus flucytosine 100 mg/kg per day divided in four doses for 2 weeks followed by fluconazole 400 mg PO per day to decrease the intracranial hypertension (i.e., >25 cm of H_2O) by either repeat lumbar punctures or temporary percutaneous lumbar drains or ventriculostomy if persistent elevations occur (Perfect, 2012). If flucytosine is not available or the patient experiences drug toxicity, the patient can be treated with a combination of amphotericin B with fluconazole either 400 mg or 800 mg once daily for 14 days. A repeat lumbar puncture should be done at the end of the 2-week period to document a negative CSF fungal culture. Intravenous amphotericin B should be continued if the patient has persistently positive CSF cultures, is clinically deteriorating or comatose, or has persistent elevated and symptomatic intracranial pressures (Perfect, 2012). A therapeutic lumbar puncture to decrease intracranial pressure was associated with a reduced risk of death in a study performed in Africa (Rolfes, 2014). The same study also documented that ART should be delayed until 5 weeks after initial presentation to avoid an increase in mortality (Boulware, 2014).

Cytomegalovirus can cause meningitis, ventriculitis, polyradiculomyopathy, retinitis, esophagitis, and colitis in patients with advanced HIV disease (CD4+ T cell count <50 cells/mm³). It is treated initially with intravenous gancyclovir 5 mg/kg every 12 hours, and then the patient is switched to oral valgancyclovir when stable (US Department of Health and Human Services (DHHS), 2016). MRI of the brain typically shows periventricular enhancement, and CSF can demonstrate a lymphocytic or a neutrophilic pleocytosis, hypoglycorrhachia, and mild elevations of the protein. A positive cytomegalovirus (CMV) PCR in the CSF makes the diagnosis.

Mycobacterial tuberculosis can occur at any stage of the HIV illness, but extrapulmonary disease (e.g., meningitis, lymphadenitis, pleuritis, and pericarditis) occurs more frequently in patients with CD4+ T cell counts <200 cells/mm³. The incidence of TB has declined in the United States, and there are fewer than 1000 cases of co-infection reported annually (DHHS, 2016). Tuberculosis and HIV must be treated together rather than sequentially, particularly in patients with low CD4 counts. Tuberculous meningitis usually has a subacute to chronic presentation, lymphocytic pleocytosis, a low CSF glucose and basilar involvement with cranial nerve palsies and altered mental status. A Thwaites' diagnostic score <4 (5 parameters—age, duration of illness, white blood cell count, total CSF white blood cell count, and percentage of CSF neutrophils) or a Lancet consensus score >6 (20 parameters divided in four categories: clinical, CSF, CNS imaging, and evidence of TB

elsewhere) indicate possible TB meningitis, and patients with these scores should be considered for empiric therapy. The CSF acid-fast bacilli smear is insensitive, and CSF cultures are positive in only 38–88% of cases (Thwaites, 2012). A CSF *M. tuberculosis* PCR and an adenosine deaminase level can also aid in the diagnosis. Duration of treatment is 1 year.

IMMUNE RECONSTITUTION SYNDROME IN HIV

IRIS occurs after the initiation of combination ART and either "unmasks" a previous subclinical infection or worsens a known infection despite appropriate therapy (paradoxical reaction). In the CNS, IRIS can develop with cryptococcal meningitis, tuberculosis meningitis, and progressive multifocal leukoencephalopathy due to JC virus and HIV (Huis in't Veld, 2012). The two most common and serious CNS IRIS events are cryptococcal and tuberculous meningitis. TB IRIS usually presents between a few weeks to 3 months after the initiation of ART, and it can present with meningitis or tuberculomas or both. Risk factors include low CD4+ cell counts, disseminated TB, and extrapulmonary TB. Treatment should consist of adjunctive steroids. CSF acid-fast bacilli cultures are typically negative. Cryptococcal IRIS can develop between 1 and 10 months after initiating ART and can present as culture-negative meningitis, cryptococcomas, pneumonitis, and/or lymphadenopathy. Adjunctive steroids should be considered. A CD8+ T cell encephalitis syndrome has been described in patients receiving ART with low or undetectable serum HIV viral loads (Lescure, 2013). These patients usually have a low CD4+ T cell nadir and a history of opportunistic infections, and they usually present with high CD4+ T cell counts. They can present with memory disturbances, headaches, diplopia, ataxia, and, sometimes, seizures. MRI of the brain shows bilateral white matter lesions, and CSF shows lymphocytic pleocytosis with detectable CSF HIV viral loads. The treatment is corticosteroids and optimizing the CNS penetration of ART.

MENINGITIS IN RESOURCE-LIMITED COUNTRIES

A review of 1303 episodes of meningitis with confirmed etiologies in HIV-infected patients in sub-Saharan Africa showed that 52% had cryptococcal meningitis, 19.6% had tuberculosis, 14.2% had bacterial meningitis, and 14.2% had other etiologies (Veltman, 2014). Mortality rates were high, ranging from 25% to 68% in the different studies.

DISTAL SYMMETRICAL POLYNEUROPATHY

WHAT'S NEW?

High-concentration capsaicin dermal patch has shown efficacy in patients with painful HIV distal symmetric polyneuropathy (SDP) and in one study produced a sustained reduction in pain over 12 weeks.

KEY POINTS

- DSP is the most common neurologic complication of HIV infection, occurring in 30–60% of patients.

- Antiretroviral toxic neuropathy is associated with use of older nucleoside reverse transcriptase inhibitor therapy, especially for didanosine and stavudine.

- Treatment includes removal of neurotoxins and management of pain/discomfort.

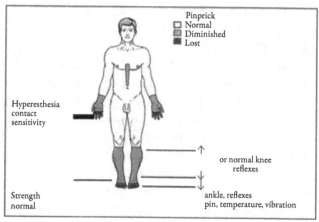

Figure 38.3 Typical Signs and Symptoms of DSP.

DSP occurs in 30–60% of all HIV-infected patients (Ellis, 2010; Evans, 2011), making it the most common neurologic complication in HIV disease. Its incidence increases to as high as 62% in advanced HIV/AIDS (Schifitto, 2002; Simpson, 2006). DSP may develop at any time after the onset of HIV infection, with a mean time of developing neuropathy at 9.5 years after HIV diagnosis (Robinson-Papp, 2009). However, a smaller study suggested that signs of neuropathy may be detected in as many as 35% of patients with a median of only 3.5 months after HIV transmission (Wang, 2014). Although the etiology of DSP is still under investigation, it is most likely an indirect result of HIV infection, probably through immune-mediated mechanisms (Pardo, 2001). Risk factors for DSP in HIV-infected individuals include increased age, Caucasian race, lower hemoglobin levels, hypertriglyceridemia, lower CD4+ cell count nadir, current combination ART use, and past use of the dideoxynucleosides drugs (didanosine, stavudine, and zalcitabine) (Banerjee, 2011; Ellis, 2010; Simpson, 2006; Tagliati, 1999).

Neuropathy associated with nucleoside reverse transcriptase inhibitors (NRTIs), especially didanosine, stavudine, and zalcitabine, is the only neurologic complication that has increased since the introduction of ART (Keswani, 2002). The risk of antiretroviral toxic neuropathy (ATN) appears to be substantially higher when didanosine and stavudine are used together, especially when combined with hydroxyurea (Moore, 2000). There are no discrete distinguishing features between DSP and ATN (Pardo, 2001; Price, 1999), and a current hypothesis is that mitochondrial dysfunction mediates NRTI toxicity (Kallianpur, 2009).

Symmetrical spontaneous and evoked pains predominantly in the feet and progressing to the upper extremities are typical symptoms, along with tingling, numbness, stabbing sensations, and burning (Figure 38.3) (Cornblath, 1988; DeVivo, 2000; Price, 1999; Wulff, 1999a). Deep tendon reflexes at the ankles are typically diminished or absent, and appreciation of temperature may be decreased (Wulff, 1999a).

The pathology of DSP includes damage to and loss of both large- and small-caliber sensory nerve fibers, with macrophage infiltration in the dorsal root ganglia and along the nerve trunks (Keswani, 2002). Sural nerve biopsies obtained from patients with ATN have shown severe axonal destruction, prominent in unmyelinated fibers (Dalakas, 1996). Different possible pathogenetic mechanisms of DSP in HIV have been studied. Activation of macrophages and production of proinflammatory cytokines appear to play a significant role (Pardo, 2001). Viral proteins such as the envelope glycoprotein gp120 that is secreted may also contribute to HIV neurotoxicity (Keswani, 2003). Mitochondrial DNA damage in the mitochondria of distal axons may also add to the distal degeneration of sensory nerve fibers (Lehmann, 2011). Prominent mitochondrial abnormalities have more significantly been noted in association with NRTIs, supporting the suggestion that neuronal mitochondrial damage underlies ATN (Chen, 1991). Further support for this concept is derived from in vitro observations of graded inhibition of gamma DNA polymerase by different NRTIs (Martin, 1994). Dideoxynucleosides (didanosine, zalcitabine, and stavudine) are the most potent inhibitors of this enzyme in vitro (Martin, 1994), and zidovudine, lamivudine, abacavir, emtricitabine, and tenofovir have only minimal effects. Mitochondrial DNA content in lymphocytes, however, does not correlate with the presence of ATN (Simpson, 2006).

The differential diagnosis of DSP/ATN includes other toxic neuropathies, including those caused by other agents commonly used in HIV/AIDS (e.g., metronidazole, dapsone, vincristine, and isoniazid) (DeVivo, 2000), and diabetes mellitus, vitamin B_{12} deficiency, diffuse infiltrative lymphocytosis syndrome, alcohol abuse, hepatitis C, and uremia (DeVivo, 2000; Williams, 2002).

DSP or ATN is usually diagnosed on clinical grounds. Marra et al. reported that a brief screening examination, performed at a single center by trained nonphysicians, correlated well with the diagnosis of DSP as made by an experienced AIDS neurologist (Marra, 1998). In a multicenter study, however, nonphysician neurological findings were less reliable (Simpson, 2006). Nerve conduction studies can be useful, typically showing axonal neuropathy, with absent or reduced sensory nerve action potentials, although they might be normal in either mild cases or when the neuropathy is restricted to small fibers (DeVivo, 2000). Punch skin biopsies have been used to identify reduced densities of unmyelinated nerve fibers in HIV-associated sensory neuropathies. Skin biopsy analysis is now available in some settings, and it is particularly helpful either when symptoms of burning pain are more prominent than actual neurologic signs or when a nonorganic cause of sensory symptoms is suspected (Polydefkis, 2002). Quantitative sudomotor axon reflex test may also be performed to document small-fiber neuropathy. In a study of 102 patients with HIV, autonomic dysfunction was present in 62% of participants (Robinson-Papp, 2013). Sural nerve biopsy is rarely indicated except when mononeuritis multiplex is present.

Diagnosis of neurotoxic neuropathy can be confirmed by withdrawal of the suspected neurotoxin and monitoring for attenuation of symptoms. Symptoms typically improve or resolve over 2–10 weeks in approximately two-thirds of patients (Blum, 1996). When antiretroviral alternatives are not available, one can "treat through"—maintain the antiretroviral regimen and add adjuvant pain-modifying agents. If the antiretroviral regimen must be switched to remove the offending agent, this is usually feasible except in heavily treated patients. Symptoms may not always subside upon stopping the offending agent—or if they do, recovery may be only partial (Price, 1999; Wulff, 1999a).

Treatment of HIV sensory neuropathies focuses on removing neurotoxins and managing pain and discomfort. One study showed that 40% of HIV-infected patients have severe pain, with a numeric pain rating scale of ≥5/10, and 90% experience some pain (Smyth, 2007). Although there is no FDA-approved treatment for the pain often associated with DSP caused by HIV, various pain-modifying agents have been used for HIV sensory neuropathies, as they have for diabetic polyneuropathy, including antidepressants, anticonvulsants, and narcotics. In mild neuropathies, over-the-counter treatments such as acetaminophen can be helpful (DeVivo, 2000; Wulff, 1999a). One randomized control study demonstrated evidence of efficacy for topical capsaicin 8% (Simpson, 2008). Night splints may also be useful in the management of neuropathic pain with improvement of sleep (Sandoval, 2010). Although pain-modifying anticonvulsants and antidepressants have been useful clinically (DeVivo, 2000; Wulff, 1999a) and can improve quality of life and function for many patients with HIV sensory neuropathies (Simpson, 2003), placebo-controlled trials on neuropathic pain have shown no significant benefit from amitriptyline, low-dose topical capsaicin, pregabalin, gabapentin, subcutaneous recombinant human nerve growth factor, subcutaneous prosapeptide, intranasal peptide T, or lamotrigine (Phillips, 2010). Lamotrigine did show some superiority to placebo in the neurotoxic ARV-exposed stratum as a secondary outcome measure of the study. Although placebo-controlled trials have been negative, tricyclic antidepressants (e.g., desipramine and amitriptyline) occasionally can be useful. Sedation is common with some, particularly amitriptyline, so these are more useful for control of nighttime neuropathic pain. Daytime sedation can generally be avoided by using small doses and escalating slowly. Pain-modifying anticonvulsants have also been useful clinically (DeVivo, 2000; Wulff, 1999a) and can improve quality of life and function for many patients with HIV sensory neuropathies (Simpson, 2003). Use of opiate medication must be approached with caution due to the prevalence of risk factors for aberrant prescription opiate use that is often found in this population (Chou, 2009). Alternative treatments include acupuncture and hypnosis (Dorfman, 2013). Further management details are provided by Verma et al. (Verma, 2004).

CONSIDERATIONS FOR RESOURCE-LIMITED SETTINGS

Cherry et al. have shown that a brief peripheral neuropathy screen, which can be easily performed in resource-limited settings, can reliably diagnose peripheral neuropathy (Cherry, 2005). Although neurotoxic dideoxynucleoside ART is declining overall, stavudine remains a common component of such therapy in less-developed areas in the world, where ATN might be expected to remain a common problem.

INFLAMMATORY DEMYELINATING POLYNEUROPATHY

LEARNING OBJECTIVE

Discuss the clinical features, differential diagnosis, and management of acute and chronic inflammatory demyelinating polyneuropathy in HIV-infected patients.

WHAT'S NEW?

The differential diagnosis of acute inflammatory demyelinating polyneuropathy (AIDP) includes disorders of the spinal cord, such as transverse myelitis, acute spinal cord compression, and acute infarction of the spinal cord; disorders affecting anterior horn cells, including poliomyelitis and West Nile virus; acute peripheral neuropathies such as tick paralysis, porphyria, Lyme disease, and lead or arsenic poisoning; and neuromuscular junction disorders such as botulism, myasthenia gravis, or Lambert–Eaton myasthenic syndrome.

KEY POINTS

- Acute and chronic inflammatory demyelinating polyneuropathies (AIDP/CIDP) are not common HIV-associated peripheral neuropathies. Their cause is autoimmune-induced inflammation and breakdown of peripheral nerve myelin.

- AIDP has rapid onset and progression and often develops during HIV seroconversion or before immunosuppression has evolved.

- AIDP/CIDP in HIV-infected patients is not associated with CSF albuminocytological dissociation. These patients often have a CSF lymphocytic pleocytosis.

- AIDP is usually treated with plasmapheresis or intravenous immunoglobulin and with ganciclovir/foscarnet/cidofovir if CMV is detected as a causative agent.

- CIDP is treated with corticosteroids or intermittent courses of either plasmapheresis or intravenous immunoglobulin that may be continued long term until therapeutic response.

Peripheral neuropathy is the most common neurologic manifestation in patients with HIV/AIDS and can manifest in a number of ways: distal symmetric polyneuropathy, inflammatory polyneuropathy (AIDP/CIDP), mononeuritis multiplex, autonomic neuropathy, and progressive polyradiculopathy (Wulff, 1999b, 2000). Distal symmetric polyneuropathy is the most common presentation and can occur secondary to direct HIV infection or as a side effect of NRTIs (Parry, 1997; Wulff, 2000). Inflammatory demyelinating neuropathies in patients with HIV are much less common (Leger, 1989).

Inflammatory demyelinating polyradiculopathies are classified as either acute or chronic based on the duration of symptom progression. AIDP, also known as Guillain–Barré syndrome (GBS), is defined as progressive, usually ascending, weakness and sensory symptoms with symptom nadir by 4 weeks. In contrast, CIDP is classified by progressive proximal and distal weakness and sensory loss with symptom progression for longer than 8 weeks.

The association between inflammatory polyneuropathies and HIV was first reported in 1985 by Lipkin et al. (Lipkin, 1985). AIDP typically occurs in the early stages of HIV infection during the seroconversion stage or during early HIV infection before seroconversion has evolved (Markarian, 1998; Mishra, 1985; Wulff 1999b). In patients with relatively intact immune function, AIDP may be the first clinical manifestation of HIV infection (Parry, 1997). Miller–Fischer/GBS overlap syndrome has been reported in advanced AIDS, with elevated anti-GQ1b antibody titer despite severe immunosuppression (Hiraga, 2007). GBS has also been reported as an immune reconstitution syndrome in patients treated with combination ART and a dramatic increase in CD4$^+$ cell counts (Piliero, 2003; Rauschkaa, 2003). CIDP generally occurs later during the advanced stage of HIV infection (Verma, 2000, 2001).

PATHOGENESIS

Both AIDP and CIDP are thought to be due to an underlying autoimmune inflammatory response against peripheral nerve myelin-associated antigens, resulting in breakdown of peripheral nerve myelin (Radziwill, 2002). Rarely, HIV infection has been reported in association with an acute axonal motor neuropathy, where the pathology is thought to be associated with an immune response against the peripheral nerve axon (Dardis, 2015; Goldstein, 2013; Jadhav, 2014; Wagner, 2007).

CLINICAL FEATURES

AIDP is frequently associated with a preceding illness, such as upper respiratory infection or acute enterocolitis. AIDP commonly presents with paresthesias, followed by back pain, ascending symmetric numbness and weakness, and absent reflexes. Patients may also experience facial weakness, ophthalmoplegia, and autonomic dysfunction (commonly labile blood pressures and tachycardia).

CIDP can present with progressive or relapsing proximal and distal weakness, sensory loss, and absent reflexes. Pain is a less common presentation (Dimachkie, 2014).

CEREBROSPINAL FLUID ANALYSIS

CSF is characteristically acellular in AIDP without HIV infection. Protein levels may be normal during the first week of the illness, but there will be an increase in protein 2 or 3 weeks after symptom onset. Elevated CSF protein has been associated mainly with increased permeability of the blood–CSF barrier (Winer, 2001). On the other hand, AIDP seen with HIV infection may be associated with lymphocytic pleocytosis. In a study of 10 patients with HIV-associated AIDP, CSF white blood cell count ranged from 2 to 17 cells/mm^3 (Brannagan, 2003). The presence of increased protein in the CSF is useful for the diagnosis, and a lymphocytic CSF pleocytosis (10–50 cells/mm^3) distinguishes HIV-associated inflammatory demyelinating neuropathies from those without HIV infection (Wulff, 1999b). However, the absence of CSF pleocytosis does not rule out HIV infection and hence warrants testing HIV in all patients with AIDP (Brannagan, 2003). In addition, either elevated protein or cell counts may be found in asymptomatic patients with HIV infection (Marshall, 1988). CSF pleocytosis is suggestive of either inflammatory/infectious etiology or underlying malignancy. Markedly elevated cell counts or the presence of CSF polymorphonuclear granulocytes in a patient with AIDP/CIDP should alert the physician to seriously consider alternative diagnoses (Hughes, 1991). Enterovirus myelitis, West Nile myelitis, European tick-borne encephalitis virus, and herpes virus infection (CMV, VZV, EBV, and HSV-1 and -2) may show an initial polymorphonuclear pleocytosis. Lyme disease and HIV infection need to be considered with a lymphocytic pleocytosis (Rauschkaa, 2003).

The mean CD4$^+$ cell count was 367 cells/mm^3 (range, 55–800 cells/mm^3) in a series of 10 HIV-infected patients with GBS as reported by Brannagan and Zhou. The etiology of an acute polyradiculapathy in patients with CD4$^+$ cell counts <50 cells/mm^3 may be secondary to CMV infection, and empiric gancyclovir is indicated (Brannagan, 2003).

ELECTROPHYSIOLOGY

Diagnosis is aided by nerve conduction studies showing features of demyelination—that is, slowing of nerve conduction velocities, prolonged distal latencies, temporal dispersion, conduction block, and prolonged F-wave latencies.

BIOPSY

Nerve biopsies are rarely done to diagnose either AIDP or CIDP, but biopsy may be considered if the clinical or physiologic picture is atypical. Pathology includes macrophage-mediated segmental demyelination and an inflammatory infiltrate (Cornblath, 1987).

DIFFERENTIAL DIAGNOSIS

The differential diagnosis of AIDP includes disorders of the spinal cord such as transverse myelitis, acute spinal cord compression, and acute infarction of the spinal cord; disorders affecting anterior horn cells, including poliomyelitis and West Nile virus; acute peripheral neuropathies such as tick paralysis, porphyria, Lyme disease, and lead or arsenic poisoning; and neuromuscular junction disorders such as botulism, myasthenia gravis, or Lambert–Eaton myasthenic syndrome (Wakerly, 2015). In patients with subacute/chronic neuropathy and HIV infection with CD4$^+$ T cell counts <50 cells/mm^3, mononeuritis multiplex, distal symmetric polyneuropathy needs to be considered in the differential diagnosis, including CMV-related polyradiculomyelitis.

TREATMENT

AIDP is treated with either high-dose IVIG therapy or plasmapheresis. These treatments enhance recovery and arrest clinical progression (Cornblath, 1987; Hadden, 1998; Plasma Exchange/Sandoglobulin Guillain–Barré Syndrome Trial Group, 1997). IVIG and plasma exchange have been shown to be equally effective in treating HIV-negative AIDP (Plasma Exchange/Sandoglobulin Guillain–Barré Trial Group, 1997; van der Meche, 1992). In 2015, Rosca et al. reported improvement in CD4$^+$ and CD8$^+$ counts and HIV RNA levels in their patient treated with IVIG for HIV-associated GBS (Rosca, 2015). Due to the possibility of CMV radiculomyelitis, patients with severe immunosuppression (CD4$^+$ T cell counts <50 cells/mm^3) should be treated with intravenous gancyclovir, foscarnet, or cidofovir or a combination of these, in addition to the standard treatment. CIDP is treated with oral prednisone, pulse intravenous high-dose methylprednisolone or dexamethasone, or intermittent courses of plasmapheresis or IVIG. A randomized controlled study confirmed the benefit of prednisone in HIV-related CIDP, although this treatment approach may worsen immunosuppression (Lindenbaum, 2001). Acute relapses in CIDP are treated with either IVIG or plasmapheresis.

PROGNOSIS

Clinical course and response to pharmacological treatment are similar in patients who are HIV seropositive or seronegative (Verma, 2001). Schreiber (2011) reported on a patient with GBS as the initial presentation of HIV infection, with full recovery using IVIG and rehabilitation without initiation of ART, suggesting that patients with GBS early in the course of HIV infection may behave like those with GBS without HIV infection. Compared to HIV-negative patients, HIV-associated GBS patients may experience relapses and may be more likely to develop CIDP (Brannagan, 2003). With CIDP, although treatment can halt the progression of the disease and remyelination of the peripheral nerves can occur, there is evidence that unrecoverable secondary axonal damage can occur in some cases (Hughes, 1991).

NEUROLOGICAL COMPLICATIONS OF HIV PATIENTS WITH CYTOMEGALOVIRUS INFECTION

LEARNING OBJECTIVE

Discuss the clinical syndromes, differential diagnosis, and management of neurological complications of CMV infection in HIV-infected patients.

KEY POINTS

- CMV CNS disease occurs late in the course of HIV and it may involve different parts of the central nervous system.

- Diagnosis is based on the clinical findings, results of imaging and virological markers.

- The treatment should be started empirically while awaiting the CSF PCR results.

CMV, a member of the herpesvirus family, is a frequent opportunistic viral infection in HIV-infected patients and occurs when the CD4+ T cell count is <100 cells/mm³ due to reactivation of latent infection. CMV infection of the nervous system accounts for <1% of CMV infections in HIV

patients (McCutchan, 1995) and often develops concurrently with other, more common CMV extraneural disease such as retinitis or gastrointestinal involvement. Clinical syndromes of CMV infection in the nervous system include encephalitis, polyradiculomyelitis, and multifocal neuropathy (Anders, 1999). Although these syndromes are uncommon, recognition, treatment with antivirals, and restoring immune response are paramount to reduce the risk of death.

CMV encephalitis is the most common manifestation of CNS infection due to CMV. Clinically, infection can present as diffuse encephalitis, ventriculoencephalitis, or focal encephalitis. Diffuse encephalitis develops over several weeks and thus presents subacutely with memory loss, attention and concentration difficulties, and delirium. Focal neurological deficits may also be seen. Pathologically, microglial nodules may be found in the cortex, brainstem, cerebellum, and basal ganglia, occurring most commonly in gray matter (Morgello, 1986). On neuroimaging, MRI may show a variety of patterns. The brain may appear normal, or it may show hyperintense T2 lesions in the areas described previously and nodular lesions with or without enhancement on T1 post-contrast images (Maschke, 2002).

Ventriculoencephalitis presents with lethargy, confusion, cranial nerve deficits, ataxia, and focal neurological deficits, and it sometimes occurs concomitantly with CMV polyradiculitis. Ventriculoencephalitis may be more insidious in onset and have a poorer prognosis (Maschke, 2002). CMV encephalitis has been reported to occur even while patients are on treatment with ganciclovir for extra-CNS disease (Bermann, 1994). Pathologically, necrotizing lesions are seen in the ventricular system, and imaging shows periventricular enhancement with or without ventriculomegaly. The third and less common type of CMV encephalitis, focal encephalitis, presents with focal neurological deficits corresponding to a cerebral mass lesion. MRI will show ring-enhancing lesions with surrounding edema.

CSF PCR for CMV DNA confirms the diagnosis of CMV encephalitis. The CSF may also show pleocytosis with either a polymorphonuclear or a mononuclear predominance, along with elevated protein and decreased glucose levels. Viral culture is rarely positive. The detection of other viruses often confounds the diagnosis; thus, the index of suspicion must be based on the presentation and imaging findings in the context of profound immunosuppression. The differential diagnosis for CMV encephalitis must include HIV encephalitis, PML, and neurosyphilis. When CMV encephalitis presents as a ring-enhancing lesion, the differential diagnosis expands to other etiologies know to present similarly, such as toxoplasmosis, primary CNS lymphoma, and tuberculous meningitis with tuberculomas (Offiah, 2006).

CMV polyradiculitis (or polyradiculomyelitis if the infection involves not only the nerve roots but also the spinal cord) typically presents as an ascending weakness beginning in the lower extremities with areflexia, sensory loss, and weakness. Patients typically experience urinary retention and decreased anal sphincter tone. MRI of the spine with contrast demonstrates enhancement of the nerve roots, often involving the cauda equina. Nerve conduction studies will show low compound muscle action potentials and mildly slowed conduction velocity corresponding to axonal involvement. Electromyography will show acute denervation with spontaneous activity and decreased recruitment. CSF studies in CMV polyradiculitis usually reveal a polymorphonuclear predominant pleocytosis, elevated protein, and decreased glucose levels. CSF PCR for CMV DNA can confirm the diagnosis.

The differential diagnosis of CMV polyradiculitis includes GBS, which may be clinically indistinguishable and only differentiated on nerve conduction studies showing a more demyelinating pattern (Corral, 1997). Other opportunistic infections, including TB, toxoplasmosis, and HSV-2, can present in a similar manner. Syphilis and lymphoma can also cause polyradiculitis. HIV can cause a vacuolar myelopathy.

Treatment for both CMV encephalitis and CMV polyradiculitis/polyradiculomyelitis is similar. Induction treatment with either intravenous ganciclovir or foscarnet is the usual first-line treatment option. Sometimes in severe encephalitis cases, combination treatment with both ganciclovir and foscarnet has been used (Portegies, 2004; Silva, 2010). Cidofovir can be used as an alternate treatment option. Empiric treatment of CMV infection is often advised because CSF results may be delayed. Maintenance treatment with ganciclovir has been recommended, but the duration of treatment has not been well studied. Of note, patients with CMV polyradiculitis/polyradiculomyelitis have been shown to be more responsive to treatment compared to CMV encephalitis patients (Cinque, 1998).

The best described CMV infection of the peripheral nervous system is an asymmetric multifocal neuropathy, observed in HIV patients with low CD4+ counts, similar to CNS CMV infection. Infection affects individual peripheral nerves, with the radial, ulnar, peroneal, and lateral cutaneous nerves of the thigh being most commonly involved (Anders, 1999). Rapid progression has been reported and can become confluent (Robinson-Papp, 2009). Electrodiagnostic studies of the nerves show multifocal sensory and motor nerve dysfunction in an axonal pattern with acute denervation. CSF studies may or may not be positive for CMV PCR, and nerve biopsy may also fail to reveal CMV. Empiric treatment is warranted when clinical suspicion is high, especially in the setting of concomitant CMV infection affecting other organs. Treatment is also with either ganciclovir or foscarnet as the first-line option. The differential diagnosis should include mononeuropathy multiplex in HIV patients with high CD4+ counts, hepatitis C with cryoglobulinemia, mononeuropathy multiplex due to vasculitis in association with B cell lymphoma, and distal sensory polyneuropathy associated with either HIV or antiretroviral treatment with dideoxynucleoside reverse transcriptase inhibitors.

Recommended Reading

Anders HJ, Goebel FD. Neurological manifestations of cytomegalovirus infection in the acquired immunodeficiency syndrome. *Int J STD AIDS*. 1999; 10:151–161.

Maschke M, Kastrup O, Diener HC. CNS manifestations of cytomegalovirus infections diagnosis and treatment. *CNS Drugs*. 2002; 16(5):303–315.

Silva CA, Penalva de Oliveira AC, Vilas-Boas L, et al. Neurologic cytomegalovirus complications in patients with AIDS: Retrospective review of 13 cases and review of the literature. *Rev Inst Med Trop Sao Paulo*. 2010; 52(6):305–310.

References

Alfahad T, Nath A. Update on HIV-associated neurocognitive disorders. *Curr Neurol Neurosci Rep*. 2013; 13:387.

American Academy of Neurology. Evaluation and management of intracranial mass lesions in AIDS: Report of the Quality Standards Subcommittee of the American Academy of Neurology. *Neurology*. 1998; 50:21–26.

American Academy of Neurology. Opportunistic infections: Toxoplasmosis. The Neurologic complications of AIDS. *Neurol Continuum*. 2000a; 6(5):128–149.

American Academy of Neurology. Primary central nervous system lymphoma in AIDS: The neurologic complications of AIDS. *Neurol Continuum*. 2000b; 6(5):177–185.

American Academy of Neurology. Opportunistic and fungal infections of the central nervous system. *Neurol Continuum*. 2002; 8(3):125.

Anders HJ, Goebel FD. Neurological manifestations of cytomegalovirus infection in the acquired immunodeficiency syndrome. *Int J STD AIDS*. 1999; 10:151–161.

Antinori A, Arendt G, Becker JT, et al. Updated research nosology for HIV-associated neurocognitive disorders. *Neurology*. 2007; 69(18):1789–1799.

Banerjee S, McCutchan JA, Ances BM, et al. Hypertriglyceridemia in combination antiretroviral-treated HIV-positive individuals: Potential impact on HIV sensory polyneuropathy. *AIDS*. 2011; 25(2):F1–F6.

Banks LT, Geraci A, Liu M, et al. A natural history of HIV myelopathy in the HAART era. *Neurology*. 2002; 58:A441.

Bermann SM, Kim RC. The development of cytomegalovirus encephalitis in AIDS patients receiving ganciclovir. *Am J Med*. 1994; 96:415–419.

Bhigjee AI, Madurai S, Bill PL, et al. Spectrum of myelopathies in HIV seropositive South African patients. *Neurology*. 2001; 57:348–351.

Birbeck G, French J, Perucca E, et al. Evidence-based guideline: Antiepileptic drug selection for people with HIV/AIDS: Report of the Quality Standards Subcommittee of the American Academy of Neurology and the Ad Hoc Task Force of the Commission on Therapeutic Strategies of the International League Against Epilepsy. *Neurology*. 2012; 78(2):139–145.

Blum AS, Dal Pan GJ, Feinberg J, et al. Low-dose zalcitabine-related toxic neuropathy: frequency, natural history, and risk factors. *Neurology.* 1996 Apr; 46(4):999–1003.

Boisse L, Gill MJ, Power C. HIV infection of the central nervous system: Clinical features and neuropathogenesis. *Neurol Clin.* 2008; 26:799–819.

Boulware DR, Meya DB, Muzoora C, et al. Timing of antiretroviral therapy after diagnosis of cryptococcal meningitis. *N Engl J Med.* 2014; 370:2487–2498.

Brannagan TH 3rd, Zhou Y. HIV associated Guillain–Barré syndrome. *J Neurol Sci.* 2003; 208(1–2):39–42.

Candy S, Chang G, Andronikous S. Acute myelopathy or cauda equine syndrome in HIV positive adults in a tuberculosis endemic setting: MRI, clinical, and pathologic findings. *AJNR.* 2014; 35(8):1634–1641.

Carvalhal A, Gill MJ, Letendre SL, et al. Central nervous system penetration effectiveness of antiretroviral drugs and neuropsychological impairment in the Ontario HIV Treatment Network Cohort Study. *J Neuroviral.* 2016 Jun; 22(3):349–357.

Chen CH, Vazquez-Padua M, Cheng YC. Effect of anti-human immunodeficiency virus nucleoside analogs on mitochondrial DNA and its implication for delayed toxicity. *Mol Pharmacol.* 1991; 39(5):625–628.

Cherner M, Masliah E, Ellis RJ, et al. Neurocognitive dysfunction predicts postmortem findings of HIV encephalitis. *Neurology.* 2002 Nov 26; 59(10):1563–1567.

Cherry CL, Wesselingh SL, Lal L, et al. Evaluation of a clinical screening tool for HIV-associated sensory neuropathies. *Neurology.* 2005; 65(11):1778–1781.

Cho T, Vaitkevicius H. Infectious myelopathies. *Continuum.* 2012; 18(6):1351–1373.

Chong J, Di Rocco A, Tagliati M, et al. MR findings in AIDS-associated myelopathy. *Am J Neuroradiol.* 1999; 20(8):1412–1416.

Chou R, Fanciullo GJ, Fine PG, et al. Opioids for chronic noncancer pain: prediction and identification of aberrant drug-related behaviors: A review of the evidence for an American Pain Society and American Academy of Pain Medicine clinical practice guideline. *J Pain.* 2009; 10(2):131–146.

Cinque P, Cleator GM, Weber T, et al. Clinical review diagnosis and clinical management of neurological disorders caused by cytomegalovirus in AIDS patients. *J NeuroVirol.* 1998; 4:120–132.

Cornblath DR, McArthur JC. Predominantly sensory neuropathy in patients with AIDS and AIDS-related complex. *Neurology.* 1988; 38(5):794–796.

Cornblath DR, McArthur JC, Kennedy PGE, et al. Inflammatory demyelinating peripheral neuropathies associated with human T-cell lymphotropic virus type III infection. *Ann Neurol.* 1987; 21:32040.

Corral I, Quereda C, Casado JL, et al. Acute polyradiculopathies in HIV-infected patients. *J Neurol.* 1997; 244:499–504.

Dal Pan GJ, Berger JR. Spinal cord disease in human immunodeficiency virus infection. In Berger JR, Levy RM (Eds.), *AIDS and the Nervous System,* 2nd ed. Philadelphia, PA: Lippincott-Raven; 1997:173–187.

Dal Pan GJ, Glass JD, McArthur JC. Clinicopathologic correlations of HIV-1-associated vacuolar myelopathy: An autopsy-based case-control study. *Neurology.* 1994; 44(11):2159–2164.

Dalakas MC, Cupler EJ. Neuropathies in HIV infection. *Baillieres Clin Neurol.* 1996; 5(1):199–218.

Dardis C. Acute motor axonal neuropathy in a patient with prolonged CD4 depletion due to HIV: A local variant of macrophage activation syndrome? *Oxford Med Case Rep.* 2015; 2:200–2002.

DeVivo DC, Percy AK, Chiriboga CA, et al. Neuromuscular disorders in HIV-1 infection. *Continuum.* 2000; 6:73–76.

Dimachkie MM, Barohn RJ. Distal myopathies. *Neurol Clin.* 2014 Aug; 32(3):817–842.

Di Rocco A. Diseases of the spinal cord in human immunodeficiency virus infection. *Semin Neurol.* 1999; 19:151–155.

Di Rocco A, Simpson, DM. AIDS-associated vacuolar myelopathy. *AIDS Patient Care STDs.* 1998; 12(6):457–461.

Dorfman D, George MC, Schnur J, et al. Hypnosis for treatment of HIV neuropathic pain: A preliminary report. *Pain Med.* 2013; 14:1048–1056.

Edén A, Fuchs D, Hagberg L, et al. HIV-1 viral escape in cerebrospinal fluid of subjects on suppressive treatment. *J Infect Dis.* 2010; 202(12):1819–1825.

Ellis R, Deutsch R, Heaton RK, et al. Neurocognitive impairment is an independent risk factor for death in HIV infection: San Diego HIV Neurobehavioral Research Center Group. *Arch Neurol.* 1997 Apr; 54(4):416–424.

Ellis RJ, Letendre SL, Vaida F, et al. Randomized trial of central nervous system targeted antiretrovirals for HIV-associated neurocognitive disorder. *Clin Infect Dis.* 2014; 58(7):1015–1022.

Ellis RJ, Rosario D, Clifford DB, et al. Continued high prevalence and adverse clinical impact of human immunodeficiency virus-associated sensory neuropathy in the era of combination antiretroviral therapy: The CHARTER Study. *Arch Neurol.* 2010; 67(5):552–558.

Evans SR, Ellis RJ, Chen H, et al. Peripheral neuropathy in HIV: Prevalence and risk factors. *AIDS.* 2011; 25(7):919–928.

Gambarin KH, Hamill RJ. Management of increased intracranial pressure in cryptococcal meningitis. *Curr Infect Dis Rep.* 2002; 4(4):332–338.

Goldstein JM, Azizi SA, Booss J, et al. Human immunodeficiency virus-associated motor axonal polyradiculoneuropathy. *Arch Neurol.* 1993; 50:1316–1319.

Hadden RD, Cornblath DR, Hughes RA, et al.; Plasma exchange/Sandoglobulin Guillain–Barré Syndrome Trial Group. Electrophysiological classification of Guillain–Barré syndrome: Clinical associations and outcome. *Ann Neurol.* 1998; 44(5): 780–788.

Hamada Y, Watanabe K, Aoki T, et al. Primary HIV infection with acute transverse myelitis. *Intern Med.* 2011; 50:1615–1617.

Hammond ER, Crum RM, Treisman GJ, et al. The cerebrospinal fluid HIV risk score for assessing central nervous system activity in persons with HIV. *Am J Epidemiol.* 2014; 180(3):297–307.

Hasbun R. The acute aseptic meningitis syndrome. *Curr Infect Dis Rep.* 2000; 2(4):345–351.

Hasbun R, Eraso J, Ramireddy S, et al. Screening for neurocognitive impairment in HIV individuals: The utility of the Montreal Cognitive Assessment Test. *J AIDS Clinic Res.* 2012; 3:10.

Hiraga A, Kuwabara S, Nakamura A, et al. Fisher/Guillain–Barré overlap syndrome in advanced AIDS. *J Neurol Sci.* 2007; 258(1–2):148–150.

Hughes RA. Inflammatory neuropathy: Sixth meeting of the Peripheral Neuropathy Association. St. Catherine's College, Oxford, England, August 14–18, 1990. *Neurology.* 1991; 41(5):758–759.

Huis in't Veld D, Sun HY, Hung CC, Colebunders R. The immune reconstitution inflammatory syndrome related to HIV co-infections: A review. *Eur J Clin Microbiol Infect Dis.* 2012 Jun; 31(6):919–927.

Ismail Z, Rajji TK, Shulman KL. Brief cognitive screening instruments: An update. *Int J Geriatr Psychiatry.* 2010; 25(2):111–120.

Jacks A, Wainwright D, Salazar L, et al. Neurocognitive deficits increase lack of retention in care among older with newly diagnosed HIV infection. *AIDS.* 2015; 29(13):1711–1714.

Jadhav S, Agrawal M, Rathi S. Acute motor axonal neuropathy in HIV infection. *Indian J Pediatr.* 2014; 81:193.

Johnson TP, Patel K, Johnson KR, et al. Induction of IL-17 and nonclassical T-cell activation by HIV-Tat protein. *Proc Natl Acad Sci USA.* 2013 Aug 13; 110:13588–13593.

Kallianpur AR, Hulgan T. Pharmacogenetics of nucleoside reverse-transcriptase inhibitor-associated peripheral neuropathy. *Pharmacogenomics.* 2009; 10(4):623–637.

Keswani SC, Pardo CA, Cherry CL, et al. HIV-associated sensory neuropathies. *AIDS.* 2002; 16(16):2105–2117.

Keswani SC, Polley M, Pardo CA, et al. Schwann cell chemokine receptors mediate HIV-1 gp120 toxicity to sensory neurons. *Arch Neurol.* 2003; 54(3):287–296.

Leger JM, Bouche P, Bolgert F, et al. The spectrum of polyneuropathies in patients infected with HIV. *J Neurol Neurosurg Psychiatry.* 1989; 52(12):1369–1374.

Lehmann HC, Chen W, Borzan J, et al. Mitochondrial dysfunction in distal axons contributes to human immunodeficiency virus sensory neuropathy. *Arch Neurol.* 2011; 69(1):100–110.

Lescure FX, Moulignier A, Savatovsky J, et al. CD8 encephalitis in HIV-infected patients receiving cART: A treatable entity. *Clin Infect Dis.* 2013; 57(1):101–108.

Letendre S. Central nervous system complications in HIV disease: HIV-associated neurocognitive disorder. *Top Antivir Med.* 2011 Nov; 19(4):137–142.

Letendre S, Fitzsimons C, Ellis R, et al. Correlates of CSF viral loads in 1221 volunteers of the CHARTER Cohort. Paper presented at the 17th Conference on Retrovirus and Opportunistic Infections, February 16–19, 2010, San Francisco, CA. Abstract 172.

Lindenbaum Y, Kissel JT, Mendell JR. Treatment approaches for Guillain–Barré syndrome and chronic inflammatory demyelinating polyradiculopathy. *Neurol Clin.* 2001; 19(1):187–204.

Lipkin WI, Parry G, Kiprov D, et al. Inflammatory neuropathy in homosexual men with lymphadenopathy. *Neurology.* 1985; 35(10):1479–1483.

Lopez Castelblanco R, Lee M, Hasbun R. Epidemiology of bacterial meningitis in the US: A population based study. *Lancet Infect Dis.* 2014; 14:813–819.

Maggiolo F, Airoldi M, Kleinloog HD, et al. Effect of adherence to HAART on virologic outcome and on the selection of resistance-conferring mutations in NNRTI- or PI-treated patients. *HIV Clin Trials.* 2007 Sep–Oct; 8(5):282–292.

Manns A, Hisada M, La Grenade L. Human T-lymphotropic virus type I infection. *Lancet.* 1999; 353(9168):1951–1958.

Markarian Y, Wulff EA, Simpson DM. Peripheral neuropathy in HIV disease. *AIDS Clin Care.* 1998; 10(12):89–91, 93, 98.

Marra C, Maxwell CL, Smith SL, et al. Cerebrospinal fluid abnormalities in patients with syphilis: Association with clinical and laboratory features. *J Infect Dis.* 2004 Feb 1; 189(3):369–376.

Marra CM, Boutin P, Collier AC. Screening for distal sensory peripheral neuropathy in HIV-infected persons in research and clinical settings. *Neurology.* 1998; 51(6):1678–1681.

Marshall DW, Brey RL, Cahill WT, et al. Spectrum of cerebrospinal fluid findings in various stages of human immunodeficiency virus infection. *Arch Neurol.* 1988; 45:954–958.

Martin F, Taylor GP. Prospects for the management of human T-cell lymphotropic virus type 1-associated myelopathy. *AIDS Rev.* 2011; 13(3):161–170.

Martin JL, Brown CE, Matthews-Davis N, et al. Effects of antiviral nucleoside analogs on human DNA polymerases and mitochondrial DNA synthesis. *Antimicrob Agents Chemother.* 1994; 38(12):2743–2749.

Maschke M, Kastrup O, Diener HC. CNS manifestations of cytomegalovirus infections diagnosis and treatment. *CNS Drugs.* 2002; 16(5):303–315.

McArthur JC, Brew BJ, Nath A. Neurological complications of HIV infection. *Lancet Neurol.* 2005; 4(9):543–555.

McCutchan JA. Cytomegalovirus infections of the nervous system in patients with AIDS. *Clin Infect Dis.* 1995 Apr; 20(4):747–754.

Mind Exchange Working Group. Assessment, diagnosis, and treatment of HIV-associated neurocognitive disorder: A consensus report of the Mind Exchange Program. *Clin Infect Dis.* 2013; 56(7):1004–1017.

Mishra BB, Sommers W, Koski CL, et al. Acute inflammatory demyelinating polyneuropathy in the acquired immune deficiency syndrome. *Ann Neurol.* 1985; 18:131–132.

Modi G, Ranchhod J, Hari K, et al. Non-traumatic myelopathy at the Chris Hani Baragwanath Hospital, South Africa—The influence of HIV. *QJM.* 2011: 104:697–703.

Moore RD, Wong WM, Keruly JC, et al. Incidence of neuropathy in HIV-infected patients on monotherapy versus those on combination therapy with didanosine, stavudine and hydroxyurea. *AIDS.* 2000; 14(3):273–278.

Morgello S, Cho ES, Nielsen S, et al. Cytomegalovirus encephalitis in patients with acquired immunodeficiency syndrome: An autopsy study of 30 cases and a review of the literature. *Hum Pathol.* 1987; 18:289–297.

Nesher L, Hadi CM, Salazar L, et al. Epidemiology of meningitis with a negative CSF Gram-stain: Underutilization of available diagnostic tests. *Epidemiol Infect.* 2016 Jan; 144(1):189–197.

Offiah CE, Turnbull IW. The imaging appearances of intracranial CNS infections in adult HIV and AIDS patients. *Clin Radiol.* 2006; 61:393–401.

Pardo CA, McArthur JC, Griffin JW. HIV neuropathy: Insights in the pathology of HIV peripheral nerve disease. *J Peripheral Nerv Syst.* 2001; 6(1):21–27.

Park H, Song Y. Multiple tuberculoma involving the brain and spinal cord in a patient with miliary pulmonary tuberculosis. *J Korean Neurosurg Soc.* 2008 Jul; 44(1):36–39.

Parry O, Mielke J, Latif AS, et al. Peripheral neuropathy in individuals with HIV infection in Zimbabwe. *Acta Neurol Scand.* 1997; 96(4):218–222.

Perfect JR, Dismukes WE, Dromer F, et al. Clinical practice guidelines for the treatment of cryptococcal disease: 2010 update from the Infectious Diseases Society of America. *Clin Infect Dis.* 2012; 50:291–322.

Petito CK, Vecchio D, Chen YT. HIV antigen and DNA in AIDS spinal cords correlate with macrophage infiltration but not with vacuolar myelopathy. *J Neuropathol Exp Neurol.* 1994; 53(1):86–94.

Phillips TJ, Cherry CL, Cox S, et al. Pharmacological treatment of painful HIV-associated sensory neuropathy: A systematic review and meta-analysis of randomised controlled trials. *PLoS One.* 2010; 5(12):e14433.

Piliero PJ, Fish DG, Preston S, et al. Guillain–Barré syndrome associated with immune reconstitution. *Clin Infect Dis.* 2003; 36(9):e111–e114.

Pillat MM, Bauer ME, de Oliveira AC, et al. HTLV-1-associated myelopathy/tropical spastic paraparesis (HAM/TSP): Still an obscure disease. *Cent Nerv Syst Agents Med Chem.* 2011; 11(4):239–245. Epub 2012/02/04.

Plasma Exchange/Sandoglobulin Guillain–Barré Syndrome Trial Group. Randomised trial of plasma exchange, intravenous immunoglobulin, and combined treatments in Guillain–Barré syndrome. *Lancet.* 1997; 349:225–230.

Polydefkis M, Yiannoutsos CT, Cohen BA, et al. Reduced intraepidermal nerve fiber density in HIV-associated sensory neuropathy. *Neurology.* 2002; 58(1):115–119.

Portegies P, Solod L, Cinque P, et al. EFNS Task Force guidelines for the diagnosis and management of neurological complications of HIV infection. *Eu J Neurol.* 2004; 11:297–304.

Price RW, Yiannoutsos CT, Clifford DB, et al. Neurological outcomes in late HIV infection: Adverse impact of neurological impairment on survival and protective effect of antiviral therapy. AIDS Clinical Trial Group and Neurological AIDS Research Consortium Study Team. *AIDS.* 1999; 13(13):1677–1685.

Radziwill AJ, Kuntzer T, Steck AJ. Immunopathology and treatments of Guillain–Barré syndrome and of chronic inflammatory demyelinating polyneuropathy. *Rev Neurol (Paris).* 2002; 158(3):301–310.

Rauschkaa H, Jellingerb K, Lassmannc H, et al. Guillain–Barré syndrome with marked pleocytosis or a significant proportion of polymorphonuclear granulocytes in the cerebrospinal fluid: Neuropathological investigation of five cases and review of differential diagnoses. *Eur J Neurol.* 2003; 10:479–486.

Robertson KR, Smurzynski M, Parsons TD, et al. The prevalence and incidence of neurocognitive impairment in the HAART era. *AIDS*. 2007; 21:1915–1921.

Robinson-Papp J, Gonzalez-Duarte A, Simpson DM, et al. The roles of ethnicity and antiretrovirals in HIV-associated polyneuropathy: A pilot study. *J Acquir Immune Defic Syndr*. 2009; 51(5):569–573.

Robinson-Papp J, Sharma S, Simpson DM, et al. Autonomic dysfunction is common in HIV and associated with distal symmetric polyneuropathy. *J Neurovirol*. 2013; 19:172–180.

Robinson-Papp J, Simpson DM. Neuromuscular diseases associated with HIV-1 infection. *Muscle Nerve*. 2009; 40(6):1043–1053.

Rolfes MA, Hullsiek KH, Rhein J, et al. The effect of therapeutic lumbar punctures on acute mortality from cryptococcal meningitis. *Clin Infect Dis*. 2014; 59(11):1607–1614.

Rosca EC, Rosca O, Simu M. Intravenous immunoglobulin treatment in a HIV-1 positive patient with Guillain–Barré syndrome. *Int Immunopharmacol*. 2015 Dec; 29(2):964–965.

Sandoval R, Runft B, Roddey T. Pilot study: Does lower extremity night splinting assist in the management of painful peripheral neuropathy in the HIV/AIDS population? *J Int Assoc Phys AIDS Care (Chic)*. 2010; 9(6):368–381.

Schifitto G, McDermott MP, McArthur JC, et al.; Dana Consortium on the Therapy of HIV Dementia and Related Cognitive Disorders. Incidence of and risk factors for HIV-associated distal sensory polyneuropathy. *Neurology*. 2002; 58(12):1764–1768.

Schreiber AL, Norbury JW, DeSousa EA. Functional recovery of untreated human immunodeficiency virus-associated Guillain–Barré syndrome: A case report. *Ann Phys Rehabil Med*. 2011; 54:519–524.

Sidtis JJ, Gatsonis C, Price RW, et al.; AIDS Clinical Trials Group. Zidovudine treatment of the AIDS dementia complex: Results of a placebo-controlled trial. *Ann Neurol*. 1993; 33:343–349.

Silva CA, Penalva de Oliveira AC, Vilas-Boas L, et al. Neurologic cytomegalovirus complications in patients with AIDS: Retrospective review of 13 cases and review of the literature. *Rev Inst Med Trop Sao Paulo*. 2010; 52(6):305–310.

Simpson DM, Brown S, Tobias J; NGX-4010 C107 Study Group. Controlled trial of high-concentration capsaicin patch for treatment of painful HIV neuropathy. *Neurology*. 2008; 70: 2305–2313.

Simpson DM, Kitch D, Evans SR, et al.; ACTG A5117 Study Group. HIV neuropathy natural history cohort study: Assessment measures and risk factors. *Neurology*. 2006; 66(11):1679–1687.

Simpson JK 3rd. Chronic neuropathic pain. *N Engl J Med*. 2003; 348(26):2688–2689; author reply 2688–2689.

Smyth K, Affandi JS, McArthur JC, et al. Prevalence of and risk factors for HIV-associated neuropathy in Melbourne, Australia 1993–2006. *HIV Med*. 2007; 8:367–373.

Tagliati M, Grinnell J, Godbold J, et al. Peripheral nerve function in HIV infection: Clinical, electrophysiologic, and laboratory findings. *Arch Neurol*. 1999; 56(1):84–89.

Tan K, Roda R, et al. PML-IRIS in patients with HIV infection: Clinical manifestations and treatment with steroids. *Neurology*. 2009; 72(17):1458–1464.

Thwaites GE. The management of suspected encephalitis. *BMJ*. 2012 Jun 6; 344.

Tunkel AR, Glaser CA, Bloch KC, et al. The management of encephalitis: Clinical practice guidelines by the Infectious Diseases Society of America. *Clin Infect Dis*. 2004; 47(3):303–327.

Tyor WR, Glass JD, Baumrind N, et al. Cytokine expression of macrophages in HIV-1-associated vacuolar myelopathy. *Neurology*. 1993; 43(5):1002–1009.

US Department of Health and Human Services, Panel on Antiretroviral Guidelines for Adults and Adolescents. Guidelines for the use of antiretroviral agents in HIV-1-infected adults and adolescents. January 28, 2016. Available at https://aidsinfo.nih.gov/guidelines/html/1/adult-and-adolescent-treatment-guidelines/0.

US Department of Health and Human Services, Panel on Opportunistic Infections in HIV-Infected Adults and Adolescents. Guidelines for the prevention and treatment of opportunistic infections in HIV-infected adults and adolescents: Recommendations from the Centers for Disease Control and Prevention, the National Institutes of Health, and the HIV Medicine Association of the Infectious Diseases Society of America. Available at https://aidsinfo.nih.gov/contentfiles/lvguidelines/adult_oi.pdf. Accessed May 11, 2016.

Valcour V, Paul R, Chiao S, et al. Screening for cognitive impairment in human immunodeficiency virus. *Clin Infect Dis*. 2011a Oct; 53(8):836–842.

Valcour VG. Evaluating cognitive impairment in the clinical setting: Practical screening and assessment tools. *Top Antivir Med*. 2011b Dec; 19(5):175–180.

Valcour V, Sithinamsuwan P, Letendre S, et al. Pathogenesis of HIV in the central nervous system. *Curr HIV/AIDS Rep*. 2011 Mar; 8(1):54–61.

Van der Meche FG, Schitz PI; Dutch Guillain–Barré Study Group. A randomized trial comparing intravenous immune globulin and plasma exchange in Guillain–Barré syndrome. *N Engl J Med*. 1992; 326(17):1123–1129.

Vanheule S, Desmet M, Groenvynck H, et al. The factor of the Beck Depression Inventory-II: An evaluation. *Assessment*. 2008; 15(2):177–187.

Veltman JA, Bristow CC, Klausner JD. Meningitis in HIV-positive patients in sub-Saharan Africa: A review. *J Int AIDS Soc*. 2014; 17:19184.

Verma A. Epidemiology and clinical features HIV-1 associated neuropathies. *J Peripheral Nerv Syst*. 2001; 6(1):8–13.

Verma A, Bradley WG. HIV-1 associated neuropathies. *CNS Spectrums*. 2000; 5(5):66–67.

Verma S, Estanislao L, Mintz L, et al. Controlling neuropathic pain in HIV. *Curr HIV/AIDS Rep*. 2004; 1(3):136–141.

Wagner JC, Bromber MB. HIV infection presenting with motor axonal variant of Guillain–Barré syndrome. *J Clin Neuromusc Disord*. 2007; 9:303–305.

Wakerly BR, Yuki N. Mimics and chameleons in Guillain–Barré and Miller–Fisher syndromes. *Practical Neurol*. 2015; 15:90–99.

Wang SX, Ho EL, Grill M, et al. Peripheral neuropathy in primary HIV infection associates with systemic and CNS immune activation. *J Acquir Immune Defic Syndr*. 2014; 66(3):303–310.

Weekly Epidemiological Record. Meningococcal disease control in countries of the African meningitis belt, 2014. *Wkly Epidemiol Rec*. 2015 Mar 27; 90(13):123–131.

Winer JB. Guillain–Barré syndrome. *J Clin Pathol*. 2001; 54:381–385.

Wulff EA, Simpson DM. Neuromuscular complications of the human immunodeficiency virus type 1 infection. *Semin Neurol*. 1999a; 19(2):157–164.

Wulff EA, Simpson DM. Neuromuscular complications of HIV-1 infection. *Curr Infect Dis Rep*. 1999b; 1(2):192–197.

Wulff EA, Wang AK, Simpson DM. HIV-associated peripheral neuropathy: Epidemiology, pathophysiology and treatment. *Drugs*. 2000; 59(6):1251–1260.

Yousem DM, Grossman RI. *The Requisites: Neuroradiology*, 3rd ed. Philadelphia, PA: Mosby; 2010:209.

39.

HIV/HEPATITIS CO-INFECTION

Ben J. Barnett and Margaret Hoffman-Terry

HIV AND HEPATITIS B CO-INFECTION

LEARNING OBJECTIVE

Discuss the clinical presentation, diagnosis, treatment, and treatment complications of hepatitis B in HIV-infected patients.

WHAT'S NEW?

All patients with HIV/hepatitis B virus (HBV) co-infection should receive treatment for both viruses, regardless of CD4⁺ T cell count or independent need for HBV treatment.

KEY POINTS

- All HIV-infected patients should have a complete evaluation for HBV infection.

- Patients without evidence of prior immunity or current HBV infection should be vaccinated against HBV.

- HBV treatment in co-infected patients should include two active agents against HBV, in the context of fully suppressive antiretroviral therapy (ART) against HIV.

HBV infection is common in people living with HIV, and all patients with HIV should be screened for HBV infection. The most common route of transmission worldwide is through perinatal or early childhood exposure, but adult transmission of HBV is often by routes similar to those for HIV, including sexual contact and injection drug use. Although it varies by exposure route, approximately 10% of HIV-positive patients also have chronic HBV infection, and up to 90% have serologic evidence of past exposure to HBV (Alter, 2006). Long-term complications of HBV infection can include cirrhosis, end-stage liver disease, and hepatocellular carcinoma (HCC).

DIAGNOSIS AND EVALUATION

Initial testing for HBV should include serologic testing for surface antigen (HBsAg), core antibody (anti-HBc total), and surface antibody (anti-HBs). HBsAg can usually be detected approximately 4 weeks after exposure. Resolution of acute HBV is characterized by negative HBsAg and the presence of anti-HBs and anti-HBc, but reactivation may recur with severe immunosuppression. Chronic HBV is defined as the presence of HBsAg for at least 6 months. For patients with chronic HBV, tests for HBV DNA, HBeAg, and anti-HBeAb are recommended.

Patients with HBeAg usually have high HBV DNA and elevated alanine aminotransferase (ALT) levels and are at high risk of future liver complications. A conversion from HBeAg to anti-HBe can imply a transition from active disease to an inactive carrier state, but this occurs less commonly in patients co-infected with HIV. This inactive carrier state is also characterized by HBV DNA <2000 IU/ml and normal ALT. These patients do remain at risk for reactivation of HBV and liver disease progression but at a lower rate than that of patients with active disease. Finally, there also exists a state of HBeAg-negative active hepatitis, which is a result of mutations in the pre-core and core promoter regions. These patients are at significant risk of progressive liver disease, and HBV DNA levels should be monitored regularly and treatment instituted as recommended (Hadziyannis, 2006).

A sometimes confusing situation, especially common in HIV co-infected patients, is the presence of anti-HBc alone, with negative results for HBsAg and anti-HBs. This may represent prior infection with subsequent loss of anti-HBs, a false-positive anti-HBc, or "occult HBV infection," with a positive HBV DNA. The clinical significance of this situation is unclear, but it may be prudent to test these patients for HBV DNA and treat if positive and vaccinate if negative. Patients with occult HBV are at increased risk of HBV reactivation, and it is also associated with increased risk of hepatocellular carcinoma (Shire, 2004).

Elevations of hepatic transaminases are suggestive of inflammation, and hepatic synthetic function is measured by serum albumin and coagulation factors. An assessment of the degree of liver fibrosis is important, and options for this include liver biopsy or noninvasive testing such as transient elastography or an increasing array of serum biomarker tests. Patients with cirrhosis should have HCC screening by ultrasound every 6–12 months, and all patients with cirrhosis should be co-managed with a hepatologist (Lok, 2009).

Authoritative guidelines have been published regarding treatment of HBV (Terrault, 2016), but it should be emphasized that current HIV guidelines recommend treatment of all HIV-infected patients, regardless of CD4 status, and that co-infected patients with HBV should be a priority group for HIV treatment. Thus, it follows that all HIV/HBV co-infected patients should be treated for both HIV and HBV, regardless of the exact stage of HBV or degree of liver fibrosis.

Symptoms and Signs

Acute hepatitis typically occurs 2–5 months after exposure and can be asymptomatic or manifest as symptoms of fatigue, fever, right upper quadrant pain, and nausea with or without jaundice. Initial studies are positive for HBsAg and immunoglobulin M (IgM) antibody to HBV core antigen (IgM anti-HBc), although IgM anti-HBc may also be seen in some patients with reactivation of chronic HBV. HBV DNA and HBeAg levels rise, and elevated levels of serum liver transaminases (ALT and aspartate aminotransferase (AST)) develop. With successful clearance of acute infection, HBV DNA, HBsAg, and HBeAg will resolve, and the antibodies anti-HBs, anti-HBe, and anti-HBc IgG will develop.

Fewer than 10% of immunocompetent adults and approximately 20% of HIV patients will fail to clear an acute HBV infection, do not produce antibody to HBsAg, and thus develop chronic infection. These patients may develop chronic fatigue or extrahepatic manifestations of hepatitis, such as glomerulonephritis or arthritis, or they may be asymptomatic until the development of cirrhosis years or decades later.

Co-infection Considerations

In general terms, the presence of HIV co-infection worsens outcomes related to HBV. HIV-infected patients are less likely to resolve acute HBV exposure and have higher levels of HBV DNA compared to patients without HIV (Colin, 1999). HIV co-infection is associated with more rapid progression of HBV-related cirrhosis, hepatocellular carcinoma, and fatal hepatic failure (Thio, 2002). Indeed, HBV infection was associated with a relative risk of 3.73 for liver-related deaths in HIV co-infected participants in the Data Collection on Adverse Events of Anti-HIV Drugs (D:A:D) study (Weber, 2006).

Because the immune response plays a key role in both HBV clearance and the immune damage associated with chronic HBV infection, HIV co-infection impacts the course of HBV infection. HIV-induced immunosuppression increases the risk of reactivation of quiescent HBV, and initiation of ART may result in exacerbation of HBV liver disease or fulminant hepatitis (Sulkowski, 2001).

Stopping antiretroviral agents with activity against HBV (lamivudine, emtricitabine, and tenofovir) may lead to frequent HBV rebound, sometimes accompanied by a severe flare of HBV and hepatocellular damage (Dore, 2010). Thus, when co-infected patients change ART regimens, it is crucial to maintain agents with anti-HBV activity. If anti-HBV treatment is discontinued, serum transaminase levels should be monitored regularly; if a hepatic flare occurs, then HBV therapy should be restarted immediately because this could be lifesaving (US Department of Health and Human Services (DHHS), Panel on Opportunistic Infections, 2015).

HBV Prevention

HIV-infected patients should be counseled about transmission risks for HBV, including sexual transmission, sharing of needles and syringes, and tattooing or body piercing. Patients at risk for HBV should be advised to avoid these behaviors associated with transmission (DHHS, Panel on Opportunistic Infections, 2015).

HBV vaccination is the most effective way to prevent HBV infection. If there is no evidence of chronic infection or previous vaccination, then a hepatitis B vaccination series should be administered (DHHS, 2015). Patients who are positive for anti-HBs and anti-HBc have a resolved infection and do not require vaccination. Patients with "isolated anti-HBc" (see previous description) who have an undetectable HBV DNA should receive a complete HBV vaccine series.

Unfortunately, the preventive HBV vaccination is less effective in people co-infected with HIV, with efficacy rates in the HIV co-infected population of approximately 65%, and those with a CD4$^+$ T cell count <350 cells/mm^3 have even lower response rates. HBV vaccination of all non-immune HIV-positive individuals is currently recommended regardless of CD4+ T cell count, and vaccination should not be deferred in patients with CD4+ T cell count <350 cells/mm³ (DHHS, Panel on Opportunistic Infections, 2015). Various revaccination strategies are available for patients who do not respond to an initial series, and research attempting to determine the optimal vaccine series for initial vaccination to improve response rates is ongoing (Launay, 2011).

The use of HBV active antiretroviral agents to prevent acquisition of HBV in HIV co-infected patients who have not responded to a vaccine series is an emerging idea. In one study, tenofovir use was particularly protective against acquisition of primary HBV infection in HIV-positive patients (Heuft, 2014).

HIV/HBV co-infected patients should also be vaccinated against hepatitis A if susceptible, and they should avoid alcohol consumption.

Goals of Treatment

The goals of treatment for HBV infection are to achieve sustained suppression of viral replication to below detectable levels and to improve or stabilize the degree of liver disease in order to prevent cirrhosis, hepatic failure, and hepatocellular carcinoma. Measurements of response to therapy include the decline in HBV DNA levels to undetectable levels, loss of HBeAg or gain of anti-HBe antibody (termed seroconversion), normalization of serum ALT, and improvement in liver histology. Functional cure is represented by an undetectable HBsAg, which may reduce progression to cirrhosis and liver cancer (Sherman, 2015).

HIV Treatment Recommendations in the Setting of HBV Co-infection

Because co-infection with HIV is associated with more rapid progression of HBV-related liver disease and there is evidence that earlier treatment of HIV may slow the development of liver disease by improving immune function and reducing HIV-related inflammation and immune activation, current HIV treatment guidelines recommend that all co-infected patients start ART and that the ART regimen include drugs with activity against both viruses (DHHS, Panel on Antiretroviral Guidelines for Adults and Adolescents, 2015). Furthermore, the Panel recommends that in settings in which it is impractical to treat all HIV-infected patients with ART, treatment should be prioritized for patients with HBV, among other high-risk conditions such as pregnancy and so on.

The Panel on Opportunistic Infections makes the following recommendations for HIV/HBV co-infected patients (DHHS, Panel on Opportunistic Infections, 2015):

- Regardless of CD4 cell count or the need for HBV treatment, ART that includes agents active against both HIV and HBV is recommended for all co-infected patients.

- ART must include two drugs active against HBV, preferably tenofovir and emtricitabine, regardless of the level of HBV DNA.

- If the patient refuses HIV treatment, then there are few options available to treat HBV because HBV drugs (including entecavir and possibly telbivudine) given without suppressive ART may result in HIV resistance. A 48-week course of pegylated interferon-α-2a can be considered in such circumstances.

- In circumstances in which tenofovir DF use is not acceptable as part of the ART regimen, the alternate recommendation is to use entecavir in addition to a fully suppressive ART.

- Chronic use of lamivudine or emtricitabine as the single active agent against HBV should be avoided because of the high rate of subsequent HBV resistance.

Patients being treated for HBV should have HBV DNA measured every 12–24 weeks. If the HBV DNA is >1000 IU/ml after 1 year, then adherence to medication should be assessed and HBV resistance testing considered. Viral failure and resistance are more common in HIV co-infected patients with HBV, especially when lamivudine is used alone for treatment. The risk of resistance has declined with the use of more potent drugs such as tenofovir and entecavir (Luetkemeyer, 2011). Unfortunately, even with long-term suppression of HBV DNA, the loss of HBsAg (functional cure) of HBV is not common in patients with HIV co-infection (Sherman, 2015), and indefinite treatment is usually recommended.

SPECIAL CONSIDERATIONS

Immune Reconstitution Inflammatory Syndrome

Immune reconstitution during the course of HIV treatment can lead to a severe flare of chronic HBV infection, with significant increases in hepatic transaminases, perhaps due to enhanced host immune responses against HBV. HBV-associated immune reconstitution inflammatory syndrome

(IRIS) is most likely to occur in the first few months after starting ART and can present as acute hepatitis. Careful monitoring of hepatic transaminases after the initiation of ART is helpful (Audsley, 2011). Development of signs of hepatic synthetic dysfunction, such as elevated prothrombin time or low albumin, should prompt evaluation by a hepatologist. Distinguishing between HBV-related IRIS and drug-induced liver toxicity can be challenging and may require examination of liver histology and consultation with a hepatologist. Very little information is available regarding the best treatment for HBV-related IRIS, and the decision regarding whether to continue, modify, or interrupt therapy should be individualized based on the severity of hepatic injury.

Treatment Interruptions

Due to the overlap in anti-HIV and HBV activity of emtricitabine, lamivudine, and tenofovir, interruption of treatment should be avoided in HIV/HBV co-infection to avoid potentially severe flares of HBV with hepatic inflammation and necrosis. In particular, when there is a need to discontinue one of the HBV-active drugs in the HIV treatment regimen, careful follow-up of liver function tests is required, and addition of a second agent with anti-HBV activity should be considered. If there is a need to change ART due to HIV resistance and HBV suppression is maintained despite HIV treatment failure, the antiretrovirals with activity against HBV should be continued for HBV treatment in addition to other appropriate antiretroviral agents.

TREATMENT OPTIONS FOR HEPATITIS B INFECTION

US Food and Drug Administration (FDA)-approved drugs for the treatment of HBV infection include interferon-α (IFN-α; standard and pegylated), lamivudine, adefovir, tenofovir DF, entecavir, and telbivudine. The fixed-dose combination of tenofovir–emtricitabine or emtricitabine alone are not FDA approved for use to treat HBV, but they have demonstrated activity (DHHS, Panel on Opportunistic Infections, 2015).

Interferons

IFN-α (standard or pegylated) is indicated for the treatment of chronic HBV, but there are limited data on the treatment of HIV/HBV co-infected patients, with lower rates of success and more toxicities compared to those of HBV mono-infected populations. Toxicities include psychiatric reactions, fatigue, headache, and cytopenias.

Nucleoside/Nucleotide Analogs

Lamivudine

Lamivudine is effective in treating HBV infection in mono-infected patients, but the development of HBV resistance to lamivudine through YMDD mutations is more common in the setting of HIV/HBV co-infection. By the fourth year of lamivudine monotherapy, greater than 90% of co-infected patients develop HBV resistance. Thus, it is recommended that lamivudine always be used in combination with another anti-HBV drug.

Emtricitabine

Emtricitabine has an overlapping resistance profile with lamivudine and a longer half-life. It is used generally in combination with tenofovir, in a fixed-dose tablet.

Tenofovir Disoproxil Fumarate

Tenofovir disoproxil fumarate (TDF) is a nucleotide analog with potent anti-HIV and anti-HBV activity. In co-infected patients, it has shown success in suppressing HBV replication, even in the presence of lamivudine resistance. It has greater activity than adefovir, in both mono-infected and co-infected populations (Peters, 2006). Tenofovir DF, in combination with emtricitabine or lamivudine, is the initial recommended treatment option as part of a fully suppressive HIV treatment regimen for co-infected patients (DHHS, Panel on Opportunistic Infections, 2015). It may be limited by renal toxicity in some patients.

Tenofovir Alafenamide

Tenofovir alafenamide (TAF) is also a prodrug of tenofovir that is preferentially concentrated in lymphoid tissue, and it is FDA approved in combination with emtricitabine, elvitegravir, and cobicistat for treatment of HIV. Late-stage studies are underway to investigate TAF in HBV infection, but results have not yet been published in peer-reviewed journals. A press release from Gilead Sciences on January 5, 2016, described the results of two phase III clinical trials evaluating the use of TAF 25 mg in treatment-naive and -experienced adults with HBeAg-negative and HBeAg-positive chronic HBV infection. The studies demonstrated that TAF was non-inferior to TDF based on viral response rates at 48 weeks of therapy.

Adefovir Dipivoxil

Adefovir dipivoxil is a nucleotide analog with modest anti-HIV activity only at higher doses (120–300 mg per day) and anti-HBV activity at a lower dose of 10 mg per day. It is less potent than other treatment choices, and resistance can develop with monotherapy (Lok, 2009).

Entecavir

Entecavir is a nucleoside analog with high anti-HBV activity. Resistance to entecavir develops at a more rapid rate in lamivudine-resistant strains of HBV. Due to rare but confirmed reports of the development of the M184V mutation in the HIV reverse transcriptase gene and evidence of anti-HIV activity in vivo, entecavir in patients with HIV/HBV co-infection must be given with a fully suppressive HIV treatment regimen.

Telbivudine

Telbivudine is a thymidine analog with little HIV activity and potent anti-HBV activity. There is a significant risk of development of resistance and cross-resistance with lamivudine with monotherapy. Few data are available regarding its use in HIV/HBV co-infected patients. It has been associated with elevations of creatine kinase and myopathy.

SUMMARY

Hepatitis B infection is a common and potentially severe comorbidity for people with HIV infection. Screening for HBV infection, vaccination, and careful assessment of chronic HBV infection are important components of HIV care. Consideration of chronic HBV status when selecting HIV treatment regimens is essential in optimizing management of both infections. Monitoring for response to treatment for HBV and screening for complications such as cirrhosis or hepatocellular carcinoma are part of the ongoing care of the HIV/HBV co-infected patient.

Recommended Reading

Terrault N, Bzowej N, Chang K-M, et al. AASLD guidelines for treatment of chronic hepatitis B. *Hepatology*. 2016; 63:261–283.

US Department of Health and Human Services, Panel on Opportunistic Infections in HIV-Infected Adults and Adolescents. Guidelines for the prevention and treatment of opportunistic infections in HIV-infected adults and adolescents: recommendations from the Centers for Disease Control and Prevention, the National Institutes of Health, and the HIV Medicine Association of the Infectious Diseases Society of America. Available at https://aidsinfo.nih.gov/contentfiles/lvguidelines/adult_oi.pdf. Accessed December 18, 2015.

HIV AND HCV CO-INFECTION

LEARNING OBJECTIVE

Discuss the clinical presentation, diagnosis, treatment, and treatment complications of hepatitis C virus (HCV) in patients co-infected with HIV.

WHAT'S NEW?

- The treatment of HCV has changed dramatically during the past few years. The emergence of new interferon-free, oral direct-acting antivirals (DAAs) is expected to cure greater than 90% of persons with chronic HCV infections. Injectable pegylated interferon (PEG-IFN) has been fully replaced by safer, more efficacious, and much better tolerated all-oral DAA combinations. HCV treatment guidelines no longer recommend use of PEG-IFN except in alternative regimens to shorten treatment.

- Because ART may slow the progression of HCV-related liver disease, it should be considered for all HIV/HCV co-infected patients, regardless of CD4+ T cell count. If treatment with the new DAAs is planned, the ART regimen may need to be modified to reduce the potential for drug–drug interactions and/or drug toxicities that may develop during the period of concurrent HIV and HCV treatment.

KEY POINTS

- Programs serving HIV/HCV co-infected patients can expect to experience an almost 70% higher rate of utilization in this group.

- The co-infection epidemic is evolving. The Swiss HIV Cohort Study (SHCS) group has observed an 18-fold increase in HIV/HCV co-infection in men who have sex with men (MSM) from 1998 to 2011, in association with a history of unsafe sex, a past syphilis history, and chronic HBV.

- Multiple DAAs have been approved by the FDA, with more in the pipeline.

- Although HCV treatment regimens are now much simpler and all oral, factors such as renal disease, drug–drug interactions, disease severity, and especially cost considerations remain. With HCV regimens typically costing $60,000–$200,000, insurance companies have many requirements for coverage.

We stand on the cusp of revolutionizing the treatment of hepatitis C (HCV). With many of the 1.2 million HIV-infected Americans already in care for their HIV, HIV providers are in a unique position to treat and likely cure HCV in the approximately one-fourth of those who are also co-infected with this virus. Rapid progress in HCV therapeutics has benefited greatly from the framework that previous

HIV research laid down during the past 30 years, rocketing along at breakneck speed and condensing into years what previously would have taken decades. HIV providers with their intimate knowledge of virology, resistance, drug–drug interactions, and the psychosocial needs of this population stand in unique stead to treat HCV.

EPIDEMIOLOGY

As ART continues to extend the lifespan of HIV-infected persons by decades, HCV co-infection has become an increasingly important cause of both morbidity and mortality. Liver disease has emerged as the leading cause of non-AIDS-related deaths in HIV-infected persons co-infected with HCV or HBV (Centers for Disease Control and Prevention (CDC), 2014). HCV co-infection places a growing burden on the HIV health care delivery system, as evidenced by an analysis conducted by the AIDS Clinical Trials Group (ACTG) Longitudinal Linked Randomized Trials (ALLRT) cohort. When controlling for age, race, sex, history of AIDS-defining events, and current CD4+ T cell count and viral load (VL), the relative risk of hospitalization, emergency department visits, and disability days for HIV/HCV co-infected versus HIV mono-infected participants was 1.8 (95% confidence interval (CI), 1.3–2.5), 1.7 (95% CI, 1.4–2.1), and 1.6 (95% CI, 1.3–1.9), respectively. Based on the ACTG's study findings, programs serving co-infected patients can expect to experience an almost 70% higher rate of utilization for this group (Linas, 2011). A study from the New York City Department of Health and Mental Hygiene using death certificate data showed HIV/HCV co-infected persons to be at exceptionally high risk for premature death (median age, 52.0 years) compared to those living with HCV alone (median age, 60.0 years) or those with neither virus (median age, 78.0 years). Decedents had an odds ratio of 2.2 for death from liver cancer and 3.1 for drug-related causes, with 53.6% of deaths attributed to HIV/AIDS and 94% occurring prematurely (defined as younger than age 65 years) (Pinchoff, 2014).

HCV is a single-stranded RNA virus transmitted primarily through blood exposure and, less commonly, through sexual or vertical transmission. Because HIV and HCV share similar routes of transmission, approximately one-fourth of all HIV-infected persons in the United States are also infected with HCV. This percentage increases to 80% for injectable drug users (IDUs) (CDC, 2014). Heterosexual transmission risk is low and generally quoted as less than 1% per year, although high-risk sex practices such as aggressive anal intercourse and multiple sex partners increase transmission risk. Vertical transmission is possible,

with pregnant women co-infected with HIV/HCV having a 15–20% chance of passing HCV to their infants compared to the 5% rate seen in infants born to HCV mono-infected mothers (Bevilacqua, 2009). Co-infected mothers receiving ART and/or undergoing cesarean section may have a lower risk of transmission. Breast-feeding is not known to transmit HCV, but because breast-feeding may transmit HIV, it is contraindicated for co-infected mothers in the United States.

In recent years, co-infection has been a changing epidemic, as evidenced by data from the Swiss Cohort Study. What was once a disease of IDUs and hemophiliacs has become a sexually transmitted disease of MSM. The 4.1 cases per 100 person-years seen in MSM in 2011 in the Swiss Cohort Study represented an 18-fold increase from 1998, with HCV seen in association with a history of unsafe anal sex, a past syphilis history, and chronic HBV (Wandeler, 2012). In 2011, a report was published that included 5-year data from 74 HIV-positive MSM who had no history of IDU and had newly elevated ALT levels with a positive HCV antibody test (Fierer, 2012). This matched case–control study was conducted beginning in July 2007 and examined men who were within 12 months of the clinical onset of HIV infection and who had no IDU history. HIV-infected MSM newly infected with HCV were significantly more likely to have had receptive anal intercourse (mOR, 24.87) or insertive anal intercourse (matched odds ratio (mOR), 2.62) with no condom use and with ejaculation, engaged in group sex (mOR, 19.2), engaged in sex while high on drugs (mOR, 11.37), previously had syphilis (mOR, 8.8), and had sex while using crystal methamphetamine (mOR, 26.8). HIV co-infection results in increased HCV RNA levels, which are thought to increase the infectiousness of HCV acquired through sexual contact. HIV-infected patients should be counseled that unprotected sex can transmit other infections, including HCV.

The connection between prescription narcotic abuse, HIV, and HCV was recently highlighted by a community outbreak of HIV linked to IDU of oxymorphone in a rural county of Indiana. Prior to this investigation, only 5 HIV cases per year were reported. As of April 21, 2015, 135 persons had confirmed or probable HIV infection in a community of 4200 persons. Mean age was 35 years, with 54.8% being males, 80% reporting IDU, and 17% who had not yet been interviewed. All reported their drug of choice was injectable crushed oxymorphone, sometimes with other illicit drugs. Of these, 7.4% were female commercial sex workers. Strikingly, co-infection with HCV was found in 84.4% of patients (Conrad, 2015). Those interviewed reported an average of 9 syringe-sharing or sex partners and social contacts who may be at risk. Of the 230 contacts tested, 109 (47.4%) were positive for HIV. IDU in this community is multigenerational, with the crushed oxymorphone (40-mg tablets are not designed to resist crushing) dissolved in nonsterile water and injected via insulin syringes with the syringes often shared. At 4–15 injections per day reported, with 1–6 injection partners per of injection event, and limited secondary education access to health care, this county is similar to many rural US counties, with this outbreak highlighting the need for community interventions at multiple levels. It also highlights the vulnerability of many resource-poor rural communities that traditionally have low rates of HIV and HCV and is a reminder of how often concomitant transmission of the two viruses continues to occur, particularly in vulnerable IDU and MSM populations.

CLINICAL COURSE

The most striking feature of HCV when acquired by a person infected with HIV is its ability to cause chronic hepatitis in as much as 90% of patients within 6 months. This occurs due to the lack of CD4$^+$ T cell responses and significantly reduced IFN-γ ELISpot responses against HCV (Elliott, 2006). Between 60% and 70% of chronically infected persons will have fluctuating serum ALT levels because this is the enzyme most associated with liver cell injury in HCV. Less than 20% have nonspecific symptoms, including fatigue and generalized weakness. There are significant similarities and differences between HIV and HCV. Both are RNA viruses with rapid replication rates (10 trillion HCV virions vs. 10 billion HIV virions produced daily). Both are prone to frequent mutations and exist as heterogeneous quasispecies to avoid the immune system. Both viruses incite abundant but ineffective antibody responses. Although both have many reservoirs in the human body, HCV exists primarily in the cytoplasm of hepatocytes and can be eradicated from the body. HIV is integrated into the nuclei of CD4$^+$ T lymphocytes and long-lived memory cell reservoirs and therefore cannot be eradicated with current ART. HCV RNA levels are only broadly predictive of long-term prognosis, whereas HIV RNA is very predictive of clinical events in untreated patients.

There are six different HCV genotypes (1–6) at various prevalence rates throughout the world. In the United States, genotype (GT) 1 accounts for two-thirds of cases, with GTs 2–4 occurring less commonly. The human genetic marker IL28B (CC polymorphism), in the region of the interleukin (IL) 28b gene on chromosome 19, has been associated with PEG-INF-α-induced clearance of HCV in co-infected patients, especially those with GTs 1 and 4

(Maheshwari, 2008). The preexisting Q80K variant within the NS3/4A protease gene confers resistance to simeprevir (SMV) and may occur in 9–48% of untreated HCV GT 1a-infected persons. The significance of this and other variants is being studied as the armamentarium of DAAs expands (Luetkemeyer, 2006).

DIAGNOSIS

HCV may be diagnosed earlier in asymptomatic HIV patients with elevated ALT/AST levels due to greater frequency of lab monitoring (Mohsen, 2003). Co-infection with HIV greatly impacts the natural history of HCV infection. Co-infected patients are less likely to spontaneously clear HCV, have increased HCV VLs, and progress more rapidly to cirrhosis and end-stage liver disease (ESLD) (Asselah, 2006). Predictors of severe liver fibrosis include age older than 40 years at time of infection, alcohol consumption >50 g/day, daily marijuana use, high body mass index, male gender, postmenopausal status, and longer duration of infection (Poynard, 1997). Although ART may slow this rate, it continues to exceed that seen in persons with HCV mono-infection. Low CD4$^+$ T cell counts also appear to magnify the progression. A meta-analysis of eight studies that examined the role of HIV with HCV found that co-infected patients had approximately two times the risk of cirrhosis on liver biopsy and six times the risk of decompensated liver disease with ascites, varices, or encephalopathy compared to HCV mono-infected patients (Poynard, 1997). A Veterans Health Administration study examined 4820 co-infected and 6079 HCV mono-infected patients in care from 1997 to 2010. All had detectable HCV RNA levels and were HCV treatment-naive. Hepatic decompensation was significantly greater at 10 years in the co-infected group (7.4% vs. 4.8%; $p < 0.001$) (Lo, 2014). Co-infected patients had a higher rate of hepatic decompensation (hazard ratio (HR) 1.56 when accounting for competing risks), even when HIV RNA levels were maintained under 1000 copies/ml (HR, 1.44). Approximately one-third of patients with chronic HCV will progress to cirrhosis at a median time of less than 20 years (Thomas, 2000). Once cirrhosis has developed, 50% will decompensate within the first 5 years, with ascites being the usual first sign. Approximately 1–4% of cirrhotic patients per year will develop HCC. Median survival time is 35 months versus 65 months for those without HIV (Beretta, 2011).

Although the average time from infection to fibrosis is shortened from 35 to 25 years in HIV-co-infected patients, Fierer's group at Mt. Sinai School of Medicine (New York City) found that HIV-positive MSM who developed HCV

Table 39.1 LIVER DISEASE PROGRESSION WHEN TREATED WITH A DIRECT-ACTING ANTIVIRAL AGENT

SCENARIO	DECOMPENSATION (%)	HEPATOCELLULAR CARCINOMA (%)	LIVER-RELATED DEATHS (%)
Treat 1 month to 1 year after diagnosis	1	2	3
Treat in F3 disease	3	8	10
Treat in F4 disease	5	20	25

had a much more rapid onset of fibrosis. In a 2008 analysis, 9 of 11 (82%) men had stage 2 (moderate) fibrosis at a median of only 4 months after diagnosis (Fierer, 2012). In 2013, Fierer et al. reported on 4 patients who developed decompensated cirrhosis and death within 2–8 years post-HCV infection (Fierer, 2013). The authors noted that the order in which the infections are acquired is important. When HCV is acquired after HIV, there is accelerated progression to fibrosis that may be proportional to the degree of immunosuppression. However, not all studies have seen such rapid progression. The European NEAT cohort evaluated fibrosis rates in 41 HIV-infected patients who subsequently developed HCV. Most were MSM on ART with a mean CD4+ T cell count of 500 cells/mm³. FibroScan transient elastometry (used to assess liver stiffness) over a maximum follow-up of 8 years found no significant hepatic changes (Boesecke, 2014).

Deferring HCV treatment in the age of DAAs may lead to increased rates of HCC and death. Data from the SHCS and published HCV data were used for mathematical modeling to predict the decrease in progression to cirrhosis, HCC, and death in the HIV/HCV co-infected population. For treatment with DAAs commenced in 100% of patients with 90% success, progression is shown in Table 39.1. If therapy was deferred to stage F3 or F4, the majority of liver-related deaths occurred after HCV cure. Important from a public health perspective, those treated between 1 month and 1 year after diagnosis remained infectious from a HCV standpoint for approximately 5 years, compared to 12 years for stage 2, 15 years for stage 3, and nearly 20 years for stage 4 (Zahnd, 2016).

DECISION TO TREAT

According to the Infectious Disease Society of America's "Primary Care Guidelines for HIV," all HIV-positive persons should be screened for HCV with antibody testing upon entry into care and annually thereafter for those at risk (Aberg, 2013). HCV RNA levels should be tested in all those with a positive antibody test to assess for active disease because antibodies persist for a lifetime even in patients who have cleared the virus. Infants born to co-infected mothers should also have antibody testing performed. Seronegative at-risk individuals, along with those with evidence of past HCV infection, should undergo annual screening. HCV transmission may be facilitated by the presence of genital erosions related to sexually transmitted diseases. Reinfection with HCV can occur, necessitating that patients be aware that high-risk behaviors put them at risk for reinfection (Danta, 2008). Patients with HCV/HIV co-infection should be advised to avoid alcohol consumption and to avoid sharing razors, toothbrushes, syringes, and so on to prevent spread of infection to others. Those who are susceptible to hepatitis A or hepatitis B should be vaccinated against these viruses because dual or triple infections are typically more severe (Low, 2008).

Although the increased likelihood of ART-associated liver toxicity with underlying HCV infection may complicate HIV treatment, this must be balanced against the increased risk of fibrosis with lower CD4+ T cell counts (Sulkowski, 2000). It should not discourage HIV providers from following DHHS treatment guidelines given the improved survival of co-infected patients on ART and the fact that newer ART agents are much less likely to cause hepatotoxicity. The benefit of HIV treatment on HCV was noted in 10,900 ART-naive HIV/HCV co-infected patients in the Veterans Aging Cohort Study's Virtual Cohort (Anderson, 2014). This study examined incident or new cases of liver decompensation occurring from 1996 to 2010. The cohort was 60% Black, median age was 47 years, and one-third had baseline CD4+ T cell counts <200 cells/mm³. During a median 3.1 years of follow-up, 69% initiated ART and 36% started IFN-based HCV treatment. During the 46,444 person-years of follow-up, 645 liver decompensation events occurred in 6% of participants. Those starting ART by prescription refill history had a significantly lower rate of liver decompensation (HR, 0.72, or 28% risk reduction). When examining those with HIV VLs >400 copies/ml at baseline (making the assumption that those with lower HIV VLs were on unreported ART), the risk reduction was even more dramatic (HR, 0.59, or 41% risk reduction). The study authors concluded that all HIV/HCV co-infected persons should receive ART to lower the risk of ESLD. This is in keeping with current DHHS treatment guidelines for ART in HIV infection.

The provider and patient must weigh many variables when deciding to treat HCV, including disease severity, extrahepatic manifestations, risk of side effects, likelihood of cure, comorbid conditions such as depression and renal disease, and likelihood of new and potentially more effective and less toxic medications in the near future. Treatment goals should include viral eradication, prevention of disease progression, improved quality of life, increased rates of survival, decreased risk of cirrhosis and HCC, and normalization of liver enzymes to simplify chronic ART. For most HIV/HCV co-infected patients, even those with cirrhosis, the potential for preservation of immune function outweighs the risk of drug-induced liver injury, so ART should always be considered. If the CD4+ T cell count is >500 cells/mm3, treatment of HCV prior to starting ART may be considered to avoid drug–drug interactions, overlapping toxicities, and high pill burden with multiple dosing. There are few data on DAAs with low CD4+ T cell counts, but patients on PEG/ribavirin (RBV) typically have more toxicity and less response to HCV treatment. If CD4+ T cell count is <200 cells/mm3, HIV treatment to improve the immune status must take precedence.

Testing for HCV RNA by polymerase chain reaction is the only reliable way to diagnose acute HCV infection because approximately 30% of patients do not have detectable antibodies at the onset of symptoms. More than 90% will have antibodies by 3 months postexposure, with less than 5% of co-infected patients (usually those with advanced immunosuppression) failing to produce detectable HCV antibodies. Acute HCV is asymptomatic in 70–80% of cases, but cure rates are significantly higher with acute disease. It is therefore important to routinely screen at-risk individuals and promptly investigate elevated hepatic transaminase levels. Acutely infected HCV patients who are symptomatic have a higher likelihood of spontaneous viral clearance, so they should be monitored for 12 weeks before initiating HCV therapy. Asymptomatic patients have a lower rate of spontaneous clearance, so they may benefit from early therapy. If HCV RNA remains elevated at 12 weeks post-seroconversion, treatment should be strongly considered. If RNA is still present at 6 months, spontaneous clearance is unlikely, and the infection is considered chronic. Due to high efficacy and safety, the same DAA regimens used to treat chronic HCV may now be used to treat acute HCV. Acute HCV infection may present with flu-like symptoms, nausea, abdominal pain, and jaundice. Infrequently, severe hepatic dysfunction with transaminases up to 10 times normal is seen, but fulminant hepatitis is rare (DHHS, Panel on Antiretroviral Guidelines for Adults and Adolescents, 2015).

Prior to initiating HCV treatment in the co-infected patient, specific baseline lab tests should be conducted. These include a complete blood count (CBC) with platelets and a chemistry panel including albumin and total bilirubin, prothrombin time/international normalized ratio (PT/INR), HIV and HCV viral levels, CD4+ T cell count, and HCV genotype. A pregnancy test is recommended for all females of childbearing potential if RBV use is planned because RBV is a known teratogen. Counseling against alcohol consumption is key because this can rapidly worsen fibrosis. HBV and hepatitis A virus vaccination should be offered to all patients without evidence of exposure to these infections.

A screening ultrasound is recommended to rule out cirrhosis and HCC in those with laboratory or clinical evidence of significant fibrosis or cirrhosis. Conventional computerized tomography, magnetic resonance imaging, or single-photon emission computed tomography (SPECT) may be used but are generally reserved for evaluation of liver masses or screening patients with more advanced fibrosis/cirrhosis. Although liver biopsy has been considered the gold standard in assessing disease stage, it is invasive, uncomfortable, and has bleeding risk (1/10,000 experience severe bleeding or fatality). Biopsies are generally scored 0–4 based on degree of inflammation (grade) and degree of fibrosis (stage). Metavir scoring is one of the most common systems for interpreting a liver biopsy and is shown in Figure 39.1.

Because of the risks associated with biopsy, alternatives such as FibroScan and FibroSURE have rapidly risen in popularity and acceptance in clinical practice. Most insurance plans now also cover the costs of these tests. FibroScan

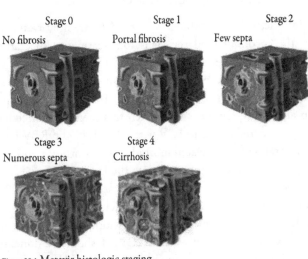

Figure 39.1 Metavir histologic staging.

utilizes a mild-amplitude, low-frequency vibration transmitted through the liver to measure tissue "stiffness." This non-invasive and less expensive monitoring tool has been used in Europe for more than a decade and has been approved in the United States since 2013 for clinical use. FibroSURE uses six blood serum tests (α_2-macroglobulin, haptoglobin, apolipoprotein A1, γ-glutamyl transferase, ALT, and total bilirubin) along with age and gender to generate a score that correlates with degree of liver disease. Other noninvasive biomarker formulas, such as APRI, which incorporates platelet counts with tests of coagulation and transaminases, may also be used to evaluate degree of fibrosis. APRI and FibroSURE have been validated in co-infection and predict no disease versus cirrhosis accurately but are not as accurate in the mid-range of the disease spectrum (Rallon, 2011; Schneider, 2014).

Several formulas are used to assess the degree of cirrhosis. The Child–Turcotte–Pugh score uses encephalopathy, ascites, bilirubin, albumin, and PT or INR to classify severity of cirrhosis (class A, 5–6 points; class B, 7–9 points; and class C, 10–15 points). The MELD (Model for End-stage Liver Disease) score uses serum creatinine, bilirubin, and INR and two or more dialysis sessions within the previous week to predict probability of survival for patients with ESLD. This is the formula currently used for liver allocation by the United Network of Organ Sharing and predicts the 3-month mortality rate. A MELD calculator is provided on the Mayo Clinic website (http://www.mayoclinic.org/medical-professionals/model-end-stage-liver-disease/meld-model). The HALT-C formula for predicting cirrhosis uses platelet count, INR, AST, and ALT to predict the probability of a biopsy demonstrating cirrhosis (Lok, 2009).

THERAPEUTIC MODALITIES

Multiple, all-oral combinations of DAAs are now available as the recommended regimens for treatment. Injectable PEG-IFN has been fully replaced by safer, more efficacious, and much better tolerated all-oral combinations, with guidelines no longer recommending its use except in alternative regimens to shorten treatment. Co-infected patients cured of their HCV with PEG-IFN and RBV had lower rates of liver-related morbidity and mortality, and we expect to see the same results with the DAAs.

Monitoring on treatment should include a week 4 HCV VL. Most HCV treatment-naive patients will be undetectable by this point unless they are cirrhotics. If detectable at 4 weeks, a follow-up at week 6 HCV VL should be done. If it is rising by 1 $\log_{10}$ or more, treatment should be stopped.

The HCV VL at 12 weeks post-treatment is crucial because this determines cure (SVR12).

Excellent cure rates result in a dramatic decrease in the rate of complications from HCV such as fibrosis and HCC, extrahepatic manifestations such as cryoglobulinemia, and debilitating symptoms such as fatigue. Evidence supports treating all patients with HCV, unless their life expectancy is less than 12 months because of a non-liver-related condition. As such, current guidelines recommend treatment for all HCV-infected persons. The guidelines also note that "immediate treatment" is assigned the highest priority in patients with advanced fibrosis/compensated cirrhosis, organ transplant, type 2/3 mixed cryoglobulinemia with end organ manifestations, and renal complications such as nephrotic syndrome. HIV places patients in the "high priority" for treatment category given the increased risk of fibrosis and HCC. Of great importance is the knowledge that treatment response is similar in co-infected and mono-infected patients. As such, HIV/ HCV co-infected persons should be treated and re-treated in the same manner as those who are not co-infected with HIV, but with constant attention to potential drug–drug interactions.

Drug–drug interactions increase the complexity of treating HCV in the HIV-infected patient on ART, as does the issue of renal function. ART switches may need to occur prior to treatment for HCV. Patients may return to their prior regimen after treatment is completed. Although choosing a regimen to avoid drug interactions may seem daunting, interrupting ART while on HCV treatment is not recommended. Treatment interruption is associated with increased cardiovascular events as well as fibrosis progression and liver-related events. Because this area is in constant flux, see "Guidelines for the Use of Antiretroviral Agents in HIV-1-Infected Adults and Adolescents" (DHHS, Panel on Antiretroviral Guidelines for Adults and Adolescents, 2015) under the HIV/HCV co-infection section for current advice on ART for HIV when treating HCV.

Resistance-associated variants (RAVs) may exist at the start of treatment in a small number of patients. Routine monitoring is recommended in (1) patients with GT 1a infection because duration of treatment with regimens such as elbasvir/grazoprevir will depend on these results and (2) patients with GT 1 infection who have failed treatment with a prior NS5A inhibitor-containing regimen and have cirrhosis or require urgent re-treatment. This area is currently in great flux, so change in these guidelines is expected. HCV resistance testing is recommended to search for RAVs that may confer decreased susceptibility to NS3/4A protease inhibitors (PIs) and NS5A complex inhibitors. For those with GT 1a with cirrhosis who are

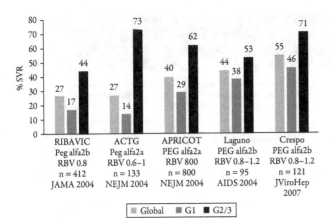

Figure 39.2 Chronic hepatitis C therapy with PEG-IFN and RBV.

- RBV typically causes a drop in hemoglobin (~2 g in the first month of treatment) and teratogenicity, cough/dyspnea, rash/pruritus, insomnia, and anorexia.

- RBV and IFN may cause flu-like symptoms, headache, myalgias, fever, fatigue, nausea, and diarrhea.

HCV treatment-naive or failed PEG/RBV in the past and in whom simeprevir/sofosbuvir (SIM/SOF) is being considered, testing for the Q80K NS3 variant is advised.

The standard of care for chronic HCV infection in HIV-infected patients was PEG-IFN-α-2a or -2b and RBV. The trials shown in Figure 39.2 demonstrate significant improvement in cure rates for chronic HCV infection in HIV patients by using PEG-IFN-α-2a or -2b with RBV. Although GT 2/3 patients consistently did better than GT 1 patients, co-infected cure rates with PEG/RBV were never as good as those in mono-infected patients.

Medication side effects are many and varied with PEG-IFN and RBV:

- IFN commonly causes depression and anxiety (and may be so severe as to require therapy cessation), neutropenia and thrombocytopenia in patients on combination regimens, reversible mild hair loss, altered thyroid or glucose metabolism, retinopathy, and/or cotton wool spots.

Fortunately, these drugs represent the past rather than the future of hepatitis C treatment. RBV is used only with SOF in certain cases, such as cirrhosis and/or re-treatment with drugs such as SOF and IFN only in genotype 3 patients. The oral DDAs represent a new direction in HCV treatment. The first two, boceprevir and telaprevir, were NS3/4A PIs. Although briefly state-of-the-art between their licensure in 2010 and 2012, they are no longer recommended in the United States because more efficacious and less toxic drugs have been developed. The previous traditional HCV therapies—PEG-IFN plus RBV—worked by nonspecifically stimulating the body's immune response. DAAs were engineered to work at multiple HCV-specific sites, such as the protease and polymerase enzymes (Figures 39.3 and 39.4). This second wave of HCV therapies has simple rules for use, shorter duration of therapy, fewer drug–drug interactions and side effects, and is highly effective in both HCV mono-infected patients and HIV/HCV co-infected patients. The results in HIV/HCV co-infected patients have been so impressive and so similar to those seen in mono-infection that many researchers are calling for a halt to separate trials in HIV-infected patients.

SOF/RBV was one of the first IFN-free combinations approved. The phase III PHOTON-1 trial enrolled 182 HCV treatment-naive HIV co-infected patients in a single-arm trial investigating SOF (400 mg once daily) plus weight-based RBV (1000–1200 mg given daily in divided doses) for

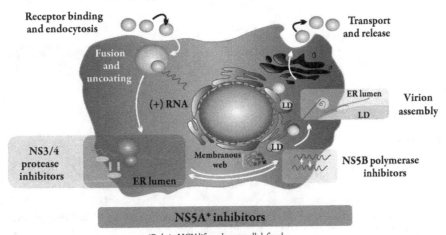

Figure 39.3 HCV life cycle and STAT-C (specifically targeted antiviral therapy for patients with HCV).

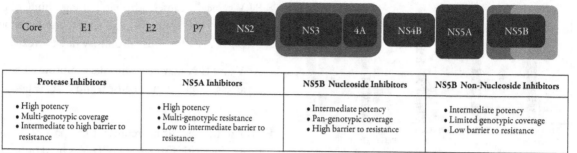

Protease Inhibitors	NS5A Inhibitors	NS5B Nucleoside Inhibitors	NS5B Non-Nucleoside Inhibitors
• High potency • Multi-genotypic coverage • Intermediate to high barrier to resistance	• High potency • Multi-genotypic resistance • Low to intermediate barrier to resistance	• Intermediate potency • Pan-genotypic coverage • High barrier to resistance	• Intermediate potency • Limited genotypic coverage • Low barrier to resistance

Figure 39.4 Therapeutic targets for direct-acting antiviral drug development. ER, endoplasmic reticulum; LD, low dermal. SOURCE: Adapted from Poordad (2012).

24 weeks in GT 1 patients and 12 weeks in GT 2/3 patients (Figures 39.5 and 39.6) (Sulkowski, 2014). Sustained virologic response at 12 weeks post-treatment (SVR12) was achieved in 76%, 88%, and 67% of GT 1, 2, and 3 patients, respectively. GT 1b was a predictor of poorer response. Cirrhotics and Blacks also exhibited trends toward lower SVR12 responses. Based on the lower response in cirrhotics, the addition of PEG-IFN to the regimen was considered for these patients. This regimen of SOF/RBV is recommended for HCV treatment-naive GT 1 patients.

The combination of SMV plus SOF with or without RBV was studied in the COSMOS trial in mono-infected patients only (Figures 39.7 and 39.8) (Lawitz, 2014). Only anecdotal data exist in HIV/HCV co-infected patients with this regimen. Similarly, no data exist for this combination in the re-treatment of HCV in patients co-infected with HIV, although data in mono-infected patients, including those with past treatment failure and advanced fibrosis, support the belief that this will be an excellent regimen in patients on compatible ART. Currently, it should be reserved for those with advanced fibrosis when treatment should not be delayed.

Study C212 was a phase III, open-label, single-arm study that investigated SMV plus PEG/RBV (fixed-dose RBV) in both HCV treatment-naive and HIV

treatment-experienced patients with GT 1 (Figures 39.9 and 39.10) (Dieterich, 2014). The study used response-guided therapy for HCV treatment-naive and prior PEG/RBV relapsers. Prior partial and null responders and all cirrhotics received 48 weeks of treatment (SMV for 24 weeks with PEG/RBV for 48 weeks). Due to diminished activity in vitro for GT 2/3 and lack of data for GT 4, this regimen cannot be recommended for these GTs.

Recommended regimens for the co-infected patient can be found at www.hcvguidelines.org (Terrault, 2016). The most recent version recommends that co-infected persons be treated the same as mono-infected persons after "recognizing and managing interactions with antiretroviral medications." Daily daclatasvir/SOF is recommended if ART changes cannot be made to accommodate alternative HCV DAA regimens as described later for HCV treatment-naive and treatment-experienced patients. When indicated, weight-based RBV is given as 1000 mg per day if <75 kg and 1200 mg per day if ≥75 kg.

Weight-based RBV may need to be added depending on the case. RBV should not be used with the older nucleoside reverse transcriptase inhibitors (NRTIs) didanosine (ddI), stavudine (d4T), or zidovudine (ZDV) due to the potential for serious toxicity such as lactic acidosis, but this

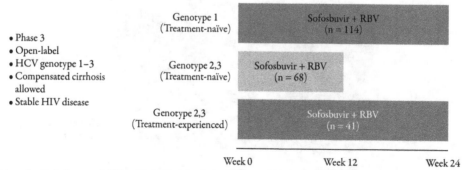

Figure 39.5 PHOTON-1 study: Sofosbuvir + RBV in HCV/HIV co-infection. Baseline demographics: Male, 83%; body mass index, 27 kg/m²; IL28B non-CC, 34%; cirrhosis, 10%; CD4+ T cell, 595–658 cells/mm³. The primary end point was a sustained virological response at week 12 (SVR12). ART regimens included emtricitabine/tenofovir plus efavirenz (36%), atazanavir (17%), darunavir (16%), raltegravir (16%), or rilpivirine (6%). SOURCE: Adapted from Naggie (2015).

- Virologic relapse
  - Treatment-naïve: GT 1 (22%); GT2 (0%), GT3 (29%)
  - Treatment-experienced: GT2 (4%); GT3 (6%)
- No S28T resistance mutations by deep sequencing in virologic failures
- HIV breakthroughs (n–2/212)
  - Not on ART (n = 11)
- Discontinuations due to adverse events: 3%
- Most common adverse events:
  - Fatigue, insomnia, headache, nausea
  - Grade ≥ 3 hyperbilirubinemia in patients receiving atazanavir versus no atazanavir (13% versus 0.8%

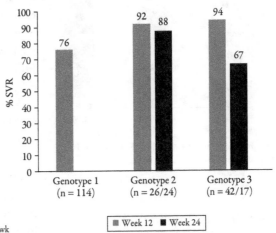

Treatment-naïve 12 wk; Treatment-experienced 24 wk

Figure 39.6 PHOTON-1 study: Treatment outcomes. SOURCE: Naggie (2015).

is very unlikely to occur with the newer NRTIs (abacavir, tenofovir DF, or tenofovir alafenamide). Administration of ddI with RBV is associated with a potential for life-threatening mitochondrial toxicity, and administration of ZDV with RBV increases anemia rates (Alvarez, 2006; Fleisher, 2004; Stock, 2013). Older antivirals, including ddI, ZDV, and tipranavir (TPV), should not be used with SOF. Cirrhotic patients should be assessed using the Child–Turcotte–Pugh system because hepatically metabolized drugs may need dose modification in those with class B and class C disease. Drug-induced liver inflammation is more common with HIV/HCV co-infection, although the highest rates are seen with drugs rarely used in clinical practice (e.g., d4T, ddI, nevirapine, and high-dose ritonavir (RTV)).

NS5B Polymerase Inhibitor(s)

SOF is a nucleotide analog inhibitor of the NS5B polymerase that is given as 400 mg once daily. It is not metabolized by the CYP450 enzyme complex and thus is an ideal candidate for use in HIV/HCV co-infection. Use with the protease inhibitor TPV is not recommended because it may induce P-glycoprotein (P-gp) and reduce SOF levels. Use with AZT and ddI is also contraindicated. The most common side effects when used with RBV are fatigue and headaches.

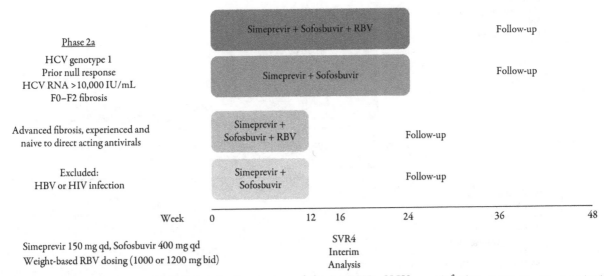

Figure 39.7 Off-label treatment options: COSMOS study: Simeprevir + sofosbuvir ± RBV in HCV mono-infection. SOURCE: Adapted from Lawitz (2014).

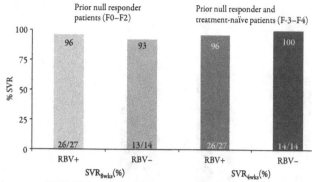

Figure 39.8 COSMOS: Sofosbuvir + simeprevir (PI) ± RBV in GT 1 week 12 treatment duration group. SOURCE: Adapted from Lawitz (2014).

NS3/4A Protease Inhibitor(s)

SMV is an HCV NS3/4A protease inhibitor given at 150 mg once daily. It is metabolized by the P450 CYP3A4 pathway and therefore is susceptible to drug interactions with inducers and inhibitors of the enzyme. It is also an inhibitor of the organic anion-transporting polypeptide (OATP) OATP1B1/3 and P-gp. Currently, most NRTIs (TDF, FTC, 3TC, and ABC), RAL, dolutegravir (DTG), RPV, enfuvirtide (ENF), and maraviroc appear to be safe with SMV. Coadministration with EFV, etravirine (ETV), HIV protease inhibitors, and cobicistat (COBI) pharmacokinetic (PK) enhancer or its co-formulations EVG/COBI/TDF/FTC is not recommended.

Rash including photosensitivity, hyperbilirubinemia, nausea, myalgias, and exertional dyspnea are the most common side effects reported.

NS5A/NS3/4A Combination Products

Zepatier (elbasvir/ grazoprevir) is a fixed-dose combination of 50 mg of elbasvir, an NS5A inhibitor, and 100 mg of grazoprevir, an NS3/4A protease inhibitor, taken once a day with or without food for the treatment of chronic HCV GT 1 or 4 infection in adults. Treatment is typically 12 weeks. RBV is added and treatment extended to 16 weeks if baseline NS5A polymorphisms are found in a GT 1a patient. RBV may be added in GT 1a or 1b patients who are PEG/RBV/PI-experienced. GT 4 patients who are PEG/IFN/RBV-experienced also receive 16 weeks of treatment. RBV is given as two daily doses depending on baseline NS5A polymorphisms and treatment experience. No dosage adjustment for Zepatier is needed for renal impairment, including those on hemodialysis, although the RBV may need adjustment per guidelines. It is contraindicated in those with Child–Pugh B or C disease. Zepatier is contraindicated with OATP1B1/3 inhibitors and strong CYP3A inducers such as EFV. Other contraindicated drugs include phenytoin and carbamazepine, rifampin, and St. John's wort. Coadministration with nafcillin, ketoconazole, bosentan, modafinil, ETV, and cobicistat-containing compounds is not recommended. The risk of ALT elevations may be elevated with ATZ, DRV, lopinavir (LPV), saquinavir, TPV, and cyclosporine. Statins also interact with Zepatier. Thus, when used with Zepatier, atorvastatin should not exceed 20 mg; rosuvastatin should not exceed 10 mg; and the lowest possible dose of fluvastatin, lovastatin, and simvastatin should be used. Tacrolimus levels may be increased by Zepatier.

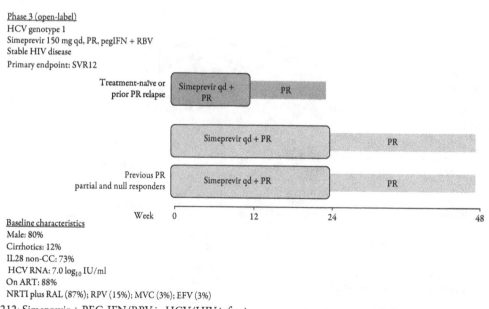

Figure 39.9 Study C212: Simeprevir + PEG-IFN/RBV in HCV/HIV infection. SOURCE: Adapted from Dieterich (2015).

- No HIV virologic failures
- Baseline factors having no impact on SVR 12 rates
  - Genotype 1 subtype, presence of Q80K, CD4 counts
- 89% of naives and relapsers met RGT criteria (24 weeks of therapy)
  - SVR12 in 87%
- Simeprevir + PR had similar safety profile in HCV-monoinfected patients
  - Fatigue (45%), headache (33%), nausea (29%)
  - Neutropenia (37%), pruritus (20%), rash (18%), photosensitivity (2%)
  - Grade 3/4 anemia (4.7%) and increased bilirubin (1.8%)

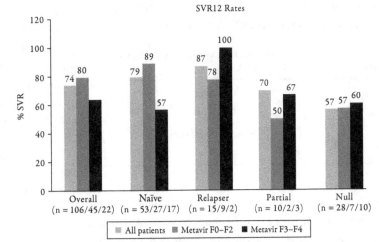

Figure 39.10 Study C212: Treatment outcomes with simeprevir + PEG-IFN/RBV in HCV/HIV infection. SOURCE: Adapted from Dieterich (2015).

In the C-EDGE Co-infection trial—a phase III, open-label trial involving 218 HCV treatment-naive HCV/HIV patients who received Zepatier one tablet daily for 12 weeks—95.0% of patients achieved a cure, with six relapses and one reinfection. The drug worked equally well in GT 1a or 1b and GT 4. Seven percent reported fatigue, 7% headache, 5% nausea, 5% insomnia, and 5% diarrhea. No serious adverse events (SAEs) occurred (Rockstroh, 2015).

NS5A Inhibitor(s)

Ledipasvir (LDV) is an NS5A inhibitor that is not metabolized by the cytochrome P450 enzyme system, so it can be used with most ART agents. LDV is a substrate and inhibitor of the drug transporters P-gp and breast cancer resistance protein and may increase intestinal absorption of coadministered substrates for these transporters. Providers should avoid using them together in patients with a creatinine clearance <60 ml/min. If coadministered, close monitoring for renal toxicity must be done.

NS5A/NS5B Combination Product

Harvoni (LDV 90 mg/SOF 400 mg), the first once-daily, single-tablet regimen for HCV, was approved by the FDA on October 14, 2014. The ION-4 study was a phase III, multicenter, open-label trial of 335 HIV/HCV co-infected patients. Seventy-five percent were infected with GT 1a, 23% GT 1b, and 2% GT 4; 82% were male, 34% Black, 20% compensated cirrhotics, and 55% had failed past HCV treatment (with 36% of this group having received DDAs). A minimum creatinine clearance of 60 ml/min was required for enrollment. Based on drug–drug interaction data available at the beginning of the trial, ARTs allowed in study patients were FTC/TDF with EFV, RPV, or RAL. Cirrhosis was determined by appropriate results via liver biopsy, FibroScan, or FibroTest. Those with a history of alcohol or drug use within the past 12 months were excluded. All patients received a fixed-dose combination tablet of the NS5A inhibitor LDV 90 mg and the NS5B polymerase inhibitor SOF 400 mg given once a day for 12 weeks. The primary end point was SVR12 post-treatment, with SVR24 as the secondary end point (Table 39.2).

In the ION-4 study, no difference in response rates at week 12 of treatment was seen with GT 1a versus GT 1b based on sex, treatment history, concomitant ART, or cirrhosis status. Thirteen patients (4%) did not achieve SVR. One person died at week 4 of treatment, 2 had breakthrough on treatment that was believed to likely be related to poor adherence by treating physicians, and 10 relapsed after treatment. All 10 relapsers were Black, with 7 having the TT allele in the gene encoding IL28B (which confers an increased risk of failure with IFN-containing regimens). Black race and the presence of the TT allele were found as a significant association in the univariate analysis. Black race alone in the multivariate analysis was significantly associated with relapse. The association of lower SVR with Black race, which comprised 34% of the study population, was not seen in the studies of LDV/SOB in HCV mono-infected persons and was not related to the CYP2B6 polymorphism, which is more common in Blacks and results in increased EFV levels (Naggie, 2015).

LDV/SOF increases exposure to TDF by approximately 40%. Patients on RTV-containing regimens may experience a relative increase of 30–60% in TDF exposure and so were excluded from the trial along with those on cobicistat-containing combinations. Although 77% of patients had an adverse event (AE), these were usually mild

Table 39.2 PERCENTAGE OF SUBJECTS IN THE ION-4 TRIAL ACHIEVING SVR12 BY GENOTYPE

GENOTYPE	% ACHIEVING SVR12 (95% CONFIDENCE INTERVAL)
Overall	96 (93–98)
GT 1a	96 (93–98)
GT 1b	96 (89–99)
GT 4	100 (63–100)

to moderate and resulted in no premature study discontinuations. Headache (25%), fatigue (21%), and diarrhea (11%) were the most common AEs. Eight patients experienced 15 SAEs, with HCC in 2 patients and portal vein thrombosis in 2 patients—all being reported in cirrhotics. Three patients experienced serious infections. Grade 3 laboratory abnormalities occurred in 9% and grade 4 laboratory abnormalities in 2% of patients, with elevations in lipase, creatinine phosphokinase, and serum glucose being most common.

Viekira Pak was approved on December 19, 2014, and involves taking two combination pills every morning (ombitasvir 12.5 mg, paritaprevir 75 mg, or RTV 50 mg) and one dose of dasabuvir 250 mg in the evening. Ombitasvir is an NS5A inhibitor, paritaprevir an NS3/4A protease inhibitor, and RTV is a CYP3A inhibitor that increases plasma concentrations of paritaprevir. Dasabuvir is a non-nucleoside NS5B polymerase inhibitor. Several CYP enzymes (3A4 and 2C8) and several drug transporters are involved in the metabolism of this drug combination; therefore, complex drug–drug interactions are likely to occur. The antiretroviral drugs least likely to cause interactions includes TDF, FTC, lamivudine, ATZ, RAL, DTG, and ENF. This combination should not be used with EFV, RPV, DRV, or LPV/RTV combination. If RTV or cobicistat is being used as a PK enhancer, it must be held during HCV treatment and the ATZ should be taken at the same time as the RTV contained in the Viekira Pak, typically in the morning. Weight-based RBV is often added to this combination. Depending on past treatment history and cirrhosis status, treatment duration may be 12 or 24 weeks.

Daclatasvir

Daclatasvir is an NS5A inhibitor that was evaluated in the ALLY-2 study, an open-label trial of 151 HCV treatment-naive and 52 treatment-experienced HIV-infected patients. HCV treatment-naive patients were randomized in a 2:1 ratio to 12 or 8 weeks at a standard dose of 60 mg per day with dose adjustment for concomitant ART as needed. All patients received SOF 400 mg once daily. All treatment-experienced patients received 12 weeks of therapy at the same doses. The primary end point was SVR12 post-treatment in the HCV GT 1 treatment-naive patients. The vast majority (87%) were male, 83% GT 1, 34% Black, and 14% cirrhotic. HCV GT 1–4 were enrolled with 83% having GT 1; 14% were compensated cirrhotics, and 98% were on ART (Table 39.3).

The most commonly reported AEs in the ALLY-2 study were fatigue (17%), nausea (13%), and headache (11%), with no study drug discontinuations due to AEs. Declines in HCV VL were rapid, with 92–98% of patients at <25 IU/ml by week 4 of treatment. No effect on HIV suppression or CD4+ T cell count was noted. On treatment, HCV responses were similar in the 8- and 12-week groups, but relapse was more common after 8 weeks of treatment. Nine of the 12 patients with HCV relapses (7 of 10 in the 8-week group) received concurrent DRV/RTV with daclatasvir at a reduced 30-mg dose. Recent data suggest that the 60-mg dose would have been ideal when given with DRV or LPV. The researchers also suggest that HIV-1 may adversely affect outcomes with the truncated course of therapy and recommend further research along these lines. They noted the following:

- Drug–drug interactions may affect dosing of this compound.

- Daclatasvir is a substrate of both CYP3A4 and P-gp.

- Strong or moderate inducers of CYP3A4 and P-gp may decrease plasma levels and the therapeutic effect of daclatasvir, so coadministration with strong inducers is contraindicated, whereas administration with moderate inducers requires dose adjustment.

- Strong inhibitors of CYP3A4 may increase plasma daclatasvir levels, so dose adjustment of daclatasvir is needed.

- Coadministration with inhibitors of P-gp is likely to have a limited effect on daclatasvir exposure.

- Daclatasvir should be decreased to 30 mg/day when given with RTV-boosted atazanavir or cobicistat, and it should be increased to 90 mg/day when given with efavirenz.

- Daclatasvir should not be given with the rifamycins or the older seizure drugs.

Table 39.3 PERCENTAGE OF SUBJECTS IN THE ALLY-2 STUDY ACHIEVING SVR12 BY GENOTYPE

GENOTYPE	12-WEEK TREATMENT ARM—SVR BY PERCENTAGE (95% CONFIDENCE INTERVAL)	8-WEEK TREATMENT ARM—SVR BY PERCENTAGE (95% CONFIDENCE INTERVAL)
GT 1 treatment-naive	96.4 (89.8–99.2)	75.6 (59.7–87.6)
GT 1 treatment-experienced	97.7 (88.0–99.9)	N/A
All GTs treatment-naive	97.0 (91.6–99.4)	76.0 (61.8–86.9)
All GTs treatment-experienced	98.1 (89.7–100)	N/A

N/A, not applicable.

TREATMENT FAILURES

For those who fail HCV treatment, assessment for disease progression should be done every 6–12 months with a hepatic function panel, CBC, and INR. If they have F3 or F4 disease, HCC surveillance every 6 months with ultrasound is advised. If cirrhotic, they should have endoscopic evaluation for varices. As new treatments become available, they should be considered for these patients.

Liver transplantation is a possibility in patients in whom HCV therapy is contraindicated due to decompensated cirrhosis. As long as the $CD4^+$ T cell count is >100 cells/mm^3 and HIV RNA levels are <400 copies/ml and without other contraindications (e.g., metastatic disease, ongoing alcohol or drug abuse, and active opportunistic infection), patients may be appropriate for referral to a transplant center for evaluation. Studies have shown higher rates of wait-list mortality and post-transplant mortality, as well as more severe recurrent HCV disease (Terrault, 2012). Data from a prospective multicenter trial showed lower 3-year survival (60% vs. 79%; $p < 0.001$) in HIV/HCV co-infected versus HCV mono-infected patients, as well as lower graft survival (53% vs. 74%; $p < 0.001$). Graft rejection was more common in co-infection (35% vs. 18%), likely related to the difficulties of managing immunosuppressive drugs in this population (Zahnd, 2015). New DAA drug therapy in HCV mono-infected and HIV/HCV co-infected individuals has shown pretransplant and post-transplant virologic responses of 70–93% in some trials.

SUMMARY

The world of HIV/ HCV co-infection is in rapid flux, with many new and exciting agents being released. Similar to HIV treatment, a combination of oral agents that disrupt the HCV virus at various sites of the life cycle has the best chance for decreasing viral replication long-term and curing infection. Questions regarding optimal combination as well as drug access and costs will need to be addressed in the next several years if the majority of HIV/HCV co-infected patients are to be effectively treated.

ACKNOWLEDGMENT

The authors acknowledge Aimee Wilkin, MD, MPH, the author of the first section of this chapter in the previous edition.

References

Aberg JA, Gallant JE, Ghanem KG, et al. Primary care guidelines for the management of persons infected with HIV: 2013 update by the HIV Medicine Association of the Infectious Diseases Society of America. *Clin Infect Dis.* 2014 Jan; 58(1):e1–e34.

Alter MJ. Epidemiology of viral hepatitis and HIV Co-infection. *J Hepatol.* 2006; 44(1 Suppl):S6–S9.

Alvarez D, Dieterich DT, Brau N, et al. Zidovudine use but not weight-based ribavirin dosing impacts anemia during HCV treatment in HIV-infected persons. *J Virol Hepatol.* 2006; 13:683–689.

American Association for the Study of Liver Diseases. Summary of recommendations for HIV/HCV-co-infected patients who are being treated for HCV, by genotype. Available at http://hcvguidelines.org/search/HIV%5CHCV. Accessed January 15, 2016.

Anderson JP, Tchetgen EJ, Lo R, et al. Antiretroviral therapy reduces the rate of hepatic decompensation among HIV and hepatitis C virus-co-infected veterans. *Clin Infect Dis.* 2014 Mar; 58(5):719–727.

Asselah T, Rubbia-Brandt L, Marcellin P, et al. Steatosis in chronic hepatitis C: Why does it really matter? *Gut.* 2006 Jan; 55(1):123–130.

Audsley J, Seaberg E, Sasadeusz J, et al. Factors associated with elevated ALT in an international HIV/HBV co-infected cohort on long-term HAART. *PLoS One.* 2011; 6(11):e26482.

Beretta M, Garlassi E, Cacopardo B, et al. Hepatocellular carcinoma in HIV-infected patients: Check early, treat hard. *The Oncologist.* 2011; 16(9):1258–1269.

Bevilacqua E, Fabris A, Floreano P, et al. Genetic factors in mother-to-child transmission of HCV infection. *Virology.* 2009 Jul 20; 390(1):64–70.

Boesecke C, Ingiliz P, Mandoerfer M, et al.; the NEAT Study Group. Is there long-term evidence of advanced liver fibrosis after acute hepatitis C in HIV coinfection? Paper presented at the 21st CROI, March 3–6, 2014. Abstract 644.

Centers for Disease Control and Prevention. HIV/AIDS and viral hepatitis fact sheet. 2014. Available at http://www.cdc.gov/hepatitis/populations/hiv.htm. Accessed January 15, 2016.

Colin J, Cazals-Hatem D, Loriot M, et al. Influence of human immunodeficiency virus infection on chronic hepatitis B in homosexual men. *Hepatology.* 1999; 29(4):1306–1310.

Conrad C, Bradley H, Broz D, et al. Community outbreak of HIV infection linked to injection drug use of oxymorphone—Indiana, 2015. *MMWR* 2015; 64(16):443–444.

Danta M, Dusheiko GM. Acute HCV in HIV-positive individuals—A review. *Curr Pharm Des*. 2008; 14(17):1690–1697.

Dieterich D, Rockstroh JK, Orkin C, et al. Simeprevir (TMC435) with pegylated interferon/ribavirin in patients co-infected with HCV genotype 1 and HIV-1: A phase 3 study. *Clin Infect Dis*. 2014 Dec 1; 59(11):1579–1587.

Dore G, Soriano V, Rockstroh J, et al. Frequent hepatitis B virus rebound among HIV-hepatitis B virus co-infected patients following antiretroviral therapy interruption. *AIDS*. 2010; 24(6):857–865.

Elliott LN, Lloyd A, Ziegler JB, et al. Protective immunity against hepatitis C virus infection. *Immunol Cell Biol*. 2006; 84:239–249.

Fierer DS, Dieterich DT, Fiel MI, et al. Rapid progression to decompensated cirrhosis, liver transplant, and death in HIV-infected men after primary hepatitis C virus infection. *Clin Infect Dis*. 2013 Apr; 56(7):1038–1043.

Fierer DS, Mullen MP, Dieterich DT, et al. Early-onset liver fibrosis due to primary hepatitis C virus infection is higher over time in HIV-infected men. *Clin Infect Dis*. 2012 Sep; 55(6):887–888; author reply, 888–889.

Fleischer R, Boxwell D, Sherman KE. Nucleoside analogues and mitochondrial toxicity. *Clin Infect Dis*. 2004; 38:e79–e80.

Hadziyannis S, Papatheodoridis G. Hepatitis B e antigen-negative chronic hepatitis B: Natural history and treatment. *Semin Liver Dis*. 2006; 26:130–141.

Heuft M, Houba S, van den Berk G, et al. Protective effect of hepatitis B virus-active antiretroviral therapy against primary hepatitis B virus infection. *AIDS*. 2014; 28(7):999–1005.

Launay O, Van der Vliet D, Rosenberg A, et al. Safety and immunogenicity of 4 intramuscular double doses and 4 intradermal low doses vs. standard hepatitis B vaccine regimen in adults with HIV-1: A randomized controlled trial. *JAMA*. 2011; 305(14):1432–1440.

Lawitz E, Ghalib R, Rodriguez-Torres M, et al. COSMOS Study: SVR4 results of a once-daily regimen of simeprevir (TMC435) plus sofosbuvir (GS-7977) with or without ribavirin in HCV genotype 1 null responders. 20th Conference on Retroviruses and Opportunistic Infections. Atlanta, GA. March 3–6, 2013. Abstract 155LB.

Lawitz E, Sulkowski M, Ghalib R, et al. Simeprevir plus sofosbuvir, with or without ribavirin, to treat chronic infection with hepatitis C virus genotype 1 in non-responders to pegylated interferon and ribavirin and treatment-naive patients: The COSMOS randomised study. *Lancet*. 2014 Nov 15; 384(9956):1756–1765.

Linas BP, Wang B, Smurzynski M, et al. The impact of HIV/HCV co-infection on health care utilization and disability: Results of the ACTG Longitudinal Linked Randomized Trials (ALLRT) Cohort. *J Viral Hepat*. 2011 Jul; 18(7):506–512.

Lo Re III V, Kallan M, Tate J, et al. Hepatic decompensation in antiretroviral-treated patients co-infected with HIV and hepatitis C virus compared with hepatitis C virus-monoinfected patients: A cohort study. *Ann Intern Med*. 2014; 160(6):369–379.

Lok AS, McMahon BJ. Chronic hepatitis B: Update 2009. *Hepatology*. 2009; 50(3):661–662.

Low E, Vogel M, Rockstroh J, et al. Acute hepatitis C in HIV-positive individuals. *AIDS Rev*. 2008 Oct–Dec; 10(4):245–253.

Luetkemeyer A, Charlebois E, Hare C, et al. Resistance patterns and response to entecavir intensification among HIV–HBV-co-infected adults with persistent HBV viremia. *J Acquir Immune Defic Syndr*. 2011; 58(3):e96–e99.

Luetkemeyer A, Hare CB, Stansell J, et al. Clinical presentation and course of acute hepatitis C infection in HIV-infected patients. *J Acquir Immune Defic Syndr*. 2006 Jan 1; 41(1):31–36.

Maheshwari A, Ray S, Thuluvath PJ. Acute hepatitis C. *Lancet*. 2008 Jul 26; 372(9635):321–332.

Mohsen AH, Easterbrook P. Hepatitis C testing in HIV infected patients. *Sex Transm Infect*. 2003 Feb; 79(1):76.

Naggie S, Cooper C, Saag M, et al. Ledipasvir and sofosbuvir for HCV in patients co-infected with HIV-1. *N Engl J Med*. 2015 Aug 20; 373(8):705–713.

Peters M, Andersen J, Lynch P, et al. Randomized controlled study of tenofovir and adefovir in chronic hepatitis B virus and HIV infection: ACTG 5127. *Hepatology*. 2006; 44(5):1110–1116.

Pinchoff J, Drobnik A, Bornschlegel K, et al. Deaths among people with hepatitis C in New York City, 2000–2011. *Clin Infect Dis*. 2014 Apr; 58(8):1047–1054.

Poordad F, Dieterich D. Treating hepatitis C: Current standard of care and emerging direct-acting antiviral agents. *J Viral Hepat*. 2012 Jul; 19(7):449–464.

Poynard T, Bedossa P, Opolon P. Natural history of liver fibrosis progression in patients with chronic hepatitis C. The OBSVIRC, METAVIR, CLINIVIR, and DOSVIRC groups. *Lancet*. 1997 Mar 22; 349(9055):825–832.

Rallon NI, Soriano V, Naggie S, et al. IL28B gene polymorphism and viral kinetics in HIV. HCV co-infected patients treated with pegylated interferon and ribavirin. *AIDS*. 2011; 25(8):1025–1033.

Rockstroh JK, Nelson M, Katlama C, et al. Efficacy and safety of grazoprevir (MK-5172) and elbasvir (MK-8742) in patients with hepatitis C virus and HIV co-infection (C-EDGE CO-INFECTION): a non-randomised, open-label, trial. *Lancet HIV*. 2015 Aug; 2(8):e319–e327.

Schneider MD, Sarrazin C. Commentary: Antiviral therapy of hepatitis C in 2014: Do we need resistance testing? *Antivir Res*. 2014; 105:64–71.

Sherman K. Management of the hepatitis B virus/HIV-co-infected patient. *Top Antivir Med*. 2015; 23(3):111–114.

Shire N, Rouster S, Rajicic N, et al. Occult hepatitis B in HIV-infected patients. *J Acquir Immune Defic Syndr*. 2004; 36(3):869–875.

Stock P. Reopening the liver transplant and HIV debate: The pros. Paper presented at the International Conference on Viral Hepatitis 2013, March 25–26, 2013, New York, NY. Debate session 1.

Sulkowski M, Thomas D, Chaisson R, et al. Reactivation of hepatitis B virus replication accompanied by acute hepatitis in patients receiving highly active antiretroviral therapy. *Clin Infect Dis*. 2001; 32(1):144–148.

Sulkowski MS, Mast EE, Seeff LB, et al. Hepatitis C virus infection as an opportunistic disease in persons infected with human immunodeficiency virus. *Clin Infect Dis*. 2000 Apr; 30(Suppl 1):S77–S84. [Review]

Sulkowski MS, Naggie S, Lalezari J, et al. Sofosbuvir and ribavirin for hepatitis C in patients with HIV co-infection. *JAMA*. 2014 Jul 23–30; 312(4):353–361. Erratum in: *JAMA*. 2014 Nov 12; 312(18):1932.

Sulkowski MS, Thomas DL, Chaisson RE, et al. Hepatotoxicity associated with antiretrovirals in adults infected with HIV and the role of hepatitis C or B infection. *JAMA*. 2000; 283:74–80.

Terrault N, Bzowej N, Chang K-M, et al. AASLD guidelines for treatment of chronic hepatitis B. *Hepatology* 2016; 63:261–283.

Terrault NA, Roland ME, Schiano T, et al. Outcomes of liver transplant recipients with hepatitis C and human immunodeficiency virus co-infection. *Liver Transpl*. 2012 Jun; 18(6):716–726.

Thio C, Seaberg E, Skolasky R Jr, et al. HIV-1, hepatitis B virus, and risk of liver-related mortality in the Multicenter Cohort Study (MACS). *Lancet* 2002; 360(9349):1921–1926.

Thomas DL, Strathdee SA, Vlahov D. Long-term prognosis of hepatitis C virus Infection. *JAMA*. 2000 Nov 22; 284(20):2592.

US Department of Health and Human Services, Panel on Antiretroviral Guidelines for Adults and Adolescents. Guidelines for the use of antiretroviral agents in HIV-1-infected adults and adolescents.

Available at https://aidsinfo.nih.gov/contentfiles/lvguidelines/AdultandAdolescentGL.pdf. Accessed January 15, 2016.

US Department of Health and Human Services, Panel on Opportunistic Infections in HIV-Infected Adults and Adolescents. Guidelines for the prevention and treatment of opportunistic infections in HIV-infected adults and adolescents: recommendations from the Centers for Disease Control and Prevention, the National Institutes of Health, and the HIV Medicine Association of the Infectious Diseases Society of America. Available at https://aidsinfo.nih.gov/contentfiles/lvguidelines/adult_oi.pdf. Accessed December 18, 2015.

Wandeler G, Gsponer T, Bregenzer A, et al. Hepatitis C virus infections in the Swiss HIV Cohort Study: A rapidly evolving epidemic. *Clin Infect Dis*. 2012 Nov 15; 55(10):1408–1416.

Weber R, Sabin CA, Friis-Moller N, et al. Liver-related deaths in persons infected with the human immunodeficiency virus: The D:A:D study. *Arch Intern Med*. 2006; 166(15):1632–1641.

Zahnd C, Salazar-Vizcaya L, Dufour JF, et al. Modelling the impact of deferring HCV treatment on liver-related complications in HIV co-infected men who have sex with men. *J Hepatol*. 2016 Jul; 65(1):26–32.

40.

OCULAR COMPLICATIONS

James P. Dunn

CYTOMEGALOVIRUS

LEARNING OBJECTIVE

Describe the incidence, screening, diagnosis, management, and referral indication for HIV-infected patients with cytomegalovirus (CMV) retinitis in the era of antiretroviral therapy (ART).

WHAT'S NEW?

As therapy for HIV has improved, CMV retinitis has become a less common opportunistic infection. However, patients with advanced HIV disease may still present with CMV retinitis. There is no evidence that routine screening can prevent disease in these patients.

KEY POINTS

- Symptoms of CMV retinitis are nonspecific and include floaters, light flashes, peripheral visual field loss, and blurred central vision. Pain, redness, and photophobia are not features, and central vision is often good.

- Immune recovery uveitis occurs in 10–15% of eyes with CMV retinitis in patients who respond to ART, with blurred vision as the most common symptom.

- Anti-CMV therapy is associated with increased survival in patients who remain immunosuppressed.

- Screening for CMV disease does not improve the diagnosis or survival of patients.

INCIDENCE AND SCREENING

Before the era of ART, CMV retinitis was the most common ocular opportunistic infection in patients with AIDS, occurring in up to 30% of patients (Jabs, 1995). The incidence of CMV retinitis, its natural history, and the indications for and response to therapy depend in part on whether at-risk patients are taking ART (Jabs, 2002). Patients taking ART, especially those with immune recovery, are at lower risk of CMV retinitis than are patients who remain profoundly immunosuppressed, and so they do not need to be screened as often.

The recent demographic shifts in the AIDS epidemic (resulting in HIV infection in more women and minorities) have been reflected by a similar demographic shift in cases of CMV retinitis (Jabs, 2002); its incidence has decreased by up to 90% in the ART era but has reached a plateau of approximately 0.2/person-year of follow-up (Sugar, 2012; Yust, 2004). A CD4$^+$ T cell count <50 cells/mm^3 at the clinical visit prior to CMV retinitis evaluation is the most important risk factor for developing retinitis (Sugar, 2012). In a large European study of patients with CMV disease, 64% had CMV retinitis, 27% had extraocular CMV disease (primarily gastrointestinal and neurologic), and 8% had both (Yust, 2004).

Primary prophylaxis for CMV retinitis is not generally recommended because of its uncertain efficacy, cost, and potential toxicity (Kaplan, 2002). Therefore, patients who have CD4$^+$ counts <100 cells/mm^3 must be educated about signs and symptoms of CMV retinitis and encouraged to seek timely evaluation if they occur (Whitley, 1998). Prompt and regular ophthalmologic screening for retinitis is appropriate for any patient with a CD4$^+$ count <50 cells/mm^3 because of the high incidence of ocular disease and the fact that most affected patients are asymptomatic (Kaplan,

2002; Nishijima, 2015; Whitley, 1998; Wohl, 2000). Routine dilated funduscopic examinations in patients at high risk may allow early diagnosis in asymptomatic patients. No study has shown, however, that regular screening improves final visual outcomes in patients with CMV retinitis compared to those who are not seen until they are symptomatic.

It is particularly important to examine CMV-seropositive children who have advanced HIV infection for possible eye disease every 4–6 months (Kaplan, 2002). Although the incidence of eye disease is low in this group (Hammond, 1997), children are less likely than adults to express symptoms of infection.

DIAGNOSIS

The majority of patients have no visual symptoms at diagnosis (Wohl, 2000), such as light flashes, loss of central or peripheral visual fields, and blurred or distorted vision (Whitley, 1998). There is typically no pain, redness, or photophobia (Jabs, 2002; Whitley, 1998). Approximately 70–80% of patients had visual acuity of 20/40 or better at the time of diagnosis in one mostly pre-ART study (Whitley, 1998). The diagnosis is based on characteristic features seen on indirect or slit-lamp funduscopy, including yellow-white areas of retinal necrosis, a dry-appearing granular border, and edema with vascular distribution, often with a hemorrhagic component (Jabs, 2002; Whitely, 1998; see Figure 40.1).

Several diagnostic screening tests have been evaluated, including quantitative plasma cytomegalovirus DNA polymerase chain reaction (PCR) (Mizushima, 2015) and CMV viral load in plasma and leukocytes (Jabs, 1999), but their cost-effectiveness remains unproven, and none is in widespread clinical use. CMV viral load has limited clinical utility because of its low positive predictive value (Jabs, 2005).

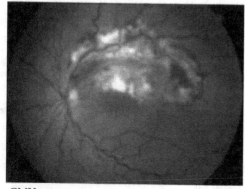

Figure 40.1 CMV retinitis. SOURCE: Reprinted and reproduced with permission from the New York State Department of Health AIDS Institute Clinical Guidelines Development Program. © 2000–2004. All rights reserved.

MANAGEMENT

Management of CMV retinitis depends on patient factors (e.g., underlying medical conditions, concomitant medications, living conditions, and lifestyle preferences), characteristics of the ophthalmic disease (e.g., location and extent of lesions), and characteristics of available therapies (e.g., their relative efficacies, risks of toxic effects and adverse outcomes, and quality-of-life issues) (Whitley, 1998). Successful management requires close collaboration between treating physicians and ophthalmologists.

The most effective treatment for CMV retinitis is an ART regimen containing a protease inhibitor, which is associated with markedly prolonged times to relapse and improved survival (Kempen, 2003). Oral valganciclovir, the prodrug of ganciclovir, has largely replaced intravenous therapy (ganciclovir, foscarnet, or cidofovir) (Martin, 2002) because of its excellent bioavailability and convenient dosing regimen. Adverse effects of valganciclovir include neutropenia, anemia, thrombocytopenia, nausea, and diarrhea. Regular monitoring of blood chemistry and hematology values is important during both induction and maintenance therapy. Foscarnet and cidofovir may still be indicated in patients with ganciclovir-resistant CMV retinitis, which is associated with worse visual outcomes (Jabs, 2003) and increased mortality (Jabs, 2010). Both drugs are nephrotoxic, and the dosage must be adjusted for renal status. Cidofovir can cause uveitis and must be given with probenecid, which itself may cause severe malaise and weakness (Whitley, 1998).

Regional anti-CMV therapy is an option in patients who cannot tolerate systemic therapy. Intravitreal ganciclovir 2 mg/0.1 ml or foscarnet 2.4 mg/0.1 ml injections are also effective and avoid the risk of systemic toxicity, but they must be repeated at least weekly (Teoh, 2012). It is important to understand, however, that systemic anti-CMV therapy, compared to only intraocular therapy, is associated with significantly lower mortality, less visceral CMV disease, and reduced risk of second-eye involvement (Jabs, 2013; Sittivarakul, 2015).

The ganciclovir ocular implant was another appropriate choice for initial therapy, and many experts chose this for patients who had immediately sight-threatening disease (Whitley, 1998). However, the implant was voluntarily taken off the market in 2013 due to poor sales.

In patients not taking ART, the combination of systemic therapy and the ganciclovir implant reduces the risk of new CMV disease and delays the progression of retinitis beyond that achieved with systemic therapy alone (Martin,1999), although either systemic or implant therapy appears comparably effective in patients with immune recovery (Kempen,

2003). The use of ART is associated with a 60% reduction in retinal detachment, with the greatest benefit among patients who have an immunologic response to highly active anti-retroviral therapy (HAART) (Kempen, 2001), and a 50% reduction in retinitis progression (Jabs, 2003). In a large retrospective series (Kempen, 2003), ART was associated with 81% lower mortality, reflecting a 98% reduction in patients with immune recovery and a 49% reduction in those without. The use of systemic anti-CMV treatment was independently associated with a 28% lower mortality rate than use of ART alone.

The most common causes of visual loss in patients with CMV retinitis are retinitis near the optic disc or fovea (zone 1 involvement), retinal detachment, cataract, and macular edema (Thorne, 2006).

Approximately 10–15% of patients who have controlled CMV retinitis have decreased vision and/or floaters after initiating ART because of immune recovery uveitis (Jabs, 2002; Kempen, 2006). Eyes with immune recovery uveitis have a significantly higher risk of cystoid macular edema and epiretinal membrane than do eyes of patients without immune recovery uveitis. Risk factors for immune recovery uveitis include large CMV lesions (25% or more of the total retinal area) and the use of intravitreous cidofovir. Reports conflict as to whether the continued use of anti-CMV therapy reduces the risk of immune recovery uveitis (Kempen, 2006; Kosobucki, 2004).

The use of ART has created distinct groups of patients based on their potential for immunologic improvement (Martin, 1999). In patients already taking ART, physicians must reevaluate this therapy if CMV retinitis develops because this can indicate progressing immune dysfunction (Martin, 1999). The previously discussed treatment options for CMV retinitis apply whether or not patients with CMV are receiving ART (Martin, 1999), but the length of therapy is affected by the response to ART. In one retrospective analysis of patients whose maintenance therapy was stopped after showing immune recovery (Curi, 2001), reactivation and progression did not occur after 20.4 months of follow-up. Maintenance anti-CMV therapy can often be discontinued in patients taking ART for at least 6 months with $CD4^+$ counts >100–150 cells/mm^3 for at least 3 months. Close follow-up is recommended, however, especially in patients with sight-threatening lesions (Wohl, 2005).

HIV RETINOPATHY

LEARNING OBJECTIVE

Discuss the diagnosis and significance of HIV retinopathy.

WHAT'S NEW?

The presence of HIV-related retinal microangiopathy is associated with the development of systemic CMV disease.

KEY POINT

- HIV retinopathy is asymptomatic, usually easily diagnosed, and serves as a marker of immunosuppression and the development of CMV retinitis.

INTRODUCTION TO HIV RETINOPATHY

Non-infectious retinal microvasculopathy, also called AIDS retinopathy or background HIV retinopathy, is the most common ocular manifestation of HIV infection, and it was present in 50% of patients in one retrospective series (Jabs, 1995). It typically occurs without CMV retinitis, and immunosuppression alone cannot account for it (Glasgow, 1994). However, given that it usually occurs only in patients who have $CD4^+$ counts <200 cells/mm^3 (Jabs, 1995), it serves as a clinical marker of advanced immunosuppression. The presence of HIV-related retinal microangiopathy is associated with the development of systemic CMV disease (Iwasaki, 2013).

Clinical features are usually limited to the posterior pole and thus are often visible on direct ophthalmoscopy. The most common findings are cotton-wool spots (Jabs, 1995). They are usually asymptomatic and often resolve spontaneously, typically within 2 months (Kuppermann, 1993). The cause is unknown. Less often noted are intra-retinal hemorrhages—which can appear as flame-shaped hemorrhages posteriorly, dot-blot hemorrhages, or punctate intraretinal hemorrhages peripherally—as well as microaneurysms, telangiectasias, and Roth spots (white-centered hemorrhages). In one study, fluorescein angiography revealed microvasculopathy in 100% of patients with AIDS (Newsome, 1984; see Figure 40.2).

Non-infectious retinal vascular occlusion (retinal vein and, less often, retinal artery occlusion) was found in 1.3% of patients with AIDS in one study (Dunn, 2005). A significant association with microvasculopathy was found. The visual prognosis is often poor.

One study described uveitis with chronic multifocal (mostly peripheral) retinal infiltrates as a distinct clinical entity of unknown cause in HIV-infected patients (Levinson, 1998). Cases of similar infiltrates with diffuse interstitial lymphocytosis syndrome have been seen,

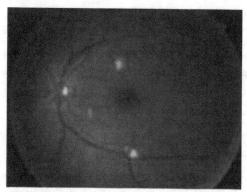

Figure 40.2 HIV microangiopathy. SOURCE: Reprinted and reproduced with permission from the New York State Department of Health AIDS Institute Clinical Guidelines Development Program. © 2000–2004. All rights reserved.

in which parotid gland swelling improved markedly with ART, but the retinal infiltrates did not. The visual prognosis is good. A similar pattern is often seen in African children with AIDS (Kestelyn, 2000).

HIV RETINOPATHY COMPARED WITH CMV RETINITIS

CMV retinitis is not thought to occur unless there is microvasculopathy, which disrupts the barrier between the blood supply and the retina, allowing CMV into the retina. There, CMV typically takes hold in parts of the retina damaged previously by HIV microvasculopathy (Ng, 1998). The diagnosis of CMV retinitis is clinical and based on the appearance of a focal necrotizing retinitis (Whitley, 1998). A small area of retinitis may resemble cotton-wool spots, a nerve-fiber layer infarct that will resolve in time. Therefore, retinal changes are more profound in HIV-infected patients who have CMV retinitis compared to those who have HIV retinopathy (including capillary destruction), and peripheral retinitis is more frequent than macular infection (Glasgow, 1994).

OTHER OCULAR INFECTIONS

LEARNING OBJECTIVE

Discuss the ocular manifestations of varicella zoster virus, including progressive outer retinal necrosis.

WHAT'S NEW?

Non-CMV ocular infections such as herpetic retinitis, toxoplasmosis retinitis, and choroiditis are less common than CMV retinitis and can occur over a wide range of CD4 counts.

KEY POINTS

- In HIV-infected patients, varicella zoster virus infection is a significant cause of ocular morbidity. Herpes zoster ophthalmicus and progressive outer retinal necrosis are the most important clinical manifestations.

- In people at risk for HIV, herpes zoster ophthalmicus may be a marker of infection; aggressive treatment with acyclovir or valacyclovir is recommended.

- Progressive outer retinal necrosis (PORN) is a rapidly progressive, necrotizing retinitis that occurs in severely immunocompromised patients; intravenous combination therapies have been successful in some cases.

Non-CMV ocular infections such as herpetic retinitis, toxoplasmosis retinitis, and choroiditis are approximately one-tenth as common as CMV retinitis, and the range of CD$^+$ counts among affected patients is also much wider than that for patients with CMV retinitis (Gangaputra, 2013). Varicella zoster virus can cause eye infections in both anterior and posterior segments of the eye in HIV-infected patients, and it is a significant cause of ocular morbidity. Herpes zoster ophthalmicus and necrotizing herpetic retinopathy are the most important clinical manifestations.

Because herpes zoster ophthalmicus can also occur in patients who are immunocompetent, it is not an AIDS-defining condition. It is more common, however, in HIV-infected patients (Hodge, 1998), and it can serve as an important early clinical marker for HIV infection when it occurs in young patients from high-risk groups (Hodge, 1998). One study found that of 112 patients with herpes zoster ophthalmicus, 29 patients (26%) were infected with HIV; all were younger than age 50 years (Sellitti, 1993). Small case series have suggested that peripheral ulcerative keratitis and neuro-ophthalmologic complications (e.g., encephalitis and cranial nerve palsies) might be more common in patients with AIDS who have herpes zoster ophthalmicus (Neves, 1996). Bilateral herpes zoster ophthalmicus has also been reported (Neves, 1996).

A study of HIV-associated herpes zoster ophthalmicus described 48 patients (Margolis, 1998). The median CD4$^+$ count at diagnosis was 48 cells/mm^3 (range, 2–490 cells/mm^3). Fifteen patients (31%) had mild or no ocular involvement, whereas 17 patients (35%) had mostly mild stromal keratitis. Serious complications occurred in 20% of patients, including postherpetic neuralgia in 2 patients (4%), chronic infectious pseudodendritic keratitis in 2 patients (4%), elevated intraocular pressure in 3 patients (6%), and central

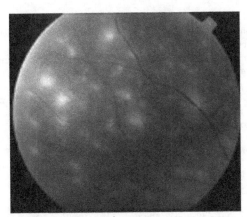

Figure 40.3 Progressive outer retinal necrosis. SOURCE: Reprinted and reproduced with permission from the New York State Department of Health AIDS Institute Clinical Guidelines Development Program. © 2000–2004. All rights reserved.

nervous system disease in 2 patients (4%). Aggressive treatment with intravenous acyclovir, high-dose oral acyclovir, or valganciclovir is recommended for all patients.

There are two forms of necrotizing herpetic retinitis, acute retinal necrosis and PORN, with substantial clinical overlap (Engstrom, 1994; Holland, 1994). Acute retinal necrosis presents as a peripheral retinitis, spreads rapidly in a centrifugal manner, and can occur at any CD4+ T cell count and in patients without immune compromise (Holland, 1994). It may be caused by either herpes simplex virus or varicella zoster virus. PORN often presents with posterior pole involvement, spreads even more rapidly, occurs largely among patients with severe immune compromise (CD4+ T cells <50 cells/mm³), and has a worse prognosis (Engstrom, 1994; Gangaputra, 2013; Margolis, 1998). Varicella zoster virus is almost always the causative agent (Engstrom, 1994). It is a rapidly progressive, necrotizing retinitis characterized by deep retinal lesions but minimal or no retinal vasculitis, vitritis, or iritis (Engstrom, 1994). A "cracked-mud" perivascular pattern may be seen (Figure 40.3). This pattern is caused by early removal of necrotic debris or edema from retinal tissue adjacent to blood vessels (Engstrom, 1994). Bilateral involvement is common. It has been emphasized that PORN is a variant of the necrotizing herpetic retinopathy that occurs in severely immunocompromised patients, whereas acute retinal necrosis tends to occur in the eyes of patients who have less severe immunosuppression (Guex-Crosier, 1997). Patients with PORN usually have a low CD4+ count, with a median of 25 cells/mm³ (Engstrom, 1994). The diagnosis of both acute retinal necrosis and PORN is usually made clinically, but it can be facilitated by PCR testing from the anterior chamber or vitreous (Knox, 1998).

One study found that 67% of patients with PORN had a history of cutaneous zoster (Engstrom, 1994). Another study found that 2 of 48 patients (4%) with herpes zoster ophthalmicus developed PORN (Margolis, 1998). Retrobulbar optic neuritis can occur before the onset of visible retinal lesions (Shayegani, 1996). In contrast to CMV retinitis, PORN progresses more rapidly and often has a dismal visual prognosis; two-thirds of affected eyes develop legal blindness within 4 weeks of diagnosis because of retrobulbar optic neuritis, retinal detachment, or central retinal necrosis (Engstrom, 1994). Some reports have linked PORN with varicella zoster virus encephalitis (Neves, 1996; van den Horn, 1996). The mortality of patients with herpetic retinitis approaches that of patients with CMV retinitis (Gangaputra, 2013).

Intravenous acyclovir alone is usually ineffective in treating PORN (Engstrom, 1994). Case reports have described successful outcomes with combined intravenous ganciclovir and foscarnet (Moorthy, 1997), intravitreal ganciclovir plus intravenous acyclovir (Meffert, 1997), ganciclovir implants (no longer available) plus intravenous acyclovir and intravitreal foscarnet injections (Roig-Melo, 2001), and intravenous cidofovir as salvage therapy (Schliefer, 1999). Most investigators recommend some type of combined therapy (Kim, 2007).

Chronic suppressive antiviral therapy is needed to prevent disease recurrence, which manifests as increased border opacification of formerly inactive lesions or the appearance of new lesions. Repair of PORN-associated retinal detachment with pars plana vitrectomy, endolaser photocoagulation, and silicone oil tamponade (along with antiviral therapy) may yield ambulatory vision in some cases (Weinberg, 1997).

Ocular complications of syphilis infection are discussed in Chapter 44.

Recommended Reading

Gangaputra S, Drye L, Vaidya V, et al.; Studies of the Ocular Complications of AIDS (SOCA) Research Group. Non-cytomegalovirus ocular opportunistic infections in patients with acquired immunodeficiency syndrome. *Am J Ophthalmol.* 2013; 155:206–212.

Kim SJ, Equi R, Belair ML, et al. Long-term preservation of vision in progressive outer retinal necrosis treated with combination antiviral drugs and highly active antiretroviral therapy. *Ocul Immunol Inflamm.* 2007; 15:425–427.

References

Ciulla TA, Danis RP. Repair of retinal detachments due to herpes varicella-zoster virus retinitis. *Ophthalmology.* 1998; 105:390–391.

Curi AL, Muralha A, Muralha L, et al. Suspension of anticytomegalovirus maintenance therapy following immune recovery due to highly active antiretroviral therapy. *Br J Ophthalmol.* 2001; 85:471–473.

Dunn JP. Viral retinitis. *Ophthalmol Clin North Am.* 1999; 12:109–121.

Dunn JP, Yamashita A, Kempen JH, et al. Retinal vascular occlusion in patients infected with human immunodeficiency virus. *Retina.* 2005; 25:759–766.

Engstrom RE Jr, Holland GN, Margolis TP, et al. The progressive outer retinal necrosis syndrome: A variant of necrotizing herpetic retinopathy in patients with AIDS. *Ophthalmology*. 1994; 101:1488–1502.

Gangaputra S, Drye L, Vaidya V, et al.; Studies of the Ocular Complications of AIDS (SOCA) Research Group. Non-cytomegalovirus ocular opportunistic infections in patients with acquired immunodeficiency syndrome. *Am J Ophthalmol*. 2013; 155:206–212.

Glasgow BJ, Weisberger AK. A quantitative and cartographic study of retinal microvasculopathy in acquired immunodeficiency syndrome. *Am J Ophthalmol*. 1994 Jul 15; 118(1):46–56.

Goldberg DE, Smithen LM, Angelilli A, et al. HIV-associated retinopathy in the ART era. *Retina*. 2005; 25:633–649.

Guex-Crosier Y, Rochat C, Herbort CP. Necrotizing herpetic retinopathies: A spectrum of herpes virus-induced diseases determined by the immune state of the host. *Ocul Immunol Inflamm*. 1997; 5:259–265.

Hammond CJ, Evans JA, Shah SM, et al. The spectrum of eye disease in children with AIDS due to vertically transmitted HIV disease: clinical findings, virology, and recommendations for surveillance. *Graefes Arch Clin Exp Opthalmol*. 1997; 235:125–129.

Hodge WG, Seiff SR, Margolis TP. Ocular opportunistic infection incidences among patients who are HIV positive compared to patients who are HIV negative. *Ophthalmology*. 1998; 105:895–900.

Holland GN. Standard diagnostic criteria for the acute retinal necrosis syndrome: Executive Committee of the American Uveitis Society. *Am J Ophthalmol*. 1994; 117:663–667.

Iwasaki Y, Yamamoto N, Kawaguchi T, et al. Human immunodeficiency virus-related retinal microangiopathy and systemic cytomegalovirus disease association. *Jpn J Ophthalmol*. 2013; 57:372–378.

Jabs DA. Ocular manifestations of HIV infection. *Trans Am Ophthalmol Soc*. 1995; 93:623–683.

Jabs DA, Ahuja A, Van Natta M, et al.; Studies of the Ocular Complications of AIDS Research Group. Comparison of treatment regimens for cytomegalovirus retinitis in patients with AIDS in the era of highly active antiretroviral therapy. *Ophthalmology*. 2013; 120:1262–1270.

Jabs DA, Forman M, Enger C, et al.; Cytomegalovirus Retinitis and Viral Resistance Study Group. Comparison of cytomegalovirus loads in plasma and leukocytes of patients with cytomegalovirus retinitis. *J Clin Microbiol*. 1999; 37:1431–1435.

Jabs DA, Martin BK, Forman MS, et al.; Cytomegalovirus Retinitis and Viral Resistance Study Group. Cytomegalovirus resistance to ganciclovir and clinical outcomes of patients with cytomegalovirus retinitis. *Am J Ophthalmol*. 2003; 135:26–34.

Jabs DA, Martin BK, Forman MS; Cytomegalovirus Retinitis and Viral Resistance Research Group. Mortality associated with resistant cytomegalovirus among patients with cytomegalovirus retinitis and AIDS. *Ophthalmology*. 2010; 117:128–132.

Jabs DA, Martin BK, Forman MS, et al. Cytomegalovirus (CMV) blood DNA load, CMV retinitis progression, and occurrence of resistant CMV in patients with CMV retinitis (published correction appears in J Infect Dis. 2004:192:1310). *J Infect Dis*. 2005; 192:640–649.

Jabs DA, Van Natta ML, Kempen JH, et al. Characteristics of patients with cytomegalovirus retinitis in the era of highly active antiretroviral therapy. *Am J Ophthalmol*. 2002; 133:48–61.

Kaplan JE, Masur H, Holmes KK; USPHS; Infectious Disease Society of America. Guidelines for preventing opportunistic infections among HIV-infected persons—2002. Recommendations of the U.S. Public Health Service and the Infectious Diseases Society of America. *MMWR Recomm Rep*. 2002 Jun 14; 51(RR-8):1–52.

Kappel PJ, Charonis AC, Holland GN, et al. Outcomes associated with ganciclovir implants in patients with AIDS-related cytomegalovirus retinitis. *Ophthalmology*. 2006; 113:673–668.

Kempen JH, Jabs DA, Dunn JP, et al. Retinal detachment risk in cytomegalovirus retinitis related to acquired immunodeficiency syndrome. *Arch Ophthalmol*. 2001; 119:33–40.

Kempen JH, Jabs DA, Wilson LA, et al. Mortality risk for patients with cytomegalovirus retinitis and the acquired immunodeficiency syndrome. *Clin Infect Dis*. 2003; 37:1365–1373.

Kempen JH, Min Y-I, Freeman WR, et al. Risk of immune recovery uveitis in patients with AIDS and cytomegalovirus retinitis. *Ophthalmology*. 2006; 113:684–694.

Kestelyn P, Lepage P, Karita E, et al. Ocular manifestations of infection with the human immunodeficiency virus in an African pediatric population. *Ocul Immunol Inflamm*. 2000; 8:263–273.

Kim SJ, Equi R, Belair ML, et al. Long-term preservation of vision in progressive outer retinal necrosis treated with combination antiviral drugs and highly active antiretroviral therapy. *Ocul Immunol Inflamm*. 2007; 15:425–427.

Knox CM, Chandler D, Short GA, et al. Polymerase chain reaction-based assays of vitreous samples for the diagnosis of viral retinitis: Use in diagnostic dilemmas. *Ophthalmology*. 1998; 105:37–45.

Kosobucki BR, Goldberg DE, Bessho K, et al. Valganciclovir therapy for immune recovery uveitis complicated by macular edema. *Am J Ophthalmol*. 2004; 137:636–638.

Kuppermann BD, Petty JG, Richman DD, et al. Correlation between CD4⁺ counts and prevalence of cytomegalovirus retinitis and human immunodeficiency virus-related noninfectious retinal vasculopathy in patients with acquired immunodeficiency syndrome. *Am J Ophthalmol*. 1993; 115:575–582.

Levinson RD, Vann R, Davis JL, et al. Chronic multifocal retinal infiltrates in patients infected with human immunodeficiency virus. *Am J Ophthalmol*. 1998; 125:312–324.

Margolis TP, Milner MS, Shama A, et al. Herpes zoster ophthalmicus in patients with human immunodeficiency virus infection. *Am J Ophthalmol*. 1998; 125:285–291.

Martin DF, Dunn JP, Davis JL, et al. Use of the ganciclovir implant for the treatment of cytomegalovirus retinitis in the era of potent antiretroviral therapy: Recommendations of the International AIDS Society–USA panel. *Am J Ophthalmol*. 1999; 127:329–339.

Martin DF, Sierra-Madero J, Walmsley S, et al.; Valganciclovir Study Group. A controlled trial of valganciclovir as induction therapy for cytomegalovirus retinitis. *N Engl J Med*. 2002; 346:1119–1126.

Meffert SA, Kertes PJ, Lim PL, et al. Successful treatment of progressive outer retinal necrosis using high-dose intravitreal ganciclovir. *Retina*. 1997; 17:560–562.

Mizushima D, Nishijima T, Yashiro S, et al. Diagnostic utility of quantitative plasma cytomegalovirus DNA PCR for cytomegalovirus end-organ diseases in patients with HIV-1 infection. *J Acquir Immune Defic Syndr*. 2015; 68:140–146.

Moorthy RS, Weinberg DV, Teich SA, et al. Management of varicella-zoster virus retinitis in AIDS. *Br J Ophthalmol*. 1997; 81:189–194.

Neves RA1, Rodriguez A, Power WJ, et al. Herpes zoster peripheral ulcerative keratitis in patients with the acquired immunodeficiency syndrome. *Cornea*. 1996; 15:446–450.

Newsome DA, Green WR, Miller ED, et al. Microvascular aspects of acquired immune deficiency syndrome retinopathy. *Am J Ophthalmol*. 1984; 98:590–601.

Nishijima T, Yashiro S, Teruya K, et al. Routine eye screening by an ophthalmologist is clinically useful for HIV-1-infected patients with CD4 count less than 200/μl. *PLoS One*. 2015; 10:e0136747.

Roig-Melo EA, Macky TA, Heredia-Elizondo ML, et al. Progressive outer retinal necrosis syndrome: Successful treatment with a new combination of antiviral drugs. *Eur J Ophthalmol*. 2001; 11:200–202.

Schliefer K, Gümbel HO, Rockstroh JK, et al. Management of progressive outer retinal necrosis with cidofovir in a human immunodeficiency virus-infected patient. *Clin Infect Dis*. 1999; 29:684–685.

Sellitti TP1, Huang AJ, Schiffman J, et al. Association of herpes zoster ophthalmicus with acquired immunodeficiency syndrome and acute retinal necrosis. *Am J Ophthalmol*. 1993; 116:297–301.

Shayegani A, Odel JG, Kazim M, et al. Varicella-zoster virus retrobulbar optic neuritis in a patient with human immunodeficiency virus. *Am J Ophthalmol.* 1996; 122:586–588.

Sittivarakul W, Benjhawaleemas T, Aui-Aree N, et al. Incidence rate and risk factors for contralateral eye involvement among patients with AIDS and cytomegalovirus retinitis treated with local therapy. *Ocul Immunol Inflamm.* 2016; 24:530–536.

Sugar EA, Jabs DA, Ahuja A, et al.; Studies of the Ocular Complications of AIDS Research Group. Incidence of cytomegalovirus retinitis in the era of highly active antiretroviral therapy. *Am J Ophthalmol.* 2012; 153:1016–1024.

Teoh SC, Ou X, Lim TH. Intravitreal ganciclovir maintenance injection for cytomegalovirus retinitis: Efficacy of a low-volume, intermediate-dose regimen. *Ophthalmology.* 2012; 119(3):588–595.

Thorne JE, Jabs DA, Kempen JH, et al.; Studies of Ocular Complications of AIDS Research Group. Causes of visual acuity loss among patients with AIDS and cytomegalovirus retinitis in the era of highly active antiretroviral therapy. *Ophthalmology.* 2006; 113:1441–1445.

van den Horn GJ, Meenken C, Troost D. Association of progressive outer retinal necrosis and varicella zoster encephalitis in a patient with AIDS. *Br J Ophthalmol.* 1996; 80:982–985.

Weinberg DV, Lyon AT. Repair of retinal detachments due to herpes varicella-zoster virus retinitis in patients with acquired immune deficiency syndrome. *Ophthalmology.* 1997; 104:279–82.

Whitley RJ, Jacobson MA, Friedberg DN, et al. Guidelines for the treatment of cytomegalovirus diseases in patients with AIDS in the era of potent antiretroviral therapy: Recommendations of an international panel. International AIDS Society–USA. *Arch Intern Med.* 1998; 158:957–969.

Wohl DA, Kendall MA, Owens S, et al. The safety of discontinuation of maintenance therapy for cytomegalovirus (CMV) retinitis and incidence of memory recovery uveitis following potent antiretroviral therapy. *HIV Clin Trials.* 2005; 6:136–146.

Wohl DA, Pedersen S, van der Horst CM. Routine ophthalmologic screening for cytomegalovirus retinitis in patients with AIDS. *J Acquir Immune Defic Syndr.* 2000; 23:438–439.

Yust I, Fox Z, Burke M, et al.; EuroSIDA. Retinal and extraocular cytomegalovirus end-organ disease in HIV-infected patients in Europe: A EuroSIDA study, 1994–2001. *Eur J Clin Microbiol Infect Dis.* 2004; 23:550–559.

41.

CARDIOVASCULAR DISEASE

David A. Wohl and Jeffrey T. Kirchner

LEARNING OBJECTIVE

Review the prevalence, prognosis, and management of cardiovascular disease in HIV-infected patients and its relationship to HIV infection and antiretroviral therapy.

WHAT'S NEW?

- Patients should be assessed for a 10-year cardiovascular risk by using the American College of Cardiology (ACC)/American Heart Association (AHA) risk calculator (atherosclerotic cardiovascular disease (ASCVD) score). Those with a risk score of ≥7.5% are eligible for medical therapy with a high- or moderate-intensity statin.

- Nonstatin therapies (e.g., fibrates, niacin, omega-3 fatty acids, and ezetimibe) are no longer routinely recommended as first-line lipid-lowering agents due to the lack of convincing data for improving cardiovascular outcomes.

KEY POINTS

- It has been known for several years that patients with HIV infection are at increased risk for cardiovascular disease (CVD), including myocardial infarction (MI) and stroke.

- Reasons for the increased risk are multiple and include a combination of traditional risk factors, chronic inflammation, immune activation, and effects of antiretroviral therapy (ART).

- Patients with HIV disease should undergo screening for cardiovascular risk factors, including hypertension, diabetes mellitus, dyslipidemia, and cigarette smoking.

- Proven interventions to lower the risk of CVD and MI include diet, exercise, smoking cessation, and the use of medical therapies including lipid-lowering agents and anti-hypertensive medications to treat modifiable risk factors.

- Changing ART to improve lipid profiles in patients with hyperlipidemia may be a consideration for some patients but should not compromise virologic or immunologic control.

There is considerable evidence that HIV-infected persons are at increased risk for CVD, including MI and stroke. Epidemiological studies have demonstrated higher rates of CVD among HIV-infected compared to HIV-uninfected patients (Triant, 2009). Premature atherosclerosis in HIV-infected patients was noted more than a decade ago in autopsy studies of HIV-infected adults (Morgello, 2002) and recently in comparative cardiac imaging studies (Post, 2014; Subramanian, 2012).

Most, but not all, of these studies acknowledge a higher prevalence of known traditional risk factors for CVD among persons living with HIV infection, and those that do so typically adjust for only a few confounding variables. The prevalence of cigarette smoking, in particular, is several-fold greater in HIV-infected individuals versus the general population. Other risks including poor diet, sedentary lifestyle, substance abuse, and even stress and mental illness—factors found to increase risk of CVD in general—may also account for some of the excess CVD burden among persons with HIV infection. Because these and other confounders are accounted in the analyses of cohort data, the association between HIV and CVD is frequently attenuated (Post, 2014).

There are, however, other biologically plausible explanations for higher CVD risk accompanying HIV. This is supported by findings of relatively higher levels of markers of immune activation and inflammation among infected patients with suppressed viremia compared to uninfected controls and a correlation between such markers and adverse events (Deeks, 2013; Hunt, 2012). Moreover, although ART has been found to consistently reduce surrogate markers for inflammation, endothelial dysfunction, and immune activation, there remains concern that some residual immune activation and inflammation persists. In addition, ART in general and specific antiretrovirals, such as lopinavir and abacavir, have been associated with CVD. It remains unclear if such associations are affected by co-confounding variables or if they are real. Are they a function of the effects of antiretrovirals on lipid levels or do they act through other, undefined, mechanisms? The heightened risk for CVD in people living with HIV infection, regardless of etiology, requires health care providers to be diligent in assessing for this risk and intervening, when appropriate, using evidence-based guidelines developed for the general population.

EVIDENCE OF EXCESS RISK FOR CARDIOVASCULAR DISEASE IN HIV

One of the largest epidemiological studies examining differential rates of CVD among HIV-infected and HIV-uninfected persons was conducted within a registry of patients receiving care in Boston that included 3851 HIV-infected and 1,044,589 HIV-uninfected patients (Triant, 2009). The difference in acute MI rates between HIV and non-HIV patients was significant, with a relative risk (RR) of 1.75 (95% confidence interval (CI), 1.51–2.02; $p < 0.0001$), adjusting for age, gender, race, hypertension, diabetes, and dyslipidemia. Complete smoking data, however, were not available, limiting the analysis given the several-fold higher rates of smoking in HIV-infected persons compared to age-matched uninfected controls (Triant, 2009).

Similar studies of the incidence of MI and stroke were conducted by the Kaiser Permanente system in California (Klein, 2014, 2015). Rates of both conditions were historically higher for HIV-infected compared to HIV-uninfected members. However, there has been a convergence over time in the rates of MI and stroke experienced by infected and uninfected patients. The adjusted MI rate ratio for HIV status declined over time, reaching 1.0 (95% CI, 0.7–1.4) in 2010–2011, the most recent study period. Improved detection and the management of CVD risk factors and more aggressive treatment of HIV infection are hypothesized to account for the decline in CVD rates in this cohort of patients.

A paper from the Veterans Aging Cohort Study that reported on 81,000 participants (33% HIV-positive) found that HIV-infected veterans had twice the risk of acute MI compared to those who were HIV-negative (Paisible, 2015).

However, it also found a low prevalence of optimization of cardiac health in this high-risk Veterans Administration population, including blood pressure control, treatment of hyperlipidemia, and smoking cessation. This alone may account for the increased risk of MI and not HIV infection.

In contrast, a retrospective cohort study from Spain examined data on 3760 HIV-infected patients who were in care from 1983 to 2011 (Echeverria, 2014). The prevalence of coronary events in this "Mediterranean cohort" was only 2.15%, which is actually lower compared to that in other similar studies of HIV-infected adults. The authors noted that the majority of patients with cardiac disease in this cohort had other CVD risk factors that were not being optimally treated, including hyperlipidemia.

Beyond cohort studies, pathophysiological evidence of excess CVD accompanying HIV infection has been pursued. Relatively high levels of inflammation within the aorta, possibly mediated by monocyte activation, were demonstrated by fluorodeoxyglucose positron emission tomography (FDG-PET) scanning in a small study of ART-receiving HIV-infected patients without known CVD compared to uninfected controls with similar CVD risks. These data were later correlated with vulnerable coronary plaques (Subramanian, 2012; Tawakol, 2014). Similarly, a larger cross-sectional study from the Multicenter AIDS Cohort Study (MACS) examined coronary calcium scores and coronary plaque morphology in HIV-infected and HIV-uninfected men who have sex with men and found that plaque was highly prevalent in both groups (Post, 2014). After adjustment for major confounders, there remained a higher prevalence of plaque in the HIV-infected men (prevalence ratio (PR), 1.13; CI, 1.04–1.23), who were also more likely to have noncalcified plaques (the most vulnerable to rupture) (PR, 1.25; CI, 1.10–1.43). Older age was associated with noncalcified plaque in HIV-infected but not HIV-uninfected men. This factor seemed to drive the overall differences between these groups. Adjustment for additional confounders reduced the association between HIV infection and noncalcified plaques.

The concept of HIV causing "accelerated" aging with CVD and other conditions accompanying growing older occurring earlier in those infected with HIV has been contradicted by data from the US Veterans Administration Aging Cohort and a study using large registries of HIV-infected and HIV-uninfected persons in Denmark (Althoff, 2015; Line 2015). In both groups, excess risk of CVD with HIV infection was observed. However, this was detected at similar ages in HIV-positive and HIV-negative persons, and over time, there was no observed increase in overall risk for those with HIV.

PROPOSED MECHANISMS

Numerous mechanistic studies have examined the association between CVD (i.e., plaque, coronary calcium, arterial inflammation, and endothelial dysfunction) and markers of inflammation, immune activation, and microbial translocation across the gut (Deeks, 2013; Hunt, 2012). In the FDG-PET study, aortic wall inflammation was significantly correlated with markers of monocyte and macrophage activation, suggesting that these cell lines play a role in the observed changes. The monocyte activation marker soluble CD163 was also correlated with noncalcified coronary plaque in HIV-infected men and women with well-controlled HIV. In the MACS coronary imaging study, as in most other cohorts, smoking rates were higher among those who were HIV-positive. That smoking interacts with HIV and aging to accelerate CVD was observed by an examination of carotid intima media thickness, suggesting HIV infection modifies the effect of smoking and age on cardiovascular health (Fitch, 2013). In a related report, smoking and obesity were each significantly associated with levels of inflammatory markers including interleukin-6 (IL-6), sCD14, and sTNFRI and -II (Krishnan, 2014). Similar findings linking smoking and inflammation were seen in the SUN cohort of HIV-infected patients (Cioe, 2014). In that study, heavy alcohol intake was also associated with elevations of the coagulation marker D-dimer.

Data from Hsue and colleagues regarding T cell activation and inflammation suggest this is yet another pathogenic means of developing vascular disease (Hsue, 2010). Residual immune activation secondary to incomplete control of HIV infection (despite undetectable viremia), co-infections (e.g., cytomegalovirus and hepatitis C virus), and irreversible translocation of microbial products across an altered gut lumen has been demonstrated in HIV-infected patients. They may collectively or individually promote a pro-inflammatory milieu that is pro-atherogenic (Deeks, 2013). Consistent findings of a relationship between nadir CD4+ T cell count and risk for CVD (as well as other end-organ diseases) add support for a role of long-term systemic inflammation in cardiovascular health of persons with HIV infection.

A number of studies have also shown that the risk of CVD among persons with HIV infection may also be influenced by immunodeficiency—specifically, low CD4+ T cell counts (Drozd, 2015). In the NA-ACCORD observational cohort, lower current CD4+ T cells, as well as a history of AIDS and detectable plasma HIV RNA levels, were predictors of primary MI in a time-updated model. This analysis also was consistent with other studies in finding a strong link between impaired renal function and CVD (Palella, 2015; Ryom, 2015).

THE EFFECT OF ANTIRETROVIRAL THERAPY ON CARDIOVASCULAR DISEASE

Multiple retrospective and prospective studies have evaluated the impact of ART on CVD. As in the epidemiological studies, these are often challenged by factors that confound analyses and/or lack an appropriate control group. The Strategies for Management of Antiretroviral Therapy (SMART) study, a randomized trial comparing continuous versus intermittent ART (based on CD4+ T cell count), found continuous ART to be significantly associated with a decreased risk of mortality. Intermittent therapy ("treatment interruption") heightened the risk for developing CVD, renal disease, and hepatic events—which led to an understanding of the adverse effects of viremia on organ function (SMART, 2006). Other work demonstrating reductions in markers of inflammation, endothelial dysfunction, and immune activation following initiation of ART has further cemented the concept that treatment of HIV, on the whole, reduces the risk of CVD (McComsey, 2012; Torriani, 2008).

Despite its benefits vis-à-vis countering the impact of ongoing viral replication on health, ART may carry an inherent risk for CVD, as suggested by the effects of some agents on lipids (e.g., increased low-density lipoprotein (LDL) cholesterol and triglyceride levels). To date, the most influential study of this issue is from the Data Collection on Adverse Events of Anti-HIV Drugs cohort (D:A:D). This is a prospective, single-arm, observational cohort study of tens of thousands of HIV-infected patients in Europe, Australia, and the United States. In 2003, D:A:D investigators reported the incidence of MI to be increased significantly with increased exposure to combination antiretroviral therapy (cART) (Friis Moller, 2003). The adjusted risk rate per year of exposure to cART ranged from 0.32 for no medication use to 2.93 for at least 6 years of use. However, although there was a significant relative risk of MI with cART, the absolute risk of MI was low (over a period of 36,199 person-years, 126 patients had an MI). Follow-up data from the cohort found that treatment-naive patients had an increased relative rate (RR = 1.16/year) of having an MI with cumulative use of protease inhibitors (PIs). The incidence of MI increased from 1.53 per 1000 person-years in those not exposed to PIs to 6.01 per 1000 person-years in those exposed to PIs for more than 6 years.

This increased risk was independent of sex and age, but it was in part related to dyslipidemia (D:A:D Study Group, 2007). The risk of MI per year of non-nucleoside reverse transcriptase inhibitor exposure was only 1.05.

D:A:D investigators also evaluated the risk of MI associated with 13 different antiretroviral agents (Worm, 2010). They assessed MI risk from both recent (past 6 months) and cumulative (per year) use of antiretroviral drugs. Overall, 580 patients with MI among 33,000 studied were examined. No associations with the use of lamivudine, tenofovir, zidovudine, zalcitabine, stavudine, nevirapine, efavirenz, or saquinavir and MI were found. However, recent exposure to abacavir or didanosine was associated with an increased relative risk (1.9 and 1.49, respectively) of experiencing an MI. Cumulative exposure to the PIs indinavir and lopinavir/ritonavir was also associated with a 1.12 and 1.13 per year relative risk of MI, respectively. In a 2012 analysis, D:A:D investigators found no association of atazanavir with cardiovascular or cerebrovascular events (Monforte, 2013). Of note, in this cohort, the relative risk per year for CVD was 1.39 for increasing age, 1.91 for male sex, 2.83 for current smoking, and 4.3 for a previous history of CVD.

The observed association of abacavir with an increased risk of MI remains controversial, with mixed findings from other cohorts and analyses (SMART/INSIGHT/D:A:D, 2008; Monforte, 2013). A 2014 repeat analysis by the D:A:D study group again found a persistent and unchanged association between abacavir use and MI. This was despite a reduction in use of abacavir in persons with higher risk for CVD that followed earlier data implicating abacavir (Sabin, 2014). However, use of abacavir in patients at low risk for CVD has remained largely unchanged over time. It was this group of patients (lower CVD risk) who were found to have the highest relative risk for MI after exposure to abacavir. Two recent analyses of cohort data have addressed the issue of abacavir and CVD—the NA-ACCORD and the Swiss HIV Cohort Study (Palella, 2015; Young, 2015). In both studies, there remained at least a signal for an association between abacavir and MI. However, the NA-ACCORD study made clear the challenge of such analyses because patients treated with abacavir were more likely to have renal disease, higher total cholesterol, low CD4$^+$ cell counts, and a history of AIDS.

Due to the conflicting studies noted previously, there is no current consensus on the association between abacavir and the risk of MI. Possible biomolecular mechanisms for this association include increased platelet reactivity and/or endothelial cell and leukocyte interactions that may be induced by abacavir, but these remain to be proven (Baum, 2011; De Pablo, 2012). For individuals who have an increased baseline risk of CVD (as calculated by the AHA or Framingham scoring system), it may be prudent to use an alternative agent to abacavir.

SCREENING AND ASSESSING CARDIOVASCULAR RISK

Given the higher risk of CVD among people living with HIV infection, the standard of HIV care must include baseline screening for traditional CVD risk factors and appropriate attention to management. This includes blood pressure control and maintaining a normal body mass index. Laboratory parameters should include a lipid panel (total cholesterol (TC), high-density lipoprotein (HDL), LDL, and triglycerides (TG)) and fasting blood glucose level or hemoglobin A1C. Baseline renal and hepatic function should be measured as well (Aberg, 2014; Dube, 2003). Patients started on ART should have a lipid profile repeated approximately 3 months after they are stabilized on therapy. If baseline and subsequent values are normal, then repeating a lipid panel yearly is recommended (Aberg, 2014; Dube, 2003). Risks for CVD and dyslipidemias should generally be managed according to the most recent ACC/AHA guidelines (Goff, 2014; Stone 2014).

Evidence suggests that the effects of smoking on CVD are magnified in those with HIV infection. Therefore, there is particular urgency for HIV care providers to incorporate evidence-based interventions to facilitate cessation of smoking into their practice. Data from the D:A:D cohort indicate a significant reduction in CVD incidence among HIV-infected individuals who quit smoking (Petoumenos, 2011). Similarly, other modifiable CVD risks (hyperlipidemia, hypertension, diabetes mellitus, and obesity) should be sought and acted on. The Framingham risk calculator (available at https://www.easycalculation.com/medical/framingham.php) has been applied to HIV-infected persons and found to generally perform well in assessing 10-year risk of CVD. However, it may underestimate risk compared to use in HIV-uninfected patients (Law, 2006). A newer 10-year CVD risk calculator has been published by the AHA and the ACC (available at http://www.cardiosource.org/science-and-quality/practice-guidelines-and-quality-standards/2013-prevention-guideline-tools.aspx) and is becoming the standard of care in the United States (Stone, 2014) (Box 41.1. Similar to the Framingham risk calculator, the ACC/AHA calculator may underestimate the risk of CVD in HIV-infected patients (Regan, 2015; Thompson, 2015). More prospective data to validate these guidelines in patients with HIV disease are needed.

Although several inflammatory biomarkers have been studied for their potential role in identifying HIV-infected persons at increased risk for coronary disease, the clinical utility of measuring these has not been determined. These markers include the highly sensitive C-reactive protein (hsCRP), D-dimer, IL-6, amyloid, and adiponectin (Triant, 2009). In several studies, such as SMART, they correlated with risk of MI and mortality. However, their predictive value for individual patients has not been established. This factor, along with the lack of specificity, leaves their role in clinical practice to be defined. Other diagnostic techniques that may be surrogate markers or provide direct evidence of coronary artery disease (CAD) in patients with HIV include carotid artery intima-media thickness and coronary artery calcification (Baker, 2010; Hsue, 2010). Similar to the inflammatory biomarkers, current utilization of these tests should follow practice standards and guidelines as applied to the general population.

INTERVENTIONS AND MANAGEMENT

There is no strong evidence that management of CVD risks in HIV-infected persons should differ from that of the general population. Modifiable risk factors, such as dyslipidemia, smoking, hypertension, diabetes mellitus, and sedentary lifestyle, are at least as important in patients who

have HIV infection, and perhaps even more so. As noted previously, the ACC/AHA and Framingham risk score probably underestimate the risk of heart disease in HIV-infected persons, but such assessments of CVD risk in this population are useful as a starting point to guide counseling, drug therapy, and other risk-reduction interventions (Stone, 2014).

Aggressively treating the patient's HIV infection with full viral suppression should remain the primary objective, even in the presence of CVD risk factors or CAD. Data from the SMART study (SMART Study Group, 2006) and the ATHENA cohort (Van Lelyveld, 2010) have shown that ongoing viremia and incomplete immune recovery increase the risk of cardiovascular events. In addition, a National Institutes of Health-sponsored study of 6517 patients, of whom 273 sustained an acute MI, determined that immunologic control was the most important HIV-related factor associated with acute MI (Triant, 2010).

The choice of ART should take into consideration a patient's individual CVD risk factors. Many, but not all, antiretroviral regimens, such as ritonavir-boosted protease inhibitors, may increase lipid subsets, including LDL cholesterol and triglycerides. However, some agents, such as non-nucleoside reverse transcriptase inhibitors and integrase strand inhibitors (elvitegravir), may actually increase the HDL ("good") cholesterol level. Abacavir increases LDL cholesterol and triglycerides, whereas tenofovir disoproxil fumarate (TDF) has been observed to lower LDL cholesterol levels (Tungsiripat, 2010). In clinical trials, the newer nucleoside reverse transcriptase inhibitor, tenofovir alafenamide (TAF), produced increases in fasting lipid parameters (TC, HDL, direct LDL, and TGs) compared to TDF (Sax, 2014). The integrase inhibitors raltegravir and dolutegravir have not been observed to significantly change lipid levels. The newer pharmacological booster, cobicistat, appears to increase LDL cholesterol, similar to ritonavir, but with a smaller impact on triglycerides.

In patients with moderated to severe dyslipidemia and increased CVD risk, switching ART to a regimen with less effects on cholesterol and/or triglycerides may be warranted. This should not be done at the expense of compromising virologic control. In the SPRIAL study, patients with stable HIV disease were switched from a ritonavir-boosted PI-based regimen to raltegravir, leading to significant improvement in patients' lipid profiles (Martinez, 2010). Similarly, in the SPIRIT study, changing from a ritonavir-boosted PI plus dual nucleoside regimen to rilpivirine plus TDF/emtricitabine led to significant reductions in LDL cholesterol (Palella, 2014).

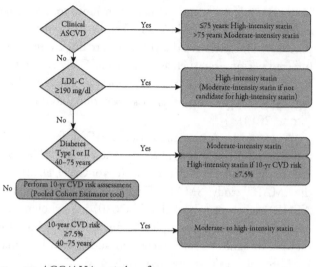

Figure 41.1 ACC/AHA statin benefit groups. SOURCE: Adapted from Stone (2014).

Management of lipid disorders in patients with HIV infection should generally follow guidelines established for the general population. Attention should be paid to the potential for drug–drug interactions between lipid-lowering and antiretroviral drugs. There are several sets of cholesterol guidelines, but most practitioners in the United States currently follow those of AHA/ACC (Figure 41.1 and Table 41.1) Pharmacologic treatment is often needed to reduce a patient's risk for CVD and is now recommended for individuals with an ASCVD calculated 10-year risk of 7.5% or greater. Depending on individual risk, this may include "high-intensity" or "moderate-intensity" dosing.

STATINS

The initial choice for CVD risk reduction is a 3-hydroxy-3-methylglutaryl coenzyme A reductase inhibitor ("statin"). Recommended statins may include pravastatin, fluvastatin, atorvastatin, and rosuvastatin and pitavastatin. All agents are effective in lowering TC and HDL cholesterol (HDL-C) but vary in potency. One retrospective cohort study of 700 HIV-infected patients taking atorvastatin, pravastatin, or rosuvastatin found that after 1 year of therapy on one of these agents, decreases in TC and LDL-C were significantly greater with atorvastatin and rosuvastatin compared to pravastatin. The likelihood of achieving treatment goals for non-HDL-C at that time was higher with rosuvastatin (odds ratio (OR), 2.3) but not atorvastatin (OR, 1.5) or pravastatin. Toxicity rates were low and were the same for all three agents (Sing, 2011). Of note, simvastatin and lovastatin should not be used in patients taking PIs. They are both metabolized by cytochrome P-34A, and inhibition of this enzyme system results in elevated drug levels and a subsequent increased risk of rhabdomyolysis and hepatic toxicity. Conversely, efavirenz reduces the level of these two agents and thus decreases efficacy. Based on current data, rosuvastatin appears to be the most effective agent in lowering total and LDL cholesterol (Table 41.2).

There are concerns regarding adverse effects of statins in the general population, including musculoskeletal symptoms and fatigue (Golumb, 2012). In addition, statin use was associated with a small increase in risk of diabetes mellitus in the JUPITER trial in HIV-uninfected patients (Ridker, 2012). There are few data regarding the tolerability of statins in HIV-infected persons. The SATURN trial randomized HIV-infected patients on ART with evidence of heightened immune activation or inflammation (hsCRP ≥2 mg/l) to rosuvastatin or placebo (McComsey, 2014). Rosuvastatin was associated with a significant decline in a number of markers of inflammation and immune activation, including monocyte activation markers, as well as increased hip bone density. However, rosuvastatin was associated with significant increases in fasting glucose, fasting insulin, and insulin resistance. Use of statins in HIV-infected patients should generally follow current ACC/AHA practice guidelines.

FIBRIC ACID DERIVATIVES

In HIV-infected patients with hypertriglyceridemia, fibric acid derivatives including clofibrate, gemfibrozil, or fenofibrate may be considered for treatment. They are generally recommended in patients with fasting triglyceride levels of ≥500 mg/dl. These drugs effectively lower triglycerides but have little effect on LDL and HDL cholesterol. Data from D:A:D suggested a very minor association between elevated triglycerides and MI, after adjusting for other lipid and nonlipid risk factors. However, the study also concluded that use of fibrates alone to lower triglycerides is unlikely to have a major impact on the incidence of MI (D:A:D, 2011). The newest US treatment guidelines do not specifically recommend this class of medication for dyslipidemia—citing a lack of data supporting any effect on CVD outcomes and noting that their role in the prevention of ASCVD is less clear and that the potential for benefit from ASCVD event reduction or triglyceride lowering must be carefully considered. The guidelines state that the combination of gemfibrozil with a statin should be avoided due to an increased risk for myopathy (Stone, 2014).

Table 41.1 SIMILARITIES AND DIFFERENCE AMONG CHOLESTEROL GUIDELINES

| RISK ASSESSMENT | ACC/AHA (2013) | ADA (2015) | GUIDELINES | |
			NICE (2014)	NLA (2014)
Screening	Fasting lipids	Fasting lipids	Fasting/nonfasting lipids	Fasting/nonfasting lipids
Eligibility for primary prevention if LDL-C <190 mg/dl	Age 40–75 years and LDL-C 70–189 mg/dl	Age >40 years (see exceptions)	Age 40–84 years (exception: type 1 diabetes)	Age ≥20 years and categorization (low, moderate, high, and very high risk)
10-year risk calculator for primary prevention	PRC	Not recommended	QRISK2 2014 risk calculator (except for type 1 diabetes)	If two major risk factors, FRS or PRC
10-year risk threshold for primary prevention	≥7.5%	None	≥10.0%	≥10.0% (FR5) ≥15% (PRC)
Lipid targets (with lifestyle therapy)				
ASCVD, FH, or LDL-C ≥190 mg/dl	High-dose statin; >50% reduction in LDL-C	High-dose statin; >50% reduction in LDL-C	High-dose statin	Non-HDL-C <100 mg/dl; LDL-C <70 mg/dl
Preferred treatment	Atorvastatin, 40–80 mg, or rosuvastatin, 20–40 mg		Atorvastatin, 80 mg	High-dose statin plus nonstatin treatment to achieve goal
Primary prevention if no FH and LDL-C <190 mg/dl				
Diabetes not present	Moderate-dose statin to lower LDL-C >30–50%		Non-HDL-C reduction ≥40% (atorvastatin, 20 mg/day)	Non-HDL-C <130 mg/dl and LDL-C <100 mg/dl for low, moderate, or high risk
Diabetes present	Type 2 or type 1: Moderate-dose statin if risk <7.5%; high-dose statin if risk ≥7.5%	If age 40–75 years, moderate-dose statin for 30–50% reduction in LDL-C if no other risk factors; high-dose statin if additional risk factors If age <40 years and other risk factors, moderate- to high-dose statin	Type 2: same as above Type 1: Same as above if age >40 years, duration >10 years, chronic kidney disease, or other risk factors	Type 2 or 1: Non-HDL-C<100 mg/dl and LDL-C <70 mg/dl if two or more risk factors or end organ damage
Older adults	Not indicated if age >75 years	Same as above for age >40 years	If age <85 years, statin per QRISK2 assessment. If age >85 years, consider statin but individualize	Not stated; follow risk categories as defined
Adherence to therapy	Initially at 4–12 weeks, then every 3–12 months (no goals for LDL-C or non-HDL-C)	Monitor as needed (no goals for LDL-C or non-HDL-C)	At 3 months to assess non-HDL-C, then yearly	Every 4–12 months to follow goals

ACC, American College of Cardiology; ADA, American Diabetes Association; AHA, American Heart Association; ASCVD, atherosclerotic cardiovascular disease; FH, familial hypercholesterolemia; FRS, Framingham risk score; non-HDL-C, non-high-density lipoprotein cholesterol; LDL-C, low-density lipoprotein cholesterol; NICE. National Institute for Health and Care Excellence; NLA, National Lipid Association; PRC, pooled risk calculator.

SOURCE: Adapted from Ganda (2015).

Table 41.2 **LEVELS OF HIGH- AND MODERATE-INTENSITY STATIN THERAPY**

HIGH-INTENSITY STATIN THERAPY	MODERATE-INTENSITY STATIN THERAPY
Lowers LDL-C by ~≥50%	Lowers LDL-C by ~30% to <50%
Atorvastatin 40*–80 mg	Atorvastatin 10 mg (*20 mg*)
Rosuvastatin 20 mg (*40 mg*)	Rosuvastatin (*5 mg*) 10 mg
	Simvastatin 20–40 mg†
	Pravastatin 40 mg (*80 mg*)
	Lovastatin 40 mg
	Fluvastatin XL 80 mg
	Fluvastatin 40 mg bid
	Pitavastatin 2-4 mg

LDL-C, low-density lipoprotein cholesterol.

SOURCE: Adapted from Stone (2014).

EZETIMIBE

Several clinical trials with ezetimibe, a cholesterol-absorption inhibitor, have been performed in patients with HIV disease. They have examined ezetimibe as both monotherapy and adjunctive therapy for lipid management (Grandi, 2014; Leyes, 2014; Saeedi, 2015). Ezetimibe appears to be safe, well tolerated, and effective in lipid lowering when added to statin therapy. However, the current ACC/AHA guidelines note that no CVD outcome trials of ezetimibe monotherapy have been conducted. These guidelines make no specific recommendations regarding its use but raise no major safety concerns apart from use of this drug in pregnancy (Stone, 2014).

OMEGA-3 FATTY ACIDS

There are data to support the use of omega-3 fatty acids (fish oils) to lower triglycerides in patients taking ART (De Truchis, 2007; Gerber, 2008; Wohl, 2005). In an ACTG trial, patients with dyslipidemia (baseline TG >650 mg/dl) were randomized to 3 g of fish oil twice daily or fenofibrate 160 mg for 8 weeks. Fish oil and fenofibrate reduced TG levels by 46% and 58%, respectively, whereas combination therapy resulted in a 65% reduction. However, only 25% of patients receiving combination therapy achieved TG levels <200 mg/dl (Gerber, 2008). Three to five grams per day of omega-3 fatty acids can produce a 30–50% reduction in triglyceride levels. Low cost, good tolerability, and lack of drug–drug interactions make these agents potentially attractive in the HIV population. However, note that current US guidelines cite a lack of any randomized controlled trials (RCTs) evaluating this class of drugs and with proof of beneficial CVD outcomes. They may prevent pancreatitis in patients with severe triglyceride elevations (>1000 mg/dl) but have been associated with adverse events, including gastrointestinal upset, skin conditions (rash and pruritus), and bleeding (Stone, 2014).

NIACIN

Niacin was previously recommended by National Cholesterol Education Program guidelines for hyperlipidemia, but there are few data on its use in HIV-infected persons (Dubé, 2006). The current ACC/AHA guidelines do not specifically recommend any formulations of oral niacin therapy for lipid lowering or CVD prevention (Stone, 2014). The current ACC/AHA guidelines note that if niacin is to be used as adjunctive therapy with a statin, the potential for CVD risk-reduction benefit should be weighed against the risks for niacin-associated adverse events, including hepatic insufficiency, peptic ulcer disease, and acute gout (Stone, 2014).

PCSK9 INHIBITORS

In 2015, the US Food and Drug Administration (FDA) approved two drugs in this class for use. Specifically, alirocumab (Praluent) and evolocumab (Repatha) are monoclonal antibodies that must be injected subcutaneously once or twice a month for treatment of high LDL cholesterol. These first-in-class medications are humanized monoclonal antibodies that inactivate proprotein convertase subtilisin-kexin type 9 (PCSK9). This inactivation results in decreased LDL-receptor degradation, increased recirculation of the receptor to the surface of hepatocytes, and consequent lowering of LDL cholesterol levels in the bloodstream (Everett, 2015). These drugs can lower LDL cholesterol by approximately 60%, which is more than that attained with statin use. They appear to be safe and generally well tolerated. However, PCSK9 inhibitors have not been proven to improve CVD outcomes, and definitive outcomes data for CVD are not expected until 2018. These agents are quite expensive, currently costing approximately $10,000 per patient/year. In general, current use of PCSK9 inhibitors is limited to add-on to statin therapy for patients with familial hypercholesterolemia (PL Detail Document, 2015).

ASPIRIN

Aspirin (ASA) is often recommended for the prevention of CVD and associated clinical events, including MI and stroke, but the evidence of benefit for *primary prevention* is limited. Moreover, there are few data specifically from

HIV-infected adults (O'Brien, 2013; Suchindran, 2014). ASA is not FDA approved for this indication, and the FDA issued an advisory in 2014 noting the lack of evidence to support ASA for this practice (Truong, 2015). However, some endorsements for ASA focus on patients at sufficiently high CVD risk to outweigh potential harms from bleeding. This may include men older than age 50 years or women older than age 60 years who have one or more additional risks, including smoking, HTN, DM, or hyperlipidemia. The AHA and American Diabetes Association recommend ASA for patients meeting various CVD/CHD 10-year risk thresholds (4–30%). Low-dose ASA (81 mg) should be used. The most recent guidelines of the US Preventive Services Task Force (USPSTF) note that in primary prevention, "aspirin modestly reduces nonfatal MI/coronary events and major CVD events, but increases major GI bleeding risk. More precise real-world estimates for bleeding events (GI, CNS) are necessary to calculate the net benefit." The USPSTF notes that at some absolute risk for 10-year CVD events, a benefit could outweigh bleeding risks, but models and studies to identify these populations are needed (Guirguis-Blake, 2015). There are at least four large, ongoing RCTs relating to ASA for primary prevention that should provide future guidance (Truong, 2015).

For *secondary prevention*, there are data demonstrating that ASA effectively reduces the risk of recurrence of vascular events in patients with a history of a previous MI, stroke, or transient ischemic attack by approximately 20%. There has been FDA-approved labeling for this indication since the 1980s (Paikin, 2012). The recommended dose is 75–325 mg/day. Because of this consistently reported benefit, which has been found to significantly outweigh the risk of major bleeding, ASA therapy for secondary prevention has gained widespread clinical acceptance.

BLOOD PRESSURE CONTROL

Hypertension becomes more prevalent as the HIV population ages. A longitudinal analysis of blood pressure changes in the D:A:D study cohort found no evidence that ART increased the risk of hypertension (Thiebault, 2005). Factors associated with elevated blood pressure in the general population predicted hypertension in this HIV-infected population. A US cross-sectional study of 707 HIV-infected adults (92% male/72% on ARV therapy) found hypertension to be common (31% prevalence) but did not find any association with use of ART (Medina-Torne, 2012). It is reasonable to screen and manage hypertension in HIV-infected adults per the current guidelines of the Joint National Commission 8

(JNC-VIII) (James, 2014). The 2015 SPRINT trial found that in older (50+ years) nondiabetic individuals, a reduction of systolic blood pressure to less than 120 mmHg was associated with fewer CVD events and all-cause mortality without an offset in adverse drug-related toxicity compared to those of patients who were treated to a target diastolic blood pressure of 140 mmHg. Because a median of three antihypertensive agents were needed to achieve the stricter goal, the feasibility of this approach in the setting of HIV, in which there is already a concern for polypharmacy, remains to be determined. Current US guidelines note that a target goal of 140/90 mmHg is recommended for most patients with CAD and hypertension. A target of 130/80 mmHg is suggested for patients with prior history of MI, stroke, or CAD risk equivalents (Rosendorff, 2015).

SMOKING CESSATION

Smoking cessation remains an important part of cardiovascular risk reduction. Getting patients to stop smoking has been shown to significantly reduce their 10-year Framingham and AHA/ACA risk scores by 50% or greater. Counseling, including the "5 A strategy" (ask, advise, assess, assist, arrange follow-up), has proven successful. In addition, pharmacologic interventions (nicotine replacement, bupropion, and varenicline) are all potentially effective therapies to assist patients with smoking cessation.

LIFESTYLE MODIFICATION

The process of atherosclerosis is thought to begin at a young age and progress over many decades before clinical CVD (e.g., acute coronary syndromes, MI, and stable or unstable angina) becomes evident. A healthy diet, increased physical activity, a healthy weight, and not smoking have been associated with improvements in ASCVD risk factors. Regarding physical activity, the ACC/AHA guidelines recommend that adults engage in three or four sessions of aerobic physical activity per week, with each session lasting an average of 40 minutes. These behaviors can also lead to improvements in TC, LDL, HDL, blood glucose, and blood pressure—and ultimately lower 10-year and lifetime rates of CVD (Stone, 2014). Because persons with HIV disease are living much longer, it is important to encourage them to combine multiple aspects of a healthy lifestyle.

References

Aberg JA, Gallant JE, Ghanem KG, et al. Primary care guidelines for the management of persons infected with HIV: 2013 update by the HIV Medicine Association of the Infectious Diseases Society of America. *Clin Infect Dis.* 2014 Jan; *58*(1):1–34.

Althoff KN, McGinnis KA, Wyatt CM, et al. Comparison of risk and age at diagnosis of myocardial infarction, end-stage renal disease, and non-AIDS defining cancer in HIV-infected versus uninfected adults. *Clin Infect Dis*. 2015; 60:627–638.

Baker JV, Henry WK, Patel P, et al.; Study to Understand the Natural History of HIV/AIDS in the Era of Effective Therapy Investigators. Progression of carotid intima-media thickness in a contemporary human immunodeficiency virus cohort. *Clin Infect Dis*. 2011 Oct; 53(8):826–835.

Baum PD, Sullam PM, Stoddart CA, et al. Abacavir increases platelet reactivity via competitive inhibition of soluble guanylyl cyclase. *AIDS*. 2011; 25(18):2243–2248.

Boden WE, Probstfield JK, Anderson T, et al. Niacin in patients with low HDL cholesterol levels receiving intensive statin therapy. *N Engl J Med*. 2011; 365(24):2255–2267.

Cioe PA, et al. Soluble CD14 and D-dimer are associated with smoking and heavy alcohol use in HIV-infected adults. Paper presented at CROI 2014, Boston, MA, March 3–6, 2014. Abstract 732.

D:A:D Study Group. Class of antiretroviral drugs and the risk of myocardial infarction. *N Engl J Med*. 2007; 356:1723–1735.

Data Collection on Adverse Events of Anti-HIV Drugs (D:A:D) Study Group. The impact of fasting on the interpretation of triglyceride levels for predicting myocardial infarction risk in HIV-positive individuals: The D:A:D study. *J Infect Dis*. 2011; 204(4):521–525.

De Pablo C, Orden S, Calatayud S, et al. Differential effects of tenofovir/emtricitabine and abacavir/lamivudine on human leukocyte recruitment. *Antivir Ther*. 2012; 17(8):1615–1619.

De Truchis P, Kirstetter M, Perier A, et al. Reduction in triglyceride level with N-3 polyunsaturated fatty acids in HIV-infected patients taking potent antiretroviral therapy: A randomized prospective study. *J Acquir Immun Defic Syndr*. 2007; 44(3):278–285.

Deeks S, Lewin SR, Havlir DA. The end of AIDS: HIV infection as a chronic disease. *Lancet*. 2013; 283(9903):1525–1533.

Drozd DR, Kitahata MM, Althoff KN, et al. Incidence and risk of myocardial infarction (MI) by type in the NA-ACCORD. Paper presented at CROI 2015, Seattle, WA, February 23–26, 2015. Abstract 748.

Dube MP, Stein JH, Aberg JA, et al. Guidelines for the evaluation and management of dyslipidemia in HIV-infected adults receiving antiretroviral therapy. *Clin Infect Dis*. 2003; 37:613–627.

Dubé W, Aberg JA, et al.; AIDS Clinical Trials Group A5148 Study Team. Safety and efficacy of extended-release niacin for the treatment of dyslipidemia in patients with HIV infection. *Antivir Ther*. 2006; 11(8):1081–1089.

Echeverria P, Domingo P, Llibre JM, et al. Prevalence of ischemic heart disease and management of coronary risk in daily clinical practice: Results from a Mediterranean cohort of HIV-infected patients. *Biomed Research Int*. 2014; 823058:1–8.

Everett BM, Smith RJ, Hiatt WR. Reducing LDL with PCSK9 Inhibitors—The clinical benefit of lipid drugs. *N Engl J Med*. 2015; 373:1588–1591.

Fitch KV, Looby SE, Rope A, et al. Effects of aging and smoking on carotid intima-media thickness in HIV-infection. *AIDS*. 2013; 27(1):49–57.

Friis-Moller, Sabin, Weber, et al.; the Data Collection on Adverse Events of Anti-HIV drugs (D:A:D) study group. *N Engl J Med*. 2003; 349:1993–2003.

Ganda OP. Deciphering cholesterol treatment guidelines: A clinician's perspective. *JAMA*. 2015; 313(10):1009–1010.

Gerber JG, Kitch DW, Fichtenbaum CJ, et al. Fish oil and fenofibrate for the treatment of hypertriglyceridemia in HIV-infected subjects on antiretroviral therapy: Results of ACTG A5186. *J Acquir Immun Defic Syndr*. 2008; 47(4):459–466.

Goff DC Jr, Lloyd-Jones DM, Bennett G, et al. 2013 ACC/AHA guideline on the assessment of cardiovascular risk: A report of the American College of Cardiology/American Heart Association Task Force on Practice Guidelines. *J Am Coll Cardiol*. 2014; 63:2935–2959.

Golomb BA, Evans MA, Dimsdale JE, et al. Effects of statins on energy and fatigue with exertion: Results from a randomized controlled trial. *Arch Intern Med*. 2012 Aug 13; 172(15): 1180–1182.

Grandi AM, Nicolini E, Rizzi L, et al. Dyslipidemia in HIV-positive patients: A randomized, controlled, prospective study on ezetimibe + fenofibrate versus pravastatin monotherapy. *J Int AIDS Soc*. 2014; 17:19004.

Guirguis-Blake JM, Evans CV, Senger CA, et al. Aspirin for the primary prevention of cardiovascular events: A systematic evidence review for the U.S. Preventive Services Task Force. Evidence Synthesis No. 131. 2015. Rockville, MD: Agency for Healthcare.

Hsue P, Hunt P, Schnell A., et al. Inflammation is associated with endothelial dysfunction among individuals with treated and suppressed HIV infection. Paper presented at CROI 2010, San Francisco, CA, 2010, Abstract 708.

Hunt PW. HIV and inflammation: Mechanisms and consequences. *Curr HIV/AIDS Rep*. 2012; 9(2):139–147.

James PA, Oparil S, Carter BL, et al. 2014 Evidence-based guideline for the management of high blood pressure in adults: Report from the panel members appointed to the Eighth Joint National Committee (JNC 8). *JAMA*. 2014; 311(5):507–520.

Klein DB, Leyden WA, Chao CR. No difference in incidence of myocardial infarction for HIV+ and HIV– individuals in recent years. *Clin Infect Dis*. 2015; 60(8):1278–1285.

Klein DB, Marcus JL, Leyden WA, et al. Infection and immunodeficiency as risk factors for ischemic stroke. Paper presented at CROI 2014, Boston, MA, March 3–6, 2014. Abstract 741.

Krishnan S, Bosch RJ, Rodriguez B, et al. Correlates of inflammatory biomarkers one year after suppressive ART. Paper presented at CROI 2014, Boston, MA, March 3–6, 2014. Abstract 757.

Law M, Friis-Moller N, El-Sadr WA, et al. The use of the Framingham equation to predict myocardial infarctions in HIV-infected patients: Comparison with observed events in the D:A:D study. *HIV Med*. 2006; 7:218–230.

Leyes P, Martinez E, Larrousse M, et al. Effects of ezetimibe on cholesterol metabolism in HIV-infected patients with protease inhibitor-associated dyslipidemia: A single-arm intervention trial. *BMC Infect Dis*. 2014; 11:14:497.

Martinez E, Larrousse M, Llibre JM, et al. Substitution of raltegravir for ritonavir-boosted protease inhibitors in HIV-infected patients: The SPIRAL study. *AIDS*. 2010; 24(11):1697–1707.

McComsey GA, Kitch D, Daar ES, et al. Inflammation markers after randomization to abacavir/lamivudine or tenofovir/emtricitabine with efavirenz or atazanavir/ritonavir. *AIDS*. 2012 Jul 17; 26(11):1371–8573.

McComsey GA, Jiang Y, Erlandson KM, et al. Rosuvastatin improves hip bone mineral density but worsens insulin resistance. Paper presented at CROI 2014, Boston, MA, March 3–6, 2014. Abstract 134.

Medina-Torne S, Ganesan A, Barahona I, et al. Hypertension is common among HIV-infected persons, but not associated with HAART. *J Int Assoc Physicians AIDS Care (Chic)*. 2012 Jan–Feb; 11(1):20–25.

Monforte A, Reiss P, Ryom L, et al. Atazanavir is not associated with an increased risk of cardio- or cerebrovascular disease events. *AIDS*. 2013 Jan 28; 27(3):407–415.

Morgello S, Mahboob R, Yakoushina T, et al. Autopsy findings in human immunodeficiency virus-infected populations over 2 decades. *Arch Path Lab Med*. 2002; 126:182–190.

O'Brien S, Montenont E, Hu L, et al. Aspirin attenuates platelet activation and immune activation in HIV-1-infected subjects on antiretroviral therapy: A pilot study. *J Acquir Immune Defic Syndr*. 2013 Jul 1; 63(3):280–288.

Paikin JS, Eikelboom JW. Cardiology patient page: Aspirin. *Circulation*. 2012 Mar 13; 125(10):e439–e442.

Paisible AL, Chang CH, So-Armah KA, et al. HIV infection, cardiovascular disease risk factor profile, and risk for acute myocardial infarction. *J AIDS*. 2015; 68:209–216.

Palella F, et al. NA-ACCORD: Recent abacavir use and risk of MI. Paper presented at CROI 2015, Seattle, WA, February 23–26, 2015. Abstract 749 LB.

Palella FJ Jr, Fisher M, Tebas P, et al. Simplification to rilpivirine/emtricitabine/tenofovir disoproxil fumarate from ritonavir-boosted protease inhibitor antiretroviral therapy in a randomized trial of HIV-1 RNA-suppressed participants. *AIDS*. 2014 Jan 28; *28*(3):335–344

Petoumenos K, Worm S, Reiss P, et al.; D:A:D Study Group. Rates of cardiovascular disease following smoking cessation in patients with HIV infection: Results from the D:A:D study. *HIV Med*. 2011 Aug; *12*(7):412–421.

PL Detail Document: PCSK9 inhibitors for high cholesterol. Pharmacist's letter/prescriber's letter, August 2015.

Post WS, et al. Associations between HIV infection and subclinical coronary atherosclerosis. *Ann Intern Med*. 2014; 160:458–467.

Rasmussen LD, May MT, Kronborg G, et al. Time trends for risk of severe age-related diseases in individuals with and without HIV infection in Denmark: A nationwide population-based cohort study. *Lancet HIV*. 2015; 2:e288–e298.

Regan S, Meigs JB, Massaro J, et al. Evaluation of the ACC/AHA CVD risk prediction algorithm among HIV-infected patients. Paper presented at CROI 2015, Seattle, WA, February 23–26, 2015. Abstract 751.

Ridker PM, Pradhan A, MacFadyen JG, et al. Cardiovascular benefits and diabetes risks of statin therapy in primary prevention: An analysis from the JUPITER trial. *Lancet*. 2012 Aug 11; *380*(9841):565–571.

Rosendorff C, Lackland DT, Allison M, et al. Treatment of hypertension in patients with coronary artery disease: A scientific statement from the AHA, ACC, and ASH. *Circulation*. 2015; *131*(19):e435–e470.

Ryom RL, Lundgren JD, Reiss P, et al. Relationship between confirmed eGFR and cardiovascular disease in HIV-positive persons. Paper presented at CROI 2015, Seattle WA, February 23–26, 2015. Abstract 742.

Sabin C, Reiss P, Ryom L, et al. Is there continued evidence for an association between abacavir and myocardial infarction risk? Paper presented at CROI 2014, Boston, MA, March 3–6, 2014. Abstract 747.

Saeedi R, Johns K, Frohlich J, et al. Lipid lowering efficacy and safety of ezetimibe combined with rosuvastatin compared with titrating rosuvastatin monotherapy in HIV-positive patients. *Lipids Health Dis*. 2015; *14*:57.

Sax PC. Zolopa A, Eleon R. Tenofovir alafenamide vs. tenofovir disoproxil fumarate in single tablet regimens for initial HIV-1 therapy: A randomized phase 2 study. *J Acquir Immune Defic Syndr*. 2014; 67(1):52–58.

Sing S, Willig JH, Mugavero MJ, et al. Comparative efficacy and toxicity among statins in HIV-infected patients. *Clin Infect Dis*. 2011; 52(3):387–395.

SPRINT Research Group. A randomized trial of intensive versus standard blood-pressure control. *N Engl J Med*. 2015; 373:2103–2116.

Stone NJ, et al. 2013 report on the treatment of blood cholesterol to reduce the risks of ASCVD in adults. *Circulation*. 2014; *129*:S1–S45.

Strategies for Management of Antiretroviral Therapy (SMART) Study Group. CD4+ count-guided interruption of antiretroviral therapy. *N Engl J Med*. 2006; 355:2283–2296.

Strategies for Management of Antiretroviral Therapy (SMART)/INSIGHT/D:A:D Study Groups. Use of nucleoside reverse transcriptase inhibitors and risk of myocardial infarction in HIV-infected patients. *AIDS*. 2008; *22*:F17–F24.

Subramanian S, Tawakol A, Burdo TH, et al. Arterial Inflammation in patients with HIV. *JAMA*. 2012; 308:379–386.

Suchindran S, Regan S, Meigs JB, et al. Aspirin use for primary and secondary prevention in human immunodeficiency virus (HIV)-infected and HIV-uninfected patients. *Open Forum Infect Dis*. 2014 Oct 20; *1*(3):ofu076.

Tawakol A, Lo J, Zanni MV, et al. Increased arterial inflammation relates to high-risk coronary plaque morphology in HIV-infected patients. *J Acquir Immune Defic Syndr*. 2014; 66(2):164–171.

Thiebaut R, El-Sadr W, Friis-Moller N, et al.; the D:A:D Study Group. Predictors of hypertension and changes in blood pressure in HIV-infected patients. *Antiviral Ther*. 2005; 10:811–823.

Thompson-Paul A, et al. Evaluation of the ACC/AHA CVD risk prediction algorithm among HIV-infected patients. Paper presented at CROI 2015, Seattle, WA, February 23–26, 2015. Abstract 747.

Torriani FJ, Komarow L, Parker RA, et al. Endothelial function in human immunodeficiency virus-infected antiretroviral naive subjects before and after starting potent antiretroviral therapy: The ACTG (AIDS Clinical Trials Group) Study 5152s. *J Am Coll Cardiol*. 2008; 52(7):569–576.

Triant V, Meig J, Grinspoon S. Association of C-reactive protein and HIV infection with acute myocardial infarction. *J Acquir Immune Defic Syndr*. 2009; 51(3):268–273.

Triant V, Regan S, Lee H, et al. Association of immunologic and virologic factors with myocardial infarction rates in the U.S. health care system. *J Acquir Immune Defic Syndr*. 2010; 55(5):615–619.

Truong C. Low-dose acetylsalicylic acid for primary prevention of cardiovascular disease: Do not misinterpret the recommendations. *Can Fam Phys*. 2015; 61(11):971–972.

Tungsiripat M, Kitch D, Glesby MJ, et al. A pilot study to determine the impact on dyslipidemia of adding tenofovir to stable background antiretroviral therapy: ACTG 5206. *AIDS*. 2010 Jul 17; *24*(11):1781–1784.

Van Lelyveld SF, Gras L, Kesselring A, et al. ATHENA national observational cohort study: Long-term complications in patients with poor immunological recovery despite virological successful HAART in Dutch ATHENA cohort. *AIDS*. 2012; 26(4):465–474.

Wohl DA, Tien HC, Busby M, et al. Randomized study of the safety and efficacy of fish oil (omega-3 fatty acid) supplementation with dietary and exercise counseling for the treatment of antiretroviral therapy associated hypertriglyceridemia. *Clin Infect Dis*. 2005; 41(10):1498–1504.

Worm S, Sabin C, Weber R, et al.; D:A:D Study Group. Risk of myocardial infarction in patients with HIV infection exposed to specific individual antiretroviral drugs from 3 major drug classes. *J Infect Dis*. 2010; 201:318–330.

Young J, Xiao Y, Moodier EE, et al. Effect of cumulating exposure to abacavir on the risk of cardiovascular disease events in patients from the Swiss HIV Cohort Study. *J AIDS*. 2015; 69(4):413–421.

42.

RENAL COMPLICATIONS

Derek M. Fine and Sana Waheed

CHAPTER GOAL

Upon completion of this chapter, the reader should be able to recognize the increasing prevalence of renal disease in HIV-infected patients, the broad spectrum of pathologic involvement including medication-induced renal injury, and potential future targets of interventions in HIV-related renal disease.

NEPHROPATHY

LEARNING OBJECTIVE

Discuss the epidemiology, risk factors, broad pathologic spectrum, and current therapeutic interventions for HIV-related renal disease.

WHAT'S NEW?

Genetic mechanisms of HIV-associated nephropathy (HIVAN) have been further elucidated, and there is growing evidence that renal transplantation is safe in these patients.

RISK FACTORS

- With improved life expectancy and antiretroviral therapy (ART)-related metabolic abnormalities, chronic kidney disease has become a significant comorbidity in HIV-infected patients.

- Risk factors for kidney disease include African American race, CD4$^+$ T cell counts <200 cells/ mm^3, HIV RNA levels >10,000 copies/ml, family history of chronic kidney disease (CKD), diabetes mellitus, hypertension, and hepatitis C co-infection.

- Compared to the general population, patients with AIDS have a 16-fold higher incidence of requiring renal replacement therapy.

PATHOLOGIC SPECTRUM OF DISEASE

- Although HIVAN used to be the predominant form of renal involvement in HIV patients a decade and a half ago, this pattern is changing and other pathologies, such as immune complex disease, diabetic glomerulosclerosis, and classic focal segmental glomerulosclerosis (vs. the collapsing form of focal segmental glomerulosclerosis (FSGS) seen in HIVAN), are being seen more frequently.

- Acute kidney injury is nearly twice as common in HIV-infected patients compared to patients without HIV, and it is associated with a sixfold increase in mortality.

PATHOGENESIS

- The *ApoL1* gene, which encodes a factor to lyse *Trypanosoma brucei*, is the key susceptibility allele in HIVAN.

- Two HIV genes, *nef* and *vpr*, appear to contribute to podocyte dysregulation in HIVAN.

TREATMENT

- ART and angiotensin inhibition slow progression of renal disease.

- Corticosteroids may have benefit in glomerular diseases, but prospective trials are lacking.

- Renal transplantation in HIV-positive patients appears to have good outcomes but requires intensive monitoring.

Renal disease is a major cause of mortality from non-AIDS-related conditions in HIV-infected patients, along with malignancy and cardiovascular and liver disease (Mocroft, 2010). Renal pathology in HIV patients was originally reported in 1984 and was called "acquired immune deficiency syndrome (AIDS) nephropathy." The histopathology on kidney biopsy showed a collapsing type of focal and segmental glomerulosclerosis, and the clinical presentation was that of proteinuria, usually nephrotic, and rapid progression to end-stage renal disease (ESRD) (Rao, 1984). Subsequently, HIVAN became more commonly recognized as a major cause of renal disease in HIV-infected patients. In the United States, the incidence of HIVAN peaked in the mid-1990s and dropped significantly with the introduction of highly active antiretroviral therapy (HAART) by the late 1990s (Ross, 2002).

EPIDEMIOLOGY

Although the incidence of HIVAN is declining, the prevalence of kidney disease in HIV-1-infected individuals is increasing as a result of improved patient survival (Mocroft, 2003). Consequently, the spectrum of kidney disease is being driven by metabolic risk factors such as obesity, diabetes, hypertension, and the use of medications with nephrotoxic potential (Waheed, 2014).

Despite widespread use of ART, HIV patients remain at a higher risk of renal insufficiency, cardiovascular disease, and overall mortality than matched cohorts of non-infected people (Kalayjian, 2011; Post, 2009). Up to 30% of patients infected with HIV are at risk of developing proteinuria. Moreover, cross-sectional cohorts from Europe, Asia, and North America have demonstrated high rates of CKD in HIV-infected patients, with 5.5% of HIV patients having stages 3–5 CKD (Post, 2009). In a large US cohort of predominantly African American HIV-infected patients with CKD, 35% progressed to ESRD (Lucas, 2008). Based on another large sample of US veterans, the incidence rate of ESRD in African Americans with HIV is even higher than that of patients with diabetes (incidence rates per 1000 person-years: 71.1 for HIV, 59.9 for diabetes mellitus, and 27.9 for patients with neither HIV nor diabetes) (Choi, 2007). Compared to the general population, patients with AIDS have a 16-fold higher risk of requiring renal replacement therapy (Lucas, 2007).

RISK FACTORS FOR NEPHROPATHY

Risk factors for the development of kidney disease in patients with HIV include African American race, diabetes mellitus, hypertension, hepatitis C co-infection, cardiovascular disease, and family history of CKD (Mocroft, 2015; Naicker, 2010).

Moreover, patients with advanced untreated HIV infection with CD 4^+ T cell counts <200 cells/mm^3 and viral load >30,000 copies/ml are at high risk for developing HIV-associated nephropathy (Bige, 2012; Lescure, 2012).

GENETIC PREDISPOSITION

The major genetic risk factor for developing HIV-associated nephropathy and non-HIVAN FSGS in patients of African descent is the presence of polymorphisms in the apolipoprotein 1 (*APOL1*) gene, which is also located on chromosome 22 (Bige, 2012; Genovese, 2010; Lescure, 2012; Tzur, 2010). Two *APOL1* risk alleles, G1 and G2, are associated with the increased susceptibility for the development of HIV-associated nephropathy (Genovese, 2010; Papeta, 2011). The association of *APOL1* genetic variation in FSGS and HIVAN has been studied by Kopp and colleagues (Kopp, 2011). Individuals carrying the high-risk alleles had 29 times higher odds of developing HIVAN and had a 17-fold higher risk of developing FSGS. In patients who carry the two APOL1 risk alleles, this alone can explain 35% of cases of HIVAN and 18% of FSGS cases (Kopp, 2011). Indeed, *APOL1* homozygosity, present in 13% of the general African American population, was noted in more than 60% of African Americans with HIVAN and non-HIVAN FSGS (Kopp, 2011). Recently, a G3 haplotype has been identified, but further studies are needed to understand its importance in the pathogenesis of HIVAN (Ko, 2013). *ApoL1* encodes a serum factor that lyses *Trypanosoma brucei*. Thus, selective mutations in Africans to counter an endemic parasite may have contributed to the current rates of HIVAN and FSGS in African American populations.

PATHOGENESIS

In animal models, HIV gene expression within kidney cells is required for the development of HIVAN (Bruggeman, 1997). Even in HIVAN patients with undetectable plasma HIV RNA levels, proviral DNA is found in the renal tissue of all patients (Izzedine, 2011). This implies that the kidney acts as a separate compartment from blood, allowing HIV to replicate in the kidney even in patients who achieve viral suppression in their plasma with treatment (Medapalli, 2011). It has been shown that the expression of nonstructural gene products of HIV, negative effector (*nef*) and viral protein r (*vpr*), in murine model results in HIVAN (Zuo, 2006). HIV induces apoptosis of cells in addition to causing cytopathic effects. These effects in combination with cytokine release are thought to play a role in the development of HIV-associated nephropathy (Kimmel, 2003).

Studies have also shown that HIV infection downregulates expression of microRNAs in human podocytes (Cheng, 2013). HIV-infected podocytes re-enter the cell cycle as evidenced by an increased expression of markers of proliferation and decreased expression of cyclin-dependent kinase inhibitors (Barisoni, 1999). These cells have increased vascular endothelial growth factor expression and persistent activation of NF-κB, which also contributes to podocyte proliferation (Korgaonkar, 2008).

MARKERS OF RENAL INJURY

Markers of renal injury include elevated creatinine, proteinuria, glycosuria, and an increased fractional excretion of uric acid (Kalayjian, 2011). Risk factors for proteinuria include older age, African American race, insulin resistance, hypertension, and a low CD4+ T cell count (Post, 2009). The presence of albuminuria and overt proteinuria is associated with increased cardiovascular morbidity and mortality in this population (George, 2010; Wyatt, 2011). In a study of HIV patients with albuminuria, the 5-year mortality rate was 20% in patients with albuminuria and 48% in patients with a glomerular filtration rate (GFR) <60 ml/min and albuminuria (Choi, 2010).

ASSESSMENT OF RENAL FUNCTION

Like the general population, kidney damage in patients with HIV is assessed by using creatinine-based estimates of glomerular filtration rate (eGFR) with the Cockcroft–Gault equation, Modification of Diet in Renal Disease (MDRD), and CKD Epidemiology Collaboration (CKD-EPI) equation, but none of these estimates have been systematically validated in patients with HIV. Cystatin C is an alternative marker of eGFR that does not depend on muscle mass and is more sensitive for kidney damage than creatinine-based formulas, but currently cystatin C is not routinely used in clinical settings. In addition, it appears that cystatin C-based eGFR is affected by HIV treatment factors and markers of T cell activation (Bhasin, 2013). It has been suggested that cystatin C levels are higher with active HIV replication and this can overestimate the GFR, limiting its usefulness in HIV patients (Mauss, 2008).

PATHOLOGIC SPECTRUM OF DISEASE

HIV-infected patients can develop multiple forms of renal involvement, including acute kidney injury (AKI), HIVAN, immune complex disease (HIVICK), thrombotic microangiopathy (TMA), and medication-induced nephrotoxicity (Box 42.1) (Cohen, 2009). Therefore, a renal biopsy is indicated in most HIV patients with kidney disease to determine the underlying renal pathology because treatment strategies often differ based on kidney biopsy findings (Fine, 2008).

Box 42.1 PATHOLOGIC SPECTRUM OF KIDNEY DISEASE IN HIV PATIENTS

Glomerular Diseases

- HIVAN—collapsing FSGS[a]
- HIVICK—HIV-associated immune complex disease[a]
  - IgA nephropathy
  - Membranoproliferative glomerulonephritis
  - Membranous nephropathy
  - Lupus-like glomerulonephritis
- Thrombotic microangiopathy[a]
- Classic FSGS (primary or secondary)
- Hypertensive nephrosclerosis
- Diabetic nephropathy
- Membranous glomerulopathy
- Membranoproliferative glomerulonephritis (frequently hepatitis C-related)
- Amyloidosis
- Minimal change disease
- Fibrillary glomerulonephritis

Tubular Diseases

- Acute tubular necrosis
- Drug-related tubular dysfunction
- Nephrolithiasis (primary or drug-related)
- Tumor lysis syndrome
- Obstruction

Interstitial Diseases

- Interstitial nephritis
- Pyelonephritis

[a]Specifically HIV virus related.

Acute Kidney Injury

Poor nutritional state of patients, use of multiple medications, and the increased risk of opportunistic infections in HIV patients predisposes them to development of AKI, with incidence rates as high as 5.9 per 100 person-years (Franceschini, 2005). In a retrospective study of HIV-infected hospitalized patients, these patients had an increased incidence of AKI in both the pre-HAART era (odds ratio (OR), 4.6) and the post-HAART era (OR, 2.8) (Franceschini, 2005). Higher incidence of AKI is associated with increased age, diabetes mellitus, chronic kidney disease, acute or chronic liver failure, CD4[+] T cell count <200 cells/mm³, HIV-1 RNA levels >10,000 copies/ml, and hepatitis co-infection (Franceschini, 2005; Wyatt, 2006). Common causes of AKI in HIV-1-infected patients are similar to those in non-infected individuals, with pre-renal states and acute tubular necrosis accounting for 39% and 37% of cases, respectively (Franceschini, 2005).

Rare causes of AKI in HIV patients include obstruction from lymphadenopathy related to malignancy, tumor lysis syndrome, and polyoma virus-induced renal dysfunction. Regardless of the etiology, AKI is associated with a sixfold increase in overall mortality in HIV patients (Kalim, 2008).

HIV-Associated Nephropathy

HIVAN is the most aggressive form of kidney disease associated with HIV infection and generally presents in patients with advanced HIV infection with rapidly declining GFR and proteinuria (Berliner, 2008). The incidence of HIVAN declined after the widespread use of ART, but it still remains a leading cause of ESRD in young African American patients. HIVAN is pathologically characterized by collapsing form of focal and segmental sclerosis, prominent tubular microcysts, and tubulointerstitial inflammation (D'Agati, 1989).

HIV-Associated Immune Complex Kidney Disease

Various immune complex kidney diseases have been reported in patients with HIV-1 infection, such as post-infectious glomerulonephritis, membranoproliferative glomerulonephritis, membranous nephropathy, immunoglobulin A nephropathy, and lupus-like glomerulonephritis, collectively referred to as HIVICK (Balow, 2005; Kalayjian, 2011). Patients with HIVICK tend to have a better prognosis with a lower incidence of ESRD compared to patients with HIVAN (Foy, 2013).

Thrombotic Microangiopathy

TMA is a rare complication of HIV-1 infection, with an incidence of isolated renal TMA as low as 0.3% (Becker, 2004). Opportunistic infections, immunosuppression, and various drugs used in advanced disease can all contribute to development of TMA (Bachmeyer, 1995).

TREATMENT

Recommendations regarding therapy are limited due to the lack of randomized prospective controlled trials. Most of the treatment options including ART, inhibition of renin–angiotensin–aldosterone system (ACE inhibitors), and corticosteroids are based on retrospective studies and non-randomized trials.

Antiretroviral Therapy

Multiple observational studies have suggested the benefit of ART in slowing the progression or reversing renal disease in patients with HIVAN (Elewa, 2011). In a large Johns Hopkins Clinic cohort of 4000 HIV-infected patients, ART was associated with a 60% risk reduction for HIVAN, with 6.8 and 26.4 episodes per 1000 patient-years in AIDS patients who did or did not receive ART, respectively. In addition, no one developed HIVAN when ART was initiated before the development of AIDS (Lucas, 2004).

Consistent evidence demonstrates preservation of renal function with ART in HIV patient populations. In the Strategies for Management of Antiretroviral Therapy (SMART) group study, continuous therapy versus episodic use of ART was evaluated in 5472 patients with CD4[+] T cell counts >350 cells/μl. In the continuous use group, fewer patients developed renal disease compared to the episodic use group (0.2 vs. 0.1 events/100 person-years) (SMART, 2006). In addition, in a prospective, multicenter cohort involving 1776 HIV patients, ART intervention in patients with CKD stage 2 or greater and low CD4[+] T cell counts led to an average increase of 9.2 ml/min in GFR at a median follow-up of 160 weeks. These results were magnified in those with a lower baseline GFR and greater decrease in viral load (Longenecker, 2009). Similar results have been demonstrated by other large African studies (Peters, 2008; Reid, 2008).

Angiotensin II Blockade

Multiple randomized controlled trials in CKD patients have demonstrated the efficacy of ACE inhibitors and angiotensin receptor blockers in slowing the progression of kidney disease, decreasing proteinuria, and decreasing the incidence of cardiovascular disease and death (Casas, 2005; Jafar, 2003). However, data regarding their use in HIV population are scarce. Kimmel et al. studied 18 patients with biopsy-proven HIVAN, of whom 9 patients treated with captopril had an enhanced renal survival compared to controls (mean renal survival, 156 ± 71 vs. 37 ± 5 days; $p < 0.002$) (Kimmel, 1996). In a study of 44 consecutive patients with biopsy-proven HIVAN, patients treated with ACE inhibition had significantly less progression to ESRD compared to those without therapy (14% vs. 100% at 5 years) (Wei, 2003). Based on these results, angiotensin II blockade is recommended for most CKD and glomerular diseases in HIV patients in the absence of contraindications.

Corticosteroids

In patients with HIVAN, tubulointerstitial inflammation improves after treatment with steroids (Briggs, 1996). However, there are no large randomized controlled trials to support steroid use in this population. In a retrospective cohort study of 21 patients, of which 13 received corticosteroids, the relative risk for progressive renal failure with corticosteroid treatment at 3 months was 0.20 ($p < 0.05$) (Eustace, 2000). This association remained significant despite adjustment in separate logistical regression analyses for baseline creatinine; 24-hour proteinuria; CD4$^+$ count; and history of intravenous drug use, hepatitis B, and hepatitis C co-infection (Eustace, 2000). However, there were 18 infections in corticosteroid-treated patients and 8 in the non-corticosteroid-treated group. In addition, steroid use has been associated with an increased risk of avascular necrosis of the femoral head (Elewa, 2011). Although larger studies are needed to further elucidate the value of steroids in patients with HIV-related kidney disease, some experts recommend a short course of corticosteroid therapy in those with a new diagnosis of HIVAN (Atta, 2008; Fine, 2008).

Novel Therapies

In animal models, all-*trans*-retinoic acid has been shown to reverse the *nef*-induced signaling pathway with improvement in proteinuria and glomerulosclerosis (Ratnam, 2011). Moreover, when phosphodiesterase inhibitors are used in combination, they increase the renal protective effect of retinoids in animal models (Zhong, 2012). However, further studies are needed before their use can be recommended.

Renal Replacement Therapy

Overall survival of HIV patients on dialysis is worse compared to that of the general ESRD population, potentially due to increased risk of infections (Atta, 2007). Older age, lower serum albumin level, lower CD4$^+$ T cell count, and lack of ART are all associated with poor survival in HIV-1-infected patients undergoing hemodialysis or peritoneal dialysis (Kimmel, 1993).

Renal Transplantation

Transplantation was considered to be risky in HIV patients because of concerns of using immunosuppression in patients with a dysregulated immune system. However, there is increasing evidence that renal transplantation is both safe and effective in patients with HIV (Qiu, 2006; Roland, 2008; Stock, 2003; van Maarseveen, 2012). In a prospective study of 150 patients, the patient survival at 1 and 3 years was 95% and 88%, respectively, with allograft survival of 90% and 74%, respectively. This rate is between the rates reported for older patients (65 years or older) and all other recipients of renal transplants. The rate of rejection was higher in these patients, with 1- and 3-year rejection rates of 31% and 41%, respectively, compared to a 1-year rejection rate of 12% as reported by the US Scientific Registry of Transplant Recipients for the general transplant population (Stock, 2010).

Recently, a single-center study examined the transplant outcomes of 16 patients with HIV infection and a renal transplant. Despite higher rates of acute rejection at 1 and 3 years (18% and 27%, respectively), 1- and 3-year graft survival rates were 100% and 81%, respectively (Waheed, 2015).

Initially, renal transplantation in HIV patients was performed without induction therapy. However, the use of antithymocyte globulin as induction therapy is associated with a 2.6-fold lower risk of rejection, as shown in a study of 516 HIV-infected patients (Locke, 2014). Many of the agents used in post-transplantation immunosuppression have antiretroviral properties. Mycophenolate mofetil has virostatic properties through depletion of guanoside nucleosides necessary for the viral life cycle. Calcineurin inhibitors (tacrolimus and cyclosporine) selectively inhibit infected cell growth, and sirolimus disrupts infective viral replication through suppression of antigen-presenting cell function. However, multiple drug interactions exist between some antiretroviral drugs and immunosuppressive therapy, particularly through the cytochrome P450 system. In particular, ritonavir and cobicistat are potent inhibitors of this system, potentially limiting their use. These interactions predispose patients to unexpected increases or decreases in drug levels, toxic side effects, organ rejection, and HIV disease breakthrough (Frassetto, 2009). Thus, although kidney transplantation appears to be effective, it requires intensive monitoring of drug levels and rejection risk.

Recommended Reading

Elewa, U., Sandri, A. M., Rizza, S. A., et al. Treatment of HIV-associated nephropathies. *Nephron Clin Pract.* 2011; 118:c346–c354.

Kalayjian, R. C. Renal issues in HIV infection. *Curr HIV/AIDS Rep.* 2011; 8:164–171.

Stock, P. G., Barin, B., Murphy, B., et al. Outcomes of kidney transplantation in HIV-infected recipients. *N Engl J Med.* 2010; 363(21):2004–2014.

ANTIRETROVIRAL THERAPY-RELATED RENAL COMPLICATIONS

LEARNING OBJECTIVE

Discuss renal complications of antiretroviral therapy.

WHAT'S NEW?

Tenofovir alafenamide fumarate, a recently US Food and Drug Administration (FDA)-approved agent, is a prodrug of tenofovir disoproxil fumarate (TDF) and has shown effective anti-HIV1 activity with fewer renal side effects in clinical trials.

KEY POINTS

- ART can contribute to renal toxicities in HIV-infected patients.

- TDF may cause acute kidney injury, chronic kidney disease, and/or proximal tubular dysfunction.

- Indinavir, atazanavir, and other protease inhibitors can cause nephrolithiasis.

- Cobicistat and dolutegravir can increase serum creatinine by inhibiting its tubular secretion, but they do not change the actual GFR.

PRESENTATION

- Elevation in serum creatinine.

- Proximal tubular renal dysfunction with decreased serum phosphorus or increased urinary phosphorus excretion.

- Hematuria and pain with nephrolithiasis.

DIAGNOSIS

- Evaluate cause of renal insufficiency.

- Monitor renal insufficiency closely.

MANAGEMENT

- The majority of renal toxicities are treated with supportive therapy.

- The offending medication should be changed in most patients.

- Evaluate the need for adjusting doses of antiretroviral medications in renal insufficiency.

Although the overall incidence is low, ART in HIV patients can cause renal dysfunction in 0.3–2% of patients (Kalyesubula, 2011). In a study by Franceschini and colleagues, drugs associated with tubular injury, interstitial nephritis, and crystalluria accounted for 32% of all cases of AKI (Franceschini, 2005). Moreover, indinavir, atazanavir, and tenofovir have been implicated in the development of chronic kidney disease (Atta, 2008).

NUCLEOS(T)IDE REVERSE TRANSCRIPTASE INHIBITORS

TDF is a nucleotide reverse transcriptase inhibitor that is commonly used in HIV patients and has often been implicated as a cause of renal disease.

Due to high renal toxicity rates of its acyclic nucleotide predecessors adefovir and cidofovir, both of which cause AKI and proximal tubular toxicity, there was concern regarding the potential renal toxicity of TDF. Initial studies did not reveal significant toxicity related to TDF, but after FDA approval, case reports emerged of Fanconi's syndrome, renal failure, and diabetes insipidus (Gaspar, 2004; Karras, 2003; Rollot, 2003). Fanconi's syndrome is characterized by proximal tubular kidney dysfunction, with decreased tubular reabsorption and urinary wasting of phosphate, glucose, amino acids, bicarbonate, and sodium. This solute loss leads to acidosis, bone disease, and electrolyte abnormalities. The exact mechanism of nephrotoxicity is unknown, but it is hypothesized that apoptosis of tubular cells and inhibition of mitochondrial DNA replication in proximal tubular cells are involved (Gitman, 2007). Fanconi's syndrome is the most common manifestation of mitochondrial diseases, which supports the hypothesis that tenofovir exposure causes mitochondrial dysfunction (Kalyesubula, 2011). Most patients do not develop the full Fanconi's syndrome but instead manifest primarily with urinary phosphate wasting and, hence, hypophosphatemia in most cases (Waheed, 2015). This may occur in isolation or in conjunction with AKI. Urinary phosphate wasting is a more sensitive marker of TDF-induced nephrotoxicity because hypophosphatemia is not present in all cases.

Patients with low CD4$^+$ T cell counts, advanced age, lower body weight, and higher serum creatinine are most at risk for developing TDF-induced nephrotoxicity (Kalyesubula, 2011).

In many clinical trials, TDF has not demonstrated significant renal toxicity, but many of these were conducted in patients without significant comorbidities and with baseline creatinine clearance >50 ml/min (Gallant, 2006). However, in a retrospective study of 948 patients with HIV, tenofovir use in 294 patients was associated with a greater decrease in calculated creatinine clearance compared to that in patients treated with a non-tenofovir-containing antiretroviral regimen (difference of 6.8 ml/min; $p = 0.02$) (Winston, 2006). In an observational cohort, use of tenofovir ($n = 344$) was associated with a greater decline in renal function (13.3 ml/min in the tenofovir group and 7.5 ml/min in the alternate group) compared to that with an alternative nucleoside analogue ($n = 314$) (Gallant, 2005). In another large study of 10,841 HIV-infected patients from the Veterans Health Administration, over a 10-year period, each year of tenofovir exposure was associated with a 33% (range, 18–51%; $p <0.0001$) increased risk of CKD (Scherzer, 2012). The HEAT trial, which compared abacavir/lamivudine or tenofovir/emtricitabine administered with lopinavir/ritonavir, showed no significant difference in renal function between the groups. However, 1% of the patients on tenofovir developed proximal tubular kidney dysfunction (Smith, 2009).

A recent long-term follow-up of 23,905 patients in the D:A:D study cohort who initiated antiretrovirals with normal eGFR (>90 ml/min/1.73 m^2) showed a significant increase in the development of CKD with exposure to tenofovir, ritonavir-boosted atazanavir, and ritonavir-boosted lopinavir but not other ritonavir-boosted protease

inhibitors or abacavir (Mocroft, 2015). These findings are similar to those of previous studies in the cohort and add to an expanding literature on the long-term effects of antiretroviral agents on the kidney (Fine, 2013).

Some studies have shown that tenofovir use in conjunction with protease inhibitors can increase the risk of renal injury (Sax, 2011). This was considered to be a result of tenofovir accumulation in renal tubular cells as a consequence of tenofovir–ritonavir interaction. Tenofovir is secreted via the multidrug resistance protein (MRP) efflux pump on the luminal side of the proximal tubular cells. It was initially believed that tenofovir secretion was through MRP2. Ritonavir is a potent inhibitor of MRP2-mediated transport, and that could have led to accumulation of tenofovir in the tubular cells (Rollot, 2003). It has since been determined that MRP4 is responsible for tenofovir secretion and is not affected by ritonavir (Ray, 2006). Because ritonavir is often used as salvage therapy, the link of ritonavir–tenofovir nephrotoxicity may actually be a reflection of advanced disease in these patients, who have a higher risk of adverse events (Winston, 2006).

Tenofovir alafenamide fumarate (TAF) is a prodrug of TDF and has demonstrated potent anti-HIV-1 activity and higher intracellular tenofovir levels compared with TDF while maintaining lower plasma tenofovir exposure at 40 mg with good tolerability (Markowitz, 2014). Tenofovir released from TDF undergoes active renal secretion via organic anion transporters (OAT1 and OAT3), leading to higher exposure of renal proximal tubules to tenofovir and a potential for renal adverse effects. Unlike tenofovir DF, TAF does not interact with renal transporters OAT1 and OAT3 and therefore is expected to have a better renal safety profile (Bam, 2014). In a recent randomized controlled trial of HIV-1-infected patients who had achieved virologic suppression (viral load <50 ml/min) on a TDF-based regimen with a GFR ≥50 ml/min, patients were randomly assigned to continue the same ART or were switched to a TAF-based regimen (in combination with elvitegravir, cobicistat, and emtricitabine). The TAF-containing regimen led to continued viral suppression with improvement in bone mineral density and renal function, making this drug an attractive option for many patients (Mills, 2016).

Based on current knowledge of TDF toxicities, biannual monitoring of serum creatinine, serum phosphate, urine glucose, and proteinuria for patients on tenofovir with GFR <90 ml/min is recommended by the Infectious Disease Society of America (Gupta, 2005). Others advocate periodic monitoring of these markers in all patients on tenofovir regardless of GFR (Fine, 2013). In those with low serum phosphate, fractional excretion of phosphate in the urine can be used to confirm decreased tubular reabsorption of phosphate (Kinai, 2005).

Although renal toxicity of TDF is mostly reversible with the cessation of this drug, patients often do not achieve their pre-TDF creatinine clearance levels (Waheed, 2015; Wever, 2010). Therefore, clinicians should be vigilant regarding monitoring patients for the renal toxicity of TDF, with early change in regimen when toxicity is identified.

PROTEASE INHIBITORS

Indinavir, ritonavir, and atazanavir are protease inhibitors (PIs) that have been used in HIV patients and can commonly induce nephrolithiasis. This was most frequently seen with indinavir but has also been observed with other PIs (Huynh, 2011; Rockwood, 2011). Indinavir is used infrequently in the current era so that its toxicity has become of historical importance.

Several studies have suggested possible nephrotoxicity associated with atazanavir use. The largest included 22,603 D:A:D cohort participants with normal baseline kidney function (eGFR >90 ml/min). The decline in eGFR by >20 ml/min to <70 ml/min was associated with the use of not only tenofovir but also ritonavir-boosted atazanavir. An earlier study of the EuroSIDA cohort (a subset of the D:A:D cohort) demonstrated similar results in a smaller population ($N = 6843$) (Mocroft, 2010). In a study of a large Veterans Health Administration population, Sherzer et al. (2011) showed an association between atazanavir use and rapid GFR decline. A plausible mechanism for this potential toxicity may be related to the predilection for atazanavir to crystallize. The formation of kidney stones with atazanavir use is well described (Chan-Tack, 2007). In a Japanese study, the use of ritonavir-boosted atazanavir was shown to be associated with a higher incidence of renal stones; however, the composition of these stones was not analyzed (Hamada, 2012). In patients developing kidney stones on atazanavir, drug discontinuation is recommended if atazanavir content is confirmed or if stone analysis cannot be performed. With an increasing number of studies showing an association of nephrotoxicity with use of boosted atazanavir, it is advisable to monitor renal function in atazanavir-treated patients. If a decline in GFR is observed, switching to an alternate agent should be considered (Fine, 2013).

INTEGRASE INHIBITORS

Several antiretrovirals are now coadministered with cobicistat, a cytochrome P450 inhibitor. This allows once-daily dosing of these drugs (Johnson, 2014). Although cobicistat has no inherent nephrotoxicity, it inhibits MATE1 (multidrug and toxin extrusion protein-efflux) at the apical membrane of the proximal tubular cells, which blocks tubular secretion of creatinine (Figure 42.1) (Lepist, 2011). This leads to an increase in plasma creatinine concentration without any effect on the actual GFR. This was evaluated in a study of 36 patients in which cobicistat use was associated with an increase in serum creatinine and an approximately 10 ml/min decrease in eGFR, but the decrease in eGFR was reversible upon discontinuation of the medication, highlighting that this drug has no adverse effect on the actual GFR (German, 2010). The timing of the increase in creatinine and subsequent resolution after discontinuation of cobicistat was consistent with altered proximal tubular creatinine secretion. A phase III study comparing elvitegravir/cobicistat/emtricitabine/TDF to emtricitabine/TDF/efavirenz showed that the increase in serum creatinine was significantly higher in the first group (Sax, 2012).

Similarly, dolutegravir (an integrase inhibitor) inhibits the tubular secretion of creatinine through the organic cation transporter (OCT) at the basolateral membrane of the proximal tubular cells, raising plasma creatinine concentration without affecting the actual GFR (Rathbun, 2014). The rise in creatinine is typically seen in the first week and then stabilizes thereafter (Stellbrink, 2013). With both cobicistat and dolutegravir, an increase in creatinine should be monitored. If the rise in creatinine is small and stable, then no further assessment is needed. Because cobicistat is combined with TDF, a known nephrotoxin, it is especially important to confirm a stable level of serum creatinine with its use.

DOSE ADJUSTMENT IN RENAL INSUFFICIENCY

Most non-nucleoside reverse transcriptase inhibitors, integrase inhibitors, and protease inhibitors can be used safely and do not require dose modification in CKD or ESRD. Although TDF should generally be avoided in those with a creatinine clearance level <50 ml/min or stopped in those with declining eGFR, there may be instances in which other options are not available and dose adjustment has to be made. Any drug containing TDF will need dose adjustment at creatinine clearance <50 ml/min. The future availability of TAF may make this less of an issue. Combination drugs may require separation of the component drugs for dosing (Kalyesubula, 2011).

In summary, renal abnormalities can develop in patients on various ART regimens and cannot always be attributed to a single drug. Renal function should be monitored on a

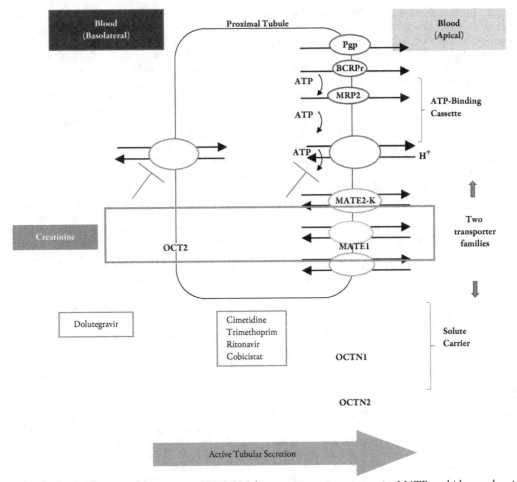

Figure 42.1 Model for effect of tested drugs on creatinine secretion. BCRP, breast cancer resistance protein; MATE, multidrug and toxin extrusion protein; MRP, multidrug resistance protein; OCT, organic cation transporter; OCTN, organic cation/ergothioneine transporter; Pgp, P-glycoprotein. SOURCE: From Lepist I, et al., ICAAC 2011, Chicago. Poster A1-1724.

regular basis in HIV patients receiving ART. Appropriate dose adjustments or changes in therapy should be made based on observed changes in serum creatinine or GFR.

Recommended Reading

Atta, M. G., Deray, G., Lucas, G. M. Antiretroviral nephrotoxicities. *Semin Nephrol.* 2008; 28(6):563–575.

Fine, D. M., Gallant, J. E. Nephrotoxicity of antiretroviral agents: Is the list getting longer? *J Infect Dis.* 2013; 207(9):1349–1351.

Kalyesubula, R., Perazella, M. A. Nephrotoxicity of HAART. *AIDS Res Treat.* 2011; 2011:562790.

References

Atta, M. G., Fine, D. M., Kirk, G. D., et al. Survival during renal replacement therapy among African Americans infected with HIV type 1 in urban Baltimore, Maryland. *Clin Infect Dis.* 2007; 45(12):1625–1632.

Atta, M. G., Lucas, G. M., Fine, D. M. HIV-associated nephropathy: Epidemiology, pathogenesis, diagnosis and management. *Expert Rev Anti Infect Ther.* 2008; 6(3):365–371.

Bachmeyer, C., Blanche, P., Sereni, D., et al. Thrombotic thrombocytopenic purpura and haemolytic uraemic syndrome in HIV-infected patients. *AIDS (London).* 1995; 9(5):532–533.

Balow, J. E. Nephropathy in the context of HIV infection. *Kidney Int.* 2005; 67(4):1632–1633.

Bam, R. A., Birkus, G., Babusis, D., et al. Metabolism and antiretroviral activity of tenofovir alafenamide in CD4+ T-cells and macrophages from demographically diverse donors. *Antivir Ther.* 2014; 19(7):669–677.

Barisoni, L., Kriz, W., Mundel, P., et al. The dysregulated podocyte phenotype: A novel concept in the pathogenesis of collapsing idiopathic focal segmental glomerulosclerosis and HIV-associated nephropathy. *J Am Soc Nephrol.* 1999; 10(1):51–61.

Becker, S., Fusco, G., Fusco, J., et al. HIV-associated thrombotic microangiopathy in the era of highly active antiretroviral therapy: An observational study. *Clin Infect Dis.* 2004; 39(Suppl 5):S267–S275.

Berliner, A. R., Fine, D. M., Lucas, G. M., et al. Observations on a cohort of HIV-infected patients undergoing native renal biopsy. *Am J Nephrol.* 2008; 28(3):478–486.

Bhasin, B., Lau, B., Atta, M. G., et al. Viremia and T-cell activation differentially affect the performance of glomerular filtration rate equations based on creatinine and cystatin C. *PloS One.* 2013; 8(12):e82028.

Bige, N., Lanternier, F., Viard, J. P., et al. Presentation of HIV-associated nephropathy and outcome in HAART-treated patients. *Nephrol Dial Transplant.* 2012; 27(3):1114–1121.

Briggs, W. A., Tanawattanacharoen, S., Choi, M. J., et al. Clinicopathologic correlates of prednisone treatment of human immunodeficiency virus-associated nephropathy. *Am J Kidney Dis.* 1996; 28(4):618–621.

Bruggeman, L. A., Dikman, S., Meng, C., et al. Nephropathy in human immunodeficiency virus-1 transgenic mice is due to renal transgene expression. *J Clin Invest.* 1997; 100(1):84–92.

Casas, J. P., Chua, W., Loukogeorgakis, S., et al. Effect of inhibitors of the renin–angiotensin system and other antihypertensive drugs on renal outcomes: Systematic review and meta-analysis. *Lancet.* 2005; 366(9502):2026–2033.

Chan-Tack, K. M., Truffa, M. M., Struble, K. A., et al. Atazanavir-associated nephrolithiasis: cases from the US Food and Drug Administration's Adverse Event Reporting System. *AIDS.* 2007 May 31; 21(9):1215–1218.

Cheng, K., Rai, P., Plagov, A., et al. MicroRNAs in HIV-associated nephropathy (HIVAN). *Exp Mol Pathol.* 2013; 94(1):65–72.

Choi, A., Scherzer, R., Bacchetti, P., et al. Cystatin C, albuminuria, and 5-year all-cause mortality in HIV-infected persons. *Am J Kidney Dis.* 2010; 56(5):872–882.

Choi, A. I., Rodriguez, R. A., Bacchetti, P., et al. The impact of HIV on chronic kidney disease outcomes. *Kidney Int.* 2007; 72(11):1380–1387.

Cohen, S. D., Kimmel, P. L. Renal biopsy is necessary for the diagnosis of HIV-associated renal diseases. *Nat Clin Pract Nephrol.* 2009; 5(1):22–23.

D'Agati, V., Suh, J., Carbone, L., et al. Pathology of HIV-associated nephropathy: A detailed morphologic and comparative study. *Kidney Int.* 1989; 35(6):1358–1370.

Elewa, U., Sandri, A. M., Rizza, S. A., et al. Treatment of HIV-associated nephropathies. *Nephron Clin Pract.* 2011; 118(4):c346–c354.

Eustace, J. A., Nuermberger, E., Choi, M., et al. Cohort study of the treatment of severe HIV-associated nephropathy with corticosteroids. *Kidney Int.* 2000; 58(3):1253–1260.

Fine, D. M., Gallant, J. E. Nephrotoxicity of antiretroviral agents: Is the list getting longer? *J Infect Dis.* 2013; 207(9):1349–1351.

Fine, D. M., Perazella, M. A., Lucas, G. M., et al. Kidney biopsy in HIV: Beyond HIV-associated nephropathy. *Am J Kidney Dis.* 2008; 51(3):504–514.

Foy, M. C., Estrella, M. M., Lucas, F., et al. Comparison of risk factors and outcomes in HIV immune complex kidney disease and HIV-associated nephropathy. *Clin J Am Soc Nephrol.* 2013; 8(9):1524–1532.

Franceschini, N., Napravnik, S., Eron, J., Jr., et al. Incidence and etiology of acute renal failure among ambulatory HIV-infected patients. *Kidney Int.* 2005; 67(4):1526–1531.

Frassetto, L. A., Tan-Tam, C., Stock, P. Renal transplantation in patients with HIV. *Nat Rev Nephrol.* 2009; 5(10):582–589.

Gallant, J. E., DeJesus, E., Arribas, J. R., et al. Tenofovir DF, emtricitabine, and efavirenz vs zidovudine, lamivudine, and efavirenz for HIV. *N Eng J Med.* 2006; 354:251–260.

Gallant, J. E., Parish, M. A., Keruly, J. C., et al. Changes in renal function associated with tenofovir disoproxil fumarate treatment, compared with nucleoside reverse-transcriptase inhibitor treatment. *Clin Infect Dis.* 2005; 40:1194–1198.

Gaspar, G., Monereo, A., Garcia-Reyne, A., et al. Fanconi syndrome and acute renal failure in a patient treated with tenofovir: a call for caution. *AIDS.* 2004; 18:351–352.

Genovese, G., Friedman, D. J., Ross, M. D., et al. Association of trypanolytic ApoL1 variants with kidney disease in African Americans. *Science.* 2010; 329(5993):841–845.

George, E., Lucas, G. M., Nadkarni, G. N., et al. Kidney function and the risk of cardiovascular events in HIV-1-infected patients. *AIDS (London).* 2010; 24(3):387–394.

German, P., Warren, D., West, S., et al. Pharmacokinetics and bioavailability of an integrase and novel pharmacoenhancer-containing single-tablet fixed-dose combination regimen for the treatment of HIV. *J Acquir Immune Defic Syndr.* 2010 Nov; 55(3):323–329.

Gitman, M.D., Hirschwerk, D., Baskin, C.H., et al. Tenofovir-induced kidney injury. *Expert Opin Drug Saf.* 2007 Mar; 6(2):155–164.

Hamada, Y., Nishijima, T., Watanabe, K., et al. High incidence of renal stones among HIV-infected patients on ritonavir-boosted atazanavir than in those receiving other protease inhibitor-containing antiretroviral therapy. *Clin Infect Dis.* 2012 Nov; 55(9):1262–1269.

Huynh, J., Hever, A., Tom, T., et al. Indinavir-induced nephrolithiasis three and one-half years after cessation of indinavir therapy. *Int Urol Nephrol.* 2011 Jun; 43(2):571–573.

Izzedine, H., Acharya, V., Wirden, M., et al. Role of HIV-1 DNA levels as clinical marker of HIV-1-associated nephropathies. *Nephrol Dial Transplant.* 2011; 26(2):580–583.

Jafar, T. H., Stark, P. C., Schmid, H., et al. Progression of chronic kidney disease: The role of blood pressure control, proteinuria, and angiotensin-converting enzyme inhibition: A patient-level meta-analysis. *Ann Intern Med.* 2003; 139(4):244–252.

Kalayjian, R. C. Renal issues in HIV infection. *Curr HIV AIDS Rep.* 2011; 8(3):164–171.

Kalyesubula, R., Perazella, M. A. Nephrotoxicity of HAART. *AIDS Res Treat.* 2011; 2011:562790.

Kalim, S., Szczech, L. A., Wyatt, C. M. Acute kidney injury in HIV-infected patients. *Semin Nephrol.* 2008; 28(6):556–562.

Karras, A., Lafaurie, M., Furco, A., et al. Tenofovir-related nephrotoxicity in human immunodeficiency virus-infected patients: three cases of renal failure, Fanconi syndrome, and nephrogenic diabetes insipidus. *Clin Infect Dis.* 2003; 36:1070–1073.

Kimmel, P. L. HIV-associated nephropathy: Virologic issues related to renal sclerosis. *Nephrol Dial Transplant.* 2003; 18(Suppl 6):vi59–vi63.

Kimmel, P. L., Mishkin, G. J., Uman, W. O. Captopril and renal survival in patients with human immunodeficiency virus nephropathy. *Am J Kidney Dis.* 1996; 28(2):202–208.

Kimmel, P. L., Umana, W. O., Simmens, S., et al. Continuous ambulatory peritoneal dialysis and survival of HIV-infected patients with end-stage renal disease. *Kidney Int.* 1993; 44(2):373–378.

Kinai, E., Hanabusa, H. Renal tubular toxicity associated with tenofovir assessed using urine-beta 2 microglobulin, percentage of tubular reabsorption of phosphate and alkaline phosphatase levels. *AIDS.* 2005 Nov 18; 19(17):2031–2033.

Ko, W. Y., Pajan, P., Gomez, F., et al. Identifying Darwinian selection acting on different human APOL1 variants among diverse African populations. *Am J Hum Genet.* 2013; 93(1):54–66.

Kopp, J. B., Nelson, G. W., Sampath, K., et al. Genetic variants in focal segmental glomerulosclerosis and HIV-associated nephropathy. *J Am Soc Nephrol.* 2011; 22(11):2129–2137.

Korgaonkar, S. N., Feng, X., Ross, M. D. HIV-1 upregulates VEGF in podocytes. *J Am Soc Nephrol.* 2008; 19(5):877–883.

Lepist, E. I., Murray, B. P., Tong, L., et al. Effect of cobicistat and ritonavir on proximal renal tubular cell uptake and efflux transporters. 51st Interscience Conference on Antimicrobial Agents and Chemotherapy (ICAAC). September 17–20, 2011. Chicago. Abstract A1-1724.

Lepist, E. I., Murray, B. P., Tong, L., et al. Effect of cobicistat and ritonavir on proximal renal tubular cell uptake and efflux transporters. 51st Interscience Conference on Antimicrobial Agents and Chemotherapy (ICAAC). September 17–20, 2011. Chicago. Abstract A1-1724.

Lescure, F. X., Flateau, C., Pacanowski, J., et al. HIV-associated kidney glomerular diseases: Changes with time and HAART. *Nephrol Dial Transplant.* 2012; 27:2349–2355.

Locke, J. E., James, N. T., Mannon, R. B., et al. Immunosuppression regimen and the risk of acute rejection in HIV-infected kidney transplant recipients. *Transplantation.* 2014; 97(4):446–450.

Longenecker, C. T., Scherzer, R., Bacchetti, P., et al. HIV viremia and changes in kidney function. *AIDS (London).* 2009; 23(9):1089–1096.

Lucas, G. M., Eustace, J. A., Sozio, S., et al. Highly active antiretroviral therapy and the incidence of HIV-1-associated nephropathy: A 12-year cohort study. *AIDS (London).* 2004; 18(3):541–546.

Lucas, G.M., Lau, B., Atta, M. G., et al. Chronic kidney disease incidence, and progression to end-stage renal disease, in HIV-infected individuals: A tale of two races. *J Infect Dis.* 2008; 197(11):1548–1557.

Lucas, G. M., Mehta, S. H., Atta, M. G., et al. End-stage renal disease and chronic kidney disease in a cohort of African-American HIV-infected and at-risk HIV-seronegative participants followed between 1988 and 2004. *AIDS (London).* 2007; 21(18):2435–2443.

Markowitz, M., Zolopa, A., Squires, K., et al. Phase I/II study of the pharmacokinetics, safety and antiretroviral activity of tenofovir alafenamide, a new prodrug of the HIV reverse transcriptase inhibitor tenofovir, in HIV-infected adults. *J Antimicrob Chemother.* 2014 May; 69(5):1362–1369.

Mauss, S., Berger, F., Kuschak, D., et al. Cystatin C as a marker of renal function is affected by HIV replication leading to an underestimation of kidney function in HIV patients. *Antiviral Ther.* 2008; 13(8):1091–1095.

Medapalli, R. K., He, J. C., Klotman, J. P. HIV-associated nephropathy: Pathogenesis. *Curr Opin Nephrol Hypertens.* 2011; 20(3):306–311.

Mills, A., Arribas, J. R., Andrade-Villanueva, J., et al. Switching from tenofovir disoproxil fumarate to tenofovir alafenamide in antiretroviral regimens for virologically suppressed adults with HIV-1 infection: a randomised, active-controlled, multicentre, open-label, phase 3, non-inferiority study. *Lancet Infect Dis.* 2016 Jan; 16(1):43–52.

Mocroft A., Kirk, O., Reiss, P., et al. Estimated glomerular filtration rate, chronic kidney disease and antiretroviral drug use in HIV-positive patients. *AIDS (London).* 2010; 24(11):1667–1678.

Mocroft, A., Ledergerber, B., Katlama, C., et al.; EUROSIDA Study Group. Decline in the AIDS and death rates in the EUROSIDA study: An observational study. *Lancet.* 2003; 362(9377):22–29.

Mocroft, A., Lundgren, J. D., Ross, M., et al.; D:A:D Study Group Royal Free Hospital Clinic Cohort, Insight Study Group, Smart Study Group and Espirit Study Group. Development and validation of a risk score for chronic kidney disease in HIV infection using protective cohort data from the D:A:D study. *PLoS Med.* 2015; 12(3):e1001809.

Naicker, S., Fabian, J. Risk factors for the development of chronic kidney disease with HIV/AIDS. *Clin Nephrol.* 2010; 74(Suppl 1):S51–S56.

Papeta, N., Kiryluk, K., Patel, A., et al. APOL1 variants increase risk for FSGS and HIVAN but not IgA nephropathy. *J Am Soc Nephrol.* 2011; 22(11):1991–1996.

Peters, P. J., Moore, D. M., Mermin, J., et al. Antiretroviral therapy improves renal function among HIV-infected Ugandans. *Kidney Int.* 2008; 74(7):925–929.

Post, F. A., Holt, S. G. Recent developments in HIV and the kidney. *Curr Opin Infect Dis.* 2009; 22(1):43–48.

Qiu, J., Terasaki, P. I., Waki, J., et al. HIV-positive renal recipients can achieve survival rates similar to those of HIV-negative patients. *Transplantation.* 2006; 81(12):1658–1661.

Rao, T. K., Filippone, E. J., Nicastri, A. D., et al. Associated focal and segmental glomerulosclerosis in the acquired immunodeficiency syndrome. *N Engl J Med.* 1984; 310(11):669–673.

Ratnam, K. K., Feng, W., Chuang, P. Y., et al. Role of the retinoic acid receptor-alpha in HIV-associated nephropathy. *Kidney Int.* 2011; 79(6):624–634.

Rathbun, R.C., Lockhart, S. M., Miller, M. M., et al. Dolutegravir, a second-generation integrase inhibitor for the treatment of HIV-1 infection. *Ann Pharmacother.* 2014 Mar; 48(3):395–403.

Ray, A. S., Cihlar, T., Robinson, K. L., et al. Mechanism of active tubular secretion of tenofovir and potential for a renal drug-drug interaction with HIV protease inhibitors. In: Program and abstracts from the 7th Workshop on Clinical Pharmacology on HIV Therapy; Lisbon, Portugal. April 20–22, 2006; Abstract 39.

Reid, A., Stohr, W., Walker, A. S., et al. Severe renal dysfunction and risk factors associated with renal impairment in HIV-infected adults in Africa initiating antiretroviral therapy. *Clin Infect Dis.* 2008; 46(8):1271–1281.

Rockwood, N., Mandalia, S., Bower, M., et al. Ritonavir-boosted atazanavir exposure is associated with an increased rate of renal stones compared with efavirenz, ritonavir-boosted lopinavir and ritonavir-boosted darunavir. *AIDS.* 2011 Aug 24; 25(13):1671–1673.

Roland, M.E., Barin, B., Carlson, M. L., et al. HIV-infected liver and kidney transplant recipients: 1- and 3-year outcomes. *Am J Transplant.* 2008; 8(2):355–365.

Rollot, F., Nazal, E. M., Chauvelot-Moachon, L., et al. Tenofovir-related Fanconi syndrome with nephrogenic diabetes insipidus in a patient with acquired immunodeficiency syndrome: the role of lopinavir-ritonavir-didanosine. *Clin Infect Dis.* 2003; 37:3174e–3176.

Ross, M. J., Klotman, P. E. Recent progress in HIV-associated nephropathy. *J Am Soc Nephrol.* 2002; 13(12):2997–3004.

Sax, P. E., DeJesus, E., Mills, A., et al. Co-formulated elvitegravir, cobicistat, emtricitabine, and tenofovir versus co-formulated efavirenz, emtricitabine, and tenofovir for initial treatment of HIV-1 infection: a randomised, double-blind, phase 3 trial, analysis of results after 48 weeks. *Lancet.* 2012 Jun 30; 379(9835):2439–2448.

Sax, P. E., Tierney, C., Collier, A. C., et al. Abacavir/lamivudine versus tenofovir DF/emtricitabine as part of combination regimens for initial treatment of HIV: final results. *J Infect Dis.* 2011 Oct 15; 204(8):1191–1201.

Scherzer, R., Estrella, M., Li, Y., et al. Association of tenofovir exposure with kidney disease risk in HIV infection. *AIDS.* 2012 Apr 24; 26(7):867–875.

Smith, K.Y., Patel, P., Fine, D., et al. Randomized, double-blind, placebo-matched, multicenter trial of abacavir/lamivudine or tenofovir/emtricitabine with lopinavir/ritonavir for initial HIV treatment. *AIDS.* 2009 Jul 31; 23(12):1547–1556.

Stellbrink, H. J., Reynes, J., Lazzarin, A., et al. Dolutegravir in antiretroviral-naive adults with HIV-1: 96-week results from a randomized dose-ranging study. *AIDS.* 2013 Jul 17; 27(11):1771–1778.

Stock, P. G., Barin, B., Murphy, B., et al. Outcomes of kidney transplantation in HIV-infected recipients. *N Engl J Med.* 2010; 363(21):2004–2014.

Stock, P. G., Roland, M. E., Carlson, L., et al. Kidney and liver transplantation in human immunodeficiency virus-infected patients: A pilot safety and efficacy study. *Transplantation.* 2003; 76(2): 370–375.

Strategies for Management of Antiretroviral Therapy (SMART) Study Group. CD4+ count-guided interruption of antiretroviral treatment. *N Engl J Med.* 2006; 355(22):2283–2296.

Tzur, S., Rosset, S., Shemer, R., et al. Missense mutations in the APOL1 gene are highly associated with end stage kidney disease risk previously attributed to the MYH9 gene. *Hum Genet.* 2010; 128(3):345–350.

Van Maarseveen, E. M., Rogers, C. C., Trofe-Clark, J., et al. Drug–drug interactions between antiretroviral and immunosuppressive agents in HIV-infected patients after solid organ transplantation: A review. *AIDS Patient Care STDs.* 2012; 26(10):568–581.

Waheed, S., Atta, M. G. Predictors of HIV-associated nephropathy. *Expert Rev Anti-Infect Ther.* 2014; 12(5):555–563.

Waheed, S., Sakr, A., Chheda, N., et al. Outcomes of renal transplantation in HIV-1 associated nephropathy. *PLoS One.* 2015; 10(6):e0129702.

Wei, A., Burns, G., Williams, C. M., et al. Long-term renal survival in HIV-associated nephropathy with angiotensin-converting enzyme inhibition. *Kidney Int.* 2003; 64(4):1462–1471.

Wever, K., van Agtmael, M. A., Carr, A. Incomplete reversibility of tenofovir-related renal toxicity in HIV-infected men. *J Acquir Immune Defic Syndr.* 2010 Sep; 55(1):78–81.

Winston, A., Amin, J., Mallon, P. W. G., et al. Minor changes in calculated creatinine clearance and anion-gap are associated with tenofovir disoproxil fumarate-containing highly active antiretroviral therapy. *HIV Med.* 2006;7:105–111.

Wyatt, C. M., Arons, R. R., Klotman, P. E., et al. Acute renal failure in hospitalized patients with HIV: Risk factors and impact on in-hospital mortality. *AIDS (London).* 2006; 20(4):561–565.

Wyatt, C. M., Hoover, D. R., Shi, Q., et al. Pre-existing albuminuria predicts AIDS and non-AIDS mortality in women initiating antiretroviral therapy. *Antiviral Ther.* 2011; 16(4):591–596.

Zhong, Y., Wu, Y., Liu, R., et al. Roflumilast enhances the renal protective effects of retinoids in an HIV-1 transgenic mouse model of rapidly progressive renal failure. *Kidney Int.* 2012; 81(9):856–864.

Zuo, Y., Matsusaka, T., Zhong, J., et al. HIV-1 genes Vpr and Nef synergistically damage podocytes, leading to glomerulosclerosis. *J Am Soc Nephrol.* 2006; 17(10):2832–2843.

43.

MUSCULOSKELETAL COMPLICATIONS OF HIV

Tanvir K. Bell

CHAPTER GOAL

This chapter discusses concepts of vitamin D deficiency in HIV-infected patients; risk factors and contributors to osteopenia and osteoporosis in HIV-infected patients; and treatment options for vitamin D deficiency, osteopenia, and osteoporosis.

LEARNING OBJECTIVES

- Discuss concepts of Vitamin D deficiency in HIV-infected patients.

- Demonstrate knowledge of the risk factors and contributors to osteopenia and osteoporosis in HIV-infected patients.

- Discuss treatment options for Vitamin D deficiency, osteopenia and osteoporosis.

VITAMIN D DEFICIENCY AND EFFECTS OF VITAMIN D

WHAT'S NEW?

- Consider checking 25-hydroxyvitamin D levels in patients with osteoporosis and patients on antiretroviral therapy (ART).

- Administration of vitamin D and calcium supplementation in patients on efavirenz, emtricitabine, and tenofovir leads to decreased bone loss.

KEY POINT

Vitamin D levels can be reduced by antiretrovirals, especially efavirenz.

Vitamin D helps set up the matrix for bone. Vitamin D levels have been observed to be low in HIV-infected patients. Vitamin D deficiency can lead to osteomalacia and rickets. Vitamin D appears to play a role in cell death and survival, which is termed autophagy; autophagy is also involved in killing intracellular organisms. Vitamin D may also play a role in autoimmune disease, cancer, cardiovascular disease, and diabetes (Spector, 2011). Vitamin D deficiency is common in both developing and developed countries. Recommendations for screening for vitamin D levels are controversial. The Endocrine Society recommends checking vitamin D levels of people who take AIDS medications (Holick, 2011).

The metabolite of vitamin D that is recommended to be measured in blood tests is 25-hydroxyvitamin D (D_2). HIV patients frequently have low vitamin D levels (Dao, 2011). Vitamin D_2 is converted to 1,25-dihydroxyvitamin D (D_3), the active form of vitamin D, in the kidneys. Sunlight assists in the process of conversion to the active form of vitamin D. Natural foods, including oily fish and egg yolks, and vitamin supplements can augment levels of D_2 or D_3. Lab tests of 25-hydroxyvitamin D should be checked to determine vitamin D levels for patients. A value less than 30 mg/ml is considered to be low (Holick, 2011).

Antiretroviral agents may influence vitamin D levels when patients are started on therapy. There is consistent evidence that efavirenz may lower vitamin D levels (Conesa-Botella, 2010; Gyllensten, 2006). The mechanism for vitamin D deficiency is inhibition of the enzymes involved in vitamin D metabolism. This is not a class effect of the non-nucleoside reverse transcriptase inhibitors; some studies have also shown that protease inhibitors lower vitamin D levels. Tenofovir disoproxil fumarate (TDF) has been associated with renal calcium and phosphate loss and higher parathyroid hormone levels. Vitamin D supplementation in adolescents with or without vitamin D deficiency at baseline led to lower levels of parathyroid hormone (Havens, 2012).

A multicenter study by the AIDS Clinical Trials Group showed that supplementation with vitamin D and calcium led to less decline in total hip and lumbar spine bone mineral density (BMD) at 48 weeks in subjects who initiated efavirenz/emtricitabine/TDF (Overton, 2015). Switching subjects from efavirenz to boosted darunavir is another strategy that has led to increased vitamin D level (Fox, 2013).

TREATMENT OF VITAMIN D DEFICIENCY

It is now common to check vitamin D levels in general medicine practice and for HIV-infected patients. Current recommended allowances for vitamin D are 600 IU for persons aged 1–70 years and 800 IU for individuals older than 70 years (Spector, 2011). If replacement of low vitamin D is warranted, initial supplementation is done with 50,000 IU of vitamin D_2 or D_3 once weekly for 8 weeks or 600 IU of vitamin D_2 or D_3 daily to achieve blood levels >30 ng/ml. This should be followed by a maintenance dosage of 1500–2000 IU/day (Holick, 2011).

Recommended Reading

McComsey GA, Tebas P, Shane E, et al. Bone disease in HIV infection: A practical review and recommendations for HIV care providers. *Clin Infect Dis.* 2010; 51(8):937–946.
Spector SA. Vitamin D and HIV: Letting the sun shine in. *Top Antivir Med.* 2011; 19(1): 6–10.

OSTEOPENIA, OSTEOPOROSIS, AND FRACTURES

WHAT'S NEW?

- The FRAX calculator should be used to determine if treatment should be initiated in HIV-infected men aged 40–49 years and HIV-infected women aged 40 years or older.

- Raltegravir has been shown to cause less BMD loss when initiating therapy compared to ritonavir-boosted atazanavir or darunavir.

- Lower baseline CD4+ cell count can lead to greater BMD loss after starting ART.

KEY POINTS

- HIV-infected patients may be at higher risk for osteopenia, osteoporosis, and fragility fractures.

- Modifiable risk factors for osteoporosis include smoking and sedentary lifestyle.

- Tenofovir and protease inhibitors may cause increased bone loss.

- Bone loss in HIV-infected patients is greatest during the first 2 years of initiation of ART (2–6%).

- Consider performing a dual-energy X-ray absorptiometry (DXA) scan in HIV-infected men older than age 50 years and postmenopausal women with a history of nontraumatic fractures.

- Postmenopausal HIV-infected women have greater BMD loss compared to HIV-uninfected postmenopausal women.

- Treatment with bisphosphonates should be considered in patients with a *T* score less than –2.5, fragility fracture, or FRAX score ≥20% and/or ≥3% for the hip.

- Tenofovir alafenamide has been shown to produce less bone loss compared to TDF.

Low BMD occurs in HIV-infected patients. Many factors contribute to osteopenia, including HIV, host characteristics, and ART. Osteopenia and osteoporosis may cause morbidity in patients with fragility fractures. As the HIV-infected population ages, osteopenia and osteoporosis have become more prevalent, and fractures have been observed more often in HIV-infected patients.

RISK FACTORS FOR BONE LOSS

Compared to controls, HIV-infected patients have a 3.7 times higher unadjusted odds ratio for osteoporosis (Brown, 2006). HIV-infected postmenopausal women have greater bone loss compared to HIV-uninfected women. In a longitudinal study of postmenopausal women, HIV-infected women had more than twofold higher rates of annualized bone loss at the lumbar spine and radius. Lower body mass index and TDF were associated with more bone loss as well (Yin, 2012). Some data on bone mineral density in HIV-infected patients may be confounded by low weight in HIV-infected patients.

Contributing factors to low BMD in HIV-infected patients are complex. Factors that dispose to osteoporosis which are pertinent to HIV patients include sedentary lifestyle, Caucasian or Asian race, steroid therapy, hepatitis C co-infection, and smoking. Drug use also contributed to bone loss in cohorts of HIV patients receiving outpatient therapy (Young, 2011). Bone loss occurs from the effects of HIV on bone metabolism and cytokine activation. Antiretrovirals can also directly affect bone cells. HIV influences bone formation through upregulating the process of bone resorption and bone formation.

Effects of Antiretroviral Drugs

The overall incidence of BMD loss with antiretroviral initiation is approximately 2–6% during the first 1 or 2 years. Starting ART at higher CD4+ cell counts, as is currently advocated by HIV treatment guidelines, may have beneficial effects on bone health. Pooled analysis of three trials starting therapy in antiretroviral treatment-naive patients showed that subjects with a CD4+ count <50 cells/mm³ had more bone loss compared to those with CD4+ count >500 cells/mm³. Multivariate analysis of this cohort found that older age, female sex, lower body mass index, and higher viral loads were associated with greater BMD decline when subjects were followed for 96 weeks after treatment initiation (Grant, 2013). Bone loss seems to stabilize after the first 2½ years on ART (Bolland, 2011).

The impact of ART on BMD has received increased scrutiny during the past decade. For example, in one study, use of TDF in macaques resulted in decreased bone density and osteomalacia. Tenofovir can cause defects in the matrix of bone by urinary calcium and phosphate wasting through proximal tubule dysfunction. Tenofovir may also influence the role of osteoclasts and osteoblasts (Grisby, 2010). The ACTG 5224 trial, a substudy of ACTG A5202, showed a greater decrease in bone density in the spine and the hip with TDF/emtricitabine versus abacavir/lamivudine (McComsey, 2011). Given the approval of TDF/emtricitabine for pre-exposure prophylaxis, bone effects of this medication in HIV-uninfected patients are a concern. Bone mineral density in the hip and spine decreased modestly after 24 weeks in a study of young men in San Francisco with the average age of 28 years. It did not decrease further after that time, and it reversed when the drug was stopped (Mulligan, 2015). Tenofovir alafenamide, a tenofovir prodrug that leads to decreased plasma tenofovir levels, has been shown to lead to significantly less bone mineral density loss at the hip and spine compared to TDF in antiretroviral treatment-naive patients (Sax, 2015). A single-tablet regimen of emtricitabine/tenofovir alafenamide/elvitegravir/cobicistat (Genvoya) was approved in the United States in November 2015.

Protease inhibitor use and low bone mineral density have been evaluated, with some studies showing a possible relationship (Tebas, 2000). Patients who underwent antiretroviral treatment and protease inhibitor treatment were more likely to have low BMD and osteoporosis compared to controls (Brown, 2006). Efavirenz was shown to lead to less bone loss in the spine compared to ritonavir-boosted atazanavir (McComsey, 2011). Integrase inhibitors may lead to less bone loss compared to protease inhibitors. In HIV antiretroviral treatment-naive patients, raltegravir versus ritonavir-boosted atazanavir or ritonavir-boosted darunavir led to less mean bone loss in the spine and hip (Brown, 2015). Data on bone effects of alternative integrase inhibitors such as dolutegravir and elvitegravir are limited.

PREVALENCE OF LOWER BONE MINERAL DENSITY IN HIV-INFECTED PATIENTS AND FRACTURES AS A CONSEQUENCE OF BONE LOSS

Fractures are observed in HIV-infected patients at higher rates than observed in HIV-uninfected individuals. Fragility fracture is a clinical manifestation of osteoporosis and is defined as a fracture from a fall from standing height or less. It usually occurs in the vertebrae, hips, or wrist. Among veterans and postmenopausal women, increased fractures occur in HIV-infected patients compared to HIV-uninfected patients. Compared to outpatients in the National Hospital Ambulatory Medical Care Survey, patients aged 25–54 years in the HIV Outpatient Study (HOPS) cohort had higher fracture rates and relative proportion of fragility fractures. In addition to older age, substance abuse, nadir CD4+ cell count <200 cells/mm³, hepatitis C co-infection, and diabetes were associated with incident fractures (Young, 2011). The Veterans Aging Cohort Study Virtual Cohort (VACS-VC) found a higher risk of fragility fractures in HIV-infected male veterans compared to uninfected male veterans, but this difference was attenuated when the model was adjusted for body mass index (Womack, 2011).

EVALUATION FOR OSTEOPENIA AND OSTEOPOROSIS

The Osteo Renal Exchange Program recommends evaluating fracture risk for HIV-infected men aged 40–49 years and women aged 40 years or older using the Fracture Risk Assessment Tool (FRAX) calculator, which is accessible on the Internet at http://www.shef.ac.uk/FRAX. (Brown, 2015). DXA scan to measure BMD is recommended in men aged 40–49 years or premenopausal women with a 10-year probability of fracture FRAX score >10%. If the 10-year risk of a major osteoporosis-related fracture on the calculator is ≥20% or a 10-year risk of hip fracture is ≥3%, in countries in which DXA scans are not available, patients should be treated for osteoporosis.

BMD is measured by DXA scan. Osteopenia and osteoporosis are defined based on T-score, which measures individual BMD by DXA and assesses the number of standard deviations compared to a young population average (30 years old), adjusted for gender and race. The World Health Organization (WHO) diagnostic criteria for categories of osteopenia and osteoporosis are listed in Table 43.1. A Z-score measures BMD compared with those of individuals of the same age, weight, ethnicity, and gender.

Table 43.1 WHO CLASSIFICATION OF BONE MINERAL DENSITY

CLASSIFICATION	*T* SCORE
Normal	Above –1
Osteopenia	Between –1 and –2.5
Osteoporosis	At or below –2.5
Severe osteoporosis	Osteoporosis with one or more fragility fractures

A *Z*-score is preferred for individuals younger than age 50 years, and a score of –2 or less is abnormal. Experts recommend DXA scans be done in HIV-infected men aged 50 years or older, postmenopausal women, patients on chronic glucocorticoid therapy, patients with a history of fragility fracture, and those with a high risk of falls. DXA should also be done in men aged 40–49 years and premenopausal women with a FRAX score >10% (Brown, 2015).

Many studies have evaluated markers of bone turnover and biomarkers and cytokines to better determine etiologies of bone loss. Markers of bone turnover include C-telopeptide, N-telopeptide, osteoprotegerin, and RANKL. Interleukin-6 and tumor necrosis factor-α are potent stimulators of osteoclast activity (Brown, 2006). Higher adiponectin, a hormone produced from adipocytes, and lower osteoprotegerin were associated in lower BMD in ART-naive HIV-infected individuals (Brown, 2013).

TREATMENT

In many trials, including an ACTG trial, alendronate has been demonstrated to be safe and effective for treatment of low BMD when diagnosed by DXA scan in patients with HIV infection (McComsey, 2007). Alendronate 70 mg weekly is usually used. Bisphosphonates are considered the first line of therapy.

Adverse effects of bisphosphonates include esophagitis. Bisphosphonates should be taken while sitting upright, without food and with water. A rare but debilitating consequence of bisphosphonate therapy is osteonecrosis of the jaw. Subtrochanteric fractures or atypical femoral shaft fractures can occur with long-term use. The optimal duration of therapy is uncertain. Benefit past 3 years of therapy is unclear. Further guidance may be available in the future. DXA scans should be followed up 1 or 2 years after initiating therapy.

If possible, underlying risks that contribute to osteoporosis should be modified. These include changing sedentary lifestyle, vitamin D level augmentation, and smoking cessation. Good bone health may be facilitated with adequate intake of vitamin D and calcium. Vitamin D levels may be checked and need to be supplemented. It is recommended that HIV-infected patients consume 1000–1500 mg of calcium per day. Increased weightbearing exercise, smoking cessation, and decreased alcohol consumption are also recommended (McComsey, 2010). Another strategy for augmenting bone health in patients with osteoporosis or bone fractures is switching antiretroviral drugs to raltegravir- or tenofovir alafenamide-containing regimens.

Recommended Reading

Brown TT, Hoy J, Borderi M, et al. Recommendations for evaluation and management of bone disease in HIV. *Clin Infect Dis.* 2015; 60(8):1242–1251.

McComsey GA, Tebas P, Shane E, et al. Bone disease in HIV infection: A practical review and recommendations for HIV care providers. *Clin Infect Dis.* 2010; 51(8):937–946.

MUSCLE DISORDERS

KEY POINTS

- HIV myopathy is a rare proximal muscle disorder that can occur in HIV-infected patients.

- Antiretroviral drugs, including zidovudine and raltegravir, can cause myopathy and elevated creatine kinase (CK)

Muscle disorders can be debilitating in HIV-infected patients. Myopathies can have a range of presentation from myalgias to rhabdomyolysis. HIV-associated myopathy and HIV-associated polymyositis are rare. This entity is slowly progressive, symmetrical proximal muscle weakness. Diagnosis is made by elevated CK, electromyography characteristics, and muscle pathology. Pathologic evaluation will show inflammatory infiltrates of CD8+ T cells and macrophages surrounding major histocompatibility complex-1-expressing muscle fibers. Treatment is with immunomodulatory regimens, including corticosteroids and intravenous immunoglobulin. HIV-associated myopathy can occur as part of the immune reconstitution inflammatory syndrome (Robinson-Papp, 2009). Myalgia and elevated CK can occur from other etiologies in HIV-infected patients, including exercising. Cocaine use and trimethoprim–sulfamethoxazole use have been associated with rhabdomyolysis.

Myopathy can also be a complication of ART. Zidovudine has classically caused HIV treatment-associated myopathy. CK levels are often checked when patients are on zidovudine, which is now less commonly used. Inhibition of DNA polymerase-γ in mitochondria has been implicated as a possible mechanism, and thus drugs that inhibit this enzyme, including stavudine, also cause myopathy. Elevated CK has been seen in HIV-infected patients on many other antiretrovirals, including protease inhibitors. Raltegravir use has been associated with muscle symptoms and elevated CK and, rarely, rhabdomyolysis. Grade 2–4 CK elevations reported in the BENCHMARK 1 and 2 trials were similar for raltegravir versus placebo when combined with optimized background regimen at 9% versus 6%, respectively (Issentress (raltegravir) package insert, https://www.merck.com/product/usa/pi_circulars/i/isentress/isentress_pi.pdf). Postmarketing evaluation in Italy among 496 patients showed that 5.2% of patients on raltegravir had muscle symptoms, and of these, 1.4% discontinued raltegravir (Madeddu, 2015). Data characterizing muscle symptoms and CK for newer integrase inhibitors such as dolutegravir and elvitegravir are lacking. When patients develop myopathy or rhabdomyolysis on a suspected HIV medication, consideration should be given to stopping that drug.

Recommended Reading

Robinson-Papp J, Simpson DM. Neuromuscular diseases associated with HIV-1 infection. *Muscle Nerve.* 2009; 40(6):1043–1053.

References

Bolland MJ, Wang TK, Gray A, et al. Stable bone density in HAART-treated individuals with HIV: A meta-analysis. *J Clin Endocrinol Metab.* 2011; 96(9):2721–2731.

Brown TT, Chen Y, Currier J, et al. Body composition, soluble markers of inflammation, and bone mineral density in antiretroviral therapy-naive HIV-1-infected individuals. *J Acquir Immune Defic Syndr.* 2013; 63(3):323–330.

Brown TT, Hoy J, Borderi M, et al. Recommendations for evaluation and management of bone disease in HIV. *Clin Infect Dis.* 2015; 60(8):1242–1251.

Brown TT, McComsey GA. Osteopenia and osteoporosis in patients with HIV: A review of current concepts. *Curr Infect Dis Rep.* 2006; 8:162–170.

Brown TT, Moser C, Currier J, et al. Changes in bone mineral density after initiation of antiretroviral treatment with tenofovir disoproxil fumarate/emtricitabine plus atazanavir/ritonavir, darunavir/ritonavir or raltegravir. *J Infect Dis.* 2015; 212(8):1241–1249.

Brown TT, Qaqish RB. Antiretroviral therapy and the prevalence of osteopenia and osteoporosis: A meta-analytic review. *AIDS.* 2006; 20(17):2165–2174.

Conesa-Botella A, Florence E, Lynen L, et al. Decrease of vitamin D concentration in patients with HIV infection on a non-nucleoside reverse transcriptase inhibitor-containing regimen. *AIDS Res Ther.* 2010; 7:40.

Dao CN, Patel P, Oveton ET, et al. Low vitamin D among HIV-infected adults: Prevalence of and risk factors for low vitamin D levels in a cohort of HIV-infected adults and comparison to prevalence among adults in the US general population. *Clin Infect Dis.* 2011; 52(3):396–405.

Fox J, Peters B, Prakash M, et al. Improvement in vitamin D deficiency following antiretroviral regimen change: Results from the MONET trial. *AIDS Res Hum Retroviruses.* 2011; 27(1):29–34.

Grant PM, Kitch D, McComsey GA, et al. Low baseline CD4[+] count is associated with greater bone mineral density loss after antiretroviral therapy initiation. *Clin Infect Dis.* 2013; 57(10):1483–1488.

Grigsby IF, Pham L, Mansky LM, et al. Tenofovir-associated bone density loss. *Ther Clin Risk Manag.* 2010; 6:41–47.

Gyllensten K, Josephson F, Lidman K, et al. Severe vitamin D deficiency diagnosed after introduction of antiretroviral therapy including efavirenz in a patient living at latitude 59 degrees N. *AIDS.* 2006; 20(14):1906–1907.

Havens PL, Stephensen CB, Hazra R, et al. Vitamin D₃ decreases parathyroid hormone in HIV-infected youth being treated with tenofovir: A randomized, placebo-controlled trial. *Clin Infect Dis.* 2012; 54(7):1013–1025.

Holick MF, Binkley NC, Heike A. Evaluation, treatment, and prevention of vitamin D deficiency: An Endocrine Society clinical practice guideline. *J Clin Endocrinol Metab.* 2011; 96:1911–1930.

Madeddu G, De Socio GVL, Ricci E, et al. Muscle symptoms and creatine phosphokinase elevations in patients receiving raltegravir in clinical practice: Results from the SCOLTA project long-term surveillance. *Int J Antimicrob Agents.* 2015; 45(3):289–294.

McComsey GA, Kendall MA, Tebas P, et al. Alendronate with calcium and vitamin D supplementation is safe and effective for treatment of decreased bone mineral density in HIV. *AIDS.* 2007; 21(18):2473–2482.

McComsey GA, Kitch D, Daar ES, et al. Bone mineral density and fractures in antiretroviral-naive persons randomized to receive abacavir–lamivudine or tenofovir disoproxil fumarate–emtricitabine along with efavirenz or atazanavir–ritonavir: AIDS Clinical Trials Group A5224s, a substudy of ACTG A5202. *J Infect Dis.* 2011; 203(12):1791–1801.

McComsey GA, Tebas P, Shane E, et al. Bone disease in HIV infection: A practical review and recommendations for HIV care providers. *Clin Infect Dis.* 2010; 51(8):937–946.

Mulligan K, Glidden DV, Anderson PL, et al. Effects of emtricitabine/tenofovir on bone mineral density in HIV-negative persons in a randomized, double-blind, placebo-controlled trial. *Clin Infect Dis.* 2015; 61(4):572–580.

Overton ET, Chan ES, Brown TT, et al. Vitamin D and calcium attenuate bone loss with antiretroviral therapy initiation: A randomized trial. *Ann Intern Med.* 2015; 162(12):815–824.

Robinson-Papp J, Simpson DM. Neuromuscular diseases associated with HIV-1 Infection. *Muscle Nerve.* 2009; 40(6):1043–1053.

Sax PE, Wohl D, Yin M, et al. Tenofovir alafenamide versus tenofovir disoproxil fumarate, coformulated with elvitegravir, cobicistat, and emtricitabine, for initial treatment of HIV-1 infection: Two randomised, double-blind, phase 3, non-inferiority trials. *Lancet.* 2015; 385(9987):2606–2615.

Spector SA. Vitamin D and HIV: Letting the sun shine in. *Top Antivir Med.* 2011; 19(1):6–10.

Tebas P, Powderly WG, Claxton S, et al. Accelerated bone mineral loss in HIV-infected patients receiving potent antiretroviral therapy. *AIDS.* 2000; 14(4):F63–F67.

Womack JA, Goulet JL, Gilbert C, et al. Increased risk of fragility fractures among HIV-infected compared to uninfected male veterans. *PLoS One.* 2011; 6(2):e17217.

Yin MT, Zhang CA, McMahon DJ, et al. Higher rates of bone loss in postmenopausal HIV-infected women: A longitudinal study. *J Clin Endocrinol Metab.* 2012; 97(2):554–562.

Young B, Dao CN, Buchacz K. Increased rates of bone fracture among HIV-infected persons in the HIV Outpatient Study (HOPS) compared with the US general population, 2000–2006. *Clin Infect Dis.* 2011; 52(8):1061–1068.

44.

SEXUALLY TRANSMITTED DISEASES

Karen J. Vigil

Upon completion of this chapter, the reader should be able to demonstrate knowledge about established and evolving science regarding the diagnosis and treatment of most prevalent sexually transmitted diseases in patients with HIV infection in order to decrease rate of transmission.

Sexually transmitted diseases (STDs) are common in HIV-infected patients. Education and counseling on changes in sexual behaviors of patients with STDs and their sexual partners, identification of asymptomatic infection, and effective diagnosis and treatment are the cornerstone for prevention.

Demonstrate knowledge about established and evolving science regarding the diagnosis and treatment of most prevalent sexual transmitted diseases in patients with HIV infection, in order to decrease rate of transmission.

SYPHILIS

- Syphilis incidence continues to increase, and it is more prevalent in HIV-infected patients and men who have sex with men (MSM).

- HIV-infected patients with syphilis should have a detailed neurologic examination. Patients with abnormal signs or symptoms should undergo cerebrospinal fluid (CSF) analysis.

- Syphilis incidence continues to increase, and it is more prevalent in HIV-infected patients and MSM.

- Clinical manifestations are similar to those of the general population, but complications may be more common (condyloma lata and lues maligna).

- Special attention to neurologic site involvement is required because laboratory-defined neurosyphilis may be more common among people with HIV.

- Although CSF abnormalities are more likely in HIV-infected patients with CD4$^+$ cell counts ≤350 cells/mm^3 and rapid plasma reagin (RPR) ≥1:32, lumbar puncture is only recommended if there is any sign or symptom of neurologic involvement.

- Penicillin is the treatment of choice for syphilis; alternatives have not been well studied in HIV-infected persons. HIV-infected persons with syphilis require more intensive clinical and serologic follow-up.

Syphilis is a systemic disease caused by *Treponema pallidum*. Between 2005 and 2013, the number of reported cases of primary and secondary syphilis nearly doubled. The annual rate increased from 2.9 to 5.3 cases per 100,000 population (Centers for Disease Control and Prevention (CDC), 2015). In 2012, MSM accounted for 83.9% of cases. Co-infection with HIV has been reported to be as much as 50–70% among MSM, with a high HIV seroconversion rate in patients with primary and secondary syphilis (Su, 2011).

CLINICAL PRESENTATION

Primary Syphilis

Primary syphilis refers to the chancre—a single, painless lesion with a clean base and indurated, raised borders. Chancres appears 1 week to 1 month after exposure. They are usually in the genital area but can occur anywhere on the body, including the oral cavity.

Secondary Syphilis

Secondary syphilis is characterized by a maculopapular erythematous rash that may involve the palms and soles. It typically occurs 3 weeks to 3 months after exposure. In HIV-infected patients, rash could present with several other forms, including papulosquamous, vesicular, and pustular forms. Condyloma lata (broad-based, fleshy wart-like lesions that occur in moist, warm body areas) and lues maligna (pustular ulceronodular syphilides) are complications of secondary syphilis and are more frequent in HIV-infected patients.

Latent Syphilis

Latent syphilis is defined by positive serological test in the absence of any clinical signs or symptoms of syphilis. Early latent syphilis is defined as that acquired within the preceding year. All other forms are either late latent syphilis or latent syphilis of unknown duration. The importance of this classification is secondary to transmission, being possible in any stage until early latent syphilis.

NEUROSYPHILIS

Central nervous system involvement may occur at any stage of syphilis. CSF laboratory abnormalities are common in persons with early syphilis, even in the absence of neurologic signs or symptoms. No evidence exists to support variation from recommended treatment for early syphilis for patients found to have such abnormalities. If clinical evidence of neurologic involvement is observed, a CSF examination should be performed.

Neurosyphilis can take any of several other forms, including cranial neuropathies (auditory dysfunction), uveitis, retinitis, or central nervous system vasculitis. A lumbar puncture and CSF examination should be performed for all patients with syphilitic eye disease to identify those with abnormalities; patients with abnormal CSF test results should be provided follow-up CSF examinations to assess treatment response.

The 2015 CDC treatment guidelines (Workowski, 2015) recommend CSF examination

- if there is evidence of neurologic symptoms;

- if there are ophthalmologic or auditory signs or symptoms;

- in patients with clinical presentation of tertiary syphilis (e.g., aortitis or gumma); and

- in patients with treatment failure.

CSF abnormalities are most likely in HIV-infected persons with syphilis of any stage when CD4+ cell count is ≤350 cells/mm^3 and a serum RPR titer is >1:32 (Libois, 2007; Marra, 2004). However, CSF examination has not been associated with improved clinical outcomes in the absence of neurologic signs and symptoms.

Other presentation of tertiary syphilis includes cardiovascular syphilis and gummatous syphilis. Cases of rapid progression after initial infection have been reported with both entities (Maharajan, 2005; Weinert, 2008).

DIAGNOSIS

Primary chancre can be diagnosed by visualization of spirochetes under dark field microscopic examination. This applies to genital lesions and not oral lesions because of the presence of nonpathogenic spirochetes in the mouth.

Nontreponemal antigen tests (Venereal Disease Research Laboratory (VDRL) and RPR) detect antibodies to antigens in the host after modification by *T. pallidum*. They become positive 4–6 weeks after infection or 1–3 weeks after the appearance of a primary lesion.

Treponemal tests (*Treponema pallidum* hemagglutination assay (TPHA), *Treponema pallidum* particle agglutination assay (TPPA), and fluorescent treponemal antibody absorption (FTA-ABS)) detect antibodies that react with *T. pallidum* antigens. They are confirmatory for syphilis.

The diagnosis of neurosyphilis in HIV-infected patients is difficult because HIV itself causes CSF abnormalities. Classic CSF findings in neurosyphilis are lymphocytic pleocytosis, total protein elevation, and a positive VDRL test. CSF VDRL may be false negative in 30–70% of cases of neurosyphilis.

TREATMENT

HIV-infected patients who have early syphilis may be at increased risk for neurologic complications (CDC, 2007) and may have higher rates of serologic treatment failure with currently recommended regimens compared to non-HIV-infected patients. No treatment regimens for syphilis have been demonstrated to be more effective in preventing neurosyphilis in HIV-infected patients than the syphilis regimens recommended for HIV-negative patients (Rolfs, 1997). Careful follow-up after therapy is essential. The recommended and alternative treatment regimens for syphilis (Workowski, 2015) in HIV-infected patients are summarized in Table 44.1.

FOLLOW-UP

HIV-infected persons should be evaluated clinically and serologically for treatment failure at 3, 6, 9, 12, and 24 months after therapy. For patients who meet the criteria

Table 44.1 RECOMMENDED AND ALTERNATIVE TREATMENT REGIMENS FOR SYPHILIS IN HIV-INFECTED PATIENTS

TYPE	RECOMMENDED REGIMEN	ALTERNATIVE REGIMEN
Primary, secondary, and early latent syphilis	Benzathine penicillin G, 2.4 million units IM in a single dose	
Late latent syphilis or syphilis of unknown duration	Benzathine penicillin G, at weekly doses of 2.4 million units for 3 weeks	
Neurosyphilis	Aqueous crystalline penicillin G, 18–24 million units per day, administered as 3–4 million units IV every 4 hours or continuous infusion for 10–14 days	Procaine penicillin 2.4 million units IM once daily *Plus* Probenecid 500 mg orally four times a day, both for 10–14 days

IM, Intramuscular; IV, Intravenous.

for treatment failure (signs or symptoms that persist or recur or persons who have a sustained fourfold increase in nontreponemal test titer), a new lumbar puncture with CSF examination should be performed and new treatment should be initiated. CSF examination and retreatment also should be strongly considered for HIV-infected patients whose nontreponemal test titers do not decrease fourfold within 6–12 months of therapy. If CSF examination is normal, treatment with benzathine penicillin G administered as 2.4 million units intramuscularly each at weekly intervals for 3 weeks is recommended.

For neurosyphilis, if CSF pleocytosis was present initially, a CSF examination should be repeated every 6 months until the cell count is normal. Research studies suggest that CSF improvement might occur much slower in HIV-infected patients, especially those with more advanced immunosuppression. If the cell count has not decreased after 6 months or if the CSF is not normal after 2 years, retreatment should be considered.

GONORRHEA

WHAT'S NEW?

Dual therapy for gonorrhea with ceftriaxone and azithromycin is recommended to hinder the development of antimicrobial-resistant *Neisseria gonorrhoeae* and to treat possible co-infection with *Chlamydia trachomatis*.

KEY POINTS

- Gonococcal infection remains an important cause of urethritis, cervicitis, pharyngitis, and proctitis in HIV-infected sexually active patients.

- Asymptomatic infection with gonorrhea and chlamydia is common at the female cervical site and male pharyngeal and rectal sites, such that routine, periodic screening for this STD is required to detect such cases.

- Nucleic acid-based testing offers high sensitivity, ease of sample collection, and use of noninvasively acquired specimens (i.e., urine), although such tests are not US Food and Drug Administration (FDA) approved for use with all specimen types.

- Antimicrobial resistance to fluoroquinolone and oral cephalosporins has been reported.

- Fewer antimicrobials are available to treat gonorrhea. Dual therapy for gonorrhea and chlamydia is recommended not only because patients usually infected with *N. gonorrhoeae* are co-infected with *C. trachomatis* but also to hinder the development of antimicrobial-resistant *N. gonorrhoeae*.

Gonorrhea is caused by *N. gonorrhoeae*. In 2014, 350,062 cases of gonorrhea were reported to the CDC (CDC, 2015)—a 10.5% increased rate since 2010. HIV-infected men are significantly more likely to have gonorrhea compared to HIV-uninfected men.

CLINICAL PRESENTATION

Acute urethritis is the main manifestation of gonorrhea. In men, urethral discharge—initially scant and later purulent—and dysuria are the major symptoms. The incubation period ranges from 1 to 10 days. Local complications include acute epididymitis, penile edema, penile lymphangitis, periurethral abscess, acute prostatitis, seminal vesiculitis, or infections of Tyson's and Cowper's glands. In women, gonorrhea presents as cervicitis and/

or asymptomatic urethritis. However, physical exam may show purulent or mucopurulent cervical exudates.

Neisseria gonorrhoeae may also cause rectal infection that could be asymptomatic or manifest as proctitis. Up to one-third of MSM who have gonorrhea have positive rectal cultures (Handsfield, 1980). In addition, pharyngeal infection has been reported but is usually asymptomatic.

Disseminated gonococcal infection results from bacteremic dissemination of *N. gonorrhoeae*. It can cause arthritis that primarily involves an asymmetric distribution in the knees, elbows, and more distal joints. A dermatitis picture with multiple discrete papules and pustules, often with a hemorrhagic component, may be present in approximately 75% of patients.

DIAGNOSIS

Urethra's discharge Gram stain reveals gram-negative diplococci during the first week after onset in men. In women, this is less common. Although cultures are the gold standard for diagnosis, nucleic acid amplification tests (NAATs) in cervical swab, urethral swab, or urine has excellent sensitivity and specificity.

TREATMENT

Quinolone-resistant *N. gonorrhoeae* strains are widely disseminated throughout the United States and the world. Treatment failure to oral cephalosporins has been reported in Asia, Europe, Africa, and Canada (Lewis, 2013; Unemo,

2012). Therefore, quinolones and oral cephalosporins are no longer recommended regimens for the treatment of gonorrhea in the United States. The recommended treatment regimens for gonorrhea infection (Workowski, 2015) in HIV-infected patients are summarized in Table 44.2. There are limited data on alternative treatments for people with cephalosporin or IgE-mediated penicillin allergy. Either gentamicin 240 mg or gemifloxacin 320 mg plus 2 g of azithromycin are possible options. However, consultation with an infectious disease specialist is recommended (Kirkcaldi, 2014).

FOLLOW-UP

If failure to ceftriaxone is suspected, patients should be retreated with at least 250 mg of ceftriaxone intramuscularly or intravenously, ensure partner treatment, and report the situation to the CDC.

CHLAMYDIA INFECTIONS

WHAT'S NEW?

Due to the high prevalence of *C. trachomatis* infection in women and men treated for chlamydial infection during the preceding several months, chlamydia-infected women and men should be retested approximately 3 months after treatment, regardless of whether they believe that their sex partners were treated.

Table 44.2 RECOMMENDED TREATMENT REGIMENS FOR GONORRHEA INFECTION IN HIV-INFECTED PATIENTS

TYPE	RECOMMENDED REGIMEN	ALTERNATIVE REGIMEN
Uncomplicated gonococcal infections of the cervix, urethra, and rectum	Ceftriaxone 250 mg IM in a single dose *Plus* Azithromycin 1 g orally in a single dose	Cefixime 400 mg PO in a single dose *Plus* Azithromycin 1 g orally in a single dose
Uncomplicated gonococcal infections of the pharynx	Ceftriaxone 250 mg IM in a single dose *Plus* Azithromycin 1 g orally in a single dose	
Disseminated gonococcal infection	Ceftriaxone 1 g IM or IV daily *Plus* Azithromycin 1 g orally in a single dose	
Gonococcal meningitis and endocarditis	Ceftriaxone 1–2 g IV every 12 hours for 10–14 days for meningitis and for at least 4 weeks for endocarditis *Plus* Azithromycin 1 g orally in a single dose	

IM, intramuscular; IV, intravenous.

Chlamydia is the most commonly reported STD in the United States in men and women. In 2014, 1,441,789 chlamydial infections were reported to the CDC from 50 states and the District of Columbia (CDC, 2015). However, underreporting might be substantial because the disease may be asymptomatic. Chlamydia infection is more frequent in younger age groups, racial/ethnic minorities, MSM, and incarcerated populations (Burstein, 1998; Rietmeijer, 2008; Satterwhite, 2008). Genital and ocular chlamydial infections are caused by serotypes D–K, whereas serotypes L1–L3 cause lymphogranuloma venereum.

CLINICAL PRESENTATION

Chlamydia genital infection secondary to serotypes D–K causes urethritis in men and cervicitis in women. Although most of the patients are asymptomatic, men may present with purulent urethral discharge (milder than gonorrhea), and women may complaint of vaginal discharge, intermenstrual bleeding, dyspareunia, and/or abdominal pain. Women may also present with symptoms exclusively of urethritis, such as dysuria.

Serovars L1–L3 cause LGV. LGV is not endemic in the United States. Southeast Asia, the Caribbean, Latin America, and Africa are areas of higher prevalence. It presents as one or more genital ulcers or papules, followed by the development of unilateral or bilateral fluctuant inguinal lymphadenopathy called buboes. Since 2003, there have been reports of outbreaks in Western Europe and in the United States of chlamydia L2 serotype proctitis, particularly in MSM.

DIAGNOSIS

NAATs for chlamydia genital infections (by polymerase chain reaction assay or transcription-mediated amplification) have great sensitivity and specificity and can be performed on first catch urine or vaginal swab without the requirement of a urethral swab. The diagnosis of LGV is challenging. Cell culture is the only diagnostic test approved by the FDA. Serology helps in the diagnosis because titers are typically elevated at the time of presentation.

Diagnosis of LGV proctitis is even more difficult. NAATs may be used if a local laboratory has validated them. The CDC recommends that when LGV is suspected, the provider should collect a specimen and send the sample to the state health department for referral to the CDC. If this is not possible, an antibiotic regimen effective against LGV should be included in empiric treatment for proctitis.

TREATMENT

Oral azithromycin 1 g single dose or doxycycline 100 mg twice a day for 7 days are the treatments of choice. For proctitis, prolonged treatment is recommended.

HUMAN PAPILLOMAVIRUS

- Persons with HIV have higher rates of HPV-related lesions; genital warts can be more aggressive and difficult to eradicate.

- A variety of patient- and provider-applied therapies are available.

- There are three types of HPV vaccines: Cervarix (a bivalent vaccine that targets HPV types 16 and 18), Gardasil (a quadrivalent HPV vaccine that targets HPV types 6, 11, 16, and 18), and Gardasil-9 (a 9-valent vaccine that targets in addition HPV types 31, 33, 45, 52, and 58, which cause approximately 20% of cervical cancers that are not covered by Gardasil). Gardasil and Gardasil-9 are indicated in females and males aged 9–26 years. Cervarix is indicated in females aged 9–25 years.

HPV is a double-stranded DNA virus that may infect the genital tract. There are more than 100 types of HPV; more than 40 may infect the genital area. HPV may cause two major clinical syndromes: genital warts (condyloma acuminata) associated mainly with types 6 and 11 and epithelial cervical or anal neoplasia linked to serotypes 16 and 18 (for more information on cervical and anal neoplasia, refer to Chapter 35).

HPV detection is significantly more common among HIV-infected women and men than among HIV-seronegative women and men (Mbulawa, 2009). Several studies have demonstrated that HPV increases the risk of HIV acquisition (Smith, 2010).

CLINICAL PRESENTATION

In most cases, HPV infection is transient and has no clinical manifestation or sequel and is self-limited. Genital warts typically present as single or multiple soft, fleshy, papillary or sessile, painless keratinized growths in the vulvovaginal area, penis, anus, urethra, or perineum. HIV-infected women have higher prevalence of genital warts, which may progress more rapidly in the presence of a declining immune status. In addition, there are higher rates of Pap smear-detected abnormalities, dysplasia, and progression to cervical cancer relative to those of uninfected women.

DIAGNOSIS

Diagnosis of warts is made clinically; laboratory confirmation is not needed.

HIV-infected patients, especially MSM, have a significantly increased risk of anal cancer due to oncogenic HPV types; therefore, routine anal Pap screening in HIV care settings is recommended.

TREATMENT

The main indications for treatment of vulvovaginal warts are bothersome symptoms and/or psychologic distress. Vulvar biopsy to exclude precancerous or cancerous lesions is indicated when warts are identified in immunocompromised or postmenopausal women, when the lesions are visually atypical, or when warts fail to respond to standard therapy. The recommended treatment regimens for HPV in HIV-infected patients are summarized in Table 44.3.

PREVENTION OR PROPHYLAXIS

There are three types of HPV vaccines: a bivalent vaccine that targets HPV types 16 and 18 (Cervarix); a quadrivalent HPV vaccine that targets HPV types 6, 11, 16, and 18 (Gardasil); and a 9-valent vaccine that prevents infection

Table 44.3 RECOMMENDED TREATMENT REGIMENS FOR HPV/WARTS IN HIV-INFECTED PATIENTS

TYPE	REGIMEN
External genital warts, patient-applied	Podofilox 0.5% solution or gel *Or* Imiquimod 5% cream *Or* Sinecatechins 15% ointment
External genital warts, provider-administered	Cryotherapy with liquid nitrogen or cryoprobe; repeat applications every 1–2 weeks *Or* Trichloroacetic acid (TCA) or bichloroacetic acid (BCA) 80–90% *Or* Surgical removal by tangential scissor excision, tangential shave excision, curettage, or electrosurgery
Vaginal warts	Cryotherapy with liquid nitrogen. *Or* TCA or BCA 80–90% applied to warts *Or* Surgical removal
Urethral meatus warts	Cryotherapy with liquid nitrogen *Or* Surgical removal
Anal warts	Cryotherapy with liquid nitrogen *Or* TCA or BCA 80–90% applied to warts *Or* Surgical removal

with HPV types 6, 11, 16, 18, 31, 33, 45, 52, and 58. Routine vaccination is recommended for boys and girls aged 11 or 12 years, although they can be vaccinated beginning at age 9 years. Women can receive any of the currently available HPV vaccines, whereas only the quadrivalent or 9-valent are recommended routinely for men. The vaccines are not licensed for use in people older than age 26 years. The CDC emphasizes that immunocompromised or immunosuppressed patients, included patients with HIV, gay and bisexual men should also be vaccinated.

GENITAL ULCERS

In the United States, most young, sexually active patients who have genital, anal, or perianal ulcers have either genital herpes or syphilis, with herpes being most prevalent. Less common causes include chancroid and donovanosis.

References

Burstein GR, Waterfield G, Joffe A, et al. Screening for gonorrhea and chlamydia by DNA amplification in adolescents attending middle school health centers: Opportunity for early intervention. *Sex Transm Dis.* 1998; 25:395.

Centers for Disease Control and Prevention. Symptomatic early neurosyphilis among HIV-positive men who have sex with men: Four cities, United States, January 2002–June 2004. *MMWR Morb Mortal Wkly Rep.* 2007; 56:625–628.

Centers for Disease Control and Prevention. Primary and secondary syphilis—United States 2005–2013. *MMWR Morbid Mortal Wkly Rep.* 2014; 63(18):402–406.

Centers for Disease Control and Prevention. *Sexually transmitted disease surveillance 2014.* Atlanta, GA: US Department of Health and Human Services; 2015.

Handsfield HH, Knapp JS, Diehr PK, et al. Correlation of auxotype and penicillin susceptibility of *Neisseria gonorrhoeae* with sexual preference and clinical manifestations of gonorrhea. *Sex Transm Dis.* 1980; 7:1–5.

Kirkcaldy RD, Weinstock HS, Moore PC, et al. The efficacy and safety of gentamicin plus azithromycin and gemifloxacin plus azithromycin as treatment of uncomplicated gonorrhea. *Clin Infect Dis.* 2014; 59:1083–1091.

Lewis DA, Sriruttan C, Muller EE, et al. Phenotypic and genetic characterization of the first two cases of extended-spectrum-cephalosporin-resistant *Neisseria gonorrhoeae* infection in South Africa and association with cefixime treatment failure. *J Antimicrob Chemother.* 2013; 68:1267–1270.

Libois A, De Wit S, Poll B, et al. HIV and syphilis: When to perform a lumbar puncture. *Sex Transm Dis.* 2007; 34:141–144.

Maharajan M. Cardiovascular syphilis in HIV infection: A case–control study at the Institute of Sexually Transmitted Diseases, Chennai, India. *Sex Transm Infect.* 2005; 81:361.

Marra CM, Maxwell CL, Smith SL, et al. Cerebrospinal fluid abnormalities in patients with syphilis: Association with clinical and laboratory features. *J Infect Dis.* 2004; 189:369–376.

Mbulawa ZZ, Coetzee D, Marais DJ, et al. Genital human papillomavirus prevalence and human papillomavirus concordance in heterosexual couples are positively associated with human immunodeficiency virus coinfection. *J Infect Dis.* 2009; 199:1514.

Rietmeijer CA, Hopkins E, Geisler WM, et al. *Chlamydia trachomatis* positivity rates among men tested in selected venues in the United States: A review of the recent literature. *Sex Transm Dis.* 2008; 35:S8.

Rolfs RT, Joesoef MR, Hendershot EF, et al. A randomized trial of enhanced therapy for early syphilis in patients with and without human immunodeficiency virus infection: The Syphilis and HIV Study Group. *N Engl J Med.* 1997; 337:307–314.

Satterwhite CL, Joesoef MR, Datta SD, et al. Estimates of *Chlamydia trachomatis* infections among men: United States. *Sex Transm Dis.* 2008; 35:S3.

Smith JS, Moses S, Hudgens MG, et al. Increased risk of HIV acquisition among Kenyan men with human papillomavirus infection. *J Infect Dis.* 2010; 201:1677.

Su JR, Weinstock H. Epidemiology of co-infection with HIV and syphilis in 34 states, United States—2009. In Proceedings of the 2011 National HIV Prevention Conference, August 13–17, 2011, Atlanta, GA.

Unemo M, Golparian D, Nicholas R, et al. High-level cefixime- and ceftriaxone-resistant *Neisseria gonorrhoeae* in France: Novel penA mosaic allele in a successful international clone causes treatment failure. *Antimicrob Agents Chemother.* 2012; 56:1273–1280.

Weinert LS, Scheffel RS, Zoratto G, et al. Cerebral syphilitic gumma in HIV-infected patients: Case report and review. *Int J STD AIDS.* 2008; 19:62.

Workowski KA, Bolan GA; Centers for Disease Control and Prevention. Sexually transmitted diseases treatment guidelines, 2015. *MMWR Recomm Rep.* 2015; 64:1–138.

45.

HIV AND BONE HEALTH

Linda A. Battalora and Benjamin Young

LEARNING OBJECTIVES

- Discuss the prevalence of diseases of bone mineral density (BMD) and fractures in HIV-infected populations.

- Describe the risk factors associated with fractures.

- Effectively communicate diagnostic and treatment strategies of bone diseases to patients.

WHAT'S NEW?

- Low BMD at the hip femoral neck was significantly more prevalent in HIV-infected persons than in matched controls from the National Health and Nutrition Examination Survey (NHANES) (47% vs. 29%; $p < 0.001$)

- Recommendations for evaluation and management of bone disease in HIV were published based on contributions from 34 HIV specialists from 16 countries.

- US Department of Health and Human Services (DHHS) HIV guidelines recommend the avoidance of tenofovir disoproxil fumarate (TDF) in patients with osteoporosis because TDF is associated with greater initial loss of BMD compared to other antiretrovirals (ARVs).

- Tenofovir alafenamide (TAF), a new prodrug of tenofovir, is associated with less BMD loss compared to TDF in both initial and antiretroviral therapy (ART) switch settings, and it may mitigate the BMD effect of TDF.

KEY POINTS

- Multiple cohort studies have found a higher than expected prevalence of low BMD in populations of adults living with HIV.

- Fracture prevalence is greater in HIV-infected women and men compared to the general population. Incident fractures rates among HIV-infected persons in the HIV Outpatient Study (HOPS) were increased nearly threefold compared to those for the U.S. general population.

- Cohort studies suggest that in addition to traditional factors such as age, smoking, and hepatitis C virus (HCV) co-infection, HIV disease-associated factors and ART factors are predictive indicators of fracture risk in HIV-infected individuals.

- ART initiation is associated with a BMD decrease of 2–6%, with the largest decrease occurring in the first 6–12 months of treatment and then stabilizing.

- Greater BMD losses occur with initiation of zidovudine, TDF, and certain protease inhibitors.

- There are limited HIV-specific evidence-based recommendations regarding screening for bone disease, although extrapolation of screening recommendations from the general population is, at a minimum, reasonable. Several organizations recommend using dual-energy X-ray absorptiometry (DXA) and/or the Fracture Risk Assessment Tool (FRAX) for screening of HIV-infected persons at risk of fractures.

With improved long-term survival among populations of people living with HIV (PLWH), it has been suggested that HIV/AIDS may hasten the aging process (Justice, 2014; Ofotokun, 2011). There is increasing evidence that cardiovascular, renal, and bone disease and neurocognitive deficits may be more common among long-term survivors of HIV infection. Revelations from cohort and prospective randomized studies suggest that PLWH are at increased risk of metabolic bone disease and related fractures (Battalora, 2016; Womack, 2011; Young, 2011).

DEFINITIONS AND EPIDEMIOLOGY

BONE MINERALIZATION ABNORMALITIES

The World Health Organization (WHO) defines two categories of bone abnormalities based on comparison with the mean BMD of young healthy women (T-score): (1) osteoporosis—low bone mass and microarchitectural deterioration of bone tissue, BMD value more than 2.5 standard deviations below the mean BMD of young adult women (BMD T-score < −2.5); and (2) osteopenia—low bone mass, BMD value between 1 and 2.5 standard deviations below the mean BMD of young adult women (−2.5 < bone mineral density T-score < −1) (WHO, 1994; Woolf, 2003). Osteomalacia is a third type of bone mineralization abnormality referring to softening of bones due to impaired bone mineralization, typically resulting from severe vitamin D deficiency (McComsey, 2010; WHO, 2002). Osteonecrosis or avascular necrosis is yet another bone mineralization abnormality resulting from interrupted blood supply to a bone or part of a bone, commonly occurring as a complication of trauma or fracture, typically located at the articular end of a bone (WHO, 2002).

In the general population, BMD peaks at approximately 22–35 years of age (Orwoll, 1995). BMD appears to decrease by 2–6% during the first 1 to 2 years of ART (Brown, 2009). Thereafter, in men and women, BMD levels stabilize or improve.

Bone strength is a function of bone density and bone quality. Bone quality refers to rate of remodeling, microarchitecture, size, shape, amount of mineralization in the bone, and matrix quality (Yin, CROI, 2012). Rate of remodeling is measured from serum levels of bone turnover markers osteocalcin (OCN; a formation marker) and N-terminal telopeptide (NTX; a resorption marker). Microarchitecture is observed with computed tomography CT imaging. Mineralization quantity and matrix quality are determined by biopsy (Yin, CROI, 2012).

PREVALENCE OF LOW BONE MINERAL DENSITY IN THE HIV POPULATION

Multiple cohort studies have found a higher than expected prevalence of low BMD in populations of adults living with HIV (Brown, 2006). Notably, these studies represent diverse populations of HIV-infected individuals, including antiretroviral treatment-naive and -experienced people (Bedimo, 2012; Escota, 2015; Looker, 1998; McComsey, 2011; Tebas, 2000).

Using data from the Study to Understand the Natural History of HIV and AIDS in the Era of Effective Therapy (SUN Study)—a prospective, observational cohort study funded by the Centers for Disease Control and Prevention (CDC)—Escota et al. determined that low BMD at the hip femoral neck was significantly more prevalent in HIV-infected persons than in matched controls from NHANES (47% vs. 29%; $p < 0.001$). In this cohort of 653 participants (77% male, 29% Black, median age 41 years, median CD4[+] T cell count 464 cells/mm[3], and 89% with HIV RNA levels <400 copies/ml), 51% of participants had osteopenia and 10% had osteoporosis at baseline (Escota, 2015).

Postmenopausal HIV-infected women demonstrate a greater decline in BMD. In a longitudinal study of bone loss in postmenopausal HIV-infected women (Yin, 2011), higher rates of bone loss at the spine and forearm were observed in postmenopausal HIV-infected women than in HIV-negative minority women. Thus, higher rates of bone loss at the spine and forearm of postmenopausal HIV-infected women described in this study coupled with increased fracture prevalence among HIV-infected individuals (Triant, 2008) suggest that an increased rate of fractures in postmenopausal HIV-infected women is a concern (Yin, 2011). Similarly, higher rates of bone loss were observed in HIV-infected men older than age 50 years (Orwoll, 1995). There are very few data on bone loss for HIV-infected women and men older than age 65 years, the period in which fractures are prevalent in the general population (Yin, 2012).

There are limited data from resource-limited setting regarding low BMD in HIV-infected populations. In one South African cohort of 444 HIV-infected individuals (median age, 35 years; interquartile range (IQR), 30–40) years; 77% women), low BMD (Z-score <−2 standard deviations (SD)) was found in 17% of participants at the lumbar spine and 5% of participants at the total hip (Dave, 2015). Dave and colleagues reported that median total hip BMD was lower among those receiving ART than in ART-naive participants (0.909 (SD 0.123) vs. 0.956 (SD 0.124) g/cm[2]; $p = 0.0001$). Similarly, femoral neck BMD was lower among ART-receiving compared to ART-naive subjects (0.796 (SD 0.130) vs. 0.844 (SD 0.120) g/cm[2]; $p = 0.0001$). In addition, vitamin D deficiency was found in 15% of cohort participants and associated with efavirenz use (adjusted odds ratio, 2.04; 95% confidence interval (CI), 101–4.13). In multivariate analysis, exposure to efavirenz or lopinavir/ritonavir-based ART was associated with lower total hip BMD; higher weight, being male, and higher vitamin D concentration were associated with higher total hip BMD (adjusted $R^2 = 0.28$). Factors independently associated with lumbar spine BMD included age, weight, sex, and efavirenz use (R^2 = 0.13) (Dave, 2015).

Hoy recently reported results from the Strategic Timing of Antiretroviral Treatment (START) Bone Mineral Density (BMD) substudy (Hoy, 2015; INSIGHT START Study Group, 2015). The primary START study enrollment consisted of 4685 HIV-infected adult participants in 35 countries with CD4+ T cell count >500 cells/mm³, median age 36 years, and 27% were female (INSIGHT START Study Group, 2015). Participants were randomized to start ART at study entry or delay therapy until CD4+ T cell count fell below 350 cells/mm³ or development of AIDS or another condition that dictated the use of ART (deferred-initiation group). In the BMD substudy of this primary START study, 193 participants were randomized to the early ART group and 204 participants to the deferred ART group (Hoy, 2015). Substudy participants underwent DXA scans of the lumbar spine, total hip, and femoral neck at baseline and annually thereafter. Mean follow-up time was 2.2 years. Hoy reported significantly greater loss of BMD at both the hip and the spine in participants randomized to early ART. There was no evidence of difference in development of osteoporosis between groups (or fractures in the main START study) (Hoy, 2015).

Ali and colleagues addressed potential research and capacity development priorities to fill gaps in data comparing the incidence of noncommunicable disease comorbidities between HIV-infected and HIV-negative populations in low- and middle-income countries (Ali, 2014).

HIGHER PREVALENCE AND INCIDENCE OF FRACTURES IN HIV POPULATION

Several recent studies have concluded that HIV-infected populations are at greater risk of bone fractures. Triant and colleagues presented findings that facture prevalence is greater in HIV-infected women and men compared to the general population (Triant, 2008). Based on an analysis of more than 11 years of data from a large US single health care database, it was determined that HIV-infected participants had a larger number of vertebral, hip, wrist, and combined fractures compared with non-HIV-infected participants. These findings were consistent across age, race and sex categories but no correlations were made as to specific risk factors due to lack of data.

Subsequently, four large observational cohort studies published findings correlating fracture incidence in HIV-infected individuals compared to control groups. Differences in population, controls, and fracture definitions

(i.e., fracture and fragility fracture definitions) were unique to each study.

The Women's Interagency HIV Study (WIHS) reported fracture incidence in 1728 HIV-infected and 663 HIV-negative predominantly premenopausal women and reported (Yin, 2010). Rates of fracture were not increased in HIV-infected patients compared to HIV-negative patients, and in the HIV-infected patients, the history of AIDS-defining illness was a more predictive indicator of fracture than ART.

Incident fractures rates among HIV-infected persons in the HOPS study were increased nearly threefold compared to rates in the US general population between 2000 and 2006 (Young, 2011). Rates of first fractures at any anatomic site were analyzed in 5826 participants (median baseline age of 40 years, 79% male, 52% white, and 73% ART). Rates of fracture were indirectly standardized to the general population by age and sex using data from outpatients in the National Hospital Ambulatory Medical Care Survey (NHAMCS-OPD). Greater proportions of fractures were located at the hip, wrist, or spine in HIV-infected subjects; fractures were associated with lower CD4+ cell count nadir, duration of HIV diagnosis, and hepatitis C co-infection. The study suggested that younger HIV-infected adults, particularly those between ages 25 and 54 years, are at an increased risk of bone fracture compared to the general population. The authors recommended regular assessment of HIV-infected persons for fracture risk and particularly those with low nadir CD4+ cell counts and other established fracture risk factors.

In the all-male Veterans Aging Cohort Study Virtual Cohort (VACS-VC) study, Womack and colleagues reported that HIV-infected men were at greater risk for fragility fracture compared to their HIV-negative counterparts (Womack, 2011). In this study of 119,318 men—of whom 33% were HIV-infected, 34% of this group were 50 years or older at baseline, and 55% were Black or Hispanic—fracture risk factors included age, race, alcohol dependency, liver disease, tobacco smoking, or current use of corticosteroids or proton pump inhibitors.

Hansen and colleagues studied the incidence of fragility fractures in HIV-infected individuals not undergoing treatment with ART and HIV-infected individuals undergoing treatment with ART in the Danish HIV Cohort Study (Hansen, 2012). In this comparative, sex- and age-matched study involving 5306 HIV-infected participants and a general population cohort of 26,530 HIV-negative participants, the HIV-infected participants were observed to have an increased overall rate of fractures, increased risk of low-energy fractures but not high-energy fractures in

HIV-infected participants without HCV co-infection, and moderate risk of low-energy fracture in HIV-infected participants undergoing ART when controlled for traditional osteoporosis risk factors of age, comorbidity, and smoking.

In the AIDS Clinical Trials Group (ACTG) A5224s, a substudy of ACTG A5202, McComsey and colleagues concluded that fracture rates increased in 269 HIV-infected patients during the first 2 years of ART initiated during the clinical trial compared to additional years of therapy. Although differences in BMD change were observed between patients who initiated different ART regimens, no significant differences in fracture rate were reported (McComsey, 2011; Yin, 2011).

Osteoporotic fractures were associated with cumulative exposure to TDF and ART in a large retrospective cohort study (56,600 patients) with a mean age of 45 years (Bedimo, 2012). Ninety-five percent of this cohort was male, limiting the ability to generalize the conclusion to females.

In addition to traditional risk factors such as older age, smoking, and HCV co-infection, HIV-associated factors ($CD4^+$ cell count nadir) and ART factors are important predictive indicators of fracture risk in HIV-infected individuals (Yin, 2012). In the 2014 *Clinician's Guide to Prevention and Treatment of Osteoporosis*, the National Osteoporosis Foundation (NOF) included AIDS/HIV as disease risk factors for osteoporosis and fragility fractures (Battalora, 2014; NOF 2014).

RECENT FINDINGS ON BONE HEALTH AND HIV

Findings from recent cohort studies have contributed to the developing field of fracture incidence in the HIV-infected population. Among 1006 participants from two CDC-funded cohorts (median age, 43 years (IQR, 36–49); 83% male; 67% non-Hispanic White; median $CD4^+$ T cell count (CD4), 461 cells/mm³ (IQR, 311–658)), osteopenia was determined in 36% ($n = 358$) of participants and osteoporosis in 4% ($n = 37$) of participants. A prior fracture was documented in 67 participants. During 4068 person-years of observation after DXA scanning, 85 incident fractures occurred, predominantly rib/sternum ($n = 18$), hand ($n = 14$), foot ($n = 13$), and wrist ($n = 11$). Low BMD (osteopenia and/or osteoporosis) was determined in nearly 40% of the participants. Factors associated with osteopenia or osteoporosis included older age, lower nadir $CD4^+$ T cell count, male–male sex HIV transmission risk, and history of fracture. Fourfold higher fracture rates were observed in

HIV-infected participants with osteoporosis compared to HIV-infected participants with normal BMD. In multivariable analyses, osteoporosis (adjusted hazard ratio (aHR), 4.02; 95% CI, 2.02–8.01) and current/prior tobacco use (aHR, 1.59; 95% CI, 1.02–2.50) were associated with incident fracture (Battalora, 2016).

Results of new fracture risk and FRAX 10-year probability of fracture among the same CDC-combined cohort of 1006 participants described previously were presented in poster format at CROI 2014. Battalora reported that increasing baseline FRAX 10-year probability was consistently associated with increased rates of incident fractures in this HIV-infected cohort. Participants with FRAX 10-year probability ≥3% compared with <3% had higher rates of major and incident fracture (Battalora, 2014).

Overton reported on results from the 48-week prospective, randomized, double-blind, placebo-controlled ACTG A5280 study evaluating the effect of high-dose vitamin D_3 (4000 IU daily) plus calcium supplementation (1000 mg calcium carbonate daily) on BMD in 142 HIV-infected subjects (90% male; 37% non-Hispanic White, 33% non-Hispanic Black, 25% Hispanic; median age, 33 years; body mass index, 24.4 kg/m²; $CD4^+$ cell count, 341 cells/mm³; HIV-1 RNA level, 4.5 $\log_{10}$ copies/ml; and 25(OH) vitamin D, 23 ng/ml) with DXA scan data at baseline and week 48 initiating ART with efavirenz/emtricitabine/tenofovir. Vitamin D/calcium supplementation mitigated the loss of BMD seen with ART initiation of efavirenz/emtricitabine/tenofovir, particularly at the total hip (Overton, 2014).

Shiau and coworkers performed a meta-analysis of all studies on bone health and HIV published through September 2012 and concluded that HIV infection is associated with a modest increase in incident fracture, and they confirmed the consistent relationship of HCV co-infection as a risk factor (Shiau, 2013).

PATHOPHYSIOLOGY AND RISK FACTORS

Bone loss in PLWH is likely multifactorial involving three common elements: the host, the virus, and ART. Lower bone density in HIV-infected persons is often attributable to host risks, including smoking, alcohol consumption, exposure to glucocorticoids, decreased activity, lipodystrophy, HCV co-infection, vitamin D deficiency, weight loss, hypogonadism, and chronic kidney disease. HLA supertype, particularly HLA-DQ3, has been associated with bone density status in one cohort study of HIV-infected adults (Haskelberg, 2014). HIV may directly affect bone cells by viral protein induction of osteoclastogenesis or by causing osteoblast apoptosis. Moreover, T cell and B cell activation during HIV infection results in increased circulating cytokines, including tumor necrosis factor-α, interleukin-6 (IL-6), and RANKL, which appear to induce osteoclast bone resorption. In a recent study, elevated levels of IL-6 were associated with risk of progression to osteoporosis among PLWH (Hileman, 2014). Similar increases in cytokine levels have been reported in other chronic inflammatory diseases—for example, rheumatoid arthritis.

ART initiation is associated with a BMD decrease of 2–6%, with the largest decrease occurring in the first 6–12 months of treatment and then stabilizing (Brown, 2009). Greater BMD losses occur with initiation of zidovudine (van Vonderen, 2009), TDF (McComsey 2011; Yin, 2011), and certain protease inhibitors (Duvivier, 2009; McComsey, 2011). Younger HIV-infected men and women on established ART had stable BMD (Yin, 2012). Among postmenopausal women, higher rates of loss of BMD were observed among the recipients of TDF-containing ART (Yin, 2011). Fracture rates, both fragility and nonfragility, are higher in HIV-infected individuals and associated with HCV co-infection and possibly ART use (Bedimo, 2012; Maalouf, 2013; Yin, 2012; Young, 2011). Currently, the fracture incidence is estimated to be approximately 3–5 per 1000 person-years, but this will likely increase as the population of HIV-infected individuals chronologically ages.

CLINICAL MANAGEMENT

SCREENING FOR BONE DISEASE

There are limited HIV-specific evidence-based recommendations regarding screening for bone disease, although extrapolation of screening recommendations from the general population is, at a minimum, reasonable.

The NOF published recommendations to clinicians for postmenopausal women and men aged 50 years or older (NOF, 2014). The reader is advised to consult the complete list of recommendations in the NOF *Clinician's Guide to Prevention and Treatment of Osteoporosis*. A brief listing of major recommendations is provided here:

- Counsel patient on risk of osteoporosis and related fractures.

- Check for secondary causes.

- Advise patient on adequate amounts of calcium (at least 1200 mg/day) and vitamin D (800–1000 IU/day), including supplements if necessary for individuals aged 50 years or older.

- Recommend regular weightbearing and muscle-strengthening exercise to reduce risk of falls and fractures.

- Advise against tobacco smoking and excessive alcohol consumption.

- Recommend BMD testing in women aged 65 years or older and men aged 70 years or older.

- In postmenopausal women and men aged 50–69 years, recommend BMD testing based on risk factor profile.

- In postmenopausal women and men older than age 50 years who have had an adult-age fracture, diagnose and determine degree of osteoporosis.

- Initiate treatment in patients with hip or vertebral (clinical or morphometric) fractures.

- Initiate therapy in patients with BMD T-scores ≤ –2.5 at the femoral neck or spine by DXA, after appropriate evaluation.

- Initiate treatment in postmenopausal women and men aged 50 years or older with low bone mass (T-score between –1.0 and –2.5, osteopenia) at the femoral neck or spine and a 10-year hip fracture probability ≥3% or a 10-year major osteoporosis-related fracture probability ≥20% based on the US-adapted WHO absolute fracture risk model FRAX.

- Current US Food and Drug Administration (FDA)-approved pharmacologic options for osteoporosis are bisphosphonates (alendronate, alendronate, ibandronate, risedronate, and zoledronic acid), calcitonin, estrogen agonist/antagonist (raloxifene), estrogens and/or hormone therapy, tissue-selective estrogen complex (conjugated estrogens/bazedoxifene), parathyroid hormone (PTH (1–34), teriparatide), and the RANKL inhibitor denosumab.

- BMD testing performed in DXA centers using accepted quality assurance measures is appropriate for monitoring bone loss.

- Patients taking FDA-approved medications should have laboratory and bone density re-evaluation after 2 years or more frequently when medically appropriate (NOF, 2014).

Brown et al. recently published recommendations for evaluation and management of bone disease in HIV infection based on contributions from 34 HIV specialists from 16 countries (Brown, 2015). Noting global variation in practice and thus difficulty in determining one set of recommendations for evaluation and management of bone disease, use of FRAX without BMD is recommended for assessment of fracture risk in resource-limited settings (Brown, 2015). The reader is referred to the publication for a complete listing of recommendations and rationale.

SCREENING FOR VITAMIN D INSUFFICIENCY

Three institutions have provided guidance for vitamin D deficiency. The Institute of Medicine (IOM) published dietary reference intakes for calcium and vitamin D, but it did not provide screening recommendations or specifically reference intakes for HIV-infected individuals (IOM, 2011). The Endocrine Society (EOS) and the European AIDS Clinical Society (EACS) recommended screening at-risk patients and those on ART and having risk factors for low vitamin D or fracture risks (EACS, 2015; EOS, 2011). There are limited data on vitamin D supplementation in HIV-infected patients, but some beneficial effects on PTH have been determined, whereas no effects on BMD have been reported (Childs, 2012).

SCREENING FOR FALL RISK

Fall Risk Assessment Tools

Fall risk assessment tools are used to determine the probability of future falls. Typical categories of the assessment tools include fall risk factors (e.g., recent falls, medications, psychological, cognitive status, vision, mobility, transfer, behaviors, activities of daily living, environment, nutrition, continence, and other risk factors).

SCREENING FOR FRACTURE RISK

FRAX

FRAX was developed by the World Health Organization Metabolic Bone Disease Group to assess fractures with more optimal predictors of fracture risk compared to T-scores (van den Bergh, 2010; WHO Metabolic Bone Disease Group, 2008). This assessment tool is not HIV specific. FRAX provides the 10-year probability of hip fracture and the 10-year probability of a major osteoporotic fracture (hip, spine, shoulder, or forearm). Probability is estimated based on clinical risk factors (CRFs) and BMD values from the femoral neck (WHO Metabolic Bone Disease Group, 2008). Models have been developed based on location (i.e., Asia, Europe, Middle East and Africa, North America,

Latin America, and Oceania) and ethnicity. CRFs included in the calculation tool are age, sex, weight (kilograms), height (centimeters), previous fracture, parent fractured hip, current tobacco smoking, exposure to glucocorticoids, rheumatoid arthritis, secondary osteoporosis, alcohol intake of three or more units per day, and BMD (g/cm^2) or, alternatively, T-score based on the NHANES III female reference data (Kanis, 2007).

The International Osteoporosis Foundation, the NOF, the American Society for Bone and Mineral Research, and the International Society for Clinical Densitometry endorse the use of FRAX (van den Bergh, 2010). NOF recommends using FRAX for postmenopausal women and men aged 50 years or older who are not on treatment, who have not had spine or hip fractures, and who have T-scores between −1.0 and −2.5 SD (NOF, 2014; van den Bergh, 2010). If the FRAX 10-year probability exceeds 20% for major osteoporotic fractures or 3% risk for hip fracture, NOF guidelines recommend drug treatment (NOF, 2014).

Increasing baseline FRAX 10-year probability was consistently associated with increased rates of incident fractures in a large cohort of HIV-infected adults (Battalora, 2014). Although FRAX may underestimate fracture risk in HIV-infected persons, EACS recommends FRAX screening in all persons older than age 40 years (EACS, 2015).

DUAL-ENERGY X-RAY ABSORPTIOMETRY

BMD measurements are widely obtained using DXA scan. Relevant measurement locations include the hip, spine, and forearm. DXA is a two-dimensional system in which the size of the specimen is directly proportional to the estimate of area density. Overestimation of BMD values obtained from larger patients is a concern (Amorosa, 2006a). Of greater concern is that DXA has not been validated for fractures among PLWH. Furthermore, fewer data exist on younger adults. Additional concerns are the application of WHO definitions for osteoporosis and osteopenia to populations and skeletal sites other than those serving as the basis for the DXA correlations on which these bone abnormality definitions are described (Amorosa, 2006b).

DXA is noninvasive and convenient, but it does not assess bone condition, bone structure, or bone quality, a factor directly linked to loadbearing strength (Ofotokun, 2011). It is suggested that DXA may underestimate fracture risk in HIV-infected persons (Ofotokun, 2011). In 2007, Nguyen and colleagues demonstrated that approximately 50% of postmenopausal women experiencing a fracture do not meet the clinical definition of osteoporosis based on DXA values (Ofotokun, 2011).

Other BMD measurement tools exist and assist in the prediction of fragility fracture risk but have inherent limitations. Quantitative CT scanning (QCT) detects volumetric density and in some clinical studies has been shown to detect a higher occurrence of osteoporosis and osteopenia (Pitukcheewanont, 2005). However, QCT costs more than DXA, requires a higher radiation dose, and is mainly used in research settings (Amorosa, 2006a). Other tools including quantitative ultrasound and analysis of biochemical and hormonal markers may prove increasingly useful in the future (Amorosa, 2006a).

NOF recommends DXA screening for osteoporosis in the general population of women aged 65 years or older and men aged 70 years or older, regardless of clinical risk factors (NOF, 2014). Postmenopausal women older than age 65 years, women in menopausal transition, and men aged 50–69 years with clinical risk factors for fracture should also be screened. Men and women aged 50 years or older who have had a fracture after age 50 years and for whom other risk factors, including rheumatoid arthritis or glucocorticoid use, are observed should be screened (NOF, 2014). NOF does not provide HIV-specific guidelines for DXA screening.

The Infectious Diseases Society of America recommends baseline DXA screening in HIV-infected postmenopausal women and men aged 50 years or older. Periodic monitoring of risk factors for premature bone loss is recommended thereafter (Aberg, 2014). Risk factors include White race, small body habitus, sedentary lifestyle, cigarette smoking, alcoholism, phenytoin therapy, corticosteroid therapy, hyperparathyroidism, vitamin D deficiency, thyroid disease, and hypogonadism (Aberg, 2014).

McComsey and colleagues recommend DXA screening in HIV-infected men and women aged 50 years or older because the majority of HIV-infected patients have an additional risk factor, and fracture data suggest that HIV and ART are linked to increased fracture risk (McComsey, 2010).

EACS recommends DXA screening for any patient with one or more of the following conditions, preferably prior to initiation of ART (EACS, 2015):

- Postmenopausal women
- Men aged 50 years or older
- History of low-impact fracture or high risk for falls
- Clinical hypogonadism
- Oral glucocorticoid use

TREATMENT

Treatment of low BMD is dependent on multiple factors, including the patient profile, risk factor reduction, and drug regimen adherence.

BEHAVIORAL AND LIFESTYLE ADVICE

Several lifestyle factors are associated with low BMD and/or fractures in the general population. Modification of diet to optimize calcium and vitamin D intake, increasing weightbearing exercise, and smoking cessation are prudent in general but especially among persons at increased risk of low BMD or fractures. In addition, because excess alcohol consumption (>3 units/daily) and substance dependency are associated with fracture risk, strategies to reduce consumption are reasonable.

IDENTIFY AND TREAT SECONDARY CAUSES OF LOW BONE MINERAL DENSITY

For persons with fragility fractures or T-scores ≤ 1, clinicians should evaluate and address secondary causes of osteoporosis, particularly in cases in which vitamin D deficiency or phosphate wasting are observed. These conditions can cause osteomalacia or bone mineralization deficiency, and they are difficult to differentiate from osteoporosis based on DXA scans (Yin, 2012).

VITAMIN D AND CALCIUM REPLACEMENT

Vitamin D deficiency is common among PLWH and may contribute to low BMD and/or fractures. Although there are no standardized guidelines for vitamin D and calcium replacement, IOM published a report brief in November 2010 (revised in March 2011) providing suggested Dietary Reference Intakes for calcium and vitamin D (IOM, 2011). It suggests 1000 mg of calcium daily for most adults aged 19–50 years and for men up to age 71 years. No more than 1200 mg of calcium per day is suggested for women older than age 50 years and for both men and women aged 71 years or older (IOM, 2011).

Assuming minimal sun exposure in geographic regions consisting of the United States and Canada, IOM suggests 600 IUs of vitamin D per day for most persons aged 1–70 years and 800 IUs for persons aged 71 years or older (IOM, 2011).

These recommendations are not specific to HIV-infected persons. However, it appears reasonable to monitor 25-hydroxyvitamin D levels in HIV-infected individuals and provide supplementation in situations of ART initiation and continued therapy (Overton, 2014; Yin, 2012).

TESTOSTERONE REPLACEMENT

Testosterone deficiency is common among men living with HIV and is associated with increased risk of low BMD in the general population. Clinicians should assess the risks and benefits of testosterone replacement in persons with low BMD and low testosterone levels.

PHARMACOLOGIC INTERVENTIONS

Currently, there are no specific guidelines for the treatment of BMD disorders among PLWH. Rather, the management of bone disease among the HIV population follows guidance from the general population. NOF recommends pharmacologic treatment of postmenopausal women and men aged 50 or older with hip or vertebral fractures or a T-score ≤-2.5 at the femoral neck or spine after evaluation to exclude secondary causes (NOF, 2014). In addition, patients with a T-score between -1.0 and -2.5 at the femoral neck or spine and 10-year probability fracture by FRAX $\geq3\%$ at the hip and $\geq20\%$ for any osteoporosis-related fracture should be considered for treatment (NOF, 2014).

Bisphosphonates are indicated for prevention and treatment of osteoporosis and other bone diseases, including Paget's disease (FDA, 2013). Bisphosphonates inhibit osteoclast resorption and have been shown to reduce vertebral and nonvertebral fractures by 25–50% in HIV-negative individuals.

The effectiveness of antiresorptive therapy in HIV-infected patients has been evaluated in six placebo-controlled randomized clinical trials. Five studies evaluated patients with T-scores not within the osteoporotic range (Bolland, 2007; Guaraldi, 2004; Huang, 2009; McComsey, 2007; Mondy, 2005), and one trial studied patients with T-scores <-2.5 (Rozenberg, 2012). Resulting data showed significant increases in BMD at the lumbar spine in all six studies and a large increase at the hip in three (Bolland, 2007; Huang, 2009; McComsey, 2007). The 2-year treatment trials (Bolland, 2007; Rozenberg, 2012) demonstrated the greatest change in BMD. Notably, an increase in BMD was detected in the placebo groups that were also given calcium and vitamin D.

Adverse effects of bisphosphonates include osteonecrosis of the jaw (<1 case per 100,000 person-years of exposure) and subtrochanteric fractures or atypical femoral shaft fractures (uncommon in patients with <5 years of treatment) (Yin, 2012). Thus, only patients with a strong indication for treatment should be administered bisphosphonates, and the FDA expert panel recommends treatment up to 5 years (Yin, 2012).

Other treatments for osteoporosis include teriparatide, which is a recombinant form of parathyroid hormone that stimulates osteoblasts and is used in patients who do not respond to bisphosphonates. However, no data exist on teriparatide's efficacy in HIV-infected individuals (Yin, 2012). Denosumab, a monoclonal RANKL antibody, blocks the RANKL/RANKL interaction but may increase the likelihood of infection (Yin, 2012). For this reason, more data are needed to determine the safety of denosumab in HIV-infected patients (NOF, 2014; Yin, 2012). Hormone replacement including estrogen and raloxifene for women may be appropriate in some cases; however, there exists a risk of cardiovascular side effects (Yin, 2012).

ROLE OF ANTIRETROVIRAL THERAPY SELECTION AND SWITCH

Because TDF is associated with greater initial loss of BMD compared to other ARVs, the DHHS HIV guidelines recommend the avoidance of TDF in patients with osteoporosis (DHHS, 2016). TAF, a new prodrug of tenofovir, is associated with less BMD loss compared to TDF in both initial and ART switch settings, and it may mitigate the BMD effect of TDF (Mills, 2016; Sax, 2014).

There are limited data on the efficacy of ART switch strategies. HIV clinicians may consider avoidance of TDF or ritonavir-boosted protease inhibitors in high-risk patients. Short-term studies showed that switching virologically suppressed patients to abacavir or raltegravir resulted in improvement in BMD compared to TDF (Haskelberg, 2012; Martin, 2009; Yin, 2012).

Recommended Reading

Battalora LA, Young B, Overton ET. Bones, fractures, antiretroviral therapy and HIV. *Curr Infect Dis Rep.* 2014 Feb; 16(2):393.

Bedimo R, Maalouf NM, Zhang S, et al. Osteoporotic fracture risk associated with cumulative exposure to tenofovir and other antiretroviral agents. *AIDS.* 2012; 26:825–831.

Brown TT, Hoy J, Borderi M, et al. Recommendations for evaluation and management of bone disease in HIV. *Clin Infect Dis.* 2015; 60:1242–1251.

Brown TT, McComsey GA, King MS, et al. Loss of bone mineral density after antiretroviral therapy initiation, independent of antiretroviral regimen. *J Acquir Immune Defic Syndr.* 2009; 51:554–561.

Brown TT, Qaqish RB. Antiretroviral therapy and the prevalence of osteopenia and osteoporosis: A meta-analytic review. *AIDS.* 2006; 20(17):2165–2174.

Maalouf NM, Zhang S, Drechsler H, et al. Hepatitis C co-infection and severity of liver disease as risk factor for osteoporotic fractures among HIV-infected patients. *J Bone Miner Res.* 2013; 28(12):2577–2583.

McComsey GA, Tebas P, Shane E, et al. Bone disease in HIV infection: A practical review and recommendations for HIV care providers. *Clin Infect Dis.* 2010 Oct 15; 51(8):937.

Triant VA, Brown TT, Lee H, et al. Fracture prevalence among human immunodeficiency virus (HIV) infected versus non-HIV-infected patients in a large U.S. healthcare system. *J Clin Endocrinol Metab.* 2008, 93(9):3499–3504.

Womack JA, Goulet JL, Gibert C, et al. Increased risk of fragility fractures among HIV-infected compared to uninfected male veterans. *PLoS One.* 2011; 6:e17217.

Yin MT, Shi Q, Hoover DR, et al. Fracture incidence in HIV-infected women: Results from the Women's Interagency HIV Study. *AIDS.* 2010; 24:2679–2686.

Young B, Dao CN, Buchacz K, et al.; HIV Outpatient Study (HOPS) Investigators. Increased rates of bone fracture among HIV-infected persons in the HIV Outpatient Study (HOPS) compared with the US general population, 2000–2006. *Clin Infect Dis.* 2011; 52:1061–1068.

References

Aberg JA, Gallant JE, Ghanem KG, et al. Primary care guidelines for the management of persons infected with HIV: 2013 update by the HIV Medicine Association of the Infectious Diseases Society of America. *Clin Infect Dis.* 2014 Jan; 58(1):e1–e34.

Ali MK, Magee MJ, Dave JA, et al. HIV and metabolic, body, and bone disorders: what we know from low- and middle-income countries. *J Acquir Immune Defic Syndr.* 2014 Sep 1; 67 Suppl 1:S27–S39.

Amorosa V, Tebas P. Bone disease and HIV infection. *Clin Infect Dis.* 2006a Jan 1; 42(1):108–114.

Amorosa V, Tebas P. Reply to Rojo and Ramos and to Vignolo et al. *Clin Infect Dis.* 2006b; 43(1):113–114.

Battalora L, Buchacz K, Armon C, et al. Low bone mineral density is associated with increased risk of incident fracture in HIV-infected adults. *Antivir Ther.* 2016; 21(1):45–54.

Battalora L, Buchacz K, Armon C, et al. New fracture risk and FRAX 10-year probability of fracture in HIV-infected adults. Presented at Poster Session P-Q5, Conference on Retroviruses and Opportunistic Infections (CROI), March 6, 2014, Boston, MA. Abstract 778.

Battalora LA, Young B, Overton ET. Bones, fractures, antiretroviral therapy and HIV. *Curr Infect Dis Rep.* 2014 Feb; 16(2):393.

Bedimo R, Maalouf NM, Zhang S, et al. Osteoporotic fracture risk associated with cumulative exposure to tenofovir and other antiretroviral agents. *AIDS.* 2012 Apr 24; 26(7):825–831.

Bolland MJ, Grey AB, Horne AM, et al. Annual zoledronate increases bone density in highly active antiretroviral therapy-treated human immunodeficiency virus-infected men: A randomized controlled trial. *J Clin Endocrinol Metab.* 2007 Apr; 92(4):1283–1288.

Brown TT, Hoy J, Borderi M, et al. Recommendations for evaluation and management of bone disease in HIV. *Clin Infect Dis.* 2015; 60:1242–1251.

Brown TT, McComsey GA, King MS, et al. Loss of bone mineral density after antiretroviral therapy initiation, independent of antiretroviral regimen. *J Acquir Immune Defic Syndr.* 2009; 51:554–561.

Brown TT, Qaqish RB. Antiretroviral therapy and the prevalence of osteoporosis and osteopenia: A meta-analytic review. *AIDS.* 2006 Nov 14; 20(17):2165–2174.

Childs K, Welz T, Samarawickrama A, et al. Effects of vitamin D deficiency and combination antiretroviral therapy on bone in HIV-positive patients. *AIDS.* 2012 Jan 28; 26(3):253–262.

Dave JA, Cohen K, Micklesfield LK, et al. Antiretroviral Therapy, Especially Efavirenz, Is Associated with Low Bone Mineral Density in HIV-Infected South Africans. *PLoS One.* 2015 Dec 3; 10(12):e0144286.

Duvivier C, Kolta S, Assoumou L, et al. Greater decrease in bone mineral density with protease inhibitor regimens compared with nonnucleoside reverse transcriptase inhibitor regimens in HIV-1 infected naïve patients. *AIDS.* 2009 Apr 27; 23(7):817–824.

Endocrine Society. Clinical guidelines—Evaluation, treatment and prevention of vitamin D deficiency: An Endocrine Society clinical practice guideline 2011. Available at http://press.endocrine.org/doi/pdf/10.1210/jc.2011-0385. Accessed December 14, 2015.

Escota GV, Mondy K, Bush T, et al.; the SUN Study Investigators. *AIDS Research and Human Retroviruses,* 2015. doi:10.1089/aid.2015.0158.

Escota GV, Mondy K, Bush T, et al. High Prevalence of Low Bone Mineral Density and Substantial Bone Loss over 4 Years Among HIV-infected Persons in the Era of Modern Antiretroviral Therapy. *AIDS Research and Human Retroviruses,* 2015.

European AIDS Clinical Society. Guidelines Version 8.0—October 2015 Available at http://www.eacsociety.org/guidelines/guidelines-archive/archive.html. Accessed December 14, 2015.

Guaraldi G, Orlando G, Madeddu G, et al. Alendronate reduces bone resorption in HIV-associated osteopenia/osteoporosis. *HIV Clin Trials.* 2004 Sep–Oct; 5(5):269–277.

Haskelberg H, Cordery DV, Amin J, et al. HLA alleles association with changes in bone mineral density in HIV-1-infected adults changing treatment to tenofovir–emtricitabine or abacavir–lamivudine. *PLoS One.* 2014 Mar 28; 9(3):e93333.

Haskelberg H, Hoy JF, Amin J, et al. Changes in bone turnover and bone loss in HIV-infected patients changing treatment to tenofovir–emtricitabine or abacavir–lamivudine. *PLoS One.* 2012; 7(6):e38377.

Hileman CO, Labbato DE, Storer NJ, et al. Is bone loss linked to chronic inflammation in antiretroviral-naïve HIV-infected adults? A 48-week matched cohort study. *AIDS.* 2014 Jul 31; 28(12):1759–1767.

Hoy J, Grund B, Roediger M, et al.; INSIGHT START Bone Mineral Density Substudy Group. Effects of immediate versus deferred initiation of antiretroviral therapy on bone mineral density: A substudy of the INSIGHT Strategic Timing of Antiretroviral Therapy (START) Study. Paper presented at the 15th European AIDS Conference and 17th International Workshop on Co-morbidities and Adverse Drug Reactions in HIV, Barcelona, Spain, October 21–24, 2015. Abstract ADRLH-62.

Huang J, Meixner L, Fernandez S, et al. A double-blinded, randomized controlled trial of zoledronate therapy for HIV-associated osteopenia and osteoporosis. *AIDS.* 2009 Jan 2; 23(1):51–57.

INSIGHT START Study Group. Initiation of antiretroviral therapy in early asymptomatic HIV infection. *N Engl J Med.* 2015; 373:795–807.

Institute of Medicine. Dietary reference intakes for calcium and vitamin D. Washington, DC: National Academies Press; 2011. Available at http://iom.nationalacademies.org/~/media/Files/Report%20Files/2010/Dietary-Reference-Intakes-for-Calcium-and-Vitamin-D/Vitamin%20D%20and%20Calcium%202010%20Report%20Brief.pdf. Accessed December 14, 2015.

Justice A, Falutz J. Aging and HIV: An evolving understanding. *Curr Opin HIV AIDS.* 2014 Jul; 9(4):291–293.

Kanis JA, on behalf of the World Health Organization Scientific Group. Assessment of osteoporosis at the primary health-care level. Technical Report. World Health Organization Collaborating Centre for Metabolic Bone Diseases, University of Sheffield, UK. 2007: Printed by the University of Sheffield. Available at https://www.shef.ac.uk/FRAX/pdfs/WHO_Technical_Report.pdf). Accessed December 14, 2015.

Looker AC, Wahner HW, Dunn WL, et al. Updated data on proximal femur bone mineral levels of US adults. *Osteoporosis Int.* 1998; 8:468–489.

Maalouf NM, Zhang S, Drechsler H, et al. Hepatitis C co-infection and severity of liver disease as risk factor for osteoporotic fractures among HIV-infected patients. *J Bone Miner Res.* 2013 Dec; 28(12):2577–2583.

Martin A, Bloch M, Amin J, et al. Simplification of antiretroviral therapy with tenofovir–emtricitabine or abacavir–lamivudine: A randomized, 96-week trial. *Clin Infect Dis.* 2009 Nov 15; 49(10):1591–1601.

McComsey GA, Kendall MA, Tebas P, et al. Alendronate with calcium and vitamin D supplementation is safe and effective for the treatment of decreased bone mineral density in HIV. *AIDS*. 2007 Nov 30; 21(18):2473–2482.

McComsey GA, Kitch D, Daar ES, et al. Bone mineral density and fractures in antiretroviral-naive persons randomized to receive abacavir–lamivudine or tenofovir disoproxil fumarate–emtricitabine along with efavirenz or atazanavir–ritonavir: Aids Clinical Trials Group A5224s, a substudy of ACTG A5202. *J Infect Dis*. 2011 Jun 15; 203(12):1791–1801.

McComsey GA, Tebas P, Shane E, et al. Bone disease in HIV infection: A practical review and recommendations for HIV care providers. *Clin Infect Dis*. 2010 Oct 15; 51(8):937–946.

Mills A, Arribas JR, Andrade-Villanueva J, et al. Switching from tenofovir disoproxil fumarate to tenofovir alafenamide in antiretroviral regimens for virologically suppressed adults with HIV-1 infection: A randomised, active-controlled, multicentre, open-label, phase 3, non-inferiority study. *Lancet Infect Dis*. 2016 Jan; 16(1):43–52.

Mondy K, Powderly WG, Claxton SA, et al. Alendronate, vitamin D, and calcium for the treatment of osteopenia/osteoporosis associated with HIV infection. *J Acquir Immune Defic Syndr*. 2005 Apr 1; 38(4):426–431.

National Osteoporosis Foundation. *Clinician's Guide to Prevention and Treatment of Osteoporosis*. Washington, DC: National Osteoporosis Foundation; 2014.

Ofotokun I, Weitzmann MN. HIV and bone metabolism. *Discov Med*. 2011 May; 11(60):385–393.

Orwoll ES, Klein RF. Osteoporosis in men. *Endocr Rev*. 1995 Feb; 16(1):87–116.

Overton ET, Chan E, Brown TT, et al. High-dose vitamin D and calcium attenuates bone loss with ART initiation: Results from ACTG A5280. Oral Abstract 133 presented at Session 0-10, Conference on Retroviruses and Opportunistic Infections (CROI), March 6, 2014, Boston, MA.

Pitukcheewanont P, Safani D, Church J, et al. Bone measures in HIV-1 infected children and adolescents: Disparity between quantitative computed tomography and dual-energy X-ray absorptiometry measurements. *Osteoporosis Int*. 2005 Nov; 16(11):1393–1396.

Rozenberg S, Lanoy E, Bentata M, et al. Effect of alendronate on HIV-associated osteoporosis: A randomized, double-blind, placebo-controlled, 96-week trial (ANRS 120). *AIDS Res Hum Retroviruses*. 2012 Sep; 28(9):972–980.

Sax PE, Zolopa A, Brar I, et al. Tenofovir alafenamide vs. tenofovir disoproxil fumarate in single tablet regimens for initial HIV-1 therapy: A randomized phase 2 study. *J AIDS*. 2014; 67(1):52–58.

Shiau S, Brown EC, Arpadi SM, et al. Incident fractures in HIV-infected individuals: A systematic review and meta-analysis. *AIDS*. 2013 Jul 31; 27(12):1949–1957.

Tebas P, Powderly WG, Claxton S, et al. Accelerated bone mineral loss in HIV-infected patients receiving potent antiretroviral therapy. *AIDS*. 2000 Mar 10; 14(4):F63–F67.

Triant VA, Brown TT, Lee H, et al. Fracture prevalence among human immunodeficiency virus (HIV)-infected versus non-HIV-infected patients in a large U.S. healthcare system. *J Clin Endocrinol Metab*. 2008 Sep; 93(9):3499–3504.

US Department of Health and Human Services, Panel on Antiretroviral Guidelines for Adults and Adolescents. Guidelines for the use of antiretroviral agents in HIV-1-infected adults and adolescents. Available at https://www.aidsinfo.nih.gov/ContentFiles/AdultandAdolescentGL.pdf. Accessed January 30, 2016.

US Food and Drug Administration. Bisphosphonates. August 15, 2013. Available at http://www.fda.gov/drugs/drugsafety/postmarketdrugsafetyinformationforpatientsandproviders/ucm124165.htm. Accessed December 14, 2015.

van den Bergh JP, van Geel TA, Lems WF, et al. Assessment of individual fracture risk: FRAX and beyond. *Curr Osteoporosis Rep*. 2010 Sep; 8(3):131–137.

van Vonderen MG, Lips P, van Agtmael MA, et al. First line zidovudine/lamivudine/lopinavir/ritonavir leads to greater bone loss compared to nevirapine/lopinavir/ritonavir. *AIDS*. 2009, Jul 17; 23(11):1367–1376.

Womack JA, Goulet JL, Gibert C, et al. Increased risk of fragility fractures among HIV infected compared to uninfected male veterans. *PloS One*. 2011; 6(2):e17217.

Woolf AD, Pfleger B. Burden of major musculoskeletal conditions. *Bull World Health Organization*. 2003; 81(9):646–656.

World Health Organization. WHO manual of diagnostic imaging. 2002. Available at http://apps.who.int/iris/bitstream/10665/42457/1/9241545550_eng.pdf. Accessed December 14, 2015.

World Health Organization. WHO Technical Report Series 843: Assessment of fracture risk and its application to screening for postmenopausal osteoporosis. Report of a WHO Study Group. *World Health Organ Tech Rep Ser*. 1994; 843:1–129. PMID: 7941614.

World Health Organization Metabolic Bone Disease Group. FRAX tool. 2008. Available at http://www.shef.ac.uk/FRAX. Accessed December 15, 2015.

Yin M. Bone loss in HIV: Virus, host or ART. Paper presented at the Conference on Retroviruses and Opportunistic Infections (CROI), March 5–8, 2012, Seattle, WA.

Yin MT, Overton ET. Increasing clarity on bone loss associated with antiretroviral initiation. *J Infect Dis*. 2011 Jun 15; 203(12):1705–1707.

Yin MT, Shi Q, Hoover DR, et al. Fracture incidence in HIV-infected women: Results from the Women's Interagency HIV Study. *AIDS*. 2010 Nov 13; 24(17):2679–2686.

Yin MT, Zhang CA, McMahon DJ, et al. Higher rates of bone loss in postmenopausal HIV-infected women: A longitudinal study. *J Clin Endocrinol Metab*. 2012 Feb; 97(2):554–562.

Young B, Dao CN, Buchacz K, et al. Increased rates of bone fracture among HIV-infected persons in the HIV Outpatient Study (HOPS) compared with the US general population, 2000–2006. *Clin Infect Dis* 2011 Apr 15; 52(8):1061–1068.

46.

HIV-ASSOCIATED LIPODYSTROPHY
AND LIPOATROPHY

Rajagopal V. Sekhar

LEARNING OBJECTIVE

Discuss the established and evolving science regarding the diagnosis and treatment of HIV-associated lipodystrophy and lipoatrophy.

WHAT'S NEW?

- HIV-associated lipodystrophy (HAL) is seen in children; for example, in a study of Indian children, lipodystrophy was observed in 33.7% of children, with lipoatrophy being the more common subtype, followed by lipohypertrophy.

- Although the utility of imaging modalities in the outpatient clinical setting is limited due to expense and availability, a study of patients on antiretroviral therapy (ART) that used dual-energy X-ray absorptiometry (DXA) for anthropometric measures proposed a fat mass ratio of 1.26, waist:thigh ratio of 1.74, and arm:trunk ratio of 2.08 to diagnose lipodystrophy.

KEY POINTS

- HIV is associated with abnormal fat distribution, which is termed lipodystrophy.

- HIV lipodystrophy can manifest as fat loss (lipoatrophy), fat gain (lipohypertrophy), or a mixed pattern.

- Therapeutic options are limited, and treatment is challenging.

- HIV lipodystrophy is associated with increased risk of developing cardiovascular disease and also fat accumulation in the liver.

For patients with HIV, the advent of ART has led to significant health benefits by reducing AIDS-related mortality and increasing life expectancy. Collateral benefits are improvement in nutritional status and a reduction in HIV-associated opportunistic infections. In parallel with these benefits, patients with HIV have also been seen to manifest unusual changes in body habitus that constitute variable combinations of peripheral fat loss (termed lipoatrophy), central fat accumulation (termed lipohypertrophy), and the condition known as HAL (Garcia-Viejo, 2001; Powderly, 2002).

Although the origins of HAL are unclear, several factors have been linked to it. Because better ART drug regimens have led to increased longevity, it is possible that the natural evolution of metabolic complications of HIV is unmasked as the lipodystrophic phenotype. The specific effects of antiretroviral medications have also been implicated, and the initial usage of ART in the 1990s was accompanied by multiple reports of abnormalities in body fat distribution variously termed the "protease paunch" and "crixivan belly," among others (Carr, 1998; Engelson, 1999; Herry, 1997; Lo, 1998; Massip, 1997; Miller, 1998). Other factors include immune phenomenon and effects mediated directly by the HIV virus. Despite intensive research to understand the mechanistic underpinnings of HIV lipodystrophy and lipoatrophy, the answers remain elusive (Bacchetti, 2005a,b; Safrin, 1999; Sattler, 2003; Tien, 2004).

LIPODYSTROPHY, LIPOHYPERTROPHY, AND LIPOATROPHY

Lipodystrophy is a broad term that collectively describes a variable combination of accumulation of fat in several regions, such as the abdomen (Engelson, 1999; Miller, 1998; Vigano, 2005; Yin, 2005), interscapular dorsocervical region (termed the "buffalo hump") (Lo, 1998; Roth, 1998; Torres, 1999), and the submental region (termed the "bull neck"), together with a simultaneous loss of fat from the limbs, face, and buttocks (Bacchetti, 2005a,b; Carr, 1998; Lichtenstein, 2003; Martin, 2005; Parruti, 2005). This "mixed" pattern of lipodystrophy incorporates a variable expression of both lipoatrophy (fat loss) and lipohypertrophy (fat gain). Other subtypes also exist, including generalized lipoatrophy and generalized obesity. These abnormalities in body habitus are often accompanied by distinct biochemical abnormalities, including dyslipidemia (mainly hypertriglyceridemia) and insulin resistance (Tsiodras, 2000; van der Valk, 2001). The US Cholesterol Education Program Adult Treatment Panel III (ATP III) defines metabolic syndrome to include three of the following five criteria: increased waist circumference (>102 cm men, >88 cm women), increased triglycerides (>150 ng/dl), reduced high-density lipoprotein cholesterol (HDL-C; <40 mg/dl men, <50 mg/dl women), high blood pressure (>130/>85 mmHg), and elevated fasting glucose (>110 mg/dl) (National Cholesterol Education Program, 2001). A study that evaluated HIV patients reported a 14% prevalence of metabolic syndrome by the International Diabetes Federation criteria and 18% by ATP III criteria (Samaras, 2007). In effect, the changes associated with HIV-associated lipodystrophy, especially with the "mixed" pattern, resemble an accelerated form of "metabolic syndrome."

DEFINITION AND PREVALENCE OF HAL

The initial description of HIV-associated lipodystrophy by Carr et al. in 1998 was followed by a flood of reports of HAL prevalence in the scientific community, but the prevalence varied widely due to the absence of a consensus case definition, leading to wide variations in the clinical diagnosis of HAL (Belloso, 2003). Therefore, it is important to have a standard and uniformly accepted "case definition" for HAL. The HIV Lipodystrophy Case Definition Study Group developed a statistical model for the diagnosis of lipodystrophy (including age, sex, duration of HIV infection, HIV disease stage, waist-to-hip ratio (WHR), anion gap, serum HDL-C concentration, trunk-to-peripheral fat ratio, percentage leg fat, and intra- and extra-abdominal fat ratio as variables), with a quantitative scale for identification (Carr 2003a,b). This model identified HIV lipodystrophy with a fair degree of accuracy, but it required multiple parameters that were not feasible or practical in a clinical outpatient setting. Thus, the field is still challenged by the lack of a standardized,

practical, clinically applicable, and relevant case definition for HIV lipodystrophy. The current practical approach appears to include identification by the treating physician of patients with central obesity, peripheral lipoatrophy, or both, together with evidence of dyslipidemia, insulin resistance, or both.

Despite these uncertainties, HIV infection is associated with an increased prevalence of lipodystrophy. One study reported increased prevalence of peripheral lipoatrophy in up to 90% of patients, abdominal obesity in 21%, and 10% of patients had a "mixed" form comprising both peripheral fat loss and central fat accumulation. Multiple additional studies have also reported an increased prevalence of central fat accumulation in HIV-infected patients (Bergersen, 2004; Bernasconi, 2002; Miller, 2002, 2003; Saint-Marc, 2000; Ward, 1999). When fat accumulation and fat loss were analyzed, it was found that the prevalence of fat accumulation was 56%, that of fat loss was 24%, and the mixed form occurred in 83% of patients infected with HIV (Safrin, 1999). More stringent analyses of the relative prevalence of the individual components of lipodystrophy have reported on average 45% central obesity, up to 62% for any lipodystrophy and 38% for peripheral lipoatrophy (Lichtenstein, 2004; Paparizos, 2000; Rozenbaum, 1999; Saves, 2002; Tien, 2004). Note that HAL is also seen in children; for example, in a study of Indian children, lipodystrophy was observed in 33.7% of children, with lipoatrophy being the most common subtype, followed by lipohypertrophy (Bhutia, 2014). These data confirm a significant presence of the lipodystrophic phenotype in the HIV-infected population. Because HAL per se is linked to an increased risk of metabolic complications, including cardiovascular disease, diabetes, and liver fat accumulation, it is important to understand the underlying contributory mechanisms.

MECHANISMS UNDERLYING THE DEVELOPMENT OF HAL

The notion of fat loss in some regions of the body concomitant with fat accumulation in other regions has led to questions of whether fat is reciprocally "redistributed" from one site to another. However, evidence to support this hypothesis is lacking, and a large cross-sectional study of HIV-infected and non-HIV patients did not find any correlation between changes in central and peripheral fat in HIV-infected men (Bacchetti, 2005a,b). These data suggest that in HIV, central fat accumulation and peripheral fat loss are independent of each other.

Several mechanistic studies using stable isotope tracer methodologies shed light on some of the fundamental biochemical defects underlying HIV (Reeds, 2003; Sekhar, 2002). It has been shown that HAL is associated with accelerated rates of adipocyte lipolysis. Although there is a significant increase in adipocyte reesterification, most of the fatty acids released by adipocyte lipolysis are released into the plasma. Oxidation of these plasma fatty acids is not increased, and therefore they are available for increased reesterification and accumulation in the liver. These fundamental defects may account for the phenotypic appearance of lipodystrophy, where lipoatrophy may be accounted for by the increased lipolysis, and lipohypertrophy in selected sites may be the result of increased adipocyte reesterification. In addition, the increased delivery of fatty acids to the liver raises the possibility of an increased risk of fatty liver disease, as discussed later in this chapter. The factors contributing to these metabolic defects are unclear, but antiretroviral drugs, immune phenomena, adipokines, and the HIV virus are involved.

CLINICAL IMPLICATIONS OF HAL

HIV patients with HAL have several clinical complications as a result of lipodystrophy. Abdominal obesity leads to the psychological discomfort of a potentially disfiguring condition (Persson, 2005; Turner, 2006) and to physical discomfort from abdominal obesity distension, umbilical herniation, and reflux disease (Miller, 2003). In addition, visceral fat accumulation is a known predictor of all-cause mortality in non-HIV-infected people (Kuk, 2006). In addition to the physical and psychological discomfort due to HAL, patients also have an elevated risk of developing increased insulin resistance, cardiovascular disease, and liver fat accumulation and fatty liver.

DYSLIPIDEMIA

The increased association with dyslipidemia is discussed in Chapter 47.

INSULIN RESISTANCE

Patients with HAL have an increased predisposition to insulin resistance. The contributing factors include antiretroviral drugs, lipotoxicity, immunocytokine factors, and hepatic steatosis. An estimated 30–90% of patients receiving protease inhibitor (PI) agents are insulin resistant, although the incidence of diabetes mellitus is less than 10% (van der Valk, 2001). Lipodystrophy (peripheral lipoatrophy and/or lipohypertrophy) and the presence of the dorsocervical fat pad or "buffalo hump" are linked to hyperinsulinemia and insulin resistance (Balasubramanyam, 2004; Calza, 2004; Hadigan, 2006; Miller, 1998). In addition, antiretroviral drugs also play a role in the development of insulin resistance in HIV. Drugs from the protease inhibitor class of agents predispose to insulin resistance by inhibiting the insulin-sensitive glucose transporter Glut4 (Mallon, 2005), and 35% of patients in a study were reported to have developed insulin resistance on PI therapy (Murata, 2002). PI drugs also predispose to impaired glucose tolerance and fasting hyperinsulinemia (Hadigan, 2001). Nucleoside reverse transcriptase inhibitor drugs, especially the thymidine analogs, also promote insulin resistance in HIV, induce lipotoxicity by disrupting mitochondrial oxidative phosphorylation, and cause defective mitochondrial fatty acid oxidation. Defective lipid kinetics together with impaired fat oxidation (Reeds, 2003; Sekhar, 2002, 2005;) promote accumulation of ectopic fat in critical metabolic sites of insulin action (e.g., liver and skeletal muscle), resulting in insulin resistance (Gan, 2002; Sutinen, 2002). Studies in rodents and humans have reported that correcting the deficiency of the endogenous antioxidant glutathione (GSH) significantly improves insulin sensitivity. One study used the gold standard hyperinsulinemic–euglycemic clamp to measure insulin sensitivity before and after GSH levels increased in HIV-infected patients and found a 32% improvement in insulin sensitivity within 2 weeks. HAL is associated with defects in adipocyte function that result in altered secretion of critical "adipokines" such as adiponectin. Deficiency of adiponectin is strongly linked to insulin resistance, and it also occurs in patients with HAL (Addy, 2003; Kim, 2007; Samaras, 2007).

CARDIOVASCULAR RISKS

Patients infected with HIV have an elevated risk of cardiovascular disease (d'Arminio, 2004; Friis-Moller, 2003) and acute myocardial infarction (Friis-Moller, 2007; Hadigan, 2003; Mary-Krause, 2003; Triant, 2007; Varriale, 2004). The mechanistic underpinnings of this increased risk are complex and involve a combination of factors, including adipocyte dysfunction, excessive lipolysis, hypertriglyceridemia, elevated low-density lipoprotein cholesterol (LDL-C) and decreased HDL-C, proatherogenic lipoprotein particle sizes with small dense LDL-C, postprandial lipemia, diabetes, adipokine, and immunokine factors (Sekhar, 2004).

SYSTEMIC STEATOSIS

There are reports of hepatic and intramyocellular fat accumulation in HAL. In HIV, fatty liver may be induced by a combination of factors, including co-infection with viral hepatitis, chronic inflammation, and metabolic defects in lipid cycling as described previously (Ristig, 2005). Interestingly, in patients with HAL, insulin resistance appears to be related to hepatic fat accumulation more than intra-abdominal fat accumulation (Sutinen, 2002). Excess circulating free fatty acids due to excessive lipolysis can be stored in other "ectopic" sites and contribute to systemic steatosis. An important site for fat deposition is skeletal muscle, and elevated levels of intramyocellular triglycerides have been reported in the soleus and tibialis anterior muscles (Luzi, 2003). An important consequence of increased myocellular fat is the development of insulin resistance in these patients.

ECTOPIC FAT ACCUMULATION

In patients with HAL, ectopic fat accumulation occurs in the interscapular dorsocervical "buffalo hump" area and the submental "bull neck" area (Lo, 1998). Such patterns of ectopic fat accumulation predispose to other co-morbidities, such as obstructive sleep apnea, limited neck motion, and neck and back discomfort (Gold, 2005; Reynolds, 2006).

METABOLIC SYNDROME

Not surprisingly, the combination of the previously discussed defects has led to an increase in metabolic syndrome in these patients. A study of HIV-positive Hispanic patients found that the presence of lipodystrophy was associated with a higher prevalence of metabolic syndrome (69%) compared to that for nonlipodystrophic patients (39%) (Ramirez-Marrero, 2014).

DIAGNOSING HAL

The clinical diagnosis of HAL is based on multiple approaches, including self-reporting, use of questionnaires, clinical scales with scores, anthropometric formulas, and radiographic techniques. Standard anthropometric tests have the advantage of being readily available to clinicians (Schwenk, 2001, 2002). Computed tomography, magnetic resonance imaging, and dual-energy X-ray absorptiometry (DXA) scans provide quantifiable data on the location and mass of visceral fat and subcutaneous adipose tissue (Schambelan, 2002) and subcutaneous limb fat (Cavalcanti, 2005). However, the usefulness of these imaging modalities in the outpatient clinical setting is limited due to considerable expense, limited availability, radiation exposure, and dependence on single-slice data instead of whole-body studies. Therefore, they are impractical for use in routine clinical practice. A study of 100 patients on ART used DXA scan for anthropometric measures and proposed a fat mass ratio of 1.26, waist:thigh ratio of 1.74, and arm:trunk ratio of 2.08 to diagnose lipodystrophy (Beraldo, 2015). Routine measurement of waist circumference and/or WHR may be helpful and is recommended for all patients.

TREATMENT OF HAL PHENOTYPE

Currently, there is no single therapy for all of the components of HAL. Medical management has included trials of underlying pathophysiological defects, including the use of thiazolidinedione drugs to increase fat deposition in lipodystrophic sites. Although data from clinical studies are conflicting (Carr, 2004; Hadigan, 2004; Sutinen, 2003), a small stable isotope-based study examining the interplay of kinetic factors suggested that rosiglitazone usage increased fat deposition, but this benefit was offset by elevated rates of lipolysis and the inability of adipocytes to retain triglycerides (Sekhar, 2011). Growth hormone (GH) has been used in an attempt to lower abdominal fat, but doses used were supraphysiological. Using GH at a physiological dose resulted in a decrease in lipolysis (D'Amico, 2006), and newer approaches using combinations of thiazolidinedione and GH could be useful and should be studied. The GH analog tesamorelin has been shown to have benefits in lowering central fat and improving dyslipidemia (Falutz, 2007).

Surgical treatment of excess fat accumulation has been attempted with liposuction, but long-term success is limited by the tendency of fat to reaccumulate. Facial lipoatrophy has been treated with lipofilling with autologous fat transfer (Uzzan, 2012), and polyalkylimide gel (De Santis, 2012) and other artificial fillers including silicone have been tried with psychological improvement in body image perception (Mori, 2006). The treatment of dyslipidemia, insulin resistance, and other complications is discussed elsewhere in this book.

CONCLUSION

HIV infection is associated with an increased prevalence of lipodystrophy and lipoatrophy. These changes in body morphology are complicated by physical symptoms due to the nature of fat accumulation, psychological discomfort due to abnormal body image perception, and metabolic complications such as dyslipidemia and insulin resistance with an increased risk of cardiovascular disease and fatty liver. Urgent therapies are needed for all these complications, and therapeutic options are limited. There is a critical need for further research to find effective therapies for HAL.

References

Addy, C.L., Gavrila, A., Tsiodras, S., et al. Hypoadiponectinemia is associated with insulin resistance, hypertriglyceridemia, and fat redistribution in human immunodeficiency virus-infected patients treated with highly active antiretroviral therapy. *J Clin Endocrinol Metab*. 2003; 88:627–636.

Bacchetti, P., Gripshover, B., Grunfeld, C., et al.; Study of Fat Redistribution and Metabolic Change in HIV Infection (FRAM). Fat distribution in men with HIV infection. *J Acquir Immune Defic Syndr*. 2005a; 40(2):121–131.

Bacchetti, P., Gripshover, B., Grunfeld, C., et al. Fat distribution in men with HIV infection. *J Acquir Immune Defic Syndr*. 2005b; 40:121–131.

Balasubramanyam, A., Sekhar, R.V., Jahoor, F., et al. Pathophysiology of dyslipidemia and increased cardiovascular risk in HIV lipodystrophy: A model of "systemic steatosis." *Curr Opin Lipidol*. 2004; 15:59–67.

Belloso, W.H., Quiros, R.E., Ivalo, S.A., et al. Agreement analysis of variables involved in lipodystrophy syndrome definition in HIV-infected patients. *J Acquir Immune Defic Syndr*. 2003; 32:104–111.

Beraldo, R.A., Vassimon, H.S., Aragon, D.C., et al. Proposed ratios and cutoffs for the assessment of lipodystrophy in HIV-seropositive individuals. *Eur J Clin Nutr*. 2015 Feb; 69(2):274–278.

Bergersen, B.M., Sandvik, L., Bruun, J.N. Body composition changes in 308 Norwegian HIV-positive patients. *Scand J Infect Dis*. 2004; 36:186–191.

Bernasconi, E., Boubaker, K., Junghans, C., et al. Abnormalities of body fat distribution in HIV-infected persons treated with antiretroviral drugs: The Swiss HIV Cohort Study. *J Acquir Immune Defic Syndr*. 2002; 31:50–55.

Bhutia, E., Hemal, A., Yadav, T.P., et al. Lipodystrophy syndrome among HIV infected children on highly active antiretroviral therapy in northern India. *Afr Health Sci*. 2014 Jun; 14(2):408–413.

Calza, L., Manfredi, R., Chiodo, F. Insulin resistance and diabetes mellitus in HIV infected patients receiving antiretroviral therapy. *Metab Syndr Relat Disord*. 2004; 2:241–250.

Carr, A., Emery, S., Law, M., et al. An objective case definition of lipodystrophy in HIV-infected adults: A case–control study. *Lancet*. 2003a; 361:726–735.

Carr, A., Law, M. An objective lipodystrophy severity grading scale derived from the lipodystrophy case definition score. *J Acquir Immune Defic Syndr*. 2003b; 33:571–576.

Carr, A., Samaras, K., Burton, S., et al. A syndrome of peripheral lipodystrophy, hyperlipidaemia and insulin resistance in patients receiving HIV protease inhibitors. *AIDS*. 1998: 12:F51–F58.

Carr, A., Workman, C., Carey, D., et al. No effect of rosiglitazone for treatment of HIV-1: Randomised, double-blind, placebo-controlled trial. *Lancet*. 2004; 363(9407):429–438.

Cavalcanti, R.B., Cheung, A.M., Raboud, J., et al. Reproducibility of DXA estimations of body fat in HIV lipodystrophy: Implications for clinical research. *J Clin Densitom*. 2005; 8:293–297.

D'Amico, S., Shi, J., Sekhar, R.V., et al. Physiologic growth hormone replacement improves fasting lipid kinetics in patients with HIV lipodystrophy syndrome. *Am J Clin Nutr*. 2006; 84(1):204–211.

d'Arminio, A., Sabin, C.A., Phillips, A.N., et al. Cardio- and cerebrovascular events in HIV-infected persons. *AIDS*. 2004; 18(13):1811–1817.

De Santis, G., Pignatti, M., Baccarani, A., et al. Long-term efficacy and safety of polyacrylamide hydrogel injection in the treatment of human immunodeficiency virus-related facial lipoatrophy: A 5-year follow-up. *Plastic Reconstruct Surg*. 2012; 129(1):101–109.

Engelson, E.S., Kotler, D.P., Tan, Y., et al. Fat distribution in HIV-infected patients reporting truncal enlargement quantified by whole-body magnetic resonance imaging. *Am J Clin Nutr*. 1999; 69:1162–1169.

Falutz, J., Allas, S., Blot, K., et al. Metabolic effects of a growth hormone-releasing factor in patients with HIV. *N Engl J Med*. 2007; 357(23):2359–2370.

Friis-Moller, N., Reiss, P., Sabin, C.A., et al. Class of antiretroviral drugs and the risk of myocardial infarction. *New Engl J Med*. 2007; 356:1723–1735.

Friis-Moller, N., Weber, R., Reiss, P., et al. Cardiovascular disease risk factors in HIV patients—Association with antiretroviral therapy. Results from the D:A:D study. *AIDS*. 2003; 17(8):1179–1193.

Gan, S.K., Samaras, K., Thompson, C.H., et al. Altered myocellular and abdominal fat partitioning predict disturbance in insulin action in HIV protease inhibitor-related lipodystrophy. *Diabetes*. 2002; 51:3163–3169.

Garcia-Viejo, M.A., Ruiz, M., Martinez, E. Strategies for treating HIV-related lipodystrophy. *Expert Opin Invest Drugs*. 2001; 10:1443–1456.

Gold, D.R., Annino, D.J., Jr. HIV-associated cervicodorsal lipodystrophy: Etiology and management. *Laryngoscope*. 2005; 115:791–795.

Hadigan, C., Kamin, D., Liebau, J., et al. Depot-specific regulation of glucose uptake and insulin sensitivity in HIV-lipodystrophy. *Am J Physiol Endocrinol Metab*. 2006; 290:E289–E298.

Hadigan, C., Meigs, J.B., Corcoran, C., et al. Metabolic abnormalities and cardiovascular disease risk factors in adults with human immunodeficiency virus infection and lipodystrophy. *Clin Infect Dis*. 2001; 32:130–139.

Hadigan, C., Meigs, J.B., Wilson, P.W., et al. Prediction of coronary heart disease risk in HIV-infected patients with fat redistribution. *Clin Infect Dis*. 2003; 36:909–916.

Hadigan, C., Yawetz, S., Thomas, A., et al. Metabolic effects of rosiglitazone in HIV lipodystrophy: A randomized, controlled trial. *Ann Intern Med*. 2004; 140(10):786–794.

Herry, I., Bernand, L., de Truchis, P., et al. Hypertrophy of the breasts in a patient treated with indinavir. *Clin Infect Dis*. 1997; 25:937–938.

Kim, R.J., Carlow, D.C., Rutstein, J.H., et al. Hypoadiponectinemia, dyslipidemia, and impaired growth in children with HIV-associated facial lipoatrophy. *J Pediatr Endocrinol Metab*. 2007; 20:65–74.

Kuk, J.L., Katzmarzyk, P.T., Nichaman, M.Z., et al. Visceral fat is an independent predictor of all-cause mortality in men. *Obesity (Silver Spring)*. 2006; 14:336–341.

Lichtenstein, K., Wanke, C., Henry, K., et al. Estimated prevalence of HIV-associated adipose redistribution syndrome (HARS)—Abnormal abdominal fat accumulation in HIV-infected patients. *Antiviral Ther*. 2004; 9:L33.

Lichtenstein, K.A., Delaney, K.M., Armon, C., et al. Incidence of and risk factors for lipoatrophy (abnormal fat loss) in ambulatory HIV-1-infected patients. *J Acquir Immune Defic Syndr*. 2003; 32:48–56.

Lo, J.C., Mulligan, K., Tai, V.W., et al. "Buffalo hump" in men with HIV-1 infection. *Lancet*. 1998; 351:867–870.

Luzi, L., Perseghin, G., Tambussi, G., et al. Intramyocellular lipid accumulation and reduced whole body lipid oxidation in HIV lipodystrophy. *Am J Physiol Endocrinol Metab*. 2003; 284:E274–E280.

Mallon, P.W., Wand, H., Law, M., et al.; HIV Lipodystrophy Case Definition Study; Australian Lipodystrophy Prevalence Survey Investigators. Buffalo hump seen in HIV-associated lipodystrophy is associated with hyperinsulinemia but not dyslipidemia. *J Acquir Immune Defic Syndr*. 2005; 38:156–162.

Martin, A., Mallon, P.W. Therapeutic approaches to combating lipoatrophy: Do they work? *J Antimicrob Chemother*. 2005; 55:612–615.

Mary-Krause, M., Cotte, L., Simon, A., et al. Increased risk of myocardial infarction with duration of protease inhibitor therapy in HIV-infected men. *AIDS*. 2003; 17(17):2479–2486.

Massip, P., Marchou, B., Bonnet, E., et al. Lipodystrophia with protease inhibitors in HIV patients. *Thérapie*. 1997; 52:615.

Miller, J., Brown, D., Amin, J., et al. A randomized, double-blind study of gemfibrozil for the treatment of protease inhibitor-associated hyper-triglyceridemia. *AIDS*. 2002; 16:2195–2200.

Miller, J., Carr, A., Emery, S., et al. HIV lipodystrophy: Prevalence, severity and correlates of risk in Australia. *HIV Med*. 2003; 4:293–301.

Miller, K.D., Jones, E., Yanovski, J.A., et al. Visceral abdominal-fat accumulation associated with use of indinavir. *Lancet*. 1998; 351:871–875.

Mori, A., Lo Russo, G., Agostini, T., et al. Treatment of human immunodeficiency virus-associated facial lipoatrophy with lipofilling and submalar silicone implants. *J Plastic Reconstruct Aesthetic Surg*. 2006; 59(11):1209–1216.

Murata, H., Hruz, P.W., Mueckler, M. Indinavir inhibits the glucose transporter isoform Glut4 at physiologic concentrations. *AIDS*. 2002; 16:859–863.

National Cholesterol Education Program. Executive summary of the third report of the National Cholesterol Education Program (NCEP) Expert Panel on Detection, Evaluation, and Treatment of High Blood Cholesterol in Adults (Adult Treatment Panel III). *JAMA*. 2001; 285:2486–2497.

Paparizos, V.A., Kyriakis, K.P., Polydorou-Pfandl, D., et al. Epidemiologic characteristics of Koebner's phenomenon in AIDS-related Kaposi's sarcoma. *J Acquir Immune Defic Syndr*. 2000; 25:283–284.

Parruti, G., Toro, G.M. Persistence of lipoatrophy after a four year long interruption of antiretroviral therapy for HIV1 infection: Case report. *BMC Infect Dis*. 2005; 5:80.

Persson, A. Facing HIV: Body shape change and the (in)visibility of illness. *Med Anthropol*. 2005; 24:237–264.

Powderly, W.G. Long-term exposure to lifelong therapies. *J Acquir Immune Defic Syndr*. 2002; 29(1):S28–S40.

Ramírez-Marrero, F.A., Santana-Bagur, J.L., Joyner, M.J., et al. Metabolic syndrome in relation to cardiorespiratory fitness, active and sedentary behavior in HIV+ Hispanics with and without lipodystrophy. *P R Health Sci J*. 2014 Dec; 33(4):163–169

Reeds, D.N., Mittendorfer, B., Patterson, B.W., et al. Alterations in lipid kinetics in men with HIV-dyslipidemia. *Am J Physiol Endocrinol Metab*. 2003; 285:E490–E497.

Reynolds, N.R., Neidig, J.L., Wu, A.W., et al. Balancing disfigurement and fear of disease progression: Patient perceptions of HIV body fat redistribution. *AIDS Care*. 2006; 18:663–673.

Ristig, M., Drechsler, H., Powderly, W.G. Hepatic steatosis and HIV infection. *AIDS Patient Care STDs*. 2005; 19:356–365.

Roth, V.R., Kravcik, S., Angel, J.B. Development of cervical fat pads following therapy with human immunodeficiency virus type 1 protease inhibitors. *Clin Infect Dis*. 1998; 27:65–67.

Rozenbaum, W., Gharakhanian, S., Salhi, Y., et al. Clinical and laboratory characteristics of lipodystrophy in a French cohort of HIV-infected patients treated with protease inhibitors. *Antiviral Ther*. 1999; 4(2):L34.

Safrin, S., Grunfeld, C. Fat distribution and metabolic changes in patients with HIV infection. *AIDS*. 1999; 13:2493–2505.

Saint-Marc, T., Partisani, M., Poizot-Martin, I., et al. Fat distribution evaluated by computed tomography and metabolic abnormalities in patients undergoing antiretroviral therapy: Preliminary results of the LIPOCO study. *AIDS*. 2000; 14:37–49.

Samaras, K., Wand, H., Law, M., et al. Prevalence of metabolic syndrome in HIV-infected patients receiving highly active antiretroviral therapy using International Diabetes Foundation and Adult Treatment Panel III Criteria: Associations with insulin resistance, disturbed body fat compartmentalization, elevated C-reactive peptide, and hypoadiponectinemia. *Diabetes Care*. 2007; 30:113–119.

Sattler, F. Body habitus changes related to lipodystrophy. *Clin Infect Dis*. 2003; 36:S84–S90.

Saves, M., Raffi, F., Capeau, J., et al. Factors related to lipodystrophy and metabolic alterations in patients with human immunodeficiency virus infection receiving highly active antiretroviral therapy. *Clin Infect Dis*. 2002; 34:1396–1405.

Schambelan, M., Benson, C.A., Carr, A., et al. Management of metabolic complications associated with antiretroviral therapy for HIV-1 infection: Recommendations of an International AIDS Society–USA panel. *J Acquir Immune Defic Syndr*. 2002; 31:257–275.

Schwenk, A. Methods of assessing body shape and composition in HIV-associated lipodystrophy. *Curr Opin Infect Dis*. 2002; 15:9–16.

Schwenk, A., Breuer, P., Kremer, G., et al. Clinical assessment of HIV-associated lipodystrophy syndrome: Bioelectrical impedance analysis, anthropometry and clinical scores. *Clin Nutr*. 2001; 20:243–249.

Sekhar, R.V., Jahoor, F., Pownall, H.J., et al. Cardiovascular implications of HIV-associated dyslipidemic lipodystrophy. *Curr Atheroscler Rep*. 2004; 6(3):173–179.

Sekhar, R.V., Jahoor, F., Pownall, H.J., et al. Severely dysregulated disposal of postprandial triacylglycerols exacerbates hypertriacylglycerolemia in HIV lipodystrophy syndrome. *Am J Clin Nutr*. 2005; 81:1405–1410.

Sekhar, R.V., Jahoor, F., White, A.C., et al. Metabolic basis of HIV lipodystrophy syndrome. *Am J Physiol Endocrinol Metab*. 2002; 283:E332–E337.

Sekhar, R.V., Patel, S.G., D'Amico, S., et al. Effects of rosiglitazone on abnormal lipid kinetics in HIV-associated dyslipidemic lipodystrophy: A stable isotope study. *Metabolism*. 2011; 60(6):754–760.

Sutinen, J., Hakkinen, A.M., Westerbacka, J., et al. Increased fat accumulation in the liver in HIV-infected patients with antiretroviral therapy-associated lipodystrophy. *AIDS*. 2002; 16:2183–2193.

Sutinen, J., Hakkinen, A.M., Westerbacka, J., et al. Rosiglitazone in the treatment of HAART-associated lipodystrophy: A randomized double-blind placebo-controlled study. *Antiviral Ther*. 2003; 8(3):199–207.

Tien, P.C., Grunfeld, C. What is HIV-associated lipodystrophy? Defining fat distribution changes in HIV infection. *Curr Opin Infect Dis*. 2004; 17:27–32.

Torres, R.A., Unger, K.W., Cadman, J.A., et al. Recombinant human growth hormone improves truncal adiposity and "buffalo humps" in HIV-positive patients on HAART. *AIDS*. 1999; 13:2479–2481.

Triant, V.A., Lee, H., Hadigan, C., et al. Increased acute myocardial infarction rates and cardiovascular risk factors among patients with HIV disease. *J Clin Endocrinol Metab*. 2007; 92:2506–2512.

Tsiodras, S., Mantzoros, C., Hammer, S., et al. Effects of protease inhibitors on hyperglycemia, hyperlipidemia, and lipodystrophy: A 5-year cohort study. *Arch Intern Med*. 2000; 160:2050–2056.

Turner, R., Testa, M.A., Su, M., et al. The impact of HIV-associated adipose redistribution syndrome (HARS) on health-related quality of life. *Antiviral Ther*. 2006; 11:L25.

Uzzan, C., Boccara, D., Lacheré, A., et al. Treatment of facial lipoatrophy by lipofilling in HIV infected patients: Retrospective study on 317 patients on 9 years. *Ann Chir Plast Esthet*. 2012, 57(3):210–216.

van der Valk, M., Bisschop, P.H., Romijn, J.A. Lipodystrophy in HIV-1-positive patients is associated with insulin resistance in multiple metabolic pathways. *AIDS*. 2001; 15:2093–2100.

Varriale, P., Saravi, G., Hernandez, E., et al. Acute myocardial infarction in patients infected with human immunodeficiency virus. *Am Heart J*. 2004; 147(1):55–59.

Vigano, A., Mora, S., Manzoni, P., et al. Effects of recombinant growth hormone on visceral fat accumulation: Pilot study in human immunodeficiency virus-infected adolescents. *J Clin Endocrinol Metab*. 2005; 90:4075–4080.

Ward, D.J., Delaney, K.M., Moorman, A.C., et al. Description of lipodystrophy in the HIV Outpatient Study (HOPS). *Antiviral Ther*. 1999; 4(2).

Yin, M.T., Glesby, M.J. Recombinant human growth hormone therapy in HIV-associated wasting and visceral adiposity. *Expert Rev Anti-Infect Ther*. 2005; 3:727–738.

47.

DYSLIPIDEMIA

Rajagopal V. Sekhar

Patients infected with HIV often develop dyslipidemia. Although lipid abnormalities have been described in HIV-infected patients from the pre-combination antiretroviral therapy (ART) era, they are most striking in patients treated with antiretroviral drugs and may even be present in those not exposed to these drugs (Fourie, 2010; Madge, 1999; Young, 2005).

The dyslipidemic profile in HIV includes abnormalities in lipids and lipoprotein, including hypertriglyceridemia, elevated plasma total LDL-C concentrations, and low levels of HDL-C. Many patients also have the phenotypic appearance of lipodystrophy, with a variable combination of centripetal fat accumulation. The consequence of an abnormal dyslipidemic profile in the HIV lipodystrophic patient is an accelerated risk of developing myocardial infarction, cardiovascular disease, nonalcoholic fatty liver disease, and type 2 diabetes (Crum-Cianflone, 2009; De Wit, 2008; Worm, 2010). Despite the urgent and aggressive treatment of dyslipidemia in these patients, effective lipid control is not achieved due to coexisting viral hepatitis and other hepatic pathologies associated with liver dysfunction that limit the use of standard lipid-lowering agents such as statin or fibrate drugs. In addition, due to drug interactions with antiretroviral agents, several drugs of the statin class are either contraindicated or restricted to lower doses (Dube, 2003; Hulgan, 2005). The use of statin drugs is also limited by a US Food and Drug Administration (FDA) advisory linking the use of these drugs to an increased risk of hyperglycemia. Furthermore, the presence of central obesity, insulin resistance, metabolic syndrome, and diabetes in this population increases the risk of dyslipidemia. The 2013 American College of Cardiology/American Heart Association (ACC/AHA) guidelines recommend the initiation of statins for primary and secondary prevention. However, there are no specific recommendations for HIV-infected patients, in whom there is a higher risk of developing coronary disease. Age is an important factor in the ACC/AHA guidelines, but HIV patients are recognized to have accelerated aging, and there are no studies to identify whether this translates to greater cardiovascular risk and what should be the treatment objectives. For these reasons, applying these guidelines to the treatment of dyslipidemia in

HIV patients has proven challenging. Thus, understanding the fundamental pathophysiology underlying dyslipidemia in HIV is important to improve clinical and therapeutic success in treating HIV-associated dyslipidemia.

MECHANISMS CONTRIBUTING TO DYSLIPIDEMIA IN HIV

NONESTERIFIED FATTY ACIDS AND TRIGLYCERIDES

Elevations in fasted triglyceride concentrations are very commonly seen in HIV-infected patients. The two important contributors to plasma triglyceride concentrations are chylomicrons (CMs) and very low-density lipoprotein (VLDL). CMs typically indicate the contribution of dietary fat, whereas VLDL-TG indicates hepatic triglyceride (TG) from de novo synthesis and recirculation of plasma free fatty acid. The mechanistic origins of triglyceride elevation are complex, and studies have shown abnormalities in the cycling of nonesterified fatty acids (NEFA) in the fasted and fed states (Reeds, 2003; Sekhar, 2002, 2005; Ware, 2002). In the fasted state, HIV-infected patients have an abnormally high rate of triglyceride lipolysis, resulting in an increased rate of release of NEFA into the plasma (Reeds, 2003; Sekhar, 2002). The increased lipolysis is associated with a futile cycle of intra-adipocyte reesterification, but a greater proportion of NEFA released by adipocyte lipolysis is released into the plasma. Despite an increased availability of NEFA, there is a lack of corresponding increase in plasma NEFA oxidation, suggesting a mitochondrial defect, and this results in elevated plasma NEFA concentrations in HIV-infected patients with lipodystrophy. Therefore, there is an increased "delivery" of NEFA to the liver, where it is a substrate available for increased hepatic reesterification into triglycerides and exported via VLDL back into plasma. It is important to note that in the fasted state most of the measured triglyceride concentrations reflect VLDL-TG, which is why fasting is necessary when the Friedewald equation is used for reporting lipid results.

HIV could be implicated in abnormalities of lipolysis. In a recent study, the role of the HIV viral protein vpr on lipolysis was investigated in transgenic mice overexpressing vpr as well as the exogenous effect of vpr infusion in wild-type mice. The results showed that exposure to vpr in both approaches led to significantly increased rates of lipolysis (Agarwal, 2013). Results from this study suggest an increased complexity for disorders of lipid kinetics in HIV that extends beyond the contribution of antiretroviral drugs. Although these mechanisms contribute to hypertriglyceridemia, they still do not fully account for the magnitude of elevated triglyceride concentrations in plasma, suggesting the presence of additional defects. A second defect exists in impaired clearance and disposal of dietary triglycerides from plasma. After a 12-hour overnight fast, HIV-infected patients had a sixfold elevation in chylomicron–triglyceride concentrations compared to matched non-HIV-infected controls, indicating a marked impairment of disposal of dietary fat from a previous meal (Ware, 2002; Sekhar, 2005). When the absorption and disposal of an orally fed triglyceride tracer labeled with palmitate were followed, it was seen that HIV-infected patients had poor disposal of palmitate from the chylomicron pool, and a greater proportion of the disposed palmitate tracer was found in the plasma. These defects likely occur due to blunted action of the adipose tissue lipoprotein lipase and defective entrapment of hydrolyzed NEFA in adipocytes (Sekhar, 2005; Ware, 2002).

In summary, a combination of increased adipocyte lipolysis, impaired oxidation of plasma NEFA, and diminished clearance of VLDL-TG in the fasted state, together with defective disposal of diet-derived chylomicron-TG in the fed state, contributes to the marked hypertriglyceridemia and increased plasma NEFA concentrations in HIV-infected patients with dyslipidemia. It is unclear whether these defects occur due to factors related to the HIV virus, to the immune/inflammatory responses associated with HIV infection, or to ART. There is evidence to support the role of the protease inhibitor (PI) ritonavir in promoting hypertriglyceridemia by increasing lipolysis (Periard, 1999) and VLDL synthesis (Purnell, 2000). From a clinical standpoint, the PI drugs are the class most frequently associated with hypertriglyceridemia (Behrens, 1999; Carr, 1999; Friis-Moller, 2003; Mulligan, 2000; Periard, 1999). For example, saquinavir, ritonavir, and nelfinavir have been associated with hypertriglyceridemia, whereas amprenavir is not as strongly associated. Altering antiretroviral regimes may be used to lower hypertriglyceridemia; for example, switching patients taking any of the previously mentioned agents to an atazanavir-based regimen led to a 46% decrease in triglyceride concentrations (Mobius, 2005).

LOW-DENSITY LIPOPROTEIN CHOLESTEROL

Elevated levels of total and LDL cholesterol are frequently seen in patients with HIV, and the incidence of new-onset hypercholesterolemia in these patients has been reported to be 24% (Tsiodras, 2000). Of the antiretroviral drugs, the PI class is closely associated with increased incidence of hypercholesterolemia as a single (60%) or dual (15%) PI-based regimen (Fellay, 2001). When otherwise healthy adult subjects without HIV took the PI drug ritonavir for 2 weeks, this resulted in elevated concentrations of plasma VLDL cholesterol, intermediate-density lipoprotein cholesterol, and apolipoprotein B (Bianchi, 2010) and a decrease in HDL-C levels (Friss-Moller, 2003). There are also differences in the potential of individual drugs to provoke hypercholesterolemia. For example, the PI agent ritonavir increased the risk of hypercholesterolemia 20-fold, but this declined to 9-fold with nelfinavir and 4-fold with indinavir (Periard, 1999). Discontinuation of antiretroviral drugs did not fully normalize the elevated cholesterol levels (Hatano, 2000), highlighting the fact that the specific mechanisms by which PI drugs promote abnormal LDL-C metabolism are still not fully understood.

In addition to the PI agents, other antiretroviral agents also contribute to hypercholesterolemia in HIV. The thymidine nucleoside reverse transcriptase inhibitor (NRTI) drugs are associated with dyslipidemia, with stavudine exerting a greater effect than zidovudine. The combination of stavudine with PI drugs is also known to significantly worsen dyslipidemia (van der Valk, 2001). In addition, combinations of two NRTI drugs with either a non-nucleoside reverse transcriptase inhibitor (NNRTI) agent or a PI drug significantly worsened hypercholesterolemia (Jones, 2005).

HIGH-DENSITY LIPOPROTEIN CHOLESTEROL

HIV-infected patients are known to have decreased concentrations of HDL-C, and lower levels of HDL particles have been shown to identify HIV-infected patients at increased risk of cardiovascular disease independent of other cardiovascular risk factors (Duprez, 2009). This was present in HIV-infected patients even prior to the combination ART era (Constans, 1994; Grunfeld, 1989, 1992). However, the association of low concentrations of HDL-C with specific antiretroviral agents is less clear than their association with hypertriglyceridemia. Although a decrease in HDL-C is known to occur with insulin resistance in non-HIV patients with metabolic syndrome, the mechanistic underpinnings of altered HDL metabolism in HIV may be different. A detailed study comparing HDL metabolism in treated and untreated HIV-infected individuals compared to uninfected individuals found increased activity and mass of cholesterol ester transfer protein, which mediates a reciprocal exchange of VLDL-TG and HDL cholesteryl esters (Rose, 2008). There is also evidence that the ATP-binding cassette transporter A1 (ABCA1)-dependent cholesterol

efflux from human macrophages is impaired in HIV-infected patients, which may lead to impaired formation of HDL-C (Mujawar, 2006). Thus, there may be unique mechanisms contributing to both abnormalities in reverse transport of cholesterol and initiation of HDL-C formation in HIV patients.

INTERVENTIONS TARGETING DYSLIPIDEMIA

Because HIV-infected patients have an increased risk of cardiovascular disease, diabetes, and hepatic fat accumulation predisposing to fatty liver and fatty liver disease, there is a critical need to develop optimal therapeutic strategies to target dyslipidemia. However, attempts at achieving lipid control with pharmacotherapeutic strategies have proven difficult due to many obstacles. For example, many HIV-infected patients have hepatic transaminitis caused by co-infection with viral hepatitis, alcohol or drug abuse, nonalcoholic fatty liver disease, or drug interactions, and the use of statin or fibrate medications in these conditions is contraindicated. Furthermore, the use of these agents has to be balanced by emerging evidence indicating an adverse effect of statin use on glycemic control. Optimal pharmacotherapy often requires combinations of different drugs, with increased risk of interactions between fibrates and statins and between statins and antiretroviral medications, predisposing to hepatic or renal dysfunction or to rhabdomyolysis (Mikhail, 2009; Schmidt, 2007). Clinical management of dyslipidemia should incorporate a combination of both lifestyle changes and optimal pharmacotherapy.

LIFESTYLE MODIFICATIONS

Patients infected with HIV should receive counseling by a certified dietitian to initiate dietary recommendations of the US Cholesterol Education Program Adult Treatment Panel III (ATP III) for management of metabolic syndrome, with periodic follow-up and reinforcement of these recommendations to encourage adherence. Although hypertriglyceridemia is recognized as a contributor to cardiac risk, and specify dietary fat reduction as a means of lowering both LDL-C and triglycerides. Patients with HIV have also been shown to have severely impaired clearance of dietary triglycerides (Sekhar, 2005). Furthermore, HIV patients with increased intake of saturated fat have been reported to develop hypertriglyceridemia (Joy, 2007). Therefore, lowering intake of dietary saturated fats should be encouraged to lower hypertriglyceridemia, and it has been shown to result in a significant improvement in dyslipidemia in this population (Lazzaretti, 2012). HIV-infected patients also benefit from exercise. Resistance training was associated with an increase in lean mass and lower fat mass compared to aerobic training. Although both types of exercise improved insulin sensitivity, increased HDL-C, and reduced inflammatory cytokines, only resistance training decreased triglyceride concentrations. An overall increase in physical activity appears to be beneficial in HIV and, together with dietary control, should complement the use of pharmacotherapy in the management of dyslipidemia.

PHARMACOTHERAPY

Consensus guidelines developed by the Infectious Diseases Society of America (Dube, 2003) recommend evaluation for cardiovascular risk and pharmacologic therapy for HIV-infected patients. The recent ACC/AHA guidelines recommend early initiation of statin therapy, but there are no specific recommendations for HIV patients, in whom there is increased risk of atherosclerotic cardiovascular disease and accelerated aging. Therapy of dyslipidemia in HIV patients commonly uses the lipid-lowering medications discussed next.

HYDROXYMETHYLGLUTARYL–COENZYME A INHIBITORS (STATIN DRUGS)

Hydroxymethylglutaryl–coenzyme A reductase (HMG-CoA) is the rate-limiting enzyme in the process of endogenous cholesterol synthesis, and the statin class of agents work by inhibiting HMG-CoA. The statin drugs are first-line therapy for treating elevations in LDL-C or non-HDL-C. Several statin drugs are metabolized by the hepatic cytochrome P450 CYP3A4 isoenzyme pathway. Because several antiretroviral agents are also eliminated by the same pathway, there is an increased risk for higher statin concentrations due to competitive inhibition of drug elimination, which is also associated with rhabdomyolysis and renal failure. The commonly used statin drugs simvastatin and atorvastatin respectively have been shown to have 517% and 122% higher steady state area under the plasma concentration–time curve when concomitantly taken with the PI drug nelfinavir (Hsyu, 2001). In general, care must be taken to confirm the precise antiretroviral combination of drugs that patients are taking before making a choice of initiating statin drugs. Because several antiretroviral combinations include a PI drug, simvastatin and lovastatin are contraindicated, and the doses of atorvastatin or rosuvastatin should be significantly lower. The FDA has advised

that statins may have deleterious effects on glycemic control. Because pravastatin, rosuvastatin, and fluvastatin are eliminated by different cytochrome P450 isoenzyme pathways (CYP2C9 or CYP2C19) (Benesic, 2004; Calza, 2005; Johns, 2007), these may be relatively safer. Statins vary in their efficacy for lowering LDL-C. Atorvastatin at a dose of 10 mg/day has been shown to lower total cholesterol by 27%, LDL-C by 37%, and triglycerides by 41% (Palacios, 2002); rosuvastatin at 10 mg/day resulted in 31.3% lower LDL-C, 29.9% lower non-HDL-C, and 34% lower triglycerides (Bottaro, 2008). However, the efficacy of pravastatin is more modest, with 17–19% lower total cholesterol, 19% lower LDL-C, no effect on HDL-C (Aberg, 2005; Baldini, 2000; Moyle, 2001), and 9% lower triglyceride concentrations. Fluvastatin induces similar reductions in total cholesterol levels (Doser, 2002). When the cholesterol-lowering abilities of pravastatin (20 mg), rosuvastatin (10 mg), and atorvastatin (10mg) were compared in HIV-infected patients taking antiretroviral drugs containing a PI, rosuvastatin had the greatest effect, with 25% lower total cholesterol, followed by atorvastatin with 19% and pravastatin with 17% (Calza, 2008).

Therefore, initiating and maintaining patients on statin drugs should be done by physicians experienced with details of interactions between statin drugs and ART. HIV-infected patients on both agents should receive education about potential risks of rhabdomyolysis and renal impairment prior to beginning therapy, and they should be aware of symptoms of rhabdomyolysis or liver dysfunction. They should be monitored periodically with tests of liver and renal functions.

FIBRIC ACID DERIVATIVES

These drugs act as agonists of the nuclear receptor peroxisome proliferator activator receptor-α (PPAR-α), which is involved in the regulation of genes of fatty acid oxidation. Commonly used fibric acid drugs are fenofibrate and gemfibrozil. Clinical studies in HIV patients have shown that fenofibrate decreases fasting plasma triglyceride concentrations by 37% (Rao, 2004) and total cholesterol concentrations by 22% (Calza, 2003). Additional benefits of fenofibrate derive from the fact that it renders LDL less atherogenic by increasing LDL particle size and enhancing LDL resistance to oxidation (Badiou, 2004). Treatment with gemfibrozil also results in lower triglyceride concentrations, but the response is not as significant as that with fenofibrate (Miller, 2002; Silverberg, 2009). A clinical trial compared the relative effects of diet, fibrate, niacin, and fibrate–niacin combination on dyslipidemia in patients with HIV and found that fenofibrate improved triglycerides, total cholesterol, and non-HDL-C, and the fenofibrate–niacin combination decreased the total cholesterol:HDL-C ratio (Balasubramanyam, 2011).

EZETIMIBE

The mechanism of action of this agent is inhibition of dietary cholesterol absorption, and ezetimibe decreases LDL-C up to 20% in patients with HIV-associated lipodystrophy (Coll, 2006). The combination of ezetimibe and statin drugs can result in a greater reduction of LDL-C compared to use of either drug alone (Gagne, 2002; Negredo, 2006; Pearson, 2005). Although some recent studies have shown little effect in HIV-negative populations, the extrapolation of these results to HIV patients is unclear, especially in light of increased risk of coronary atherosclerotic disease in HIV patients. Further studies are needed to clarify the role of ezetimbe in primary and secondary prevention of atherosclerotic cardiovascular disease in HIV patients.

NIACIN

Nicotinic acid (niacin) is used to treat low HDL-C. Treating patients who had HIV-associated lipodystrophy and elevated fasting triglyceride concentrations with extended-release niacin at 2 g/dl resulted in increased HDL-C concentrations and lower concentrations of fasting triglycerides, total cholesterol, and non-HDL-C (Dube, 2006). In a randomized, double-blind, placebo-controlled trial, niacin use was shown to increase HDL-C when used as monotherapy, and it increased HDL-C and adiponectin, in addition to lowering triglyceride concentrations and non-HDL-C, when used in combination with fenofibrate, diet, and exercise (Balasubramanyam, 2011). However, niacin should be used with caution because it can induce insulin resistance and cause hepatotoxicity (Dube, 2006). Furthermore, in a significant departure from the ATP III guidelines, the current ACC/AHA guidelines do not address the role of HDL-C treatment or Niaspan, and clinical studies are needed in the HIV population to determine whether elevations in HDL-C can prevent atherosclerotic cardiovascular disease.

THIAZOLIDINEDIONES

Thiazolidinedione drugs were used to treat HIV-associated lipodystrophy based on their effect on adipogenesis. The use of pioglitazone in HIV-associated lipodystrophy has been shown to improve HDL-C (Slama, 2008) and

triglyceride levels. Rosiglitazone has been associated with negative effects on dyslipidemia, with increases in the concentration of small, dense LDL (Hadigan, 2007), increased LDL-C concentrations, and lower HDL-C (Hadigan, 2007; Mulligan, 2007) and triglyceride concentrations (Kovacic, 2005; Mulligan, 2007).

OMEGA-3 FATTY ACIDS

Fish oils are known to lower serum triglyceride concentrations in HIV-infected patients (Carter, 2006; Wohl, 2005). The AHA recommends 2–4 g per day of eicosapentanoic acid and docosahexanoic acid for patients with hypertriglyceridemia. When used as monotherapy in hypertriglyceridemic HIV patients, fish oil usage led to a 22–46% reduction in triglyceride levels (DeTruchis, 2007; Gerber, 2008). Other studies have confirmed the benefit of omega fish oils compared to placebo on lowering triglyceride concentrations in 70 HIV-infected patients (Amador-Licona, 2016; Metkus, 2012).Omega fish oils have been associated with gastrointestinal disturbances, including nausea, vomiting, and a "fishy" taste, and their usage is contraindicated in patients with active gastrointestinal bleeding.

ACIPIMOX

A key pathophysiological defect in HIV-associated lipodystrophy is increased rates of lipolysis (Reeds, 2003; Sekhar, 2002). Acipimox, a niacin derivative drug known to decrease lipolysis, has been studied in patients with HIV-associated lipodystrophy. When subjects took acipimox at a dose of 250 mg three times daily for 3 months, lipolytic rates decreased significantly, along with reductions in triglyceride and fatty acid concentrations (Hadigan, 2006). Acipimox is not currently approved for clinical use in the United States.

GROWTH HORMONE AND TESAMORELIN

Patients with HIV have an increased prevalence of growth hormone (GH) deficiency, especially when associated with increased abdominal fat, and diminished GH secretion is independently associated with dyslipidemia (Lo, 2009). Patients with GH deficiency have been reported to have elevated lipolysis, and replacement of GH to maintain serum insulin-like growth factor-1 levels in the physiological range lowered lipolytic rates (D'Amico, 2006). The use of tesamorelin, a GH-releasing factor, in HIV-infected subjects led to lower triglyceride and total cholesterol concentrations and higher HDL-C concentrations (Falutz, 2007).

LEPTIN

Leptin is an adipocyte-secreted hormone that is implicated as an important regulator of fatty acid and energy metabolism. The use of leptin in patients with HIV-associated lipodystrophy, leptin deficiency, and hypertriglyceridemia was associated with increases in HDL-C concentrations; reductions in total cholesterol, non-HDL cholesterol, and triglycerides; and improved insulin sensitivity (Lee, 2006; Mulligan, 2009). In a randomized placebo-controlled, double-blind trial, correcting leptin deficiency in hypoleptinemic patients using escalating doses of leptin did not result in improvement of abnormal lipid kinetics, but it did improve glycemia and non-HDL-C (Sekhar, 2012). Currently, recombinant human leptin is not approved by the FDA for treatment of dyslipidemia in individuals with HIV-associated lipodystrophy.

GLUTATHIONE

Glutathione (GSH) is an endogenous tripeptide intracellular antioxidant composed of cysteine, glycine, and glutamic acid that combats oxidative stress. Patients with HIV are reported both to be deficient in GSH and to have elevated oxidative stress (Nakamura, 2002; Nguyen, 2014; Srabana, 2004). A small study found that correcting GSH deficiency in HIV-infected patients who were taken off their lipid-lowering medications for the study significantly lowered LDL-C concentrations (by 10%) and resulted in a significant reduction in circulating free fatty acid concentrations (Nguyen, 2014). The study also found that the cause of GSH deficiency in these patients was diminished availability of cysteine and glycine, and these deficiencies were corrected by oral dietary supplementation of cysteine (as *N*-acetylcysteine) and glycine (Nguyen, 2014). Additional work is needed to understand the role of GSH in improving dyslipidemia in larger cohorts of patients.

CONCLUSION

The therapeutic approach to dyslipidemia in HIV-infected patients should consist of a combination of patient education, implementation of dietary recommendations (usually a low-fat diet), initiation of exercise where appropriate, and careful use of pharmacotherapy. Patients must have periodic follow-up visits with careful monitoring of lipid profiles, liver and renal functions, and muscle breakdown markers (when indicated) to assess clinical improvement and adverse reactions.

References

Aberg JA, Zackin RA, Brobst SW, et al. A randomized trial of the efficacy and safety of fenofibrate versus pravastatin in HIV-infected subjects with lipid abnormalities: AIDS Clinical Trials Group Study 5087. *AIDS Res Hum Retroviruses*. 2005; 21:757–767.

Agarwal N, Iyer D, Patel SG, et al. HIV-1 Vpr induces adipose dysfunction in vivo through reciprocal effects on PPAR/GR co-regulation. *Sci Transl Med*. 2013 Nov 27; 5(213):213ra164.

Amador-Licona N, Díaz-Murillo TA, Gabriel-Ortiz G, et al. Omega 3 fatty acids supplementation and oxidative stress in HIV-seropositive patients: A clinical trial. *PLoS One*. 2016 Mar 25; 11(3):e0151637.

Badiou S, Merle De Boever C, Dupuy AM, et al. Fenofibrate improves the atherogenic lipid profile and enhances LDL resistance to oxidation in HIV-positive adults. *Atherosclerosis*. 2004; 172:273–279.

Balasubramanyam A, Coraza I, Smith EO, et al. Combination of niacin and fenofibrate with lifestyle changes improves dyslipidemia and hypoadiponectinemia in HIV patients on antiretroviral therapy: Results of "Heart Positive," a randomized, controlled trial. *J Clin Endocrinol Metab*. 2011 Jul; 96(7):2236–2247.

Baldini F, Di Giambenedetto S, Cingolani A, et al. Efficacy and tolerability of pravastatin for the treatment of HIV-1 protease inhibitor-associated hyperlipidaemia: A pilot study. *AIDS*. 2000; 14:1660–1662.

Behrens G, Dejam A, Schmidt H, et al. Impaired glucose tolerance, beta cell function and lipid metabolism in HIV patients under treatment with protease inhibitors. *AIDS*. 1999; 13:F63–F70.

Benesic A, Zilly M, Kluge F, et al. Lipid lowering therapy with fluvastatin and pravastatin in patients with HIV infection and antiretroviral therapy: Comparison of efficacy and interaction with indinavir. *Infection*. 2004; 32:229–233.

Bianchi G, Marchesini C, Conte R., et al. Non-alcoholic fatty liver disease and aging: Prevalence and associated factors. Paper presented at the 45th annual meeting of the European Association for the Study of the Liver 2010 (EASL).

Bottaro EG, Caravello O, Scapellato PG, et al. Rosuvastatin for the treatment of dyslipidemia in HIV-infected patients receiving highly active antiretroviral therapy: Preliminary experience. *Enferm Infecc Microbiol Clin*. 2008; 26:325–329.

Calza L, Colangeli V, Manfredi R, et al. Rosuvastatin for the treatment of hyperlipidaemia in HIV-infected patients receiving protease inhibitors: A pilot study. *AIDS*. 2005; 19:1103–1105.

Calza L, Manfredi R, Chiodo F. Statins and fibrates for the treatment of hyperlipidaemia in HIV-infected patients receiving HAART. *AIDS*. 2004; 17:851–859.

Calza L, Manfredi R, Colangeli V, et al. Rosuvastatin, pravastatin, and atorvastatin for the treatment of hypercholesterolaemia in HIV-infected patients receiving protease inhibitors. *Curr HIV Res*. 2008; 6:572–578.

Carr A, Samaras K, Thorisdottir A, et al. Diagnosis, prediction, and natural course of HIV-1 protease-inhibitor associated lipodystrophy, hyperlipidaemia, and diabetes mellitus: A cohort study. *Lancet*. 1999; 353:2093–2099.

Carter VM, Woolley I, Jolley D, et al. A randomised controlled trial of omega-3 fatty acid supplementation for the treatment of hypertriglyceridemia in HIV-infected males on highly active antiretroviral therapy. *Sex Health*. 2006; 3:287–290.

Constans J, Pellegrin JL, Peuchant E, et al. Plasma lipids in HIV-infected patients: A prospective study in 95 patients. *Eur J Clin Invest*. 1994; 24:416–420.

Crum-Cianflone N, Dilay A, Collins G, et al. Nonalcoholic fatty liver disease among HIV-infected persons. *J Acquir Immune Defic Syndr*. 2009; 50:464–473.

D'Amico S, Shi J, Sekhar RV, et al. Physiologic growth hormone replacement improves fasting lipid kinetics in patients with HIV lipodystrophy syndrome. *Am J Clin Nutr*. 2006; 84:204–211.

De Truchis P, Kirstetter M, Perier A, et al. Reduction in triglyceride level with N-3 polyunsaturated fatty acids in HIV-infected patients taking potent antiretroviral therapy: A randomized prospective study. *J Acquir Immune Defic Syndr*. 2007; 44:278–285.

De Wit S, Sabin CA, Weber R, et al. Incidence and risk factors for new-onset diabetes in HIV-infected patients: The Data Collection on Adverse Events of Anti-HIV Drugs (D:A:D) study. *Diabetes Care*. 2008; 31:1224–1229.

Doser N, Kubli S, Telenti A, et al. Efficacy and safety of fluvastatin in hyperlipidemic protease inhibitor-treated HIV-infected patients. *AIDS*. 2002; 16:1982–1983.

Dube MP, Stein JH, Aberg JA, et al. Guidelines for the evaluation and management of dyslipidemia in human immunodeficiency virus (HIV)-infected adults receiving antiretroviral therapy: Recommendations of the HIV Medical Association of the Infectious Disease Society of America and the Adult AIDS Clinical Trials Group. *Clin Infect Dis*. 2003; 37:613–627.

Dube MP, Wu JW, Aberg JA, et al. Safety and efficacy of extended-release niacin for the treatment of dyslipidaemia in patients with HIV infection: AIDS Clinical Trials Group Study A5148. *Antivir Ther*. 2006; 11:1081–1089.

Duprez DA, Kuller LH, Tracy R, et al. Lipoprotein particle subclasses, cardiovascular disease and HIV infection. *Atherosclerosis*. 2009 Dec; 207(2):524–529.

Falutz J, Allas S, Blot K, et al. Metabolic effects of a growth hormone-releasing factor in patients with HIV. *N Engl J Med*. 2007; 357:2359–2370.

Fellay J, Boubaker K, Ledergerber B, et al. Prevalence of adverse events associated with potent antiretroviral treatment: Swiss HIV Cohort Study. *Lancet*. 2001; 358:1322–1327.

Fourie CM, Van Rooyen JM, Kruger A, et al. Lipid abnormalities in a never-treated HIV-1 subtype C-infected African population. *Lipids*. 2010; 45:73–80.

Friis-Moller N, Weber R, Reiss P, et al. Cardiovascular disease risk factors in HIV patients—Association with antiretroviral therapy: Results from the D:A:D study. *AIDS*. 2003; 17:1179–1193.

Gagne C, Bays HE, Weiss SR, et al. Efficacy and safety of ezetimibe added to ongoing statin therapy for treatment of patients with primary hypercholesterolemia. *Am J Cardiol*. 2002; 90:1084–1091.

Gerber JG, Kitch DW, Fichtenbaum CJ, et al. Fish oil and fenofibrate for the treatment of hypertriglyceridemia in HIV-infected subjects on antiretroviral therapy: Results of ACTG A5186. *J Acquir Immune Defic Syndr*. 2008; 47:459–466.

Grunfeld C, Kotler DP, Hamadeh R, et al. Hypertriglyceridemia in the acquired immunodeficiency syndrome. *Am J Med*. 1989; 86:27–31.

Grunfeld C, Pang M, Doerrler W, et al. Lipids, lipoproteins, triglyceride clearance, and cytokines in human immunodeficiency virus infection and the acquired immunodeficiency syndrome. *J Clin Endocrinol Metab*. 1992; 74:1045–1052.

Hadigan C, Liebau J, Torriani M, et al. Improved triglycerides and insulin sensitivity with 3 months of acipimox in human immunodeficiency virus-infected patients with hypertriglyceridemia. *J Clin Endocrinol Metab*. 2006; 91:4438–4444.

Hadigan C, Mazza S, Crum D, et al. Rosiglitazone increases small dense low-density lipoprotein concentration and decreases high-density lipoprotein particle size in HIV-infected patients. *AIDS*. 2007; 21:2543–2546.

Hatano H, Miller KD, Yoder CP, et al. Metabolic and anthropometric consequences of interruption of highly active antiretroviral therapy. *AIDS*. 2000; 14:1935–1942.

Hsyu PH, Schultz-Smith MD, Lillibridge JH, et al. Pharmacokinetic interactions between nelfinavir and 3-hydroxy-3-methylglutaryl coenzyme A reductase inhibitors atorvastatin and simvastatin. *Antimicrob Agents Chemother*. 2001; 45:3445–3450.

Hulgan T, Sterling TR, Daugherty J, et al. Prescribing of contraindicated protease inhibitor and statin combinations among HIV-infected persons. *J Acquir Immune Defic Syndr*. 2005; 38:277–282.

Johns KW, Bennett MT, Bondy GP. Are HIV+ patients resistant to statin therapy? *Lipids Health Dis*. 2007; 6:27.

Jones R, Sawleshwarkar S, Michailidis C, et al. Impact of antiretroviral choice on hypercholesterolaemia events: The role of the nucleoside reverse transcriptase inhibitor backbone. *HIV Med*. 2005; 6:396–402.

Joy T, Keogh HM, Hadigan C, et al. Dietary fat intake and relationship to serum lipid levels in HIV-infected patients with metabolic abnormalities in the HAART era. *AIDS*. 2007; 21:1591–1600.

Kovacic JC, Martin A, Carey D, et al. Influence of rosiglitazone on flow-mediated dilation and other markers of cardiovascular risk in HIV-infected patients with lipoatrophy. *Antivir Ther*. 2005; 10:135–143.

Lazzaretti RK, Kuhmmer R, Sprinz E, et al. Dietary intervention prevents dyslipidemia associated with highly active antiretroviral therapy in human immunodeficiency virus type 1-infected individuals: A randomized trial. *J Am Coll Cardiol*. 2012 Mar 13; 59(11):979–988.

Lee JH, Chan JL, Sourlas E, et al. Recombinant methionyl human leptin therapy in replacement doses improves insulin resistance and metabolic profile in patients with lipoatrophy and metabolic syndrome induced by the highly active antiretroviral therapy. *J Clin Endocrinol Metab* 2006; 91:2605–2611.

Lo J, You SM, Wei J, et al. Relationship of peak growth hormone to cardiovascular parameters, waist circumference, lipids and glucose in HIV-infected patients and healthy adults. *Clin Endocrinol (Oxford)*. 2009; 71(6):815–822.

Madge S, Kinloch-de-Loes S, Mercey D, et al. Lipodystrophy in patients naive to HIV protease inhibitors. *AIDS*. 1999; 13:735–737.

Metkus TS, Timpone J, Leaf D, et al. Omega-3 fatty acid therapy reduces triglycerides and interleukin-6 in hypertriglyeridemic HIV patients. *HIV Med*. 2013 Oct; 14(9):530–539.

Mikhail N, Iskander E, Cope D. Rhabdomyolysis in an HIV-infected patient on anti-retroviral therapy precipitated by high-dose pravastatin. *Curr Drug Saf*. 2009; 4:121–122.

Miller J, Brown D, Amin J, et al. A randomized, double-blind study of gemfibrozil for the treatment of protease inhibitor-associated hypertriglyceridaemia. *AIDS*. 2002; 16:2195–2200.

Mobius U, Lubach-Ruitman M, Castro-Frenzel B, et al. Switching to atazanavir improves metabolic disorders in antiretroviral experienced patients with severe hyperlipidemia. *J Acquir Immune Defic Syndr*. 2005; 39:174–180.

Moyle GJ, Lloyd M, Reynolds B, et al. Dietary advice with or without pravastatin for the management of hypercholesterolaemia associated with protease inhibitor therapy. *AIDS*. 2001; 15:1503–1508.

Mujawar Z, Rose H, Morrow MP, et al. Human immunodeficiency virus impairs reverse cholesterol transport from macrophages. *PLoS Biol*. 2006; 4:e365.

Mulligan K, Grunfeld C, Tai VW, et al. Hyperlipidemia and insulin resistance are induced by protease inhibitors independent of changes in body composition in patients with HIV infection. *J Acquir Immune Defic Syndr*.2000; 23:35–43.

Mulligan K, Khatami H, Schwarz JM, et al. The effects of recombinant human leptin on visceral fat, dyslipidemia, and insulin resistance in patients with human immunodeficiency virus-associated lipoatrophy and hypoleptinemia. *J Clin Endocrinol Metab*. 2009; 94:1137–1144.

Mulligan K, Yang Y, Wininger DA, et al. Effects of metformin and rosiglitazone in HIV-infected patients with hyperinsulinemia and elevated waist/hip ratio. *AIDS*. 2007; 21:47–57.

Nakamura H, Masutani H, Yodoi J. Redox imbalance and its control in HIV infection. *Antioxid Redox Signal*. 2002; 4(3):455–464.

Negredo E, Molto J, Puig J, et al. Ezetimibe, a promising lipid-lowering agent for the treatment of dyslipidaemia in HIV-infected patients with poor response to statins. *AIDS*. 2006; 20:2159–2164.

Nguyen D, Hsu JW, Jahoor F, et al. Effect of increasing glutathione with cysteine and glycine supplementation on mitochondrial fuel oxidation, insulin sensitivity, and body composition in older HIV-infected patients. *J Clin Endocrinol Metab*. 2014 Jan; 99(1):169–177.

Palacios R, Santos J, Gonzalez M, et al. Efficacy and safety of atorvastatin in the treatment of hypercholesterolemia associated with antiretroviral therapy. *J Acquir Immune Defic Syndr*. 2002; 30:536–537.

Pearson TA, Denke MA, McBride PE, et al. A community-based, randomized trial of ezetimibe added to statin therapy to attain NCEP ATP III goals for LDL cholesterol in hypercholesterolemic patients: The Ezetimibe Add-on to Statin for Effectiveness (EASE) trial. *Mayo Clin Proc*. 2005; 80:587–595.

Periard D, Telenti A, Sudre P, et al. Atherogenic dyslipidemia in HIV-infected individuals treated with protease inhibitors: The Swiss HIV Cohort Study. *Circulation*.1999; 100:700–705.

Purnell JQ, Zambon A, Knopp RH, et al. Effect of ritonavir on lipids and post-heparin lipase activities in normal subjects. *AIDS*. 2000; 14:51–57.

Rao A, D'Amico S, Balasubramanyam A, et al. Fenofibrate is effective in treating hypertriglyceridemia associated with HIV lipodystrophy. *Am J Med Sci*. 2004; 327:315–318.

Reeds DN, Mittendorfer B, Patterson BW, et al. Alterations in lipid kinetics in men with HIV-dyslipidemia. *Am J Physiol Endocrinol Metab*. 2003; 285:E490–E497.

Rose H, Hoy J, Woolley I, et al. HIV infection and high density lipoprotein metabolism. *Atherosclerosis*. 2008; 199:79–86.

Schmidt GA, Hoehns JD, Purcell JL, et al. Severe rhabdomyolysis and acute renal failure secondary to concomitant use of simvastatin, amiodarone, and atazanavir. *J Am Board Fam Med*. 2007; 20:411–416.

Sekhar RV, Jahoor F, Iyer D, et al. Leptin replacement therapy does not improve the abnormal lipid kinetics of hypoleptinemic patients with HIV-associated lipodystrophy syndrome. *Metabolism*. 2012; 61(10):1395–1403.

Sekhar RV, Jahoor F, Pownall HJ, et al. Severely dysregulated disposal of postprandial triacylglycerols exacerbates hypertriacylglycerolemia in HIV lipodystrophy syndrome. *Am J Clin Nutr*. 2005; 81:1405–1410.

Sekhar RV, Jahoor F, White AC, et al. Metabolic basis of HIV-lipodystrophy syndrome. *Am J Physiol Endocrinol Metab*. 2002; 283:E332–E337.

Silverberg MJ, Leyden W, Hurley L, et al. Response to newly prescribed lipid-lowering therapy in patients with and without HIV infection. *Ann Intern Med*. 2009; 150:301–313.

Slama L, Lanoy E, Valantin MA, et al. Effect of pioglitazone on HIV-1-related lipodystrophy: A randomized double-blind placebo-controlled trial (ANRS 113). *Antivir Ther*. 2008; 13:67–76.

Tsiodras S, Mantzoros C, Hammer S, et al. Effects of protease inhibitors on hyperglycemia, hyperlipidemia, and lipodystrophy: A 5-year cohort study. *Arch Intern Med*. 2005; 160:2050–2056.

Ware LJ, Wootton SA, Morlese JM, et al. The paradox of improved antiretroviral therapy in HIV: Potential for nutritional modulation? *Proc Nutr Soc*. 2002; 61:131–136.

Wohl DA, Tien HC, Busby M, et al. Randomized study of the safety and efficacy of fish oil (omega-3 fatty acid) supplementation with dietary and exercise counseling for the treatment of antiretroviral therapy-associated hypertriglyceridemia. *Clin Infect Dis*. 2005; 41:1498–1504.

Worm SW, Sabin C, Weber R, et al. Risk of myocardial infarction in patients with HIV infection exposed to specific individual antiretroviral drugs from the 3 major drug classes: The Data Collection on Adverse Events of Anti-HIV Drugs (D:A:D) study. *J Infect Dis*. 2010; 201:318–330.

van der Valk M, Gisolf EH, Reiss P, et al. Increased risk of lipodystrophy when nucleoside analogue reverse transcriptase inhibitors are included with protease inhibitors in the treatment of HIV-1 infection. *AIDS*. 2001; 15:847–855.

Young J, Rickenbach M, Weber R, et al. Body fat changes among antiretroviral-naive patients on PI- and NNRTI-based HAART in the Swiss HIV cohort study. *Antivir Ther*. 2005; 10:73–81.

48.

IMMUNE RECONSTITUTION INFLAMMATORY SYNDROME

Dagan Coppock and William R. Short

LEARNING OBJECTIVE

Review the current status of research in the field of immune reconstitution inflammatory syndrome (IRIS).

WHAT'S NEW?

Earlier initiation of antiretroviral therapy (ART) in tuberculosis co-infected patients shows a reduction in mortality. Standard clinical practice has changed to reflect this finding.

KEY POINTS

- IRIS is associated with either worsening of a recognized infection (paradoxical IRIS) or an unrecognized infection (unmasking IRIS), which occurs in the setting of improved immunologic function.

- Most patients presenting with IRIS should be maintained on ART along with treatment for the associated infection.

The hallmark of HIV pathogenesis is the gradual destruction of the cell-mediated immune system over a period of many years, as evidenced by a progressive and profound decline in CD4+ T-helper lymphocytes, leading to increased susceptibility to opportunistic infections (OIs), malignancies, and the development of AIDS. ART can suppress HIV replication, preventing further deterioration, and it allows for regeneration of the immune system. Even patients with advanced AIDS have a marked improvement in both quantity and quality of their immune system after starting ART. In a subset of those initiating ART, the harmonious, gradual reconstitution of the immune system does not occur; rather, there is a rapid immunologic recovery with an abrupt transition to a pathologic inflammatory state often causing clinical deterioration. Opportunistic and other infections, previously unrecognized or tolerated by the failing immune system, suddenly become the targets of this overzealous immunologic recovery. In this inflammatory state, patients can clinically worsen, despite an otherwise excellent response to ART, as evidenced by a decreased viral load and increased CD4+ T cell counts. This paradoxical inflammatory response has been termed immune reconstitution inflammatory syndrome or IRIS (French, 2004).

The term IRIS is used to describe two clinical entities:

1. Paradoxical IRIS: An exacerbation of a known OI

2. Unmasking IRIS: A flare of an undiagnosed (subclinical) OI

INCIDENCE AND CLINICAL CHARACTERISTICS OF IRIS

The incidence of IRIS is dependent on the patient population being studied, occurring more frequently in persons with more previous and concurrent OIs, greater burden of HIV infection (higher viral load), and more advanced HIV disease (CD4+ T cell count <50 cells/mm^3) (Müller, 2010). The HIV Outpatient Study—an eight-city, US-wide, prospective, observational cohort study—evaluated 2610 patients with 370 cases of IRIS (occurring in 276 patients) who initiated or resumed ART and, during the next 6 months, demonstrated a decline in plasma HIV RNA viral load of at least 0.5 log$_{10}$ copies/ml or had an increase of at least 50% in CD4+ cell count per microliter; it reported that the incidence of IRIS was 10.6%. The most common IRIS-defining diagnoses were candidiasis (23%), cytomegalovirus infection (3.5%), disseminated *Mycobacterium avium* intracellulare (3.2%), *Pneumocystis* pneumonia (2.7%), *Varicella zoster* (2.4%), Kaposi's sarcoma (2.4%), non-Hodgkin's lymphoma (2.2%), and *Mycobacterium tuberculosis* (0.3%). IRIS was independently associated with CD4$^+$ T cell counts less than 50 cells/ml versus at least 200 cells/ml (odds ratio (OR), 5.0) and a viral load of at least 5.0 log$_{10}$ copies/ml versus less than 4.0 log$_{10}$ copies/ml (OR, 2.3) (Novak, 2012). In contrast, a study from the University of Washington HIV Cohort demonstrated a higher rate of IRIS in patients with Kaposi's sarcoma (KS; 29%), with no evident cases in patients with cytomegalovirus disease or *Candida* esophagitis. In this study, the highest IRIS-associated morbidity was in cases of visceral KS. The differences in clinical characteristics between these two studies alone may reflect population and geographic variability. Just as the presentation of IRIS may vary within the United States, predominant presentations of IRIS likely vary based on global regions.

In addition to the potential demographic factors that might affect the presentation of IRIS, the choice of highly active antiretroviral therapy (HAART) may also play a role. The AIDS Clinical Trial Group (ACTG) reported the incidence and associations with IRIS in ACTG 5202, which was a phase IIIb, randomized clinical trial conducted in the United States that compared the safety, tolerability, and efficacy of four commonly used, once-daily, initial ART regimens. Two dual nucleoside/nucleotide reverse transcriptase inhibitor fixed-dose combinations (tenofovir DF/emtricitabine or abacavir/lamivudine) were compared when used in combination with either a non-nucleoside reverse transcriptase inhibitor (efavirenz) or a ritonavir-boosted protease inhibitor (atazanavir/ritonavir). Among 1848 eligible subjects who initiated in this study, IRIS events occurred in 52 subjects by week 48, with 4 subjects having two events. Incidence rates were 6.05 (95% confidence interval (CI), 4.57–8.00) and 3.30 (95% CI, 2.51–4.33) cases/100 person-years through 24 and 48 weeks, respectively. IRIS occurred 1–298 days after the initiation of ART, with 75% of cases occurring within 67 days and 3 cases after 24 weeks. IRIS events included the following associated OIs or other clinical diagnoses: *Mycobacterium avium* complex (MAC) ($n = 11$); *Varicella zoster* virus ($n = 11$); herpes simplex virus ($n = 8$); KS ($n = 5$); hepatitis C virus (HCV), tuberculosis (TB), and *Pneumocystis jirovecii* pneumonia (PCP) ($n = 4$ each); toxoplasmosis and cryptococcosis ($n = 2$ each); and cytomegalovirus-associated colitis, progressive multifocal leukoencephalopathy (PML), *Mycobacterium kansasii*,

eosinophilic folliculitis, and swollen lymph node ($n = 1$ each). The most commonly reported symptoms were fever and pain. There were no deaths from IRIS in this cohort. Among subjects with IRIS, median baseline HIV RNA was 4.9 log$_{10}$ copies/ml, median CD4$^+$ T cell count was 49 cells/mm^3, and 50% had prior AIDS illness. In univariate Cox proportional hazards models, increased risk of IRIS was associated with baseline prior AIDS illness, higher HIV RNA level, lower CD4$^+$ T cell count and percentage, lower CD8$^+$ T cell count and higher percentage, and lower CD4$^+$:CD8$^+$ T cell ratio (all $p \leq 0.01$). No significant association was observed with sex, age, or race/ethnicity ($p > 0.19$). Of interest is the finding that IRIS events were more common with abacavir/lamivudine relative to tenofovir/emtricitabine for subjects with low CD4$^+$ T cell counts. This finding may reflect the observed more rapid CD4$^+$ T cell increases with abacavir/lamivudine regimens (Fischl, 2010).

ETIOLOGY AND PATHOGENESIS

Recovery of pathogen-specific T cell responses and an increased production of pro-inflammatory chemokines and cytokines produced by the innate immune response after commencing ART may contribute to the immunopathogenesis of IRIS. Higher T cell responses to nonstructural antigens of HCV in enzyme-linked immunosorbent spot assays and higher serum levels of antibodies to a mixture of virus proteins were demonstrated in patients with HIV and HCV co-infection who experienced an increase in serum liver enzyme levels after commencing ART (Cameron, 2011). Patients who develop TB-IRIS have lower plasma levels of the chemokine CCL2 before commencing ART (Oliver, 2010).

The identification of biomarkers could be used to diagnose IRIS in the future and predict which patients might be at risk. A cohort of 45 HIV-1-infected, treatment-naive patients with baseline CD4$^+$ T cell counts ≤100 cells/µl who were started on ART, suppressed HIV RNA to <50 copies/ml, and seen every 1–3 months for 1 year were retrospectively evaluated for suspected or confirmed IRIS. Pre-ART levels of both D-dimer and the inflammatory biomarker C-reactive protein (CRP) were higher in IRIS cases versus controls (Porter, 2010). In another study, individuals with elevated baseline levels of CRP and the fibrosis biomarker hyaluronic acid were more likely to progress to AIDS, develop IRIS, or die within the first month after starting ART (Boulware, 2011). Large prospective studies to elucidate the predictive and diagnostic values of IRIS biomarkers are needed.

STARTING ART IN THE SETTING OF AN ACUTE OPPORTUNISTIC INFECTION: RISK OF IRIS

No universally accepted consensus of opinion on the optimal timing for the initiation of ART in the setting of all acute OIs has been defined. Rather, it is increasingly clear that this is an OI-specific decision. Previous reports have been based primarily on retrospective data, as well as case reports in the literature. In the ACTG 5164 study, 282 subjects with an acute OI and a baseline median CD4$^+$ T cell count of 29 cells/mm^3 were prospectively randomized to immediate (<14 days) versus delayed (>28 days) initiation of ART. In this study, which included subjects diagnosed with PCP (63%), cryptococcal meningitis (12%), and bacterial infections (12%), earlier initiation of ART resulted in less progression to AIDS and/or death and no increase in adverse events or loss of virologic response compared to deferred ART. Subjects with or on treatment for TB were excluded. Rates of IRIS in this study were low (7%) and did not differ by timing of ART (Zolopa, 2009). IRIS was reported in 23 cases and confirmed in 20: 8 subjects in the immediate arm and 12 in the deferred arm. There was no evidence of an association of IRIS with the entry OI/bacterial infection: 13 (65%) IRIS cases were in subjects with PCP who comprised 63% of the study population. IRIS developed a median of 33 days (interquartile range, 26–72 days) after initiation of ART. There was no significant difference in the frequency of IRIS between subjects who received corticosteroids during the treatment of their OI and those who did not receive corticosteroids: 9/150 (6%) versus 11/112 (9.8%), respectively ($p = 0.35$).

Approximately 25% of patients with HIV and treated cryptococcal meningitis will experience IRIS after commencing ART (Haddow, 2010). It is associated with mortality in more than 25% of patients from resource-poor countries, and it is an important cause of early mortality after starting ART in patients with HIV from these countries. Early initiation of ART in patients with treated cryptococcal meningitis was associated with a higher rate of mortality in one study (Makadzange, 2010).

JC polyoma virus reactivation can lead to PML in patients with advanced HIV infection. However, approximately 15% of patients experience an exacerbation of PML after ART is commenced (Martin-Blondel, 2011).

Up to 25% of patients with HIV and hepatitis B virus (HBV) or HCV co-infection experience a flare of hepatitis and/or elevation of serum liver enzyme levels after commencing ART (Cameron, 2011; Crane, 2009). Hepatitis flares in patients with HIV and HBV co-infection are associated with a higher plasma HBV DNA level before ART (Crane, 2009), suggesting that pathogen load is an important determinant of disease. US Department of Health and Human Services (DHHS) guidelines recommend initiating ART for HIV/HBV co-infected and HIV/HCV co-infected patients, regardless of CD4$^+$ T count. However, the guidelines do recognize that some clinicians consider completing treatment for HCV prior to initiating ART in HCV/HIV co-infected patients with CD4$^+$ T counts >500 cells/mm^3.

TUBERCULOSIS IRIS

For individuals with HIV and TB co-infection, unmasking and paradoxical IRIS can lead to two distinct clinical scenarios. In the context of TB, unmasking IRIS is the development of overt TB in patients who initially screened negative for this infection, typically seen within the first 60 days following ART initiation (Dheda, 2004; Shelburne, 2006). It is thought to be due to an increase in circulating memory T cells, which were sequestered in lymphatic tissue prior to therapy. Alternatively, paradoxical IRIS involves worsening of signs and symptoms of TB in individuals with a known history of TB after they have been started on ART.

The HIV-CAUSAL Collaboration demonstrated that the incidence of TB decreased after ART initiation but not among persons older than age 50 years or those with a CD4$^+$ T cell count <50 cells/mm^3. Despite an overall decrease in TB incidence, the increased rate during 3 months of ART suggests unmasking IRIS. This is a multinational cohort study among HIV-positive patients from high-income countries. Among 65,121 individuals, 712 developed TB during 28 months of median follow-up (incidence, 3.0 cases per 1000 person-years). The hazard ratio (HR) for TB for ART versus no ART was 0.56 (95% CI, 0.44–0.72) overall, 1.04 (95% CI, 0.64–1.68) for individuals aged >50 years, and 1.46 (95% CI, 0.70–3.04) for people with a CD4+ cell count <50 cells/mm^3. Compared with people who had not started ART, HRs differed by time since ART initiation: 1.36 (95% CI, 0.98–1.89) for initiation <3 months previously and 0.44 (95% CI, 0.34–0.58) for initiation ≥3 months previously. Compared with people who had not initiated ART, HRs <3 months after ART initiation were 0.67 (95% CI, 0.38–1.18), 1.51 (95% CI, 0.98–2.31), and 3.20 (95% CI, 1.34–7.60) for people younger than age 35, 35–50, and older than age 50 years, respectively, and 2.30 (95% CI, 1.03–5.14) for people with a CD4$^+$ cell count <50 cells/mm^3 (HIV-CAUSAL Collaboration, 2012).

In a South African cohort of 498 persons with advanced HIV, symptomatic patients were screened for TB by chest X-ray and/or sputum examination. Patients who screened positive were initiated on anti-TB therapy prior to starting ART. Individuals who screened negative and went on to develop unmasking IRIS were found to have significantly elevated levels of interferon-γ and CRP at baseline prior to ART compared to non-IRIS, non-TB controls. These results suggest the presence of subclinical TB infection despite negative screening that was done prior to the initiation of ART (Haddow, 2009). Persons who exhibit paradoxical IRIS have been reported to have elevated tuberculin-specific effector memory CD4$^+$ T cells prior to initiation of ART. Following the commencement of ART, increased levels of Th1-associated cytokines, interferon-γ, and tumor necrosis factor-α most likely contribute to the overwhelming inflammatory reaction to the TB antigen present (Bourgarit, 2009). Persons with HIV and latent TB (defined as >5 mm skin test induration or positive interferon-γ release assay) are at increased risk for progression to active TB compared to the HIV-negative population, which underscores the need to identify and treat patients with latent disease. Active TB in HIV-infected patients requires immediate treatment. However, optimal timing of ART has yet to be established. Potential for multiple adverse drug reactions, drug–drug interactions, and IRIS reactions has led to increased difficulty in defining the proper timing of ART.

TIMING OF ART WITH TB IRIS

In recent years, there has been debate on the timing of ART initiation relative to the initiation of TB treatment in known co-infected patients. However, based on a number of trials, as discussed here, current DHHS guidelines recommend an early, integrative approach to ART and TB treatment initiation.

In the SAPiT trial, there were no differences in rates of AIDS or death between patients who started ART within 4 weeks after initiating TB treatment and those who started ART at 8–12 weeks (i.e., within 4 weeks after completing the intensive phase of TB treatment) (Abdool Karim, 2010). However, in patients with baseline CD4$^+$ counts <50 cells/mm^3, the rate of AIDS or death was lower in the earlier therapy group than in the later therapy group (8.5 vs. 26.3 cases per 100 person-years, a strong trend favoring the earlier treatment arm ($p = 0.06$)). For all patients, regardless of CD4$^+$ cell count, earlier therapy was associated with a higher incidence of IRIS and of adverse events that

required a switch in antiretroviral drugs compared to those who started therapy later. In this study, two deaths were attributed to IRIS.

In the CAMELIA study, patients who had CD4$^+$ counts <200 cells/mm^3 were randomized to initiate ART at 2 or 8 weeks after initiation of TB treatment (Blanc, 2011). Study participants had a median CD4$^+$ count of 25 cells/mm^3 and high rates of disseminated TB disease. ART initiated at 2 weeks resulted in a 38% reduction in mortality ($p = 0.006$) compared with that of therapy initiated at 8 weeks. A significant reduction in mortality was seen in patients with CD4$^+$ counts ≤50 cells/mm^3 and in patients with CD4$^+$ counts of 51–200 cells/mm^3. Overall, six deaths were associated with TB IRIS.

The ACTG 5221 (STRIDE) trial, a multinational study, randomized ART-naive patients with confirmed or probable TB and CD4$^+$ counts <250 cells/mm^3 to earlier (<2 weeks) or later (8–12 weeks) ART (Havlir, 2011). At study entry, the participants' median CD4$^+$ count was 77 cells/mm^3. The rates of mortality and AIDS diagnoses were not different between the earlier and later arms, although higher rates of IRIS were seen in the earlier arm. However, a significant reduction in AIDS or death was seen in the subset of patients with CD4$^+$ counts <50 cells/mm^3 who were randomized to the earlier ART arm ($p = 0.02$).

Given the previously discussed data, DHHS guidelines recommend the initiation of HAART within 2 weeks when an individual's CD4$^+$ count is <50 cells/mm^3 and by 8–12 weeks for all others. This reflects the observation that earlier ART initiation in TB-infected patients improves mortality.

TREATMENT OF IRIS

Although the nonsteroidal anti-inflammatory agents or steroids are commonly used in clinical practice, the dosage and timing have not been well-established in the medical literature. A double-blind, placebo-controlled, randomized clinical trial, including patients receiving both ART and anti-TB therapy and experiencing paradoxical IRIS, evaluated a tapering course of prednisone over 4 weeks. Individuals on steroid therapy had a significantly decreased length of hospitalization and marked improvement of symptoms related to IRIS, suggesting a potential role for steroids in the management of paradoxical IRIS (Meintjes, 2010). In the previously described ACTG 5164 study, 63% of subjects reported having pneumocystis pneumonia as an OI. There was no significant difference in the frequency of IRIS between subjects who received corticosteroids during the treatment and those who did not receive corticosteroids: 9/150 (6%) versus 11/112 (9.8%), respectively ($p = 0.35$).

In other forms of IRIS, such as MAC, surgical drainage of necrotic lymphadenitis may be of benefit. In patients with cryptococcal meningitis IRIS, cerebrospinal fluid drainage may provide relief of increased intracranial pressure. Corticosteroid or other anti-inflammatory therapies may also be effective for treating some forms of IRIS, such as PML-associated IRIS (Martin-Blondel, 2011).

As a general approach, in unmasking IRIS, management should focus on diagnosis of the OI and instituting appropriate treatment. Screening for latent TB infection should be undertaken in all HIV-infected patients. In paradoxical IRIS, it is crucial to exclude alternate diagnoses and ensure the patient is receiving appropriate treatment for the condition. In the majority of cases, ART is continued, but on rare occasions cessation of ART is warranted in severe IRIS, particularly when it is life-threatening.

References

Abdool Karim SS. Timing of initiation of antiretroviral drugs during tuberculosis therapy. *N Engl J Med.* 2010 Feb 5; 362(8):697–706.

Blanc FX, Sok T, Laureillard D, et al. Earlier versus later start of antiretroviral therapy in HIV-infected adults with tuberculosis. *N Engl J Med.* 2011 Oct 20; 365(16):1471–1481.

Boulware DR, Hullsiek KH, Puronen CE, et al.; INSIGHT Study Group. Higher levels of CRP, D-dimer, IL-6, and hyaluronic acid before initiation of antiretroviral therapy (ART) are associated with increased risk of AIDS or death. *J Infect Dis.* 2011 Jun 1; 203(11):1637–1646.

Bourgarit A, Carcelain G, Samri A, et al. TB-associated immune restoration syndrome in HIV-1-infected patients involves tuberculin-specific CD4 Th1 cells and can be predicted by KIR-negative gammadelta T cells. Paper presented at the 16th Conference on Retroviruses and Opportunistic Infections, February 8–11, 2009, Montréal, Canada. Abstract 772.

Cameron BA, Emerson CR, Workman C, et al. Alterations in immune function are associated with liver enzyme elevation in HIV and HCV co-infection after commencement of combination antiretroviral therapy. *J Clin Immunol.* 2011; 31:1079–1083.

Crane M, Oliver B, Matthews G, et al. Immunopathogenesis of hepatic flare in HIV/hepatitis B virus (HBV)-coinfected individuals after the initiation of HBV-active antiretroviral therapy. *J Infect Dis.* 2009; 199:974–981.

Dheda K, Lampe FC, Johnson MA, et al. Outcome of HIV-associated tuberculosis in the era of highly active antiretroviral therapy. *J Infect Dis.* 2004; 190(9):1670.

Fischl M, Mollan K, Pahwa S, et al. IRIS among US subjects starting ART in AIDS Clinical Trials Group Study A5202. Paper presented at the 15th Conference on Retroviruses and Opportunistic Infections, February 16–19, 2010, San Francisco, CA. Abstract 791.

French MA, Price P, Stone SF. Immune restoration disease after antiretroviral therapy. *AIDS.* 2004; 18:1615–1627.

Haddow L, Borrow P, Dibben O, et al. Cytokine profiles predict unmasking TB immune reconstitution inflammatory syndrome and are associated with unmasking and paradoxical presentations of TB immune reconstitution inflammatory syndrome. Paper presented at the 16th Conference on Retroviruses and Opportunistic Infections, February 8–11, 2009, Montréal, Canada. Abstract 773.

Haddow LJ, Colebunders R, Meintjes G, et al. Cryptococcal immune reconstitution inflammatory syndrome in HIV-1-infected individuals: Proposed clinical case definitions. *Lancet Infect Dis* 2010; 10:791–802.

Havlir DV, Kendall MA, Ive P, et al. Timing of antiretroviral therapy for HIV-1 infection and tuberculosis. *N Engl J Med.* 2011 Oct 20; 365(16):1482–1491.

HIV-CAUSAL Collaboration. Impact of antiretroviral therapy on tuberculosis incidence among HIV-positive patients in high-income countries. *Clin Infect Dis.* 2012 May; 54(9):1364–1372.

Makadzange AT, Ndhlovu CE, Takarinda K, et al. Early versus delayed initiation of antiretroviral therapy for concurrent HIV infection and cryptococcal meningitis in sub-Saharan Africa. *Clin Infect Dis.* 2010; 50:1532–1538.

Martin-Blondel G, Delobel P, Blancher A, et al. Pathogenesis of the immune reconstitution inflammatory syndrome affecting the central nervous system in patients infected with HIV. *Brain.* 2011; 134:928–946.

Meintjes G, Wilkinson RJ, Morroni C, et al. Randomized placebo-controlled trial of prednisone for paradoxical tuberculosis-associated immune reconstitution inflammatory syndrome. *AIDS.* 2010 Sep 24; 24(15):2381–2390.

Müller M, Wandel S, Colebunders R, et al. Immune reconstitution inflammatory syndrome in patients starting antiretroviral therapy for HIV infection: A systematic review and meta-analysis. *Lancet Infect Dis.* 2010; 10:251–261.

Novak RM, Richardson JT, Buchacz K, et al.; HIV Outpatient Study (HOPS) Investigators. Immune reconstitution inflammatory syndrome: Incidence and implications for mortality. *AIDS.* 2012 Mar 27; 26(6):721–730.

Oliver BG, Elliott JH, Price P, et al. Mediators of innate and adaptive immune responses differentially affect immune restoration disease associated with *Mycobacterium tuberculosis* in HIV patients beginning antiretroviral therapy. *J Infect Dis.* 2010; 202:1728–1737.

Porter BO, Ouedraogo GL, Hodge JN, et al. d-Dimer and CRP levels are elevated prior to antiretroviral treatment in patients who develop IRIS. *Clin Immunol.* 2010 Jul; 136(1):42–50.

Shelburne SA, Montes M, Hamill RJ Immune reconstitution inflammatory syndrome: More answers, more questions. *J Antimicrob Chemother.* 2006; 57(2):167.

US Department of Health and Human Services. DHHS guidelines for the use of antiretroviral agents in HIV-1 infected adults and adolescents. Available at https://aidsinfo.nih.gov/guidelines. Accessed November 3, 2015.

Zolopa AR, Anderson J, Komarow L, et al. Early antiretroviral therapy reduces AIDS progression/death in individuals with acute opportunistic infections: A multicenter randomized strategy trial. *PLoS One.* 2009; 4(5):e5575.

49.

US HEALTH CARE SYSTEMS, HIV PROGRAMS, AND COVERAGE POLICY ISSUES

Holly Kilness Packett, MA

LEARNING OBJECTIVE

Discuss the issues related to the coverage and reimbursement for HIV services following the implementation of the Affordable Care Act.

WHAT'S NEW?

Following the implementation of the Affordable Care Act, availability of health coverage for HIV patients is greatly expanded in the United States. However, challenges such as affordability and access to treatments still remain. In addition, the landscape of coverage options, including Medicaid, varies widely between states.

KEY POINTS

- Since 2014, all US citizens are required by law to have health coverage.

- Coverage and reimbursement for HIV services vary widely based on payer or coverage source and also state.

- Access to treatment varies greatly between payers, as does affordability.

- Most states now offer Medicaid coverage to all citizens under 138% federal poverty level (FPL). However, some states still do not, leaving a pool of very poor individuals with little to no access to affordable health coverage options in those states.

- Health coverage systems are evolving rapidly based largely on politics.

- The Ryan White Program is a federal "wrap-around" program designed to provide services to HIV patients with insufficient coverage and benefits.

HIV-related health care services have historically been covered or provided by a patchwork of federal, state, and local programs, such as Medicare, Medicaid, the Ryan White Program, and state and local health programs. AIDS service organizations (ASOs) and private and charitable health organizations also provided services for HIV patients without coverage. These programs represent the long-standing pathways to insurance coverage, access to care, and access to treatment for people with HIV. Some of these programs also supply coverage for or access to medications that treat co-occurring conditions for people with HIV.

Recent public policy changes, including the passage of a health reform law, have effected significant changes in availability of private insurance coverage to HIV patients. In 2010, the Patient Protection and Affordable Care Act (the "Affordable Care Act" or "ACA") was passed by Congress and signed into law by President Obama (Levy, 2015). The law, aimed at reforming health care coverage in the United States, represented the broadest reform to the US health care systems since the 1960s. The law has many aspects; however, among the reforms with greatest impact for HIV patients were prohibited discrimination against individuals with preexisting conditions by insurers, a requirement for all US citizens to obtain health insurance coverage, the expansion of the Medicaid program to cover all individuals under 138% of FPL, and the creation of individual and small group insurance markets (exchanges) in each state along with federal tax credits for low-income individuals in order to purchase insurance affordably.

Many provisions of the law were scheduled to be implemented during the following decade, with the most significant changes scheduled for 2014 ("Health Care Reform Timeline"). However, lawmakers and other opponents of the law have undertaken regular efforts at altering, defunding, or overturning the law and likely will continue these efforts.

In addition, the constitutionality of the law was challenged in several cases that reached the US Supreme Court (Duignan, "Affordable Care Act Cases"). In 2012, a key provision of the law was struck down by the Court in part, effectively making Medicaid expansion optional to states. That, coupled with significant flexibility provided to state lawmakers and insurers in the state insurance markets, has created significant variability among coverage options available to HIV patients in each state. Because the Ryan White Program is a safety net program designed to wrap around other forms of health coverage, this has created wide variability and challenges for that program as well.

PRIVATE INSURANCE

Private health insurance in the United States is typically offered by private for-profit or nonprofit companies to various markets. One of the largest markets has been employment-based insurance in the United States (US Census Bureau, 2010), in which health insurance is offered as a benefit or form of compensation to employees by their employer. Individual insurance plans were less common before the health care law in 2014.

Some common forms of private insurance are indemnity plans, preferred provider plans, and health maintenance organizations. With indemnity plans, individuals can generally choose any health care provider and have a portion of the fees paid by the insurance. With preferred provider plans, individuals must choose from a defined network of clinicians, but the clinicians are generally employed by different groups. With health maintenance plans, individuals receive care from one or a small number of clinician groups.

Reimbursement to clinicians varies widely with private insurance policies, with lower rates generally paid by managed care organizations. The provider networks within insurance plans can affect reimbursement levels, as can plan benefits, co-pays, and cost-sharing mechanisms. Coverage of particular medications and treatments for patients varies widely under private insurance plans.

The Affordable Care Act prohibited health insurance discrimination based on health status or gender, as well as lifetime limits on coverage, preexisting condition exclusions, and charging higher premiums based on gender or health status ("Obamacare Pre-Existing Conditions"; "Obamacare No Discrimination"). The Affordable Care Act created a so-called "individual mandate" requiring all US citizens to obtain health coverage beginning in 2014 or face federal tax penalties ("Obamacare Individual Mandate"; "If You Don't Have Health Insurance: How Much You'll Pay"). Individuals who did not have access to employer-based insurance, or other insurance coverage, and did not qualify for public health coverage programs such as Medicaid could purchase individual insurance through the state insurance exchanges (marketplaces).

STATE INSURANCE EXCHANGES (MARKETPLACES)

One of the most significant accomplishments of the Affordable Care Act was the creation of marketplaces for individual and small group insurance plans in each state ("State Health Insurance Marketplaces"). Each state insurance exchange (marketplace) is simply a market forum where private insurance companies offer various qualified health plans (QHPs) to residents of that state ("Health Insurance Marketplace"). Individuals can access the marketplace online, by phone, or in person through assisters, and they can also use the marketplace to determine eligibility for Medicaid or CHIP benefits ("Health Insurance Marketplace").

The Affordable Care Act also made tax credit subsidies available to some low- and medium-income individuals in order to purchase insurance through the state exchanges (Kaiser Family Foundation). Tax credits of gradated amounts are available to those with income levels between 138% and 400% FPL, and they are taken as upfront subsidies to the plan premium ("Premium Tax Credit").

The plans offered within the markets vary in cost as well as coverage and benefit design. The Essential Health Benefits (EHBs) include services within the following 10 categories: ambulatory patient services, emergency services, hospitalization, maternity and newborn care, mental health and substance use disorder services (including behavioral health treatment), prescription drugs, rehabilitative and habilitative services and devices, laboratory services, preventive and wellness services and chronic disease management, and pediatric services (including oral and vision care) ("Essential Health Benefits"; "10 Health Care Benefits Covered in the Health Insurance Marketplace").

In addition, all plans in the state exchanges are required to include a minimum percentage of all the Essential Community Providers (ECPs) in a geographic area in their provider network. ECPs are providers that serve predominately low-income medically underserved individuals. This includes Ryan White HIV/AIDS providers.

MEDICAID

The Medicaid program has long been the nation's public health insurance program for those with low-income status, limited resources, and disability. Originally, the program covered only certain populations, such as the medically disabled and pregnant women, infants, and children of poverty status.

The Affordable Care Act sought to expand the program's coverage to include all citizens below 138% FPL regardless of other categorizations. However, in 2012, the requirement for states to expand their Medicaid program in this regard was struck down by the US Supreme Court (Duignan, "Affordable Care Act Cases"). In effect, this made the Medicaid expansion optional to states (Rudowitz, 2015). Many states have selected to expand the state Medicaid program in whole, as envisioned by the law. Other states have partially expanded their Medicaid program in a variety of ways via the use of a state program amendment or waiver, which must be approved by the US Department of Health and Human Services (DHHS) (Rudowitz, 2015). Some states have declined to expand altogether, for political reasons. In states in which Medicaid has not been expanded fully, some low-income individuals are left without affordable health insurance coverage options. However, individuals in those states are exempt from the tax penalties under the individual mandate ("Obamacare Mandate: Exemption and Tax Penalty").

Medicaid has continually been estimated to be the single largest source of coverage for people with HIV in the United States, estimated to account for roughly half of people with HIV in regular care (Kates, 2011). Medicaid covers inpatient, ambulatory care, and skilled nursing care. Medicaid also covers prescription medications except for persons who also have Medicare (dual eligibles) ("Dual Eligibles"). Coverage levels, eligibility criteria, and program benefits vary widely from state to state ("Benefits").

Medicaid is financed jointly by the federal government and states and is administered by state governments in accordance with certain basic federal eligibility and benefit standards ("Financing & Reimbursement"). At the federal level, the Medicaid program is run by the Centers for Medicare and Medicaid Services (CMS) under the DHHS. Medicaid is the third largest domestic program in the federal budget, after Social Security and Medicare (Rudowitz, 2015). It is also the second largest program in most state budgets. The federal government matches state spending in Medicaid, paying for 56% of the program's spending overall (Rudowitz, 2015). The Affordable Care Act law initially paid for 100% of the cost of a state's expansion of Medicaid, with that amount decreasing over time.

In recent years, some states have tried to mitigate Medicaid budgetary costs through reductions of benefits, limitations to drug formularies, and other efforts. Many states also offer managed care-type programs to particular populations in efforts to reduce costs.

Medicaid managed care has grown significantly in recent decades, with more than half of Medicaid beneficiaries now receiving care and services through Medicaid managed care organizations (MCOs). MCOs contract directly with the state to provide services and benefits in a variety of capacities ("Medicaid Managed Care Market Tracker"). Some MCOs are operated by a parent firm that also participates in the private insurance market.

Traditional Medicaid programs offer provider reimbursement through fee-for-service rates that are determined by the state. MCOs make agreements for provider reimbursement based on monthly capitation rates.

MEDICARE

Medicare is the federal health insurance program for seniors older than age 65 years and also for people younger than age 65 years with permanent disabilities, including people living with AIDS. The Medicare program is administered by the CMS under the DHHS.

Eligibility is tied to work history and contributions to Medicare through employment-based withholding. Some individuals are eligible for both Medicare and Medicaid (dual eligibles), given their income and disability status. The number of persons living with HIV/AIDS who access Medicare has increased due to increased survival rates from antiretroviral therapies and the aging of the population living with HIV/AIDS. Medicare covers inpatient and outpatient care, some skilled nursing and home care, and medications. Medicare also covers HIV testing for beneficiaries.

In 2006, Medicare began providing prescription drug coverage under the Medicare Part D drug benefit. Most Medicare-eligible individuals can decide whether to participate through enrollment in one of several prescription drug plans that are marketed as stand-alone coverage or as part of managed care plans (called Medicare Advantage). In addition, those dually eligible for both Medicare and Medicaid must participate. Medicare requires that each plan cover six categories of drugs, one of which is antiretroviral drugs. Medicare Part D includes an exceptions and appeals process that can be used to request coverage of drugs not covered by the plan.

Individual Medicare Part D plans differ widely in terms of premiums and other cost-sharing requirements. Medicare Part D includes a sequence of cost-sharing requirements, including an initial deductible and subsequent "out-of-pocket" costs. Most Medicare Part D plans also have a coverage gap (or "donut hole") in which, after a certain amount of costs have been paid through the coverage plan, any additional costs become the responsibility of the individual ("Costs in the Coverage Gap") until the costs reach the catastrophic coverage threshold ("Catastrophic Coverage"). At that point, nearly all costs are then covered by Medicare. The Affordable Care Act law closes the "donut hole" gap in coverage gradually by 2020, and it provides some rebates for those who encounter the coverage gap in the interim ("Costs in the Coverage Gap").

Medicare reimbursement rates are similar to those of private insurance. Clinicians who accept Medicare reimbursement are subject to federal audits of their charts to check billed amounts against services documented.

THE RYAN WHITE PROGRAM

The Ryan White HIV/AIDS Program is a federal program designed specifically for the care, treatment, and support services for people with HIV/AIDS in the United States. The Ryan White Program was first enacted in 1990, and it is administered by the Health Resources and Services Administration under the DHHS ("About the Ryan White HIV/AIDS Program").

The Ryan White Program is a "safety net" program for people with HIV/AIDS who have no other source of coverage or face coverage limits ("The Ryan White Program"). The program is designed to wrap around other forms of coverage and is "payer of last resort" as required by law. This designation means that if an individual is eligible for any other program, he or she must access its coverage and benefits before accessing the Ryan White Program ("Eligible Individuals & Allowable Uses of Funds for Discretely Defined Categories of Services,").

It is the third largest source of federal funding for HIV care in the United States after Medicare and Medicaid. It is estimated to reach more than half a million people with HIV each year ("The Ryan White Program"). Funding for the Ryan White Program is subject to Congressional appropriations each year. In addition to federal funding, some states and localities also provide funding to their Ryan White services through state matching funds requirements.

Part A of the Ryan White Program provides funding to Eligible Metropolitan Areas and Transitional Grant Areas hardest hit by the HIV/AIDS epidemic for a wide range of services and efforts. Part B of the program provides funding to states and territories ("About the Ryan White HIV/AIDS Program").

A vitally important part of the program for HIV patients is the AIDS Drug Assistance Program (ADAP), which is funded through allocations to the states under Part B of the program along with state funding. The ADAP in each state provides HIV-related prescription drugs to low-income individuals with limited or no prescription drug coverage ("AIDS Drug Assistance Programs"). Many states also use ADAP funding to purchase health insurance and/or pay insurance premiums, copayments, or deductibles for people with HIV/AIDS. All ADAPs participate in the 340B program, enabling them to purchase drugs at or below the statutorily defined 340B ceiling price.

Part C of the Ryan White Program funds providers and medical clinics that deliver comprehensive medical care and treatment to people with HIV who have no other source for care ("About the Ryan White HIV/AIDS Program"). Part C also funds early intervention services, ambulatory care, and primary health care services for people with HIV or who are at risk of infection in underserved or rural communities and communities of color. Finally, Part C also provides planning grants and capacity grants to support organizations in the delivery of high-quality effective HIV care ("The Ryan White Program").

Part D of the program grants support services for women, infants, children, and youth ("About the Ryan White HIV/AIDS Program").

Part F of the program provides funding for a variety of programs, including the Special Projects of National Significance, AIDS Education & Training Centers, dental programs, and the Minority AIDS Initiative ("About the Ryan White HIV/AIDS Program").

The Ryan White Program is a "payer of last resort" program, meaning that patients who have access to other forms of coverage must access those benefits first. For this reason, the Affordable Care Act heralded major changes for the future of the Ryan White Program. Thousands of patients who previously received care and treatment primarily through the Ryan White Program became eligible to receive primary coverage through Medicaid or the state insurance marketplaces under the law.

NETWORKS OF CARE

For HIV providers, inclusion in networks of care for health programs is of great importance. Most patients' health coverage limits them to seeing only certain providers who are "in network" or charges substantially higher fees or declines payment for services by providers not included in the network.

The Affordable Care Cat required that all plans in the state exchanges include a minimum percentage of all the ECPs in a geographic area in their provider network. ECPs are providers that serve predominately low-income, medically underserved individuals ("Definition of Essential Community Providers (ECPs) in Marketplaces"). This includes Ryan White HIV/AIDS providers.

Reimbursement rates and schedules for providers who are part of the network are set by or negotiated with health coverage issuers and entities.

PROVIDER REIMBURSEMENT

Reimbursement for medical procedures highly depends on thorough and accurate documentation of the medical encounter, diagnosis, treatment, and services as recorded and submitted through coding claims. The level of complexity and severity of the medical encounter—and thus the level of reimbursement—is defined by the level of complexity of the problem(s), the number of problems at issue, the amount of time spent with the patient, and other factors. To ensure adequate and appropriate reimbursement, careful documentation of these factors, as well as the specific elements of the medical history, the physical examination, and the medical decision-making, is essential. Documenting time spent on prevention efforts (e.g., counseling the patient about consistent condom use or disclosure to partners) and promoting other behavioral changes (e.g., quitting smoking or avoiding substance abuse) is also essential for reimbursement of these services.

CODING

Standardized coding systems are used in the United States to process billing claims to private and public insurers. The two principal systems used for coding medical information in the United States are the International Classification of Diseases (ICD) and the Current Procedural Terminology (CPT) codes that make up the Healthcare Common Procedure Coding System (HCPCS). In general, CPT/HCPCS codes identify the services rendered, whereas ICD codes focus more on the diagnosis.

The CPT codes are created, maintained, and trademarked by the American Medical Association (AMA) ("Coding with CPT for Proper Reimbursement").

The HCPCS was created by the federal CMS. The HCPCS is based on the CPT codes but provides for two levels of coding. Level I consists of AMA's CPT codes and provides for medical services and procedures furnished by clinicians. Level I codes are numeric. Level II codes are alphanumeric and apply primarily to medical devices and nonclinician services, such as ambulatory care, immunizations, diagnostic procedures, family counseling, and services provided by other health professionals (e.g., clinical nurses, psychologists, and pharmacists) ("HCPCS—General Information"). Medicaid and Medicare services are reimbursed by CMS on the basis of the HCPCS codes for clinician activities.

The ICD is the international standard diagnostic classification for all epidemiological, health, and clinical use. It is a coding and classification system of diseases, symptoms, injuries, abnormal findings, and also the social circumstances and external causes of injury or diseases, as classified by the World Health Organization (WHO). The most recent iteration of these codes, ICD-10, was endorsed by the 43rd World Health Assembly in May 1990 and came into use in WHO member states in 1994 ("International Classification of Diseases (ICD)"). The United States, however, delayed transition to the ICD-10 system until 2014 ("ICD 10"). The ICD-11 codes set is scheduled for release in 2018 ("International Classification of Diseases (ICD)").

In the context of reimbursement, ICD codes are used in conjunction with CPT codes to classify vital records and health conditions codes associated with outpatient, inpatient, medical office utilization, and hospital charges.

References

Levy M. "Patient Protection and Affordable Care Act (PPACA)," Encyclopedia Britannica, June 26, 2015, https://www.britannica.com/topic/Patient-Protection-and-Affordable-Care-Act. Accessed January 14, 2016.

"Health Care Reform Timeline," Obamacare Facts, http://obamacarefacts.com/health-care-reform-timeline. Accessed January 14, 2016.

"Obamacare Pre-Existing Conditions," Obamacare Facts, http://obamacarefacts.com/pre-existing-conditions. Accessed January 14, 2016.

"Obamacare No Discrimination," Obamacare Facts, http://obamacarefacts.com/no-discrimination. Accessed January 14, 2016.

"Obamacare Individual Mandate," Obamacare Facts, http://obamacarefacts.com/obamacare-individual-mandate. Accessed January 14, 2016.

"If You Don't Have Health Insurance: How Much You'll Pay," HealthCare.gov, https://www.healthcare.gov/fees. Accessed January 14, 2016.

"State Health Insurance Marketplaces," Center for Consumer Information & Oversight, https://www.cms.gov/cciio/resources/fact-sheets-and-faqs/state-marketplaces.html. Accessed January 14, 2016.

"Health Insurance Marketplace," HealthCare.gov, https://www.health-care.gov/glossary/health-insurance-marketplace-glossary. Accessed January 14, 2016.

"Premium Tax Credit" Glossary, HeathCare.gov, https://www.health-care.gov/glossary/premium-tax-credit. Accessed January 14, 2016.

"Essential Health Benefits" Glossary, HeathCare.gov, https://www.healthcare.gov/glossary/essential-health-benefits. Accessed January 14, 2016.

"10 Health Care Benefits Covered in the Health Insurance Marketplace" Blog, HeathCare.gov, August 22, 2013, https://www.healthcare.gov/blog/10-health-care-benefits-covered-in-the-health-insurance-marketplace.

Duignan B, "Affordable Care Act Cases," Encyclopedia Britannica, http://www.britannica.com/event/Affordable-Care-Act-cases. Accessed January 14, 2016.

Rudowitz R, Musumeci M, "The ACA and Medicaid Expansion Waivers," The Henry J. Kaiser Family Foundation, November 20, 2015, http://kff.org/medicaid/issue-brief/the-aca-and-medicaid-expansion-waivers.

"Obamacare Mandate: Exemption and Tax Penalty," Obamacare Facts, http://obamacarefacts.com/obamacare-mandate-exemption-penalty. Accessed January 14, 2016.

Kates J, "Medicaid and HIV: A National Analysis," The Henry J. Kaiser Family Foundation, October 2011, http://kff.org/hivaids/report/medicaid-and-hiv-a-national-analysis.

"Dual Eligibles," Medicaid.Gov, https://www.medicaid.gov/affordablec-areact/provisions/dual-eligibles.html. Accessed January 14, 2016.

"Benefits," Medicaid.gov, https://www.medicaid.gov/medicaid-chip-program-information/by-topics/benefits/medicaid-benefits.html. Accessed January 14, 2016.

"Financing & Reimbursement," Medicaid.gov, https://www.medicaid.gov/medicaid-chip-program-information/by-topics/financing-and-reimbursement/financing-and-reimbursement.html. Accessed January 14, 2016.

Rudowitz R, Snyder L, "The ACA and Medicaid Expansion Waivers," The Henry J. Kaiser Family Foundation, May 20, 2015, http://kff.org/medicaid/issue-brief/medicaid-financing-how-does-it-work-and-what-are-the-implications/.

"Medicaid Managed Care Market Tracker," The Henry J. Kaiser Family Foundation, http://kff.org/data-collection/medicaid-managed-care-market-tracker. Accessed January 14, 2016.

"Costs in the Coverage Gap," Medicare.gov, https://www.medicare.gov/part-d/costs/coverage-gap/part-d-coverage-gap.html. Accessed January 14, 2016.

"Catastrophic Coverage," Medicare.gov, https://www.medicare.gov/part-d/costs/catastrophic-coverage/drug-plan-catastrophic-coverage.html. Accessed January 14, 2016.

"About the Ryan White HIV/AIDS Program," HRSA HIV AIDS Programs, http://hab.hrsa.gov/abouthab/aboutprogram.html. Accessed January 14, 2016.

"The Ryan White Program," The Henry J. Kaiser Family Foundation, March 5, 2013, http://kff.org/hivaids/fact-sheet/the-ryan-white-program.

"Eligible Individuals & Allowable Uses of Funds for Discretely Defined Categories of Services," HRSA.gov, http://hab.hrsa.gov/managey-ourgrant/pinspals/eligible1002.html. Accessed January 14, 2016.

"AIDS Drug Assistance Programs," The Henry J. Kaiser Family Foundation, April 8, 2014, http://kff.org/hivaids/fact-sheet/aids-drug-assistance-programs/

"Definition of Essential Community Providers (ECPs) in Marketplaces," The Henry J. Kaiser Family Foundation, http://kff.org/other/state-indicator/definition-of-essential-community-providers-ecps-in-marketplaces. Accessed January 14, 2016.

"Coding with CPT for Proper Reimbursement," American Medical Association, http://www.ama-assn.org/ama/pub/physician-resources/solutions-managing-your-practice/coding-billing-insurance/cpt.page. Accessed January 14, 2016.

"HCPCS—General Information," Centers for Medicare and Medicaid Services, https://www.cms.gov/medicare/coding/medhcpcsgen-info/index.html. Accessed January 14, 2016.

"International Classification of Diseases (ICD)," World Health Organization, http://www.who.int/classifications/icd/en. Accessed January 14, 2016.

"ICD 10," Centers for Medicare and Medicaid Services, https://www.cms.gov/medicare/Coding/ICD10/index.html. Accessed January 14, 2016.

50.

LEGAL ISSUES[a]

Jeffrey T. Schouten

CHAPTER GOAL

Upon completion of this chapter, the reader should be able to demonstrate knowledge about legal issues surrounding HIV health care and to interact more effectively, professionally, and sensitively with patients and their families.

ROUTINE HIV TESTING (WITH CONSENT)

LEARNING OBJECTIVE

Discuss the Centers for Disease Control and Prevention's (CDC) recommendations for routine HIV testing in various health care settings.

WHAT'S NEW?

The US Preventive Services Task Force (USPSTF) gave an "A" level recommendation in April 2013 to the CDC's recommendations for routine HIV testing for all adolescents and adults aged 15–65 years.

KEY POINTS

- It is estimated that the 12.8% of people who do not know they are HIV-infected account for 50% of new cases of HIV infection.

- The CDC recommends that all people aged 13–65 years receive an HIV test at least once as part of routine health care. Persons identified as high risk for HIV infection should be retested at least annually.

- Routine testing delinks pre- and post-test counseling from testing.

The CDC estimates that more than 1.2 million people in the United States are living with HIV infection. One in eight (12.8%) of those people are unaware of their infection (CDC, 2015). A meta-analysis of 11 independent studies showed that the prevalence of high-risk sexual behavior is reduced substantially after people become aware they are HIV-infected (Marks, 2006). Estimated transmission is 3.5 times higher among persons who are unaware of their infection than among persons who are aware of their infection, which contributes disproportionately to the number of new HIV infections each year in the United States (Marks, 2006). Updated modeling data showed that an estimated 49% of transmissions were from the 20% of persons living with HIV unaware of their infection (Hall, 2012).

A study in South Carolina found that among the persons identified as late testers (persons who received an AIDS diagnosis within 1 year of HIV diagnosis), approximately three-fourths had visited a South Carolina health care facility prior to their HIV diagnosis. In addition, most of the late testers had made multiple visits, and most of their visits occurred 1 year or more before diagnosis of HIV infection. According to the report, the majority of diagnoses for these previous visits probably would not have prompted HIV testing under a risk-based testing strategy (CDC, 2006). The CDC published revised recommendations concerning routine HIV testing in health care settings in September 2006. The major revisions in the recommendations are as follows:

- For patients in all health care settings

  - HIV screening is recommended for patients in all health care settings after patients are notified that

---

[a] The author wrote or revised text from previous editions and takes responsibility for it; however, the work represents a group product including previous authors.

testing will be performed, unless patients decline (opt-out screening).

- Persons at high risk for HIV infection should be screened for HIV at least annually.

- Separate written consent for HIV testing should not be required; general consent for medical care should be considered sufficient to encompass consent for HIV testing.

- Prevention counseling should not be required as part of HIV diagnostic testing or HIV screening programs in health care settings.

- For pregnant women

  - HIV screening should be included in the routine panel of prenatal screening tests for all pregnant women.

  - HIV screening is recommended after the patient is notified that testing will be performed, unless the patient declines (opt-out screening).

  - Separate written consent for HIV testing should not be required; general consent for medical care should be considered sufficient to encompass consent for HIV testing.

  - Repeat screening in the third trimester is recommended in certain jurisdictions with elevated rates of HIV infection among pregnant women.

Although the CDC recommends that prevention counseling should not be required with HIV diagnostic testing in health care settings, the elements of informed consent include some of the information communicated during pretest counseling. Also, risk assessment is needed to identify patients at high risk for HIV infection who should be screened for HIV at least annually. The CDC recommendations define informed consent as follows (CDC, 2006):

A process of communication between patient and provider, through which, an informed patient can choose whether to undergo HIV testing or decline to do so. Elements of informed consent typically include providing oral or written information regarding HIV, the risks and benefits of testing, the implications of HIV test results, how test results will be communicated, and the opportunity to ask questions.

Routine testing means that HIV testing is offered to all patients. Testing requires informed consent, but that consent can be included in the general consent to care agreements. Patients can choose to "opt out" of routine testing if they do not want to be tested.

Laws governing consent for HIV testing are state specific. Although all states require consent for an HIV test, many states that had required explicit written consent prior to the 2006 CDC revised HIV testing recommendations have changed their laws (*JAMA*, 2011). This remains a dynamic area of law and regulation. A good resource is the Compendium of State HIV Testing Laws maintained by the Nations HIV/AIDS Clinicians' Consultation Center, although it is no longer updated.

Challenges in implementing routine HIV testing include the cost of testing, follow-up notification of positive results in emergency departments and in-patient settings, and adoption of rapid testing. The USPSTF recommends that clinicians screen for HIV infection in adolescents and adults aged 15–65 years. Younger adolescents and older adults who are at increased risk should also be screened.

Recommended Reading

AMA Code of Ethics: Opinion 2.23—HIV Testing. Available at http://www.ama-assn.org/ama/pub/physician-resources/medical-ethics/code-medical-ethics/opinion223.page. Accessed November 28, 2015.

Centers for Disease Control and Prevention. Revised recommendations for HIV testing of adults, adolescents, and pregnant women in health-care settings. *MMWR Morbid Mortal Wkly Rep.* 2006; 55(RR14):1–17. Available at www.cdc.gov/mmwr/preview/mmwrhtml/rr5514a1.htm. Accessed November 30, 2015.

Hall HI, Holtgrave D, Maulsby C. HIV transmission rates from persons living with HIV who are aware and unaware of their infection. *AIDS.* 2012; 26:893–896.

Hughes C. ICD-10 simplifies preventive care coding, sort of. *Fam Pract Manag.* 2014 Jul–Aug; 21(4):OA1–OA4. Available at http://www.aafp.org/fpm/2014/0700/oa1.html. Accessed November 28, 2015.

Marks G, Crepaz N, Janssen RS. Estimating sexual transmission of HIV from persons aware and unaware that they are infected with the virus in the USA. *AIDS.* 2006; 20:1447–1450.

HIV TESTING WITHOUT CONSENT

LEARNING OBJECTIVE

Discuss the circumstances under which it is allowable to test a patient for HIV without consent, including reference to applicable legal regulations.

WHAT'S NEW?

The information on HIV testing without consent has remained consistent during the past few years.

Although all states require consent for HIV testing (Halpern, 2005), there are situations in which it is possible to obtain an HIV test without the consent of the person to be tested. In some cases, non-consented HIV testing may be standard practice. For example, in New York, newborn infants are tested without parental consent if their mother did not consent to HIV testing during pregnancy. Some states require HIV testing of convicted sexual offenders (e.g., Revised Code of Washington RCW 70.24.340).

A minority of states provide explicit exceptions for consent for HIV testing in emergency medical situations (Halpern, 2005). Some states allow for testing of source patients when there has been a potential exposure to HIV in a health care setting or when a public safety officer has had potential exposure. California allows for non-consented testing of blood samples but will not permit the ordering of a blood draw specifically for HIV testing after an occupational exposure without the consent of the local public health officer or a court (California Health and Safety Code 120260-120263). In most health care settings, when there has been an occupational exposure capable of transmitting blood-borne pathogens, the source patient will consent to testing and allow access to his or her medical record (Maryland Department of Health and Mental Hygiene, 2003).

California and several other states allow for HIV testing of persons accused of a criminal act capable of transmitting HIV. California requires a court hearing showing there is probable cause to believe that the accused committed the offense and that blood, semen, or another bodily fluid capable of transmitting HIV (as identified in State Department of Health Services regulations) has been transferred from the accused to the victim (California Penal Code 1524.1(b)(3)(A)). A major challenge with non-consented testing is getting the required order from the appropriate authority so that testing and initiation of post-exposure prophylaxis can take place in a timely manner (Chapter 3). A survey showed that intensivists' decisions to pursue non-consented testing,

a not uncommon situation, are associated with their personal ethics and often erroneous perceptions of state laws but not with the laws themselves (Halpern, 2007). Because laws and regulations vary by state, the clinician is responsible for knowing the appropriate rules in the state in which he or she practices. Consultation with the local public health officer is advised whenever non-consented HIV testing is believed to be necessary.

Recommended Reading

Halpern SD. HIV testing without consent in critically ill patients. *JAMA*. 2005; 294(6):734–737.

Halpern SD, Metkus TS, Fuchs BD, et al. Nonconsented human immunodeficiency virus testing among critically ill patients: Intensivists' practices and the influence of state laws. *Arch Intern Med*. 2007 Nov 26; 167(21):2323–2328.

DISEASE REPORTING SYSTEM

AIDS SURVEILLANCE

Since HIV/AIDS was first recognized as a disease, most state and city departments of health have used the reporting of AIDS cases to track the incidence and prevalence of HIV infections and HIV-related complications. Data on AIDS cases are reported in a standardized format to the CDC by all 50 states, the District of Columbia, and US dependencies and possessions.

HIV/AIDS SURVEILLANCE

In 1991, some states began implementing standardized HIV case reporting, in addition to AIDS case reporting. The reauthorization of the Ryan White CARE Act in 2000 gave states 6 years to adopt named-based HIV reporting or risk losing federal funds. Most states complied with this mandate. Integrated AIDS and HIV case reporting among adults, adolescents, and children had been implemented in 33 states, the Virgin Islands, and Guam by July 2005. Seven states (California, Hawaii, Illinois, Maryland, Massachusetts, Rhode Island, and Vermont) and the District of Columbia implemented a code-based system to conduct case surveillance for HIV infection (not AIDS); five other states (Delaware, Maine, Montana, Oregon, and Washington) implemented a name-to-code system. In 2005, the CDC recommended that name-based HIV reporting be implemented using the same approach that is used for nationwide AIDS surveillance. All states successfully implemented confidential name-based HIV infection reporting by April 2008.

BENEFITS OF HIV SURVEILLANCE

The rationale frequently cited for using HIV rather than AIDS case surveillance is that it allows for a more thorough and accurate characterization of the populations in which HIV infection has been newly diagnosed and helps in the prioritization of prevention services (CDC, 2005b; Holtgrave, 2004). Significant changes in HIV transmission and behavior can be achieved by appropriate programs. For example, aggressive efforts to prevent maternal–fetal transmission have been credited with the steep decline in mother-to-child HIV transmission, the increase in the proportion of HIV-infected pregnant women who have been tested prior to delivery, and the high proportion of HIV-infected pregnant women who accept antiretroviral prophylaxis (Wortley. 2001). Lab-based reporting of CD4 counts and HIV RNA for surveillance has become a helpful tool to assess engagement, linkage, and retention in care (Lubelchek, 2015; Wiewel, 2015).

ANONYMOUS AND CONFIDENTIAL HIV TESTING

Although most studies have not shown a decrease in HIV testing in states that have adopted name-based reporting, data indicate that some people prefer anonymous HIV testing to name-based confidential testing (CDC, 1998; Charlebois, 2005). Many people are understandably reluctant to have their name entered in a database of persons with HIV infection. Although the states have established elaborate precautions to prevent breaches of security, the risk of revelation of HIV status can be intimidating. Therefore, in many areas, individuals can choose to be tested for HIV either anonymously (without giving any identifying information) or confidentially (with the HIV test result linked to identifying information, such as patient name).

In states that require HIV case reporting, only confidential testing results must be reported to public health authorities. Test results from anonymous testing are not reportable. However, they do provide the clinician with an important opportunity for educating and counseling patients about reducing high-risk behaviors and HIV management.

REPORTABLE HIV-RELATED DISEASES

Most states require reporting of conditions that commonly occur or are associated with HIV infection, including syphilis and other sexually transmitted diseases (STDs), tuberculosis, acute hepatitis (A, B, or C), histoplasmosis, and HIV-related opportunistic infections. Certain microbiologic diagnoses that are made by culture or serology are reported directly by the laboratory to the appropriate state or local health authority.

THE CLINICIAN'S ROLE

Health care providers should know which illnesses and complications must be reported to their state health department and the time frame within which reporting is required. They should understand that reporting of notifiable conditions is dependent on the jurisdiction, that a legal obligation is imposed upon practitioners by those states, and that sanctions (e.g., fines) can be imposed upon practitioners for failure to report.

Recommended Reading

Lubelchek RJ, Finnegan KJ, Hotton AL, et al. Assessing the use of HIV surveillance data to help gauge patient retention-in-care. *J Acquir Immune Defic Syndr*. 2015; 69:S25–S30.

US Department of Health and Human Services, Office for Civil Rights. HIPAA. Medical Privacy—National standards to protect the privacy of personal health information. Washington, DC: US Department of Health and Human Services. Available at http://www.hhs.gov/ocr/privacy/index.html.

Wiewel E, Braunstein SL, Xiaet Q, et al. Monitoring outcomes for newly diagnosed and prevalent HIV cases using a care continuum created with New York City surveillance data. *J Acquir Immune Defic Syndr*. 2015; 68:217–226.

Wortley PM, Lindegren ML, Fleming PL. Successful implementation of perinatal HIV prevention guidelines: A multistate surveillance evaluation. *MMWR Morbid Mortal Wkly Rep.* 2001; 50(RR-6):17–28.

PARTNER NOTIFICATION AND PREVENTION FOR POSITIVES

LEARNING OBJECTIVE

Describe the requirements for partner notification practices in HIV disease.

WHAT'S NEW?

Major efforts are ongoing at the national, state, and local levels in many communities to encourage HIV-infected individuals to take a proactive approach to preventing the spread of HIV.

KEY POINTS

- Many states require health care providers to discuss partner notification options with their HIV-infected patients. The federal 1996 Ryan White CARE Act requires all states to adopt laws requiring notification of spouses of HIV-infected patients.

- Many HIV-infected individuals do not disclose their HIV status to their partners out of fear of rejection, loss of financial support, and/or abuse. Their partners then remain unaware of their potential HIV exposure.

- Partner notification programs typically allow HIV-infected persons to anonymously inform their sexual and needle-sharing partners that they may have been exposed to HIV.

PARTNER NOTIFICATION LEGAL REQUIREMENTS

In many states, health care providers are required to discuss partner notification options with HIV-infected patients. This is not only a legal requirement, carrying the possibility of civil and/or legal sanctions for violation of partner notification laws, but also an ethical issue. Amendments to the federal Ryan White CARE Act in 1996 require states to take "administrative or legislative action to require that a good faith effort" is made to notify the spouse of a known HIV-infected patient of the spouse's potential exposure to HIV. This action must be taken by states in order to be eligible for CARE Act funds (Webber, 2004).

States can be categorized into three groups based on their rules and regulations for partner notification programs: (1) States that require health care providers to provide the contact's name to the local health officer, and the public health official then notifies the contact; (2) states that give the health care provider the choice of notifying either the local health officer or the contacts named by the source patient directly; and (3) states that make such disclosures to a state agency discretionary or optional (Lin, 2005). Health care providers should seek advice from local public health departments and their own attorneys to specifically understand their legal responsibilities.

THE CLINICIAN'S ROLE

Preventing harm not only to the patient but also to others should be the goal of every clinician. The CDC has recommended an increased emphasis on prevention efforts in the primary care of HIV-infected people (Box 50.1).

In general, an HIV-infected person should be given the option of directly informing his or her sexual or needle-sharing contacts. A study of men who have sex with men found that knowledge of HIV status resulted in a significant decrease in behaviors capable of transmitting HIV; however, the behavioral changes were not permanent (Colfax, 2002).

Many HIV-infected individuals do not disclose their HIV status to their partners, fearing that they would be threatened, harmed, or abandoned. Non-disclosers, however, are not more likely than disclosers to use condoms or other disease prevention measures (Stein, 1998; Wolitski, 1998). When individuals are reluctant to disclose their HIV status to their partners themselves, partner notification programs can assist.

PARTNER NOTIFICATION PROGRAMS

Partner notification programs are designed to allow HIV-infected individuals to inform their sexual and needle-sharing partners that they may have been exposed to HIV. For HIV-infected persons who opt not to inform their partners themselves, these programs typically provide counselors who will inform the at-risk persons of possible

HIV exposure without revealing the identity of the HIV-
infected person who may have exposed them.

Partner notification programs maximize the opportunity for persons to become aware of their HIV exposure
and to access HIV testing and counseling. Partner notification may prevent an at-risk individual from acquiring HIV
or, if he or she already has HIV, allow him or her to receive
appropriate treatment and learn how to prevent the transmission of HIV infection to others.

Recommended Reading

Centers for Disease Control and Prevention. Incorporating HIV
prevention into the medical care of persons living with HIV.
Recommendations of CDC, the Health Resources and Services
Administration, the National Institutes of Health, and HIV
Medicine Association of the IDSA. *MMWR Morbid Mortal Wkly
Rep*. 2003; 52:1–24. Available at http://www.cdc.gov/mmwr/pre-
view/mmwrhtml/rr5212a1.htm.

Colfax GN, Buchbinder SP, Cornelisse PGA, et al. Sexual risk behaviors
and implications for secondary HIV transmission during and after
HIV seroconversion. *AIDS*. 2002; 16:1529–1535.

Laar AK, DeBruin DA, Craddock S. Partner notification in the context
of HIV: An interest-analysis. *AIDS Res Ther*. 2015; 12:15. Available
at http://www.biomedcentral.com/content/pdf/s12981-015-0057-
8.pdf. Accessed November 30, 2015.

Lin L, Liang BA. HIV and health law: Striking the balance between legal
mandates and medical ethics. *Virtual Mentor AMA J Ethics*. 2005;
7(10). Available at http://journalofethics.ama-assn.org/2005/10/
hlaw1-0510.html.

Stein MD, Freedberg KA, Sullivan LM, et al. Sexual ethics: Disclosure
of HIV-positive status to partners. *Arch Intern Med*. 1998;
158:253–257.

Webber DW. Self-incrimination, partner notification, and the criminal law: Negatives for the CDC's "prevention for positives" initiative. *AIDS Public Policy J*. 2004; 19:54–66. Available at http://
www.hivlawandpolicy.org/resources/self-incrimination-partner-
notification-and-criminal-law-negatives-cdc%E2%80%99s-
%E2%80%9Cprevention. Accessed November 30, 2015.

ISSUES IN DISCLOSURE

LEARNING OBJECTIVE

Discuss the health care provider's legal responsibilities to
HIV-infected patients who do not disclose their HIV status
to sexual and needle-sharing partners.

WHAT'S NEW?

Information regarding disclosure issues has remained consistent during the past few years.

KEY POINTS

- The obligation of health care providers to maintain patient
  confidence may be overridden to protect the public health or
  individuals who are endangered by HIV-infected persons.

- Health care providers should consult an attorney or
  their state laws and regulations before making any such
  disclosures.

- Health care providers may have a "duty to warn" if there is an
  ongoing exposure to potential HIV infection. Conversely,
  there may be criminal actions brought against patients based
  on information provided to local health departments about
  ongoing behaviors endangering the public health.

Information disclosed by a patient to a health care provider
during the course of the provider–patient relationship is
considered confidential. This confidentiality is essential for
a full and free disclosure of information so that effective
counseling and therapy can be provided. In general, unless
required by the law to do so, a health care provider is ethically barred from revealing confidential communications or
information without the patient's consent.

The obligation to maintain patient confidence is not
without limits, however, and it may be overridden by exceptions that are ethically and legally justified. Such justification may occur when a patient threatens to inflict bodily
harm to another person or to him- or herself and there is
a reasonable probability that the patient may carry out the
threat and also when reports are required by law, such as
with communicable diseases and gunshot and knife wounds.
California established a physician's duty to warn third parties if there is an imminent threat of serious harm to a known
third party (Tarasoff, 1976). Subsequent to the *Tarasoff*
case, many other states have adopted this duty-to-warn

requirement and even expanded it to the unknown third parties. However, it is still not clear whether the duty to warn as identified in the *Tarasoff* case would apply to a sexual or needle-sharing partner of an HIV-infected patient who had not disclosed his or her HIV status.

It is important to differentiate "permissive" disclosures allowed under state laws, usually to local public health officers, from "mandatory" disclosures as required by law. A mandatory disclosure is one that a health care provider must make, such as disclosure of reportable diseases or suspected child abuse. In a permissive disclosure, local regulations allow a health care provider to discuss a specific patient with local public health officials (e.g., to seek their assistance in modifying a patient's behavior).

It is within this legal and ethical framework that providers should consider their obligations when they are aware that an HIV-infected patient is endangering others by engaging in acts that may lead to transmission of HIV. American Medical Association (AMA) guidelines issued in 1992 and updated in 1994, while recognizing a physician's obligation to protect the patient's confidentiality whenever possible, acknowledge that there are exceptions to this confidentiality:

> When necessary to protect the public health or when necessary to protect individuals, including healthcare workers, who are endangered by persons infected with HIV. If a physician knows that a seropositive individual is endangering a third party, the physician should, within the constraints of the law: (1) attempt to persuade the infected patient to cease endangering the third party; (2) if persuasion fails, notify authorities; and (3) if the authorities take no action, notify the endangered third party.

Given the legal implications of divulging a person's HIV status, health care providers should consult an attorney or become familiar with state laws and regulations before making any such disclosures.

Recommended Reading

AIDS.gov. Do you have to tell? Available at https://www.aids.gov/hiv-aids-basics/just-diagnosed-with-hiv-aids/talking-about-your-status/do-you-have-to-tell. Accessed December 2, 2015.

Downs L. The duty to protect a patient's right to confidentiality: Tarasoff, HIV, and confusion. *J Forensic Psychol Pract*. 2015; 15(2):160–170. Available at http://dx.doi.org/10.1080/15228932.2015.1007776.

Lin L, Liang BA. HIV and health law: Striking the balance between legal mandates and medical ethics. *Virtual Mentor Am Med Assoc J Ethics*. 2005; 7(10).

Obermeyer CM, Baijal P, Pegurri E. Facilitating HIV disclosure across diverse settings: A review. *Am J Pub Health*. 2011; 101(6):1011–1023.

Richardson R, Golden S, Hanssens C. Ending & defending against HIV criminalization—A manual for advocates: Vol. 1. State and federal laws and prosecutions, 2nd ed., Winter 2015. Available at http://www.hivlawandpolicy.org/sites/www.hivlawandpolicy.org/files/HIV%20Crim%20Manual%20%28updated%205.4.15%29.pdf.

Webber DW. Self-incrimination, partner notification, and the criminal law: Negatives for the CDC's "prevention for positives" initiative. *AIDS Public Policy J*. 2004; 19:54–66.

HIV CRIMINALIZATION

LEARNING OBJECTIVE

Describe recommendations from the *National HIV/AIDS Strategy* (NHAS) concerning criminal laws regarding HIV transmission and prevention.

WHAT'S NEW?

This section has been separated from the Issues in Disclosure section due to the increased concerns about criminalization of HIV non-disclosure and/or exposure.

KEY POINTS

- Stigma and discrimination continue to be major challenges to the comprehensive response necessary to address the HIV public health crisis.

- NHAS recommends that evidence-based public health approaches to HIV prevention and care be implemented and that state legislatures should review HIV-specific criminal statutes to ensure that they are consistent with current scientific knowledge of HIV transmission and support public health approaches to preventing and treating HIV.

In an attempt to limit the spread of HIV, many states have enacted laws that criminalize willful or knowing exposure of another person to HIV infection (Gostin, 1989). Some statutes do not require proof of intent to harm—only proof that the person knew that he or she was HIV-infected and despite that knowledge failed to inform at-risk contacts or use appropriate precautions (e.g., safer sex or clean needles) to prevent contacts from becoming infected. These laws have also been applied to HIV-positive people who solicited sex for money, a prisoner who bit a prison guard, and individuals who spat on another person. Although these statutes have been challenged on the alleged grounds of unconstitutional vagueness or violations of free speech or free association, most have been upheld. In addition to these laws, prosecutors have brought other criminal charges against HIV-infected individuals who unreasonably risk transmission of HIV through such acts as attempted murder, assault or assault with a dangerous or deadly weapon, and reckless endangerment (Gostin, 1989; Webber, 2004). The tension between the public health approach versus a criminal justice approach and effect on disclosure continues as applied to HIV transmission (Csete, 2011; Obermeyer, 2011).

Criminalization of potential HIV exposure is largely a matter of state law. An analysis by CDC and US Department of Justice researchers found that through 2011, a total of 67 laws explicitly focused on persons living with HIV had been enacted in 33 states. These laws vary as to what behaviors are criminalized or result in additional penalties. In 24 states, laws require persons who are aware that they have HIV to disclose their status to sexual partners, and 14 states require disclosure to needle-sharing partners. Twenty-five states criminalize one or more behaviors that pose a low or negligible risk for HIV transmission. As noted by Lehman et al., many of these laws criminalize behaviors that pose low or negligible risk for HIV transmission (Lehman, 2014). The majority of laws were passed before studies showed that antiretroviral therapy (ART) reduces HIV transmission risk, and most laws do not account for HIV prevention measures that reduce transmission risk, such as condom use, ART, or preexposure prophylaxis. Punishing people for behavior that is either consensual or poses no risk of HIV transmission only serves to further stigmatize already marginalized communities while missing opportunities for prevention education.

The American Academy of HIV Medicine (AAHIVM) and its members are opposed to laws that distinguish HIV disease from other comparable diseases or that create disproportionate penalties for disclosure, exposure, or transmission of HIV disease beyond normal public health ordinances. The AAHIVM supports nonpunitive prevention approaches to HIV centered on current scientific understanding and evidence-based research. The HIV Medicine Association (HIVMA) urged repeal of HIV-specific criminal statutes and noted that stigma and discrimination continue to be major impediments to the comprehensive response necessary to address the HIV public health crisis. HIVMA noted that policies and laws that create HIV-specific crimes or that impose penalties for persons who are HIV-infected are unjust and harmful to public health throughout the world.

NHAS, released by the White House in July 2010 and updated in 2015, recommends that federal and state governments should ensure that federal and state criminal laws reflect current scientific information regarding HIV transmission and prevention. NHAS also recommends evidence-based public health approaches to HIV prevention and care. The document notes that state legislatures should review HIV-specific criminal statutes to ensure that they are consistent with current scientific knowledge of HIV transmission and support public health approaches to preventing and treating HIV.

Recommended Reading

Adam BD, Corriveau P, Elliott R, et al. HIV disclosure as practice and public policy. *Crit Public Health*. 2015; 25(4):386–397. Available at http://dx.doi.org/10.1080/09581596.2014.980395.

American Civil Liberties Union. State criminal statutes on HIV transmission—2008. Available at https://www.aclu.org/state-criminal-statutes-hiv-transmission?redirect=lgbt-rights_hiv-aids/state-criminal-statutes-hiv-transmission. Accessed December 2, 2015.

Francis LP, Francis JG. Criminalizing health-related behaviors dangerous to others? Disease transmission, transmission-facilitation, and the importance of trust. *Criminal Law Philosophy*. 2012; 6:47–63.

Haire B, Kaldor J. HIV transmission law in the age of treatment-as-prevention. *J Med Ethics*. 2015; 41:982–986.

Lehman JS, Carr MH, Nichol AJ, et al. Prevalence and public health implications of state laws that criminalize potential HIV exposure in the United States. *AIDS Behav* 2014; 18(6):997–1006. Available at http://rd.springer.com/article/10.1007/s10461-014-0724-0/fulltext.html.

Mykhalovskiy E. The public health implications of HIV criminalization: Past, current, and future research directions. *Crit Public Health*. 2015; 25(4):373–385. Available at http://dx.doi.org/10.1080/09581596.2015.1052731.

TREATING MINORS

LEARNING OBJECTIVE

Describe legal issues related to treatment of minors with HIV infection.

WHAT'S NEW?

Information on treating minors has remained consistent during the past few years.

KEY POINTS

- Medical treatment of minors (persons younger than age 18 years) must generally be authorized by a parent or legal guardian, with specific exceptions that vary across states.

- This area of law is often complex and variable. Health care providers unsure of their state laws and regulations should seek legal advice before treating minors for HIV.

The medical care of a minor—defined in most states as a person younger than age 18 years—must generally be authorized by his or her parent or legal guardian. This usually means that a parent or guardian of a minor is required to give informed consent on behalf of the minor for most medical decisions. However, there are exceptions to this rule, and certain minors can consent to certain types of medical care without the authority of a parent or legal guardian.

CONSENT FOR STD SERVICES AND MEDICAL TREATMENT

STD Services

All 50 states and the District of Columbia explicitly allow minors to consent to STD services, although 11 states require that a minor be of a certain age (generally age 12 or 14 years) before being allowed to consent. Thirty states explicitly include HIV testing and treatment in the package of STD services to which minors may consent.

Medical Treatment

Most states have laws that authorize all minors to consent to certain types of medical treatment, such as care for pregnancy; contraception and abortion care; treatment for contagious diseases, STDs, rape, sexual assault, mental health, and drug or alcohol abuse; and HIV testing. In many states, absent exceptional circumstances, a minor is not able to consent to HIV treatment, and consent must be obtained from the parent or legal guardian (e.g., see New York State Public Health Law 2504).

Exceptions

Almost all states have laws that authorize minors who have attained a certain status to make the majority of their own health care decisions. These may include minors who are married (or divorced), on active duty with the US Armed Forces, emancipated by a court order, or self-sufficient such that they have attained a designated age and live away from home and manage their own financial affairs.

LAWS RELATED TO INFORMING PARENTS

Eighteen states allow health care providers to inform a minor's parents that he or she is seeking or receiving STD services. With the exception of one state (Iowa requires parental notification in the case of a positive HIV test), no state requires that providers notify parents (Guttmacher Institute, 2007; Ho, 2005). In some states, health care providers are prohibited from telling the minor's parent(s) or legal guardian about any test-related medical care unless the minor authorizes it (e.g., see New York State Public Health Law 2780.5).

SEEKING LEGAL ADVICE

Health care providers should be aware that this area of the law is very complex, highly variable by state, and rife with legal risks and exposure if an incorrect decision regarding treatment is made. Therefore, it is highly advisable that health care providers who are unsure of the law in their state consult a lawyer before providing HIV testing or treatment to a minor. Health care providers must be acutely aware of the importance of consulting and obtaining the informed consent of a parent or legal guardian of the minor when required by law.

Recommended Reading

Guttmacher Institute. Minors' access to STD services. State Polices in Brief, April 1, 2007. Available at http://www.guttmacher.org/state-center/spibs/spib_MASS.pdf.

Ho WW, Brandfield J, Retkin R, et al. Complexities in HIV consent in adolescents. *Clin Pediatr (Phil)*. 2005; 44:473-478.

CONFIDENTIALITY

LEARNING OBJECTIVE

Discuss legal issues related to confidentiality and HIV, including health information protected under HIPAA's Privacy Rule and HIPAA's impact on communicating a patient's personal health information.

KEY POINTS

- There are many reasons for maintaining strict confidentiality in the medical setting, including the need to maintain effective clinician–patient relationships.

- Various state and federal regulations govern confidentiality of medical information. Non-compliance carries the risk of civil and/or criminal penalties.

- Federal provisions governing confidentiality were established in the Health Insurance Portability and Accountability Act of 1996 (HIPAA). The act defines which health entities are covered, the types of medical information covered, how information can be used, and requirements for notifying patients. The deadline for compliance with the HIPAA Privacy Rule was April 14, 2003.

- The HIPAA Security Standards dictate that "administrative, physical, and technical" safeguards must be in place to protect confidential information and its transmission and storage. Health care providers had to comply with the HIPAA Security Standards by April 21, 2005, with a 1-year extension permitted for small health plans.

- Available resources may assist clinicians in complying with HIPPA and other confidentiality provisions.

The rationale for confidentiality in the medical setting is that an effective clinician–patient relationship is based on trust and strict confidentiality regarding the patient's medical information. Maintaining patient confidentiality has particular importance when the patient is infected with HIV. The patient may choose to keep his or her status private in order to avoid significant emotional, social, and financial stigmatization, isolation, and loss that many HIV-infected persons encounter when their status becomes known. Therefore, every clinician should seek to respect the privacy of his or her patients, including persons living with HIV, and their wishes not to have personal information about themselves made available to others.

The Hippocratic Oath and other ethical guidelines instruct providers that information gained through the provider–patient relationship is confidential. Confidentiality requirements are also underscored by various state laws and federal provisions. HIPAA has implications for nearly all health care providers and facilities, including federally funded facilities that provide substance abuse treatment services.

In general, both state and federal confidentiality requirements address the areas discussed in the following sections.

HANDLING OF MEDICAL INFORMATION

State laws require patient consent for releasing information to all or only certain requestors. The HIPAA provide criteria to oversee transmission of information within the current interrelated health care system for purposes of treatment, payment, or other health care functions. HIPAA regulates the sharing of information among multiple providers and payers.

PROCEDURES FOR HANDLING EXCEPTIONAL SITUATIONS

State laws typically provide for disclosure of information for public health purposes, such as the "duty to warn" an individual facing imminent harm from a patient. Assaults and communicable diseases are reportable, and their reporting may be legally mandated (AMA, 2005). Physician–patient confidentiality is not absolute under the law of most states. The courts and legislators in many states have attempted to strike a balance between competing rights: those of patients to confidentiality and those of others to information about the significant dangers they may face. It seems reasonable that the patient's right to privacy should be breached only when it is necessary to avoid imminent and serious harm. If the chance of contracting HIV from contact with the patient is remote (i.e., a household contact), then the right to confidentiality should be considered paramount. However, if the chance of contracting HIV is high (i.e., through sexual contact), then the duty to warn may take precedence (see Objective 60.5, Issues in Disclosure).

PENALTIES

Providers treating HIV-infected patients must seek to balance these legal and ethical obligations. There is no guarantee that the balance struck by the clinician will be the same struck by a court should the matter end up in litigation. Almost half of the states have provisions for revoking a health care provider's medical license or exercising other disciplinary action when confidential patient information is inappropriately or unlawfully disclosed. HIPAA also contains penalty provisions. When in doubt, the clinician should consult an attorney before taking any action or making any disclosure without consent.

HIPAA

In 2003, Boyle and colleagues described the HIPAA regulations on privacy and disclosure of medical information (i.e., the "Privacy Rule"). HIPAA places the burden on health care providers and others who have access to confidential medical information to keep that information private and protected. HIPAA outlines who must comply, what information is protected, and what providers must do to comply. Similar state laws take precedence if they are more stringent than HIPAA.

The Privacy Rule definition of who must comply ("covered entities") covers most clinicians and health plans because it essentially applies to anyone who bills for services electronically. "Protected health information" (PHI) also is broadly defined (i.e., medical records and other identifying information). Covered entities were required to comply with the Privacy Rule by April 14, 2003.

The Privacy Rule stipulates in great detail how information may be used and disclosed. A key example of allowed uses is the release of information to the patient in question. Patients must have access to their medical records along with information about who has been granted access to them. Information also can be used in treatment and payment processes. HIPAA contains provisions for special circumstances in which medical information can be released, such as the "duty to warn" provisions cited previously.

Patients consent must be obtained for most disclosures of medical information. Covered entities are also required to provide patients with a written "Notice of Privacy Practices" that clearly explains the provider's privacy policy—and must document that their patients received it (Boyle, 20003). In general, health care providers must institute reasonable measures to prevent incidental disclosure of patient information. Such measures include ensuring that unauthorized persons cannot wander into record rooms, access computer databases, or overhear names during in-person or telephone communications. However, HIPAA is not intended to impede customary communications, nor does it require protection against any conceivable incidental disclosure, such as when a visitor glimpses patient names on a sign-in sheet.

In addition to the Privacy Rule, HIPAA also requires clinicians and health plans to protect the security of patients' medical information that is stored or transmitted electronically (the "Security Standards"). The Security Standards call for all covered entities to enact administrative, physical, and technical safeguards for electronic data. Examples of such safeguards in an office setting are policies that limit access to database software to those who require it (physical safeguard), sanctions for employees who violate the standards (administrative safeguard), and the maintenance of electronic "audit logs" on computer systems that are equipped to access PHI (technical safeguard).

The compliance date for the Security Standards was April 21, 2005. Small health plans had an additional year to comply with the rules.

IDEAS FOR COMPLIANCE

Clinicians should establish compliance provisions not only to fulfill HIPAA requirements but also to be prepared to handle confidentiality in a responsible manner. Among the methods used is the securing of written informed consent from patients (required by HIPAA for certain situations) and formulation of clear procedures for handling patient information (e.g., secure storage, definitions of what information is to be protected and with whom it can be shared, and strategies for handling special circumstances). Other options include designating a privacy officer who is knowledgeable about the details of HIPAA and providing staff training on confidentiality.

For handling situations in which a "duty to warn" another individual arises, such as a sex partner or injection drug-using partner, clinicians can seek assistance. Most local or state health departments have partner notification programs that do this work. A number of Internet resources can assist clinicians in complying with HIPAA and other confidentiality provisions (Table 50.1).

The Patient Safety and Quality Improvement Act of 2005 (PSQIA) establishes a voluntary reporting system to enhance the data available to assess and resolve patient safety and health care quality issues. To encourage the reporting and analysis of medical errors, PSQIA provides federal privilege and confidentiality protections for patient safety information called patient safety work product. Patient safety work product includes information collected and created during the reporting and analysis of patient safety events. The regulation implementing the PSQIA became effective on January 19, 2009 (42 C.F.R. Part 3).

PSQIA establishes a voluntary reporting system designed to enhance the data available to assess and resolve patient safety and health care quality issues. To encourage the reporting and analysis of medical errors, PSQIA provides federal privilege and confidentiality protections for patient safety information, called patient safety work product. PSQIA authorizes DHHS to impose civil money penalties for violations of patient safety confidentiality. PSQIA also authorizes the Agency for Healthcare Research and Quality (AHRQ) to list patient safety organizations (PSOs). PSOs are the external experts that collect and review patient safety information.

The Administrative Simplification provisions of HIPPA (Title II) require the DHHS to adopt national standards for electronic health care transactions and national identifiers from providers, health plans, and employers. To date, the implementation of HIPPA standards has increased the use of electronic data interchange. Provisions under the Affordable Care Act of 2010 include requirements to adopt the following:

- Operating rules for each of the HIPPA-covered transactions

Table 50.1 WEB-BASED HIPAA AND PRIVACY COMPLIANCE RESOURCES FOR HEALTH CARE PROVIDERS

ORGANIZATION	URL	CONTENTS
American Medical Association	http://www.ama-assn.org/ama/pub/physician-resources/solutions-managing-your-practice/coding-billing-insurance/hipaahealth-insurance-portability-accountability-act.page?	• HIPAA information • FAQ page • Sample documents • Links to other resources • Complaint form for out-of-compliance health plans and other payers
US Department of Health and Human Services Office of Civil Rights	www.hhs.gov/ocr/hipaa	• HIPAA information for clinicians and patients • Fact sheets • Sample documents • Educational materials
Centers for Medicare and Medicaid Services	https://www.cms.gov/Regulations-and-Guidance/Administrative-Simplification/HIPAA-ACA/index.html	• Standards • Educational materials

- A unique, standard Health Plan Identifier (HPID)

- Standard and operating rules for electronic funds transfer and electronic remittance advice and claims attachments

In addition, health plans will be required to certify their compliance. The Act provides for substantial penalties for failures to comply with the new standards and operation rules.

Recommended Reading

American Medical Association (AMA). The AMA Code of Medical Ethics' opinions on confidentiality of patient information. Available at http://journalofethics.ama-assn.org/2012/09/coet1-1209.html.

American Medical Association (AMA). The AMA Code of Medical Ethics' opinions on confidentiality of patient information. Opinion 9.124—Professionalism in the use of social media. Available at http://journalofethics.ama-assn.org/2011/07/coet1-1107.html.

ADVANCE PLANNING

LEARNING OBJECTIVE

Discuss the use of advance directives, durable power of attorney, health proxy, and arranging for custody of minors for HIV-infected patients.

WHAT'S NEW?

Information regarding advance planning has remained consistent during the past few years.

People newly diagnosed with HIV infection (or any potentially life-threatening illness) face a myriad of legal concerns that affect almost every facet of their lives. At times, this may seem overwhelming to patient and provider alike. However, legal planning can greatly benefit HIV-infected patients and their families. Providers can play an important role in informing patients of the benefits of planning ahead.

Every provider should advise their patients to investigate and prepare three essential tools of effective legal planning:

1. A durable power of attorney for medical decision-making

2. An advance directive ("living will")

3. A will

DURABLE POWER OF ATTORNEY

A durable power of attorney makes legal provision for someone to make decisions in a patient's stead if he or she is no longer able to do so. Patients should consider two such documents to best protect their legal interests: one for health care decisions and one for legal and financial decisions. A patient may choose a single person to fill both roles, but the responsibilities are different. A durable power of attorney for financial issues may cover any and all financial concerns or may stipulate only specific tasks, such as paying standard household expenses or filing tax returns (Nolo, 2002a). A durable power of attorney for health care may cover any and all medical decisions or may stipulate only specific decisions can be made, such as consenting to or refusing any medical treatment. These documents are particularly important for couples who are not legally married, including gay and lesbian couples, because without a durable power of attorney, hospitals and courts frequently look to the closest biological relative to make decisions.

A power of attorney may take effect immediately when a patient signs it, or it may become effective only at a time or circumstance that the patient designates—for example, upon the patient's incapacity or other disability that hinders medical or financial decision-making (Nolo, 2002a). Patients must state in the document that a power of attorney is durable, or it will automatically end if the patient becomes incapacitated. In all cases, a power of attorney ends when the patient dies. Patients may choose to revoke the power of attorney at any time. If married patients grant power of attorney to a spouse, in some states (e.g., California, Illinois, and Texas) the power terminates if the couple divorces (Nolo, 2002a). Patients should consult an attorney in drafting a durable power of attorney to ensure that it is drawn up correctly.

ADVANCE DIRECTIVES

An advance directive is a document in which patients provide instructions about the kind of health care they do or do not want in the event that they have an incapacity that makes them unable to make or communicate medical decisions. These instructions are commonly referred to as a "living will." However, there is an important distinction: Living wills generally are limited to cases of terminal illness, whereas advance directives may apply to any situation in which a patient is incapacitated, even temporarily. This distinction is especially compelling regarding HIV-infected patients, who may experience AIDS-related dementia or other complications that may impair rational decision-making, but they may subsequently have improved executive function as a result of ART. Patients should know that an advance directive "may be the most convincing evidence of your wishes you can create" (American Association of Retired Persons, 1995). However, in a large national study of HIV-infected patients, fewer than half reported having advance directives. The most important factor associated with having an advance directive was whether their practitioner had discussed end-of-life issues (Wenger, 2001).

Advance directives are valid in every US state and the District of Columbia, but the specifics of the law vary from state to state. Therefore, patients who spend significant time in more than one state or who move to another state should have directives adjusted to follow each state's guidelines (Caring Connections, 2006). In creating an advance directive, the patient should consult an expert and should attempt to answer three important questions:

- What are my goals for treatment? Among other things, patients should consider their values relative to independence and their environment and their religious beliefs.

- How specific should I be? No directive can cover all eventualities, but it is suggested that patients address anything that is especially important to them.

- How can I make sure that health care providers will follow my advance directive?

Most states give health care providers the right to refuse to honor directives on grounds of conscience. In such cases, health care providers generally are obligated to refer patients to other health care providers who will honor the directive. It is important to ask patients about their wishes. Generally, patients need both a durable power of attorney and an advance directive. In essence, the advance directive expresses a patient's specific wishes, and the durable power of attorney grants someone the authority to execute those wishes or to make health care decisions that could not be anticipated by the advance directive.

Although patients are urged to draft durable powers of attorney and advance directives in every state, legal arrangements are especially critical in New York, Michigan, and Massachusetts. In New York, families are not authorized to make medical decisions for patients who cannot make decisions for themselves (New York, 1991). Therefore, an incapacitated patient may have health care decisions made for him or her by health care providers or lawyers. To avoid that situation, patients in New York must have a health care proxy. The health care proxy combines elements of an advance directive and a durable power of attorney; the proxy is a form that patients must sign. Two witnesses (other than the person named in the proxy to make decisions on the patient's behalf) are required (New York State Department of Health, 2003).

Massachusetts and Michigan do not have statutes allowing for living wills, but they do allow for health care proxies, which can serve a similar function (FindLaw, 2006). Massachusetts requires a specific health care proxy form, which clinicians should make available to patients.

A 2001 study by Stein and Bonuck found that gay men and lesbians were more likely than the general population to have executed advance directives (Stein, 2001). However, given the importance of these documents to HIV-infected patients, and because fewer than half of those studied had executed formal directives, health care providers are urged to assume a larger role in educating patients about advance care planning. Another study in 2000 affirmed previous results that intervention in an outpatient setting significantly increased the likelihood that HIV-infected patients would execute advance care planning (Ho, 2000).

Although the focus of advance care planning is usually on the health care and legal value of the process, another study showed that advance care planning also increased patients' sense of control and strengthened their relationships with their loved ones (Martin, 1999). However, more than 75% of all respondents in the Stein and Bonuck study said that their health care provider had never asked who should make medical decisions if patients were unable to do so themselves (Stein, 2001). Health care providers are encouraged to discuss these issues with patients.

WILLS

A will determines what happens to a person's property after his or her death. Despite considerable attention to wills in the popular press, do not assume that your patients have one—half of all Americans die without one (MCEC, 2006). Without a will, the courts will distribute a person's assets according to state laws. Wills are particularly important for people with minor children because without a will, the state will decide the children's guardianship (Nolo, 2002b). Wills are also important in situations in which the person is not legally married to his or her partner (e.g., common law marriage and gay and lesbian couples) because without a will, a survivor may inherit nothing and, worse, may lose personal property because he or she cannot prove ownership (HRC, 2004).

Many people mistakenly believe that they do not need wills because they do not have large estates. In truth, everyone needs a will to ensure that their wishes are followed when their assets are distributed. Handwritten, unwitnessed wills (called holographic wills) are valid in approximately 25 states, but more formal wills are preferable. A valid, legal will must include the following elements:

- It must be typewritten or computer generated (except holographic wills, described previously).

- The document must expressly state that it is a "Will."

- The person making the will must date and sign it.

- The will must be signed by at least two or, in some states, three witnesses who will not inherit anything under the terms of the will.

Health care providers should be aware that legal planning is vital for all patients but especially for HIV-infected patients. By focusing on the three documents discussed previously (durable power of attorney, advance directives, and wills) and by obtaining appropriate legal advice, the planning should not be difficult or confusing.

ARRANGING FOR CUSTODY OF MINORS

A major concern for HIV-infected parents is the welfare of their children (or grandchildren) in the event of the death of the parents. Several legal mechanisms help to address this concern, but the underlying principle is that the court will look to the best interest of the child, taking into account the parent's desires. A statement in a will about child custody will help inform the court of the parent's wishes. In addition, guardianships with a springing clause for incapacity (standby guardianship) can be used to appoint a guardian if a single parent becomes incapacitated. Adoption is a less attractive choice because it requires the parent(s) to surrender all parental rights. Because it is common for parents not to make formal legal arrangements for custody of their children in the event of the parents' death, providers can be helpful in urging patients to consider custody arrangements in advance.

Recommended Reading

American Association of Retired Persons, American Bar Association Commission on Legal Problems of the Elderly, and American Medical Association. Shape your health care future with health care advance directives. 1995. Available at http://www.americanbar.org/content/dam/aba/migrated/publiced/practical/books/wills/appendix_b.authcheckdam.pdf.

Human Rights Campaign. Last will and testament. Available at http://www.hrc.org/resources/entry/last-will-and-testament.

Human Rights Campaign. Health care proxy. Available at http://www.hrc.org/resources/entry/health-care-proxy.

Nolo website. http://www.nolo.com/about.html.

Simoni JM, Davis ML, Drossman JA, et al. Mothers with HIV/AIDS and their children: Disclosure and guardianship issues. *Women Health*. 2000; 31:39–54.

References

American Academy for HIV Medicine. HIV criminalization. Available at http://www.aahivm.org/hivcriminalization. Accessed December 2, 2015.

Boyle BA, Bradley T, Bradley H, et al. Health Insurance Portability and Accountability Act of 1996: new national medical privacy standards. *AIDS Read*. 2003; 13:261–262, 265–266.

Center for HIV Law and Policy. Criminal law. Available at http://www.hivlawandpolicy.org/issues/criminal-law. Accessed November 30, 2015.

Centers for Disease Control and Prevention. HIV/AIDS statistics overview. Available at http://www.cdc.gov/hiv/statistics/overview/index.html. Accessed November 28, 2015.

Centers for Disease Control and Prevention. State HIV laws. Available at http://www.cdc.gov/hiv/policies/law/states/index.html. Accessed November 28, 2015.

Centers for Disease Control and Prevention. HIV surveillance report. Available at http://www.cdc.gov/hiv/library/reports/surveillance/index.html#panel0. Accessed November 30, 2015.

Centers for Disease Control and Prevention (CDC). HIV testing among populations at risk for HIV infection – nine states. November 1995-December 1996. MMWR Morb Mortal Wkly Rep. 1998; 47(50):1086–1091.

Centers for Disease Control and Prevention. HIV-specific criminal law. Available at http://www.cdc.gov/hiv/policies/law/states/exposure. html. Accessed November 30, 2015.

Charlebois ED, Maiorana A, McLaughlin M, et al. Potential deterrent effect of name-based HIV infection surveillance. *J Acquir Immune Defic Syndr*. 2005; 39:219–227.

Csete J, Elliott R. Criminalization of HIV transmission and exposure: in search of rights-based public health alternatives to criminal law. *Future Virology*. Vol 62011:941.

Gostin L. The politics of AIDS: compulsory state powers, public health and civil liberties. *Ohio State Law J*. 1989; 49:1017–1058.

HIV Medicine Association. HIVMA urges repeal of HIV-specific criminal statutes. Available at http://www.hivma.org/upload-edFiles/IDSA/Careers_and_Training/Opportunities_for_ Students_Residents/ID_Career_Paths/HIVMA%20Policy%20 Statement%20on%20HIV%20Criminalization.pdf. Accessed December 2, 2015.

Massachusetts Medical Society. Health care proxies and end of life care. Available at http://www.massmed.org/Patient-Care/Health-Topics/ Health-Care-Proxies-and-End-of-Life-Care/Health-Care-Proxies-and-End-of-Life-Care/#.Vl9Xmzfru70. Accessed December 2, 2015.

The Kaiser Foundation. Minors' authority to consent to STI services. Available at http://kff.org/hivaids/state-indicator/minors-right-to-consent. Accessed November 28, 2015.

University of California San Francisco Clinical Consultation Center. State testing laws. Available at http://www.cdc.gov/hiv/policies/ law/states/index.html. Accessed November 30, 2015.

US Department of Health and Human Services, Office for Civil Rights Privacy Rule. Available at http://www.hhs.gov/ocr/privacy/psa/ understanding/index.html. Accessed December 2, 2015.

US Preventative Services Task Force. Recommendations for screening. Available at http://www.uspreventiveservicestaskforce.org/ BrowseRec/Search?s=hiv+screening. Accessed November 30, 2015.

American Association of Retired Persons, American Bar Association Commission on Legal Problems of the Elderly, and American Medical Association. Shape your health care future with health care advance directives. 1995. Available at http://www.americanbar.org/ content/dam/aba/migrated/publiced/practical/books/wills/appen-dix_b.authcheckdam.pdf.

Caring Connections. Advance Care Planning. Caring Connections web site. www.caringinfo.org/i4a/pages/index.cfm?pageid=3278. Accessed March 14, 2006.

Centers for Disease Control and Prevention. Revised recommenda-tions for HIV testing of adults, adolescents, and pregnant women in health-care settings. *MMWR Morbid Mortal Wkly Rep*. 2006; 55(RR14):1–17. Available at www.cdc.gov/mmwr/preview/ mmwrhtml/rr5514a1.htm. Accessed November 30, 2015.

Centers for Disease Control and Prevention. Trends in HIV/AIDS diagnosis-33 States, 2001–2004. MMWR Morb Mortal Wkly Rep. 2005b; 54(45):1149–1153.

Colfax GN, Buchbinder SP, Cornelisse PGA, et al. Sexual risk behaviors and implications for secondary HIV transmission during and after HIV seroconversion. *AIDS*. 2002; 16:1529–1535.

FindLaw. State laws: living wills. FindLaw Web site. http://estate.find-law.com/estate-planning/living-wills/estate-planning-law-state-liv-ing-wills.html. Accessed Dec 1, 2015.

Guttmacher Institute. Minors' access to STD services. State Polices in Brief. April 1, 2007. Available at http://www.guttmacher.org/state-center/spibs/spib_MASS.pdf.

Hall HI, Holtgrave D, Maulsby C. HIV transmission rates from persons living with HIV who are aware and unaware of their infection. *AIDS*. 2012; 26:893–896.

Halpern SD. HIV testing without consent in critically ill patients. *JAMA*. 2005; 294(6):734–737.

Halpern SD, Metkus TS, Fuchs BD, et al. Nonconsented human immu-nodeficiency virus testing among critically ill patients: intensivists' practices and the influence of state laws. *Arch Intern Med*. 2007 Nov 26; 167(21):2323–2328.

Ho WW, Brandfield J, Retkin R, et al. Complexities in HIV consent in adolescents. *Clin Pediatr (Phil)*. 2005; 44:473–478.

Ho VW, Thiel EC, Rubin HR, et al. The effect of advance care planning on completion of advance directives and patient satisfaction in peo-ple with HIV/AIDS. *AIDS Care*. 2000; 12:97–108.

Holtgrave DR, Anderson T. Utilizing HIV transmission rates to assist in prioritizing HIV prevention services. *Int J STD AIDS*. 2004; 15:7890792.

Human Rights Campaign (HRC), Last will and testament. Human Rights Campaign Web site. Available at www.hrc.org/Template. cfm?Section=Home&Template=/ContentManagement/ ContentDisplay.cfm&ContentID=18673. Published 2004. Accessed Dec 1, 2015.

Lehman JS, Carr MH, Nichol AJ, et al. Prevalence and public health implications of state laws that criminalize potential HIV exposure in the United States. *AIDS Behav* 2014; 18(6):997–1006. Available at http://rd.springer.com/article/10.1007/s10461-014-0724-0/full-text.html.

Lin L, Liang BA. HIV and health law: Striking the balance between legal mandates and medical ethics. *Virtual Mentor AMA J Ethics*. 2005; 7(10). Available at http://journalofethics.ama-assn.org/2005/10/ hlaw1-0510.html.

Lubelchek RJ, Finnegan KJ, Hotton AL, et al. Assessing the use of HIV surveillance data to help gauge patient retention-in-care. *J Acquir Immune Defic Syndr*. 2015; 69:S25–S30.

Marks G, Crepaz N, Janssen RS. Estimating sexual transmission of HIV from persons aware and unaware that they are infected with the virus in the USA. *AIDS*. 2006; 20:1447–1450.

Martin DK, Thiel EC, Singer PA. A new model of advance care plan-ning: observations from people with HIV. *Arch Intern Med*. 1999; 159:86–92.

Met Life Consumer Education Center (MCEC). Making a will. www. thebody.com/metlife/will.html. Accessed Dec 1, 2015.

Neff S, Goldschmidt, R. Centers for Disease Control and Prevention 2006 human immunodeficiency virus testing recommendations and state testing laws. *JAMA*. 2011; 305(17):1767–1768.

New York State Department of Health (NYSDOH). New York State Task Force on Life and the Law. The Health Care Proxy Law: A Guidebook for Health Professionals. New York: New York State Department of Health; 1991. Accessed Dec 1, 2015. October 2001 revisions available at: www.health.state.ny.us.nysdoh/consumer/ patient/hcproxy.htm.

New York State Department of Health (NYSDOH). Frequently asked questions: why should I choose a health care agent? New York State Department of Health Web site. www.health.state.ny.us/nys-doh/hospital/healthcareproxy/faq/htm. Published January 2003. Accessed December 1, 2015.

Nolo. How a financial power of attorney works. Nolo.com web site. www.nolo.com/lawcenter/ency/article.cfm?objectID=8DB3E0EC-D6CA-4479-B3FA7E9174E0827A/catID/EDC82D5A-7723-4A77-9E10DDB947D1F801. Published 2002a. Accessed Dec 1, 2015.

Nolo. Wills FAQ. Nolo.com Web Site. www.nolo.com/lawcenter/ency/ article.cfm/objectid/10689FA1-E24C-4849-BEA73FE77F295A5F/ catID/F251EA55-13A9-4EE0-85D21CEB27636030#C6722A8D-33C5-4A8E-A49D330568AACE2F. Published 2002b. Accessed Dec 1, 2015.

Obermeyer CM, Baijal P, Pegurri E. Facilitating HIV disclo-sure across diverse settings: A review. *Am J Pub Health*. 2011; 101(6):1011–1023.

Stein GL, Bonuck KA. Attitudes on end-of-life care and advance care planning in the lesbian and gay community. *J Palliat Med.* 2001; 4:173–190.

Stein MD, Freedberg KA, Sullivan LM, et al. Sexual ethics: Disclosure of HIV-positive status to partners. *Arch Intern Med.* 1998; 158:253–257.

Tarasoff v Regents of U. of California, 131 Cal. Rptr. 14, 551 P.2d 334 (1976).

Webber DW. Self-incrimination, partner notification, and the criminal law: Negatives for the CDC's "prevention for positives" initiative. *AIDS Public Policy J.* 2004; 19:54–66. Available at http://www.hivlawandpolicy.org/resources/self-incrimination-partner-notification-and-criminal-law-negatives-cdc%E2%80%99s-%E2%80%9Cprevention. Accessed November 30, 2015.

Wenger NS, Kanouse DE, Collins RL, et al. End-of-life discussions and preferences among persons with HIV. *JAMA.* 2001; 285:2880–2887.

Wiewel E, Braunstein SL, Xiaet Q, et al. Monitoring outcomes for newly diagnosed and prevalent HIV cases using a care continuum created with New York City surveillance data. *J Acquir Immune Defic Syndr.* 2015; 68:217–226.

Wortley PM, Lindegren ML, Fleming PL. Successful implementation of perinatal HIV prevention guidelines: A multistate surveillance evaluation. *MMWR Morbid Mortal Wkly Rep.* 2001; 50(RR-6):17–28.

Wolitski RJ, Rietmeijer CA, Goldbaum GM, et al. HIV serostatus disclosure among gay and bisexual men in four American cities: general patterns and relation to sexual practices. *AIDS Care.* 1998; 10:599–610.

51.

RESEARCH DESIGN AND ANALYSIS

Christian B. Ramers

CHAPTER GOAL

Upon completion of this chapter, the reader should be able to demonstrate basic knowledge regarding the interpretation of results of medical research related to HIV in order to better incorporate emerging scientific concepts into the provision of optimal patient care.

EVALUATING THE STATISTICAL ANALYSIS OF CLINICAL TRIALS

LEARNING OBJECTIVES

Differentiate between on-treatment (OT) and intent-to-treat (ITT) analyses and between time-to-loss of virologic response (TLOVR) analysis and SNAPSHOT analysis. Give an example of when non-inferiority analysis might be used.

KEY POINTS

- Because of inherent differences in approach, the OT analysis will frequently report better outcomes than will the ITT analysis.

- Therapeutic responses to antiretroviral therapy (ART) regimens may be evaluated using various approaches, such as TLOVR and SNAPSHOT analyses; each method may be more appropriate in certain study populations than in others.

- New ART regimens are usually compared to existing standard-of-care regimens using a type of statistical comparison called a non-inferiority analysis.

- A common error in reporting clinical trial results is not correctly distinguishing between clinical and statistical significance.

- To properly interpret the results of scientific studies, the reader must understand the difference between a statistical association and causality.

ON-TREATMENT VERSUS INTENT-TO-TREAT

In randomized trials, an OT analysis (also known as "as-treated analysis" or "observed analysis") examines outcomes in only those patients who remain on their assigned study regimen for the duration of the trial or, in the case of an interim analysis, up to a particular time point. An ITT analysis evaluates each patient according to the treatment group to which he or she was originally randomized, regardless of whether that patient received the treatment or completed the study. Both ITT and OT analyses are valuable in understanding the findings of a clinical trial.

By removing from the analysis those patients who are lost to follow-up, do not complete the study (for any reason), or do not stay on their prescribed regimen, the OT analysis selects for the patients who have been able to tolerate study medication(s). This analysis method is intrinsically biased toward a best-case scenario, and it may systematically bias results such that bad outcomes associated with a treatment that is not well tolerated may be hidden. The value of the ITT analysis is that it limits bias by evaluating the entire population of patients randomized to a given drug regimen. It encompasses efficacy, tolerability, adverse events, and the myriad other reasons why patients do not remain on or deviate from the prescribed drug regimen; therefore, it accounts for the influence of these factors on outcomes (Lang, 1997). The more rigorous ITT approach conveys a truer sense of a regimen's overall efficacy and is considered to be less subject to bias.

Because of the inherent differences in these approaches, the OT analysis will frequently report better outcomes than will the ITT analysis (e.g., a higher proportion of patients achieving a specified level of HIV-1 RNA reduction). OT analysis excludes patients who are non-compliant with study medications, procedures, and/or study visits and also those who drop out due to intolerance of the assigned regimen. If more patients are excluded from one treatment arm than another, the OT analysis may report a clinical difference that is quite different than the actual treatment difference obtained when all subjects are analyzed.

TIME TO LOSS OF VIROLOGIC RESPONSE VERSUS SNAPSHOT ANALYSIS

End points such as HIV RNA levels (viral load) are often accepted as being relevant for predicting the effect of antiretroviral regimens on clinically important end points that may be rare or take years to occur (e.g., progression to AIDS and death). As such, drug regimens in HIV clinical trials are frequently evaluated over time by assessing the percentage of subjects achieving low (suppressed) plasma levels of HIV-1 RNA. Because assays that detect HIV RNA have different limits of detection, it is important to know which level of HIV RNA was considered "suppressed" or "undetectable." In addition to measuring failure to achieve or maintain HIV-1 RNA suppression, the TLOVR analysis also considers the introduction of a new antiretroviral drug, death, or loss to follow-up as failures (US Food and Drug Administration (FDA), 2002). Recently, the FDA introduced the SNAPSHOT method of analyzing results with the goal of simplifying the evaluation of study results. SNAPSHOT differs from TLOVR in that it primarily focuses on a visit of interest (e.g., only if a subject is a responder with an HIV RNA <50 copies/ml at week 48) (Qaqish, 2010). Both methods of analysis have value, and clinical trials will typically report results in both forms.

NON-INFERIORITY ANALYSIS

In contrast to analyses used to demonstrate superiority, new drug regimens may be evaluated with the aim of demonstrating equivalence or non-inferior efficacy relative to a standard drug regimen. The non-inferiority trial is used mainly when the added value of a new drug/regimen is due to issues such as improved convenience, better tolerability, simpler dosing schedule, lower toxicity, or lower cost (Wittkop, 2010). Guidance given by the FDA to industry regarding procedures for accelerated and traditional new drug approval is helping to standardize the statistical methods used in major clinical trials. The proportion of treatment responders at 48 weeks is often used to assess non-inferiority (FDA, 2002). In practical terms, a non-inferiority analysis is a statistically rigorous way in which a clinical trial can show that a new regimen is at least as good as a currently available option. Trials are often powered differently, with larger numbers of participants if they aim to show superiority of one regimen over another.

CLINICAL VERSUS STATISTICAL SIGNIFICANCE

When evaluating research, it is important to be aware of the difference between a statistically significant finding and a clinically significant finding. One of the most common errors made in reporting clinical trial results is not correctly distinguishing between clinical and statistical significance (Braitman, 1991). A clinically significant finding is one that has important implications for patient care. A statistically significant finding is a conclusion that there is evidence against the null hypothesis; that is, a low probability exists of getting a result as extreme or more extreme than the one observed in the data by chance alone. Statistical significance, when applied to the terms non-inferiority or superiority, means that the result of a clinical trial would be unlikely to occur by chance. It does not necessarily mean that the result will be important for treating patients (Braitman, 1991; Lang, 1997).

Recommended Reading

Friedman LM, Furberg CD, DeMets DL. *Fundamentals of Clinical Trials*, 3rd ed. New York, NY: Springer-Verlag; 1998.

Pocock SJ. *Clinical Trials: A Practical Approach*. New York, NY: Wiley; 1983.

DETERMINING CAUSE-AND-EFFECT ASSOCIATIONS

LEARNING OBJECTIVE

Discuss the difficulties of drawing cause-and-effect conclusions about associated factors identified in research studies, including the limitations of observational studies and cross-study comparisons.

KEY POINTS

- Randomized clinical trials and observational cohorts provide different but equally valuable information.

- Cohort studies frequently follow large numbers of HIV-infected people for prolonged periods and have greater representation of "real-world" populations (e.g., women and minorities) than do typical randomized studies.

> • Cohort studies lack randomization and controls but are useful in generating hypotheses and demonstrating associations that can be further evaluated in randomized, prospective trials.

Randomized controlled trials (RCTs) are the gold standard of modern clinical research because they randomly assign equivalent groups of patients to different treatments, thus eliminating many types of bias that might influence outcome. If randomization works, the different arms of an RCT should be equivalent in all aspects except for the treatment administered, allowing conclusions to be drawn regarding the causality of the intervention and a given outcome. However, RCTs are expensive, time-consuming, and typically must include a large number of patients in order to show results that are generalizable across patient populations. Although considered to provide a less rigorous level of evidence, observational cohort studies, cross-sectional analyses, and case–control studies have also played a major role in HIV research and can add value to our general scientific understanding of a particular problem.

From the earliest findings of the Multicenter AIDS Cohort Study (MACS) to other ongoing national and international cohorts, these databases have provided crucial insights into the natural history of HIV and the efficacy and toxicity of HIV treatment. Lipodystrophy, cardiovascular disease, renal and bone complications, treatment interruptions, and the timing of initiation of highly active antiretroviral therapy (HAART) are areas with recent contributions from observational studies. Analyses involving cohorts are no more or less valuable than are prospective, randomized clinical trials; they are simply different vehicles designed to answer different types of questions.

Cohort studies are able to follow large numbers of patients for prolonged periods of time and often better reflect the "real world" of HIV-infected patients, in contrast to patients who are able and willing to participate in randomized trials. Cohort studies frequently have greater representation of women, minorities, and those with comorbid conditions than do typical randomized studies.

Cohort studies, however, do have biases. First, the quality of the results is only as good as the quality, consistency, and completeness of the data from participants in the cohort. Second, a lack of randomization or control of treatments administered to patients can significantly impact interpretation of the results through introduction of selection bias. For example, patients starting a particular treatment in a cohort study may be selected by clinicians so as

to avoid a perceived toxicity or selected so as to gain a perceived benefit, and this in turn could lead to results favoring one agent over another that may or may not be correct. Similarly, large changes in policy, availability of treatment advances, or other confounding disease states—so-called historical bias—can influence outcomes and may be more important than the specific variables being assessed. Cohort studies are very useful for generating hypotheses, where an observation may lead to the undertaking of a randomized clinical trial to confirm or refute the observations made in the cohort analysis. Cohort studies may detect associations between certain treatments or factors with an outcome that prompts a more rigorous evaluation to help determine causality. They can provide preliminary information about long-term clinical end points, survival, complications, and the role of comorbid conditions that may be tested later in an RCT. Thus, the observational cohort study and the RCT are complementary rather than competitive.

Focused observational studies can be valuable for evaluating factors associated with rare diseases or outcomes. In a case–control study, a set of individuals (cases) with the condition of interest is assembled (Schulz, 2002). A corresponding set of individuals (controls) without the condition is then selected. Controls are frequently matched to be similar to the cases, and they should be selected from the same population.

Information on risk factors is then collected and analyzed to identify factors that are more (or less) common in the cases compared to the controls. For example, thresholds used to define the appropriate use of prophylaxis for opportunistic infections are largely derived from case–control studies that showed increased risk for these infections in groups of patients with lower CD4 counts than those patients with higher counts. Careful design and implementation are needed to minimize bias, particularly to select appropriate controls and to collect unbiased information on risk factors.

Cross-study comparisons of randomized trials—that is, trying to relate efficacy of one particular treatment to that of another when they have not been directly compared—must be undertaken with caution because patient characteristics as well as study management may differ considerably between studies that share the same primary end point. A meta-analysis of related studies is more reliable than a simplistic comparison because researchers can carefully analyze data to avoid misleading conclusions, and they can thoroughly explain what they did and why.

In summary, when attempting to determine causality between an intervention or risk factor and an outcome,

RCTs provide the highest level of evidence. Observational studies such as cohort, case–control, and cross-sectional studies are useful to generate hypothesis, to show preliminary associations, and to guide the design of future clinical trials. Most of what is known about HIV natural history, treatment response, and associated clinical risk factors for progression or virologic control is derived from these types of studies.

Recommended Reading

Collins R, MacMahon S. Reliable assessment of the effects of treatment on mortality and major morbidity: I. Clinical trials. *Lancet.* 2001; 357:373–380.

Ioannidis JPA, Haidich A, Pappa M, et al. Comparison of evidence of treatment effects in randomized and nonrandomized studies. *JAMA.* 2001; 286:821–830.

MacMahon S, Collins R. Reliable assessment of the effects of treatment on mortality and major morbidity: II. Observational studies. *Lancet.* 2001; 357:455–462.

References

Braitman LE. Confidence intervals assess both clinical significance and statistical significance. *Ann Intern Med.* 1991; 114:515–517.

Lang TA, Secic M. *How to Report Statistics in Medicine: Annotated Guidelines for Authors, Editors, and Reviewers.* Philadelphia, PA: American College of Physicians; 1997.

Qaqish R, van Wyk J, & King M. JIAS. 2010; 13:P58. doi:10.1186/1758-2652-13-S4-P58.

Schulz KF, Grimes DA. Case–control studies: Research in reverse. *Lancet.* 2002; 359:431–434.

US Food and Drug Administration. Guidance for industry. Antiretroviral drugs using plasma HIV RNA measurements—Clinical considerations for accelerated and traditional approval. Washington, DC: US Department of Health and Human Services; 2002. Available at www.fda.gov/cder/guidance/3647fnl.pdf.

52.

ETHICAL CONDUCT OF CLINICAL TRIALS, INSTITUTIONAL REVIEW BOARDS, INFORMED CONSENT, AND FINANCIAL CONFLICTS OF INTEREST

Christian B. Ramers

LEARNING OBJECTIVE

Describe the essential components of the ethical conduct of research, the role of the institutional review board, the process of informed consent, the potential areas of conflict of interest for clinicians participating in research, and other ethical issues related to research in HIV medicine.

Treatment advances in the management of HIV-infected patients have been a direct result of decades of research initiatives involving tens of thousands of patients. The ethical considerations when performing research include basic ethical principles (e.g., autonomy, confidentiality, nonmaleficence, informed consent, beneficence, justice, and utility), as well as nuances such as appropriate study designs, investigator conflict of interests, and bias in all its forms. To help guide clinicians, a number of professional and governmental organizations have posted guidelines and recommendations on various aspects of clinical research (e.g., the American Medical Association, the National Institutes of Health, and the US Food and Drug Administration (FDA)).

The *Declaration of Helsinki* and the *Belmont Report* are important historical benchmarks that have laid the foundation of currently accepted ethical standards in the treatment of patients participating in clinical trials. The *Declaration of Helsinki*, first adopted in 1964 and updated in 2013, stresses that it is the duty of the physician to promote and safeguard the health of patients and that the well-being of the individual research subjects must take precedence over all other interests (World Medical Association, 2013). Although the document does not highlight individual diseases or research initiatives, the following points have particular importance to HIV-infected patients: (1) Participation in clinical trials must be completely voluntary and without undue coercion or influence, (2) it is the duty of the physician to maintain privacy and confidentiality of personal information, and (3) populations that are underrepresented in medical research should be provided appropriate access to participation in research. Similarly, the *Belmont Report* (US Department of Health and Welfare, 1979) highlights three fundamental ethical principles relating specifically to the conduct of research: (1) The principle of *respect for persons* acknowledges the dignity and autonomy of individuals, (2) the principle of *beneficence* protects individuals by maximizing anticipated benefits and minimizing possible harms, and (3) the principle of *justice* requires that all subjects are treated fairly.

There are seven requirements for determining whether a research trial is ethical, which are discussed next.

SEVEN REQUIREMENTS FOR DETERMINING WHETHER A RESEARCH TRIAL IS ETHICAL

Emanuel and colleagues described the following requirements for determining whether a clinical trial is ethical (Emanual, 2000):

1. Value: Enhancements of health or knowledge must be derived from the research.

2. Scientific validity: The research must be methodologically rigorous.

3. Fair subject selection: Scientific objective, not vulnerability or privilege, and the potential for and distribution of risks and benefits should determine the communities selected for study sites and the inclusion criteria for individual subjects.

4. Favorable risk:benefit ratio: Within the context of standard clinical practices and the research protocol, risk must be minimized and potential benefits enhanced, and the potential benefits to individuals and the knowledge gained for society must outweigh the risks.

5. Independent review: Unaffiliated individuals must review the research and approve, amend, or terminate it.

6. Informed consent: Individuals should be informed about the research and provide their voluntary consent.

7. Respect for enrolled subjects: Subjects should have their privacy protected, the opportunity to withdraw from the research without penalty, and their well-being monitored.

Facing ethical dilemmas during the conduct of a clinical trial is not uncommon. A survey of physicians engaged in clinical research found that almost all of them had recently faced such issues (DuVal, 2005). They can arise at any stage of the research process, from trial design through execution and the final publication of the research report. Notably, this survey found that most ethical dilemmas occurred after institutional review board (IRB) approval, suggesting that ethical consideration should be continuous rather than a one-time process. Approximately half of the physicians requested an ethical consultation before resolving the issue, and many institutions are beginning to offer such services outside of the IRB process.

INSTITUTIONAL REVIEW BOARDS

IRBs are charged with (1) the review of protocols and consent documents and any modifications to them prior to their implementation and (2) monitoring those trials to ensure ethical conduct. IRBs do not have primary responsibility for the safety issues of a trial; that responsibility resides with the principal investigator(s), the safety officer designated by the study sponsor, and the regulatory affairs office responsible for adverse event reporting to the FDA and other regulatory agencies. However, IRBs must be informed of safety concerns as they arise because safety issues may impact the ethical conduct of the trial. Multicenter trials may utilize an independent, central IRB chosen by the trial sponsor as well as local IRBs established by participating research centers. IRB composition and responsibilities are guided by the *US Code of Federal Regulations* (21 CFR 56.107-111), which provides minimum standards for subject safety and information.

Although some forms of research (e.g., retrospective chart reviews) may be considered "low risk" and thus eligible for an IRB exemption or waiver, when in doubt regarding the ethical merits of a particular research effort, an investigator or clinician should always err on the side of caution and engage a local IRB or ethics committee.

INFORMED CONSENT

The FDA provides a comprehensive review on the informed consent process and guidance for development of the informed consent document (FDA, 2016). The informed consent procedure is more than just a signature on a form; it is a process of information exchange that may include, in addition to reading and signing the informed consent document, subject recruitment materials, verbal instructions, a question/answer session, and measures of subject understanding. Researchers must provide potential participants with full disclosure of anticipated benefits, risks, and alternatives to the study intervention. That obligation extends throughout the course of the study to include updating volunteer participants in a timely manner on emerging knowledge that might change their perception of the risks and benefits of continued participation in the trial. The informed consent document should be in a language and level understandable to the subject (or subject's representative) and provide the subject with sufficient opportunity to consider whether or not to participate without the possibility of coercion or undue influence. In addition, the document must state that participation is completely voluntary and subjects can withdrawal from the study at any point in time without loss of benefits or penalty.

CONFLICTS OF INTERESTS IN THE CONDUCT OF CLINICAL TRIALS

As research has expanded to include centers outside academic health institutions, partnerships between pharmaceutical companies and private practice research sites have grown. As such, physicians may play dual roles of both investigator and clinician. This could lead to a conflict of interest to enroll subjects in trials when financial incentives are in place. The American Medical Association (AMA) has posted recommendations to safeguard against conflict of interests during clinical trials. Only physicians with medical expertise in the areas of the research being performed should be investigators. When financial compensation is offered from trial sponsors, it should be at fair market value, with the rate commensurate with the efforts of the physician performing the research; should not vary according to the volume of subjects enrolled by the physician; and must be disclosed to a potential participant as part of the informed consent process. In addition, the AMA states that it is unethical for physicians to accept payment solely for referring patients to research studies. Finally, both the AMA and the *Declaration of Helsinki* (2008) make specific statements about the publication of study results. The AMA states that physicians should ensure that the publications of study results not be unduly delayed or otherwise obstructed by the sponsoring company, and the most recent update of the *Declaration of Helsinki* highlights that negative and inconclusive as well as positive results should be published or otherwise be made publicly available.

PERCEPTIONS AND MISPERCEPTIONS

Altruism often is a core but seldom a sole reason for volunteering to participate in a study (Kass, 1996). Many people participate in clinical trials for very pragmatic reasons, such as having inadequate or no health insurance, or they may have exhausted or found no relief from currently approved therapies (Council of Public Representatives, 2001; Kass, 1996). A trial may represent their only perceived access to care or hope for relief. These mixed motives can exacerbate the "therapeutic misconception," wherein volunteers believe that they are receiving care rather than engaging in research.

With an increasing number of clinical trials being performed and expansion of their conduct from research medical centers to private practice settings, the distinction between research and care can become blurred (Morin, 2002). It may be difficult for individual physicians to separate their roles of health care provider and researcher (Miller, 1998), both within their own minds and in communicating with patients who are potential subjects in a study. This also may lead investigators to circumvent strict enrollment criteria or bypass the randomization process (Morin, 2002). This can heighten the potential for a volunteer's "therapeutic misconception." The two roles that the physician plays often result in a tension that is ethically complex and ambiguous, and if it cannot be avoided, it must be managed (Miller, 1998).

The AMA has taken the position that the physician who has treated a patient on an ongoing basis should not be responsible for obtaining informed consent. Rather, once a patient has been identified as meeting trial eligibility, a non-treating person should conduct the formal consent procedure (Morin, 2002). This is particularly important when studies are performed in institutional settings, including correctional facilities, in which broad supervision may impact upon the free will and autonomy of the potential volunteer.

Clinicians must be mindful of the trust that patients place in them in helping to make health care decisions, including participation in a clinical research trial, and clinicians must be clear in distinguishing between providing care and offering participation in a clinical trial (Kass, 1996). Many clinician–researchers find it helpful to separate clinical care visits temporally and geographically from research study visits in order to clearly separate the goals of each interaction.

ETHICAL CONSIDERATIONS IN INTERNATIONAL RESEARCH

Advances in the treatment of HIV have produced anti-retroviral regimens that are highly potent, well tolerated, and easy to take. As a result, the interest in patient participation in clinical trials of novel agents and regimens in industrialized countries has declined. This in turn has caused many biotechnology and pharmaceutical companies to shift a large portion of their research initiatives to regions of the world that are lacking in infrastructure and/or resources to provide standard of care treatments. In an editorial in *The New England Journal of Medicine* in 2001, Shapiro and Meslin highlighted the following key issues regarding research in developing countries (Shapiro, 2001):

1. Clinical trials conducted abroad should meet all ethical standards for trials based in the United States.

2. Studies should be sensitive to the local customs, conditions, and culture of the region.

3. Careful consideration must be undertaken in areas that have high rates of illiteracy or where signing a form may be considered dangerous in countries with oppressive political regimes.

4. It is unethical to ask persons to participate in a trial in which the intervention being tested is not likely affordable in the host country or the health care infrastructure cannot support its proper distribution and use.

5. The experimental intervention should be normally compared with an established, effective treatment.

6. Research participants should not be made worse off by their inability to have continued access to a successful intervention after the trial has ended.

7. A review by ethics committees in both host and sponsoring countries should be performed.

CONCLUSION

HIV-related biomedical research has resulted in a large body of therapeutic advancements and vast improvements in our scientific knowledge and understanding of the biology, pathogenesis, natural history, and epidemiology of HIV infection. Foundational ethical principles such as autonomy, confidentiality, non-maleficence, informed consent, beneficence, justice, and utility must be continually applied to the conduct of research in order to maintain ethically sound research programs. Institutional review boards and ethics consultation services can serve as resources for researchers and clinicians in need of consultation.

References

Council of Public Representatives. Human research protections in clinical trials: A public perspective. Report to the Director of the National Institutes of Health. Bethesda, MD: National Institutes of Health; October 2001.

DuVal G, Gensler G, Danis M. Ethical dilemmas encountered by clinical researchers. *J Clin Ethics*. 2005; 16(3):267–276.

Emanuel EJ, Wendler D, Grady C. What makes clinical research ethical? *JAMA*. 2000; 283(20):2701–2711.

Kass NE, Sugarman J, Faden R, et al. Trust, the fragile foundation of contemporary biomedical research. *Hastings Cent Rep*. 1996; 26(5):25–29.

Miller FG, Rosenstein DL, DeRenzo EG. Professional integrity in clinical research. *JAMA*. 1998; 280(16):1449–1454.

Morin K, Rakatansky H, Riddick FA, et al. Managing conflicts of interest in the conduct of clinical trials. *JAMA*. 2002; 287:78–84.

Shapiro HT, Mesline EM. Ethical issues in the design and conduct of clinical trials in developing countries. *N Engl J Med*. 2001; 345(2):139–142.

US Department of Health and Welfare, National Commission for the Protection of Human Subjects of Biomedical and Behavioral Research. The Belmont report: Ethical principles and guidelines for the protection of human subjects of research. April 18, 1979. Available at http://www.hhs.gov/ohrp/humansubjects/guidance/belmont.html.

US Food and Drug Administration. A guide to informed consent—Information sheet: Guidance for institutional review boards and clinical investigators. 2016. Available at www.fda.gov/RegulatoryInformation/Guidances/ucm126431.htm.

World Medical Association. World Medical Association Declaration of Helsinki: Ethical principles for medical research involving human subjects. *JAMA*. 2013; 310(20):2191–2194.

INDEX